The Complete
Mental Health
Directory

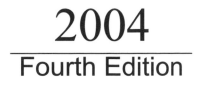

2004
Fourth Edition

The Complete Mental Health Directory

A Comprehensive
Source Book for
Individuals and Professionals

A SEDGWICK PRESS Book

Grey House
Publishing

PUBLISHER:	Leslie Mackenzie
EDITORIAL DIRECTOR:	Laura Mars-Proietti
MEDICAL EDITOR:	Nada Stotland, MD
PRODUCTION MANAGER:	Karen Stevens
ASSISTANT PRODUCTION MANAGER:	Cecilia Acerbo
PRODUCTION ASSISTANTS:	Vicki Barker, Stephanie Capozzi, Elizabeth Corteville, Debra Giordano, Alison Import, Megan McClune, Meghan Mead, Nicole Richards
MARKETING DIRECTOR:	Jessica Moody

A Sedgwick Press Book
Grey House Publishing, Inc.
185 Millerton Road
Millerton, NY 12546
518.789.8700
FAX 518.789.0545
www.greyhouse.com
e-mail: books @greyhouse.com

3 1561 00172 6961

First edition published 1999
Fourth edition published 2004

Printed in the USA
The complete mental health directory. — 1999-
   v. 27.5 cm.
   Annual
   "A comprehensive source book for individuals and professionals."
   Includes index.
   ISSN: 1538-0556

1. Mental health services--United States--Directories.

RA790.6 .C625
362—dc21   2001-233121
ISBN 1-59237-046-2   softcover

Table of Contents

Each of the above chapters includes a description and the following sections:

> Association & Agencies
> Books
> Periodicals & Pamphlets
> Research Centers
> Support Groups & Hot Lines
> Video & Audio
> Web Sites

SECTION TWO
Mental Health Associations & Organizations

SECTION THREE
Government Agencies

SECTION FOUR
Professional Support & Services

SECTION FIVE
Facilities

SECTION SIX
Clinical Management

SECTION SEVEN
Pharmaceutical Companies

Indexes

Introduction

Welcome to the fourth edition of *The Complete Mental Health Directory* published by Sedgwick Press, an imprint of Grey House Publishing. This unique reference directory provides comprehensive coverage of 26 specific mental health disorders, from Adjustment Disorders to Tic Disorders, including a separate section devoted to Pediatric and Adolescent issues. It is designed to offer valuable information for those suffering from these disorders, their families and support systems, as well as mental health professionals. It combines, in a single volume, disorder descriptions written by industry professionals in clear, easy-to-understand language, and a wide variety of resources, including Associations, Publications, Support Groups, Web Sites, State Agencies and Facilities. Here's where you'll find where to go and who to ask – for the most prevalent mental health disorders in the country.

Whether you simply browse through these pages to confirm something you're already aware of, or search the more than 5,000 listings for new resources, you will find data that reflects the latest findings in the mental health community. For example, it's easy to understand how Eating Disorders can be triggered by cultural pressure, but did you know that there are a number of web sites that actually promote anorexia as a "lifestyle"? And, despite the recent publicity on the supposed dangers of antidepressants for children, Prozac is still considered safe and effective in the younger population.

Amidst the ongoing controversy over whether or not to allow psychologists, who lack medical degrees, to prescribe psychotropic drugs, this edition has added to the Drug chapter several new drugs that are now being used to treat a variety of conditions. These include Aricept for Alzheimer's Disease, Lexapro for Depression, and Provigil for Sleep Disorders, as well as the companies who manufacturer them.

The Complete Mental Health Directory is organized into seven sections, outlined below.

SECTION ONE
This section consists of 26 chapters dealing with specific mental health disorders from Adjustment Disorders to Tic Disorders. Each chapter begins with a description, written in clear, accessible language that includes symptoms, prevalence and treatment options. Many of the disorder descriptions include information on specific syndromes within a general category, such as Panic Disorder and Social Anxiety Disorder within the Anxiety Disorder chapter.

Following the descriptions are specific resources relevant to the disorder, including Associations, Books, Agencies, Periodicals, Pamphlets, Support Groups, Hot Lines, Resource Centers, Audio & Video Tapes, and Web Sites.

SECTIONS TWO & THREE
More than 1,000 National Associations, and Federal and State Agencies are profiled in these sections that offer general mental health services and support for patients and their families.

SECTION FOUR
This section provides resources that support the many different professionals in the mental heath field. Included are specific chapters on Accreditation and Quality Assurance, Associations, Books, Conferences and Meetings, Periodicals, Training and Recruitment, Audio & VideoTapes, Web Sties, and Workbooks and Manuals.

SECTION FIVE

This section lists major facilities and hospitals, arranged by state that provide treatment for persons with mental health disorders.

SECTION SIX

Here you will find products and services that support the Clinical Management aspect of the mental health industry, including Directories and Databases, Management Companies, and Information Services, which provide patient and medical data, as well as marketing information.

SECTION SEVEN

This section offers information on the pharmaceutical companies that manufacture drugs to treat many mental health disorders. This information is presented in two ways, depending on research criteria. One format lists the companies alphabetically by name and includes address, phone, fax, web site, and a list of specific drugs they manufacture. The second arrangement lists the drugs alphabetically by name, gives the disorder it typically is prescribed for, and references the company or companies that manufacture it.

INDEXES

Disorder Index lists all entries by dozens of terms – a combination of disorders and a number of topics relevant to the mental health community.

Entry Index is an alphabetical list of all entries.

Geographic Index lists entries by state, making is easy to find all available resources in a desired state.

Web Sites Index categorizes all web sites listed in the directory by disorder name or related topic.

Grey House Publishing thanks Nada Stotland, M.D., for her careful review and important updates to this material. The editors also acknowledge the hundreds of people in the mental health community who responded to a fax or phone call.

This data is also available as **The Complete Mental Health Directory – Online Database.** Using powerful search and retrieval software, this interactive Online Database quickly accesses the information in the print version, searchable by dozens of criteria. Visit www.greyhouse.com for a free search.

User's Guide

Below is a sample listing illustrating the kind of information that is or might be included in an Association entry, with additional fields that apply to publication and trade show listings. Each numbered item of information is described in the paragraphs on the following page.

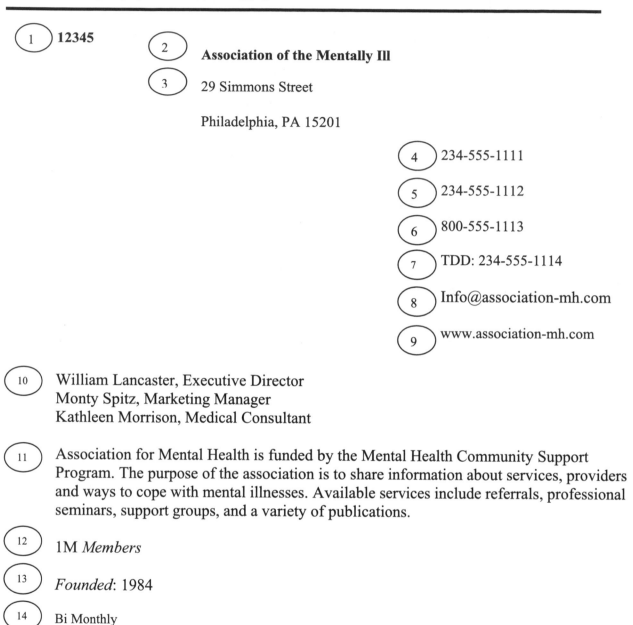

(1) **12345**

(2) **Association of the Mentally Ill**

(3) 29 Simmons Street

Philadelphia, PA 15201

(4) 234-555-1111

(5) 234-555-1112

(6) 800-555-1113

(7) TDD: 234-555-1114

(8) Info@association-mh.com

(9) www.association-mh.com

(10) William Lancaster, Executive Director
Monty Spitz, Marketing Manager
Kathleen Morrison, Medical Consultant

(11) Association for Mental Health is funded by the Mental Health Community Support Program. The purpose of the association is to share information about services, providers and ways to cope with mental illnesses. Available services include referrals, professional seminars, support groups, and a variety of publications.

(12) 1M *Members*

(13) *Founded*: 1984

(14) Bi Monthly

(15) $59.00

(16) 110,000

User's Key

(1) Record Number: Entries are listed alphabetically within each category and numbered sequentially. The entry number, rather than the page number, are used in the indexes to refer to listings.

(2) Title: Formal name of association or publication. Where names are completely capitalized, the listing will appear at the beginning of the section. If listing is a publication or trade show, the publisher or sponsoring organization will appear below the title.

(3) Address: Location or permanent address of the association.

(4) Phone Number: The listed phone number is usually for the main office of the association, but may also be for the sales, marketing, or public relations office as provided.

(5) Fax Number: This is listed when provided by the association.

(6) Toll-Free Number: This is listed when provided by the association.

(7) TDD: This is listed when provided by the association. It refers to Telephone Device for the Deaf.

(8) E-Mail: This is listed when provided by the association.

(9) Web Site: This is listed when provided by the association and is also referred to as an URL address. These web sites are accessed through the Internet by typing http:// before the URL address.

(10) Key Executives: Lists key contacts of the association, publication or sponsoring organization.

(11) Description: This paragraph contains a brief description of the association, their purpose and services.

(12) Members: Total number of association members.

(13) Founded: Year association was founded.

(14) Frequency, if listing is a publication.

(15) Subscription price, if listing is a publication.

(16) Circulation, if listing is a publication.

Introduction

The experience of stress in life is inevitable and begins in utero. When we are faced with a painful event or situation, we do our best to cope, get through it, and move on. How we cope and how long it takes varies according to the stressful situation. In most situations, we respond appropriately to the stressful event or situation and show an adaptive response.

Adjustment Disorders are maladaptive reactions to a stressful event or situation. The adjustment is to a real event or situation (e.g.,the breaking up of a relationship, the threat of being laid off), and the disorder signifies that the adjustment is more extreme than would be warranted considering the stressor, or it keeps the individual from functioning as usual.

SYMPTOMS

•The development of emotional or behavioral symptoms is in response to an identifiable stressor except bereavement within three months of the appearance of the stressor;
•The emotions or behaviors are significant either because the distress is more extreme than would normally be caused by the stressor, or because the emotions or behaviors are clearly impairing the person's social, school, or work functioning;
•Once the stressor has ended, the emotions or behaviors continue for more than six months.
A disturbance that lasts less than six months is acute, one lasting longer than six months is chronic.
•Adjustment Disorders are divided into several subtypes:

•**Depressed Mood** - predominant mood is depression, with symptoms such as tearfulness, hopelessness, sadness, sleep disturbances;
•**Anxiety** - predominant symptoms are edginess, nervousness, worry, or in children, fears of separation from important attachment figures;
•**Anxiety and Depressed Mood** - chief manifestation is a combination of depression and anxiety;
•**Disturbance of Conduct** - predominant symptoms are conduct which involves either a violation of other people's rights (e.g., reckless driving, fighting), or the violation of social norms and rules;
•**Disturbance of Emotions and Conduct** - chief symptoms are both emotional (e.g., depression, anxiety) and a disturbance of conduct.

ASSOCIATED FEATURES

Many commonplace events can be stressful (e.g., first day of school, changing jobs). If the stressor is an acute event (like an impending operation), the onset of the disturbance is usually immediate but may not last more than six months after the stressor ends. If the stressor or its consequences continue (such as a long-term illness), the Adjustment Disorder may also continue. Whatever the nature of the event, the person can feel overwhelmed. A person may be reacting to one or many stressors; the stressor may affect one person or the whole family. The more severe the stressor, the more likely that an Adjustment Disorder will develop. If a person is already vulnerable, e.g., is suffering from a disability or a mental disorder, an Adjustment Disorder is more likely.

The diagnosis of an Adjustment Disorder is called a residual category, meaning that other possible diagnoses must be ruled out first. For example, symptoms that are part of a personality disorder and become worse under stress are not usually considered to be Adjustment Disorders unless they are new types of symptoms for the individual.

There are three questions to consider in diagnosing Adjustment Disorder: How out-of-proportion is the response to the stressor? How long does it go on? To what extent does it impair the person's ability to function in social, workplace, and school settings?

The emotional response may show itself in excessive worry and edginess, excessive sadness and hopelessness or abination of these. There may also be changes in behavior in response to the stressful event or situation, where the person is violating

1

other people's rights or is breaking agreed-upon rules and regulations. The emotional response and the changes in behavior persist, even after the stressful event or circumstances have ended. Finally, the response significantly affects the person's normal functioning in social, school and work settings.

Adjustment Disorders increase the risk of suicidal behavior and completed suicide, and they also complicate the course of other medical conditions (for example, patients may not take their medication, eat properly, etc).

PREVALENCE

Men and women of all ages, as well as children, can suffer from this disorder. In outpatient mental health centers the diagnosis of Adjustment Disorder ranges from five percent to twenty percent. In a general hospital setting, ten percent of people seeking a consultation were diagnosed with Adjustment Disorder.

TREATMENT OPTIONS

Anyone who is experiencing one or more stressful events or circumstances and feels overwhelmed or markedly distressed and cannot function normally, should seek help. A psychiatrist or other mental health professional should make an evaluation including a referral for physical examination if necessary. Treatment prescribed is often psychotherapy and, depending on the circumstances, can include individual, couple, or family therapy. Medication is sometimes prescribed for a few weeks or months. In most instances long-term therapy will not be necessary and the person can expect marked improvement within 8 to 12 sessions.

Associations & Agencies

2 Center for Family Support (CFS)

333 7th Avenue
New York, NY 10001-5004   212-629-7939
Fax: 212-239-2211
www.cfsny.org

Steven Vernickofs, Executive Director

Service agency devoted to the physical well-being and development of the retarded child and the sound mental health of the parents. Helps families with retarded children with all aspects of home care including counseling, referrals, home aide service and consultation. Offers intervention for parents at the birth of a retarded child with in-home support, guidance and infant stimulation. Pioneered training of nonprofessional women as home aides to provide supportive services in homes.

3 Center for Mental Health Services Knowledge Exchange Network

US Department of Health and Human Services
PO Box 42490
Washington, DC 20015-4800
800-789-2647
Fax: 301-984-8796
E-mail: ken@mentalhealth.org
www.mentalhealth.org

Information about resources, technical assistance, research, training, networks, and other federal clearing houses, and fact sheets and materials. Information specialists refer callers to mental health resources in their communities as well as state, federal and non-profit contacts. Staff available Monday through Friday, 8:30 AM - 5:00 PM, EST, excluding federal holidays. After hours, callers may leave messages and an information specialist will return their call.

4 National Association for the Dually Diagnosed: NADD

NADD Press
132 Fair Street
Kingston, NY 12401-4802   845-331-4336
800-331-5362
Fax: 845-331-4569
E-mail: info@thenadd.org
www.thenadd.org

Dr. Robert Fletcher, Executive Director

Nonprofit organization designed to promote interest of professional and parent development with resources for individuals who have the coexistence of mental illness and mental retardation. Provides conference, educational services and training materials to professionals, parents, concerned citizens, and service organizations.

5 National Mental Health Consumer's Self-Help Clearinghouse

1211 Chestnut Street
Suite 1207
Philadelphia, PA 19107   215-751-1810
800-553-4539
Fax: 215-636-6312
E-mail: info@mhselfhelp.org
www.mhselfhelp.org

Alex Morrsey, Information/Referral

Funded by the National Institute of Mental Health Community Support Program, the purpose of the Clearinghouse is to encourage the development and growth of consumer self-help groups.

Year Founded: 1992

6 National SIDS Foundation

2 Metro Plaza, Suite 700
8240 Professional Place
Landover, MD 20785
800-211-7437

Devoted to individuals who have lost an infant to Sudden Infant Death Syndrome. Offers support groups, referrals, publications and more.

7 Sudden Infant Death Syndrome Alliance

1314 Bedford Avenue
Suite 210
Baltimore, MD 21208   410-653-8226
800-221-7437
Fax: 410-653-8709
E-mail: info@sidsalliance.org
www.sidsalliance.org

For parents and siblings who have suffered the loss of an infant through SIDS. Offers workshops, community outreach programs, books, videos.

Books

8 1-2-3 Magic: Training Your Children to Do What You Want

ADD WareHouse
300 NW 70th Avenue
Suite 102
Plantation, FL 33317   954-792-8100
800-233-9273
Fax: 954-792-8545
E-mail: sales@addwarehouse.com
www.addwarehouse.com

Learn about a new, no-nonsense discipline program that enables parents to manage children ages 2-12 without arguing, yelling or hitting. The 1-2-3 Magic program tells you exactly how to handle screaming, tantrums and fighting, as well as how to encourage positive behavior. *$14.95*

192 pages Year Founded: 1995 ISBN 0-963386-19-0

9   Columbia University College of Physicians and Surgeons Complete Guide to Mental Health

Henry Holt & Company
115 W 18th Street
New York, NY 10011-4113   212-886-9200
                                 Fax: 212-633-0748

A compendium of information on all aspects of mental health; written primarily for the lay reader. *$35.00*

476 pages Year Founded: 1995

10   Consumer's Guide to Psychiatric Drugs

New Harbinger Publications
5674 Shattuck Avenue
Oakland, CA 94609-1662   510-652-2002
                                800-748-6273
                          Fax: 510-652-5472
E-mail: customerservice@newharbinger.com
                   www.newharbinger.com

Helps consumers understand what treatment options are available and what side effects to expect. Covers possible interactions with other drugs, medical conditions and other concerns. Explains how each drug works, and offers detailed information about treatments for depression, bipolar disorder, anxiety and sleep disorders, as well as other conditions. *$16.95*

340 pages ISBN 1-572241-11-X

11   Don't Despair on Thursdays: the Children's Grief-Management Book

ADD WareHouse
300 NW 70th Avenue
Suite 102
Plantation, FL 33317   954-792-8100
                                800-233-9273
                          Fax: 954-792-8545
E-mail: sales@addwarehouse.com
                   www.addwarehouse.com

Children are sure to be comforted by the friendly manner and sensitivity that this book imparts as it explains the grief process to children and helps them understand that grieving is a normal response. For children ages 4-10. *$18.95*

61 pages Year Founded: 1996 ISBN 0-933849-60-5

12   Don't Feed the Monster on Tuesdays: The Children's Self-Esteem Book

ADD WareHouse
300 NW 70th Avenue
Suite 102
Plantation, FL 33317   954-792-8100
                                800-233-9273
                          Fax: 954-792-8545
E-mail: sales@addwarehouse.com
                   www.addwarehouse.com

Strikes right at the heart of the basic elements of self-esteem. He presents valuable information to children that will help them understnad the importance of their self worth. A friendly book that children ages 4 to 10 will love. *$18.95*

55 pages Year Founded: 1991 ISBN 0-933849-38-9

13   Don't Pop Your Cork on Mondays: The Children's Anti-Stress Book

ADD WareHouse
300 NW 70th Avenue
Suite 102
Plantation, FL 33317   954-792-8100
                                800-233-9273
                          Fax: 954-792-8545
E-mail: sales@addwarehouse.com
                   www.addwarehouse.com

This book explores the causes and effects of stress and offers children techniques for dealing with everyday stress factors. Bold and colorful cartoons project a blend of sensitivity and broad humor. Ages 4-10. *$18.95*

48 pages Year Founded: 1988 ISBN 0-933849-18-4

14   Don't Rant and Rave on Wednesdays: The Children's Anger-Control Book

ADD WareHouse
300 NW 70th Avenue
Suite 102
Plantation, FL 33317   954-792-8100
                                800-233-9273
                          Fax: 954-792-8545
E-mail: sales@addwarehouse.com
                   www.addwarehouse.com

A book that will delight both children and adults. Explains the causes of anger and offers methods that can help children reduce the amount of anger they feel. Gives effective techniques to help young people control their behavior even when they are angry. Ages 5-12. *$18.95*

61 pages Year Founded: 1994 ISBN 0-933849-54-0

15   Don't Tell a Whopper on Fridays: The Children's Truth-Control Book

ADD WareHouse
300 NW 70th Avenue
Suite 102
Plantation, FL 33317   954-792-8100
                                800-233-9273
                          Fax: 954-792-8545
E-mail: sales@addwarehouse.com
                   www.addwarehouse.com

Discusses the problems of lying and the importance of telling the truth in a very clear and understandable narrative. Suggests ways that can help children to choose to tell the truth, instead of lying. Informative text and colorful, funny illustrations. Ages 4-10. *$18.95*

61 pages Year Founded: 1999 ISBN 0-933849-76-1

16 **Preventing Maladjustment from Infancy Through Adolescence**

Sage Publications
2455 Teller Road
Thousand Oaks, CA 91320
805-499-9774
800-818-7243
Fax: 800-583-2665
E-mail: info@sagepub.com
www.sagepub.com

Hardcover. Paperback also available. *$92.95*

156 pages Year Founded: 1987 ISBN
0-803928-68-8

17 **Stressors and the Adjustment Disorders**

John Wiley & Sons
111 River Street
Hoboken, NJ 07030-5774
201-748-6000
Fax: 201-748-6088
E-mail: info@wiley.com
www.wiley.com

Clinically oriented investigation into the sources of stress, the forms of stress reponse and the current array of treatment possibilities. Brings together contributions from many of the country's leading psychiatrists who possess expertise in the various syndromes associated with human stress. A provocative collection of professional perspectives in this controversial area of modern psychiatric thinking, it will also serve as a solid foundation for future research activities. *$300.00*

693 pages Year Founded: 1990 ISBN
0-471621-86-2

18 **Treatment of Stress Response Syndromes**

American Psychiatric Publishing
1000 Wilson Boulevard
Suite 1825
Arlington, VA 22209-3901
703-907-7322
800-368-5777
Fax: 703-907-1091
E-mail: appi@psych.org
www.appi.org

A comprehensive clinical guide to treating patients with disorders related to loss, trauma and terror. Author Mardi J Horowitz, MD, is the clinical researcher who is largely responsible for modern concepts of posttraumatic stress disorder (PTSD). In this book he reveals the latest strategies for treating PTSD and expands the coverage to include several related diagnoses. *$26.00*

134 pages Year Founded: 2003 ISBN
1-585621-07-2

Periodicals & Pamphlets

19 **National Association for the Dually Diagnosed: NADD Newsletter**

NADD Press
132 Fair Street
Kingston, NY 12401-4802
845-331-4336
800-331-5362
Fax: 845-331-4569
E-mail: info@thenadd.org
www.thenadd.org

Dr. Robert Fletcher, Executive Director

Bi-monthly publication designed to promote interest of professional and parent development with resources for individuals who have the coexistence of mental illness and mental retardation.

ISSN 1065-25-74

20 **Treatment of Children with Mental Disorders**

National Institute of Mental Health
6001 Executive Boulevard
Room 8184
Bethesda, MD 20892-9663
866-615-6464
Fax: 301-443-4279
TTY: 301-443-8431
E-mail: nimhinfo@nih.gov
www.nimh.nih.gov

Ruth Dubois, Assistant Chief

A short booklet that contains questions and answers about therapy for children with mental disorders. Includes a chart of mental disorders and medications used.

Support Groups & Hot Lines

21 **Compassionate Friends**

PO Box 3696
Oak Brook, IL 60522-3696
708-990-0010
877-969-0010
Fax: 708-990-0246
www.compassionatefriends.org

For parents suffering the loss of a child.

22 **Friends for Survival**

PO Box 214463
Sacramento, CA 95821
916-392-0664
800-646-7322

Assists family, friends, and professionals following a suicide death.

23 **Parents of Murdered Children**

100 E Street
B-41
Cincinnati, OH 45202
513-721-5683

Parents supporting parents who have suffered the loss of a murdered child.

24 Rainbows

1111 Tower Road
Schaumburg, IL 60173   708-310-1880

Peer support groups for adults and children who are grieving.

25 SHARE Office

St. Joseph Health Center
300 1st Capitol Drive
Saint Charles, MO 63301-2893   636-947-6164
800-821-6819
Fax: 636-947-7486
E-mail: share@nationalshareoffice.com
www.NationalSHAREOffice.com

Pregnancy and infant loss support.

26 SOLOS-Survivors of Loved Ones' Suicides

PO Box 1716
Springfield, VA 22151-0716
www.1000deaths.com

For the families and friends who have suffered the suicide loss of a loved one.

Web Sites

27 www.DivorceNet.com
DivorceNet

Legally oriented, searchable site.

28 www.compassionatefriends.org
Compassionate Friends

Organization for those having lost a child.

29 www.couns.uiuc.edu/grief.htm
Grief and Loss

Guidelines for explaining the grief process.

30 www.counselingforloss.com
Counseling for Loss and Life Changes

Look under articles for reprints of writings and links.

31 www.cyberpsych.org
CyberPsych

Hosts the American Psychoanalyists Foundation, American Association of Suicideology, Society for the Exploration of Psychotherapy Intergration, and Anxiety Disorders Association of America. Also subcategories of the anxiety disorders, as well as general information, including panic disorder, phobias, obsessive compulsive disorder (OCD), social phobia, generalized anxiety disorder, post traumatic stress disorder, and phobias of childhood. Book reviews and links to web pages sharing the topics.

32 www.death-dying.com
Death and Dying Grief Support

Information on grief and loss.

33 www.divorceasfriends.com
Bill Ferguson's How to Divorce as Friends

Useful information on how to eliminate the anger usually associated with divorce.

34 www.divorcecentral.com/lifeline/life_ans
Surviving the Emotional Trauma of Divorce

Offers helpful advice and suggestions on what to expect emotionally, and how to deal with the emotional effects of divorce.

35 www.divorcedfather.com
Still a Dad

For divorced fathers.

36 www.divorceinfo.com
Divorceinfo.com

Simply written and covers all the issues.

37 www.divorcemag.com
Divorce Magazine

The printed magazine's commercial site.

38 www.divorcesupport.com
Divorce Support

Covers all aspects of divorce.

39 www.fortnet.org/WidowNet
WidowNet

Help for someone suffering the loss of a spouse.

40 **www.grieftalk.com/help1.html**
Grief Journey

Short readings for clients.

41 **www.home.clara.net/spig/guidline.htm**
Guidelines for Separating Parents

Useful information that helps to decrease the stress associated with separation.

42 **www.misschildren.org**
Mothers in Sympathy and Support

Help for mothers suffering the loss of a child.

43 **www.planetpsych.com**
Planetpsych.com

Learn about disorders, their treatments and other topics in psychology. Articles are listed under the related topic areas. Ask a therapist a question for free, or view the directory of professionals in your area. If you are a therapist sign up for the directory. Current features, self-help, interactive, and newsletter archives.

44 **www.prividence.org/safecrossings**
Safe Crossings

For children facing a loved one's death.

45 **www.psychcentral.com**
Psych Central

Personalized one-stop index for psychology, support, and mental health issues, resources, and people on the Internet.

46 **www.psycom.net/depression.central.grief. html**
Grief and Bereavement

Helpful information for those grieving from the loss of a loved one.

47 **www.rcpsych.ac.uk/public/help/bereav/**
Bereavement

Overview for general readers.

48 **www.realtionshipjourney.com**
Relationship and Personal Development Center

Articles on divorce, among other articles.

49 **www.rivendell.org**
GriefNet

Useful information on coping with loss.

50 **www.ubalt.edu/www/bereavement**
Bereavement and Hospice Support Netline

Lists of support groups.

51 **www.utexas.edu/student/cmhc/grief.html**
Life after Loss: Dealing with Grief

Six page overview for college students.

52 **www.walnet.org**
Lunatics' Liberation Front

Alternatives to psychiatry, forced treatment. Civil rights of individuals are considered, as well as suggestions on helping those who may need some form of therapy.

Directories & Databases

53 **After School And More: After School, Weekend and Holiday Programs for Children and Youth With Disabilities**
Resources for Children with Special Needs
116 E 16th Street
5th Floor
New York, NY 10003   212-677-4650
Fax: 212-254-4070
E-mail: info@resourcenyc.org
www.resourcenyc.org

The most complete directory of after school programs for children with disabilities and special needs in the metropolitan New York area. *$25.00*

ISBN 0-967836-57-3

54   **Camps 2004: A Directory of Camps and Summer Programs for Children and Youth With Special Needs and Disabilities**

Resources for Children with Special Needs
116 E 16th Street
5th Floor
New York, NY 10003   212-677-4550
                                 Fax: 212-254-4070
                        E-mail: info@resourcenyc.org
                             www.resourcenyc.org

Our guide includes profiles of more than 300 day camps, recreation, tutoring, and travel programs, museums, nature experience and summer employment in New York City, sleep away programs in the northeast, and travel programs throughout the U.S. that serve both special and mainstream children. *$22.00*

1 per year Year Founded: 2004 ISBN 0-967836-57-3

Introduction

Substance abuse and addictive disorders are among the most destructive mental disorders in America today, contributing to a host of social problems and to widespread individual suffering. Alcohol, a drug that is widely available and socially approved, is unquestionably the most abused of all substances, and alcohol addiction is a pervasive mental disorder. Like all addictive disorders, alcohol addiction is characterized by repeated use despite repeated adverse consequences, and by physical and psychological craving.

Alcohol addiction can be treated, but successful recovery is dependent on acceptance by the patient that he or she has an illness; it is this acceptance that is often the greatest stumbling block to treatment.

Relapse is common due to several reasons: lack of acceptace of a diagnosis; genetic vulnerability; and social factors. In addition, although many people relapse, so that it takes about three tries at treatment before the results are fairly permanent, most people do eventually respond to treatment.

Scientific understanding of how alcohol works on the body and the brain, and the underlying physiology of addiction, has advanced remarkably in recent years. Successful treatment very often requires involvement by the patient in some form of self-help group, such as Alcoholics Anonymous or another 12-step program.

SYMPTOMS

Alcohol addiction is diagnosed according to criteria established for all substance abuse disorders.
•Tolerance, as defined by either a need for markedly increased amounts of the substance to achieve intoxication or desired effect, or markedly diminished effect with continued use;
•Withdrawal, and use of alcohol to relieve or avoid withdrawal symptoms; alcohol is often used in larger amounts over a longer period than was intended;
•A persistent desire or unsuccessful efforts to cut down or control alcohol use;
•A great deal of time is spent in activities necessary to obtain alcohol or recover from its effects;
•Important social, occupational, or recreational activites are given up or reduced because of alcohol use;
•Alcohol use is continued despite knowledge of having a persistent or recurrent physical or psychological problem that is likely to have been caused or exacerbated by alcohol.

ASSOCIATED FEATURES

Frequently, alcohol abuse and dependence occur together with dependence on other substances, and alcohol may be used to counteract the ill effects of these substances. Depression, anxiety, and sleep disorders are common in alcohol dependence.

Typically, accidents, injuries and suicide accompany alcohol dependence, and it is estimated that half of all traffic accidents involve alcoholic intoxication. Absenteeism, low work productivity and injuries on the job may often be attributed to alcohol dependence. Alcohol is also the most common cause of preventable birth defects, including fetal alcohol syndrome, according to the American Psychiatric Association.

PREVALENCE

Alcohol dependence and abuse are among the most prevalent mental disorders in the general population. One community study in the US found that about eight percent of the adult population had alcohol dependence and about five percent had alcohol abuse at some time in their lives. Approximately six percent had alcohol dependence or abuse during the preceding year.

TREATMENT OPTIONS

Diagnosis and treatment of alcohol dependence has improved as understanding of the physiology of addiction has advanced. But successful treatment still relies on acceptance by the patient that he or she has an illness, as well as support from other people who have gone through the same thing. For this reason, medical treatment is most often successful when it is accompanied by involvement in a support group, for both the patient and family members; these may include Alcoholics Anonymous and Al-Anon, 12-step spiritual programs that have gained enormous popularity over the years. Local groups can be found in almost every community by looking in the phone book.

Recently, similar groups have formed that do not emphasize spirituality, but do rely on group support for sobriety.

Medical treatment of alcohol dependence may include Anabuse, a drug that makes an individual violently ill if alcohol is used. Group or hospital-based treatment may also be useful, and psychotherapy can be beneficial to help the patient more effectively deal with underlying conflicts, as well as interpersonal problems.

Associations & Agencies

56 Alcoholics Anonymous (AA): Worldwide

475 Riverside Drive
11th Floor
New York, NY 10115   212-870-3400
                                      Fax: 212-870-3003
                                      E-mail: cr@aa.org
                                      www.aa.org

A fellowship of men and women who share their experience, strenght and hope with each other that they may solve their common problem and help others to recover from alcoholism.

57 American Council on Alcoholism

PO Box 25126
Arlington, VA 22203-1612   703-248-9005
                                      800-527-5344
                                      Fax: 703-248-9007
                                      www.aca-usa.org

Referrals to DWI classes and treatment centers.

58 American Public Human Services Association

810 1st Street NE
Suite 500
Washington, DC 20002   202-682-0100
                                      Fax: 202-289-6555
                                      www.aphsa.org

Nonprofit, bipartisan organization of individuals and agencies concerned with human services. Members include all state and many territotiral human service agencies, more than 1,200 local agencies and thousands of individuals.

59 Association of Behavioral Healthcare Management

12300 Twinbrook Parkway
Suite 320
Rockville, MD 20852   301-984-6200
                                      Fax: 301-881-7159
                          E-mail: administration@nccbh.org
                                      www.nccbh.org

Jeannie Campbell, CEO
David Schuerholz, Marketing/Communications

Promotes professionalism among those working in healthcare management. Serves as a network for sharing information and fellowship among members. Provides technical assistance to members and functions as a liaison to related professional organizations.

60 Center for Family Support (CFS)

333 7th Avenue
New York, NY 10001-5004   212-629-7939
                                      Fax: 212-239-2211
                                      www.cfsny.org

Steven Vernickofs, Executive Director

Service agency devoted to the physical well-being and development of the retarded child and the sound mental health of the parents. Helps families with retarded children with all aspects of home care including counseling, referrals, home aide service and consultation. Offers intervention for parents at the birth of a retarded child with in home support, guidance and infant stimulation. Pioneered training of nonprofessional women as home aides to provide supportive services in homes.

61 Center for Mental Health Services Knowledge Exchange Network

US Department of Health and Human Services
PO Box 42557
Washington, DC 20015-4800
                                      800-789-2647
                                      Fax: 301-984-8796
                          E-mail: ken@mentalhealth.org
                                      www.mentalhealth.samsa.gov

Information about resources, technical assistance, research, training, networks, and other federal clearing houses, and fact sheets and materials. Information specialists refer callers to mental health resources in their communities as well as state, federal and nonprofit contacts. Staff available Monday through Friday, 8:30 AM - 5:00 PM, EST, excluding federal holidays. After hours, callers may leave messages and an information specialist will return their call.

62 National Association of Alcohol and Drug Abuse Counselors

901 N Washington Street
Suite 600
Alexandria, VA 22314-1535   703-741-7686
                                      800-548-0497
                                      Fax: 800-377-1136
                          E-mail: rdavis@naadac.org
                                      www.naadac.org

Pat Ford-Roegner, Executive Director

The only professional membership organization that serves counselors who specialize in addiction treatment. With 14,000 members and 47 state affiliates representing more than 80,000 addiction counselors, it is the nation's largest network of alcoholism and drug abuse treatment professionals. Among the organization's national certifaction programs are the National Certified Addiction Counselor and the Masters Addiction Counselor designations.

63 National Clearinghouse for Alcohol and Drug Information

PO Box 2345
Rockville, MD 20847-2345   301-468-2600
                                      800-729-6686
                                      Fax: 301-468-6433
                                      TDD: 800-487-4889
                                      www.health.org

One-stop resource for information about abuse prevention and addiction treatment.

64 National Institute on Alcohol Abuse and Alcoholism

6000 Executive Boulevard
Willco Building
Bethesda, MD 20892-7003   301-443-3860
                                 Fax: 301-443-8774
                                 www.niaaa.nih.gov

Ting-Kai Li, Director

Federal agency that supports research nationwide on alcohol abuse and alcoholism. Includes investigator-initiated research on homeless persons.

65 National Mental Health Consumer's Self-Help Clearinghouse

1211 Chestnut Street
Suite 1207
Philadelphia, PA 19107   215-751-1810
                                800-553-4539
                                Fax: 215-636-6312
                                E-mail: info@mhselfhelp.org
                                www.mhselfhelp.org

Alex Morrsey, Information/Referral

Funded by the National Institute of Mental Health Community Support Program, the purpose of the Clearinghouse is to encourage the development and growth of consumer self-help groups.

Year Founded: 1992

66 National Organization on Fetal Alcohol Syndrome

900 17th Street NW
Suite 910
Washington, DC 20006   202-785-4585
                              800-666-6327
                              Fax: 202-466-6456
                              E-mail: information@nofas.org
                              www.nofas.org

Tom Donaldson, Executive Director
Kathleen Mitchell, Program Director/Spokesperson

Develops and implements innovative prevention and education strategies assessing fetal alcohol syndrome - the leading known preventable cause of mental retardation - including information, resource and referral clearinghouse, a medical and allied health curriculum, training workshops, and national community-based awareness campaigns.

Books

67 Alcohol and the Community

Cambridge University Press
40 W 20th Street
New York, NY 10011-4211   212-924-3900
                                 800-872-7423
                                 Fax: 212-691-3239
                                 E-mail: marketing@cup.org
                                 www.cup.org

The authors challenge the current implicit models used in alcohol problem prevention and demonstrate an ecological perspective of the community as a complex adaptive systems composed of interacting subsystems. This volume represents a new and sensible approach to the prevention of alcohol dependence and alcohol-related problems. *$85.00*

197 pages ISBN 0-521591-87-2

68 Alcoholism Sourcebook

Omnigraphics
PO Box 625
Holmes, PA 19043
                                 800-234-1340
                                 Fax: 800-875-1340
                                 E-mail: info@omnigraphics.com
                                 www.omnigraphics.com

Omnigraphics is the publisher of the Health Reference Series, a growing consumer health information resource with more than 100 volumes in print. Each title in the series features an easy to understand format, nontechnical language, comprehensive indexing, and resources for further information. Material in each book has been collected from a wide range of government agencies, professional accociations, periodicals, and other sources. *$78.00*

613 pages ISBN 1-780803-25-6

69 Elephant in the Living Room: Leader's Guide for Helping Children of Alcoholics

Hazelden
15251 Pleasant Valley Road
PO Box 176
Center City, MN 55012-0176   651-213-4000
                                    800-328-9000
                                    Fax: 651-213-4590
                                    www.hazelden.org

Practical guidance for education and health professionals who help young people cope with a family member's chemical dependency. *$12.00*

88 pages ISBN 1-568380-34-8

70 Eye Opener

Hazelden
15251 Pleasant Valley Road
PO Box 176
Center City, MN 55012-0176   651-213-4000
                                    800-328-9000
                                    Fax: 651-213-4590
                                    www.hazelden.org

These daily meditations support core concepts of the AA program and help clients review key recovery ideas. *$12.00*

381 pages ISBN 0-894860-23-2

71 Fetal Alcohol Syndrome & Fetal Alcohol Effect

Hazelden
15251 Pleasant Valley Road
PO Box 176
Center City, MN 55012-0176   651-213-4000
                                    800-328-9000
                                    Fax: 651-213-4590
                                    www.hazelden.org

If you're a chemical dependency counselor or work with women in pregnancy planning or self-care, this resource is filled with facts to help you better meet your clients needs. *$5.25*

48 pages ISBN 0-894869-51-5

72 Getting Hooked: Rationality and Addiction

Cambridge University Press
40 W 20th Street
New York, NY 10011-4221   **212-924-3900**
                              Fax: 212-691-3239
                    E-mail: marketing@cup.org
                                      www.cup.org

The essays in this volume offer thorough and up-to-date discussion on the relationship between addiction and rationality. Includes contributions from philosophers, psychiatrists, neurobiologists, sociologists and economists. Offers the neurophysiology of addiction, examination of the Becker theory of rational addiction, an argument for a visceral theory of addiction, a discussion of compulsive gambling as a form of addiction, discussions of George Ainslie's theory of hyperbolic discounting, analyses of social causes and policy implications and an investigation into relapse. *$75.00*

296 pages Year Founded: 1999 ISBN 0-521640-08-3

73 Getting Involved in AA

Hazelden
15251 Pleasant Valley Road
PO Box 176
Center City, MN 55012-0176   **651-213-4000**
                              800-328-9000
                        Fax: 651-213-4590
                            www.hazelden.org

Twelve specific suggestions help clients through their early days in the AA fellowship. Topics include different types of meetings, expectations, common pitfalls, as well as do's and don'ts. *$1.95*

24 pages ISBN 0-894861-36-0

74 Inside a Support Group

Rosen Publishing Group
29 E 21st Street
New York, NY 10010-6209   **212-777-3017**
                              800-237-9932
                        Fax: 888-436-4643
                E-mail: info@rosenpub.com
                      www.rosenpublishing.com

Lists support organizations for children of alcoholics. Explains what to expect at Alateen meetings and support groups for teenagers. *$25.25*

64 pages

75 Living Skills Recovery Workbook

Elsevier Science
11830 Westline Industrial Drive
St. Louis, MO 63146   **314-453-7010**
                              800-545-2522
                        Fax: 314-453-7095
                E-mail: custserv@elsevier.com
                          www.elsevier.com

Katie Hennessy, Medical Promotions Coordinator

Provides clinicians with the tools necessary to help patients with dual diagnoses acquire basic living skills. Focusing on stress management, time management, activities of daily living, and social skills training, each living skill is taught in relation to how it aids in recovery and relapse prevention for each patient's individual lifestyle and pattern of addiction. *$36.95*

224 pages ISBN 0-750671-18-1

76 Mother's Survival Guide to Recovery: All About Alcohol, Drugs & Babies

New Harbinger Publications
5674 Shattuck Avenue
Oakland, CA 94609-1662   **510-652-0215**
                              800-748-6273
                        Fax: 510-652-5472
        E-mail: customerservice@newharbinger.com
                      www.newharbinger.com

Offers a strong message of hope to help women cope with the challenges of recovering, deal with prenatal care and parenting issues, and take steps toward creating the healthy, happy families they want to have. A must read textbook for healthcare professionals and children's service workers. *$12.95*

138 pages ISBN 1-572240-49-0

77 Relapse Prevention for Addictive Behaviors: a Manual for Therapists

Blackwell Publishing
350 Main Street
Malden, MA 02148   **781-388-8200**
                        Fax: 781-388-8210
                E-mail: appi@psych.org
                            www.appi.org

Katie Duffy, Marketing Assistant

$34.95

224 pages ISBN 0-632024-84-4

78 Selfish Brain: Learning from Addiction

Hazelden
15251 Pleasant Valley Road
PO Box 176
Center City, MN 55012-0176   **651-213-4000**
                              800-328-9000
                        Fax: 651-213-4590
                            www.hazelden.org

Helps clients or loved ones face addiction and recovery by exploring the biological, historical and cultural aspects of addiction and its destructiveness. *$18.95*

544 pages ISBN 0-880486-86-4

79 Seven Points of Alcoholics Anonymous

Hazelden
15251 Pleasant Valley Road
PO Box 176
Center City, MN 55012-0176   **651-213-4000**
                              800-328-9000
                        Fax: 651-213-4590
                            www.hazelden.org

By the author of Twenty-Four Hours a Day. *$9.95*

103 pages ISBN 0-934125-16-3

80 Treating Alcoholism

Jossey-Bass Publishers
10475 Crosspoint Blvd
Indianapolis, IN 46256
877-762-2974
Fax: 800-597-3299
www.josseybass.com

$37.00

448 pages ISBN 0-787938-76-9

81 Twenty-Four Hours a Day

Hazelden
15251 Pleasant Valley Road
PO Box 176
Center City, MN 55012-0176
651-213-4000
800-328-9000
Fax: 651-213-4590
www.hazelden.org

Daily meditation in this classic book helps clients develop a solid foundation in a spiritual program, learn to relate the Twelve Steps to their everyday lives and accomplish their treatment and aftercare goals. Includes 366 daily meditations with special consideration and extra encouragement given during holidays. Helps clients find the power to stay sober each day and not to take that first drink. Hardcover - $12.00, Softcover - $10.00. *$10.00*

400 pages ISBN 0-894868-34-9

82 Why Haven't I Been Able to Help?

Hazelden
15251 Pleasant Valley Road
PO Box 176
Center City, MN 55012-0176
651-213-4000
800-328-9000
Fax: 651-213-4590
www.hazelden.org

Discusses how spouses of alcoholics are also trapped by deteriorating self-image, unconscious defense, destructive behavior, and offers change, especially through intervention. *$2.75*

12 pages ISBN 0-935908-40-4

Periodicals & Pamphlets

83 5 Smart Steps to Safer Drinking

ETR Associates
4 Carbonero Way
Scotts Valley, CA 95066
831-438-4060
800-321-4407
Fax: 800-435-8433
E-mail: customerservice@etr.org
www.etr.org

John Henry Ledwith, Sales

Steps to making healthy decisions about alcohol include: make choices, learn about alcohol, know your limits, have a plan, and watch for problems.

84 About Alcohol

ETR Associates
4 Carbonero Way
Scotts Valley, CA 95066
831-438-4060
800-321-4407
Fax: 800-435-8433
E-mail: customerservice@etr.org
www.etr.org

What it is, why it's dangerous, and its negative effects on the body and in prenatal development.

85 Al-Anon Speaks Out

Al-Anon Family Group Headquarters
1600 Corporate Landing Parkway
Virginia Beach, VA 23454-5617
757-563-1600
888-425-2666
Fax: 757-563-1655
E-mail: wso@al-anon.org
www.al-anon.alateen.org

Caryn Johnson, Communications

A newsletter for professionals who help families and friends of alcoholics. Explains the Al-Anon/Alateen program, how it works, new developments and items of interest and how Al-Anon/Alateen serves as a community resource.

86 Al-Anon/Alateen Lone Member Letter Box

Al-Anon Family Group Headquarters
1600 Corporate Landing Parkway
Virginia Beach, VA 23454-5617
757-563-1600
800-356-9996
Fax: 757-563-1655
E-mail: wso@al-anon.org
www.al-anon.alateen.org

Mary Ann Keller, Members Services

Provides a forum for members of Al-Anon and Alateen who cannot regularly attend meetings. Develops support correspondence with other Al - Anon and Alateen members.

4 pages 3 per year

87 Alateen Talk

Al-Anon Family Group Headquarters
1600 Corporate Landing Parkway
Virginia Beach, VA 23454-5617
757-563-1600
800-425-2666
Fax: 757-563-1655
E-mail: wso@al-anon.org
www.al-anon.alateen.org

Mary Ann Keller, Director Member Services

Newsletter with articles and drawings created by teenage and preteen Alateen members. Material relates to members' application of twelve step, and principles of Alateen program. Also includes articles by Alateen sponsors. *$2.50*

4 pages 4 per year ISSN 1054-1411

88 Alcohol ABC's

ETR Associates
4 Carbonero Way
Scotts Valley, CA 95066   831-438-4060
800-321-4407
Fax: 800-435-8433
E-mail: customerservice@etr.org
www.etr.org

Presents the consequenes of drinking and explains the difference between use and abuse in a straightforward, matter-of-fact way.

89 Alcohol Issues Insights

Beer Marketer's Insights
PO Box 264
W Nyack, NY 10994-0264   845-624-2337
Fax: 845-624-2340
E-mail: eric@beerinsights.com
www.beerinsights.com

Benjamin Steinman, Publisher

Provides information on the use and misuses of alcohol. Covers such topics as misrepresentation in the media, minimum age requirements, advertising bans, deterrence of drunk driving, and the effects of tax increases on alcoholic beverage consumption. *$255.00*

4 pages 12 per year ISSN 1067-3105

90 Alcohol Self-Test

ETR Associates
4 Carbonero Way
Scotts Valley, CA 95066   831-438-4060
800-321-4407
Fax: 800-435-8433
E-mail: customerservice@etr.org
www.etr.org

Thought provoking questions include: What do I know about alcohol? How safely do I drink? When and why do I drink?

91 Alcohol: Incredible Facts

ETR Associates
4 Carbonero Way
Scotts Valley, CA 95066   831-438-4060
800-321-4407
Fax: 800-435-8433
E-mail: customerservice@etr.org
www.etr.org

Strange but true facts to trigger discussion about alcohol use, social consequences, and risks involved.

92 Alcoholism: a Merry-Go-Round Named Denial

Hazelden
15251 Pleasant Valley Road
PO Box 176
Center City, MN 55012-0176   651-213-4000
800-328-9000
Fax: 651-213-4590
www.hazelden.org

This pamphlet provides a clear description of alcoholism and defines the roles of the alcoholic and those affected by chemical dependency. *$2.25*

20 pages ISBN 0-894860-22-4

93 Alcoholism: a Treatable Disease

Hazelden
15251 Pleasant Valley Road
PO Box 176
Center City, MN 55012-0176   651-213-4000
800-328-9000
Fax: 651-213-4590
www.hazelden.org

A hard look at the disease of chemical dependence, the confusion and delusion that go with it, intervention and a hopeful conclusion - alcoholism is treatable. *$2.75*

18 pages ISBN 0-935908-37-4

94 Binge Drinking: Am I At Risk?

ETR Associates
4 Carbonero Way
Scotts Valley, CA 95066   831-438-4060
800-321-4407
Fax: 800-435-8433
E-mail: customerservice@etr.org
www.etr.org

Easy-to-follow checklists help students decide if they have a problem with binge drinking, make a plan, and get help.

95 Chalice

Calix Society
2555 Hazelwood Avenue
Saint Paul, MN 55109-2030   651-773-3117
800-398-0524
Fax: 651-777-3069
www.calixsociety.org

Directed toward Catholic and non-Catholic alcoholics who are maintaining their sobriety through affiliation with and participation in Alcoholics Anonymous. Emphasizes the virtue of total abstinence, through contributed stories regarding spiritual and physical recovery. Recurring features include statistics, book announcements, and research. *$15.00*

4-6 pages 24 per year

96 Children and Youth Funding Report

CD Publications
8204 Fenton Street
Silver Spring, MD 20910-4509   301-588-6380
800-666-6380
Fax: 301-588-6385
E-mail: fsr@cdpublications.com
www.cdpublications.com

Mark Sherman, Editor

Helps social service professionals stay up-to-date on changing federal priorities and legislative develpments in Washington, with insight from agency officials, Congressional staff, and advocates on what's likely to happen in the months ahead. Also provides updates on national and local news, with in-depth reports on welfare reform, the federal budget, and entitlement programs. Features program ideas from around the country, to help children and youth service providers learn about innovative new strategies they can implement in their communities. *$269.00*

18 pages 24 per year ISSN 1524-9484

97 Crossing the Thin Line: Between Social Drinking and Alcoholism

Hazelden
15251 Pleasant Valley Road
PO Box 176
Center City, MN 55012-0176   651-213-4000
800-328-9000
Fax: 651-213-4590
www.hazelden.org

This pamphlet explores the physical predisposition to alcoholism, as well as behavioral and emotional changes. *$2.50*

20 pages ISBN 0-894860-77-1

98 Disease Concept of Alcoholism and Other Drug Addiction

Hazelden
15251 Pleasant Valley Road
PO Box 176
Center City, MN 55012-0176   651-213-4000
800-328-9000
Fax: 651-213-4590
www.hazelden.org

This pamphlet gives a close examination of the history of the disease concept and the nature of addiction as a disease. *$4.50*

35 pages ISBN 0-894866-91-5

99 Drug and Alcohol Dependence

Customer Support Services
PO Box 945
New York, NY 10159-0945   212-633-3730
888-437-4636
Fax: 212-633-3680
www.elsevier.nl/locate/drugalcdep

$200.00

12 per year ISSN 0376-8716

100 Getting Started in AA

Hazelden
15251 Pleasant Valley Road
PO Box 176
Center City, MN 55012-0176   651-213-4000
800-328-9000
Fax: 651-213-4590
www.hazelden.org

The principles and working of Alcoholics Anonymous provide an excellent resource for clients in early treatment and as a aftercare tool to provide ongoing support. *$10.00*

160 pages ISBN 1-568380-91-7

101 Getting What You Want From Drinking

ETR Associates
4 Carbonero Way
Scotts Valley, CA 95066   831-438-4060
800-321-4407
Fax: 800-435-8433
E-mail: customerservice@etr.org
www.etr.org

Practical ideas for drinking more safely, preventing hangovers, weight gain, and injuries; blood alcohol chart shows the effect of alcohol on the mind and body.

102 I Can't Be an Alcoholic Because...

Hazelden
15251 Pleasant Valley Road
PO Box 176
Center City, MN 55012-0176   651-213-4000
800-328-9000
Fax: 651-213-4590
www.hazelden.org

This pamphlet describes fallacies and misconceptions about alcoholism and includes facts and figures about alcohol, its use, and its abuse. Available in Spanish. *$1.75*

9 pages ISBN 0-894861-58-1

103 Miles of Heart

White House Press
PO Box 211
Hamburg, NY 14075-0211   716-648-6191
Fax: 716-648-6192
www.sobertimes.com/AboutUs.htm

Tom Claunch, Editor

Addresses alcoholism, chemical dependency and other addictions, prevention, treatment, and recovery. Recurring features include letters to the editor, interviews, a calendar of events, news of educational opportunities, job listings, book reviews, and notices of publications available. *$17.50*

20-32 pages 12 per year

104 Motivational Interviewing: Preparing People to Change Addictive Behavior

Guilford Publications
72 Spring Street
New York, NY 10012-4019   212-431-9800
800-365-7006
Fax: 212-966-6708
E-mail: info@guilford.com
www.guilford.com

A nonauthoritarian approach to helping people free up their own motivations and resources, overcome ambivalence and help 'unstuck.' Presents a practical, research-tested approach to effecting change in persons with addictive behaviors. Paperback also available. $36.00

419 pages ISBN 1-572305-63-0

105 Real World Drinking

ETR Associates
4 Carbonero Way
Scotts Valley, CA 95066   831-438-4060
                                 800-321-4407
                            Fax: 800-435-8433
       E-mail: customerservice@etr.org
                                 www.etr.org

Credible young people talk about benefits of not drinking and risks of drinking.

106 Teens and Drinking

ETR Associates
4 Carbonero Way
Scotts Valley, CA 95066   831-438-4060
                                 800-321-4407
                            Fax: 800-435-8433
       E-mail: customerservice@etr.org
                                 www.etr.org

Includes common sense messages about drinking, binge drinking, and important things to know about drinking.

107 When Someone You Care About Abuses Drugs and Alcohol: When to Act, What to Say

Hazelden
15251 Pleasant Valley Road
PO Box 176
Center City, MN 55012-0176   651-213-4000
                                 800-328-9000
                            Fax: 651-213-4590
                            www.hazelden.org

This pamphlet shows family, friends, and co-workers how to confront someone who may be abusing alcohol or other drugs. *$2.00*

16 pages

Support Groups & Hot Lines

108 Adult Children of Alcoholics World Services Organization

PO Box 3216
Torrance, CA 90510   310-534-1815
       E-mail: info@adultchildren.org
                            www.adultchildren.org

A 12-Step and 12-Tradition program for adults raised in an environment including alcohol or other dysfunctions.

109 Al-Anon Family Group Headquarters

1600 Corporate Landing Parkway
Virginia Beach, VA 23454-5617   212-302-7240
                                 888-425-2666

For relatives and friends of persons with alcohol problems. Includes Alateen.

110 Al-Anon Family Group National Referral Hotline

1600 Corporate Landing Parkway
Virginia Beach, VA 23454   757-563-1600
                                 888-425-2666
                            Fax: 757-563-1655
       E-mail: wso@al-anon.org
                            www.al-anon.alateen.org

Al-Anon's purpose is to help families and friends of alcoholics recover from the effects of living with the problem drinking of a relative or friend.

111 Alateen and Al-Anon Family Groups

1600 Corporate Landing Parkway
Virginia Beach, VA 23454-5617   757-563-1600
                                 888-425-2666
                            Fax: 757-563-1655
       E-mail: wso@al-anon.org
                            www.al-anon.org

Mary Ann Keller, Director Members Services

A fellowship of youth affected by another person's drinking.

112 Alcoholics Anonymous (AA): Worldwide

475 Riverside Drive
New York, NY 10115   212-870-3400
                            Fax: 212-870-3137
                            E-mail: cr@aa.org
                                 www.aa.org

For men and women who share the common problems of alcoholism.

113 Mothers Against Drunk Drivers

511 E John Carpenter Freeway
Suite 700
Irving, TX 75062   214-744-6233
                                 800-438-6233
                                 www.madd.org

114 Rational Recovery

PO Box 800
Lotus, CA 95651   530-621-2667
                            www.rational.org/recovery

Abstinence-based.

115 SADD-Students Against Drunk Drivers

PO Box 800
Marlboro, MA 01752   508-481-3568
                                 www.saddonline.org

116 Self Management and Recovery Training

7537 Mentor Avenue, Suite 306
Mentor, OH 44060
440-951-5357
Fax: 440-951-5358
E-mail: srmail1@aol.com
www.smartrecovery.org

Cognitive behavioral abstinence-based approach.

Video & Audio

117 Alcohol: the Substance, the Addiction, the Solution

Hazelden
15251 Pleasant Valley Road
PO Box 176
Center City, MN 55012-0176
651-213-4000
800-328-9000
Fax: 651-213-4590
www.hazelden.org

Weaves dramatic personal stories of recovery from alcoholism with essential facts about alcohol itself. Emphasizes the impact of using and abusing alcohol in conjunction with other drugs. Educates about the dangers of this legally sanctioned drug, including the myth of safer versions such as wine and beer. *$225.00*

118 Disease of Alcoholism Video

Hazelden
15251 Pleasant Valley Road
PO Box 176
Center City, MN 55012-0176
651-213-4000
800-328-9000
Fax: 651-213-4590
www.hazelden.org

This video is used daily in treatment, corporations, and schools. Dr. Ohlms discusses startling and convincing information on the genetic and physiological aspects of alcohol addiction. *$395.00*

119 Fetal Alcohol Syndrome and Effect, Stories of Help and Hope

Hazelden
15251 Pleasant Valley Road
PO Box 176
Center City, MN 55012-0176
651-213-4000
800-328-9000
Fax: 651-213-4590
www.hazelden.org

Provides clients with a factual defintion of the medical diagonosis of fetal alcohol syndrome and its effects, including how children are diagnosed and the positive prognosis possible for these children. *$225.00*

120 I'll Quit Tomorrow

Hazelden
15251 Pleasant Valley Road
PO Box 176
Center City, MN 55012-0176
651-213-4000
800-328-9000
Fax: 651-213-4590
www.hazelden.org

Show clients the progressive nature of alcoholism through one of the most powerful films ever made about this disease. This three-part video series and facilitator's guide use a dramatic personal story to provide a clear and thorough introduction to the disease concept of alcoholism, enabling the intervention process, treatment and the hope of healing and recovery. Facilitator's guide costs $14.00. *$300.00*

121 Twenty-Four Hours a Day Audio

Hazelden
15251 Pleasant Valley Road
PO Box 176
Center City, MN 55012-0176
651-213-4000
800-328-9000
Fax: 651-213-4590
www.hazelden.org

Clients gain the wisdom of the book Twenty-Four Hours a Day in a convenient audio format. Clients develop a deeper connection with their spiritual nature and with the Twelve Steps. Two audio tapes. *$17.95*

ISBN 1-574532-65-0

Web Sites

122 Join Together Online

1 Appleton Street
4th Floor
Boston, MA 02116
617-437-1500
Fax: 617-437-9394
E-mail: editor@jointogether.org
www.jointogether.org

A project of the Boston University School of Public Health, this association's mission is to help reduce substance abuse and gun violence.

123 www.Al-Anon-Alateen.org

Al-Anon and Alateen

AA literature may serve as an introduction.

124 www.addictionresourceguide.com

Addiction Resource Guide

Descriptions of inpatient, outpatient programs.

125 www.alcoholism.about.com/library

Alcohol and the Elderly

Links to other pages relevant to overuse of alcohol and drugs in the elderly.

126 **www.alcoholismhelp.com**

Another Empty Bottle

Links to health, organizations, drunk driving, support, treatment, etc.

127 **www.jacsweb.org**

JACS

Ten articles dealing with denial and ignorance.

128 **www.mayohealth.org/mayo/9707/htm/alcohol.htm**

Alcohol-An Interactive Assessment

Test and feedback guide to 12 step programs.

129 **www.mckinley.uiuc.edu/health-info/drug-alc/ drug-alc.html**

Drug/Alcohol Brochures

Single page handouts with basic information.

130 **www.naadac.org**

National Association of Alcohol and Drug Abuse Counselors

Its mission is to lead, unify and empower global addiction focused professionals to achieve excellence through education, advocacy, knowledge, standards of practice, ethics, professional development and research. Advocates on behalf of addiction professionals and the people they serve. Establishes and promotes the highest possible standards of practice and qualifications for addiction professionals.

131 **www.psychcentral.com**

Psych Central

Personalized one-stop index for psychology, support, and mental health issues, resources, and people on the Internet.

132 **www.pta.org/commonsense**

Common Sense: Strategies for Raising Alcoholic/Drug Free Children

Drug facts, warning signs, and guidance.

133 **www.smartrecovery.org**

SMART: Self-Management and Recovery Training

Four-Point program includes maintaining motivation, coping with urges, managing feelings and behavior, balancing momentary/enduring satisfactions.

134 **www.soulselfhelp.on.ca/coda.html**

The Issues of Codependency

Discusses self-help, mental health, issues of co-dependency.

135 **www.unhooked.com/toolbox/index.html**

LifeRing

Offers nonreligious approach with links to groups.

136 **www.well.com/user/woa/**

Web of Addictions

Links to fact sheets from trustworthy sources.

Introduction

It is perfectly normal to feel worried or nervous sometimes, especially if there is an obvious reason: a loved one is late coming home; your yearly evaluation meeting; an important social event is looming. Even when you are nervous or anxious with good cause, you continue performing life's functions adequately. Indeed, some anxiety is not only normal, it is necessary, helping us to avoid trouble and danger - like making sure your child is safely buckled in a car. But if you can't rid yourself of your worry, if people close to you comment that you seem bothered and unlike yourself, or if your nervousness is affecting important relationships in your personal and work life, it is time to seek help. Sometimes a person who suffers from persistent anxiety turns to alcohol or other drugs in an effort to seek relief.

Different kinds of Anxiety Disorders have been identified. Several of the most prevalent are discussed in detail below. Treatment is tailored to the particular disorder and has become more effective as a result.

SYMPTOMS

Agoraphobia
•Usually involves fears connected with being outside the home and alone;
•Anxiety about being in places or situations from which it is difficult or embarrassing to escape (e.g., in the middle seat of a row in a theatre) or in which help may not be immediately available (as in an airplane);
•Such situations are avoided or endured with distress and fear of having a panic attack.

Social Anxiety Disorder
•Fear of being humiliated or embarrassed in a social situation with strangers or where other people are watching;
•Being in the situation causes intense anxiety, sometimes with panic attacks;
•Realizing that the fear is irrational;

•The fear leads to avoidance of social situations and interferes with the ability to function at work or with friends and family.

General Anxiety Disorder
•Excessive worry and anxiety on most days for at least six months about several events or activities such as work or school performance;
•Difficulty in controlling the worry;
•The anxiety is connected with at least three of the following: restlessness/feeling on edge; being easily tired; difficulty concentrating; irritability; muscle tension; difficulty falling/staying asleep or restless sleep;
•The anxiety or physical symptoms seriously affect the person's social life, work life, or other important areas.

Panic Disorder
Repeated panic attacks, followed by continuous anxiety that another attack will occur, fear of terrible consequences (e.g., a heart attack or going crazy), and behavior that is markedly changed because of the attacks. A panic attack is a period of intense fear in which four or more of the following symptoms escalate suddenly, reaching a peak within ten minutes, after which they diminish:
•Palpitations and pounding;
•Rapid heartbeat;
•Sweating;
•Trembling or shaking;
•Shortness of breath;
•Feeling of choking;
•Chest pain;
•Nausea;
•Feeling dizzy or faint;
•Feelings of unreality, or being detached;
•Fear of losing control or going crazy;
•Fear of dying;
•Numbness or tingling;
•Chills or hot flashes.

Phobias
•Persistent, unreasonable, and exaggerated fear of the presence or anticipated presence of a particular object or situation (e.g., snake, flying, blood);
•The presence of such an object or situation triggers immediate anxiety which may be a panic attack;

•Knowledge that the fear is exaggerated and unreasonable;

•The phobic situation is either avoided or experienced with extreme distress;

•The avoidance, fearful anticipation, and distress seriously affects the person's normal routine, work and social activities, and relationships.

ASSOCIATED FEATURES

Anxiety can be extremely intense such as the fear of imminent death in a panic attack or it can be experienced as state of chronic nagging worry for those suffering from Generalized Anxiety Disorder. Whatever its intensity or frequency, it persists over time. One of the hallmarks of Anxiety Disorders is that the person is unable to control the anxiety, even when he or she knows it is exaggerated and unreasonable. To other people, the person may seem edgy, irritable, fearful, or have unexpected outbursts of anger. For the anxious person, the problem can take up time and effort and can become a major preoccupation. In addition to the psychological effects (and entangled with them) are the physical effects, that is, a frequent or constant state of physical arousal and tension. Using alcohol or drugs to resolve the problem is ineffective and dangerous. Anxiety Disorders negatively affect all aspects of life-family, work, and friends.

PREVALENCE

Anxiety Disorders are the most common psychiatric disorders in the U.S. In any six-month period, one out of 20 Americans — children, adults, the elderly, men and women will suffer from an Anxiety Disorder that should be treated professionally. Anxiety Disorders are approximately twice as common in women as in men.

TREATMENT OPTIONS

It is very important to have a psychiatric evaluation so that a proper diagnosis can be made. Self medication with alcohol, tranquilizers, or other drugs is dangerous and can lead to serious drug abuse. Many people who abuse drugs are suffering from an underlying Anxiety Disorder. Treatment will vary depending on which of the Anxiety Disorders is diagnosed. Drugs, psychotherapy or both will be prescribed. Effective treatments have been developed for various Anxiety Disorders. People with Agoraphobia, Panic Disorder, and the Phobias generally respond very well to medication and a specially tailored course of psychotherapy. Paxil has proved to be specifically effective for Social Anxiety Disorder. Generalized Anxiety Disorder is treated with psychotherapy or a combination of therapy and drugs. Some psychotherapies which have proven helpful in certain cases are cogitive-behavioral therapies, such as exposure therapy, as well as other types including the fairly controversial eye movement desensitization therapy. Selective Serotonin Reuptake Inhibitors, or SSRIs, which were originally developed as Antidepressants, have proved to be effective in several Anxiety Disorders as well. Suddenly stopping an SSRI can cause rebound symptoms including sleeplessness, headaches, and irritability. Medications should be tapered under the care of a physician.

Associations & Agencies

138 Agoraphobics in Motion
1719 Crooks Road
Royal Oak, MI 48067-1306   248-547-0400
E-mail: anny@ameritech.net
www.aim-hq.org

AIM is a nationwide, nonprofit, support group organization, committed to the support and recovery of those suffering with anxiety disorders, and their families.

139 Anxiety Disorders Association of America
8730 Georgia Avenue
Suite 600
Silver Spring, MD 20910   240-485-1001
Fax: 240-485-1035
E-mail: AnxDis@adaa.org
www.adaa.org

Alies Muskin, COO
Jerilyn Ross, President/CEO

A national non profit organization dedicated exclusively to promoting the prevention, treatment, and cure of anxiety disorders and improving the lives of all people touched by these disorders. ADAA provides educational and advocacy services, supports research, self help, and access to care. ADAA serves consumers, health care professionals, researchers, educators and other interested individuals and organizations. The association publishes a bimonthly newsletter, hosts an annual conference, and maintains an extensive online bookstore.

140 Anxiety Disorders Institute
1 Dunwoody Park
Suite 112
Atlanta, GA 30338-6539   770-395-6845

Karen Strickland RN

Provides support, training, and services for those suffering from anxiety disorders, and their families.

141 Anxiety and Phobia Treatment Center
White Plains Hospital Center
Davis Avenue at E Post Road
White Plains, NY 10601   914-681-1038
Fax: 914-681-2284
E-mail: questions@phobia-anxiety.com
www.healthanxiety.org

Fredrick J Neumen MD, Director

Treatment groups for individuals suffering from phobias. Deals with fears through contextual therapy, a treatment and study of the phobia in the actual setting in which the phobic reactions occur. Conducts Intensive Courses, Phobia Self-Help Groups, 8-week Phobia Clinics and individual treatment. Publications: PM Newsletter, bimonthly. Articles and papers. Annual conference.

142 Career Assessment & Planning Services
Goodwill Industries-Suncoast
10596 Gandy Boulevard
PO Box 14456
St. Petersburg, FL 33733   727-523-1512
Fax: 727-563-9300
E-mail: gw.marketing@goodwill-suncoast.com
www.goodwill-suncoast.org

R Lee Waits, President/CEO
Gary Hebert, VP/Treasurer
Dan Johnson, Secretary

Provides a comprehensive assessment, which can predict current and future employment and potential adjustment factors for physically, emotionally, or developmentally disabled persons who may be unemployed or underemployed. Assessments evaluate interests, aptitudes, academic achievements, and physical abilities (including dexterity and coordination) through coordinated testing, interviewing, and behavioral observations.

143 Center for Family Support (CFS)
333 7th Avenue
New York, NY 10001-5004   212-629-7939
Fax: 212-239-2211
www.cfsny.org

Steven Vernickofs, Executive Director

Service agency devoted to the physical well-being and development of the retarded child and the sound mental health of the parents. Helps families with retarded children with all aspects of home care including counseling, referrals, home aide service and consultation. Offers intervention for parents at the birth of a retarded child with in-home support, guidance and infant stimulation. Pioneered training of nonprofessional women as home aides to provide supportive services in homes.

144 Center for Mental Health Services Knowledge Exchange Network
US Department of Health and Human Services
PO Box 42490
Washington, DC 20015-4800
800-789-2647
Fax: 301-984-8796
E-mail: ken@mentalhealth.org
www.mentalhealth.org

Information about resources, technical assistance, research, training, networks, and other federal clearing houses, and fact sheets and materials. Information specialists refer callers to mental health resources in their communities as well as state, federal and nonprofit contacts. Staff available Monday through Friday, 8:30 AM-5:00 PM, EST, excluding federal holidays. After hours, callers may leave messages and an information specialist will return their call.

145 Freedom From Fear
308 Seaview Avenue
Staten Island, NY 10305   718-351-1717
Fax: 718-667-8893
www.freedomfromfear.com

The mission of Freedom From Fear is to aid and counsel individuals and their families who suffer from anxiety and depressive illness.

146 International Critical Incident Stress Foundation

10176 Baltimore National Park
Unit 201
Ellicott City, MD 21042   410-750-9600
                                Fax: 410-750-9601
                                www.icisf.org

A nonprofit, open membership foundation dedicated to the prevention and mitigation of disabling stress by education, training and support services for all emergency service professionals. Continuing education and training in emergency mental health services for psychologists, psychiatrists, social workers and licensed professional counselors.

147 NADD: Association for Persons with Developmental Disabilities and Mental Health Needs

132 Fair Street
Kingston, NY 12401-4802   845-334-4336
                                800-331-5362
                                Fax: 845-331-4569
                                E-mail: nadd@mhv.net
                                www.thenadd.org

Dr. Robert Fletcher, Executive Director

Nonprofit organization designed to promote interest of professional and parent development with resources for individuals who have the coexistence of mental illness and mental retardation. Provides conference, educational services and training materials to professionals, parents, concerned citizens and service organizations. Formerly known as the National Association for the Dually Diagnosed.

148 National Alliance for the Mentally Ill

2107 Wilson Boulevard
Suite 300
Arlington, VA 22201-3042   703-524-7600
                                800-950-6264
                                Fax: 703-524-9094
                                TDD: 703-516-7227
                                E-mail: helpline@nami.org
                                www.nami.org

Laurie Flynn, Executive Director

Nation's leading self-help organization for all those affected by severe brain disorders. Mission is to bring consumers and families with similar experiences together to share information about services, care providers, and ways to cope with the challenges of schizophrenia, manic depression, and other serious mental illnesses.

149 National Anxiety Foundation

3135 Custer Drive
Lexington, KY 40517-4001   859-272-7166
                                www.lexington-on-line.com/naf.html

To alleviate suffering and to save lives by educating the public about anxiety disorders.

150 National Mental Health Consumer's Self-Help Clearinghouse

1211 Chestnut Street
Suite 1207
Philadelphia, PA 19107   215-751-1810
                                800-553-4539
                                Fax: 215-636-6312
                                E-mail: info@mhselfhelp.org
                                www.mhselfhelp.org

Alex Morrsey, Information/Referral

Funded by the National Institute of Mental Health Community Support Program, the purpose of the Clearinghouse is to encourage the development and growth of consumer self-help groups.

Year Founded: 1992

151 Selective Mutism Foundation

PO Box 1198
Medford, NY 11763   305-748-7714
                          Fax: 305-748-7714
                          E-mail: sue@selectivemutismfoundation.org
                          www.selectivemutismfoundation.org

Sue Newman, Co-Founder/Director

Promote awareness and understanding for individuals and families affected by selective mutism, an inherited anxiety disorder in which children with normal or deficient language skills are unable to speak in school or social situations. SM is often mistaken for normal shyness and may go undetected for as long as two years. Encourages research and treatment. Maintains speakers' bureau. Publications: Let's Talk, annual newsletter. Selective Mutism, A Silent Cry for Help, brochure.

152 Special Interest Group on Phobias and Related Anxiety Disorders (SIGPRAD)

245 E 87th Street
New York, NY 10028-1320   212-860-5560
                                Fax: 212-744-5751
                                E-mail: lindy@interport.net
                                www.cyberpsych.org

Carol Lindemann PhD, CEO

For psychologists, psychiatrists, social workers and other individuals interested in treatment of anxiety disorders. Objectives are to increase knowledge, facilitate communication, and support research and treatment of phobias and related anxiety disorders. Conducts programs at professional meetings. Affiliated with the Association for Advancement of Behavior Therapy. Periodic symposiums and workshops.

153 Suncoast Residential Training Center/Developmental Services Program

Goodwill Industries-Suncoast
10596 Gandy Boulevard
St. Petersburg, FL 33733   727-523-1512
                                888-279-1988
                                Fax: 727-563-9300
                                E-mail: gw.marketing@goodwill-suncoast.com
                                www.goodwill-suncoast.org

R Lee Waits, President/CEO
Loreen M Spencer, Chair Person

A large group home which serves individuals diagnosed as mentally retarded with a secondary diagnosis of psychiatric difficulties as evidenced by problem behavior. Providing residential, behavioral and instructional support and services that will promote the development of adaptive, socially appropriate behavior, each individual is assessed to determine, socialization, basic academics and recreation. The primary intervention strategy is applied behavior analysis. Professional consultants are utilized to address the medical, dental, psychiatric and pharmacological needs of each individual. One of the most popular features is the active community integration component of SRTC. Program customers attend an average of 15 monthly outings to various community events.

154 Territorial Apprehensiveness (TERRAP) Programs

932 Evelyn Street
Menlo Park, CA 94025-4710

800-274-6242

Crucita V Hardy, Director

Territorial Apprehensiveness was formed to disseminate information concerning the recognition, causes, and treatment of anxieties, fears and phobias especially agoraphobia. Provides information and counseling for those with phobias. Sponsors service centers and training for psychotherapists and counselors. Publications: TERRAP Manual, audiotapes, booklets, monographs, and videos.

155 Women Helping Agoraphobia

PO Box 4900
S Framingham, MA 01701   508-620-0300

Constance Fitzpatrick, Director

Organization of women dedicated to support women who suffer from this disorder and their families.

Books

156 An End to Panic: Breakthrough Techniques for Overcoming Panic Disorder

New Harbinger Publications
5674 Shattuck Avenue
Oakland, CA 94609-1662   510-652-2002
                              800-748-6273
                          Fax: 510-652-5472
E-mail: customerservice@newharbinger.com
              www.newharbinger.com

A state of the art treatment program covers breathing retraining, taking charge of fear fueling thoughts, overcoming the fear of physical symptoms, coping with phobic situations, avoiding relapse, and living in the here and now. *$18.95*

230 pages ISBN 1-572241-13-6

157 Anxiety & Phobia Workbook

New Harbinger Publications
5674 Shattuck Avenue
Oakland, CA 94609-1662   510-652-2002
                              800-748-6273
                          Fax: 510-652-5472
E-mail: customerservice@newharbinger.com
              www.newharbinger.com

This comprehensive guide is recommended to those struggling with anxiety disorders. Includes step by step instructions for the crucial cognitive - behavioral techniques that have given real help to hundreds of thousands of readers struggling with anxiety disorders. *$19.95*

448 pages ISBN 1-572240-03-2

158 Anxiety Cure: Eight Step-Program for Getting Well

John Wiley & Sons
605 3rd Avenue
New York, NY 10058-0180   212-850-6000
                          Fax: 212-850-6008
              E-mail: info@wiley.com
                      www.wiley.com

Anxiety disorders are the most common type of emotional trouble and among the most treatable. Dupont provides a practical guide featuring a step-by-step program for curing the six kinds of anxiety. *$14.95*

256 pages ISBN 0-471247-01-4

159 Anxiety Disorders

Cambridge University Press
40 W 20th Street
New York, NY 10011-4211   212-924-3900
                              800-872-7423
                          Fax: 212-691-3239
          E-mail: marketing@cup.org
                      www.cup.org

Stephen Bourne, Chief Press Executive / Director

This comprehensive text covers all the anxiety disorders found in the latest DSM and ICD classifications. Provides detailed information about seven principal disorders, including anxiety in the medically ill. For each disorder, the book covers diagnosis criteria, epidemiology, etiology and pathogenesis, clinical features, natural history and different diagnosis. Describes treatment approaches, both psychological and pharmacological. *$74.95*

354 pages

160 Anxiety Disorders: Practioner's Guide

John Wiley & Sons
605 3rd Avenue
New York, NY 10058-0180   212-850-6000
                          Fax: 212-850-6008
              E-mail: info@wiley.com
                      www.wiley.com

$135.00

210 pages ISBN 0-471931-12-8

161 Anxiety and Its Disorders

Guilford Publications
72 Spring Street
New York, NY 10012　　212-431-9800
　　　　800-365-7006
　　　　Fax: 212-966-6708
E-mail: info@guilford.com
www.guilford.com

Incorporating recent advances from cognitive science and neurobiology on the mechanisms of anxiety and using emotion theory as basic theoretical framework. Ties theory and research of emerging clinical knowledge to create a new model of anxiety with profound implications for treatment. *$75.00*

700 pages ISBN 1-572304-30-8

162 Anxiety and Phobia Workbook

Anxiety Disorders Association of America
8730 Georgia Avenue
Suite 600
Silver Spring, MD 20910　　301-231-9350
Fax: 301-231-7392
E-mail: AnxDis@adaa.org
www.adaa.org

Alies Muskin, COO
Michelle Alonso, Communications/Membership

Comprehensive guide offering help to anyone who is struggling with panic attacks, agoraphobia, social fears, generalized anxiety, obsessive - compulsive behavior or other anxiety disorders.

163 Anxiety and the Anxiety Disorders

Lawrence Erlbaum Associates
10 Industrial Avenue
Mahwah, NJ 07430-2262　　201-258-2200
　　　　800-926-6579
Fax: 201-236-0072
E-mail: orders@erlbaum.com
www.erlbaum.com

Hardcover. *$160.00*

1172 pages Year Founded: 1985 ISBN 0-898595-32-0

164 Anxiety, Phobias, and Panic: a Step-By-Step Program for Regaining Control of Your Life

Time Warner Books
3 Center Plaza
Boston, MA 02108
　　　　800-759-0190
E-mail: sales@aoltwbg.com
www.twbookmark.com

Helps you identify stress and reduce stress anxiety, recognize and change distorted mental habits, stop thinking and acting like a victim, eliminate the excessive need for approval, make anger your friend and ally, stand up for yourself and feel good about yourself, and conquer your fears and take charge of your life. *$11.00*

363 pages ISBN 0-446670-53-7

165 Check Up from the Neck Up, Ensuring your Mental Health in the New Millennium

Hope Press
PO Box 188
Duarte, CA 91009-0100　　818-303-0644
　　　　800-321-4039
Fax: 818-358-3520
www.hopepress.com

Provides concise coping techniques for adults who have difficulties due to anxiety, depression, short temper, irritability, rage-attacks, compulsions, obsession and attention deficit hyperactivity disorder. *$19.95*

550 pages ISBN 1-878267-09-4

166 Cognitive Therapy for Depression and Anxiety

American Psychiatric Publishing
1000 Wilson Boulevard
Suite 1825
Arlington, VA 22209-3901　　703-907-7322
　　　　800-368-5777
Fax: 703-907-1091
E-mail: appi@psych.org
www.appi.org

Katie Duffy, Marketing Assistant

Detailed guide to using cognitive therapy in the treatment of patients suffering from depression and anxiety - two of the most prevalent disorders encountered in the community. *$44.95*

240 pages ISBN 0-632039-86-8

167 Cognitive Therapy of Anxiety Disorders: Practice Manual & Conceptual Guide

John Wiley & Sons
605 3rd Avenue
New York, NY 10058-0180　　212-850-6000
Fax: 212-850-6008
E-mail: info@wiley.com
www.wiley.com

168 Comorbidity of Mood and Anxiety Disorders

American Psychiatric Publishing
1000 Wilson Boulevard
Suite 1825
Arlington, VA 22209-3901　　703-907-7322
　　　　800-368-5777
Fax: 703-907-1091
E-mail: appi@psych.org
www.appi.org

Katie Duffy, Assistant Editor

Presents a systematic examination of the concurrence of different symptoms and syndromes in patients with anxiety or mood disorders. *$75.00*

868 pages ISBN 0-880483-24-5

169 Concise Guide to Anxiety Disorders

American Psychiatric Publishing
1000 Wilson Boulevard
Suite 1825
Arlington, VA 22209-3901
703-907-7322
800-368-5777
Fax: 703-907-1091
E-mail: appi@psych.org
www.appi.org

Robert S Pursell, Marketing

Concise Guide to Anxiety Disorders summarizes the latest research and translates it into practical treatment strategies for the best clinical outcomes. Designed for daily use in the clinical setting, it serves as an instant library of current information, quick to access and easy to understand. Every clinician who diagnoses and treats patients with anxiety disorders-including psychiatrists, residents and medical students, psychologists, and mental health professionals-will find this book invaluable for making informed treatment decisions. *$29.95*

272 pages Year Founded: 2003 ISBN 1-585620-80-7

170 Consumer's Guide to Psychiatric Drugs

New Harbinger Publications
5674 Shattuck Avenue
Oakland, CA 94609-1662
510-652-2002
800-748-6273
Fax: 510-652-5472
E-mail: customerservice@newharbinger.com
www.newharbinger.com

Helps consumers understand what treatment options are available and what side effects to expect. Covers possible interactions with other drugs, medical conditions and other concerns. Explains how each drug works, and offers detailed information about treatments for depression, bipolar disorder, anxiety and sleep disorders, as well as other conditions. *$16.95*

340 pages ISBN 1-572241-11-X

171 Coping with Anxiety and Panic Attacks

Rosen Publishing Group
29 E 21st Street
New York, NY 10010-6209
800-237-9932
Fax: 888-436-4643
E-mail: info@rosenpub.com
www.rosenpublishing.com

Strategies to get on with your life. *$26.50*

ISBN 0-823932-02-8

172 Coping with Trauma: A Guide to Self Understanding

Anxiety Disorders Association of America
8730 Georgia Avenue
Suite 600
Silver Spring, MD 20910
301-231-9350
Fax: 301-231-7392
E-mail: AnxDis@adaa.org
www.adaa.org

Alies Muskin, COO
Michelle Alonso, Communications/Membership

Book will appeal to and including survivors of traumatic stress, as well as mental health professionals.

173 Don't Panic: Taking Control of Anxiety Attacks

Anxiety Disorders Association of America
8730 Georgia Avenue
Suite 600
Silver Spring, MD 20910
301-231-9350
Fax: 301-231-7392
E-mail: AnxDis@adaa.org
www.adaa.org

Alies Muskin, COO
Michelle Alonso, Communications/Marketing

Book on overcoming panic and anxiety.

174 Dying of Embarrassment: Help for Social Anxiety and Social Phobia

New Harbinger Publications
5674 Shattuck Avenue
Oakland, CA 94609-1662
510-652-2002
800-748-6273
Fax: 510-652-5472
E-mail: customerservice@newharbinger.com
www.newharbinger.com

Clear, supportive instructions for assessing your fears, improving or developing new social skills, and changing self defeating thinking patterns. *$13.95*

204 pages ISBN 1-879237-23-7

175 EMDR: Breakthrough Therapy for Overcoming Anxiety, Stress and Trauma

Basic Books/Perseus Books Group
5500 Central Avenue
Boulder, CO 80301
800-386-5656
Fax: 720-406-7336
E-mail: westview.orders@perseusbooks.com
www.perseusbooksgroup.com

Sonya Harris, Specialty Wholesale
Jim Cook, Specialty Retail

EMDR-Eye Movement Desensitization and Reprocessing, has successfully relieved symptoms like depression, phobias and nightmares of PTSD survivors, with a rapidity that almost defies belief. In this book for general audiences, Shapiro, the originator of EMDR, explains how she created the groundbreaking therapy, how it works and how it can help people who feel stuck in negative reactions and behaviors. Included with the text are a variety of compelling case studies. *$17.00*

304 pages ISSN 04301-1ISBN 0-465043-01-1

176 Encyclopedia of Phobias, Fears, and Anxieties

Facts on File
132 West 31st Street
17th Floor
New York, NY 10001-2006

800-322-8755
Fax: 800-678-3633
E-mail: custserv@factsonfile.com
www.factsonfile.com

Providing the basic information on common phobias and anxieties, some 2000 entries explain the nature of anxiety disorders, panic attacks, specific phobias, and obsessive-complusive disorders. *$71.50*

576 pages Year Founded: 2000 ISBN 0-816039-89-5

177 Five Weeks to Healing Stress: the Wellness Option

New Harbinger Publications
5674 Shattuck Avenue
Oakland, CA 94609-1662

510-652-2002
800-748-6273
Fax: 510-652-5472
E-mail: customerservice@newharbinger.com
www.newharbinger.com

This workbook presents a quick and effective, body oriented program for regaining inner strength and calming stress. *$17.95*

216 pages ISBN 1-572240-55-5

178 Flying Without Fear

New Harbinger Publications
5674 Shattuck Avenue
Oakland, CA 94609-1662

510-652-2002
800-748-6273
Fax: 510-652-5472
E-mail: customerservice@newharbinger.com
www.newharbinger.com

Program to confront fears of flying and guides you through first takeoff and later flights. *$13.95*

176 pages ISBN 1-572240-42-3

179 Free from Fears: New Help for Anxiety, Panic and Agoraphobia

Anxiety Disorders Association of America
8730 Georgia Avenue
Suite 600
Silver Spring, MD 20910

301-231-9350
Fax: 301-231-7392
E-mail: AnxDis@adaa.org
www.adaa.org

Alies Muskin, COO
Michelle Alonso, Communications/Membership

Book shows you how to recognize the avoidance trap, combat fears, and modify your behavior for a lasting cure.

180 Healing Fear: New Approaches to Overcoming Anxiety

New Harbinger Publications
5674 Shattuck Avenue
Oakland, CA 94609-1662

510-652-2002
800-748-6273
Fax: 510-652-5472
E-mail: customerservice@newharbinger.com
www.newharbinger.com

Covers a wide range of healing strategies that help you learn how to relinquish control, discover a unique purpose that is bigger than your particular fears, and find ways to restructure your work and home environments to make them more congruent with the real you. *$ 16.95*

416 pages ISBN 1-572241-16-0

181 How to Help Your Loved One Recover from Agoraphobia

Anxiety Disorders Association of America
8730 Georgia Avenue
Suite 600
Silver Spring, MD 20910

301-231-9350
Fax: 301-231-7392
E-mail: AnxDis@adaa.org
www.adaa.org

Alies Muskin, COO
Michelle Alonso, Communications/Membership

Book is helpful for sufferer and family members to understand what a sufferer is going through.

182 It's Nobody's Fault: New Hope and Help for Difficult Children and Their Parents

ADD WareHouse
300 NW 70th Avenue
Suite 102
Plantation, FL 33317

954-792-8100
800-233-9273
Fax: 954-792-8545
E-mail: sales@addwarehouse.com
www.addwarehouse.com

This book explains that neither the parents nor children are causes of mental disorders and related problems. *$15.00*

320 pages Year Founded: 1997

183 It's Not All In Your Head: Now Women Can Discover the Real Causes of their Most Misdiagnosed Health Problems

Anxiety Disorders Association of America
8730 Georgia Avenue
Suite 600
Silver Spring, MD 20910

301-231-9350
Fax: 301-231-7392
E-mail: AnxDis@adaa.org
www.adaa.org

Alies Muskin, COO
Michelle Alonso, Communications/Membership

This book will present you with information about when, how and from whom to see treatment.

184 Master Your Panic and Take Back Your Life

Anxiety Disorders Association of America
8730 Georgia Avenue
Suite 600
Silver Spring, MD 20910   301-231-9350
                          Fax: 301-231-7392
                   E-mail: AnxDis@adaa.org
                              www.adaa.org

Alies Muskin, COO
Michelle Alonso, Communications/Membership

This book will help those suffering from panic and agoraphobia.

185 Master Your Panic and Take Back Your Life: Twelve Treatment Sessions to Overcome High Anxiety

Impact Publishers
PO Box 6016
Atascadero, CA 93423-6016   805-466-5917
                                 800-246-7228
                            Fax: 805-466-5919
              E-mail: info@impactpublishers.com
                     www.impactpublishers.com

Practical, self empowering book on overcoming agoraphobia and debilitating panic attacks is now completely revised and expanded to include the latest information and research findings on relaxation, breathing, medication and other tratments. *$15.95*

304 pages Year Founded: 1998 ISBN 1-886230-08-0

186 No More Butterflies: Overcoming Shyness, Stagefright, Interview Anxiety, and Fear of Public Speaking

New Harbinger Publications
5674 Shattuck Avenue
Oakland, CA 94609-1662   510-652-2002
                                 800-748-6273
                            Fax: 510-652-5472
          E-mail: customerservice@newharbinger.com
                      www.newharbinger.com

Demonstrates how to pinpoint fears, refute fear - provoking thoughts, and exhibit confidence at interviews and auditions. *$13.95*

176 pages ISBN 1-572240-41-5

187 Panic Disorder and Agoraphobia: A Guide

Madison Institute of Medicine
7617 Mineral Point Road
Suite 300
Madison, WI 53717-1623   608-827-2470
                            Fax: 608-827-2479
                    E-mail: mim@miminc.org
                              www.miminc.org

Learn about the causes of panic disorder and agoraphobia and how patients can overcome these disabling disorders with medications and behavior therapy in this booklet written by leading experts on the subject. *$5.95*

69 pages

188 Panic Disorder: Critical Analysis

Guilford Publications
72 Spring Street
New York, NY 10012   212-431-9800
                                 800-365-7006
                            Fax: 212-966-6708
                   E-mail: info@guilford.com
                              www.guilford.com

Provides a comprehensive, integrative exploration of panic disorder. Discusses the phenomenology of the disorder, with extensive reviews of the epidemiology, biological aspects and psychopharmacalogic treatments, followed by detailed explorations of psychological aspects, including predictability and controllability and psychological treatments including cognitive behavioral techniques. *$38.00*

276 pages ISBN 0-898622-63-8

189 Perfectionism: What's Bad About Being Too Good

Free Spirit Publishing
217 5th Avenue N
Suite 200
Minneapolis, MN 55401-1299   612-338-2068
                                 800-735-7323
                            Fax: 612-337-5050
             E-mail: help4kids@freespirit.com
                              www.freespirit.com

Revised and updated edition includes new research and statistics on the causes and consequenses of perfectionisim and new strategies for avoiding or escaping the perfectionism trap. *$12.95*

144 pages ISBN 1-575420-62-7

190 Relaxation & Stress Reduction Workbook

New Harbinger Publications
5674 Shattuck Avenue
Oakland, CA 94609-1662   510-652-2002
                                 800-748-6273
                            Fax: 510-652-5472
        E-mail: customerservice@newharbinger.com
                      www.newharbinger.com

Matthew McKay, Editor

Step by step instructions cover progressive muscle relaxation, meditation, autogenics, visualization, thought stopping, refuting irrational ideas, coping skills training, job stress management, and much more. *$17.95*

256 pages ISBN 1-879237-82-2

191 Self-Esteem Revolutions in Children: Understanding and Managing the Critical Transition in Your Child's Life

ADD WareHouse
300 NW 70th Avenue
Suite 102
Plantation, FL 33317   954-792-8100
                                 800-233-9273
                            Fax: 954-792-8545
              E-mail: sales@addwarehouse.com
                      www.addwarehouse.com

As youngsters grow up, they experience sweeping changes in self-esteem. This book explains why these occur, offering easily understood, step-by-step methods for parents to help young children and teens gain self-respect. Also available in audiotape. *$13.00*

180 pages ISBN 1-889140-01-5

192 Social Anxiety Disorder: A Guide

Madison Institute of Medicine
7617 Mineral Point Road
Suite 300
Madison, WI 53717-1623   **608-827-2470**
                                           Fax: 608-827-2479
                             E-mail: mim@miminc.org
                                   www.miminc.org

Do you fear public speaking or do you avoid social situations because you worry you may do something embarassing or humiliating? Learn how social anxiety disorder, also known as social phobia, is diagnosed and treated in this thorough publication written by leading experts on the subject. *$5.95*

61 pages

193 Social Phobia: From Shyness to Stage Fright

Anxiety Disorders Association of America
8730 Georgia Avenue
Suite 600
Silver Spring, MD 20910   **301-231-9350**
                                           Fax: 301-231-7392
                            E-mail: AnxDis@adaa.org
                                   www.adaa.org

Alies Muskin, COO
Michelle Alonso, Communications/Membership

Book on social phobia.

194 Stop Obsessing: How to Overcome Your Obsessions and Compulsions

Anxiety Disorders Association of America
8730 Georgia Avenue
Suite 600
Silver Spring, MD 20910   **301-231-9350**
                                           Fax: 301-231-7392
                            E-mail: AnxDis@adaa.org
                                   www.adaa.org

Alies Muskin, COO
Michelle Alonso, Communications/Membership

Book provides knowledgeable descriptions of the steps, the challenges, and the value of self-treatment.

195 Stress and Mental Health: Contemporary Issues and Prospects for the Future

Kluwer Academic/Plenum Publishers
233 Spring Street
New York, NY 10013   **212-620-8000**
                                       Fax: 212-463-0742
                                 www.kluweronline.com

Providing fresh insights into the complex relationship between stress and mental health, internationally recognized contributors identifie emerging conceptual issues, highlight promising avenues for further study, and detail novel methodological techniques for addressing contemporary empirical problems. Specific coverage includes stressful life events, chronic strains, psychosocial resources and mediators, vulnerability to stress, and mental health outcomes -thus providing researchers with a tool to take stock of the past and future of this field. *$84.00*

358 pages ISBN 0-306446-87-1

196 Stress-Related Disorders Sourcebook

Omnigraphics
PO Box 625
Holmes, PA 19043
                                       800-234-1340
                                       Fax: 800-875-1340
                         E-mail: info@omnigraphics.com
                                  www.omnigraphics.com

Omnigraphics is the publisher of the Health Reference Series, a growing consumer health information resource with more than 100 volumes in print. Each title in the series features an easy to understand format, nontechnical language, comprehensive indexing and resources for further information. Material in each book has been collected from a wide range of government agencies, professional associations, periodicals, and other sources. *$78.00*

600 pages ISBN 0-780805-60-7

197 Textbook of Anxiety Disorders

American Psychiatric Publishing
1000 Wilson Boulevard
Suite 1825
Arlington, VA 22209-3901   **703-907-732**
                                             800-368-5777
                                           Fax: 703-907-1091
                          E-mail: appi@psych.org
                                   www.appi.org

Katie Duffy, Marketing Assistant

US and international experts cover every major anxiety disorder, compare it with animal behavior and the similarities in the brain that exist, how disorders can relate to age specific groups, and covers the latest developments in understanding and treating these disorders. *$77.00*

544 pages ISBN 0-880488-29-8

198 Treatment Plans and Interventions for Depression and Anxiety Disorders

Guilford Publications
72 Spring Street
New York, NY 10012   **212-431-9800**
                                       800-365-7006
                                     Fax: 212-966-6708
                          E-mail: info@guilford.com
                                   www.guilford.com

Provides information on treatments for seven frequently encountered disorders: major depression, generalized anxiety, panic, agoraphobia, PTSD, social phobia, specific phobia and OCD. Serving as ready to use treatment packages, chapters describe basic cognitive behavioral therapy techniques and how to tailor them to each disorder. Also featured are diagnostic decision trees, therapist forms for assessment and record keeping, client handouts and homework sheets. *$ 55.00*

320 pages ISBN 1-572305-14-2

199 Triumph Over Fear: a Book of Help and Hope for People with Anxiety, Panic Attacks, and Phobias

Anxiety Disorders Association of America
8730 Georgia Avenue
Suite 600
Silver Spring, MD 20910   301-231-9350
                          Fax: 301-231-7392
              E-mail: AnxDis@adaa.org
                          www.adaa.org

Alies Muskin, COO
Michelle Alonso, Communications/Marketing

Resource and guide for both lay and professional readers.

200 Worry Control Workbook

New Harbinger Publications
5674 Shattuck Avenue
Oakland, CA 94609-1662   510-652-2002
                          800-748-6273
                  Fax: 510-652-5472
E-mail: customerservice@newharbinger.com
              www.newharbinger.com

Self help program that shares experiences of people who have developed ways to overcome chronic worry. Step by step format helps identify areas likely to reoccur and develop new skills. *$15.95*

266 pages ISBN 1-572241-20-9

201 Trichotillomania: A Guide

Madison Institute of Medicine
7617 Mineral Point Road
Suite 300
Madison, WI 53717-1623   608-827-2470
                          Fax: 608-827-2479
              E-mail: mim@miminc.org
                          www.miminc.org

Learn more about compulsive hair pulling and its treatment with medications and behavior therapy in this informative guide. *$5.95*

49 pages

Periodicals & Pamphlets

202 101 Stress Busters

ETR Associates
4 Carbonero Way
Scotts Valley, CA 95066   831-438-4060
                          800-321-4407
                  Fax: 800-435-8433
        E-mail: customerservice@etr.org
                          www.etr.org

These 101 stress busters were written by students to help fellow students relieve stress: tell a joke, laugh out loud, beat a pillow to smitherines. *$16.00*

203 5 Smart Steps to Less Stress

ETR Associates
4 Carbonero Way
Scotts Valley, CA 95066-1200   831-438-4060
                          800-321-4407
                  Fax: 800-435-8433
        E-mail: customerservice@etr.org
                          www.etr.org

Steps to managing stress include: know what stresses you, manage your stress, take care of your body, take care of your feelings, ask for help. *$16.00*

204 Anxiety Disorders

National Institute of Mental Health
6001 Executive Boulevard
Room 8184
Bethesda, MD 20892-9663
                          866-615-6464
                  Fax: 301-443-4279
                  TTY: 301-443-8431
          E-mail: nimhinfo@nih.gov
                  www.nimh.nih.gov

This brochure helps to identify the symptoms of anxiety disorders, explains the role of research in understanding the causes of these conditions, describes effective treatments, helps you learn how to obtain treatment and work with a doctor or therapist, and suggests ways to make treatment more effective.

205 Anxiety Disorders Fact Sheet

Center for Mental Health Services: Knowledge Exchange Network
PO Box 42490
Washington, DC 20015
                          800-789-2647
                  Fax: 301-984-8796
                  TDD: 866-889-2647
          E-mail: ken@mentalhealth.org
                  www.mentalhealth.org

This fact sheet presents basic information on the symptoms, formal diagnosis, and treatment for generalized anxiety disorder, panic disorders, phobias, and post-traumatic stress disorder.

3 pages

206 Facts About Anxiety Disorders

National Institute of Mental Health
6001 Executive Boulevard
Room 8184
Bethesda, MD 20892-9663

866-615-6464
Fax: 301-443-4279
TTY: 301-443-8431
E-mail: nimhinfo@nih.gov
www.nimh.nih.gov

Series of fact sheets that provide overviews and descriptions of generalized anxiety disorder, obsessive-compulsive disorder, panic disorder, post-traumatic stress disorder, social phobia, and the Anxiety Disorders Education Program.

207 Families Can Help Children Cope with Fear, Anxiety

Center for Mental Health Services: Knowledge Exchange Network
PO Box 42490
Washington, DC 20015

800-789-2647
Fax: 301-984-8796
TDD: 866-889-2647
E-mail: ken@mentalhealth.org
www.mentalhealth.org

This fact sheet defines conduct disorder, identifies risk factors, discusses types of help available, and suggests what parents or other caregivers to common signs of fear and anxiety.

208 Getting What You Want From Stress

ETR Associates
4 Carbonero Way
Scotts Valley, CA 95066-4200

831-438-4060
800-321-4407
Fax: 800-435-8433
E-mail: customerservice@etr.org
www.etr.org

Includes signs of stress, some stress can be healthy, and when to change, when to adapt. *$16.00*

209 Journal of Anxiety Disorders

Elsevier Publishing
360 Park Avenue South
New York, NY 10010-1710

212-633-3730
888-437-4636
Fax: 212-633-3680
E-mail: usinfo-e@elsevier.com
www.elsevier.nl/locate/janxdis

Year Founded: 1987 ISSN 0887-6185

210 Let's Talk Facts About Anxiety Disorders

American Psychiatric Publishing
1000 Wilson Boulevard
Suite 1825
Arlington, VA 22209-3901

703-907-7322
800-368-5777
Fax: 703-907-1091
E-mail: appi@psych.org
www.appi.org

Katie Duffy, Marketing Assistant

$12.50

8 pages ISBN 0-890423-60-1

211 Let's Talk Facts About Panic Disorder

American Psychiatric Publishing
1000 Wilson Boulevard
Suite 1825
Arlington, VA 22209-3901

703-907-7322
800-368-5777
Fax: 703-907-1091
E-mail: appi@psych.org
www.appi.org

Katie Duffy, Marketing Assistant

$12.50

8 pages ISBN 0-890423-57-1

212 Panic Attacks

ETR Associates
4 Carbonero Way
Scotts Valley, CA 95066

831-438-4060
800-321-4407
Fax: 800-435-8433
E-mail: customerservice@etr.org
www.etr.org

Describes causes of panic attacks, including genetics, stress, and drug use; prevention and treatment, and how to stop a panic attack in its tracks. *$16.00*

213 Real Illness: Generalized Anxiety Disorder

National Institute of Mental Health
6001 Executive Boulevard
Room 8184
Bethesda, MD 20892-9663

866-615-6464
Fax: 301-443-4279
TTY: 301-443-8431
E-mail: nimhinfo@nih.gov
www.nimh.nih.gov

If you worry and feel tense a lot, even though others may assure you there are no real problems, you have a treatable disorder. Read this easy pamphlet to learn more.

9 pages

214 Real Illness: Panic Disorder

National Institute of Mental Health
6001 Executive Boulevard
Room 8184
Bethesda, MD 20892-9663

866-615-6464
Fax: 301-443-4279
TTY: 301-443-8431
E-mail: nimhinfo@nih.gov
www.nimh.nih.gov

Do you often have feelings of sudden fear that don't make sense? If so, you may have panic disorder. Read this pamplet of simple information about getting help.

9 pages

215 Real Illness: Social Phobia Disorder

National Institute of Mental Health
6001 Executive Boulevard
Room 8184
Bethesda, MD 20892-9663

866-615-6464
Fax: 301-443-4279
TTY: 301-443-8431
E-mail: nimhinfo@nih.gov
www.nimh.nih.gov

Are you terrified of talking in groups or even going to parties because you're afraid people will think badly of you? This simple pamphlet describes how to get help.

9 pages

216 Stress

ETR Associates
4 Carbonero Way
Scotts Valley, CA 95066

831-438-4060
800-321-4407
Fax: 800-435-8433
E-mail: customerservice@etr.org
www.etr.org

Includes common changes that cause stress, symptoms of stress, and effects on feelings, actions and physical health.

Support Groups & Hot Lines

217 Agoraphobics Building Independent Lives

3805 Cutshaw Avenue
Suite 415
Richmond, VA 23230

804-353-3964
E-mail: abil1996@aol.com

218 Agoraphobics in Action

PO Box 1662
Antioch, TN 37011-1662

615-831-2383

219 Pass-Group

6 Mahogany Drive
Williamsville, NY 14221-2419

716-689-4399

Shirley Swede, Program Coordinator

Offers three-month telephone counseling program for panic attack suffers (angoraphobia). 'The Panic Attack Recovery Book' explains the cause and cure for panic attacks.

220 Phobics Anonymous

PO Box 1180
Palm Springs, CA 92263

619-322-2673

Twelve-step program for panic disorders and anxiety. Publications available.

221 Recovery

802 N Dearborn Street
Chicago, IL 60610-3364

312-337-5661
Fax: 312-337-5756
E-mail: inquiries@recovery-inc.com
www.recovery-inc.com

Kelly Garcia, Executive Director
Maurine Pyle, Assistant Director

Techniques for controlling behavior, changing attitudes for recovering mental patients. Systematic method of self-help offered.

Video & Audio

222 Acquiring Courage: Audio Cassette Program for the Rapid Treatment of Phobias

New Harbinger Publications
5674 Shattuck Avenue
Oakland, CA 94609-1662

510-652-2002
800-748-6273
Fax: 510-652-5472
E-mail: customerservice@newharbinger.com
www.newharbinger.com

$14.95

Year Founded: 1991 ISBN 1-879237-03-2

223 Anxiety Disorders

American Counseling Association
5999 Stevenson Avenue
Alexandria, VA 22304-3300

703-823-9800
800-347-6647
Fax: 703-823-0252
E-mail: webmaster@counseling.org
www.counseling.org

Increase your awareness of anxiety disorders, their symptoms, and effective treatments. Learn the effect these disorders can have on life and how treatment can change the quality of life for people presently suffering from these disorders. Includes 6 audiotapes and a study guide. *$124.00*

ISSN 74238

224 Clinical Hypnosis for Stress & Anxiety Reduction

New Harbinger Publications
5674 Shattuck Avenue
Oakland, CA 94609-1662

510-652-2002
800-748-6273
Fax: 510-652-5472
E-mail: customerservice@newharbinger.com
www.newharbinger.com

45 minute videotape explains the nature of hypnosis and why it is such a valuable aid to relaxation. *$24.95*

Year Founded: 1988 ISBN 0-934986-69-X

225 Driving Far from Home

New Harbinger Publications
5674 Shattuck Avenue
Oakland, CA 94609-1662   510-652-2002
                               800-748-6273
                          Fax: 510-652-5472
E-mail: customerservice@newharbinger.com
                    www.newharbinger.com

120 minute videotape that reduces fear associated with leaving the safety of your home base. $11.95

Year Founded: 1995 ISBN 1-572240-14-8

226 Driving Freeways

New Harbinger Publications
5674 Shattuck Avenue
Oakland, CA 94609-1662   510-652-2002
                               800-748-6273
                          Fax: 510-652-5472
E-mail: customerservice@newharbinger.com
                    www.newharbinger.com

120 minute videotape that reduces fear of driving freeways so you can get where you need to go without long trips on surface streets. $11.95

Year Founded: 1994 ISBN 1-879237-88-1

227 FAT City: How Difficult Can This Be?

ADD WareHouse
300 NW 70th Avenue
Suite 102
Plantation, FL 33317   954-792-8100
                               800-233-9273
                          Fax: 954-792-8545
E-mail: sales@addwarehouse.com
                    www.addwarehouse.com

Teachers and parents will understand the anxiety felt by students with learning disabilities after viewing this remarkable video. Presents a series of striking simulations to teachers, counselors and parents designed to emulate the daily experience of children with learning disabilities. Includes a discussion guide for group presentations. 70 minutes. $56.00

228 Fear of Illness

New Harbinger Publications
5674 Shattuck Avenue
Oakland, CA 94609-1662   510-652-2002
                               800-748-6273
                          Fax: 510-652-5472
E-mail: customerservice@newharbinger.com
                    www.harbinginger.com

120 minute videotape that reduces fears arising from unexplained pain or symptoms; learn to relax while you desensitize to strange body sensations. $11.95

Year Founded: 1995 ISBN 1-572240-15-6

229 Flying

New Harbinger Publications
5674 Shattuck Avenue
Oakland, CA 94609-1662   510-652-2002
                               800-748-6273
                          Fax: 510-652-5472
E-mail: customerservice@newharbinger.com
                    www.newharbinger.com

120 minute videotape that reduces fear to the point where you can take longer and longer flights; desensitize to the sensations of flying. $11.95

Year Founded: 1994 ISBN 1-879237-90-3

230 Giving a Talk

New Harbinger Publications
5674 Shattuck Avenue
Oakland, CA 94609-1662   510-652-2002
                               800-748-6273
                          Fax: 510-652-5472
E-mail: customerservice@newharbinger.com
                    www.newharbinger.com

120 minute videotape that makes you feel more confident and safe as you speak to small, or even large groups. $11.95

Year Founded: 1994 ISBN 1-879237-86-5

231 Heights

New Harbinger Publications
5674 Shattuck Avenue
Oakland, CA 94609-1662   510-652-2002
                               800-748-6273
                          Fax: 510-652-5472
E-mail: customerservice@newharbinger.com
                    www.newharbinger.com

120 minute videotape that makes you feel more comfortable in high - rise buildings, on bridges, and on mountain roads. $11.95

Year Founded: 1994 ISBN 1-879237-91-1

232 Shopping in a Supermarket

New Harbinger Publications
5674 Shattuck Avenue
Oakland, CA 94609-1662   510-652-2002
                               800-748-6273
                          Fax: 510-652-5472
E-mail: customerservice@newharbinger.com
                    www.newharbinger.com

120 minute videotape that reduces fear of panicking or losing control while shopping or waiting in line at the market. $11.95

Year Founded: 1994 ISBN 1-879237-89-X

Web Sites

233 www.algy.com/anxiety/files/barlow.html
Causes of Anxiety and Panic Attacks

Overview by noted experts.

234 www.algy.com/anxiety/index.shtml
Anxiety Panic Internet Resource

Chat and good quality links.

235 www.algy.com/anxiety/panicfaq.html

FAQ: Panic Disorder

Excellent overview with resources.

236 www.algy.com/anxiety/registry/index.html

Tapir Registry

Search engine for support groups.

237 www.amwa-doc.org/publications/WCHealthbook/ stressamwa-ch09.html

How Stress Affects the Body

238 www.anxietypanic.com/menuunderstanding.html

Menu for Understanding Panic Attacks

239 www.apa.org/pubinfo/panic.html

Answers to Your Questions about Panic Disorder

Four-page overview American Psychological Association publication.

240 www.couns.uiuc.edu/stress.htm

Stress Management

241 www.cyberpsych.org

CyberPsych

Hosts the American Psychoanalyists Foundation, American Association of Suicideology, Society for the Exploration of Psychotherapy Intergration, and Anxiety Disorders Association of America. Also subcategories of the anxiety disorders, as well as general information, including panic disorder, phobias, obsessive compulsive disorder (OCD), social phobia, generalized anxiety disorder, post traumatic stress disorder, and phobias of childhood. Book reviews and links to web pages sharing the topics.

242 www.dstress.com/guided.htm

Basic Guided Relaxation: Advanced Technique

Devoted to stress management for organizations and individuals, and information to enhance your levels of Health/Wellness and Productivity.

243 www.eadd.com/~berta/

How to Treat Your Own Panic Disorder

244 www.factsforhealth.org

Madison Institute of Medicine

Resource to help identify, understand and treat a number of medical conditions, including social anxiety disorder and posttraumatic stress disorder.

245 www.icisf.org

International Critical Incident Stress Foundation

A nonprofit, open membership foundation dedicated to the prevention and mitigation of disabling stress by education, training and support services for all emergency service professionals. Continuing education and training in emergency mental health services for psychologists, psychiatrists, social workers and licensed professional counselors.

246 www.intelihealth.com

Mastering Your Stress Demons

247 www.jobstresshelp.com

Job Stress Help

248 www.klis.com/chandler/pamphlet/panic/

Panic Disorder, Separation, Anxiety Disorder, and Agoraphobia

249 www.lexington-on-line.com

Panic Disorder

Explains development and treatment of panic disorder.

250 www.members.aol.com/avpsyrich/stress.htm

Progressive Muscle Relaxation

251 www.npadnews.com

National Panic/Anxiety Disorder Newsletter

This resource was founded by Phil Darren who collects and collates information of recovered anxiety disorder sufferers who want to distribute some of the lessons that they learned with a view to helping others.

252 www.npadnews.com/support.htm

For the Support Person: Helping Your Partner Do In-Vivo Exposure

253 www.omhrc.gov/ctg/mhm-02.htm

Coping with Racial Stress

254 www.pacificcoast.net/~kstrong

Anxiety Disorders-Caregiver

Offers advice, support, information.

255 www.panicattacks.com.au/

Panic and Anxiety Hub

Informations, resources and support.

256 www.panicdisorder.about.com/

Agoraphobia: For Friends/Family

257 www.planetpsych.com

Planetpsych.com

Learn about disorders, their treatments and other topics in psychology. Articles are listed under the related topic areas. Ask a therapist a question for free, or view the directory of professionals in your area. If you are a therapist sign up for the directory. Current features, self-help, interactive, and newsletter archives.

258 www.psych.ac.uk/public/help/anxiety/

Anxiety and Phobias

Introductory brochure.

259 www.psych.org/public_info/anxiety.cfm

Anxiety Disorders

American Psychiatric Association publication diagnostic criteria and treatment.

260 www.psychcentral.com

Psych Central

Personalized one-stop index for psychology, support, and mental health issues, resources, and people on the Internet.

261 www.queendom.com/selfhelp/index.html

Self-Help Corner: Anxiety

On-line tests, books, case studies, advice, chat, organizations and articles.

262 www.shpm.com/articles/stress

Meditation, Guided Fantasies, and Other Stress Reducers

263 www.virtualpsych.com/stress/stressframe set. htm

Stress

264 www2.mc.duke.edu/pcaad

Duke University's Program in Child and Adolescent Anxiety Disorder

Introduction

Attention-Deficit/Hyperactivity Disorder (AD/HD) includes the following persistent, wide-ranging general conditions: (1) a pervasive pattern of inattention, (2) difficulty in controlling impulses including the impulse to be constantly on the move. Both of these conditions are more severe than is typical for a person at a comparable developmental level, and the symptoms must appear before age seven.

The problems of hyperactivity show themselves in constant movement, especially among younger children. Preschool children with hyperactivity cannot sit still, are always on the move, run rather than walk, and jump on furniture. In older children the intensity of the hyperactivity is reduced but fidgeting, getting up during meals or homework, and excessive talking continue to occur.

People with Attention-Deficit/Hyperactivity Disorder have great difficulty controlling all their impulses, not just the craving for movement and stimulation. They have little sense of time (five minutes seems like hours), and waiting for something is intolerable. Thus, they are impatient, interrupt, make comments out of turn, grab objects from others, clown around, and cause trouble at home, in school, work, and in social settings.

From a young age, people with Attention-Deficit/Hyperactivity Disorder may experience failure repeatedly, including rejection by peers. The consequences are low self-esteem and sometimes more serious problems.

SYMPTOMS

Inattention
•Often fails to attend to details, or makes careless mistakes in schoolwork, work or other activities;
•Often finds it difficult to maintain attention in tasks or play activities;
•Often does not seem to listen when spoken to;
•Often doesn't follow through on instructions and doesn't finish schoolwork, chores, or tasks;
•Often has difficulty organizing tasks or activities;
•Often avoids tasks that demand sustained mental effort, such as schoolwork or homework;
•Often loses things needed for tasks or activities, such as toys and school assignments;
•Often is easily distracted;
•Often is forgetful in daily activities.

Hyperactivity
•Often fidgets with hands or feet, or squirms in chair;
•Often leaves seat in classroom or other situations where remaining seated is expected;
•Often runs or climbs about in situations in which it is inappropriate (among adolescents or adults, this may be a feeling of restlessness);
•Often has difficulty playing or handling leisure activities quietly;
•Often is on the go, moving excessively;
•Often talks excessively.

Impulsivity
•Often blurts out answers before questions are finished;
•Often has difficulty waiting in turn;
•Often interrupts or intrudes on others' games, activities, or conversations.
Three distinctions are made in the diagnosis:

Attention-Deficity/Hyperactivity Disorder, Combined Type if six or more items from List (1) and 6 or more from List (2) are applicable;

Attention-Deficit/Hyperactivity Disorder, Predominantly Inattentive Type if six or more items from List (1) only are applicable;

Attention-Deficit/Hyperactivity Disorder, Predominantly Hyperactive-Impulsive Type if six or more items from List (2) only are applicable.

ASSOCIATED FEATURES

Certain behaviors often go along with Attention-Deficity/Hyperactivity Disorder. The person is often frustrated and angry, exhibiting outbursts of temper and bossiness. To others, the lack of application and inability to finish tasks may look like laziness or irresponsibility. Other conditions may also be associated with the disorder, including Hyperthyroidism (an overactive thyroid). There may be a higher prevalence of anxiety, depression, and learning disorders among people with AD/HD.

PREVALENCE

AD/HD occurs in various cultures. It is much more frequent in males than females, with male to female ratios at 4:1 in the general population, and 9:1 in clinic populations. The prevalence among school-age children is from three percent to five percent.

There is emerging literature concerning adult AD/HD, and evidence that some adults can benefit from the same treatments used for children.

TREATMENT OPTIONS

A careful assessment and diagnosis by a professional familiar with AD/HD are essential, especially since some of the typical AD/HD behaviors may resemble those of other disorders. This is a lifelong disorder, though sometimes attenuated in adulthood.

The diagnosis is especially difficult to establish in young children, e.g., at the toddler and preschool level, because behavior that is typical at that age is similar to the symptoms of AD/HD. Children at that age may be extremely active but do not develop the disorder. Current treatments can have a positive impact and, in some cases, transform behaviors so that a formerly chaotic life becomes one over which the person has much greater control and more frequent experience of success. Treatment should be based on an understanding that Attention-Deficit/Hyperactivity Disorder is not intentional, and punishment is not a cure.

The AD/HD person has great need for external motivation, consistency, and structure. This should be provided by a professional who is familiar with the disorder. For a school-aged child, it is important to enlist the help of the school in designing a treatment plan which should include con-

crete steps aimed at developing specific compentencies (e.g., handling time, sequencing, problem-solving, and social interaction).

Medication is often prescribed but should not be the only treatment. Newer preparations of medications, such as Concerta, offer once or twice a day dosing, so that children do noted to take medication during the school day. Since this condition affects all members of the family, the family needs help in providing consistency and structure, and in changing the role of the AD/HD person as the family member who always gets into trouble.

Associations & Agencies

266 Attention Deficit Disorder Association

PO Box 1303
Northbrook, IL 60065-1303

E-mail: mail@add.org
www.add.org

Provides children, adolescents and adults with ADD information, support groups, publications, videos, and referrals.

267 Center for Family Support (CFS)

333 7th Avenue
New York, NY 10001-5004

212-629-7939
Fax: 212-239-2211
www.cfsny.org

Steven Vernickofs, Executive Director

Service agency devoted to the physical well-being and development of the retarded child and the sound mental health of the parents. Helps families with retarded children with all aspects of home care including counseling, referrals, home aide service and consultation. Offers intervention for parents at the birth of a retarded child with in-home support, guidance and infant stimulation. Pioneered training of nonprofessional women as home aides to provide supportive services in homes.

268 Center for Mental Health Services Knowledge Exchange Network

US Department of Health and Human Services
PO Box 42490
Washington, DC 20015-4800

800-789-2647
Fax: 301-984-8796
E-mail: ken@mentalhealth.org
www.mentalhealth.org

Information about resources, technical assistance, research, training, networks, and other federal clearing houses, and fact sheets and materials. Information specialists refer callers to mental health resources in their communities as well as state, federal and non-profit contacts. Staff available Monday through Friday, 8:30 AM-5:00 PM, EST, excluding federal holidays. After hours, callers may leave messages and an information specialist will return their call.

269 Children and Adults with AD/HD

8181 Professional Place
Suite 150
Landover, MD 20785

301-306-7070
800-233-4050
Fax: 301-306-7090
www.chadd.org

National nonprofit organization representing children and adults with attention deficit/hyperactivity disorder (AD/HD).

270 Children and Adults with Attention Deficit Disorders

CHADD
8181 Professional Place
Suite 150
Landover, MD 20785

301-306-7070
800-233-4050
Fax: 301-306-7090
www.chadd.org

This organization can provide parents, professionals and adults disgnosed with ADD with information, support and educational materials dealing with this disorder. CHADD has over 600 chapters across the country and over 28,000 active members of their organization.

271 Learning Disability Association of America

4156 Library Road
Pittsburgh, PA 15234-1349

412-341-1515
Fax: 412-344-0224
E-mail: info@ldaamerica.org
www.ldanatl.org

John E Muench, National Executive Director

272 NADD: Association for Persons with Developmental Disabilities and Mental Health Needs

132 Fair Street
Kingston, NY 12401-4802

845-334-4336
800-331-5362
Fax: 845-331-4569
E-mail: nadd@mhv.net
www.thenadd.org

Dr. Robert Fletcher, Executive Director

Nonprofit organization designed to promote interest of professional and parent development with resources for individuals who have the coexistence of mental illness and mental retardation. Provides conference, educational services and training materials to professionals, parents, concerned citizens and service organizations. Formerly known as the National Association for the Dually Diagnosed.

273 National Alliance for the Mentally Ill

2107 Wilson Boulevard
Suite 300
Arlington, VA 22201-3042

703-524-7600
800-950-6264
Fax: 703-524-9094
TDD: 703-516-7227
E-mail: helpline@nami.org
www.nami.org

Laurie Flynn, Executive Director

Nation's leading self-help organization for all those affected by severe brain disorders. Mission is to bring consumers and families with similar experiences together to share information about services, care providers, and ways to cope with the challenges of schizophrenia, manic depression, and other serious mental illnesses.

274 National Attention Deficit Disorder Association

PO Box 543
Pottstown, PA 19464
484-945-2101
Fax: 610-970-7520
E-mail: mall@add.org
www.add.org

The mission of ADDA is to provide information, resources and networking to adults with AD/HD and to the professionals working with them. In doing so, ADDA generates hope, awareness, empowerment and connections worldwide in the field of AD/HD through bringing together science and the human experience.

275 National Information Center for Children and Youth with Disabilities

PO Box 1492
Washington, DC 20013
800-695-0285

Provides support and services for children and youth with physical and mental disabilities, as well as education and training services for their families.

276 National Mental Health Consumer's Self-Help Clearinghouse

1211 Chestnut Street
Suite 1207
Philadelphia, PA 19107
215-751-1810
800-553-4539
Fax: 215-636-6312
E-mail: info@mhselfhelp.org
www.mhselfhelp.org

Alex Morrsey, Information/Referral

Funded by the National Institute of Mental Health Community Support Program, the purpose of the Clearinghouse is to encourage the development and growth of consumer self-help groups.

Year Founded: 1992

Books

---

277 1-2-3 Magic: Training Your Children to Do What You Want

ADD WareHouse
300 NW 70th Avenue
Suite 102
Plantation, FL 33317
954-792-8100
800-233-9273
Fax: 954-792-8545
E-mail: sales@addwarehouse.com
www.addwarehouse.com

Learn about a new, no-nonsense discipline program that enables parents to manage children ages 2-12 without arguing, yelling or hitting. The 1-2-3 Magic program tells you exactly how to handle screaming, tantrums and fighting, as well as how to encourage positive behavior. *$13.00*

192 pages

278 AD/HD Forms Book: Identification, Measurement, and Intervention

Research Press
Dept 24 W
PO Box 9177
Champaign, IL 61826
217-352-3273
800-519-2707
Fax: 217-352-1221
E-mail: rp@researchpress.com
www.researchpress.com

Russell Pense, VP Marketing

A collection of intervention procedures and over 30 reproducible forms and checklists for use with any AD/HD program for children or adolescents. Each item is prefaced by a brief description of its purpose and use. The AD/HD Forms Book helps educators, mental health professionals and parents translate their knowledge into action. *$25.95*

128 pages ISBN 0-878223-78-9

279 ADD & Learning Disabilities: Reality, Myths, & Controversial Treatments

Bantam Doubleday Dell Publishing
1745 Broadway
New York, NY 10019
212-782-9000
Fax: 212-782-9700

For parents of children with learning disabilities and attention deficit disorder - and for educational and medical professionals who encounter these children - two experts in the field have devised a handbook to help identify the very best treatments. *$10.36*

256 pages ISBN 0-385469-31-4

280 ADD & Romance

ADD WareHouse
300 NW 70th Avenue
Suite 102
Plantation, FL 33317
954-792-8100
800-233-9273
Fax: 954-792-8545
E-mail: sales@addwarehouse.com
www.addwarehouse.com

Romantic relationships are hard enough, but sustaining a stimulating and satisfying romantic relationship can be even more challenging if one partner has ADD. This book discusses how ADD can influence vital aspects of one's romantic life, such as intimacy and communication and provides effective techniques for communication, conflict resolution and ways to cope with ADD in a relationship. *$12.95*

230 pages

281 ADD Hyperactivity Handbook for Schools

ADD WareHouse
300 NW 70th Avenue
Suite 102
Plantation, FL 33317
954-792-8100
800-233-9273
Fax: 954-792-8545
E-mail: sales@addwarehouse.com
www.addwarehouse.com

A must read for anyone interested in learning evaluation methods for ADD and ways to effectively assist children with ADD in regular and special education. Contains an overview of the important facts about ADD and provides practical and proven techniques teachers can use in the classroom to help students and their families. *$29.00*

330 pages

282 ADD Kaleidoscope: The Many Facets of Adult Attention Deficit Disorder

Hope Press
PO Box 188
Duarte, CA 91009-0188
818-303-0644
800-321-4039
Fax: 818-358-3520
www.hopepress.com

A comprehensive presentation of all aspects of attention deficit disorder in adults. While often thought of as a childhood disorder, ADD symptoms usually continue into adulthood where they can cause a wide range of problems with personal interactions, work performance, attitude towards one's employer, and interactions with spouses and children. *$24.95*

ISBN 1-878267-03-5

283 ADD Success Stories: Guide to Fulfillment for Families with Attention Deficit Disorder

ADD WareHouse
300 NW 70th Avenue
Suite 102
Plantation, FL 33317
954-792-8100
800-233-9273
Fax: 954-792-8545
E-mail: sales@addwarehouse.com
www.addwarehouse.com

Real-life stories of people with ADD who achieved success in school, at work, in marriages and relationships. Thousands of interviews and histories as well as new research show children and adults from all walks of life how to reach the next-step, a fulfilling, successful life with ADD. Discover which occupations are best for people with ADD. *$12.00*

250 pages

284 ADD and Adolescence: Strategies for Success

CHADD
8181 Professional Place
Suite 150
Landover, MD 20785
301-306-7070
800-233-4050
Fax: 301-306-7090
www.chadd.org

A diversity of national experts present new information on the nature of ADD during adolescence; possible comorbid conditions that will be seen in many cases; strategies for parents and clinicians on the management of teens with ADD. Includes advice on school management, parent and teen counseling, and psychopharmacological treatment; and needed guidance for preparing the adolescent with ADD for college and the workplace. *$15.00*

136 pages

285 ADD in the Workplace: Choices, Changes and Challenges

ADD WareHouse
300 NW 70th Avenue
Suite 102
Plantation, FL 33317
954-792-8100
800-233-9273
Fax: 954-792-8545
E-mail: sales@addwarehouse.com
www.addwarehouse.com

It's one thing to deal with ADD in the doctor's office or at home, but quite another 'out there' in the workplace. This unique guide focuses on adults living with ADD, and illustrates various ways to initiate and maintain the best possible work situation. *$24.00*

248 pages

286 ADD/ADHD Checklist: an Easy Reference for Parents & Teachers

ADD WareHouse
300 NW 70th Avenue
Suite 102
Plantation, FL 33317
954-792-8100
800-233-9273
Fax: 954-792-8545
E-mail: sales@addwarehouse.com
www.addwarehouse.com

This resource for parents and teachers is packed with up-to-date facts, findings and proven strategies and techniques for understanding and helping children and adolescents with attention deficit problems and hyperactivity. *$12.00*

150 pages

287 ADHD Monitoring System

ADD WareHouse
300 NW 70th Avenue
Suite 102
Plantation, FL 33317
954-792-8100
800-233-9273
Fax: 954-792-8545
E-mail: sales@addwarehouse.com
www.addwarehouse.com

Provides a simple, cost effective way to carefully monitor how well a student with ADHD is doing at school. Parents and teachers will be able to easily track behavior, academic performance, quality of student classwork and homework. Contains monitoring forms along with instructions for use. *$8.95*

288 ADHD Survival Guide for Parents and Teachers

Hope Press
PO Box 188
Duarte, CA 91009-0188
818-303-0644
800-321-4039
Fax: 818-358-3520
www.hopepress.com

ISBN 1-878267-43-4

289 ADHD and Teens: Parent's Guide to Making it Through the Tough Years

ADD WareHouse
300 NW 70th Avenue
Suite 102
Plantation, FL 33317
954-792-8100
800-233-9273
Fax: 954-792-8545
E-mail: sales@addwarehouse.com
www.addwarehouse.com

Unlike the parents of elementary school children with ADHD, parents of ADHD teens must focus on gaining and keeping control of the situation because the risks are increased in severity and consequence. A manual of practical advice to help parents cope with the problems that can arise during these years. *$13.00*

208 pages

290 ADHD and the Nature of Self-Control

Guilford Publications
72 Spring Street
New York, NY 10012
212-431-9800
800-365-7006
Fax: 212-966-6708
E-mail: info@guilford.com
www.guilford.com

Provides a radical shift of perspective on ADHD, arguing that the disorder is a developmental problem of self control and that a deficit attention is a secondary characteristic. Combines neuropsychological research and the theory on the executive functions, illustrating how normally functioning individuals are able to bring behavior under the control of time and orient their actions toward the future. *$46.00*

410 pages ISBN 1-572302-50-X

291 ADHD in the Young Child: Driven to Redirection

ADD WareHouse
300 NW 70th Avenue
Suite 102
Plantation, FL 33317
954-792-8100
800-233-9273
Fax: 954-792-8545
E-mail: sales@addwarehouse.com
www.addwarehouse.com

The authors sensitively and effectively describe what life is like living with a young child with ADHD. With the help of over 75 cartoon illustrations they provide practical solutions to common problems found at home, in school and elsewhere. *$18.95*

202 pages

292 Adventures in Fast Forward: Life, Love and Work for the ADD Adult

ADD WareHouse
300 NW 70th Avenue
Suite 102
Plantation, FL 33317
954-792-8100
800-233-9273
Fax: 954-792-8545
E-mail: sales@addwarehouse.com
www.addwarehouse.com

For all adults with ADD, this book is designed to be a practical guide for day-to-day life. No matter where you are in the scenario - curious about ADD, just diagnosed or experiencing particular problems, this book will give you effective strategies to help anticipate and negotiate the challenges that come with the condition. Filled with important tools and tactics for self-care and success. *$23.00*

210 pages

293 All About Attention Deficit Disorder: Revised Edition

ADD WareHouse
300 NW 70th Avenue
Suite 102
Plantation, FL 33317
954-792-8100
800-233-9273
Fax: 954-792-8545
E-mail: sales@addwarehouse.com
www.addwarehouse.com

A practical and comprehensive manual for parents and teachers interested in understanding the facts about ADD. Chapters on home management, the 1-2-3 Magic discipline method, facts about medication management and practical ideas for teachers to use in managing learning and classroom behavior. *$13.00*

165 pages

294 All Kinds of Minds

ADD WareHouse
300 NW 70th Avenue
Suite 102
Plantation, FL 33317
954-792-8100
800-233-9273
Fax: 954-792-8545
E-mail: sales@addwarehouse.com
www.addwarehouse.com

Primary and elementary students with learning disorders can now gain insight into the difficulties they face in school. This book helps all children understand and respect all kinds of minds and can encourage children with learning disorders to maintain their motivation and keep from developing behavior problems stemming from their learning disorders. *$31.00*

283 pages

295 Answers to Distraction

ADD WareHouse
300 NW 70th Avenue
Suite 102
Plantation, FL 33317
954-792-8100
800-233-9273
Fax: 954-792-8545
E-mail: sales@addwarehouse.com
www.addwarehouse.com

A user's guide to ADD presented in a question and answer format ideal for parents of children and adolescents with ADD, adults with ADD and teachers who work with students who have ADD. *$13.00*

334 pages

296 Attention Deficit Disorder and Learning Disabilities

Bantam Doubleday Dell Publishing
1745 Broadway
New York, NY 10019   212-782-9000
                                  Fax: 212-782-9700

Discusses ADHD and learning disabilities as well as their effective treatments. Warns against nutritional and other alternative treatments. *$12.95*

256 pages ISBN 0-385469-31-4

297 Attention Deficit Hyperactivity Disorder in Children: A Medication Guide

Madison Institute of Medicine
7617 Mineral Point Road
Suite 300
Madison, WI 53717-1623   608-827-2470
                                  Fax: 608-827-2479
                            E-mail: mim@miminc.org
                                     www.miminc.org

Written for parents, this explains the various medications used commonly to treat ADHD/ADD. It includes a review of the symptoms of ADHD, medication therapy, commonly asked questions, and side effects of medications. *$5.95*

41 pages

298 Attention Deficit Hyperactivity Disorder: Questions and Answers for Parents

Research Press
Dept 24 W
PO Box 9177
Champaign, IL 61826   217-352-3273
                                      800-519-2707
                                  Fax: 217-352-1221
                      E-mail: rp@researchpress.com
                                www.researchpress.com

Russell Pense, VP Marketing

In question and answer format, an overview (syptoms, causes, evaluation, and diagnosis) and a review of treatments (psychostimulant medication and cognitive behavior therapy) are followed by detailed strategies for improving behavior. *$12.95*

144 pages ISBN 0-878228-22-3

299 Attention Deficit/Hyperactivity Disorder

American Psychiatric Publishing
1000 Wilson Boulevard
Suite 1825
Arlington, VA 22209-3901   703-907-7322
                                      800-368-5777
                                  Fax: 703-907-1091
                         E-mail: appi@psych.org
                                     www.appi.org

Katie Duffy, Marketing Assistant

Addressing day to day management issues faced by physicians and mental health professionals who see patients with ADHD, this how to guidebook discusses such practical concerns as how to make a differential diagnosis, work with children and families in a multimodal treatment setting, manage a medication regimen, and explain ADHD to parents. Covering ways to work with the school system as well as new and controversial therapies, this up to the minute book is essential reading for all who care. *$29.95*

320 pages ISBN 0-880489-40-5

300 Attention Deficits and Hyperactivity in Children: Developmental Clinical Psychology and Psychiatry

Sage Publications
2455 Teller Road
Thousand Oaks, CA 91320   805-499-9774
                                      800-818-7243
                                  Fax: 800-583-2665
                         E-mail: info@sagepub.com
                                     www.sagepub.com

Provides background information and evaluates key debates and questions that remain unanswered about ADHD. Includes what tools can be used to gain optimal information about this disorder and which factors predict subsequent functioning in adolescence and adulthood. Advances, challenges and unresolved problems in diverse but relevant areas are analyzed and placed in context. Paperback also available. *$43.95*

161 pages Year Founded: 1993 ISBN 0-803951-96-5

301 Beyond Ritalin: Facts About Medication and Other Strategies for Helping Children, Adolescents and Adults with Attention Deficit Disorders

ADD WareHouse
300 NW 70th Avenue
Suite 102
Plantation, FL 33317   954-792-8100
                                      800-233-9273
                                  Fax: 954-792-8545
                   E-mail: sales@addwarehouse.com
                                www.addwarehouse.com

The authors respond to concerns all parents and individuals have about using medication to treat disorders such as ADHD, explain the importance of a treatment program for those with this condition and discuss fads and fallacies in current treatments. *$13.50*

254 pages

302 Check Up from the Neck Up, Ensuring your Mental Health in the New Millennium

Hope Press
PO Box 188
Duarte, CA 91009-0188   818-303-0644
                                      800-321-4039
                                  Fax: 818-358-3520
                                     www.hopepress.com

Provides concise coping techniques for adults who have difficulties due to anxiety, depression, short temper, irritability, rage-attacks, compulsions, obsession and attention deficit hyperactivity disorder. *$19.95*

550 pages ISBN 1-878267-09-4

303 Complete Learning Disabilities Handbook

ADD WareHouse
300 NW 70th Avenue
Suite 102
Plantation, FL 33317   954-792-8100
800-233-9273
Fax: 954-792-8545
E-mail: sales@addwarehouse.com
www.addwarehouse.com

Provides a wealth of useful, practical suggestions and ready-to-use materials for meeting the special needs of students with learning disabilities and attention deficit disorders. Outlines an effective referral and identification process utilizing the concept of student study teams to provide data and formulate effective intervention strategies to assist the student in class. *$30.00*

206 pages

304 Conduct Disorders in Children and Adolesents

American Psychiatric Publishing
1000 Wilson Boulevard
Suite 1825
Arlington, VA 22209-3901   703-907-7322
800-368-5777
Fax: 703-907-1091
E-mail: appi@psych.org
www.appi.org

Katie Duffy, Marketing Assistant

Examines the phenomenology, etiology, and diagnosis of conduct disorders, and describes therapeutic and preventive interventions. Includes the range of treatments now availaable, including individual, family, group, and behavior therapy; hospitalization; and residential treatment. *$52.00*

448 pages ISBN 0-880485-17-5

305 Consumer's Guide to Psychiatric Drugs

New Harbinger Publications
5674 Shattuck Avenue
Oakland, CA 94609-1662   510-652-2002
800-748-6273
Fax: 510-652-5472
E-mail: customerservice@newharbinger.com
www.newharbinger.com

Helps consumers understand what treatment options are available and what side effects to expect. Covers possible interactions with other drugs, medical conditions and other concerns. Explains how each drug works, and offers detailed information about treatments for depression, bipolar disorder, anxiety and sleep disorders, as well as other conditions. *$16.95*

340 pages ISBN 1-572241-11-X

306 Daredevils and Daydreamers: New Perspectives on Attention Deficit/Hyperactivity Disorder

ADD WareHouse
300 NW 70th Avenue
Suite 102
Plantation, FL 33317   954-792-8100
800-233-9273
Fax: 954-792-8545
E-mail: sales@addwarehouse.com
www.addwarehouse.com

Summarizes what has been learned about ADHD in the past ten years and explains how parents can use this knowledge to help their child. Explains how to obtain a good evaluation, how to spot coexisting problems like depression and learning disabilities, how to find the right professional to treat your child and answers many other questions about caring for a child with ADHD. *$11.00*

260 pages

307 Disruptive Behavior Disorders in Children and Adolescents

American Psychiatric Publishing
1000 Wilson Boulevard
Suite 1825
Arlington, VA 22209-3901   703-907-7322
800-368-5777
Fax: 703-907-1091
E-mail: appi@psych.org
www.appi.org

Katie Duffy, Marketing Assistant

Discusses attention - deficit hyperactivity disorder, conduct disorder, substance abuse and disruptive behavior disorders. Examines the relationship between violence and mental illness in adolescence.

240 pages ISBN 0-880489-60-X

308 Distant Drums, Different Drummers: A Guide for Young People with ADHD

ADD WareHouse
300 NW 70th Avenue
Suite 102
Plantation, FL 33317   954-792-8100
800-233-9273
Fax: 954-792-8545
E-mail: sales@addwarehouse.com
www.addwarehouse.com

Barbara Ingersoll PhD

This book presents a positive perspective of ADHD - one that stresses the value of individual differences. Written for children and adolescents struggling with ADHD, it offers young readers the opportunity to see themselves in a positive light and motivates them to face challenging problems. Ages 8-14. *$16.00*

48 pages

309 Don't Give Up Kid

ADD WareHouse
300 NW 70th Avenue
Suite 102
Plantation, FL 33317   954-792-8100
800-233-9273
Fax: 954-792-8545
E-mail: sales@addwarehouse.com
www.addwarehouse.com

Alex, the hero of this book, is one of two million children in the US who have learning disabilities. This book gives children with reading problems and learning disabilities a clear understanding of their difficulties and the necessary courage to learn to live with them. Ages 5-12. *$13.00*

310 Down and Dirty Guide to Adult Attention Deficit Disorder

ADD WareHouse
300 NW 70th Avenue
Suite 102
Plantation, FL 33317   954-792-8100
800-233-9273
Fax: 954-792-8545
E-mail: sales@addwarehouse.com
www.addwarehouse.com

A book about ADD that is immensely entertaining, informative and uncomplicated. Describes concepts essential to understanding how this disorder is best identified and treated. You'll find a refreshing absence of jargon and an abundance of common sense, practical advice and healthy skepticism. *$17.00*

194 pages

311 Driven to Distraction: Recognizing and Coping with Attention Deficit Disorder from Childhood through Adulthood

ADD WareHouse
300 NW 70th Avenue
Suite 102
Plantation, FL 33317   954-792-8100
800-233-9273
Fax: 954-792-8545
E-mail: sales@addwarehouse.com
www.addwarehouse.com

Edward M Hallowell MD
John J Ratey MD

Through vivid stories of the experiences of their patients (both adults and children), this books shows the varied forms ADD takes - from the hyperactive search for high stimulation to the floating inattention of daydreaming - and the transforming impact of precise diagnosis and treatment. The authors explain when and how medication can be helpful, and since both authors have ADD, their advice on effective behavior-modification techniques is enriched by their own experience. Also available on audiotape for $16.00. *$13.00*

319 pages

312 Eagle Eyes: A Child's View of Attention Deficit Disorder

ADD WareHouse
300 NW 70th Avenue
Suite 102
Plantation, FL 33317   954-792-8100
800-233-9273
Fax: 954-792-8545
E-mail: sales@addwarehouse.com
www.addwarehouse.com

Jeanne Gehret

This book helps readers of all ages understand ADD and gives practical suggestions for organization, social cues and self calming. Expressive illustrations enhance the book and encourage reluctant readers. Ages 5-12. *$13.00*

313 Eukee the Jumpy, Jumpy Elephant

ADD WareHouse
300 NW 70th Avenue
Suite 102
Plantation, FL 33317   954-792-8100
800-233-9273
Fax: 954-792-8545
E-mail: sales@addwarehouse.com
www.addwarehouse.com

Cliff Corman MD
Esther Trevino

A story about a bright young elephant who is not like all the other elephants. Eukee moves through the jungle like a tornado, unable to pay attention to the other elephants. He begins to feel sad, but gets help after a visit to the doctor who explains why Eukee is so jumpy and hyperactive. With love, support and help, Eukee learns ways to help himself and gain renewed self-esteem. Ideal for ages 3-8. *$15.00*

22 pages

314 Facing AD/HD: A Survival Guide for Parents

Research Press
Dept 24 W
PO Box 9177
Champaign, IL 61826   217-352-3273
800-519-2707
Fax: 217-352-1221
E-mail: rp@researchpress.com
www.researchpress.com

Russell Pense, VP Marketing

Provides parents with the skills they need to help minimize the everyday struggles and frustrations associated with AD/HD. The book addresses structure, routines, setting goals, using charts, persistency with consistency, teamwork, treatment options, medication and more. *$ 14.95*

232 pages ISBN 0-878223-81-9

315 First Star I See

ADD WareHouse
300 NW 70th Avenue
Suite 102
Plantation, FL 33317

954-792-8100
800-233-9273
Fax: 954-792-8545
E-mail: sales@addwarehouse.com
www.addwarehouse.com

Jaye Andras Caffrey

This entertaining and funny look at ADD without hyperactivity is a must-read for middle grade girls with ADD, their teachers and parents. *$11.00*

150 pages

316 Gene Bomb-Does Higher Education and Advanced Technology Accelerate the Selection of Genes for Learning Disorders, Addictive and Disruptive Behaviors?

Hope Press
PO Box 188
Duarte, CA 91009-0188

818-303-0644
800-321-4039
Fax: 818-358-3520
www.hopepress.com

Explores the hypothesis that autism, learning disorders, alcoholism, drug abuse, depression, attention deficit disorder, and other disruptive behavioral disorders are increaseing in frequency because of an increasing selection, in the 20th century, for the genes associated with these conditions. *$29.95*

304 pages ISBN 1-878267-38-8

317 Give Your ADD Teen a Chance: A Guide for Parents of Teenagers with Attention Deficit Disorder

ADD WareHouse
300 NW 70th Avenue
Suite 102
Plantation, FL 33317

954-792-8100
800-233-9273
Fax: 954-792-8545
E-mail: sales@addwarehouse.com
www.addwarehouse.com

Lynn Weiss PhD

Parenting teenagers is never easy, especially if your teen suffers from ADD. This book provides parents with expert help by showing them how to determine which issues are caused by 'normal' teenager development and which are caused by ADD. *$15.00*

299 pages

318 Grandma's Pet Wildebeest Ate My Homework (and other suspect stories)

ADD WareHouse
300 NW 70th Avenue
Suite 102
Plantation, FL 33317

954-792-8100
800-233-9273
Fax: 954-792-8545
E-mail: sales@addwarehouse.com
www.addwarehouse.com

Tom Quinn

Parents and teachers dealing with hyperactive or daydreaming kids will find this book outstanding. As an ADHD adult himself, Quinn draws upon his own experience, making use of straightforward, creative behavioral management techniques, along with a keen sense of humor. A highly informative and enlightened book. *$16.95*

272 pages

319 Healing ADD: Simple Exercises That Will Change Your Daily Life

ADD WareHouse
300 NW 70th Avenue
Suite 102
Plantation, FL 33317

954-792-8100
800-233-9273
Fax: 954-792-8545
E-mail: sales@addwarehouse.com
www.addwarehouse.com

Thom Hartmann

Presents simple methods involving visualization and positive thinking that can be readily picked up by adults and taught to children with ADD. *$10.00*

178 pages

320 Help 4 ADD@High School

ADD WareHouse
300 NW 70th Avenue
Suite 102
Plantation, FL 33317

954-792-8100
800-233-9273
Fax: 954-792-8545
E-mail: sales@addwarehouse.com
www.addwarehouse.com

This new book was written for teenagers with ADHD. Designed like a web site, it has short, easy-to-read information packed sections which tell you what you need to know about how to get your life together - for yourself, not for your parents or your teachers. Includes tips on studying, ways your high school can help you succeed, tips on getting along better at home, on dating, exercise and much more. *$19.95*

119 pages

321 HomeTOVA: Attention Screening Test

ADD WareHouse
300 NW 70th Avenue
Suite 102
Plantation, FL 33317

954-792-8100
800-233-9273
Fax: 954-792-8545
E-mail: sales@addwarehouse.com
www.addwarehouse.com

Screen yourself or your child (ages 4 to 80 plus) for attention problems. After a simple installation on your home computer (Windows 95/98 OS only), the Home TOVA program runs with use of a mouse. Takes 21.6 minutes and measures how fast, accurate and consistent a person is in responding to squares flashing on a screen. Each program is limited to two administrators. *$29.95*

322 How to Do Homework without Throwing Up

ADD WareHouse
300 NW 70th Avenue
Suite 102
Plantation, FL 33317

954-792-8100
800-233-9273
Fax: 954-792-8545
E-mail: sales@addwarehouse.com
www.addwarehouse.com

Cartoons and witty insights teach important truths about homework and strategies for getting it done. Learn how to make a homework schedule, when to do the hardest homework, where to do homework, the benefits of homework and more. Useful in motivating students with ADD. For ages 8-13. *$9.00*

67 pages

323 Hyperactive Child, Adolescent, and Adult

Oxford University Press
198 Madison Avenue
New York, NY 10016

212-726-6000
800-451-7556
Fax: 919-677-1303
www.oup-usa.org/orbs/

Discusses symptoms and treatment of ADD/ADHD in children and adults with practical suggestions for the management of children. *$27.00*

172 pages ISBN 0-195042-91-3

324 Hyperactive Children Grown Up: ADHD in Children, Adolescents, and Adults

Guilford Publications
72 Spring Street
New York, NY 10012

212-431-9800
800-365-7006
Fax: 212-966-6708
E-mail: info@guilford.com
www.guilford.com

Explores what happens to hyperactive children when they grow to adulthood. Based on the McGill prospective studies, which spans more than 30 years, the volume reports findings on the etiology, treatment and outcome of attention deficits and hyperactivity at all stages of development. Paperback also available. *$44.95*

473 pages ISBN 0-898620-39-2

325 I'm Somebody, Too!

ADD WareHouse
300 NW 70th Avenue
Suite 102
Plantation, FL 33317

954-792-8100
800-233-9273
Fax: 954-792-8545
E-mail: sales@addwarehouse.com
www.addwarehouse.com

Jeanne Gehret

Because it is written for an older, non-ADD audience, this book explains ADD in depth and explains methods to handle the feelings that often result from having a family member with ADD. For children ages 9 and older. *$13.00*

159 pages

326 Is Your Child Hyperactive? Inattentive? Impulsive? Distractible?

ADD WareHouse
300 NW 70th Avenue
Suite 102
Plantation, FL 33317

954-792-8100
800-233-9273
Fax: 954-792-8545
E-mail: sales@addwarehouse.com
www.addwarehouse.com

Written with compassion and hope, this parent guide prepares you for the process of determining if your child has ADD and guides you in your dealings with educators, doctors and other professionals. *$13.00*

235 pages

327 It's Nobody's Fault: New Hope and Help for Difficult Children and Their Parents

ADD WareHouse
300 NW 70th Avenue
Suite 102
Plantation, FL 33317

954-792-8100
800-233-9273
Fax: 954-792-8545
E-mail: sales@addwarehouse.com
www.addwarehouse.com

Patrick J Kilcatt PhD
Patricia O Quinn MD

This book explains that neither the parents nor children are causes of mental disorders and related problems. *$20.00*

184 pages

328 Kids with Incredible Potential

Active Parenting Publishers
1955 Vaughn Road NW
Suite 108
Kennesaw, GA 30144-7808

770-429-0565
800-825-0060
Fax: 770-429-0334
E-mail: cservice@activeparenting.com
www.activeparenting.com

An ADHD curriculum to supplement the Active Parenting Today parenting education program. *$39.95*

329 Learning to Slow Down and Pay Attention

ADD WareHouse
300 NW 70th Avenue
Suite 102
Plantation, FL 33317

954-792-8100
800-233-9273
Fax: 954-792-8545
E-mail: sales@addwarehouse.com
www.addwarehouse.com

Written for children to read, and illustrated with charming cartoons and activity pages, the book helps children identify problems and explains how their parents, teachers and doctors can help. For children 6-14. *$10.00*

70 pages

330 Living with Attention Deficit Disorder: a Workbook for Adults with ADD

New Harbinger Publications
5674 Shattuck Avenue
Oakland, CA 94609-1662   510-652-2002
800-748-6273
Fax: 510-652-5472
E-mail: customerservice@newharbinger.com
www.newharbinger.com

Includes strategies for handling common problems at work and school, dealing with intimate relationships, and finding support. *$17.95*

176 pages ISBN 1-572240-63-6

331 Medications for Attention Disorders and Related Medical Problems: Comprehensive Handbook

ADD WareHouse
300 NW 70th Avenue
Suite 102
Plantation, FL 33317   954-792-8100
800-233-9273
Fax: 954-792-8545
E-mail: sales@addwarehouse.com
www.addwarehouse.com

ADHD and ADD are medical conditions and often medical intervention is regarded by most experts as an essential component of the multimodal program for the treatment of these disorders. This text presents a comprehensive look at medications and their use in attention disorders. *$37.00*

420 pages

332 Meeting the ADD Challenge: A Practical Guide for Teachers

Research Press
Dept 24 W
PO Box 9177
Champaign, IL 61826   217-352-3273
800-519-2707
Fax: 217-352-1221
E-mail: rp@researchpress.com
www.researchpress.com

Russell Pense, VP Marketing

Information on the needs and treatment of children and adolescents with ADD. The book addresses the defining characteristics of ADD, common treatment approaches, myths about ADD, matching intervention to student, use of behavior rating scales and checklists, evaluating interventions, regular versus special class placement, helping students regulate their own behavior and more. Includes case examples. *$17.95*

196 pages ISBN 0-878223-45-2

333 Misunderstood Child: Understanding and Coping with Your Child's Learning Disabilities

ADD WareHouse
300 NW 70th Avenue
Suite 102
Plantation, FL 33317   954-792-8100
800-233-9273
Fax: 954-792-8545
E-mail: sales@addwarehouse.com
www.addwarehouse.com

In this revised and updated edition you will find promising treatment options for children, adolescents and adults with learning disabilities, discussion of ADHD, pros and cons of using medication, revision to federal and state laws covering discrimination and educational rights, new approaches for those of college age and older. *$15.00*

403 pages

334 My Brother's a World Class Pain: a Sibling's Guide to ADHD

ADD WareHouse
300 NW 70th Avenue
Suite 102
Plantation, FL 33317   954-792-8100
800-233-9273
Fax: 954-792-8545
E-mail: sales@addwarehouse.com
www.addwarehouse.com

While they frequently bear the brunt of the ADHD child's impulsiveness and distractibility, siblings usually are not afforded opportunities to understand the nature of the problem and to have their own feelings and thoughts addressed. This story shows brothers and sisters how they can play an important role in the family's quest for change. *$12.00*

34 pages

335 Negotiating the Special Education Maze

ADD WareHouse
300 NW 70th Avenue
Suite 102
Plantation, FL 33317   954-792-8100
800-233-9273
Fax: 954-792-8545
E-mail: sales@addwarehouse.com
www.addwarehouse.com

Revised and updated, this book offers parents and teachers a wide range of current information about programs and legislation. The authors present a step-by-step process complete with planning guides, personalized checklists and exercises to guide parents toward the special education programs that will be most beneficial for their child. *$17.00*

264 pages

336 Other Me: Poetic Thoughts on ADD for Adults, Kids and Parents

ADD WareHouse
300 NW 70th Avenue
Suite 102
Plantation, FL 33317   954-792-8100
                             800-233-9273
                        Fax: 954-792-8545
        E-mail: sales@addwarehouse.com
                        www.addwarehouse.com

Arnold C Fellman, Illustrator

A collection of poems for adults and kids with ADD and parents of children with ADD. Within the highly serious world of diagnosis and treatment of a painful disorder, this book provides a lighter, sensitive look at the manifestations of ADD. *$16.00*

136 pages

337 Out of the Fog

ADD WareHouse
300 NW 70th Avenue
Suite 102
Plantation, FL 33317   954-792-8100
                             800-233-9273
                        Fax: 954-792-8545
        E-mail: sales@addwarehouse.com
                        www.addwarehouse.com

Gives adults with ADD and their families everything they need to understand and live with ADD, including practical advice on how to cope with its symptoms and current methods for treating this often debilitating condition. *$13.00*

300 pages

338 Out-of-Sync Child

Perigee
375 Hudson Street
New York, NY 10014   212-366-2000
                        Fax: 212-366-2679
                   www.penguinputnam.com

A new explanation and a new hope for parents whose children have been labled with words like difficult, picky, clumsy, or inattentive. Discusses Sensory Integration (SI) Dysfunction, often confused with ADD, learning disabilities, and other problems and subtle develpmental difficulties that prevent children from interpreting sensory signals coming from their bodies and the world around them. *$14.00*

277 pages

339 Overcoming Underachieving: an Action Guide to Helping Your Child Succeed in School

ADD WareHouse
300 NW 70th Avenue
Suite 102
Plantation, FL 33317   954-792-8100
                             800-233-9273
                        Fax: 954-792-8545
        E-mail: sales@addwarehouse.com
                        www.addwarehouse.com

Two nationally recognized experts in children's school problems show you how to become your child's advocate, coach and guide through the educational process. They help you pinpoint your child's unique learning patterns and the problems that interfere with learning, behavior and achievement. Learn proven methods to learning and behavior. *$16.95*

312 pages

340 Performance Breakthroughs for Adolescents with Learning Disabilities or ADD

Research Press
Dept 24 W
PO Box 9177
Champaign, IL 61826   217-352-3273
                             800-519-2707
                        Fax: 217-352-1221
        E-mail: rp@researchpress.com
                        www.researchpress.com

Russell Pense, VP Marketing

Covers program planning, assessment procedures, self-management strategies, the instructional process, reading and writing skills, test taking, homework, crisis intervention and more. *$23.95*

336 pages ISBN 0-878223-49-5

341 Psychoses and Pervasive Developmental Disorders in Childhood/Adolescents

American Psychiatric Publishing
1000 Wilson Boulevard
Suite 1825
Arlington, VA 22209-3901   703-907-7322
                             800-368-5777
                        Fax: 703-907-1091
        E-mail: appi@psych.org
                        www.appi.org

Katie Duffy, Marketing Assistant

Provides a concise summary of current knowledge of psychoses and pervasive developmental disorders of childhood and adolescence. Discusses recent changes in aspects of diagnosis and definition of these disorders, advances in knowledge, and aspects of treatment. *$46.50*

368 pages ISBN 1-882103-01-7

342 Put Yourself in Their Shoes: Understanding Teenagers with Attention Deficit Hyperactivity Disorder

ADD WareHouse
300 NW 70th Avenue
Suite 102
Plantation, FL 33317   954-792-8100
                             800-233-9273
                        Fax: 954-792-8545
        E-mail: sales@addwarehouse.com
                        www.addwarehouse.com

Contains up-to-date information on how ADHD affects the lives of adolescents at home, in school, in the workplace and in social relationships. Chapters discuss how to get a good assessment, controversial treatments and medications for ADHD, building positive communication at home, problem-solving strategies to resolve family conflict, ADHD and the military, study strategies to improve learning, ADHD and delinquency, two hundred educational accommodations for ADHD teens and more. *$19.00*

249 pages

343 RYAN: A Mother's Story of Her Hyperactive/ Tourette Syndrome Child

Hope Press
PO Box 188
Duarte, CA 91009-0188   818-303-0644
800-321-4039
Fax: 818-358-3520
www.hopepress.com

A moving and informative story of how a mother struggled with the many behavioral problems presented by her son with Tourette syndrome, ADHD and oppositional defiant disorder. *$9.95*

302 pages ISBN 1-878267-25-6

344 Scoutmaster's Guide to Attention Deficit Disorder

ADD WareHouse
300 NW 70th Avenue
Suite 102
Plantation, FL 33317   954-792-8100
800-233-9273
Fax: 954-792-8545
E-mail: sales@addwarehouse.com
www.addwarehouse.com

We all want Scouting to be the best possible experience for our children. However, Scouts with ADD are not often equipped with the skills necessary for their Scouting, no matter how badly they may want to succeed. This unique book is for adults working with youth with ADD in Scouting and other youth activities. *$14.95*

177 pages

345 Self-Esteem Revolutions in Children: Understanding and Managing the Critical Transition in Your Child's Life

ADD WareHouse
300 NW 70th Avenue
Suite 102
Plantation, FL 33317   954-792-8100
800-233-9273
Fax: 954-792-8545
E-mail: sales@addwarehouse.com
www.addwarehouse.com

As youngsters grow up, they experience sweeping changes in self-esteem. This book explains why these 'revolutions' occur, offering easily understood, step-by-step methods for parents to help young children and teens gain self-respect. Also available in audiotape. *$13.00*

180 pages

346 Shelley, The Hyperative Turtle

ADD WareHouse
300 NW 70th Avenue
Suite 102
Plantation, FL 33317   954-792-8100
800-233-9273
Fax: 954-792-8545
E-mail: sales@addwarehouse.com
www.addwarehouse.com

Deborah Moss

The story of a bright young turtle who's not like all the other turtles. Shelley moves like a rocket and is unable to sit still for even the shortest periods of time. Because he and the other turtles are unable to understand why he is so wiggly and squirmy, Shelley begins to feel naughty and out of place. But after a visit to the doctor, Shelley learns what 'hyperactive' means and that it is necessary to take special medicine to control that wiggly feeling. Ideal for ages 3-7. *$14.00*

24 pages

347 Sometimes I Drive My Mom Crazy, But I Know She's Crazy About Me

ADD WareHouse
300 NW 70th Avenue
Suite 102
Plantation, FL 33317   954-792-8100
800-233-9273
Fax: 954-792-8545
E-mail: sales@addwarehouse.com
www.addwarehouse.com

This warm and humorous story of a young boy with ADHD addresses the many difficult and frustrating issues kids like him confront every day - from sitting still in the classroom, to remaining calm, to feeling 'different' from other children. This book is an amusing look at how a youngster with ADHD can develop a sense of self-worth through better understanding of this disorder. Ages 6-12. *$16.00*

129 pages

348 Succeeding in College with Attention Deficit Disorders: Issues and Strategies for Students, Counselors and Educators

ADD WareHouse
300 NW 70th Avenue
Suite 102
Plantation, FL 33317   954-792-8100
800-233-9273
Fax: 954-792-8545
E-mail: sales@addwarehouse.com
www.addwarehouse.com

Written for college students, their couselors and educators. Based on the real life experiances of adults who were interviewed as part of a research study, this book offers a vivid picture of how college students with ADD can cope and find success in school. *$18.00*

189 pages

349 Survival Guide for College Students with ADD or LD

ADD WareHouse
300 NW 70th Avenue
Suite 102
Plantation, FL 33317

954-792-8100
800-233-9273
Fax: 954-792-8545
E-mail: sales@addwarehouse.com
www.addwarehouse.com

A useful guide for high school or college students diagnosed with attention deficit disorder of learning disabilities. Provides the information needed to survive and thrive in a college setting. Full of practical suggestions and tips from an experienced specialist in the field and from college students who also suffer from these difficulties. *$10.00*

56 pages

350 Survival Strategies for Parenting Your ADD Child: Dealing with Obsessions, Compulsions, Depression, Explosive Behavior and Rage

Underwood Books
PO Box 1609
Grass Valley, CA 95945

Fax: 530-274-7179
E-mail: timunderwd@cs.com
www.underwoodbooks.com

Provides parents with methods which can heal the fractures and pain that occur in families with troubled children. *$12.95*

268 pages ISBN 1-887424-19-9

351 Taking Charge of ADHD: Complete, Authoritative Guide for Parents

ADD WareHouse
300 NW 70th Avenue
Suite 102
Plantation, FL 33317

954-792-8100
800-233-9273
Fax: 954-792-8545
E-mail: sales@addwarehouse.com
www.addwarehouse.com

Written for parents who are ready to take charge of their child's life. Strong on advocacy and parental empowerment, this book provides step-by-step methods for managing a child with ADHD in a variety of everyday situations, gives information on medications and discusses numerous techniques for enhancing a child's school performance. *$18.00*

350 pages

352 Teaching the Tiger, a Handbook for Individuals Involved in the Education of Students with Attention Deficit Disorders, Tourette Syndrome, or Obsessive - Compulsive Disorder

Hope Press
PO Box 188
Duarte, CA 91009-0188

818-303-0644
800-321-4039
Fax: 818-358-3520
www.hopepress.com

Innovative methods of teaching children with ADD, Tourette Syndrome, Obsessive-Compulsive Disorders *$35.00*

ISBN 1-878267-34-5

353 Teenagers with ADD: A Parent's Guide

Woodbine House
6510 Bells Mill Road
Bethesda, MD 20817

301-897-3570
800-843-7323
Fax: 301-897-5838
E-mail: info@woodbinehouse.com
www.woodbinehouse.com

Double-column book full of information, suggestions and case studies. Lively, upbeat, comprehensive and well targeted to the problems parents face with ADD teenagers. *$18.95*

370 pages ISBN 0-933149-69-7

354 Understanding Girls with Attention Deficit Hyperactivity Disorder

ADD WareHouse
300 NW 70th Avenue
Suite 102
Plantation, FL 33317

954-792-8100
800-233-9273
Fax: 954-792-8545
E-mail: sales@addwarehouse.com
www.addwarehouse.com

Symptoms of ADHD are often overlooked or misunderstood in girls who are often diagnosed much later, and their ADHD symptoms may go untreated. This groundbreaking book reveals how ADHD affects girls from preschool through high school years. Gender differences are discussed along with issues related to school success, medication treatment, family relationships and susceptibility to other disorders such as anxiety, depression and learning problems. *$19.95*

291 pages

355 Voices From Fatherhood: Fathers, Sons and ADHD

ADD WareHouse
300 NW 70th Avenue
Suite 102
Plantation, FL 33317

954-792-8100
800-233-9273
Fax: 954-792-8545
E-mail: sales@addwarehouse.com
www.addwarehouse.com

Patrick J Kilcatt PhD
Patricia O Quinn MD

Written to specifically help fathers navigate the complex world of parenting and ADHD, this book helps fathers enhance and deepen their relationships with their sons while providing them with strategies for guiding their sons. *$20.00*

184 pages

356 What Makes Ryan Tick? A Family's Triumph over Tourette's Syndrome and Attention Deficit Hyperactivity Disorder

Hope Press
PO Box 188
Duarte, CA 91009-0188
818-303-0644
800-321-4039
Fax: 818-358-3520
www.hopepress.com

A moving and informative story how a mother struggled with the many behavioral problems presented by her son with Tourettes syndrome, ADHD and oppositional defiant disorder. *$15.95*

303 pages ISBN 1-878267-35-3

357 Women with Attention Deficit Disorder

ADD WareHouse
300 NW 70th Avenue
Suite 102
Plantation, FL 33317
954-792-8100
800-233-9273
Fax: 954-792-8545
E-mail: sales@addwarehouse.com
www.addwarehouse.com

Combines real-life histories, treatment experiences and recent clinical research to highlight the special challenges facing women with Attention Deficit Disorder. After describing what to look for and what to look out for in treatment and counseling, this book outlines empowering steps that women living with ADD may use to change their lives. Also available on audiotape. 3 hours on 2 cassettes for $20.00. *$12.00*

288 pages

358 You Mean I'm Not Lazy, Stupid or Crazy?

ADD WareHouse
300 NW 70th Avenue
Suite 102
Plantation, FL 33317
954-792-8100
800-233-9273
Fax: 954-792-8545
E-mail: sales@addwarehouse.com
www.addwarehouse.com

Katie Kelly
Peggy Ramundo

This book is the first written by ADD adults for ADD adults. A comprehensive guide, it provides accurate information, practical how-to's and moral support. Readers will also get information on unique differences in ADD adults, the impact on their lives, treatment options available for adults, up-to-date research findings and much more. Also available on audiotape. *$14.00*

426 pages

359 Your Defiant Child: Eight Steps to Better Behavior

ADD WareHouse
300 NW 70th Avenue
Suite 102
Plantation, FL 33317
954-792-8100
800-233-9273
Fax: 954-792-8545
E-mail: sales@addwarehouse.com
www.addwarehouse.com

This book helps concerned parents understand what causes child defiance, when it becomes a problem and how it can be resolved. Its clear eight-step program stresses consistency and cooperation, promoting changes through a system of praise, rewards and mild punishment. Readers benefit from concrete guidelines for establishing clear patterns of discipline, communicating with children on a level they can understand and reducing family stress overall. *$14.95*

240 pages

360 Attention-Deficit Hyperactivity Disorder in Adults: A Guide

Madison Institute of Medicine
7617 Mineral Point Road
Suite 300
Madison, WI 53717-1623
608-827-2470
Fax: 608-827-2479
E-mail: mim@miminc.org
www.miminc.org

This guide provides an overview of adult ADHD and how it is treated with medications and other treatment approaches. *$5.95*

58 pages

Periodicals & Pamphlets

361 ADHD Report

Guilford Publications
72 Spring Street
New York, NY 10012
212-431-9800
800-365-7006
Fax: 212-966-6708
E-mail: info@guilford.com
www.guilford.com

This accessible newsletter provides a single reliable guide to the latest developments, newest topics, and current trends in ADHD. An indispensibe resource, the ADHD Report examines the nature, definition, diagnosis, developmental course, outcomes and etiologies associated with ADHD, as well as changes occuring in the fields of education and clinical management. It includes handouts for clinicians and parents, as well as annotated research findings.

6 per year

362 Add-Up

Listening
214 Main Street
Hobart, IN 46342

219-938-6962
Fax: 219-938-7435
E-mail: addup@crown.net

Provides information about treating and reversing attention deficit disorder. Recurring features include letters to the editor, interviews, news of research, a calendar of events and book reviews. *$12.00*

4-6 pages 24 per year

363 Attention Deficit/Hyperactivity Disorder in Children and Adolescents

Center for Mental Health Services: Knowledge Exchange Network
PO Box 42490
Washington, DC 20015

800-789-2647
Fax: 301-984-8796
TDD: 866-889-2647
E-mail: ken@mentalhealth.org
www.mentalhealth.org

This fact sheet defines attention-deficit/hyperactivity disorder, describes the warning signs, discusses types of help available, and suggests what parents or other caregivers can do.

3 pages Year Founded: 1997

364 Treatment of Children with Mental Disorders

National Institute of Mental Health
6001 Executive Boulevard
Room 8184
Bethesda, MD 20892-9663

866-615-6464
Fax: 301-443-4279
TTY: 301-443-8431
E-mail: nimhinfo@nih.gov
www.nimh.nih.gov

Ruth Dubois, Assistant Chief

A short booklet that contains questions and answers about therapy for children with mental disorders. Includes a chart of mental disorders and medications used.

Research Centers

365 Health Research Institute and Pfeiffer Treatment Center

1804 Centre Point Circle
Suite 102
Naperville, IL 60563-1440

630-505-0300
Fax: 630-505-1907
www.hriptc.org

William Walsh PhD, Founder

Strives to serve the public at low cost, identifies specific chemical imbalances through extensive chemical testing and provides individualized treatments for balancing body chemistry.

Support Groups & Hot Lines

366 AD-IN: Attention Deficit Information Network

58 Prince Street
Needham, MA 02494-1200

781-455-9895
Fax: 781-449-1332
E-mail: adin@gis.net
www.addinfonetwork.org

Libby Ostrofsky, President

We offer support and information to families of children with ADD, adults with ADD and professionals through a network of AD-IN chapters. AD-IN was founded in 1988. AD-IN is a community resource for information on training programs and speakers for those who work with individuals with ADD. The organization also presents conferences and workshops for parents and professionals on current issues, research and treatments for ADD and makes an annual, post-secondary scholarship award. Video cassette, paperback, audio cassette.

367 CHADD: Children and Adults with AD/HD

8181 Professional Place
Suite 150
Landover, MD 20785

301-306-7070
800-233-4050
Fax: 301-306-7090
www.chadd.org

Video & Audio

368 ADHD: What Can We Do?

ADD WareHouse
300 NW 70th Avenue
Suite 102
Plantation, FL 33317

954-792-8100
800-233-9273
Fax: 954-792-8545
E-mail: sales@addwarehouse.com
www.addwarehouse.com

Can serve as a companion to ADHD: What Do We Know?, this video focuses on the most effective ways to manage ADHD, both in the home and in the classroom. Scenes depict the use of behavior management at home and accommodations and interventions in the classroom which have proven to be effective in the treatment of ADHD. Thirty five minutes. *$95.00*

369 ADHD: What Do We Know?

ADD WareHouse
300 NW 70th Avenue
Suite 102
Plantation, FL 33317

954-792-8100
800-233-9273
Fax: 954-792-8545
E-mail: sales@addwarehouse.com
www.addwarehouse.com

This video provides an overview of the disorder and introduces the viewer to three young people who have ADHD. Discusses how ADHD affects the lives of the children and adults, causes of the disorder, associated problems, outcome in adulthood and provides vivid illustrations of how individuals with ADHD function at home, at school and on the job. Thirty five minutes. *$95.00*

370 Adults with Attention Deficit Disorder: ADD Isn't Just Kids Stuff

ADD WareHouse
300 NW 70th Avenue
Suite 102
Plantation, FL 33317   954-792-8100
800-233-9273
Fax: 954-792-8545
E-mail: sales@addwarehouse.com
www.addwarehouse.com

Explains this often misunderstood condition and the effects it has on one's work, home and social life. With the help of a panel of six adults, four ADD adults and two of their spouses, the book addresses the most common concerns of adults with ADD and provides information that will help families who are experiancing difficulties. *$47.00*

371 Educating Inattentive Children

ADD WareHouse
300 NW 70th Avenue
Suite 102
Plantation, FL 33317   954-792-8100
800-233-9273
Fax: 954-792-8545
E-mail: sales@addwarehouse.com
www.addwarehouse.com

Samuel Goldstein PhD
Michael Goldstein MD

This two-hour video is ideal for in-service to regular and special educators concerning problems experienced by inattentive elementary and secondary students. Provides educators with information necessary to indentify and evaluate classroom problems caused by inattention and a well-defined set of practical guidelines to help educate children with ADD. *$49.00*

372 Medication for Attention Deficit Disorder: All You Need to Know

ADD WareHouse
300 NW 70th Avenue
Suite 102
Plantation, FL 33317   954-792-8100
800-233-9273
Fax: 954-792-8545
E-mail: sales@addwarehouse.com
www.addwarehouse.com

This comprehensive video describes the nomal concerns that parents and ADD adults have when faced with the decision of medication. ADD experts describe some of the myths about medication and treatment as well as the different medications available for treating attention deficit disorder. *$47.00*

373 New Look at ADHD: Inhibition, Time and Self Control

Guilford Publications
72 Spring Street
New York, NY 10012   212-431-9800
800-365-7006
Fax: 212-966-6708
E-mail: info@guilford.com
www.guilford.com

Steve Lerner, Producer

This video provides an accessible introduction to Russell A Barkley's influential theory of the nature and origins of ADHD. The program brings to life the conceptual framework delineated in Barkley's other books. Discusses concrete ways that our new understanding of the disorder might facilitate more effective clinical interventions. This lucid, state of the art program is ideal viewing for clinicians, students and inservice trainees, parents of children with ADHD and adults with the disorder. *$95.00*

Year Founded: 2000 ISBN 1-572304-97-9

374 Understanding and Treating the Hereditary Psychiatric Spectrum Disorders

Hope Press
PO Box 188
Duarte, CA 91009-0188   818-303-0644
800-321-4039
Fax: 818-358-3520
www.hopepress.com

David E Comings MD, Presenter

Learn with 10 hours of audio tapes from a two day seminar given in May 1997 by David E Comings, MD. Tapes cover: ADHD, Tourette Syndrome, Obsessive-Compulsive Disorder, Conduct Disorder, Oppositional Defiant Disorder, Autism and other Hereditary Psychiatric Spectrum Disorders. Eight audio tapes. *$75.00*

Year Founded: 1997

375 Understanding the Defiant Child

Guilford Publications
72 Spring Street
New York, NY 10012   212-431-9800
800-365-7006
Fax: 212-966-6708
E-mail: info@guilford.com
www.guilford.com

Presents information on Oppositional Defiant Disorder and Conduct Disorder with scenes of family interactions, showing the nature and causes of these disorders and what can and should be done about it. Thirty five minutes with a manual that contains more information. *$ 95.00*

ISBN 1-572301-66-X

376 Why Won't My Child Pay Attention?

ADD WareHouse
300 NW 70th Avenue
Suite 102
Plantation, FL 33317   954-792-8100
                             800-233-9273
                       Fax: 954-792-8545
          E-mail: sales@addwarehouse.com
                   www.addwarehouse.com

Provides an easy-to-follow explanation concerning the effect ADD has on children at school, home and in the community. Provides guidelines to help parents and professionals successfully and happily manage the problems these behaviors can cause. *$38.00*

Web Sites

377 www.CHADD.org

CHADD: Children/Adults with Attention Deficit/Hyperactivity Disorder

378 www.LD-ADD.com

Attention Deficit Disorder and Parenting Site

379 www.aap.org/policy/AC0002.html

American Academy of Pediatrics Practice Guidelines on ADHD

Site serves the purpose of giving the public guidelines for diagnosing and evaluating children with possible ADHD.

380 www.abcparenting.com

ABCs of Parenting

381 www.add-plus.com/forms.html

Forms

Data collection forms including: Medication Effectiveness Report Form; Academic Problem Identification Checklist; Social/Academic/Emotional Adjustment Checklist; and Hyperactivity Screening Checklist.

382 www.add.about.com

Attention Deficit Disorder

Hundreds of sites.

383 www.add.about.com/msubjobs.htm

Job Information for People with ADD

384 www.add.org

Psychoeducational Materials for Clients and Families

National Attention Deficit Disorder Association publication.

385 www.add.org/content/group1.htm

Attention Deficit Disorder Association

386 www.add.org/content/menu1.html

National Attention Deficit Disorder Association

Offers articles under ABCs, Research, and Treatment.

387 www.additudemag.com

ADDitude: Happy Healthy Lifestyle Magazine for People with ADD

388 www.addvance.com

ADDvance Magazine

Site for women and girls has links, chat, and support groups.

389 www.adhdnews.com.ssi.htm

Social Security

Applying for disability benefits for children with ADHD.

390 www.adhdnews.com/Advocate.htm

Advocating for Your Child

391 www.adhdnews.com/sped.htm

Special Education Rights and Responsibilities

Writing IEP's and TIEPS. Pursuing special education services.

392 www.amenclinic.com/ac/addtests/default.asp

Amen Clinic ADD Subtype Test

Interactive test diagnoses five ADD subtypes, also provides an adult ADD checklist.

393 www.babycenter.com/rcindex.html

BabyCenter

394 www.bobseay.com/littlecorner/newurl/

Bob's Little Corner of the Web

Sections include Traits of ADDers, How Are We Different, and Secret Lives of ADDers.

395 www.catalog.com/chadd/doe/doe_myth.ht
m

Attention Deficit Disorder: Beyond the Myths

Facts and myths.

396 www.chadd.org

Children and Adults with Attention Deficit/Hyperactivity Disorder

Covers everything on ADHD and provides links to other credible sources.

397 www.cyberpsych.org

CyberPsych

Hosts the American Psychoanalyists Foundation, American Association of Suicideology, Society for the Exploration of Psychotherapy Intergration, and Anxiety Disorders Association of America. Also subcategories of the anxiety disorders, as well as general information, including panic disorder, phobias, obsessive compulsive disorder (OCD), social phobia, generalized anxiety disorder, post traumatic stress disorder, and phobias of childhood. Book reviews and links to web pages sharing the topics.

398 www.focusas.com/AttentionalDisorders.ht
ml

Focus Adolescent Services

Information about attention disorders and many differing approaches plus valuable book information.

399 www.healthatoz.com/atoz/adhd/aindex.ht
ml

HealthAtoZ.com on ADHD

Reliable information on ADHD.

400 www.hometown.aol.com/BevKPrice/HTM
L/index

A Journey into Attention Deficit Disorder

Under Strategies and Intervention there are pages on modifying school settings and coping at home.

401 www.kidsource.com

Kidsource Online on ADHD

Site run by parents of ADHD kids.

402 www.kidsource.com./LDA-CA/ADD_WO.
html

ADD without Hyperactivity: ADHD, Predominately Inattentive Type

403 www.klis.com/chandler/pamphlet/adhd/

Attention Deficit Hyperactivity Disorder

404 www.mentalhealth.org/publications/allpu
bs/

Attention-Deficit/Hyperactiviy Disorder in Children and Adolescents

Lists symptoms very fully.

405 www.nichcy.org

National Information Center for Children and Youth with Disabilities

Excellent information in English and Spanish.

406 www.nimh.nih.gov/publicat/adhd.cfm

Attention Deficit Hyperactivity Disorder

Thirty page booklet.

407 www.nimh.nih.gov/publicat/adhdmenu.cf
m

National Institute of Mental Health on ADHD

Covers the basics and latest in research.

408 www.nimh.nih.gov/publicat/spadhd.htm

Attention Deficit Hyperactivity Disorder

Thirty 30 page booklet - Spanish.

409 www.oneaddplace.com

One ADD Place

410 **www.planetpsych.com**

Planetpsych.com

Learn about disorders, their treatments and other topics in psychology. Articles are listed under the related topic areas. Ask a therapist a question for free, or view the directory of professionals in your area. If you are a therapist sign up for the directory. Current features, self-help, interactive, and newsletter archives.

411 **www.psychcentral.com**

Psych Central

Personalized one-stop index for psychology, support, and mental health issues, resources, and people on the Internet.

412 **www.sciam.com/1998/0998issue/0998barkley**

Attention-Deficit Hyperactivity Disorder

New theory suggesting ADHD may arise because key brain circuits fail to develop properly, perhaps due to an altered gene.

413 **www.svr.com/addhelp/index.htm**

ADHD Assessment Service

Evaluation materials, diagnosis, outcomes, educational rights, behavioral treatments and medication.

414 **www.svr.com/addhelp/over.htm**

What Is ADHD? a General Overview

Questions and answers.

415 **www.users.aol.com:80/jimams/answers1.html**

Questions from Younger Children about ADD

Responses to children's questions.

416 **www.users.aol.com:80/jimams/answers2.html**

Questions from Adolescents about ADD

Responses to children's questions.

417 **www3.sympatico.ca/frankk**

ADD FAQ

Good information on Attention Deficit Disorder.

Introduction

Autistic Disorder is a pervasive developmental disorder whose main symptoms are a marked lack of interest in connecting, interacting, or communcating with others. People with this disorder cannot share something of interest with other people, rarely make eye contact with others, avoid physical contact, show little facial expression, and do not make friends. Autistic Disorder is a profound, lifelong condition with wide ranging and severe disabilities, often including additional behavior problems, such as hyperactivity, obsessive compulsive behavior, self injury, and tics. Although present before age three, the disorder may not show itself right away. Parents often sense that there is something wrong because of their child's marked lack of interest in social interaction. Very young children with autism not only show no desire for affection and cuddling, but show actual aversion to it. There is no socially directed smiling or facial responsiveness, and no responsiveness to the voices of parents and siblings. As a result, parents may sometimes worry that their child is deaf. Later, the child may be more willing to interact socially, but the quality of interaction is unusual, usually inappropriately intrusive with little understanding of social rules and boundaries. The autistic child seems not to have the abilities and desires that would make it possible for him or her to become a social being. Instead, the child seems locked up in an alien interior world which is both incomprehesible and inaccessible to parents, siblings, and others.

SYMPTOMS

Impairment in the Quality of Social Interaction
•Gross lack of nonverbal behavior (e.g., eye contact, facial expression, body postures, and gestures), which gives meaning to social interaction and social behavior;
•Failure to make friends in age-appropriate ways;
•Lack of spontaneously seeking to share interests or achievements with others (e.g., not showing things to others, not pointing to, or bringing interesting objects to others);
•Lack of social or emotional give and take (e.g., not joining in social play or simple games with others);
•Notable lack of awareness of others. Oblivious of other children (including siblings), of their excitement, distress, or needs.

Marked Impairment in the Quality of Communication
•Delay in, or lack of, spoken language development. Those who speak cannot initiate or sustain comunication with others;
•Lack of spontaneous make-believe or imitative play common among young children;
•When speech does develop, it may be abnormal and monotonous;
•Repetitive use of language.

Restricted Repetitive Patterns or Behavior
•Restricted range of interests often fixed on one subject and its facts (e.g., baseball);
•A great deal of exact repetition in play, (e.g., lining up play objects in the same way again and again);
•Resistance and distress if anything in the environment is changed, (e.g., a chair moved to a different place);
•Insistence on following certain rules and routines (e.g., walking to school by the same route each day);
•Repeated body movements (e.g., body rocking, hand clapping);
•Persistent preoccupation with details or parts of objects (e.g., buttons).

ASSOCIATED FEATURES

Autism seems to bring with it an increased risk of other disorders. In most cases of autism, retardation is also present; seventy-five percent of autistic children are retarded. Yet that means that a large minority (twenty-five percent), have cognitive abilities at or above average. Twenty-five percent of cases also have seizure disorders. The development of intellectual skills is usually uneven. An autistic child may be able to read extremely early, but may have few comprehension skills. There may be other symptoms, such as hyperactivity, short attention span, impulsivity, aggressiveness, and self injury, such as head banging, hair pulling, and arm biting (particularly in young children). There may be unusual physiological responses in which there is much less than normal sensitivity to pain but extreme sensitivity to sounds or to being touched. There may be abnormalities in emotional expression, giggling or weeping for no apparent reason, and little or no emotional reaction when one would be expected. Similar abnormal responses may be shown in relation to fear; an absence of fear in response to real danger, but great fearfulness in the presence of harmless objects.

In adolescence or adulthood, people with Autistic Disorder who have the capacity for insight may become depressed when they realize how seriously impaired they are.

Autistic Disorder sometimes follows medical and obstetrical problems, such as encephalitis, anoxia (absence of oxygen) during birth, and maternal rubella during pregnancy.

The disorder is not caused by inappropriate parenting.

Some new, intensive, multi-dimensional treatments are quite promising, but few people have access to them at this time.

PREVALENCE

By definition, Autistic Director is present before age three. There are two to five cases of the disorder per 10,000 births. Rates of autism are four to five times greater among males than females. Females with Autistic Disorder are more likely to be severely retarded than are males with Autistic Disorder. Follow-up studies suggest that only a small percentage of people with Autistic Disorder live independent adult lives. Even the highest functioning adults continue to have problems in social interaction and communication, together with greatly restricted interests and activities. The siblings of people with the disorder are at increased risk.

TREATMENT OPTIONS

It is difficult or unusual to be able to eradicate all the symptoms of Autistic Disorder, but there are many intervention and education programs which help to improve functioning. It is extremely important, however, that a proper assessment and diagnosis be made. Since the disturbance in behavior is so wide ranging, this can require an array of professional skills - psychological, langugage development, neuropsychological, and medical. Such a multiple assessment establishes the presence of other disorders, the level of intellectual functioning, together with individual strengths and weaknesses, and the child's capacity for social and personal self-sufficiency. Since the symptoms of Autistic Disorder vary widely from individual to individual, a proper assessment becomes the foundation for designing and planning an individually tailored intervention program.

The autistic person may benefit from a combination of educational and behavioral interventions, which may reduce many of the behavioral disturbances, and improve the quality of life for the person and his or her family. In some cases, medication may also be prescribed. The diagnosis of Autistic Disorder can be a shattering experience for any family. The outcome of the diagnosis is open-ended and uncertain and includes a lifetime of care. Every member of the family is affected and it is vital to work with and support them.

Associations & Agencies

419 ARRISE
205 W Wacker
Suite 701
Chicago, IL 60606   847-451-2740

Provides information about autism.

420 Asperger Syndrome Education Network (ASPEN)
9 Aspen Circle
Edison, NJ 08820   732-321-0880
E-mail: LoriSue59@aol.com
www.aspennj.org

Regionally based nonprofit organization headquarted in New Jersey, with 12 local chapters, providing families and those individuals affected with Asperger Syndrome, PDD-NOS, High Function Autism and related disorders. Provides education about the issues surrounding Asperger Syndrome and other related disorders. Support in knowing that they are not alone and in helping individuals with AS achieve their maximum potential. Advocacy in areas of appropriate educational programs and placement, medical research funding and increased public awareness and understanding.

421 Autism Network International
PO Box 35448
Syracuse, NY 13235-5448
E-mail: ani@calcentral.com
www.ani.ac

Jim Sinclair, Coordinator

This organization is run by and for the autistic people. The best advocates for autistic people are autistic people themselves. Provides a forum for autistic people to share information, peer support, tips for coping and problem solving, as well as providing a social outlet for autistic people to explore and participate in autistic social experiences. In addition to promoting self advocacy for high functioning autistic adults, ANI also works to improve the lives of autistic people who, whether they are too young or because they do not have the communication skills, are not able to advocate for themselves. Helps autistic people by providing information and referrals for parenting and teachers. Also strives to educate the public about autism.

422 Autism Research Foundation
c/o Moss-Rosene Lab, W701
715 Albany Street
Boston, MA 02118   617-414-7012
Fax: 617-414-7207
E-mail: tarf@ladders.org
www.ladders.org

Anne Booker, Project Manager/Coordinator

A nonprofit, tax-exempt organization dedicated to researching the neurological underpinnings of autism and other related developmental brain disorders. Seeking to rapidly expand and accelerate research into the pervasive developmental disorders. To do this, time and effort goes into investigating the neuropathology of autism in their laboratories, collecting and redistributing brain tissue to promising research groups for use by projects approved by the Tissue Resource Committee, studies frozen autistic brain tissue collected by TARF. They believe that only aggressive scientific and medical research will reveal the cure for this lifelong disorder.

423 Autism Research Institute
4182 Adams Avenue
San Diego, CA 92116-2536   619-281-7165
Fax: 619-563-6840
www.autismresearchinstitute.com
Dr. Bernard Rimland, Director/Editor

A nonprofit organization which was established in 1967. ARI is primarily devoted to conducting research on the causes of autism and on methods of preventing, diagnosing and treating autism and other severe behavioral disorders of childhood. We provide information based on research to parents and professionals throughout the world. Relies primarily on the generosity of donors for its support. Publishes a quarterly newsletter called the Autism Research Review International, that covers various issues in autism, including Asperger's.

4 per year ISBN 0-893847-4 -

424 Autism Services Center
929 4th Avenue
PO Box 507
Huntington, WV 25710-0507   304-525-8014
Fax: 304-525-8026
www.autismservicescenter.org
Ruth C Sullivan PhD, Executive Director

Service agency for individuals with autism and other developmental disabilities and their families. Makes available technical assistance in designing programs. Provides supervised apartments, group homes, respite services, independent living programs and job-coached employment. Provides case management services for a four-county area in West Virginia. Publishes bi-annual newsletter and offers video cassettes for sale.

425 Autism Society of America
7910 Woodmont Avenue
Suite 300
Bethesda, MD 20814-3067   301-657-0881
Fax: 301-657-0869
www.autism-society.org

Promotes lifelong access and opportunities for persons within the autism spectrum and their families, to be fully included, participating members of their communities through advocacy, public awareness, education and research related to autism.

426 Autistic Services

4444 Bryant Stratton Way
Williamsville, NY 14221   716-631-5777
888-288-4764
Fax: 716-631-9234
www.autisticservices.com

Agency exclusively dedicated to serving the unique lifelong needs of autistic individuals. Also a regional resource for parents, school districts, physicians and other professionals.

427 Center for Family Support (CFS)

333 7th Avenue
New York, NY 10001-5004   212-629-7939
Fax: 212-239-2211
www.cfsny.org

Steven Vernickofs, Executive Director

Service agency devoted to the physical well-being and development of the retarded child and the sound mental health of the parents. Helps families with retarded children with all aspects of home care including counseling, referrals, home aide service and consultation. Offers intervention for parents at the birth of a retarded child with in-home support, guidance and infant stimulation. Pioneered training of nonprofessional women as home aides to provide supportive services in homes.

428 Center for Mental Health Services Knowledge Exchange Network

US Department of Health and Human Services
PO Box 42490
Washington, DC 20015-4800
800-789-2647
Fax: 301-984-8796
E-mail: ken@mentalhealth.org
www.mentalhealth.org

Information about resources, technical assistance, research, training, networks, and other federal clearing houses, and fact sheets and materials. Information specialists refer callers to mental health resources in their communities as well as state, federal and non-profit contacts. Staff available Monday through Friday, 8:30 AM - 5:00 PM, EST, excluding federal holidays. After hours, callers may leave messages and an information specialist will return their call.

429 Center for the Study of Autism (CSA)

PO Box 4538
Salem, OR 97302

www.autism.org

Located in the Salem/Portland, Oregon area. Provides information about autism to parents and professionals, and conducts research on the efficacy of various therapeutic interventions. Much of our research is in collaboration with the Autism Research Institute in San Diego, California.

430 Community Services for Autistic Adults and Children

751 Twinbrook Parkway
Rockville, MD 20851-1400   301-762-1650
Fax: 301-762-5230
TTY: 800-735-2258
E-mail: csaac@csaac.org
www.csaac.org

431 Families for Early Autism Treatment

PO Box 255722
Sacramento, CA 95865-5722   916-843-1536
E-mail: feat@feat.org
www.feat.org

Nancy Fellmeth, President
Kathleen Berry, VP
Gordon Hall, Treasurer
Meg Lambert, Secretary

A nonprofit organization of parents and professionals, designed to help families with children who are diagnosed with autism or pervasive developmental disorder. It offers a network of support for families. FEAT has a Lending Library, with information on autism and also offers Support Meetings on the third Wednesday of each month.

432 Indiana Institute on Disability and Community

Indiana University
2853 E Tenth Street
Bloomington, IN 47408-2696   812-855-6508
800-280-7010
Fax: 812-855-9630
TTY: 812-855-9396
E-mail: uap@indiana.edu
www.iidc.indiana.edu

David M Mank PhD, Director
Joel F Fosha, Information/Public Relations

Committed to providing disability-related information and services that touch the entire life span, from birth through older adulthood. Through collaborative efforts with institutions of higher education, state and local governmental agencies, community service providers, persons with disabilities and their families, and advocacy oganizations. Institute facility and staff work to increase community capacity in disability through academic instruction, research, information, dissemination training and technical assistance. The work of the Indiana Institute carried out in our centers addresses early intervention and education, school improvement and inclusion, transition, employment, aging issues, planning and policy studies, autism and disability issues.

433 More Advanced Autistic People

PO Box 524
Crown Point, IN 46308-0524   219-662-1311
Fax: 219-662-0638

434 NADD: Association for Persons with Developmental Disabilities and Mental Health Needs

132 Fair Street
Kingston, NY 12401-4802   845-334-4336
800-331-5362
Fax: 845-331-4569
E-mail: nadd@mhv.net
www.thenadd.org

Dr. Robert Fletcher, Executive Director

Nonprofit organization designed to promote interest of professional and parent development with resources for individuals who have the coexistence of mental illness and mental retardation. Provides conference, educational services and training materials to professionals, parents, concerned citizens and service organizations. Formerly known as the National Association for the Dually Diagnosed.

435 National Alliance for the Mentally Ill

2107 Wilson Boulevard
Suite 300
Arlington, VA 22201-3042   703-524-7600
800-950-6264
Fax: 703-524-9094
TDD: 703-516-7227
E-mail: helpline@nami.org
www.nami.org

Laurie Flynn, Executive Director

Nation's leading self-help organization for all those affected by severe brain disorders. Mission is to bring consumers and families with similar experiences together to share information about services, care providers, and ways to cope with the challenges of schizophrenia, manic depression, and other serious mental illnesses.

436 National Mental Health Consumer's Self-Help Clearinghouse

1211 Chestnut Street
Suite 1207
Philadelphia, PA 19107   215-751-1810
800-553-4539
Fax: 215-735-0275
E-mail: info@mhselfhelp.org
www.mhselfhelp.org

Alex Morrsey, Information/Referral

Funded by the National Institute of Mental Health Community Support Program, the purpose of the Clearinghouse is to encourage the development and growth of consumer self-help groups.

Year Founded: 1992

437 New England Center for Children

33 Turnpike Road
Southborough, MA 01772-2108   508-481-1015
Fax: 508-485-3421
E-mail: info@necc.org
www.necc.org

Serving students between the ages of 3 and 22 diagnosed with autism, learning disabilities, language delays, mental retardation, behavior disorders and related disabilities; educational curriculum encompasses both the teaching of functional life skills and traditional academics; communication skills are taught throughout all activities in the school, residence and community. Tuition and fees are set by the state. Consulting services also available.

438 Schools for Children With Autism Spectrum Disorders: A Directory of Educational Programs in NYC and The Lower Hudson Valley

Resources for Children with Special Needs
116 E 16th Street
Fifth Floor
New York City, NY 10003   212-677-4650
Fax: 212-254-4070
E-mail: info@resourcesnyc.org
www.resourcesnyc.org

Detailed descriptions of more than 300 public and private schools with programs for children with Autism and Autism Spectrum Disorders. In addition, a general introduction on autism, educational approaches, available resources, supplementary services, definitions, and other related services are included. *$20.00*

ISBN 0-967836-53-0

439 Son-Rise Autism Treatment Center of America

2080 S Undermountain Road
Sheffield, MA 01257   413-229-2100
Fax: 413-229-3202
www.son-rise.org

Training center for autism professionals and parents of autistic children. Programs focuses on the design and implementation of home-based/child-centered alternatives. Offers publications and other resource materials to educate parents, sufferers and professionals.

Books

440 A Book: A Collection of Writings from the Advocate

Autism Society of North Carolina Bookstore
505 Oberlin Road
Suite 230
Raleigh, NC 27605-1345   919-743-0204
800-442-2762
Fax: 919-743-0208
www.autismsociety-nc.org

A collection of articles and writings from the Advocate, the national newsletter of the Autism Society of America. *$12.00*

441 Activities for Developing Pre-Skill Concepts in Children with Autism

Autism Society of North Carolina Bookstore
505 Oberlin Road
Suite 230
Raleigh, NC 27605-1345
919-743-0204
800-442-2762
Fax: 919-743-0208
www.autismsociety-nc.org

Chapters include auditory development, concept development, social development and visual-motor integration. *$34.00*

442 Adults with Autism

Cambridge University Press
40 W 20th Street
New York, NY 10011-4221
212-924-3900
Fax: 212-691-3239
E-mail: marketing@cup.org
www.cup.org

$50.00

312 pages Year Founded: 1996 ISBN 0-521456-83-5

443 Are You Alone on Purpose?

Autism Society of North Carolina Bookstore
505 Oberlin Road
Suite 230
Raleigh, NC 27605-1345
919-743-0204
800-442-2762
Fax: 919-743-0208
www.autismsociety-nc.org

This is the story of Alison, the twin sister of an autistic boy, who develops a friendship with a boy who has become paralyzed. Alison's feelings of isolation from her family and brother are discussed as she develops a true friendship. *$14.95*

444 Aspects of Autism: Biological Research

Autism Society of North Carolina Bookstore
505 Oberlin Road
Suite 230
Raleigh, NC 27605-1345
919-743-0204
800-442-2762
Fax: 919-743-0208
www.autismsociety-nc.org

Reviews the evidence for a physical cause of autism and the roles of genetics, magnesium and vitamin B6. *$15.00*

445 Asperger Syndrome

Guilford Publications
72 Spring Street
New York, NY 10012
212-431-9800
800-365-7006
Fax: 212-966-6708
E-mail: info@guilford.com
www.guilford.com

Brings together preeminent scholars and practitioners to offer a definitive statement of what is currently known about Asperger syndrome and to highlight promising leads in research and clinical practice. Sifts through the latest developments in theory and research, discussing key diagnostic and conceptual issues and reviewing what is known about behavioral features and neurobiology. The effects of Asperger syndrome on social development, learning and communication are examined. *$48.00*

484 pages ISBN 1-572305-34-7

446 Asperger Syndrome: A Practical Guide for Teachers

ADD WareHouse
300 NW 70th Avenue
Suite 102
Plantation, FL 33317
954-792-8100
800-233-9273
Fax: 954-792-8545
E-mail: sales@addwarehouse.com
www.addwarehouse.com

A clear and concise guide to effective classroom practice for teachers and support assistants working with children with Asperger Syndrome in school. The authors explain characteristics of children with Asperger Syndrome, discusses methods of assessment and offers practical strategies for effective classroom interventions. *$24.95*

90 pages

447 Asperger's Syndrome: A Guide for Parents and Professionals

ADD WareHouse
300 NW 70th Avenue
Suite 102
Plantation, FL 33317
954-792-8100
800-233-9273
Fax: 954-792-8545
E-mail: sales@addwarehouse.com
www.addwarehouse.com

Providing a description and analysis of the unusual characteristics of Asperger's syndrome, with strategies to reduce those that are most conspicuous or debilitating. This guide brings together the most relevant and useful information on all aspects of the syndrome, from language and social behavior to motor clumsiness. *$18.95*

223 pages

448 Aspergers Syndrome: A Guide for Educators and Parents, Second Edition

Pro-Ed Publications
8700 Shoal Creek Boulevard
Austin, TX 78757-6816
512-451-3246
800-897-3202
Fax: 800-397-7633
E-mail: info@proedinc.com
www.proedinc.com

Packed with the current knowledge of a syndrome only recently applied in this country to individuals with significant social and language peculiarities. Will assist special education professionals and parents in understanding the special needs of children with AS, as well as how to address them in the classroom. For families, it offers helpful planning strategies for post secondary schooling. *$28.00*

130 pages

449 Autism

Autism Society of North Carolina Bookstore
505 Oberlin Road
Suite 230
Raleigh, NC 27605-1345   **919-743-0204**
800-442-2762
Fax: 919-743-0208
www.autismsociety-nc.org

In a question-and-answer format, the authors respond to questions about autism asked by countless parents and family members of children and youths with autism. *$26.00*

450 Autism & Asperger Syndrome

Cambridge University Press
40 W 20th Street
New York, NY 10011-4211   **212-924-3900**
800-872-7423
Fax: 212-691-3239
www.cup.org

Six clinician-researchers present aspects of Asperger Syndrome, one form of autism. Research summaries are enlivened by case studies. *$24.00*

247 pages

451 Autism & Sensing: The Unlost Instinct

Jessica Kingsley Publishers
325 Chestnut Street
Philadelphia, PA 19106   **215-625-8900**
Fax: 215-625-2940
www.jkp.com

Available in paperback. *$26.95*

200 pages Year Founded: 1998 ISBN 1-853026-12-3

452 Autism Bibliography

TASH
29 W Susquehanna Avenue
Suite 210
Baltimore, MD 21204   **410-828-8274**
Fax: 410-828-6706
E-mail: info@tash.org
www.tash.org

Three hundred recent references to publications on autism along with brief abstracts. *$9.00*

453 Autism Handbook: Understanding & Treating Autism & Prevention Development

Oxford University Press
198 Madison Avenue
New York, NY 10016   **212-726-6000**
800-451-7556
Fax: 919-677-1303
www.oup-usa.org

$25.00

320 pages ISBN 0-195076-67-2

454 Autism Spectrum

Autism Society of North Carolina Bookstore
505 Oberlin Road
Suite 230
Raleigh, NC 27605-1345   **919-743-0204**
800-442-2762
Fax: 919-743-0208
www.autismsociety-nc.org

An excellent publication for new parents and professionals. *$28.95*

455 Autism Treatment Guide

Autism Society of North Carolina Bookstore
505 Oberlin Road
Suite 230
Raleigh, NC 27605-1345   **919-743-0204**
800-442-2762
Fax: 919-743-0208
www.autismsociety-nc.org

A comprehensive book covering treatments and methods used to help individuals with autism. *$12.75*

456 Autism and Pervasive Developmental Disorders

Cambridge University Press
40 W 20th Street
New York, NY 10011-4221   **212-924-3900**
Fax: 212-691-3239
E-mail: marketing@cup.org
www.cup.org

Featuring contributions from leading authorities in the clinical and social sciences, this volume reflects recent progress in the understanding of autism and related conditions, and offers an international perspective on the present state of the discipline. Chapters cover current approaches to definition and diagnosis; prevalence and planning for service delivery; cognitive, genetic and neurobiological features and pathophysiological mechanisms. *$75.00*

294 pages Year Founded: 1998 ISBN 0-521553-86-5

457 Autism in Adolescents and Adults

Kluwer Academic/Plenum Publishers
233 Spring Street
New York, NY 10013   **212-620-8000**
Fax: 212-463-0742
www.kluweronline.com

$63.00

456 pages ISBN 0-306410-57-5

458 Autism: Explaining the Enigma

Autism Society of North Carolina Bookstore
505 Oberlin Road
Suite 230
Raleigh, NC 27605-1345   **919-743-0204**
                                     800-442-2762
                                Fax: 919-743-0208
                         www.autismsociety-nc.org

Explains the nature of autism. *$27.95*

459 Autism: From Tragedy to Triumph

Branden Publishing Company
PO Box 812094
Wellesley, MA 02482
                             Fax: 781-790-1056
                  E-mail: branden@branden.com
                              www.branden.com

A new book that deals with the Lovaas method and includes a foreward by Dr. Ivar Lovaas. The book is broken down into two parts, the long road to diagnosis and then treatment. *$12.95*

Year Founded: 1998 ISBN 0-828319-65-0

460 Autism: Identification, Education and Treatment

Autism Society of North Carolina Bookstore
505 Oberlin Road
Suite 230
Raleigh, NC 27605-1345   **919-743-0204**
                                     800-442-2762
                                Fax: 919-743-0208
                         www.autismsociety-nc.org

Chapters include medical treatments, early intervention and communication and development in autism. *$36.00*

461 Autism: Nature, Diagnosis and Treatment

Guilford Publications
72 Spring Street
Department 4E
New York, NY 10012-4019   **212-431-9800**
                                     800-365-7006
                      E-mail: exam@guilford.com
                             www.guilford.com

Foremost experts explore new perspectives on the nature and treatment of autism. Covering theory, research and the development of hypotheses and models, this book provides a balance between depth and breadth by focusing on questions most central to the field. For each question, an expert examines theoretical issues as well as empirical findings to offer new directions and testable hypotheses for future research. *$52.00*

417 pages ISBN 0-898627-24-9

462 Autism: Strategies for Change

Groden Center
86 Mount Hope Avenue
Providence, RI 02906   **401-274-6310**
                                Fax: 401-421-3280
           E-mail: grodencenter@grodencenter.org
                          www.grodencenter.org
Andrea Pingitore, Administrative Assistant

A comprehensive approach to the education and treatment of children with autism and related disorders. Clinicians, parents, and students of autism who are, or want to be advocates for change will find in this book a blueprint, and much detail, on how to bring change about. This applies at the level of program planning and management as well as of clinical or education practice. *$21.95*

463 Autism: an Inside-Out Approach

Jessica Kingsley Publishers
325 Chestnut Street
Philadelphia, PA 19106   **215-625-8900**
                                Fax: 215-625-2940
                                     www.jkp.com
Marisa Kitsock, Marketing Representative

Available in paperback. *$23.95*

336 pages ISBN 1-853023-87-6

464 Autism: an Introduction to Psychological Theory

Harvard University Press
79 Garden Street
Cambridge, MA 02138   **800-405-1619**
                                Fax: 800-406-9145
          E-mail: CONTACT_HUP@harvard.edu
                           www.hup.harvard.edu

$32.00

160 pages Year Founded: 1998 ISBN 0-674053-12-5

465 Autism: the Facts

Oxford University Press
198 Madison Avenue
New York, NY 10016   **212-726-6000**
                                     800-451-7556
                                Fax: 919-677-1303
                                 www.oup-usa.org

$19.95

128 pages ISBN 0-192623-28-1

466 Autistic Adults at Bittersweet Farms

Haworth Press
10 Alice Street
Binghamton, NY 13904-1580   **607-722-5857**
                                     800-429-6784
                                Fax: 607-722-1424
           E-mail: getinfo@haworthpressinc.com
                          www.haworthpress.com

A touching view of an inspirational residential care program for autistic adolescents and adults. *$17.95*

212 pages ISBN 1-560240-57-1

467 Avoiding Unfortunate Situations

Autism Society of North Carolina Bookstore
505 Oberlin Road
Suite 230
Raleigh, NC 27605-1345   919-743-0204
                                800-442-2762
                           Fax: 919-743-0208
                        www.autismsociety-nc.org

A collection of tips and information from and about people with autism and other developmental disabilities. *$5.00*

468 Beyond Gentle Teaching

Autism Society of North Carolina Bookstore
505 Oberlin Road
Suite 230
Raleigh, NC 27605-1345   919-743-0204
                                800-442-2762
                           Fax: 919-743-0208
                        www.autismsociety-nc.org

A nonaversive approach to helping those in need. *$35.00*

469 Biology of the Autistic Syndromes

Autism Society of North Carolina Bookstore
505 Oberlin Road
Suite 230
Raleigh, NC 27605-1345   919-743-0204
                                800-442-2762
                           Fax: 919-743-0208
                        www.autismsociety-nc.org

A revision of the original, classic text in the light of new developments and current knowledge. This book covers the epidemiological, genetic, biochemical, immunological and neuropsychological literature on autism. *$74.95*

470 Children with Autism

Taylor & Francis
325 Chestnut Street
Philadelphia, PA 19106   215-625-8900
                           Fax: 215-625-2940
                        www.taylorandfrancis.com

Hilary Selznick

471 Children with Autism: Parents' Guide

Woodbine House
6510 Bells Mill Road
Bethesda, MD 20817   301-897-3570
                                800-843-7323
                           Fax: 301-897-5838
              E-mail: info@woodbinehouse.com
                        www.woodbinehouse.com

Recommended as the first book parents should read, this completely revised volume offers information and a complete introduction to autism, while easing the family's fears and concerns as they adjust and cope with their child's disorder. *$14.95*

456 pages ISBN 1-890627-04-6

472 Children with Autism: a Developmental Perspective

Harvard University Press
79 Garden Street
Cambridge, MA 02138   800-405-1619
                          Fax: 800-406-9145
          E-mail: CONTACT_HUP@harvard.edu
                          www.hup.harvard.edu

473 Communication Unbound: How Facilitated Communication Is Challenging Views

Baker & Taylor International
2709 Water Ridge Parkway
Charlotte, NC 28217   704-357-3500
                               800-775-1800
                               www.btol.com

Addresses the ways in which we receive persons with autism in our society, our community and our lives. *$18.95*

240 pages

474 Diagnosis and Treatment of Autism

Autism Society of North Carolina Bookstore
505 Oberlin Road
Suite 230
Raleigh, NC 27605-1345   919-743-0204
                                800-442-2762
                           Fax: 919-743-0208
                        www.autismsociety-nc.org

Various chapters written by professionals working with autistic children and adults. *$110.00*

475 Discovering My Autism

Taylor & Francis
325 Chestnut Street
Philadelphia, PA 19106   215-625-8900
                           Fax: 215-625-2940
                        www.taylorandfrancis.com

Hilary Selznick

476 Facilitated Communication and Technology Guide

Autism Society of North Carolina Bookstore
505 Oberlin Road
Suite 230
Raleigh, NC 27605-1345   919-743-0204
                                800-442-2762
                           Fax: 919-743-0208
                        www.autismsociety-nc.org

Chapters include technology and facilitated communication, augmentative and alternative communication, spelling boards, speech synthesizers and software. *$20.00*

477 Fighting for Darla: Challenges for Family Care & Professional Responsibility

Baker & Taylor International
2709 Water Ridge Parkway
Charlotte, NC 28217   704-357-3500
                               800-775-1800
                               www.btol.com

Follows the story of Darla, a pregnant adolescent with autism. *$18.95*

176 pages ISBN 0-807733-56-3

478 Fragile Success - Ten Autistic Children, Childhood to Adulthood

Autism Society of North Carolina Bookstore
505 Oberlin Road
Suite 230
Raleigh, NC 27605-1345
919-743-0204
800-442-2762
Fax: 919-743-0208
www.autismsociety-nc.org

A book about the lives of autistic children, whom the author has followed from their early years at the Elizabeth Ives School in New Haven, CT, through to adulthood. *$24.95*

479 Getting Started with Facilitated Communication

Syracuse University, Facilitated Communication Institute
370 Huntington Hall
Syracuse, NY 13244-2340
315-443-9657
Fax: 315-443-2274
E-mail: fcstaff@sued.syr.edu
www.soeweb.syr.edu/thefci

Describes in detail how to help individuals with autism and/or severe communication difficulties get started with facilitated communication.

480 Handbook of Autism and Pervasive Developmental Disorders

ADD WareHouse
300 NW 70th Avenue
Suite 102
Plantation, FL 33317
954-792-8100
800-233-9273
Fax: 954-792-8545
E-mail: sales@addwarehouse.com
www.addwarehouse.com

A comprehensive view of all information presently available about autism and other pervasive developmental disorders, drawing on findings and clinical experience from a number of related disciplines psychiatry, psychology, neurobiology and pediatrics. *$95.00*

1092 pages

481 Helping People with Autism Manage Their Behavior

Autism Society of North Carolina Bookstore
505 Oberlin Road
Suite 230
Raleigh, NC 27605-1345
919-743-0204
800-442-2762
Fax: 919-743-0208
www.autismsociety-nc.org

Covers the broad topic of helping people with autism manage their behavior. *$7.00*

482 Hidden Child: The Linwood Method for Reaching the Autistic Child

Woodbine House
6510 Bells Mill Road
Bethesda, MD 20817
301-897-3570
800-843-7323
Fax: 301-897-5838
E-mail: info@woodbinehouse.com
www.woodbinehouse.com

Chronicle of the Linwood Children's Center's successful treatment program for autistic children. *$14.95*

286 pages ISBN 0-933149-06-9

483 History of Childhood and Disability

Baker & Taylor International
2709 Water Ridge Parkway
Charlotte, NC 28217
704-357-3500
800-775-1800
www.btol.com

This book presents an interdisciplinary perspective on children considered exceptional and how services have evolved in reponse to their diverse needs. *$36.00*

352 pages

484 How to Teach Autistic & Severely Handicapped Children

Autism Society of North Carolina Bookstore
505 Oberlin Road
Suite 230
Raleigh, NC 27605-1345
919-743-0204
800-442-2762
Fax: 919-743-0208
www.autismsociety-nc.org

Book provides procedures for effectively assessing and teaching autistic and other severely handicapped children. *$9.00*

485 I Don't Want to Be Inside Me Anymore: Messages from an Autistic Mind

Basic Books
387 Park Avenue S
New York, NY 10016
212-340-8100

$22.00

240 pages ISBN 0-465031-72-2

486 I'm Not Autistic on the Typewriter

TASH
29 W Susquehanna Avenue
Suite 210
Baltimore, MD 21204
410-828-8274
Fax: 410-828-6706
E-mail: info@tash.org
www.tash.org

Donna Gilles, President
Nancy Weiss, Executive Director
Jorge Pineda, Treasurer
Barbara Ransom, Secretary

An introduction to the facilitated communication training method. *$25.00*

487 Inner Life of Children with Special Needs

Taylor & Francis
325 Chestnut Street
Philadelphia, PA 19106   215-625-8900
                                Fax: 215-625-2940
                                www.taylorandfrancis.com

488 Joey and Sam

Autism Society of North Carolina Bookstore
505 Oberlin Road
Suite 230
Raleigh, NC 27605-1345   919-743-0204
                                800-442-2762
                                Fax: 919-743-0208
                                www.autismsociety-nc.org

A beautifully illustrated storybook for children, focusing on a family with two sons, one of whom suffers from autism. *$16.95*

489 Keys to Parenting the Child with Autism

Autism Society of North Carolina Bookstore
505 Oberlin Road
Suite 230
Raleigh, NC 27605-1345   919-743-0204
                                800-442-2762
                                Fax: 919-743-0208
                                www.autismsociety-nc.org

This book explains what autism is and how it is diagnosed. *$7.95*

490 Kristy and the Secret of Susan

Autism Society of North Carolina Bookstore
505 Oberlin Road
Suite 230
Raleigh, NC 27605-1345   919-743-0204
                                800-442-2762
                                Fax: 919-743-0208
                                www.autismsociety-nc.org

This book discusses Kristy and her new baby-sitting charge, Susan. Susan can't speak but sings beautifully. Susan is autistic. *$ 3.50*

491 Learning and Cognition in Autism

Kluwer Academic/Plenum Publishers
233 Spring Street
New York, NY 10013   212-620-8000
                                Fax: 212-463-0742
                                www.kluweronline.com

Collection of papers written by experts in the field of autism. Describes the cognitive and educational characteristics of people with autism and explains intervention techniques and strategies. Topics include motivating communication in children with autism and a chapter by a high-functioning woman with autism who discusses special learning problems and unique learning strengths that characterize their development and offers specific suggestions for working with people like herself. *$59.00*

368 pages ISBN 0-306448-71-8

492 Let Community Employment Be the Goal For Individuals with Autism

Autism Society of North Carolina Bookstore
505 Oberlin Road
Suite 230
Raleigh, NC 27605-1345   919-743-0204
                                800-442-2762
                                Fax: 919-743-0208
                                www.autismsociety-nc.org

A guide designed for people who are responsible for preparing individuals with autism to enter the work force. *$7.00*

493 Let Me Hear Your Voice

Autism Society of North Carolina Bookstore
505 Oberlin Road
Suite 230
Raleigh, NC 27605-1345   919-743-0204
                                800-442-2762
                                Fax: 919-743-0208
                                www.autismsociety-nc.org

The Maruice family's second and third children were diagnosed with autism. This book recounts their experience with a home program using behavior therapy. *$13.95*

494 Letting Go

Autism Society of North Carolina Bookstore
505 Oberlin Road
Suite 230
Raleigh, NC 27605-1345   919-743-0204
                                800-442-2762
                                Fax: 919-743-0208
                                www.autismsociety-nc.org

A book of poems about a journey, an emotional road of placing a child in a residential group home for children with autism. *$7.50*

495 Management of Autistic Behavior

Pro-Ed Publications
8700 Shoal Creek Boulevard
Austin, TX 78757-6816   512-451-3246
                                800-897-3202
                                Fax: 800-397-7633
                                E-mail: info@proedinc.com
                                www.proedinc.com

Comprehensive and practical book that tells what works best with specific problems. *$41.00*

450 pages ISBN 0-890791-96-1

496 Mindblindness: An Essay on Autism and Theory of Mind

Autism Society of North Carolina Bookstore
505 Oberlin Road
Suite 230
Raleigh, NC 27605-1345   919-743-0204
                                800-442-2762
                                Fax: 919-743-0208
                                www.autismsociety-nc.org

Interpretations and research into the theory of mindblindness in children with autism. *$19.95*

300 pages ISBN 0-262023-84-9

497 Mixed Blessings

Autism Society of North Carolina Bookstore
505 Oberlin Road
Suite 230
Raleigh, NC 27605-1345   **919-743-0204**
                                    800-442-2762
                            Fax: 919-743-0208
                      www.autismsociety-nc.org

A real-life family discusses the raising of their autistic son. *$19.95*

498 More Laughing and Loving with Autism

Autism Society of North Carolina Bookstore
505 Oberlin Road
Suite 230
Raleigh, NC 27605-1345   **919-743-0204**
                                    800-442-2762
                            Fax: 919-743-0208
                      www.autismsociety-nc.org

A collection of warm and humorous parent stories about raising a child with autism. *$9.95*

499 Neurobiology of Autism

Johns Hopkins University Press
2715 N Charles Street
Baltimore, MD 21218-4363   **410-516-6900**
                                      800-537-5487
                              Fax: 410-516-6968
                    www.press.jhu.edu/index.html

This book discusses recent advances in scientific research that point to a neurobiological basis for autism and examines the clinical implications of this research. *$44.95*

272 pages Year Founded: 1997 ISBN 0-801856-80-9

500 News from the Border: a Mother's Memoir of Her Autistic Son

Houghton Mifflin Company
222 Berkeley Street
Boston, MA 02116   **617-351-5000**
                        www.hmco.com

A searingly honest account of the author's family experiences with autism. Raising an autistic child is the central, ongoing drama of her married life in this riveting account of acceptance and coping. *$22.95*

384 pages

501 Nobody Nowhere

Autism Society of North Carolina Bookstore
505 Oberlin Road
Suite 230
Raleigh, NC 27605-1345   **919-743-0204**
                                    800-442-2762
                            Fax: 919-743-0208
                      www.autismsociety-nc.org

An autobiography giving readers a tour of the author's life with autism. *$14.00*

502 Parent Survival Manual

Autism Society of North Carolina Bookstore
505 Oberlin Road
Suite 230
Raleigh, NC 27605-1345   **919-743-0204**
                                    800-442-2762
                            Fax: 919-743-0208
                      www.autismsociety-nc.org

Compiled from three hundred fifty anecdotes told by parents of autistic and developmentally disabled children. *$38.50*

503 Parent's Guide to Autism

Autism Society of North Carolina Bookstore
505 Oberlin Road
Suite 230
Raleigh, NC 27605-1345   **919-743-0204**
                                    800-442-2762
                            Fax: 919-743-0208
                      www.autismsociety-nc.org

An essential handbook for anyone facing autism. *$14.00*

504 Please Don't Say Hello

Human Sciences Press
233 Spring Street
New York, NY 10013-1522   **212-620-8000**
                            Fax: 212-807-1047

Paul and his family moved into a new neighborhood. Paul's brother was autistic. The children thought that Eddie was retarded until they learned that there were skills that he could do better than they could. *$10.95*

47 pages ISBN 0-898851-99-8

505 Preschool Issues in Autism

Kluwer Academic/Plenum Publishers
233 Spring Street
New York, NY 10013   **212-620-8000**
                        Fax: 212-463-0742
                      www.kluweronline.com

Combines some of the most important theory and data related to the early identifiction and intervention in autism and related disorders. Addresses clinical aspects, parental concerns and legal issues. Helps professionals understand and implement state-of-the-art services for young children and their families. *$54.00*

294 pages ISBN 0-306444-40-2

506 Psychoeducational Profile

Autism Society of North Carolina Bookstore
505 Oberlin Road
Suite 230
Raleigh, NC 27605-1345   **919-743-0204**
                                    800-442-2762
                            Fax: 919-743-0208
                      www.autismsociety-nc.org

The PEP-R is a revision of the popular instrument that has been used for over twenty years to assess skills and behavior of autistic and communication-handicapped children who function between the ages of 6 months and 7 years. *$74.00*

507 Reaching the Autistic Child: a Parent Training Program

Brookline Books/Lumen Editions
PO Box 97
Newton Upper Falls, MA 02464
800-666-2665
Fax: 617-558-8011
www.brooklinebooks.com

Detailed case studies of social and behavioral change in autistic children and their families show parents how to implement the principles for improved socialization and behavior. Revised and updated 1998. *$15.95*

ISBN 1-571290-56-7

508 Record Books for Individuals with Autism

Indiana Institute on Disability and Community
Indiana University
2853 E Tenth Street
Bloomington, IN 47408-2696
812-855-6508
800-280-7010
Fax: 812-855-9630
TTY: 812-855-9396
E-mail: uap@indiana.edu
www.iidc.indiana.edu

This book was developed with parent information about an autistic child so that it is organized, easily accessible and can be copied as needed. *$5.00*

37 pages

509 Russell Is Extra Special

Autism Society of North Carolina Bookstore
505 Oberlin Road
Suite 230
Raleigh, NC 27605-1345
919-743-0204
800-442-2762
Fax: 919-743-0208
www.autismsociety-nc.org

A sensitive portrayal of an autistic boy written by his father. *$8.95*

510 Sex Education: Issues for the Person with Autism

Indiana Institute on Disability and Community
Indiana University
2853 E Tenth Street
Bloomington, IN 47408-2696
812-855-6508
800-280-7010
Fax: 812-855-9630
TTY: 812-855-9396
E-mail: uap@indiana.edu
www.iidc.indiana.edu

Discusses issues of sexuality and provides some methods of instruction for persons with autism. *$3.00*

18 pages

511 Siblings of Children with Autism: A Guide for Families

Autism Society of North Carolina Bookstore
505 Oberlin Road
Suite 230
Raleigh, NC 27605-1345
919-743-0204
800-442-2762
Fax: 919-743-0208
www.autismsociety-nc.org

Offers information on the needs of a child with autism. *$16.95*

512 Somebody Somewhere

Autism Society of North Carolina Bookstore
505 Oberlin Road
Suite 230
Raleigh, NC 27605-1345
919-743-0204
800-442-2762
Fax: 919-743-0208
www.autismsociety-nc.org

Offers a revealing account of the author's battle with autism. *$15.00*

513 Son-Rise: the Miracle Continues

HJ Kramer
PO Box 1082
Tiburon, CA 94920-7002
415-435-5367
Fax: 415-435-5364
E-mail: monique@nwlib.com
www.newworldlibrary.com

Monique Muhlenkamp, Marketing Director/Publicity

This book is written about the astonishing account of Raun Kaufman's development from autistic child into an active, loving little boy. *$12.95*

372 pages ISBN 0-915811-61-8

514 Soon Will Come the Light

Autism Society of North Carolina Bookstore
505 Oberlin Road
Suite 230
Raleigh, NC 27605-1345
919-743-0204
800-442-2762
Fax: 919-743-0208
www.autismsociety-nc.org

Offers new perspectives on the perplexing disability of autism. *$19.95*

515 Teaching Children with Autism: Strategies to Enhance Communication

Autism Society of North Carolina Bookstore
505 Oberlin Road
Suite 230
Raleigh, NC 27605-1345
919-743-0204
800-442-2762
Fax: 919-743-0208
www.autismsociety-nc.org

This valuable new book describes teaching strategies and instructional adaptations which promote communication and socialization in children with autism. *$34.95*

516 Teaching and Mainstreaming Autistic Children

Love Publishing Company
9101 E Kenyon Avenue
Suite 2200
Denver, CO 80237   303-221-7333
                        Fax: 303-221-7444
        E-mail: lpc@lovepublishing.com
              www.lovepublishing.com

Dr Knoblock advocates a highly organized, structured environment for autistic children, with teachers and parents working together. His premise is that the learning and social needs of autistic children must be analyzed and a daily program be designed with interventions that respond to this functional analysis of their behavior. *$39.95*

Year Founded: 1982 ISBN 0-891081-11-9

517 Ultimate Stranger: The Autistic Child

Autism Society of North Carolina Bookstore
505 Oberlin Road
Suite 230
Raleigh, NC 27605-1345   919-743-0204
                              800-442-2762
                        Fax: 919-743-0208
              www.autismsociety-nc.org

Delacato's thesis is that autism is neuro-genic and not psycho-genic in origin. *$10.00*

518 Understanding Autism

Fanlight Productions
4196 Washington Street
Boston, MA 02130   617-469-4999
                              800-937-4113
                        Fax: 617-469-3379
        E-mail: fanlight@fanlight.com
              www.fanlight.com

Parents of children with autism discuss the nature and symptoms of this lifelong disability, and outline a treatment program based on behavior modification principles. *$195.00*

ISBN 1-572951-00-1

519 Understanding Other Minds: Perspectives from Autism

Oxford University Press
198 Madison Avenue
New York, NY 10016   212-726-6000
                              800-451-7556
                        Fax: 919-677-1303
              www.oup-usa.org

$35.00

544 pages ISBN 0-192620-56-8

520 Until Tomorrow: A Family Lives with Autism

Autism Society of North Carolina Bookstore
505 Oberlin Road
Suite 230
Raleigh, NC 27605-1345   919-743-0204
                              800-442-2762
                        Fax: 919-743-0208
              www.autismsociety-nc.org

The central theme of this book is an effort to show what it is like to live with a child who cannot communicate. *$10.00*

521 When Snow Turns to Rain

Woodbine House
6510 Bells Mill Road
Bethesda, MD 20817   301-897-3570
                              800-843-7323
                        Fax: 301-897-5838
        E-mail: info@woodbinehouse.com
              www.woodbinehouse.com

A gripping personal account of one family's experiences with autism. Chronicles a family's journey from parental bliss to devastation, as they learn that their son has autism. This book delves into diagnosis, treatments, and attitudes toward persons with autism. *$14.95*

250 pages ISBN 0-933149-63-8

522 Wild Boy of Aveyron

Autism Society of North Carolina Bookstore
505 Oberlin Road
Suite 230
Raleigh, NC 27605-1345   919-743-0204
                              800-442-2762
                        Fax: 919-743-0208
              www.autismsociety-nc.org

$15.95

523 Winter's Flower

Autism Society of North Carolina Bookstore
505 Oberlin Road
Suite 230
Raleigh, NC 27605-1345   919-743-0204
                              800-442-2762
                        Fax: 919-743-0208
              www.autismsociety-nc.org

The story of Ranae Johnson's quest to rescue her son from a world of silence. A story of love, patience and dedication. *$12.95*

524 Without Reason

Autism Society of North Carolina Bookstore
505 Oberlin Road
Suite 230
Raleigh, NC 27605-1345   919-743-0204
                              800-442-2762
                        Fax: 919-743-0208
              www.autismsociety-nc.org

A story of a family coping with two generations of autism. *$19.95*

Periodicals & Pamphlets

525 Autism Newslink

Autism Society Ontario
1179A King Street W
Suite 004
Toronto, ON   416-246-9592
                          Fax: 416-246-9417
          E-mail: mail@autismsociety.on.ca
                  www.autismsociety.on.ca

Covers society activities and contains information on autism. Recurring features include news of research, a calendar of events, reports of meetings, and book reviews. *$30.00*

10 pages 4 per year

526 Autism Research Review

Autism Research Institute
4182 Adams Avenue
San Diego, CA 92116-2536   619-281-7165
                          Fax: 619-563-6840
          www.autisimresearchinstitute.com

Dr. Bernard Rimland, Director/Editor

Discusses current research and provides information about the causes, diagnosis, and treatment of autism and related disorders.

8 pages 4 per year

527 Autism Society News

Utah Parent Center
2290 E 4500 S
Suite 110
Salt Lake City, UT 84117-4428   801-272-1051
                                      800-468-1160
                          Fax: 801-272-8907
                  www.utahparentcenter.org

Kim Moody, Director

Presents news, research information, and legislative updates regarding autism. Recurring features include a calendar of events and columns titled Parent Meetings, What's On in the News, Research News, Parent Corner, Legislative Summary, and A Big Thank You!

8 pages

528 Autism Spectrum Disorders in Children and Adolescents

Center for Mental Health Services: Knowledge Exchange Network
PO Box 42490
Washington, DC 20015
                                      800-789-2647
                          Fax: 301-984-8796
                          TDD: 866-889-2647
          E-mail: ken@mentalhealth.org
                  www.mentalhealth.org

This fact sheet defines autism, describes the signs and causes, discusses types of help available, and suggests what parents or other caregivers can do.

2 pages Year Founded: 1997

529 Facts About Autism

Indiana Institute on Disability and Community
Indiana University
2853 E Tenth Street
Bloomington, IN 47408-2696   812-855-6508
                                      800-280-7010
                          Fax: 812-855-9630
                          TTY: 812-855-9396
          E-mail: uap@indiana.edu
                  www.iidc.indiana.edu

Marci Wheeler
Suzie Rimstidt
Susan Gray
Valerie DePalma

Provides concise information describing autism, diagnosis, needs of the person with autism from diagnosis through adulthood. Information on the Autism Society of America chapters in Indiana are listed in the back, along with a description of the Indiana Resource Center for Autism and suggested books to look for in the local library. Also available in Spanish. *$1.00*

17 pages

530 Journal of Autism and Developmental Disorders

Kluwer Academic/Plenum Publishers
233 Spring Street
New York, NY 10013   212-620-8000
                          Fax: 212-463-0742
                  www.kluweronline.com

$98.00

6 per year   ISSN 0162-3257

531 Learning Together

Indiana Institute on Disability and Community
Indiana University
2853 E Tenth Street
Bloomington, IN 47408-2696   812-855-6508
                                      800-280-7010
                          Fax: 812-855-9630
                          TTY: 812-855-9396
          E-mail: uap@indiana.edu
                  www.iidc.indiana.edu

Introduces preschool and early elementary school children to a classmate who has autism. Also available in Spanish and Korean. *$2.00*

27 pages

532 Learning to be Independent and Responsible

Indiana Institute on Disability and Community
Indiana University
2853 E Tenth Street
Bloomington, IN 47408-2696   812-855-6508
                                      800-280-7010
                          Fax: 812-855-9630
                          TTY: 812-855-9396
          E-mail: uap@indiana.edu
                  www.iidc.indiana.edu

People with autism build trust in people and environments through successful interactions. Individualized, supportive programs utilizing positive instructional and environmental supports that lead to increased opportunities, choice and motivation are described in this booklet. *$3.00*

11 pages

533 MAAP

MAAP Services
PO Box 524
Crown Point, IN 46307   219-662-1311
                                Fax: 219-662-0638
                        E-mail: chart@netnitco.net
                           www.maapservices.org

This quarterly newsletter provides the opportunity for parents and professionals to network with families of more advanced individuals with Autism, Asperger's syndrome, and Pervasive developmental disorder. Helps you to learn about more advanced individuals within the autism spectrum.

534 Sex Education: Issues for the Person with Autism

Autism Society of North Carolina Bookstore
505 Oberlin Road
Suite 230
Raleigh, NC 27605-1345   919-743-0204
                                800-442-2762
                          Fax: 919-743-0208
                        www.autismsociety-nc.org

Discusses issues of sexuality and provides methods of instruction for people with autism. *$4.00*

535 Treatment of Children with Mental Disorders

National Institute of Mental Health
6001 Executive Boulevard
Room 8184
Bethesda, MD 20892-9663
                                866-615-6464
                          Fax: 301-443-4279
                          TTY: 301-443-8431
                     E-mail: nimhinfo@nih.gov
                           www.nimh.nih.gov

Ruth Dubois, Assistant Chief

A short booklet that contains questions and answers about therapy for children with mental disorders. Includes a chart of mental disorders and medications used.

Research Centers

536 Facilitated Learning at Syracuse University

Syracuse University, Facilitated Communication Institute
370 Huntington Hall
Syracuse, NY 13244-2340   315-443-9657
                          Fax: 315-443-2274
                     E-mail: fcstaff@sued.syr.edu
                        www.soeweb.syr.edu/thefci

College offering facilitated learning research into communication with persons who have autism or severe disabilities. Offers books, videos and public awareness on research projects.

537 TEACCH

CB#7180, 100 Renee Lynne Court
University of NC at Chapel Hill
Chapel Hill, NC 27599-7180   919-966-2174
                                Fax: 919-966-4127
                                 www.teacch.com

This organization is the division for the treatment and education of autistic and related communication handicapped children.

Support Groups & Hot Lines

538 Autism Services Center

929 4th Avenue
PO Box 507
Huntington, WV 25710-0507   304-525-8014
                                Fax: 304-525-8026
                        www.autismservicescenter.org

Ruth Sullivan PhD, Executive Director

ASC is a nonprofit, licensed bahavioral health center providing services to individuals with developmental disabilities in a four-county area in West Virginia. We also have an outside hotline (9-5) (M-F), which provides information to parents and other individuals.

539 Autism Society of America

7910 Woodmont Avenue
Suite 300
Bethesda, MD 20814-3067   301-657-0881
                                800-328-8476
                          Fax: 301-657-0869
                   E-mail: info@autism-society.org
                         www.autism-society.org

The mission of the Autism Society of America is to promote lifelong access and opportunities for persons within the autism spectrum and their families, to be fully included, participating members of their communities through advocacy, public awareness, education, and research related to autism.

540 Autism Treatment Center of America Sun-Rise Program

2080 S Undermountain Road
Sheffield, MA 01257   413-229-2100
                          Fax: 413-229-3202
                            www.son-rise.org

Teaches parents and professionals caring for children and adults challenged by Autism how to design and implement home-based/child-centered programs.

Video & Audio

541 Autism: A Strange, Silent World

Filmakers Library
124 E 40th Street
New York, NY 10016   212-808-4980
                          Fax: 212-808-4983
                  E-mail: info@filmakers.com
                            www.filmakers.com

Sue Oscar, Co-President

British educators and medical personnel offer insight into autism's characteristics and treatment approaches through the cameos of three children.

542 Autism: Being Friends

Indiana Institute on Disability and Community
Indiana University
2853 E Tenth Street
Bloomington, IN 47408-2696   812-855-6508
                              800-280-7010
                         Fax: 812-855-9630
                         TTY: 812-855-9396
                  E-mail: uap@indiana.edu
                          www.iidc.indiana.edu

This autism awareness videotape was produced specifically for use with young children. The program portrays the abilities of the child with autism and describes ways in which peers can help the child to be a part of the everyday world. *$10.00*

Year Founded: 1991

543 Autism: Learning to Live

Indiana Institute on Disability and Community
Indiana University
2853 E Tenth Street
Bloomington, IN 47408-2696   812-855-6508
                              800-280-7010
                         Fax: 812-855-9630
                         TTY: 812-855-9396
                  E-mail: uap@indiana.edu
                          www.iidc.indiana.edu

Filmed throughout the state of Indiana, this public television documentary focuses on children and young adults with autism as they learn in community settings. Sites vary from a family home, to a bakery, to a classroom. Teachers, friends, a principal, a speech clinician, a job coach, and parents talk about the ways they have helped specific individuals with autism learn, and about what they have learned from these individuals. *$30.00*

Year Founded: 1990

544 Autism: a World Apart

Fanlight Productions
4196 Washington Street
Suite 2
Boston, MA 01231   617-469-4999
                              800-937-4113
                         Fax: 617-469-3379
                  E-mail: fanlight@fanlight.com
                            www.fanlight.com

Kelli English, Publicity Coordinator

In this documentary, three families show us what the textbooks and studies cannot; what it's like to live with autism day after day, raise and love children who may be withdrawn and violent and unable to make personal connections with their families. #039. Video cassette. *$195.00*

ISBN 1-572950-39-0

545 Breakthroughs: How to Reach Students with Autism

ADD WareHouse
300 NW 70th Avenue
Suite 102
Plantation, FL 33317   954-792-8100
                              800-233-9273
                         Fax: 954-792-8545
                  E-mail: sales@addwarehouse.com
                            www.addwarehouse.com

Karen Sewell

This video is designed for instructors of children with autism, K-12. The program provides a fully-loaded teacher's manual with reproducible lesson plans that will take you through an entire school year as well as an award-winning video that demonstrates the instrudtional and behavioral techniques recommended in the manual. Covers math, reading, fine motor, self-help, vocational, social and life skills. Features a veteran instructor who was named 'Teacher of the Year' by the Autism Society of America. Book - 243 pages. Video - 25 minutes. *$99.00*

546 Going to School with Facilitated Communication

Syracuse University, Facilitated Communication Institute
370 Huntington Hall
Syracuse, NY 13244-2340   315-443-9657
                         Fax: 315-443-2274
                  E-mail: fcstaff@sued.syr.edu
                            www.soeweb.syr.edu/thefci

A video in which students with autism and/or severe disabilities illustrate the use of facilitated communication focusing on basic principles fostering facilitated communication.

547 Health Care Desensitization

Indiana Institute on Disability and Community
Indiana University
2853 E Tenth Street
Bloomington, IN 47408-2696   812-855-6508
                              800-280-7010
                         Fax: 812-855-9630
                         TTY: 812-855-9396
                  E-mail: uap@indiana.edu
                          www.iidc.indiana.edu

Mark Robinson, Producer/Editor

Training videotape for teachers, parents, health professionals and group home staff showing how the desensitization procedure to medical, dental and optometric exams was applied to preschool and adolescent students with autism and thier successful cooperation with the subsequent health care. *$25.00*

Year Founded: 1989

548 I'm Not Autistic on the Typewriter

Syracuse University, Facilitated Communication Institute
370 Huntington Hall
Syracuse, NY 13244-2340   315-443-9657
                                     Fax: 315-443-2274
                         E-mail: fcstaff@sued.syr.edu
                         www.soeweb.syr.edu/thefci

A video introducing facilitated communication, a method by which persons with autism express themselves.

549 Introduction to Autism

Indiana Institute on Disability and Community
Indiana University
2853 E Tenth Street
Bloomington, IN 47408-2696   812-855-6508
                                        800-280-7010
                                   Fax: 812-855-9630
                                   TTY: 812-855-9396
                           E-mail: uap@indiana.edu
                           www.iidc.indiana.edu

Bill Scroggie
Chris Lewis

Training tape covers key points from the Introduction to Autism: Self - Instructional Module. It contains portions of the Autism series, but narrates specifically to provide a clear, accurate introduction to the disability. *$25.00*

Year Founded: 1991

550 Managing Behaviors in Community Settings

Indiana Institute on Disability and Community
Indiana University
2853 E Tenth Street
Bloomington, IN 47408-2696   812-855-6508
                                        800-280-7010
                                   Fax: 812-855-9630
                                   TTY: 812-855-9396
                           E-mail: uap@indiana.edu
                           www.iidc.indiana.edu

Nancy Dalrymple
Misha Angrist

This training videotape is for teachers, parents, paraprofessionals, group homes, and recreational staff. Takes the viewer through the development of a philosophy, searching for the purpose of behaviors, environmental plans, and reactive plans. Students with autism are the stars as they are involved in community life, from trips to the dentist and work at Holiday Inn to the ski slopes and lakes. *$25.00*

Year Founded: 1988

551 Program Development Associates

Perry Como
PO Box 2038
Syracuse, NY 13220-2038   315-452-0643
                                     800-543-2119
                                Fax: 315-452-0710
                        E-mail: pda@pdassoc.com
                        www.disabilitytraining.com

Perry Como, President

Distributor of video, CD-ROM and book resources for professionals in the disability field.

552 Sense of Belonging: Including Students with Autism in Their School Community

Indiana Institute on Disability and Community
Indiana University
2853 E Tenth Street
Bloomington, IN 47408-2696   812-855-6508
                                        800-280-7010
                                   Fax: 812-855-9630
                                   TTY: 812-855-9396
                           E-mail: uap@indiana.edu
                           www.iidc.indiana.edu

Kim Davis
Cathy Pratt

Highlights the efforts of two elementary and one middle school students with autism in general education settings. Illustrates the value of inclusion and importance it plays for the future of all students. Practical strategies for teaching students with autism are described. *$40.00*

Year Founded: 1997

553 Straight Talk About Autism

ADD WareHouse
300 NW 70th Avenue
Suite 102
Plantation, FL 33317   954-792-8100
                                  800-233-9273
                             Fax: 954-792-8545
                    E-mail: sales@addwarehouse.com
                    www.addwarehouse.com

These revealing videos contain intimate interviews with parents of kids with autism and the young people themselves. Topics discussed include friends and social isolation, communication difficulties, hypersensitivities, teasing, splinter skills, parent support groups and more. One video focuses on childhood issues, while the second covers adolescent issues. Two 40 minute videos. *$129.00*

554 Understanding and Treating the Hereditary Psychiatric Spectrum Disorders

Hope Press
PO Box 188
Duarte, CA 91009-0188   818-303-0644
                                   800-321-4039
                              Fax: 818-358-3520
                              www.hopepress.com

David E Comings MD, Presenter

Learn with ten hours of audio tapes from a two day seminar given in May 1997 by David E Comings, MD. Tapes cover: ADHD, Tourette Syndrome, Obsessive-Compulsive Disorder, Conduct Disorder, Oppositional Defiant Disorder, Autism, and other Hereditary Psychiatric Spectrum Disorders. Eight audio tapes. *$75.00*

Year Founded: 1997

Web Sites

555   www.aane.autistics.org

Asperger's Association of New England

Working advocacy group of Massachusetts parents of adults and teens with AS who have come together with the goal of getting state funding for residential supports for adults with AS. At the present time no state agency will provide these needed supports. Interested parents and AS adults are welcome to join this working group.

556   www.ani.ac

Autism Network International

This organization is run by and for the autistic people. The best advocates for autistic people are autistic people themselves. Provides a forum for autistic people to share information, peer support, tips for coping and problem solving, as well as providing a social outlet for autistic people to explore and participate in autistic social experiances. In addition to promoting self advocacy for high-functioning autistic adults, ANI also works to improve the lives of autistic people who, whether they are too young or because they do not have the communication skills, are not able to advocate for themselves. Helps autistic people by providing information and referrals for parenting and teachers. Also strives to educate the public about autism.

557   www.aspennj.org

Asperger Syndrome Education Network (ASPEN)

Regionally-based non-profit organization headquartered in New Jersey, with 11 local chapters, providing families and thouse individuals affected with Asperger Syndrome, PDD-NOS, High Function Autism, and related disorders. Provides education about the issues surrounding Asperger Syndrome and other related disorders. Support in knowing that they are not alone and in helping individuals with AS achieve their maximum potential. Advocacy in areas of appropriate educational programs and placement, medical research funding, and increased public awareness and understanding.

558   www.autism-society.org

Promotes lifelong access and opportunities for persons within the autism spectrum and their families, to be fully included, participating members of their communities through advocacy, public awareness, education and research related to autism.

559   www.autism.org

Center for the Study of Autism (CSA)

Located in the Salem/Portland, Oregon area. Provides information about autism to parents and professionals, and conducts research on the efficacy of various therapeutic interventions. Much of our research is in collaboration with the Autism Research Institute in San Diego, California.

560   www.cyberpsych.org

CyberPsych

Hosts the American Psychoanalyists Foundation, American Association of Suicideology, Society for the Exploration of Psychotherapy Intergration, and Anxiety Disorders Association of America. Also subcategories of the anxiety disorders, as well as general information, including panic disorder, phobias, obsessive compulsive disorder (OCD), social phobia, generalized anxiety disorder, post traumatic stress disorder, and phobias of childhood. Book reviews and links to web pages sharing the topics.

561   www.feat.org

Families for Early Autism Treatment

A nonprofit organization of parents and professionals, designed to help families with children who are diagnosised with autism or pervasive developmental disorder. It offers a network of support for families. FEAT has a Lending Library, with information on autism and also offers Support Meetings on the third Wednesday of each month.

562   www.ladders.org

The Autism Research Foundation

A nonprofit, tax-exempt organization dedicated to researching the neurological underpinnings of autism and other related developmental brain disorders. Seeking to rapidly expand and accelerate research into the pervasive developmental disorders. To do this, time and efforts goes into investigating the neuropathology of autism in their laboratories, collecting and redistributing brain tissue to promising research groups for use by projects approved by the Tissue Resource Committee, studies frozen autistic brain tissue collected by TARF. They believe that only aggressive scientific and medical research will reveal the cure for this lifelong disorder.

563   www.naar.org

National Alliance for Autism Research (NAAR)

National nonprofit, tax-exempt organization dedicated to finding the causes, preventions, effective treatments and, ultimately, a cure for the autism spectrum disorders. NAAR's mission is to fund, promote and support biomedical research into autism. Aims to have an aggressive and far-reaching research program. Seeks to encourage scientists outside the field of autism to apply their insights and experience to autism. Publishes a newsletter that focuses on developments in autism research. Supports brain banks and tissue consortium development.

564   **www.planetpsych.com**

Planetpsych.com

Learn about disorders, their treatments and other topics in psychology. Articles are listed under the related
topic areas. Ask a therapist a question for free, or view
the directory of professionals in your area. If you are a
therapist sign up for the directory. Current features,
self-help, interactive, and newsletter archives.

Introduction

Bipolar Disorder (Manic Depression) is the name for a group of severe mental illnesses characterized by alterations between extreme depression and manic euphoria or irritability.

The two states are not independent of each other, but part of the same illness. Individuals in the manic phase of Bipolar Disorder may feel exuberant, invincible, or even immortal. They may be awake for days at a time, and be able to work tirelessly; they may rush from one idea to the next carried by a nearly uncontrollable burst of energy that leaves others bewildered and unable to keep up. (Some extraordinarily creative people, Vincent Van Gogh, for example, have had Bipolar Disorder.)

In the depressed phase which follows a manic high, the patient may be nearly suicidal. The depressed phase of the illness mirrors a major depressive episode. There are three forms of Bipolar Disorders: Bipolar I Disorder, Bipolar II Disorder, and Cyclothymic Disorder.

A number of researchers are closing in on genetic links to the illness. Like all mental disorders, however, the relationship between genetic, physiologic, psychological, and environmental causes is complex. While medication (especially Lithium) is quite effective, patients with Bipolar Disorder often need psychotherapy as well, in order to address issues like compliance with medication, noting early signs of relapse and environmental life stressors.

SYMPTOMS

A **manic episode** consists of the following:

•A distinct period of abnormally and persistently elevated, expansive, or irritable mood, lasting at least one week;
•Inflated self-esteem or grandiosity; decreased need for sleep;

•More talkative than usual;
•Flight of ideas or a subjective experience that thoughts are racing;
•Distractibility;
•Increase in goal-directed activity;
•Excessive involvement in activities that have a high potential for painful consequences;
•The mood disturbances are severe enough to cause impairment in social or occupational functioning;
•The symptoms are not due to the direct physiological effects of a substance.

The **depressive phase** of Bipolar Disorder consists of the following:

•Depressed mood most of the day, nearly every day, as indicated by either subjective report or observation;
•Markedly diminished interest or pleasure in almost all activities most of the day;
•Significant weight loss when not dieting, or weight gain, or decrease or increase in appetite nearly every day;
•Insomnia or hypersomnia nearly every night;
•Psychomotor agitation or retardation nearly every day;
•Fatigue or loss of energy nearly every day;
•Feelings of worthlessness or excessive or inappropriate guilt nearly every day.

ASSOCIATED FEATURES

Bipolar Disorder is a severe mental illness that can cause extreme distruption to individual lives and careers, and to whole families. Suicide is a risk factor in the illness, and an estimated ten percent to fifteen percent of individuals with Bipolar I Disorder complete a suicide attempt. Abuse of children, spouses or other family members, or other types of violence, may occur during the manic phase of the illness.

It is important for patients with depression to be carefully screened for any manic or hypomanic symptoms so that Bipolar Disorder can be diagnosed and the appropriate treatment prescribed. The cycles of mood changes tend to become more frequent, shorter, and more intense as the patient gets older.

Disturbances in work, school or social functioning are common, resulting in frequent school truancy or failure, occupational failure, divorce, or episodic antisocial behavior. A variety of other mental disorders may accompany Bipolar Disorder; these include Anorexia Nervosa, Bulimia Nervosa, Attention Deficit/Hyperactivity Disorder, Panic Disorder, Social Phobia, Substance-Abuse Related Disorder.

PREVALENCE

The prevalence of Bipolar I Disorder varies from 0.4 percent to 0.6 percent in the community. Community prevalence of Bipolar II Disorder is approximately 0.5 percent. The prevalence of Cyclothymic Disorder is estimated at 0.4 percent to one percent, and from three percent to five percent in clinics specializing in mood disorders.

TREATMENT OPTIONS

Lithium is the most commonly prescribed drug for Bipolar Disorder and is effective for stabilizing patients in the manic phase of the illness and preventing mood swings. However, compliance is a problem among patients both because of the nature of the condition (some patients may actually miss the high of their mood swings) and because of the side effects associated with the drug. These include weight gain, excessive thirst, tremors and muscle weakness. Lithium is also very toxic in overdose. The distruptive nature of the condition also necessitates the use of psychotherapy and family therapy to help patients rebuild relationships, to maintain compliance with treatment and a positive attitude toward living with chronic illness, and to restore confidence and self-esteem.

Anticonvulsants/mood stabilizers have also become first-line treatments, such as Valproate, Carbamazepine, Lamotrigine, Gabapentin, and Topiramate.

Education of the family is crucial for successful treatment, as is education of patients about the disorder and treatment.

Associations & Agencies

566 Bipolar Disorders Treatment Information Center

Madison Institute of Medicine
7617 Mineral Point Road
Suite 300
Madison, WI 53717-1623   608-827-2470
Fax: 608-827-2479
E-mail: mim@miminc.org
www.miminc.org

Provides information on mood stabilizers other than lithium for bipolar disorder. With more than 4,000 references on file, the Center collects and disseminates information about all medications and other forms of treatment of bipolar disorder, including divalproex sodium (valproate), carbamazepine, lamotrigine, gabapentin and topiramate.

567 Career Assessment & Planning Services

Goodwill Industries-Suncoast
10596 Gandy Boulevard
PO Box 14456
St. Petersburg, FL 33702   727-523-1512
888-279-1988
Fax: 727-563-9300
www.goodwill-suncoast.org

R Lee Waits, President/CEO
Chris Ward, Marketing Media Manager

Provides a comprehensive assessment, which can predict current and future employment and potential adjustment factors for physically, emotionally, or developmentally disabled persons who may be unemployed or underemployed. Assessments evaluate interests, aptitudes, academic achievements, and physical abilities (including dexterity and coordination) through coordinated testing, interviewing and behavioral observations.

568 Center for Family Support (CFS)

333 7th Avenue
New York, NY 10001-5004   212-629-7939
Fax: 212-239-2211
www.cfsny.org

Steven Vernickofs, Executive Director

Service agency devoted to the physical well-being and development of the retarded child and the sound mental health of the parents. Helps families with retarded children with all aspects of home care including counseling, referrals, home aide service and consultation. Offers intervention for parents at the birth of a retarded child with in-home support, guidance and infant stimulation. Pioneered training of nonprofessional women as home aides to provide supportive services in homes.

569 Center for Mental Health Services Knowledge Exchange Network

US Department of Health and Human Services
PO Box 42490
Washington, DC 20015-4800
800-789-2647
Fax: 301-984-8796
E-mail: ken@mentalhealth.org
www.mentalhealth.org

Information about resources, technical assistance, research, training, networks, and other federal clearing houses, and fact sheets and materials. Information specialists refer callers to mental health resources in their communities as well as state, federal and nonprofit contacts. Staff available Monday through Friday, 8:30 AM - 5:00 PM, EST, excluding federal holidays. After hours, callers may leave messages and an information specialist will return their call.

570 Depression & BiPolar Support Alliance

730 N Franklin Street
Suite 501
Chicago, IL 60610-7204   312-642-0049
800-826-3632
Fax: 312-642-7243
www.ndmda.org

Lydia Lewis, President
Laura Hoofnagle, Publications

Educates patients, families, professionals, and the public concerning the nature of depressive and manic-depressive illnesses as treatable medical diseases, fosters self-help for patients and families, eliminates discrimination and stigma, improves access to care, advocates for research toward the elimination of these illnesses.

571 Lithium Information Center

Madison Institute of Medicine
7617 Mineral Point Road
Suite 300
Madison, WI 53717-1623   608-827-2470
Fax: 608-827-2479
E-mail: mim@miminc.org
www.miminc.org

A resource for information on lithium treatment of bipolar disorders and on the other medical and biological applications of lithium. The Center currently has more than 32,000 references on file.

572 NADD: Association for Persons with Developmental Disabilities and Mental Health Needs

132 Fair Street
Kingston, NY 12401-4802   845-334-4336
800-331-5362
Fax: 845-331-4569
E-mail: nadd@mhv.net
www.thenadd.org

Dr. Robert Fletcher, Executive Director

Nonprofit organization designed to promote interest of professional and parent development with resources for individuals who have the coexistence of mental illness and mental retardation. Provides conference, educational services and training materials to professionals, parents, concerned citizens and service organizations. Formerly known as the National Association for the Dually Diagnosed.

573 National Alliance for the Mentally Ill

2107 Wilson Boulevard
Suite 300
Arlington, VA 22201-3042   703-524-7600
                             800-950-6264
                        Fax: 703-524-9094
                        TDD: 703-516-7227
               E-mail: helpline@nami.org
                            www.nami.org

Laurie Flynn, Executive Director

Nation's leading self-help organization for all those affected by severe brain disorders. Mission is to bring consumers and families with similar experiences together to share information about services, care providers, and ways to cope with the challenges of schizophrenia, manic depression, and other serious mental illnesses.

574 National Mental Health Consumer's Self-Help Clearinghouse

1211 Chestnut Street
Suite 1207
Philadelphia, PA 19107   215-751-1810
                             800-553-4539
                        Fax: 215-735-0275
            E-mail: info@mhselfhelp.org
                       www.mhselfhelp.org

Alex Morrsey, Information/Referral

Funded by the National Institute of Mental Health Community Support Program, the purpose of the Clearinghouse is to encourage the development and growth of consumer self-help groups.

Year Founded: 1992

575 Suncoast Residential Training Center/Developmental Services Program

Goodwill Industries-Suncoast
10596 Gandy Boulevard
PO Box 14456
St. Petersburg, FL 33702   727-523-1512
                        Fax: 727-577-2749
                www.goodwill-suncoast.org

R Lee Waits, President/CEO
Jay McCloe, Director Resource Development

Large group home which serves individuals diagnosed as mentally retarded with a secondary diagnosed of psychiatric difficulties as evidenced by problem behavior. Providing residential, behavioral and instructional support and services that will promote the development of adaptive, socially appropriate behavior, each individual is assessed to determine socialization, basic academics and recreation. The primary intervention strategy is applied behavior analysis. Professional consultants are utilized to address the medical, dental, psychiatric and pharmacological needs of each individual. One of the most popular features is the active community integration component of SRTC. Program customers attend an average of 15 monthly outings to various community events.

Books

576 A Story of Bipolar Disorder (Manic-Depressive Illness) Does this Sound Like You?

National Institute of Mental Health
6001 Executive Boulevard
Room 8184
Bethesda, MD 20892-9663
                             866-615-6464
                        Fax: 301-443-4279
                        TTY: 301-443-8431
               E-mail: nimhinfo@nih.gov
                          www.nimh.nih.gov

Feeling really down sometimes and really up other times? Are these mood changes causing problems at work, school, or home? If yes, you may have bipolar disorder, also called manic-depressive illness.

20 pages

577 Bipolar Disorders: A Guide to Helping Children and Adolescents

ADD WareHouse
300 NW 70th Avenue
Suite 102
Plantation, FL 33317   954-792-8100
                             800-233-9273
                        Fax: 954-792-8545
          E-mail: sales@addwarehouse.com
                     www.addwarehouse.com

Mitzi Waltz

A million children and adolescents in the US may have childhood-onset bipolar disorder-including a significant number with ADHD. This new book helps parents and professionals recognize, treat and cope with bipolar disorders. It covers diagnosis, family life, medications, talk therapies, school issues, and other interventions. *$24.95*

340 pages

578 Bipolar Disorders: Clinical Course and Outcome

American Psychiatric Publishing
1000 Wilson Boulevard
Suite 1825
Arlington, VA 22209-3901 703-907-7322
800-368-5777
Fax: 703-907-1091
E-mail: appi@psych.org
www.appi.org

Katie Duffy, Marketing Assistant

Provides a concise, up to date summary of affective relapse, comorbid psychopathalogy, functional disability, and psychosocial outcome in contemporary bipolar disorders. *$49.95*

312 pages ISBN 0-880487-68-2

579 Bipolar Puzzle Solution

National Alliance for the Mentally Ill
2107 Wilson Boulevard
Suite 300
Arlington, VA 22201-3042 703-524-7600
800-950-6264
Fax: 703-524-9094
TDD: 703-516-7227
www.nami.org

An informative book on bipolar illness in a 187 question-and-answer format. *$17.00*

580 Carbamazepine and Manic Depression: A Guide

Madison Institute of Medicine
7617 Mineral Point Road
Suite 300
Madison, WI 53717-1623 608-827-2470
Fax: 608-827-2479
E-mail: mim@miminc.org
www.miminc.org

A concise guide to the use of carbamazepine for the treatment of manic depression with information about dosing, monitoring and side effects. *$5.95*

32 pages

581 Consumer's Guide to Psychiatric Drugs

New Harbinger Publications
5674 Shattuck Avenue
Oakland, CA 94609-1662 510-652-2002
800-748-6273
Fax: 510-652-5472
E-mail: customerservice@newharbinger.com
www.newharbinger.com

Helps consumers understand what treatment options are available and what side effects to expect. Covers possible interactions with other drugs, medical conditions and other concerns. Explains how each drug works, and offers detailed information about treatments for depression, bipolar disorder, anxiety and sleep disorders, as well as other conditions. *$16.95*

340 pages ISBN 1-572241-11-X

582 Covert Modeling & Covert Reinforcement

New Harbinger Publications
5674 Shattuck Avenue
Oakland, CA 94609-1662 510-652-2002
800-748-6273
Fax: 510-652-5472
E-mail: customerservice@newharbinger.com
www.newharbinger.com

$11.95

ISBN 0-934986-29-0

583 Divalproex and Bipolar Disorder: A Guide

Madison Institute of Medicine
7617 Mineral Point Road
Suite 300
Madison, WI 53717-1623 608-827-2470
Fax: 608-827-2479
E-mail: mim@miminc.org
www.miminc.org

Written by leading experts on bipolar disorder (manic depression) and its treatment, this concise, up-to-date guide includes the most important information every patient taking divalproex (valproate) for bipolar disorder needs to know about this medication. *$5.95*

32 pages

584 Guildeline for Treatment of Patients with Bipolar Disorder

American Psychiatric Publishing
1000 Wilson Boulevard
Suite 1825
Arlington, VA 22209-3901 703-907-7322
800-368-5777
Fax: 703-907-1091
E-mail: appi@psych.org
www.appi.org

Katie Dufffy, Marketing Assistant

Provides guidance to psychiatrists who treat patients with bipolar I disorder. Summarizes the pharmacologic, somatic, and psychotherapeutic treatments used for patients. *$22.50*

96 pages ISBN 0-890423-02-4

585 Lithium and Manic Depression: A Guide

Madison Institute of Medicine
7617 Mineral Point Road
Suite 300
Madison, WI 53717-1623 608-827-2470
Fax: 608-827-2479
E-mail: mim@miminc.org
www.miminc.org

A concise, up-to-date guide written by a leading expert on manic depression (bipolar disorder) and its treatment. This publication includes the most important information every patient taking lithium needs to know about lithium dosing, monitoring and side effects. *$5.95*

31 pages

586 Living Without Depression & Manic Depression: a Workbook for Maintaining Mood Stability

New Harbinger Publications
5674 Shattuck Avenue
Oakland, CA 94609-1662   510-652-2002
                               800-748-6273
                          Fax: 510-652-5472
E-mail: customerservice@newharbinger.com
                    www.newharbinger.com

Outlines a program that helps people achieve breakthroughs in coping and healing. Contents include: self advocacy, building a network of support, wellness lifestyle, symptom prevention strategies, self-esteem, mood stability, a career that works, trauma resolution, dealing with sleep problems, diet, vitamin and herbal therapies, dealing with stigma, medication side effects, psychotherapy, and counseling alternatives. $18.95

263 pages ISBN 1-879237-74-1

587 Management of Bipolar Disorder: Pocketbook

American Psychiatric Publishing
1000 Wilson Boulevard
Suite 1825
Arlington, VA 22209-3901   703-907-7322
                                  800-368-5777
                             Fax: 703-907-1091
                   E-mail: appi@psych.org
                             www.appi.org

Katie Duffy, Marketing Assistant

Contains the need for treatment, what defines bipolar disorders, spectrum of the disorder, getting the best out of treatment, treatment of mania and bipolar depression, preventing new episodes, special problems in treatment, mood stabilizers and case studies. $14.95

96 pages ISBN 1-853172-74-X

588 Mania: Clinical and Research Perspectives

American Psychiatric Publishing
1000 Wilson Boulevard
Suite 1825
Arlington, VA 22209-3901   703-907-7322
                                  800-368-5777
                             Fax: 703-907-1091
                   E-mail: appi@psych.org
                             www.appi.org

Katie Duffy, Marketing Assistant

Diagnostic considerations, biological aspects, and treatment of mania. $59.95

478 pages ISBN 0-880487-28-3

589 Oxcarbazepine and Bipolar Disorder: A Guide

Madison Institute of Medicine
7617 Mineral Point Road
Suite 300
Madison, WI 53717-1623   608-827-2470
                           Fax: 608-827-2479
                   E-mail: mim@miminc.org
                             www.miminc.org

This 31 page booklet provides patients with the information they need to know about the use of oxcarbazepine in the treatment of bipolar disorder, including information about proper dosing, medication management, and possible side effects. $5.95

31 pages

Periodicals & Pamphlets

590 Bipolar Disorder

National Institute of Mental Health
6001 Executive Boulevard
Room 8184
Bethesda, MD 20892-9663
                               866-615-6464
                          Fax: 301-443-4279
                          TTY: 301-443-8431
                 E-mail: nimhinfo@nih.gov
                          www.nimh.nih.gov

Bipolar disorder, also known as manic-depressive illness, is a brain disorder that causes unusual shifts in a person's mood, energy, and ability to function. Different from the normal ups and downs that everyone goes through, the symptoms of bipolar disorder are severe. They can result in damaged relationships, poor job or school performance, and even suicide. But there is good news: bipolar disorder can be treated, and people with this illness can lead full and productive lives.

24 pages

591 Child and Adolescent Bipolar Disorder: An Update from the National Institute of Mental Health

National Institute of Mental Health
6001 Executive Boulevard
Room 8184
Bethesda, MD 20892-9663
                               866-615-6464
                          Fax: 301-443-4279
                          TTY: 301-443-8431
                 E-mail: nimhinfo@nih.gov
                          www.nimh.nih.gov

Research findings, clinical experience, and family accounts provide substantial evidence that bipolar disorder, also called manic-depressive illness, can occur in children and adolescents. Bipolar disorder is difficult to recognize and diagnose in youth. Better understanding of the diagnosis and treatment is urgently needed. In pursuit of this goal, the NIMH is conducting and supporting research on child and adolescent bioplar disorder.

3 pages Year Founded: 2000

592 Coping With Unexpected Events: Depression & Trauma

Depression & BiPolar Support Alliance
730 N Franklin Street
Suite 501
Chicago, IL 60610-7204   312-642-0049
                                800-826-3632
                           Fax: 312-642-7243
         E-mail: programs@dbsalliance.org
                             www.ndmda.org

Lydia Lewis, President
Laura Hoofnagle, Publications

How to cope with depression after trauma, helping others and preventing suicide.

593 Mood Disorders

Center for Mental Health Services: Knowledge Exchange Network
PO Box 42490
Washington, DC 20015

800-789-2647
Fax: 301-984-8796
TDD: 866-889-2647
E-mail: ken@mentalhealth.org
www.mentalhealth.org

This fact sheet provides basic information on the symptoms, formal diagnosis, and treatment for bipolar disorder.

3 pages

Research Centers

594 Epidemiology-Genetics Program in Psychiatry

John Hopkins University School of Medicine
1820 Lancaster Street
Suite 300
Baltimore, MD 21231

410-955-0455
888-289-4095
Fax: 410-955-0644
E-mail: familystudy@jhmi.edu
www.hopkinsmedicine.org

Ann Pulver

The research program is to help characterize the genetic (biochemical) developmental, and environmental components of bipolar disorder. The hope is that once scientists understand the biological causes of this disorder new medications and treatments can be developed.

Video & Audio

595 Families Coping with Mental Illness

Mental Illness Education Project
PO Box 470813
Brookline Village, MA 02247-0244

617-562-1111
800-343-5540
Fax: 617-779-0061
E-mail: info@miepvideos.org
www.miepvideos.org

Christine Ledoux, Executive Director

Ten family members share their experiences of having a family member with schizophrenia or bipolar disorder. Designed to provide insights and support to other families, the tape also profoundly conveys to professionals the needs of families when mental illness strikes. In two versions: a 22-minute version ideal for short classes and workshops, and a richer 43-minute version with more examples and details. Discounted price for families/consumers. *$68.95*

Web Sites

596 www.bpso.org

BPSO-Bipolar Significant Others

597 www.bpso.org/nomania.htm

How to Avoid a Manic Episode

598 www.chandra.astro.indiana.edu/bipolar/physical.html

Primer on Depression and Bipolar Disorder

Useful for those struggling with committing to treatment.

599 www.cyberpsych.org

CyberPsych

Hosts the American Psychoanalyists Foundation, American Association of Suicideology, Society for the Exploration of Psychotherapy Intergration, and Anxiety Disorders Association of America. Also subcategories of the anxiety disorders, as well as general information, including panic disorder, phobias, obsessive compulsive disorder (OCD), social phobia, generalized anxiety disorder, post traumatic stress disorder, and phobias of childhood. Book reviews and links to web pages sharing the topics.

600 www.dbsalliance.org

Depression & Bi-Polar Support Alliance

Mental health news updates and local support group information.

601 www.geocities.com/EnchantedForest/1068

Bipolar Kids Homepage

Set of links.

602 **www.healthguide.com/english/brain.bipolar**

Bipolar Disorder

Covers symptoms, diagnoses, and medications.

603 **www.hometown.aol.com/DrgnKprl/BPCAT.html**

Bipolar Children and Teens Homepage

604 **www.klis.com/chandler/pamphlet/bipolar/bipolarpamphlet.html**

Bipolar Affective Disorder in Children and Adolescents

An introduction for families.

605 **www.med.jhu.edu/drada/creativity.html**

Creativity and Depression and Manic-Depression

606 **www.mhsource.com/wb/thow9903.html**

Steven Thos Mental Health Resources-Depression and Bipolar Disorder

About 40 questions asked by patients.

607 **www.moodswing.org/bdfaq.html**

Bipolar Disorder Frequently Asked Questions

Excellent for those newly diagnosed.

608 **www.pendulum.org/alternatives/lisa_alternatives.htm**

Alternative Approaches to the Treatment of Manic-Depression

Introduction to uses of nutrients.

609 **www.planetpsych.com**

Planetpsych.com

Learn about disorders, their treatments and other topics in psychology. Articles are listed under the related topic areas. Ask a therapist a question for free, or view the directory of professionals in your area. If you are a therapist sign up for the directory. Current features, self-help, interactive, and newsletter archives.

610 **www.psychcentral.com**

Psych Central

Personalized one-stop index for psychology, support, and mental health issues, resources, and people on the Internet.

611 **www.psychguides.com/bphe.html**

Expert Consensus Treatment Guidelines for Bipolar Disorder

612 **www.tcnj.edu/~ellisles/BipolarPlanet**

Bipolar Planet

Links to sites on mood disorders.

Introduction

Cognitive disorders are a group of conditions characterized by impairments in the ability to think, reason, plan and organize. There are three types of cognitive disorders; delirium, dementia (of which Alzheimer's Disease is the most common) and amnestic disorder.

Delirium is a relatively short-term condition in which conciousness waxes and wanes, common in patients after surgery or who are acutely ill, as with high fever. It resolves when the underlying problem resolves. There are three categories of causes of delirium: that which is due to a general medical condition, delirium that is substance-induced, and delirium due to multiple causes. An amnestic disorder, in contrast to delirium or dementia, is a condition in which only memory is impaired; for instance a person may be unable to recall important facts or events, making it difficult to function normally. Dementia is a chronic disorder; it is an impairment of multiple cognitive functions; a person with dementia may have severe memory loss and also be unable to plan or prepare for events or to care for oneself.

Dementia, Alzheimer's type, is a progressive disorder that slowly kills nerve cells in the brain. While definitive treatments are lacking, there is a prodigious amount of research on the condition, some which suggests the near-future possiblity of a vaccine preventing onset of the condition. Though such hopeful breakthroughs remain distant, there is much that families and patients can do when the condition is recognized and care and support are sought early in the disorder's progression. Since other, serious, treatable disorders can resemble Alzeimer's Disease, it is very important for individuals who are losing cognitive functions to be evaluated by a physician. Early detection of Alzheimer's Disease, with early treatment, may improve the chances for slowing the rate of decline.

Here we will describe only Alzheimer's dementia, the most prevalent Cognitive Disorder.

SYMPTOMS

•Langugage disorders;
•Impaired ability to carry out motor activities despite intact motor function;
•Failure to recognize or identify objects despite intact sensory perception;
•Disturbance in executive functioning (planning, organizing, sequencing, abstracting);
•The deficits cause impairment in social or occupational functioning and represent a decline from previous level of functioning;
•The course is gradual and continuous;
•The deficits are not due to central nervous system conditions such as Parkinson's Disease, other conditions known to cause dementia, and are not substance-induced;
•The deficits do not occur during the course of delirium and are not better accounted for by severe depression or schizophrenia.

ASSOCIATED FEATURES

Dementia, Alzheimer's type, is liable to begin gradually, not with deficits in cognition but with a marked change in personality. For instance, a person may suddenly become given to fits of anger for no apparent reason.

Soon, however, family and acquaintances may notice that the individual begins to mix up facts, or may get lost driving to a familiar place. One of the terrifying aspects of the condition is that in the early stages the afflicted individual may become aware of slipping cognitive functions, adding to confusion, fright and depression. After a period, lapses in memory grow more obvious; patients with Alzheimer's are liable to repeat themselves, and may forget the names of grandchildren or longtime friends. They may also be increasingly agitated and combative as family members try to correct them or help with accustomed tasks. The memory lapses in patients with Alzheimer's differ markedly from those in normal aging: a patient with Alzheimer's may often forget entire experiences and rarely remembers them later; the patient also only grudgingly acknowledges lapses. Skills deteriorate and a patient is increasingly unable to follow directions, or care for him/herself.

PREVALENCE

An estimated two percent to four percent of the population over age 65 has dementia, Alzheimer's type. Other types of dementia are believed to be much less common. Prevalance of the condition increases with age, particularly after age 75; in persons over 85, an estimated twenty percent have dementia, Alzheimer's type.

TREATMENT OPTIONS

There is no known cure or definitive treatment for dementia, Alzheimer's type. However, research has suggested avenues that involve drugs, such as THA, Donepezil, and Rivastigmine, for regulating acetylcholine, seratonin or norepinephrine in the brain. According to the American Psychiatric Association, some progress has been seen in slowing the death rate among nerve cells using a chemical known as Alcar (acetyl-l-carnitine). Psychiatrists treating patients with dementia, Alzheimer's type, may also be able to prescribe medications that can treat the depression and anxiety that accompanies the condition. And families are strongly encouraged to take advantage of adjunctive services including support groups, counseling and psychotherapy.

Associations & Agencies

614 Alzheimer's Association National Office

225 N Michigan Avenue
Suite 1700
Chicago, IL 60601-7633   312-335-8700
                               800-272-3900
                          Fax: 312-335-1110
                     E-mail: info@alz.org
                               www.alz.org

Chuck Meredith, Public Information

Headquarters for the nation's leading organization for all those suffering with alzheimer's disease and their families and support network. Offers referrals, support groups, workshops, training seminars, publications.

615 Alzheimer's Disease Education and Referral Center

PO Box 8250
Silver Spring, MD 20907-8250   301-495-3311
                                 800-438-4380
                            Fax: 301-495-3334
                  E-mail: adear@alzheimers.org
                               www.alzheimers.org

The ADEAR Center provides information about Alzheimer's Disease and related disorders to health professionals, patients and their families, and the public. We are a service of The National Institute on Aging, one of The Federal Government's National Institutes of Health. The majority of our publications are free.

616 Alzheimer's Disease and Related Disorders Association

919 N Michigan Avenue
Suite 1000
Chicago, IL 60611-8700   312-335-8700
                               800-272-3900
                          Fax: 312-335-1110
                               www.alz.org

Association dedicated to supporting the caregivers of individuals with alzheimer's disease.

617 Alzheimer's Hospital Association

919 N Michigan Avenue
Suite 1000
Chicago, IL 60611-1696   312-335-5720
                          Fax: 312-335-1110

618 American Health Assistance Foundation

22512 Gateway Center Drive
Clarksburg, MD 20871   301-948-3244
                               800-437-2423
                          Fax: 301-258-9454
                   E-mail: jwilson@ahaf.org
                               www.ahaf.org

Jarmal Wilson, Alzheimer's Family Relief

Provides information on treatment, medication medical referrals regarding Alzheimer's disease.

619 Center for Family Support (CFS)

333 7th Avenue
New York, NY 10001-5004   212-629-7939
                          Fax: 212-239-2211
                               www.cfsny.org

Steven Vernickofs, Executive Director

Service agency devoted to the physical well-being and development of the retarded child and the sound mental health of the parents. Helps families with retarded children with all aspects of home care including counseling, referrals, home aide service and consultation. Offers intervention for parents at the birth of a retarded child with in-home support, guidance and infant stimulation. Pioneered training of nonprofessional women as home aides to provide supportive services in homes.

620 Center for Mental Health Services Knowledge Exchange Network

US Department of Health and Human Services
PO Box 42490
Washington, DC 20015-4800   800-789-2647
                          Fax: 301-984-8796
               E-mail: ken@mentalhealth.org
                               www.mentalhealth.org

Information about resources, technical assistance, research, training, networks, and other federal clearing houses, and fact sheets and materials. Information specialists refer callers to mental health resources in their communities as well as state, federal and nonprofit contacts. Staff available Monday through Friday, 8:30 AM - 5:00 PM, EST, excluding federal holidays. After hours, callers may leave messages and an information specialist will return their call.

621 NADD: Association for Persons with Developmental Disabilities and Mental Health Needs

132 Fair Street
Kingston, NY 12401-4802   845-334-4336
                               800-331-5362
                          Fax: 845-331-4569
                   E-mail: nadd@mhv.net
                               www.thenadd.org

Dr. Robert Fletcher, Executive Director

Nonprofit organization designed to promote interest of professional and parent development with resources for individuals who have the coexistence of mental illness and mental retardation. Provides conference, educational services and training materials to professionals, parents, concerned citizens and service organizations. Formerly known as the National Association for the Dually Diagnosed.

622 National Association of Developmental Disabilities Councils

1234 Massachusetts Avenue NW
Suite 103
Washington, DC 20005-4504   202-347-1234
                          Fax: 202-347-4023
                   E-mail: naddc@naddc.org
                               www.naddc.org

Donna Heuneman, Executive Director
Mary Kelly, Governmental Affairs

Covers about 55 state and territorial councils on developmental disabilities.

623 National Family Caregivers Association

10400 Connecticut Avenue
Suite 500
Kensington, MD 20895-3944

800-896-3650
Fax: 301-942-2302
E-mail: info@nfcacares.org
www.nfcacares.org

Suzanne Mintz, President

Acts as a support and an advocate for family caregivers.

624 National Institute of Neurological Disorders and Stroke

Neurological Institute
PO Box 5801
Bethesda, MD 20911

301-496-5751
800-352-9424
Fax: 301-402-2186
www.ninds.nih.gov

Federal agency that supports research nationwide on disorders of the brain and nervous system. Website has updated neuroscience news and articles.

625 National Mental Health Consumer's Self-Help Clearinghouse

1211 Chestnut Street
Suite 1207
Philadelphia, PA 19107

215-751-1810
800-553-4539
Fax: 215-636-6312
E-mail: info@mhselfhelp.org
www.mhselfhelp.org

Alex Morrsey, Information/Referral

Funded by the National Institute of Mental Health Community Support Program, the purpose of the Clearinghouse is to encourage the development and growth of consumer self-help groups.

Year Founded: 1992

626 National Niemann-Pick Disease Foundation

22201 Riverpoint Trail
Carrollton, VA 23314

804-357-6774

Offers support and funding for individuals with cognitive disorders and their support network.

Books

627 36-Hour Day: a Guide to Caring for Persons with Alzheimer's Disease, Related Dementing Illnesses and Memory Loss in Later Life

Time Warner Books
3 Center Plaza
Boston, MA 02108

800-759-0190
E-mail: sales@aoltwbg.com
www.twbookmark.com

Combining practical advice with specific examples, this is a newly revised, updated and comprehensive edition of a helpful guide for people dealing with victims of Alzheimer's disease. Provides the basic facts about dementia and shows readers how to deal with daily care, get outside help, and handle financial issues. *$7.50*

427 pages ISBN 0-446361-04-6

628 Agitation in Patients with Dementia: a Practical Guide to Diagnosis and Management

American Psychiatric Publishing
1000 Wilson Boulevard
Suite 1825
Arlington, VA 22209-3901

703-907-7322
800-368-5777
Fax: 703-907-1091
E-mail: appi@psych.org
www.appi.org

Appealing to a wide audience of geriatric psychiatrists, primary case physicians and internists, general practitioners, nurses, social workers, psychologists, pharmacists and mental health care workers and practitioners in hospitals, nursing homes and clinics, this remarkable monograph offers practical direction on assessing and managing agitation in patients with dementia. *$43.95*

288 pages Year Founded: 2003 ISBN 0-880488-43-3

629 Alzheimer's Disease Sourcebook

Omnigraphics
PO Box 625
Holmes, PA 19043

800-234-1340
Fax: 800-875-1340
E-mail: info@omnigraphics.com
www.omnigraphics.com

Omnigraphics is the publisher of the Health Reference Series, a growing consumer health information resource with more than 100 volumes in print. Each title in the series features an easy to understand format, nontechnical language, comprehensive indexing and resources for further information. Material in each book has been collected from a wide range of government agencies, professional associations, periodicals, and other sources. *$78.00*

524 pages ISBN 0-780802-23-3

630 Alzheimer's Disease: Activity-Focused Care

Theraputic Resources
PO Box 16814
Cleveland, OH 16814   440-331-7114
                             888-331-7114
                        Fax: 440-331-7118
E-mail: contactus@theraputicresources.com
www.theraputicresources.com

Katie Hennessy, Medical Promotions Coordinator

Provides practical and innovative strategies for care of people with Alzheimer's disease, emphasizing the activities that make up daily living - dressing, toileting, eating, exercising, and communication. The text is written from the viewpoint that activity-focused care promotes the resident's cognitive, physical, psychosocial, and spiritual well-being.

436 pages ISBN 0-750699-08-6

631 Alzheimer's, Stroke & 29 Other Neurolgical Disorders Sourcebook

Omnigraphics
PO Box 625
Holmes, PA 19043
                             800-234-1340
                        Fax: 800-875-1340
E-mail: info@omnigraphics.com
www.omnigraphics.com

Omnigraphics is the publisher of the Health Reference Series, a growing consumer health information resource with more than 100 volumes in print. Each title in the series features an easy to understand format, nontechnical language, comprehensive indexing and resources for further information. Material in each book has been collected from a wide range of goverment agencies, professional associations, periodicals and other sources. *$78.00*

579 pages ISBN 1-558887-48-2

632 American Psychiatric Association Practice Guideline for the Treatment of Patients with Delirium

American Psychiatric Publishing
1000 Wilson Boulevard
Suite 1825
Arlington, VA 22209-3901   703-907-7322
                             800-368-5777
                        Fax: 703-907-1091
E-mail: appi@psych.org
www.appi.org

James Scully MD, President
Katie Duffy, Marketing

Best practices examined from the group whose vision is a society that has available, accessible quality psychiatric diagnosis and treatment. *$22.50*

64 pages ISBN 0-890423-13-X

633 Behavioral Complications in Alzheimer's Disease

Health Source
1404 K Street NW
Washington, DC 20005-2401   202-789-7303
                             800-713-7122
                        Fax: 202-789-7899
E-mail: healthsource@appi.org
www.healthsourcebooks.org

Practical management strategies for the identification, measurement and treatment of behavioral symptoms in patient with Alzheimer's disease. *$36.50*

272 pages ISBN 0-880484-77-2

634 Care That Works: a Relationship Approach to Persons With Dementia

Johns Hopkins University Press
2715 N Charles Street
Baltimore, MD 21218-4319   410-516-6936
                             800-537-5487
                        Fax: 410-516-6998
www.press.jhu.edu

Adam Glazer, Promotion Manager

Real life strategies for a challenging task. *$58.00*

ISBN 0-801860-25-3

635 Cognitive Behavior Therapy for Children and Families

Cambridge University Press
40 W 20th Street
New York, NY 10011-4221   212-924-3900
                        Fax: 212-691-3239
E-mail: marketing@cup.org
www.cup.org

Cognitive behavior therapy is a relatively new treatment approach that has been demonstrated to be the most effective form of treatment for many childhood disorders. This volume provides a comprehensive approach to psychological problems in children, adolescents and their families and is structured developmentally, covering preschool through adolescence. Multimodal therapy is also highlighted along with the direction of future research. *$110.00*

310 pages

636 Cognitive Vulnerability to Depression

Guilford Publications
72 Spring Street
New York, NY 10012   212-431-9800
                             800-365-7006
                        Fax: 212-966-6708
E-mail: info@guilford.com
www.guilford.com

Cognitive Disorders/Books

Explores what makes some people more vulnerable to recurrence of depressive episodes following successful treatments. Combines the most current research and theory on cognitive vulnerability. Covering methodoligical, theoretical and empirical issues, the authors review cognitive theories of depression, explicate and assess the vulnerability approach to psychopathology and formulate an integrative view of the key proximal and distal antecedents of depression in adults. $37.95

307 pages ISBN 1-572303-04-2

637 Cognitive-Behavioral Strategies in Crisis Intervention

Guilford Publications
72 Spring Street
New York, NY 10012

212-431-9800
800-365-7006
Fax: 212-966-6708
E-mail: info@guilford.com
www.guilford.com

This text brings together leading cognitive-behavioral practitioners to describe effective intervention for a broad crisis situations. Covers panic disorder, Cluster B personality disorders, suicidal depression, substance abuse, rape, sexual abuse, family crises, natural disasters, medical problems, problems of the elderly and much more. This book presents proven short term approaches to helping patients weather the immediate crisis and build needed coping and problem solving skills. $46.95

470 pages ISBN 1-572305-79-7

638 Delusions and Hallucinations in Old Age

American Psychiatric Publishing
1000 Wilson Boulevard
Suite 1825
Arlington, VA 22209-3901

703-907-7322
800-368-5777
Fax: 703-907-1091
E-mail: appi@psych.org
www.appi.org

Katie Duffy, Marketing Assistant

$32.00

248 pages

639 Dementia: a Clinical Approach

Elsevier Health Sciences
11830 Westline Industrial Drive
St. Louis, MO 63146

314-453-7010
800-568-5136
Fax: 314-453-7095
E-mail: orders@bhusa.com or
custserv@bhusa.com
www.bh.com

This is both a scholarly review of the dementias and a practical guide to their diagnosis and trcatment. $89.95

560 pages ISBN 0-750690-65-8

640 Dementias: Diagnosis, Management, and Research

American Psychiatric Publishing
1000 Wilson Boulevard
Suite 1825
Arlington, VA 22209-3901

703-907-7322
800-368-5777
Fax: 703-907-1091
E-mail: appi@psych.org
www.appi.org

Designed to met the needs of clinicians dealing with persons with dementing illness and to serve as an introduction to the pathophysiology of dementing illness and a resource of clinical investigators.

280 pages Year Founded: 2003 ISBN 1-585620-43-2

641 Disorders of Brain and Mind

Cambridge University Press
40 W 20th Street
New York, NY 10011-4221

212-924-3900
Fax: 212-691-3239
E-mail: marketing@cup.org
www.cup.org

Discusses various neuropsychiatry topics where the brain and mind come together. $50.00

388 pages Year Founded: 1999 ISBN 0-521778-51-4

642 Guidelines for the Treatment of Patients wit h Alzheimer's Disease and Other Dementias of Late Life

American Psychiatric Publishing
1000 Wilson Boulevard
Suite 1825
Arlington, VA 22209-3901

703-907-7322
800-368-5777
Fax: 703-907-1091
E-mail: appi@psych.org
www.appi.org

Katie Duffy, Marketing Assistant

$22.50

40 pages ISBN 0-890423-04-0

643 Language in Cognitive Development: the Emergence of the Mediated Mind

Cambridge University Press
40 W 20th Street
New York, NY 10011-4221

212-924-3900
Fax: 212-691-3239
E-mail: marketing@cup.org
www.cup.org

Katherine Nelson

Discusses the articulation between cognition, language and culture. An experimental theoretical view of cognitive development. Brings together the fields of cognitive development and linguistic development. $33.00

448 pages Year Founded: 1998

644 Practice for the Treatment of Patients with Alzheimer's Disease and Other Dementia

American Psychiatric Publishing
1000 Wilson Boulevard
Suite 1825
Arlington, VA 22209-3901   703-907-7322
                                   800-368-5777
                              Fax: 703-907-1091
                      E-mail: appi@psych.org
                                www.appi.org

Katie Duffy, Marketing Assistant

$22.50

112 pages

645 Progress in Alzheimer's Disease and Similar Conditions

American Psychiatric Publishing
1000 Wilson Boulevard
Suite 1825
Arlington, VA 22209-3901   703-907-7322
                                   800-368-5777
                              Fax: 703-907-1091
                      E-mail: appi@psych.org
                                www.appi.org

Katie Duffy, Marketing Assistant

Details advances in research on human genetics that is broadening our knowledge of Alzheimer's disease and other related afflictions. Describes disease mechanisms, including prions, that provide insight into the role environment plays in the development of disease. Includes stories about the pain inflicted by this disease on the patients and their family and friends as well as current efforts in management and treatment. *$47.50*

368 pages ISBN 0-880487-60-7

646 Victims of Dementia: Service, Support, and Care

Haworth Press
10 Alice Street
Binghamton, NY 13904-1580   607-722-5857
                                    800-342-9678
                               Fax: 607-722-6362
              E-mail: getinfo@haworthpressinc.com
                         www.haworthpress.com

Jackie Blakeslee, Advertising/Journal Liaison

Provides an in depth look at the concept, construction and operation of Wesley Hall, a special living area at the Chelsea United Methodist retirement home in Michigan. *$39.95*

155 pages ISBN 1-560242-64-7

647 What You Need To Know About Alzheimer's

New Harbinger Publications
5674 Shattuck Avenue
Oakland, CA 94609-1662   510-652-2002
                                 800-748-6273
                            Fax: 510-652-5472
       E-mail: customerservice@newharbinger.com
                         www.newharbinger.com

John Medina

Provides a detailed overview of the symptoms, explains th underlying biology, provides information about the latest medications and other treatments, also offers practical guidance for coping with the hardship of caring for an Alzheimer's patient. *$15.95*

165 pages ISBN 1-572241-27-6

Periodicals & Pamphlets

648 Alzheimer's Disease Research and the American Health Assistance Foundation

American Health Assistance Foundation
22512 Gateway Center Drive
Clarksburg, MD 20871   301-948-3244
                               800-437-2423
                          Fax: 301-258-9454
                  E-mail: jwilson@ahaf.org
                            www.ahaf.org

Jarmal Wilson, Alzheimer's Family Relief

Provides information on treatment, medication, medical referrals.

Web Sites

649 www.aan.com

American Academy of Neurology

Provides information for both professionals and the public on neurology subjects, covering Alzheimer's and Parkinson's diseases to stroke and migraine, includes comprehensive fact sheets.

650 www.acsu.buffalo.edu/drstall/hndbk0/html

Caregiver's Handbook

100 pages with practical ideas about emotions, nutrition, personal care, financial and legal issues.

651 www.agelessdesign.com/alz.htm

Ageless Design

Information on age related diseases such as Alzheimer's disease.

652 www.ahaf.org/alzdis/about/adabout.htm

American Health Assistance Foundation

Alzheimer's resource for patients and caregivers.

653 www.alz.co.uk

Alzheimer's Disease International

Umbrella organization of associations that support people with dementia.

654 www.alz.org

Alzheimer's Organization

Locate an Alzheimer's Association chapter near you and learn about recent research advances.

655 www.alzforum.org

Alzheimer Research Forum

Information in layman's terms, plus many references and resources listed.

656 www.alzheimers.org

Alzheimer's Disease Education and Referral

A division of the National Institute on Aging of the National Institute of Health. Solid information and a list of federally funded centers for evaluation, referral, treatment.

657 www.alzheimersbooks.com/

Alzheimer's Disease Bookstore

658 www.alzheimersupport.Com

AlzheimerSupport.com

Information and products for people dealing with Alzheimer's Disease.

659 www.alznsw.asn.au.library/libtoc.htm

Alzheimer's Association of NSW

Information for people diagnosed and caregivers.

660 www.alzwell.com

ALZwell Alzheimer's Caregivers' Page

Many resources designed to support caregivers.

661 www.biostat.wustl.edu/alzheimer

Washington University - Saint Louis

Page on Alzheimer's information, from basic care to friends and family networking experiences for support.

662 www.cbshealthwatch.medscape.com/ alzheimerscenter

CBS News

Backround information articles, community features, resources and related links concerning Alzheimer's disease.

663 www.cyberpsych.org

CyberPsych

Hosts the American Psychoanalyists Foundation, American Association of Suicideology, Society for the Exploration of Psychotherapy Intergration, and Anxiety Disorders Association of America. Also subcategories of the anxiety disorders, as well as general information, including panic disorder, phobias, obsessive compulsive disorder (OCD), social phobia, generalized anxiety disorder, post traumatic stress disorder, and phobias of childhood. Book reviews and links to web pages sharing the topics.

664 www.depression.com/health_library/treat ments /cognitive.html

Cognitive Therapy

A complete introduction.

665 www.geocities.com/~elderly-place

Elderly Place

Includes Caregiver's Guide to Alzheimer's.

666 www.habitsmart.com/cogtitle.html

Cognitive Therapy Pages

Offers accessible explanations.

667 www.mayohealth.org/mayo/common/htm/

Alzeimer's Center Reference List

668 www.mentalhealth.com

Internet Mental Health

On-line information and a virtual encyclopedia related to mental disorders, possible causes and treatments. News, articles, on-line diagnostic programs and related links. Designed to improve understanding, diagnosis and treatment of mental illness throughout the world. Awarded the Top Site Award and the NetPsych Cutting Edge Site Award.

669 www.mentalhealth.org/search/DoSearch.a sp
Center for Mental Health Services

US Department of Health and Human Services website with current Alzheimer's information.

670 www.mindstreet.com/synopsis.html
Cognitive Therapy: A Multimedia Learning Program

The basics of cognitive therapy are presented.

671 www.ninds.nih.gov
National Institute of Neurological Disorders & Stroke

Neuroscience updates and articles.

672 www.noah-health.org/english/aging/aging. html
Ask NOAH About: Aging and Alzheimer's Disease

Links to brochures on medical problems of the elderly.

673 www.ohioalzcenter.org/facts.html
Alzheimer's Disease Fact Page

674 www.planetpsych.com
Planetpsych.com

Learn about disorders, their treatments and other topics in psychology. Articles are listed under the related topic areas. Ask a therapist a question for free, or view the directory of professionals in your area. If you are a therapist sign up for the directory. Current features, self-help, interactive, and newsletter archives.

675 www.psych.org/clin_res/pg_dementia.cfm
Practice Guidelines for the Treatment of Patients with Alzheimer's

American Psychiatric Association.

676 www.psychcentral.com
Psych Central

Personalized one-stop index for psychology, support, and mental health issues, resources, and people on the Internet.

677 www.rcpsych.ac.uk/public/help/memory/
Memory and Dementia

678 www.usc.edu/isd/locations/science/
Caregiving-Special Topics

Unannotated list of books.

679 www.zarcrom.com/users/alzheimers
Alzheimer's Outreach

Detailed and practical information.

680 www.zarcrom.com/users/yeartorem
Year to Remember

A memorial site covering many aspects of Alzheimer's disease.

Introduction

Conduct disorder is a diagnosis given to children who demonstrate a repetitive and persistent pattern of behavior in which societal norms and the basic rights of others are violated. These behaviors can include physical harm to people or animals, damage to property, deceitfulness or theft, and extreme violations of rules. It is important to note that troublesome behavior can also result from adverse circumstances, and that the circumstances need to be fully investigatied, and attempts to rectify adversity made, before Conduct Disorder is diagnosed. The diagnosis can be divided into two types, depending on the age of diagnosis: childhood-onset type and adolescent-onset type.

SYMPTOMS

•Aggression to people and animals, including bullying, picking fights, using weapons, physical cruelty to people and animals, stealing or forcing someone into sexual activity;
•Destruction of property;
•Deceitfulness or theft, including breaking into someone's house, lying to obtain goods or favors, or shoplifting;
•Violations of rules, including staying out past curfews, running away from home, and truancy from school.

ASSOCIATED FEATURES

Conduct disorder is often associated with early onset of sexual activity, drinking and smoking. The disorder can lead to school disruption, problems with the police, sexually transmitted diseases, unplanned pregnancy, and injury from accidents and fights. Suicide and suicidal attempts are more common among adolescents with Conduct Disorder. Individuals with Conduct Disorder appear to have little remorse for their acts, though they may learn that expressing guilt can diminish punishment; and they often show little or no empathy for the feelings, wishes, and well-being of others.

PREVALENCE

Prevalence of Conduct Disorder appears to have increased in recent years. For males under 18 years of age, rates range from six percent to sixteen percent; for females, rates range from two percent to nine percent.

TREATMENT OPTIONS

Both psychotherapy and medication can be useful in treating Conduct Disorder. As with many mental disorders, family members are often affected and it is crucial that they are supported and involved in the treatment.

Associations & Agencies

682 Association for Advancement of Behavior Therapy

305 Seventh Avenue
16th Floor
New York, NY 10001-6008   212-647-1890
Fax: 212-647-1865
E-mail: mebrown@aabt.org
www.aabt.org

Mary Jane Eimer, Executive Director
Mary Ellen Brown, Administration/Convention
Rosemary Park, Membership

Membership listing of mental health professionals focusing in behavior therapy.

683 Career Assessment & Planning Services

Goodwill Industries-Suncoast
10596 Gandy Boulevard
St. Petersburg, FL 33702   727-523-1512
Fax: 727-563-9300
www.goodwill-suncoast.org

R Lee Waits, President/CEO
Jay McCloe, Resource Development

Provides a comprehensive assessment, which can predict current and future employment and potential adjustment factors for physically, emotionally, or developmentally disabled persons who may be unemployed or underemployed. Assessments evaluate interests, aptitudes, academic achievements, and physical abilities (including dexterity and coordination) through coordinated testing, interviewing and behavioral observations.

684 Center for Family Support (CFS)

333 7th Avenue
New York, NY 10001-5004   212-629-7939
Fax: 212-239-2211
www.cfsny.org

Steven Vernickofs, Executive Director

Service agency devoted to the physical well-being and development of the retarded child and the sound mental health of the parents. Helps families with retarded children with all aspects of home care including counseling, referrals, home aide service and consultation. Offers intervention for parents at the birth of a retarded child with in-home support, guidance and infant stimulation. Pioneered training of nonprofessional women as home aides to provide supportive services in homes.

685 NADD: Association for Persons with Developmental Disabilities and Mental Health Needs

132 Fair Street
Kingston, NY 12401-4802   845-334-4336
800-331-5362
Fax: 845-331-4569
E-mail: nadd@mhv.net
www.thenadd.org

Dr. Robert Fletcher, Executive Director

Nonprofit organization designed to promote interest of professional and parent development with resources for individuals who have the coexistence of mental illness and mental retardation. Provides conference, educational services and training materials to professionals, parents, concerned citizens and service organizations. Formerly known as the National Association for the Dually Diagnosed.

686 National Mental Health Consumer's Self-Help Clearinghouse

1211 Chestnut Street
Suite 1207
Philadelphia, PA 19107   215-751-1810
800-553-4539
Fax: 215-636-6312
E-mail: info@mhselfhelp.org
www.mhselfhelp.org

Alex Morrsey, Information/Referral

Funded by the National Institute of Mental Health Community Support Program, the purpose of the Clearinghouse is to encourage the development and growth of consumer self-help groups.

Year Founded: 1992

687 Suncoast Residential Training Center/Developmental Services Program

Goodwill Industries-Suncoast
10596 Gandy Boulevard
PO Box 14456
St. Petersburg, FL 33702   727-523-1512
Fax: 727-563-9300
www.goodwill-suncoast.org

Jay McCloe, Director Resource Development

Large group home which serves individuals diagnosed as mentally retarded with a secondary diagnosis of psychiatric difficulties as evidenced by problem behavior. Providing residential, behavioral and instructional support and services that will promote the development of adaptive, socially appropriate behavior, each individual is assessed to determine, socialization, basic academics and recreation. The primary intervention strategy is applied behavior analysis. Professional consultants are utilized to address the medical, dental, psychiatric and pharmacological needs of each individual. One of the most popular features is the active community integration component of SRTC. Program customers attend an average of 15 monthly outings to various community events.

Books

688 1-2-3 Magic: Training Your Children to Do What You Want

ADD WareHouse
300 NW 70th Avenue
Suite 102
Plantation, FL 33317   954-792-8100
800-233-9273
Fax: 954-792-8545
E-mail: sales@addwarehouse.com
www.addwarehouse.com

Learn about a new, no-nonsense discipline program that enables parents to manage children ages two - twelve without arguing, yelling or hitting. The 1-2-3 Magic program tells you exactly how to handle screaming, tantrums and fighting, as well as how to encourage positive behavior. *$13.00*

192 pages

689 Antisocial Behavior by Young People

Cambridge University Press
40 W 20th Street
New York, NY 10011-4221   212-924-3900
                              Fax: 212-691-3239
                    E-mail: marketing@cup.org
                              www.cup.org

Michael Rutter, MRC Child Psychiarty Unit
Ann Hagell
Henri Giller

Written by a child psychiatrist, a criminologist and a social psychologist, this book is a major international review of research evidence on anti-social behavior. Covers all aspects of the field, including descriptions of different types of delinquency and time trends, the state of knowledge on the individuals, social-psychological and cultural factors involved and recent advances in prevention and intervention. *$25.00*

496 pages

690 Bad Men Do What Good Men Dream: a Forensic Psychiatrist Illuminates the Darker Side of Human Behavior

American Psychiatric Publishing
1000 Wilson Boulevard
Suite 1825
Arlington, VA 22209-3901   703-907-7322
                              800-368-5777
                         Fax: 703-907-1091
                    E-mail: appi@psych.org
                              www.appi.org

Katie Duffy, Marketing Assistant

$16.00

376 pages ISBN 0-880489-95-2

691 Black Like Kyra, White Like Me

Childs Work/Childs Play
135 Dupont Street
PO Box 760
Plainville, NY 11803-0760
                              800-962-1141
                         Fax: 800-262-1886
                    E-mail: info@Childswork.com
                              www.Childswork.com

Helping children understand racisim. Ages 6 - 10. *$5.95*

692 Check Up from the Neck Up, Ensuring your Mental Health in the New Millennium

Hope Press
PO Box 188
Duarte, CA 91009-0188   818-303-0644
                              800-321-4039
                         Fax: 818-358-3520
                              www.hopepress.com

Provides concise coping techniques for adults who have difficulties due to anxiety, depression, short temper, irritability, rage-attacks, compulsions, obbsession and attention defict hyperactivity disorder. *$19.95*

550 pages ISBN 1-878267-09-4

693 Conduct Disorders in Childhood and Adolescence, Developmental Clinical Psychology and Psychiatry

Sage Publications
2455 Teller Road
Thousand Oaks, CA 91320   805-499-9774
                              800-818-7243
                         Fax: 800-583-2665
                    E-mail: info@sagepub.com
                              www.sagepub.com

Conduct disorder is a clinical problem among children and adolescents that includes aggressive acts, theft, vandalism, firesetting, running away, truancy, defying authority and other antisocial behaviors. This book describes the nature of conduct disorder and what is currently known from research and clinical work. Topics include psychiatric dignosis, parent psychopathology and child-rearing processes. Paperback also available. *$43.95*

160 pages

694 Creative Therapy 2: Working with Parents

Impact Publishers
PO Box 6016
Atascadero, CA 93423-6016   805-466-5917
                              800-246-7228
                         Fax: 805-466-5919
                    E-mail: info@impactpublishers.com
                              www.impactpublishers.com

Sequel and companion volume to the authors' highly successful Creative Therapy with Children and Adolesents. Creative Therapy 2 offers practicing therapists a wealth of resources for working with parents whose children are experiencing emotional and/or behavioral problems. The procedures and exercises are carefully crafted to provide help even when the parents have been less than understanding - or perhaps even abusive toward their children. Therapists will find dozens of creative ways to form good working relationships with parents, and to prepare them to help their children. *$21.95*

192 pages ISBN 1-886230-42-0

695 Difficult Child

Bantam Doubleday Dell Publishing
1745 Broadway
New York, NY 10019   212-782-9000
                                             Fax: 212-782-9700
                E-mail: books@randomhouse.com
                             www.randomhouse.com

Help for parents dealing with behavioral problems. *$15.95*

696 Disruptive Behavior Disorders in Children and Adolescents

American Psychiatric Publishing
1000 Wilson Boulevard
Suite 1825
Arlington, VA 22209-3901   703-907-7322
                                              800-368-5777
                             Fax: 703-907-1091
                E-mail: appi@psych.org
                             www.appi.org

Katie Duffy, Marketing Assistant

$26.50

240 pages ISBN 0-880489-60-X

697 Dysinhibition Syndrome How to Handle Anger and Rage in Your Child or Spouse

Hope Press
PO Box 188
Duarte, CA 91009-0188   818-303-0644
                                              800-321-4039
                             Fax: 818-358-3520
                             www.hopepress.com

How to understand and handle rage and anger in your children or spouse. The book presents behavioral approaches that can be very effective and an understanding that can be family saving. *$24.95*

271 pages ISBN 1-878267-08-6

698 Helping Parents, Youth, and Teachers Understand Medications for Behavioral and Emotional Problems: Resource Book of Medication Information Handouts, Second Edition

American Psychiatric Publishing
1000 Wilson Boulevard
Suite 1825
Arlington, VA 20009-3901   703-907-7322
                                              800-368-5777
                             Fax: 703-907-1091
                E-mail: appi@psych.org
                             www.appi.org

Valuable resource for anyone involved in evaluating psychiatric disturbances in children and adolescents. Provides a compilation of information sheets to help promote the dialogue between the patient's family, caregivers and the treating physician. *$54.00*

224 pages Year Founded: 2003 ISBN 1-585620-41-6

699 How to Handle a Hard to Handle Kid: Parent's Guide to Understanding and Changing Problem Behaviors

Active Parenting Publishers
1955 Vaughn Road NW
Suite 108
Kennesaw, GA 30144-7808   770-429-0565
                                              800-825-0060
                             Fax: 770-429-0334
                E-mail: cservice@activeparenting.com
                             www.activeparenting.com

Some children are simply more challenging than others. In this book you'll learn why this is true, specific strategies for handling everyday problems, how to be an authoritative parent, how to respond effectively to certain behaviors and how to take care of yourself. *$15.95*

216 pages   ISSN Q8301

700 It's Nobody's Fault: New Hope and Help for Difficult Children and Their Parents

ADD WareHouse
300 NW 70th Avenue
Suite 102
Plantation, FL 33317   954-792-8100
                                              800-233-9273
                             Fax: 954-792-8545
                E-mail: sales@addwarehouse.com
                             www.addwarehouse.com

This book explains that neither the parents nor children are causes of mental disorders and related problems. *$20.00*

184 pages

701 Preventing Antisocial Behavior Interventions from Birth through Adolescence

Guilford Publications
72 Spring Street
New York, NY 10012   212-431-9800
                                              800-365-7006
                             Fax: 212-966-6708
                E-mail: info@guilford.com
                             www.guilford.com

Establishes the crucial link between theory, measurement, and intervention. Brings together a collection of studies that utilize experimental approaches for evaluating intervention programs for preventing deviant behavior. Demonstrates both the feasibility and necessity of independent evaluation. Also shows how the information obtained in such studies can be used to test and refine prevailing theories about human behavior in general and behavior changes in particular. *$45.00*

391 pages ISBN 0-898628-82-2

702 Skills Training for Children with Behavior Disorders

Courage to Change
PO Box 1268
Newburgh, NY 12551
                                              800-772-6499
                             Fax: 800-440-4003

Written for both parents and therapists, this book provides backround, instructions, and many reproducible worksheets. Academic success, anger management, emotional well being and compliance/following rules are covered. *$32.95*

272 pages

Periodicals & Pamphlets

703 Conduct Disorder in Children and Adolescents

Center for Mental Health Services: Knowledge Exchange Network
PO Box 42490
Washington, DC 20015

800-789-2647
Fax: 301-984-8796
TDD: 866-889-2647
E-mail: ken@mentalhealth.org
www.mentalhealth.org

This fact sheet defines conduct disorder, identifies risk factors, discusses types of help available, and suggests what parents or other caregivers can do.

2 pages

704 Mental, Emotional, and Behavior Disorders in Children and Adolescents

Center for Mental Health Services: Knowledge Exchange Network
PO Box 42490
Washington, DC 20015

800-789-2647
Fax: 301-984-8796
TDD: 866-889-2647
E-mail: ken@mentalhealth.org
www.mentalhealth.org

This fact sheet describes mental, emotional, and behavioral problems that can occur during childhood and adolescence and discusses related treatment, support services, and research.

4 pages

705 Treatment of Children with Mental Disorders

National Institute of Mental Health
6001 Executive Boulevard
Room 8184
Bethesda, MD 20892-9663

866-615-6464
Fax: 301-443-4279
TTY: 301-443-8431
E-mail: nimhinfo@nih.gov
www.nimh.nih.gov

Ruth Dubois, Assistant Chief

A short booklet that contains questions and answers about therapy for children with mental disorders. Includes a chart of mental disorders and medications used.

Research Centers

706 Child & Family Center

Menninger Clinic Department of Research
PO Box 829
Topeka, KS 66601-0829

713-275-5000
800-351-9058
Fax: 713-275-5107
www.menninger.edu

The Center's goals: to further develop emerging understanding of the impact of childhood maltreatment and abuse; to chart primary prevention strategies that will foster healthy patterns of caregiving and attachment and reduce the prevalence of maltreatment and abuse; to develop secondary prevention strategies that will promote early detection of attachment-related problems and effective interventions to avert the development of chornic and severe disorders; and to develop more effective treatment approaches for those individuals whose early attachment problems have eventuated in severe psychopathology.

Video & Audio

707 Active Parenting Today

Active Parenting Publishers
1955 Vaughn Road NW
Suite 108
Kennesaw, GA 30144-7808

770-429-0565
800-825-0060
Fax: 770-429-0334
E-mail: cservice@activeparenting.com
www.activeparenting.com

A complete video-based parenting education program curriculum. Helps parents of children ages two to twelve raise responsible, courageous children. Emphasizes nonviolent discipline, conflict resolution and improved communication. With Leader's Guide, videotapes, Parent's Guide and more. Also available in Spanish. *$ 349.00*

708 Managing the Defiant Child

Courage to Change
PO Box 1268
Newburgh, NY 12551

800-440-4003
Fax: 800-772-6499

Enhanced parenting skills can truly improve the parent child relationship. A partner video to Understanding the Defiant Child, this title is perfect for parents and professionals dealing with a child who is defiant, and/or has Oppositional Defiant Disorder or Conduct disorders. *$99.00*

709   Understanding and Treating the Hereditary Psychiatric Spectrum Disorders

Hope Press
PO Box 188
Duarte, CA 91009-0188
818-303-0644
800-321-4039
Fax: 818-358-3520
www.hopepress.com

David E Comings MD, Presenter

Learn with ten hours of audio tapes from a two day seminar given in May 1997 by David E Comings, MD. Tapes cover: ADHD, Tourette Syndrome, Obsessive-Compulsive Disorder, Conduct Disorder, Oppositional Defiant Disorder, Autism and other Hereditary Psychiatric Spectrum Disorders. Eight audio tapes. *$75.00*

Year Founded: 1997

710   Understanding the Defiant Child

Courage to Change
PO Box 1268
Newburgh, NY 12551
800-440-4003
Fax: 800-772-6499

Presents information on Oppositional Defiant Disorder and Conduct Disorder with scenes of family interactions, showing the nature and causes of these disorders and what can and should be done about it. 35 minutes with a manual that contains more information. *$99.00*

Web Sites

711   www.cyberpsych.org

CyberPsych

Hosts the American Psychoanalyists Foundation, American Association of Suicideology, Society for the Exploration of Psychotherapy Intergration, and Anxiety Disorders Association of America. Also subcategories of the anxiety disorders, as well as general information, including panic disorder, phobias, obsessive compulsive disorder (OCD), social phobia, generalized anxiety disorder, post traumatic stress disorder, and phobias of childhood. Book reviews and links to web pages sharing the topics.

712   www.planetpsych.com

Planetpsych.com

Learn about disorders, their treatments and other topics in psychology. Articles are listed under the related topic areas. Ask a therapist a question for free, or view the directory of professionals in your area. If you are a therapist sign up for the directory. Current features, self-help, interactive, and newsletter archives.

713   www.psychcentral.com

Psych Central

Personalized one-stop index for psychology, support, and mental health issues, resources, and people on the Internet.

Introduction

Feelings of sadness are common to everyone, and quite natural in reaction to appropriate circumstances. The death of a loved one, the end of a relationship, or other traumatic life experiences are bound to bring on the blues. But when feelings of sadness and despair persist beyond a reasonable period, arise for no particular reason, or begin to affect our ability to function, help is needed. Depression is a diagnosis made by a psychiatrist or other mental health professional to describe serious and prolonged symptoms of sadness or despair. While it is quite common, it is also a disease that no one should take lightly: Depression can be deadly. Some people who are deeply depressed think about or actually try to commit suicide. An even relatively mild depression, if untreated, can disrupt marriages and relationships or impede careers.

After giving birth, women may suffer from a spectrum of psychiatric disorders related to the demands of new motherhood and the abrupt hormonal changes that occur after delivery. A common postpartum condition is baby blues which begins within a few days of birth and causes increased emotional sensitivity to events, sometimes demonstrated by happy or sad tears. Reassurance is the only treatment required and the condition goes away spontaneously.

More serious is Postpartum Depression which often begins before birth, during pregnancy. The symptoms are the same as those of depression at any other time, but the mother's thoughts are preocced with concerns about whether she is a good mother. Unlike an average, tired new mother, the depressed woman cannot rest even when the baby is sleeping, loses her appetite and cannot enjoy her baby. She feels guilty about this and reluctant to tell her family about it. Severe Postpartum Depression, or Postpartum Psychosis, is a serious medical condition demanding professional attention, that causes confusion, disorienta-

tion, delusions, and hallucinations, and can cause suicide or infanticide.

SYMPTOMS

Depression is diagnosed when an individual experiences 1) persistent feelings of sadness or 2) loss of interest or pleasure in usual activities, in addition to five of the following symptoms for at least two weeks:
•Significant weight gain or loss unrelated to dieting;
•Inability to sleep or, conversely, sleeping too much;
•Restlessness and agitation;
•Fatigue or loss of energy;
•Feelings of worthlesness or guilt;
•Diminished ability to think or concentrate;
•Recurrent thoughts of death or suicide;
•Distress is not caused by a medication or the symptoms of a medical illness.

Postpartum Depression (in addition to symptoms above)
•Preoccupation with concerns of being a good mother;
•Inability to rest while the baby is sleeping;
•Inability to enjoy her baby accompanied with feeling of guilt;
•Reluctance to discuss her feelings with friends and family.

ASSOCIATED FEATURES

Because Depression can range from moderate to severe, people who are depressed may exhibit a variety of behaviors. Often, people who are depressed are tearful, irritable, or brooding. Problems sleeping (either insomnia or sleeping too much) are common. People with Depression may worry unnecessarily about being sick or having a disease, or they may report physical symptoms such as headaches or other pains. Depression can seriously affect people's friendships and intimate relationships.

Depression can make people worry about having a disease, but this is not a central symptom. Depression very frequently coexists with one or another anxiety disorder, and there is a genetic predisposition in some people.

Abuse of alcohol, prescription drugs, or illegal drugs is also common among people who are depressed. The most serious risk associated with Depression is the risk of suicide: people who have tried to commit suicide in the past, or who have family members who have commited suicide are especially at risk. Individuals who have another mental disorder, such as Schizophrenia, in addition to Depression are also more likely to commit suicide.

PREVALENCE

Every year more than 17 million Americans suffer some type of depressive illness. Depression does not discriminate; anyone can have it. Children, adults and the elderly are susceptible. Nevertheless, studies do indicate that women are twice as likely to have Depression as men. Depression has significant adverse effects on children's functioning and development; among adolescents, suicide is believed to be the fifth leading cause of death. Depression is also common among the elderly, and can be treated as an illness distinct from the loneliness or sadness that may accompany old age.

Very mild depression after delivery, or baby blues, affects over half, perhaps up to 90% of postpartum women. Baby blues is actually not depression at all; rather it is a common condition characterized by sensitivity and emotionality, both happy and sad. Postpartum Depression affects approximately 10% of new mothers. Much postpartum depression is a continuation of depression that was already present during pregnancy. The use of antidepressant drugs both during and after pregnancy, for nursing mothers, can be discussed with a patient's psychiatrist. There is an increasing amount of literature on the safety of medications at those times. Untreated depression has adverse consequences for fetus, mother and baby. Women who have had depression following one birth have a 50% chance of becoming depressed after a second delivery, and those who have had Postpartum Depression twice have a 75% likelihooder having a third baby. Postpartum Psychosis, a rare permu-

tation of postpartum conditions, affects fewer than 1% of women.

TREATMENT OPTIONS

Depression is a medical disease and does not respond to the usual ways we have of cheering up ourselves or others. In fact, attempts to cheer depressed invidiuals may have the opposite and unfortunate consequence of making them feel worse, often because they are frustrated and feel guilty that others' well-meaning efforts do not help. If a person experiences the symptoms of Depression, he or she should seek treatment from a qualified professional. The vast majority of people with Depression get better when they are treated properly, and virtually everyone gets some relief from their symptoms.

A psychiatrist or other mental health professional should conduct a thorough evaluation, including an interview; a physical examination should be done by a primary care provider. On the basis of a complete evaluation, the appropriate treatment will be prescribed. Most likely, the treatment will be medication or psychotherapy, or both. Antidepressants usually take effect within three to six weeks after treatment has begun; usually the prescribing psychiatrist will recommend that patients continue to take medication at least nine months to a year after symptoms have improved.

The natural course of depression is about nine months and then, even though patients may feel better on the medication, the depression is likely to come back if they discontinue their medication too early. In addition, depression recurs later in about 50% of patients after one episode, and more frequently if there is a second or third episode, so that some patients choose to remain on medication indefinitely to decrease their risk of recurrence. Dysthymic disorder is more low-level and chronic than major depressive episodes which last about nine months. Dysthymia can be treated with medication and psychotherapy as well.

Psychotherapy, or talk therapy, may be used to help the patient improve the way he or she thinks about things and deals with specific life problems.

Individual, family or couples therapy may be recommended, depending on the patient's life experiences. If the depression is not severe, treatment can take a few weeks; if the Depression has been a longstanding problem, it may take much longer, but in many cases, a patient will experience improvement in 10-15 sessions.

Treatment for Postpartum Depression is similar to treatment for depression in general. Possible risks of medications taken during pregnancy and breast-feeding have to be weighed against the risks of leaving the depression untreated.

Associations & Agencies

715 **Center for Family Support (CFS)**

333 7th Avenue
New York, NY 10001-5004
212-629-7939
Fax: 212-239-2211
www.cfsny.org

Steven Vernickofs, Executive Director

Service agency devoted to the physical well being and development of the retarded child and the sound mental health of the parents. Helps families with retarded children with all aspects of home care including counseling, referrals, home aide service and consultation. Offers intervention for parents at the birth of a retarded child with in-home support, guidance and infant stimulation. Pioneered training of nonprofessional women as home aides to provide supportive services in homes.

716 **Center for Mental Health Services Knowledge Exchange Network**

US Department of Health and Human Services
PO Box 42490
Washington, DC 20015-4800
800-789-2647
Fax: 301-984-8796
E-mail: ken@mentalhealth.org
www.mentalhealth.org

Information about resources, technical assistance, research, training, networks, and other federal clearing houses, and fact sheets and materials. Information specialists refer callers to mental health resources in their communities as well as state, federal and nonprofit contacts. Staff available Monday through Friday, 8:30 AM - 5:00 PM, EST, excluding federal holidays. After hours, callers may leave messages and an information specialist will return their call.

717 **Depression & Bi-Polar Support Alliance**

730 N Franklin Street
Suite 501
Chicago, IL 60610-7204
800-826-3632
Fax: 312-642-7243
www.dbsalliance.org

Lydia Lewis, President
Ingrid Deetz, Program Manager

Educates patients, families, professionals, and the public concerning the nature of depressive and manic-depressive illnesses as treatable medical diseases, fosters self-help for patients and families, works to eliminate discrimination and stigma, improves access to care, advocates for research toward the elimination of these illnesses.

718 **Depression & Related Affective Disorders Association: DRADA**

410-583-2919
E-mail: drada@jhmi.edu
www.drada.org

Catherine Pollock, Executive Director
Elizabeth Boyce, Director Development

Non profit association whose mission is to alleviate the suffering arising from depression and manic depression by assisting self - help groups, providing education and information and lending support to research programs.

719 **Depression After Delivery**

91 E Somerset Street
Raritan, NJ 08869-2129
908-575-9121
800-944-4773
Fax: 908-541-9713
www.depressionafterdelivery.com

Donna Cangialosi, Office Manager

Twenty four information request line. Free information packet of referrals and volunteer contacts nationwide for women with postpartum disorders.

720 **Depression and Bi-Polar Alliance**

730 N Franklin Street
Suite 501
Chicago, IL 60610-7204
800-826-3632
Fax: 312-642-7243
www.ndmda.org

Lydia Lewis, Executive Director
Julie Bremer, External Relations Director
Ann Spehal, Development Director

Previously called the National Depressive and Manic Depressive Association, the Depression and Bi-Polar Alliance publishes a variety of educational materials for adults and teens on mood disorders, all available free of charge or for a nominial fee. Because the Alliance focuses on the consumer living with a mood disorder, their publications are written in language free from medical and scientific jargon and everything they produce conveys a strong message of hope and optimism.

721 **Emotions Anonymous International Service Cen ter**

PO Box 4245
Saint Paul, MN 55104-0245
651-647-9712
Fax: 651-647-1593
E-mail: eaisc@mtn.org
www.EmotionsAnonymous.org

Karen Mead, Executive Director

Fellowship of men and women who share their experience, strength and hope with each other, that they may solve their common problem and help others recover from emotional illness. Uses the Twelve Steps of Alcoholics Anonymous, adapted to emotional problems. Disseminates literature and information, provides telephone referrals to local chapters. Publications: Emotions Anonymous Membership, book. New Message, quarterly magazine. Annual EA International Convention in September.

722 **Freedom From Fear**

308 Seaview Avenue
Staten Island, NY 10305
718-351-1717
Fax: 718-667-8893
www.freedomfromfear.com

Depression/Associations & Agencies

The mission of Freedom From Fear is to aid and counsel individuals and their families who suffer from anxiety and depressive illness.

723 NADD: Association for Persons with Developmental Disabilities and Mental Health Needs

132 Fair Street
Kingston, NY 12401-4802
845-334-4336
800-331-5362
Fax: 845-331-4569
E-mail: nadd@mhv.net
www.thenadd.org

Dr Robert Fletcher, Executive Director

Nonprofit organization designed to promote interest of professional and parent development with resources for individuals who have the coexistence of mental illness and mental retardation. Provides conference, educational services and training materials to professionals, parents, concerned citizens and service organizations. Formerly known as the National Association for the Dually Diagnosed.

724 National Alliance for Research on Schizophrenia and Depression

60 Cutter Mill Road
Suite 404
Great Neck, NY 11021-3104
516-487-6930
800-829-8289
Fax: 516-487-6930
E-mail: info@narsad.org
www.narsad.org

Constance Lieber, President
Steven G Doochin, Executive Director

Nonprofit corporation and registered public charity. Raises and distributes funds for scientific research into the causes, cures, treatments and prevention of brain disorders.

725 National Alliance for the Mentally Ill

2107 Wilson Boulevard
Suite 300
Arlington, VA 22201-3042
703-524-7600
800-950-6264
Fax: 703-524-9094
TDD: 703-516-7227
E-mail: helpline@nami.org
www.nami.org

Laurie Flynn, Executive Director

Nation's leading self-help organization for all those affected by severe brain disorders. Mission is to bring consumers and families with similar experiences together to share information about services, care providers, and ways to cope with the challenges of schizophrenia, manic depression, and other serious mental illnesses.

726 National Foundation for Depressive Illness: NAFDI

PO Box 2257
New York, NY 10116-2257
800-239-1265
www.depression.org

Peter Ross, Executive Director
Amy C Rusell, Administrator

NAFDI's purpose is to inform the public, primary health care providers, other health care professionals and corporations about depression, and provide the information about correct diagnosis and treatment and the availability of qualified doctors and support groups.

727 National Institute of Mental Health

6001 Executive Boulevard
Room 8184
Bethesda, MD 20892-9663
866-615-6464
Fax: 301-443-4279
TTY: 301-443-8431
E-mail: nimhinfo@nih.gov
www.nimh.nih.gov

Information and resources concerning depression, manic depression, bi-polar disorder and other mental health issues.

728 National Mental Health Consumer's Self-Help Clearinghouse

1211 Chestnut Street
Suite 1207
Philadelphia, PA 19107
215-751-1810
800-553-4539
Fax: 215-636-6312
E-mail: info@mhselfhelp.org
www.mhselfhelp.org

Alex Morrsey, Information/Referral

Funded by the National Institute of Mental Health Community Support Program, the purpose of the Clearinghouse is to encourage the development and growth of consumer self-help groups.

Year Founded: 1992

729 National Organization for Seasonal Affective Disorder (SAD)

PO Box 40133
Washington, DC 20016
www.nosad.com

Increases awareness of effects of seasonal affective disorder and offers support and information on treatment for those individuals diagnosed with the condition.

730 New York City Depressive & Manic Depressive Group

100 LaSalle Street
Suite 5A
New York, NY 10027
917-445-2399
E-mail: nycdmdg@aol.com
www.columbia.edu/~jgg17/DMDA/PAGE_1.html

Support groups meets regularly at Mt. Siani Hospital. Web page has helpful information and links to mental health sites.

731 Postpartum Support International

927 N Kellogg Avenue
Santa Barbara, CA 93111
805-967-7636

104

Increases awareness of emotional changes in women while pregnant and after childbirth.

732 Suncoast Residential Training Center/Developmental Services Program

Goodwill Industries-Suncoast
10596 Gandy Boulevard
PO Box 14456
St. Petersburg, FL 33702   727-523-1512
                                  Fax: 727-577-2749
                          www.goodwill-suncoast.org

Jay McCloe, Director Resource Development

A large group home which serves individuals diagnosed as mentally retarded with a secondary diagnosed of psychiatric difficulties as evidenced by problem behavior. Providing residential, behavioral and instructional support and services that will promote the development of adaptive, socially appropriate behavior, each individual is assessed to determine, socialization, basic academics and recreation. The primary intervention strategy is applied behavior analysis. Professional consultants are utilized to address the medical, dental, psychiatric and pharmacological needs of ech individual. One of the most popular features is the active community integration component of SRTC. Program customers attend an average of 15 monthly outings to various community events.

Books

---

733 Anxiety and Depression in Adults and Children, Banff International Behavioral Science Series

Sage Publications
2455 Teller Road
Thousand Oaks, CA 91320   805-499-9774
                                 800-818-7243
                           Fax: 800-583-2665
                      E-mail: info@sagepub.com
                               www.sagepub.com

Collection of papers by well respected researchers in the field of anxiety and depression. Brings together desparate areas of research and integrates them in an informative and interesting way. Focuses on recent advances in treating anxiety and depression in adults and children. Topics include self-management therapy, assessing and treating sexually abused children and unipolar depression. Integrates empirical research with clinical applications. Paperback also available. *$46.95*

296 pages ISBN 0-803970-20-X

734 Breaking the Patterns of Depression

Random House
1745 Broadway
New York, NY 10019   212-782-9000
                                 800-733-3000
                           Fax: 212-572-6066
                        www.randomhouse.com

Presents skills that enable readers to understand and ultimately avert depression's recurring cycles. Focusing on future prevention as well as initial treatment, the book includes over one hundred structured activities to help sufferers learn the skills necessary to become and remain depression-free. Translates the clinical literature on psychotherapy and antidepressant medication into understandable language. Defines what causes depression and clarifies what can be done about it. With this knowledge in hand, readers can control their depression, rather than having depression control them. *$13.95*

362 pages ISBN 0-385483-70-8

735 Broken Connection: On Death and the Continuity of Life

American Psychiatric Publishing
1000 Wilson Boulevard
Suite 1825
Arlington, VA 22209   703-907-7322
                                 800-368-5777
                           Fax: 703-907-1091
                    E-mail: appi@psych.org
                               www.appi.org

Katie Duffy, Marketing Assistant

Exploration of the inescapable connections between death and life, the psychiatric disorders that arise from these connections, and the advent of the nuclear age which has jeopardized any attempts to ensure the perpetuation of the self beyond death. *$38.00*

474 pages ISBN 0-880488-74-3

736 Check Up from the Neck Up, Ensuring your Mental Health in the New Millennium

Hope Press
PO Box 188
Duarte, CA 91009-0188   818-303-0644
                                 800-321-4039
                           Fax: 818-358-3520
                         www.hopepress.com

Provides concise coping techniques for adults who have difficulties due to anxiety, depression, short temper, irritability, rage-attacks, compulsions, obsession and attention deficit hyperactivity disorder. *$19.95*

550 pages ISBN 1-878267-09-4

737 Clinical Guide to Depression in Children and Adolescents

American Psychiatric Publishing
1000 Wilson Boulevard
Suite 1825
Arlington, VA 22209-3901   703-907-7322
                                 800-368-5777
                           Fax: 703-907-1091
                    E-mail: appi@psych.org
                               www.appi.org

Katie Duffy, Marketing Assistant

Integrates advances in the recognition, diagnosis, management, and treatment of depressive disorders and bipolar disorders in infancy, childhood, and adolescence. *$39.50*

304 pages ISBN 0-880483-56-3

738 Cognitive Vulnerability to Depression

Guilford Publications
72 Spring Street
New York, NY 10012   212-431-9800
800-365-7006
Fax: 212-966-6708
E-mail: info@guilford.com
www.guilford.com

Explores what makes some people more vulnerable to recurrence of depressive episodes following successful treatments. Combines the most current research and theory on cognitive vulnerability. Covering methodligical, theoretical and empirical issues, the authors review cognitive theories of depression, explicate and assess the vulnerability approach to psychopathology and formulate an integrative view of the key proximal and distal antecedents of depression in adults. *$37.95*

307 pages ISBN 1-572303-04-2

739 Comorbid Depression in Older People

American Psychiatric Publishing
1000 Wilson Boulevard
Suite 1825
Arlington, VA 22209-3901   703-907-7322
800-368-5777
Fax: 703-907-1091
E-mail: appi@psych.org
www.appi.org

Katie Duffy, Marketing Assistant

Contents include how common depression is in older people with physical illness, who will become depressed, depression in specific physical illness, recognizing depression in older people, detection of depression by clinical staff, improving detection, depression and suicide in older mentally ill patients, and depression and outcome. *$14.95*

88 pages ISBN 1-853175-71-4

740 Consumer's Guide to Psychiatric Drugs

New Harbinger Publications
5674 Shattuck Avenue
Oakland, CA 94609-1662   510-652-2002
800-748-6273
Fax: 510-652-5472
E-mail: customerservice@newharbinger.com
www.newharbinger.com

Helps consumers understand what treatment options are available and what side effects to expect. Covers possible interactions with other drugs, medical conditions and other concerns. Explains how each drug works, and offers detailed information about treatments for depression, bipolar disorder, anxiety and sleep disorders, as well as other conditions. *$16.95*

340 pages ISBN 1-572241-11-X

741 Depression & Anxiety Management

New Harbinger Publications
5674 Shattuck Avenue
Oakland, CA 94609-1662   510-652-2002
800-748-6273
Fax: 510-652-5472
E-mail: customerservice@newharbinger.com
www.newharbinger.com

Offers step-by-step help for identifying the thoughts that make one anxious and depressed, confronting unrealistic and distorted thinking, and replacing negative mental patterns with healthy, realistic thinking. *$11.95*

ISBN 1-879237-46-6

742 Depression Workbook: a Guide for Living with Depression

New Harbinger Publications
5674 Shattuck Avenue
Oakland, CA 94609-1662   510-652-2002
800-748-6273
Fax: 510-652-5472
E-mail: customerservice@newharbinger.com
www.newharbinger.com

Based on responses of participants sharing their insights, experiences, and strategies for living with extreme mood swings. *$18.95*

320 pages ISBN 1-879237-32-6

743 Depression and Anxiety

American Psychiatric Publishing
1000 Wilson Boulevard
Suite 1825
Arlington, VA 22209-3901   703-907-7322
800-368-5777
Fax: 703-907-1091
E-mail: appi@psych.org
www.appi.org

Katie Duffy, Marketing Assistant

$14.95

88 pages ISBN 1-853170-56-9

744 Depression and Its Treatment

Time Warner Books
3 Center Plaza
Boston, MA 02108   800-759-0190
E-mail: sales@aoltwbg.com
www.twbookmark.com

A layman's guide to help one understand and cope with America's number one mental health problem. *$19.95*

157 pages

745 Depression in General Practice

American Psychiatric Publishing
1000 Wilson Boulevard
Suite 1825
Arlington, VA 22209-3901   703-907-7322
800-368-5777
Fax: 703-907-1091
E-mail: appl@psych.org
www.appi.org

Katie Duffy, Marketing Assistant

Contents include explanation of depression, treatment and management of depression, suicide, and skills and training requirements of general practitioners in mental health. *$14.95*

64 pages ISBN 1-853172-88-X

746 Depression, Anxiety and the Mixed Condition

American Psychiatric Publishing
1000 Wilson Boulevard
Suite 1825
Arlington, VA 22209-3901   703-907-7322
                                  800-368-5777
                              Fax: 703-907-1091
                      E-mail: appi@psych.org
                                  www.appi.org

Katie Duffy, Marketing Assistant

Contents include diagnosis and classification, general principles of treatment, treament of depression suicide, DSH and anxiety, mixed anxiety and depression, and treating difficult cases. *$14.95*

72 pages ISBN 1-853173-59-2

747 Depression, the Mood Disease

Johns Hopkins University Press
2715 N Charles Street
Baltimore, MD 21218-4319   410-516-6900
                                  800-537-5487
                              Fax: 410-516-6998

Explores the many faces of an illness that will affect as many as 36 million Americans at some point in their lives. Updated to reflect state-of-the-art treatment. *$12.76*

240 pages ISBN 0-801851-84-X

748 Depression: How it Happens, How it's Healed

New Harbinger Publications
5674 Shattuck Avenue
Oakland, CA 94609-1662   510-652-2002
                                800-748-6273
                            Fax: 510-652-5472
          E-mail: customerservice@newharbinger.com
                      www.newharbinger.com

Explains how chemical changes in the brain contribute to feelings of depression, details the facts about the drugs used to treat depression, and suggests ways to make psychotherapy a helpful component of the healing process. *$14.95*

160 pages ISBN 1-572241-00-4

749 Diagnosis and Treatment of Depression in Late Life: Results of the NIH Consensus Development Conference

American Psychiatric Publishing
1000 Wilson Boulevard
Suite 1825
Arlington, VA 22209-3901   703-907-7322
                                  800-368-5777
                              Fax: 703-907-1091
                      E-mail: appi@psych.org
                                  www.appi.org

Katie Duffy, Marketing Assistant

Provides comprehensive studies in early life depression versus late life depression, the prevalence of depression in elderly people and the risk factors involved. *$21.95*

536 pages ISBN 0-880485-56-6

750 Emotions Anonymous Membership Book

Emotions Anonymous
PO Box 4245
Saint Paul, MN 55104-0245   651-647-9712
                               Fax: 651-647-1593
                       E-mail: eaisc@mtn.org
                      www.emotionsanonymous.org

Karen Mead, Executive Director

Fellowship of men and women who share their experience, strength and hope with each other, that they may solve their common problem and help others recover from emotional illness. Uses the Twelve Steps of Alcoholics Anonymous, adapted to emotional problems. Hardcover also available. *$10.15*

260 pages ISBN 0-960735-65-8

751 Encyclopedia of Depression

Facts on File
132 W 31st Street
17th Floor
New York, NY 10001
                                  800-322-8755
                              Fax: 800-678-3633
              E-mail: custserv@factsonfile.com
                              www.factsonfile.com

This volume defines and explains all terms and topics relating to depression. *$58.50*

170 pages

752 Everything You Need To Know About Depression

Rosen Publishing Group
29 E 21st Street
New York, NY 10010
                                  800-237-9932
                              Fax: 888-436-4643
              E-mail: info@rosenpub.com
                      www.rosenpublishing.com

An important resource for teens who are looking for help with depression. *$25.25*

Year Founded: 2001 ISBN 0-823934-39-X

753 Growing Up Sad: Childhood Depression and Its Treatment

WW Norton & Company
500 5th Avenue
New York, NY 10100   212-354-5500
                            800-233-4830
                        Fax: 212-869-0856
              E-mail: npb@wwnorton.com
                      www.wwnorton.com

The authors have updated their classic study, Why Isn't Johnny Crying? that looks at the symptoms and treatment of childhood - onset depression. The authors give an authoritative summary of research, counsel prompt diagnosis, and assert that the disorder is treatable. *$25.00*

216 pages ISBN 0-393317-88-9

754 Help Me, I'm Sad: Recognizing, Treating, and Preventing Childhood and Adolescent Depression

Penguin Putnam
375 Hudson Street
New York, NY 10014-3658

212-366-2000
800-227-9604
Fax: 201-896-8569
www.pengiunputnam.com

Especially helpful to parents and other caregivers in recognizing the warning sigins of depression whatever the development stage. Offers case histories to illustrate what childhood-onset depression looks like at different ages. *$14.00*

200 pages

755 Helping Your Depressed Teenager: a Guide for Parents and Caregivers

John Wiley & Sons
605 3rd Avenue
New York, NY 10058-0180

212-850-6000
Fax: 212-850-6008
E-mail: info@wiley.com
www.wiley.com

The authors, a psychologist and a social worker, contrast clinical depression with normal adolescent mood changes. They deal realistically with teenage suicide and urge prompt intervention. *$ 16.95*

184 pages ISBN 0-471621-84-6

756 Herbs for the Mind: What Science Tells Us about Nature's Remedies for Depression, Stress, Memory Loss and Insomnia

Guilford Publications
72 Spring Street
New York, NY 10012

212-431-9800
800-365-7006
Fax: 212-966-6708
E-mail: info@guilford.com
www.guilford.com

Offers an authoritive guide to the most popular herbs for the mind, St. John's wort, kava, valerian and ginkgo. Clear guidelines are provided for developing an herbal self-help regimen, evaluating its ongoing effectiveness, and recognizing when professional intervention may be necessary. A reliable scientific source for answers to frequently asked questions about herbal remedies. *$14.95*

260 pages ISBN 1-572304-76-6

757 How to Cope with Mental Illness In Your Family: Guide for Siblings and Offspring

Health Source
1404 K Street NW
Washington, DC 20005-2401

202-789-7303
800-713-7122
Fax: 202-789-7899
E-mail: healthsource@appi.org
www.healthsourcebooks.org

Illnesses such as schizophrenia, manic depression and major depression are discussed. Also provides the tools to overcome the devastating effects of growing up or living in a family where these disorders exist. Covers the essential stages of recovery and how to reclaim their life. *$13.95*

240 pages ISBN 0-874779-23-5

758 Inside Manic Depression

Sunnyside Press
PO Box 1717
San Marcos, CA 92079-1717

619-424-3348

The true story of one victim's triumph over despair. A first person account. *$13.95*

176 pages

759 Interpersonal Psychotherapy for Dysthymic Di sorder

American Psychiatric Publishing
1000 Wilson Boulevard
Suite 1825
Arlington, VA 22209-3901

703-907-7322
800-368-5777
Fax: 703-907-1091
E-mail: appi@psych.org
www.appi.org

Katie Duffy, Marketing Assistant

Examines the use of psychotherapy for dysthymic disorder, or chronic depression. Contains case examples that illustrate how to use this treatment approach. *$32.50*

176 pages ISBN 0-880489-14-6

760 Is Full Recovery from Depression Possible?

American Psychiatric Publishing
1000 Wilson Boulevard
Suite 1825
Arlington, VA 22209-3901

703-907-7322
800-368-5777
Fax: 703-907-1091
E-mail: appi@psych.org
www.appi.org

Katie Duffy, Marketing Assistant

Analyzes the efficacy and econonic benefits of the correct therapeutic treatment of depressed patients. *$14.95*

56 pages ISBN 1-853177-49-0

761 Is That All There Is? Balancing Expectation and Disappointment in Your Life

Impact Publishers
PO Box 6016
Atascadero, CA 93423-6016

805-466-5917
800-246-7228
Fax: 805-466-5919
E-mail: info@impactpublishers.com
www.impactpublishers.com

Offers an antidote for those whose hopes and expectations exceed reality. The book explains the psychology of disappointment, the social influences that contribute to it, the variety of ways we deal with it, and how each of us can convert it to a force for positive growth in our lives. *$15.95*

224 pages ISBN 1-886230-13-7

762 It's Nobody's Fault: New Hope and Help for Difficult Children and Their Parents

ADD WareHouse
300 NW 70th Avenue
Suite 102
Plantation, FL 33317   **954-792-8100**
                                   800-233-9273
                          Fax: 954-792-8545
              E-mail: sales@addwarehouse.com
                      www.addwarehouse.com

This book explains that neither the parents nor children are causes of mental disorders and related problems. *$20.00*

184 pages

763 Lonely, Sad, and Angry: a Parent's Guide to Depression in Children and Adolescents

ADD Warehouse
300 NW 70th Avenue
Suite 102
Plantation, FL 33317   **954-792-8100**
                                   800-233-9273
                          Fax: 954-792-8545
                      www.addwarehouse.com

Covers the symptoms of depression, its diagnosis, causes, treatment (including medication), suicide, and management strategies at home and at school. For parents and teenagers. *$14.95*

225 pages

764 Loss and Beveavement: Managing Change

American Psychiatric Publishing
1000 Wilson Boulevard
Suite 1825
Arlington, VA 22209-3901   **703-907-7322**
                                     800-368-5777
                           Fax: 703-907-1091
                    E-mail: appi@psych.org
                             www.appi.org

Katie Duffy, Marketing Assistant

Practical guide for all involved in teaching and learning about bereavement, loss and managing change. *$34.95*

288 pages ISBN 0-632047-87-

765 Management of Depression

American Psychiatric Publishing
1000 Wilson Boulevard
Suite 1825
Arlington, VA 22209-3901   **703-907-7322**
                                     800-368-5777
                           Fax: 703-907-1091
                    E-mail: appi@psych.org
                             www.appi.org

Katie Duffy, Marketing Assistant

Comprehensive text all the important issues in the management of depression. *$39.95*

136 pages ISBN 1-853175-47-1

766 Managing Depression

American Counseling Association
5999 Stevenson Avenue
Alexandria, VA 22304-3300
                                     800-347-6647
                           Fax: 703-823-0252
             E-mail: webmaster@counseling.org
                        www.counseling.org

Offers hands-on methods for helping depressed clients. Explores the roots and causes of depression, different approaches to treatment, strategies for managing various forms, the manner in which depression affects certain populations and treatment considerations for administering antidepressant medications. *$29.95*

305 pages ISBN 1-886330-10-7

767 Medical Management of Depression

EMIS Medical Publishers
PO Box 820062
Dallas, TX 75382-0062
                                     800-225-0694
                           Fax: 214-349-2266
              E-mail: emis@redriverrok.com
                          www.emispub.com

Mark Gibson, VP Operations

Provides a comprehensive, but user-friendly guide for healthcare professionals to the growing number of options in the medical assessment and treatment of depression. Paperback. *$17.95*

272 pages ISBN 0-929240-83-9

768 Mood Apart

Basic Books
387 Park Avenue S
New York, NY 10016   **212-340-8100**

An overview of depression and manic depression and the available treatments for them. *$24.00*

363 pages

769 Mood Apart: Thinker's Guide to Emotion & It' s Disorders

Harper Collins
10 E 53rd Street
New York, NY 10022   **212-207-7000**
              E-mail: sales@harpercollins.com
                        www.harpercollins.com

Discussion of depression and mania includes symptoms, human costs, biological underpinnings, and therapies. Authoritatively written, it uses case histories, appendices, and historical references. *$15.00*

ISBN 0-060977-40-X

770 Natural History of Mania, Depression and Schizophrenia

American Psychiatric Publishing
1000 Wilson Boulevard
Suite 1825
Arlington, VA 22209-3901   **703-907-7322**
                                      800-368-5777
                          Fax: 703-907-1091
                E-mail: appi@psych.org
                          www.appi.org

Katie Duffy, Marketing Assistant

An unusual look at the course of mental illness, based on data from the Iowa 500 Research Project. *$42.50*

336 pages ISBN 0-880487-26-7

771 On the Edge of Darkness

Doubleday
666 5th Avenue
New York, NY 10103-0001   **212-765-6500**
                          Fax: 212-492-9700
                www.randomhouse.com

Multiple brief descriptions, primarily by celebrities, of their experiences with depression. *$22.50*

352 pages

772 Overcoming Depression

Harper Collins
10 E 53rd Street
New York, NY 10022   **212-207-7000**
                    Fax: 800-822-4090
          www.harpercollins.com

Described as one of the most comprehensive books available for the layperson on depression. Covers the full range of mood disorders. *$15.00*

ISBN 0-060927-82-8

773 Pain Behind the Mask: Overcoming Masculine Depression

Haworth Press
10 Alice Street
Binghamton, NY 13904-1580   **607-722-5857**
                                800-429-6784
                    Fax: 607-722-1424
          E-mail: getinfo@haworthpress.com
                    www.haworthpress.com

Presents a model of masculinity based on the premise that men express depression through behaviors that distort the feelings and human conflicts they experience. *$39.95*

ISBN 0-789005-57-3

774 Pastoral Care of Depression

Haworth Press
10 Alice Street
Binghamton, NY 13904-1503   **607-722-5857**
                                800-429-6784
                          Fax: 800-895-0582
          E-mail: getinfo@haworthpressinc.com
                          www.haworthpress.com

Helps caregivers by overcoming the simplistic myths about depressive disorders and probing the real issues. *$14.95*

ISBN 0-789002-65-5

775 Post-Natal Depression: Psychology, Science and the Transition to Motherhood

Routledge
2727 Palisade Avenue
Suite 4H
Bronx, NY 10463-1020   **888-765-1209**
                          Fax: 718-796-0971
                E-mail: vd6@columbia.edu

$23.95

ISBN 0-415163-62-5

776 Postpartum Mood Disorders

American Psychiatric Publishing
1000 Wilson Boulevard
Suite 1825
Arlington, VA 22209-3901   **703-907-7322**
                                      800-368-5777
                          Fax: 703-907-1091
                E-mail: appi@psych.orgg
                          www.appi.org

Katie Duffy, Marketing Assistant

Provides thorough coverage of a highly prevalent, but often misunderstood subject. *$38.50*

280 pages ISBN 0-880489-29-4

777 Practice Guideline for Major Depressive Disorders in Adults

American Psychiatric Publishing
1000 Wilson Boulevard
Suite 1825
Arlington, VA 22209-3901   **703-907-7322**
                                      800-368-5777
                          Fax: 703-907-1091
                E-mail: appi@psych.org
                          www.appi.org

Katie Duffy, Marketing Assistant

Summarizes the specific forms of somatic, psychotherapeutic, psychosocial, and educational treatments developed to deal with major depressive order and its various subtypes. *$22.50*

51 pages ISBN 0-890423-01-6

778 Predictors of Treatment Response in Mood Disorders

American Psychiatric Publishing
1000 Wilson Boulevard
Suite 1825
Arlington, VA 22209-3901   703-907-7322
    800-368-5777
Fax: 703-907-1091
E-mail: appi@psych.org
www.appi.org

Katie Duffy, Marketing Assistant

Helps clinicians and managed care administrators assign the correct somatic therapy. *$29.00*

224 pages ISBN 0-880484-94-2

779 Prozac Nation: Young & Depressed in America, a Memoir

Houghton Mifflin Company
222 Berkeley Street
Boston, MA 02116   617-351-5000
www.hmco.com

Struck with depression at 11, Wurtzel, now 27, chronicles her struggle with the illness. Witty, terrifying and sometimes funny, it tells the story of a young life almost destroyed by depression. *$19.95*

317 pages

780 Questions & Answers About Depression & Its Treatment

Charles Press Publishers
117 S 17th Street
Suite 310
Philadelphia, PA 19103   215-496-9616
Fax: 215-496-9637
E-mail: mailbox@charlespresspub.com
www.charlespresspub.com

All the questions you'd like to ask, with answers.

136 pages

781 Seasonal Affective Disorder and Beyond: Light Treatment for SAD and Non-SAD Conditions

American Psychiatric Publishing
1000 Wilson Boulevard
Suite 1825
Arlington, VA 22209-3901   703-907-7322
    800-368-5777
Fax: 703-907-1091
E-mail: appi@psych.org
www.appi.org

Katie Duffy, Marketing Assistant

Summarizes issues around the therapeutic uses of light treatment. *$45.00*

320 pages ISBN 0-880488-67-0

782 Stories of Depression: Does this Sound Like You?

National Institute of Mental Health
6001 Executive Boulevard
Room 8184
Bethesda, MD 20892-9663   866-615-6464
Fax: 301-443-4279
TTY: 301-443-8431
E-mail: nimhinfo@nih.gov
www.nimh.nih.gov

Are you feeling really sad, tired, and worried most of the time? Are these feelings lasting more than a few days? If yes, you may have depression.

20 pages

783 Today Meditation Book

Emotions Anonymous
PO Box 4245
Saint Paul, MN 55104-0245   651-647-9712
Fax: 651-647-1593
E-mail: eaisc@mtn.org
www.EmotionsAnonymous.org

Karen Mead, Executive Director

Paperback. *$8.00*

400 pages ISBN 0-960735-62-3

784 Treatment Plans and Interventions for Depression and Anxiety Disorders

Guilford Publications
72 Spring Street
New York, NY 10012   212-431-9800
    800-365-7006
Fax: 212-966-6708
E-mail: info@guilford.com
www.guilford.com

Provides information on treatments for seven frequently encountered disorders: major depression, generalized anxiety, panic, agoraphobia, PTSD, social phobia, specific phobia and OCD. Serving as ready to use treatment packages, chapters describe basic cognitive behavioral therapy techniques and how to tailor them to each disorder. Also featured are diagnostic decision trees, therapist forms for assessment and record keeping, client handouts and homework sheets. *$ 49.50*

332 pages ISBN 1-572305-14-2

785 Treatment for Chronic Depression: Cognitive Behavioral Analysis System of Psychotherapy (CBASP)

Guilford Publications
72 Spring Street
New York, NY 10012   212-431-9800
    800-365-7006
Fax: 212-966-6708
E-mail: info@guilford.com
www.guilford.com

This book describes CBASP, a research based psychotherapeutic approach designed to motivate chronically depressed patients to change and help them develop needed problem solving and relationship skills. Filled with illustrative case material that brings challenging clinical situations to life, this book now puts the power of CBASP in the hands of the clinician. Readers are provided with two essential assets: an innovative framework for understanding the patient's psychopathology and a disciplined plan for helping the individual overthrow depression. *$35.00*

326 pages ISBN 1-572305-27-4

786 When Nothing Matters Anymore: a Survival Guide for Depressed Teens

Free Spirit Publishing
217 5th Avenue N
Suite 200
Minneapolis, MN 55401-1299   **612-338-2068**
                                         800-735-7323
                              Fax: 612-337-5050
              E-mail: help4kids@freespirit.com
                          www.freespirit.com

Betsy Gabler, Sales Manager

Written for teens with depression and those who feel despondent, dejected or alone. This powerful book offers help, hope, and potentially lifesaving facts and advice. *$13.98*

176 pages ISBN 1-575420-36-8

787 Winter Blues

Guilford Publications
72 Spring Street
New York, NY 10012   **212-431-9800**
                                800-365-7006
                        Fax: 212-966-6708
              E-mail: info@guilford.com
                          www.guilford.com

Complete information about Seasonal Affective Disorder and its treatment. *$14.95*

788 Yesterday's Tomorrow

Hazelden
15251 Pleasant Valley Road
Center City, MN 55012-9640   **612-257-4010**
                                         800-822-0080
                              Fax: 612-257-4449
                          www.hazelden.org

Meditation book that shows why and how recovery works, from the author's own experiences. *$12.00*

432 pages ISBN 1-568381-60-3

789 You Can Beat Depression: Guide to Prevention and Recovery

Impact Publishers
PO Box 6016
Atascadero, CA 93423-6016   **805-466-5917**
                                        800-246-7228
                             Fax: 805-466-5919
              E-mail: info@impactpublishers.com
                          www.impactpublishers.com

Includes material on prevention of depression, prevention of relapse after treatment, brief therapy interventions, exercise, other non medical approaches and the Prozac controversy. Helps readers recognize when and how to help themsevles, and when to turn to professional treatment. *$14.95*

176 pages ISBN 1-886230-40-4

Periodicals & Pamphlets

790 Depression

National Institute of Mental Health
6001 Executive Boulevard
Room 8184
Bethesda, MD 20892-9663
                                        866-615-6464
                              Fax: 301-443-4279
                              TTY: 301-443-8431
                  E-mail: nimhinfo@nih.gov
                          www.nimh.nih.gov

This brochure gives descriptions of major depression, dysthymia and bipolar disorder (manic depression). It lists symptoms, gives possible causes, tells how depression is diagnosed and discusses available treatments. This brochure provides help and hope for the depressed person, family and friends.

23 pages

791 Depression in Children and Adolescents: A Fact Sheet for Physicians

National Institute of Mental Health
6001 Executive Boulevard
Room 8184
Bethesda, MD 20892-9663
                                        866-615-6464
                              Fax: 301-443-4279
                              TTY: 301-443-8431
                  E-mail: nimhinfo@nih.gov
                          www.nimh.nih.gov

Discusses the scope of the problem and the screening tools used in evaluating children with depression.

8 pages

792 Depression: Help On the Way

ETR Associates
4 Carbonero Way
Scotts Valley, CA 95066   **831-438-4060**
                                      800-321-4407
                           Fax: 800-435-8433
              E-mail: customerservice@etr.org
                          www.etr.org

Includes symptoms of minor depression, major depression, and seasonal affective depression; treatment options and medication, and the importance of exercise and laughter. Sold in lots of 50.

793 Depression: What Every Woman Should Know

National Institute of Mental Health
6001 Executive Boulevard
Room 8184
Bethesda, MD 20892-9663

866-615-6464
Fax: 301-443-4279
TTY: 301-443-8431
E-mail: nimhinfo@nih.gov
www.nimh.nih.gov

This booklet discusses the symptoms of depression and some of the reasons that make women so vulnerable. It also discusses the types of therapy and where to go for help.

24 pages

794 Let's Talk About Depression

National Institute of Mental Health
6001 Executive Boulevard
Room 8184
Bethesda, MD 20892-9663

866-615-6464
Fax: 301-443-4279
TTY: 301-443-8431
E-mail: nimhinfo@nih.gov
www.nimh.nih.gov

Facts about depression, and ways to get help. Target audience is teenaged youth.

795 Major Depression in Children and Adolescents

Center for Mental Health Services: Knowledge Exchange Network
PO Box 42490
Washington, DC 20015

800-789-2647
Fax: 301-984-8796
TDD: 866-889-2647
E-mail: ken@mentalhealth.org
www.mentalhealth.org

This fact sheet defines depression and its signs, identifies types of help available, and suggests what parents or other caregivers can do.

2 pages

796 Men and Depression

National Institute of Mental Health
6001 Executive Boulevard
Room 8184
Bethesda, MD 20892-9663

866-615-6464
Fax: 301-443-4279
TTY: 301-443-8431
E-mail: nimhinfo@nih.gov
www.nimh.nih.gov

Have you known a man who is grumpy, irritable, and has no sense of humor? Maybe he drinks too much or abuses drugs. Maybe he physically or verbally abuses his wife and his kids. Maybe he works all the time, or compulsively seeks thrills in high-risk behavior. Or maybe he seems isolated, withdrawn, and no longer interested in the people or activities he used to enjoy. Perhaps this man is you. Talk to a healthcare provider about how you are feeling, and ask for help.

36 pages

797 New Message

Emotions Anonymous
PO Box 4245
Saint Paul, MN 55104-0245

651-647-9712
Fax: 651-647-1593
E-mail: eaisc@mtn.org
www.EmotionsAnonymous.org

Karen Mead, Executive Director

Quarterly magazine. *$8.00*

4 per year

798 Recovering Your Mental Health: a Self-Help Guide

Center for Mental Health Services: Knowledge Exchange Network
PO Box 42490
Washington, DC 20015

800-789-2647
Fax: 301-984-8796
TDD: 866-889-2647
E-mail: ken@mentalhealth.org
www.mentalhealth.org

This booklet offers tips for understanding symptoms of depression and other conditions and getting help. Also details the advantages of counseling, medications available, options for professional help, relaxation techniques and paths to positive thinking.

32 pages

799 Storm In My Brain

Depression & Bi-Polar Support Alliance
730 N Franklin Street
Suite 501
Chicago, IL 60610-7204

800-826-3632
Fax: 312-642-7243
www.dbsalliance.org

Lydia Lewis, President
Ingrid Deetz, Program Director

Pamphlet free on the Internet or by mail. Discusses child or adolescent Bi-Polar symptoms.

800 What Do These Students Have in Common?

National Institute of Mental Health
6001 Executive Boulevard
Room 8184
Bethesda, MD 20892-9663

866-615-6464
Fax: 301-443-4279
TTY: 301-443-8431
E-mail: nimhinfo@nih.gov
www.nimh.nih.gov

Provides college sutdents with clear descriptions of the most prevalent forms of depression. Discusses symptoms, causes and treatment options. Includes information about suicide and resources for help that are available to most college students.

4 pages

801 What to do When a Friend is Depressed: Guide for Students

National Institute of Mental Health
6001 Executive Boulevard
Room 8184
Bethesda, MD 20892-9663

866-615-6464
Fax: 301-443-4279
TTY: 301-443-8431
E-mail: nimhinfo@nih.gov
www.nimh.nih.gov

This brochure offers information on depression and its symptoms and suggests things a young person can do to guide a depressed friend in finding help. Especially good for health fairs, health clinics and school health units.

3 pages

Research Centers

802 National Alliance for Research on Schizophrenia and Depression

60 Cutter Mill Road
Suite 200
Great Neck, NY 11021-3104

516-487-6930
800-829-8289
E-mail: info@narsad.org
www.narsad.org

Constance Lieber, President

NARSAD raises funds for research on schizophrenia, depression, and other serious brain disorders.

803 Sid W Richardson Institute for Preventive Medicine of the Methodist Hospital

6565 Fannin Street
Houston, TX 77030-2704

713-790-3136

Alan Herd MD, Director

804 University of Pennsylvania: Depression Research Unit

School of Medicine, Department of Psychiatry
3600 Spruce Street
Philadelphia, PA 19104-4211

215-662-3462
Fax: 215-662-6443

Jay D Amsterdam MD, Director

Focuses on mental health and depression.

805 University of Texas: Mental Health Clinical Research Center

5323 Harry Hines Boulevard
Dallas, TX 75235-7208

214-648-5343
Fax: 214-648-5340

Dr A John Rush, Director

Research activity of major and atypical depression.

806 Yale University: Depression Research Program

Yale University Department of Psychiatry
25 Deer Park Street
Room 613
New Haven, CT 06519

203-764-9131
E-mail: gerard.sanacora@yale.edu
www.info.med.yale.edu/ysm

Hoyle Leigh MD, Director

Successfuly treating people with depression for over three decades. Operated jointly by the Connecticut Mental Health Center and the Yale University School of Medicine, Department of Psychiatry.

Support Groups & Hot Lines

807 Depressed Anonymous

PO Box 17414
Louisville, KY 40217

502-569-1989
E-mail: info@depressedanon.com
www.depressedanon.com

Individuals suffering from depression or anxiety. A self-help organization with meetings and sharing of experiences. Similar to the 12 step program, uses mutual aid as a theraputic healing force. Website offers information on how to form groups in your area.

808 Recovery

802 N Dearborn Street
Chicago, IL 60610

312-337-5661
Fax: 312-337-5756
E-mail: inquiries@recovery-inc.com
www.recovery-inc.com

Kelly Garcia, Executive Director
Maurine Pyle, Assistant Director

Techniques for controlling behavior, changing attitudes for recovering mental patients. Systematic method of self-help offered.

Video & Audio

809 Coping with Depression

New Harbinger Publications
5674 Shattuck Avenue
Oakland, CA 94609-1662

510-652-2002
800-748-6273
Fax: 510-652-5472
E-mail: customerservice@newharbinger.com
www.newharbinger.com

60 minute videotape that offers a powerful message of hope for anyone struggling with depression. *$39.95*

Year Founded: 1994 ISBN 1-879237-62-8

810 Day for Night: Recognizing Teenage Depression

DRADA-Depression and Related Affective Disorders Association
2330 W Joppa Road
Suite 100
Lutherville, MD 21097
410-583-2919
Fax: 410-583-2964
E-mail: drada@jhmi.edu
www.drada.org

Catherine Pollock, Executive Director
Sallie Mink, Director Education

Award winning video that provides an in depth look at teenage depression and offers educational support and hope for those who suffer this treatable condition. *$22.50*

811 Depression and Manic Depression

Fanlight Productions
47 Halifax Street
Boston, MA 02131
617-524-0980
800-937-4113
Fax: 617-524-8838
E-mail: info@fanlight.com
www.fanlight.com

Explores the realities of depression and manic depression, as well as provides an overview of available treatments, and a listing of other resources. *$149.00*

812 Living with Depression and Manic Depression

New Harbinger Publications
5674 Shattuck Avenue
Oakland, CA 94609-1662
510-652-2002
800-748-6273
Fax: 510-652-5472
E-mail: customerservice@newharbinger.com
www.newharbinger.com

Describes a program based on years of research and hundreds of interviews with depressed persons. Warm, helpful, and engaging, this tape validates the feelings of people with depression while it encourages positive change. *$11.95*

Year Founded: 1994 ISBN 1-879237-63-6

813 Why Isn't My Child Happy? Video Guide About Childhood Depression

ADD WareHouse
300 NW 70th Avenue
Suite 102
Plantation, FL 33317
954-792-8100
800-233-9273
Fax: 954-792-8545
E-mail: sales@addwarehouse.com
www.addwarehouse.com

The first of its kind, this new video deals with childhood depression. Informative and frank about this common problem, this book offers helpful guidance for parents and professionals trying to better understand childhood depression. 110 minutes. *$55.00*

814 Women and Depression

Fanlight Productions
47 Halifax Street
Boston, MA 02131
617-524-0980
800-937-4113
Fax: 617-524-8838
E-mail: info@fanlight.com
www.fanlight.com

Clinical depression affects 19 million Americans, about 10 million of these are women. 28 minute video features women who talk about their own depression, and how it is viewed and handled in the African American community, and a therapist who deals with her own depression. Treatments are explored and practical strategies are offered. *$129.00*

Year Founded: 2000

Web Sites

815 www.apa.org/journals/anton.html

Psychotherapy versus Medication for Depression

Article reviews range of studies comparing psychological with pharmacological treatments.

816 www.befrienders.org

Samaritans International

Support, helplines, and advice.

817 www.blarg.net/~charlatn/voices/voices.html

Voices of Depression

Compilation of writings by people suffering from depression.

818 www.cyberpsych.org

CyberPsych

Hosts the American Psychoanalyists Foundation, American Association of Suicideology, Society for the Exploration of Psychotherapy Intergration, and Anxiety Disorders Association of America. Also subcategories of the anxiety disorders, as well as general information, including panic disorder, phobias, obsessive compulsive disorder (OCD), social phobia, generalized anxiety disorder, post traumatic stress disorder, and phobias of childhood. Book reviews and links to web pages sharing the topics.

819 www.depressedteens.com

Depression and Related Affective Disorders Association: DRADA

115

Educational site dedicated to helping teens, parents and teachers understand symptoms of teenage depression. Provides resources for those ready to seek help.

820 **www.depression.org**

National Foundation for Depressive Illness

Support, helplines, and advice.

821 **www.drada.org**

Depressive and Related Affective Disorders Association

National organization provides facts on depressive disorders, support for the depressed individual and also their families.

822 **www.emdr.com**

EMDR Institute

Discusses EMDR-Eye Movement Desensitization and Reprocessing-as an innovative clinical treatment for trauma, including sexual abuse, domestic violence, combat, crime, and those suffering from a number of other disorders including depressions, addictions, phobias and a variety of self-esteem issues.

823 **www.klis.com/chandler/pamphlet/dep/depressionpamphlet.htm**

Jim Chandler MD

White paper on depression in children and adolesents.

824 **www.mentalhealth.com/story/p52-dps2.html**

How to Help a Person with Depression

Valuable family education.

825 **www.mhsource.com/wb/thow9903.html**

Steven Thos Mental Health Resources-Depression and Bipolar Disorder

About 40 questions asked by patients.

826 **www.nimh.nih.gov/publicat/depressionmenu.cfm**

National Institute of Mental Health

National Institute of Mental Health offers brochures organized by topic. Depression discusses symptoms, diagnosis, and treatment options.

827 **www.nimh.nih.gov/publist/964033.htm**

National Institute of Mental Health

Discusses depression in older years, symptoms, treatment, going for help.

828 **www.planetpsych.com**

Planetpsych.com

Learn about disorders, their treatments and other topics in psychology. Articles are listed under the related topic areas. Ask a therapist a question for free, or view the directory of professionals in your area. If you are a therapist sign up for the directory. Current features, self-help, interactive, and newsletter archives.

829 **www.psychcentral.com**

Psych Central

Personalized one-stop index for psychology, support, and mental health issues, resources, and people on the Internet.

830 **www.psychologyinfo.com/depression**

Psychology Information On-line: Depression

Information on diagnosis, therapy, and medication.

831 **www.psycom.net/depression.central.html**

Dr. Ivan's Depression Central

Medication-oriented site. Clearinghouse on all types of depressive disorders.

832 **www.queendom.com/selfhelp/depression/depression.html**

Queendom

Articles, information on medication and support groups.

833 **www.shpm.com**

Self Help Magazine

Articles and discussion forums, resource links.

834 **www.wingofmadness.com**

Wing of Madness: A Depression Guide

Accurate information, advice, support, and personal experiences.

Introduction

Dissociative Disorders are a cluster of mental disorders, united by a profound change in consciousness or a disruption in continuity of consciousness. People with a Dissociative Disorder may abruptly take on different personalities, or they may undergo long periods in which they do not remember anything that happened; in some cases, individuals may embark on lengthy international travels, returning home with no recollection of where they have been or why they had gone.

Dissociative Disorders are uncommon, mysterious and somewhat controversial; reports of Dissociative Disorders have grown more frequent in recent years and a degree of debate surrounds the validity of these reports. Some professionals say the disorder is far more rare than is reported, and that many individuals diagnosed with a Dissociative Disorder while they may indeed be mentally or emotionally disturbed are highly suggestible, taking on symptoms subtly suggested by others.

Dissociative Disorders are believed to be related in many cases to severe trauma, although the historical validity of these cases is difficult to determine. Nevertheless, Dissociative Disorders are quite real and severe. There are five types of Dissociative Disorders: Dissociative Amnesia; Dissociative Fugue; Dissociative Identity Disorder; Depersonalization Disorder; and Dissociative Disorder Not Otherwise Specified.

SYMPTOMS

Dissociative Amnesia

•One or more episodes of inability to recall important personal information, usually of a traumatic or stressful nature, that is too extensive to be explained by ordinary forgetfulness;
•The disturbance does not occur exclusively during the course of any other Dissociative Disorder and is not due to the direct physiological effects of a substance abuse or general medical condition;

•The symptoms cause clinically significant distress or impairment in social, occupational or other important areas of functioning.

Dissociative Fugue

•A sudden, unexpected travel away from home or work, with inability to recall one's past;
•Confusion about personal identity or assumption of a new identity;
•The disturbance does not occur exclusively during the course of any other Dissociative Disorder and is not due to the direct physiological effects of a substance or a general medical condition;
•The symptoms cause clinically significant distress or impairment in social, occupational, or other important areas of functioning.

Dissociative Identity Disorder

•The presence of two or more distinct identities or personality states that take control of the person's behavior;
•Inability to recall important personal information;
•The disturbance is not due to the direct physiological effects of a substance or a general medical condition.

Depersonalization Disorder

•Persistent or recurrentxperiences of feeling detached from one's body and mental processes;
•During the depersonalization experience, reality testing remains intact;
•The depersonalization causes clinically significant distress or impairment in social, occupational, or other important areas of functioning;
•The depersonalization does not occur during the course of another Dissociative Disorder or as a direct physiological effect of a substance or general medical condition;
•Akin to depersonalization (feeling one is not real) is derealization, which is feeling that one's environment and/or perceptions are not real.

ASSOCIATED FEATURES

Patients with any of the Dissociative Disorders may be depressed, and may experience depersonalization, or a feeling of not being in their own body. They will often experience impairment work or interpersonal relationships, and they may practice self-mutilation or have aggressive and suicidal impulses. They may also have symptoms typical of a Mood or Personality Disorder. Individuals with Dissociative Amnesia and Dissociative Identity Disorder (sometimes known as multiple personality disorder) often report severe physical and/or sexual abuse in childhood. Controversy surrounds the accuracy of these reports, in part because of the unreliability of some childhood memories. Individuals with Dissociative Identity Disorder may have symptoms typical of Post-Traumatic Stress Disorder, as well as Mood, Substance Abuse Related, Sexual, Eating or Sleep Disorders.

PREVALENCE

The prevalence of Dissociative Disorders in most cases is either unknown, difficult to ascertain, or subject to controversy. The recent rise in the US in reports of Dissociative Amnesia and Dissociative Identity Disorder related to traumatic childhood abuse has been very controversial. Some say these disorders are overreported, the result of suggestibility in individuals and the unreliability of childhood memories. Others say the disorders are underreported, given the propensity for children and adults to dismiss or forget abusive memories and the tendency of perpetrators to deny or obscure their abusive actions. For Dissociative Fugue, a prevalence rate of 0.2 percent of the population has been reported. Dissociative Identity Disorder tends to be far more common in females than in males: the disorder is diagnosed three to nine times more frequently in females than in males.

Associations & Agencies

836 Center for Family Support (CFS)

333 7th Avenue
New York, NY 10001-5004
212-629-7939
Fax: 212-239-2211
www.cfsny.org

Steven Vernickofs, Executive Director

Service agency devoted to the physical well-being and development of the retarded child and the sound mental health of the parents. Helps families with retarded children with all aspects of home care including counseling, referrals, home aide service and consultation. Offers intervention for parents at the birth of a retarded child with in home support, guidance and infant stimulation. Pioneered training of nonprofessional women as home aides to provide supportive services in homes.

837 Center for Mental Health Services Knowledge Exchange Network

US Department of Health and Human Services
PO Box 42490
Washington, DC 20015-4800
800-789-2647
Fax: 301-984-8796
E-mail: ken@mentalhealth.org
www.mentalhealth.org

Information about resources, technical assistance, research, training, networks, and other federal clearing houses, and fact sheets and materials. Information specialists refer callers to mental health resources in their communities as well as state, federal and nonprofit contacts. Staff available Monday through Friday, 8:30 AM 5:00 PM, EST, excluding federal holidays. After hours, callers may leave messages and an information specialist will return their call.

838 International Society for the Study of Dissociation

Haworth Press
60 Revere Drive
Suite 500
Northbrook, IL 60062
847-480-0899
Fax: 847-480-9282
E-mail: issd@issd.org
www.issd.org

Steven N. Gold PhD, President
Ruth Blizard PhD, Director
Frances Waters DCSW LMFT, Secretary/Treasurer
Eli Somer PhD, International Director

The society is a nonprofit professional association organized for the porposes of: information sharing and international networking of clinicians and researchers; providing professional and public education; promoting research and theory about dissociation; and promoting research and training in the identification, treatment, and prevention of dissociative disorders.

839 NADD: Association for Persons with Developmental Disabilities and Mental Health Needs

132 Fair Street
Kingston, NY 12401-4802
845-334-4336
800-331-5362
Fax: 845-331-4569
E-mail: nadd@mhv.net
www.thenadd.org

Dr. Robert Fletcher, Executive Director

Nonprofit organization designed to promote interest of professional and parent development with resources for individuals who have the coexistence of mental illness and mental retardation. Provides conference, educational services and training materials to professionals, parents, concerned citizens and service organizations. Formerly known as the National Association for the Dually Diagnosed.

840 National Mental Health Consumer's Self-Help Clearinghouse

1211 Chestnut Street
Suite 1207
Philadelphia, PA 19107
215-751-1810
800-553-4539
Fax: 215-636-6312
E-mail: info@mhselfhelp.com
www.mhselfhelp.org

Alex Morrsey, Information/Referral

Funded by the National Institute of Mental Health Community Support Program, the purpose of the Clearinghouse is to encourage the development and growth of consumer self-help groups.

Year Founded: 1992

Books

841 Amongst Ourselves: A Self-Help Guide to Living with Dissociative Identity Disorder

New Harbinger Publications
5674 Shattuck Avenue
Oakland, CA 94609-1662
510-652-2002
800-748-6273
Fax: 510-652-5472
E-mail: customerservice@newharbinger.com
www.newharbinger.com

Tracy Alderman PhD
Karen Marshall LCSW

First person perspective of Dissociative Identity Disorder and practical suggestions to come to terms with and improve their lives. $14.95

240 pages ISBN 1-562241-22-5

842 Dissociation

American Psychiatric Publishing
1000 Wilson Boulevard
Suite 1825
Arlington, VA 22209-3901   703-907-7322
                                  800-368-5777
                         Fax: 703-907-1091
                    E-mail: appi@psych.org
                                  www.appi.org

Katie Duffy, Marketing Assistant

Combines cultural anthropology, congitive psychology, neurophysiology, and the study of psychosomatic illness to present the latest information on the dissociative process. Designed for professionals in cross cultural psychiatry and the influence of the mind on the body. *$33.50*

227 pages ISBN 0-880485-57-4

843 Dissociative Child: Diagnosis, Treatment and Management

200 E Joppa Road
Suite 207
Baltimore, MD 21286   410-825-8888
                             888-825-8249
                    Fax: 410-337-0747
               E-mail: sidran@sidran.org
                             www.sidran.org

This second groundbreaking edition addresses all aspects of caring for the dissociative child and adolescents. Contributors include experienced and eminent practitioners in the field of childhood DID. The section on diagnosis offers comprehensive coverage of various aspects of diagnosis, including diagnosis taxonomy, differential diagnosis, interviewing, testing and the special problems of male children and adolescents with DID. The section on treatment covers factors associated with positive theraputic outcome, therapeutic phases, the five-domain crisis model, promoting intergration in dissociative children, art therapy and group therapy. Includes ways school personnel can act to help the dissociative child, multiculturalism and other important information. *$45.00*

400 pages

844 Handbook for the Assessment of Dissociation: a Clinical Guide

American Psychiatric Publishing
1000 Wilson Boulevard
Suite 1825
Arlington, VA 22209-3901   703-907-7322
                                  800-368-5777
                         Fax: 703-907-1091
                    E-mail: appi@psych.org
                                  www.appi.org

Katie Duffy, Marketing Assistant

Offers guidelines for the systematic assessment of dissociation and posttraumatic syndromes for clinicians and researchers. Provides a comprehensive overview of dissociative symptoms and disorders and an introduction to the use of the SCID-D, a diagnostic interview for the dissociative disorders. *$54.00*

433 pages ISBN 0-880486-82-1

845 Lost in the Mirror: An Inside Look at Borderline Personality Disorder

200 E Joppa Road
Suite 207
Baltimore, MD 21286   410-825-8888
                             888-825-8249
                    Fax: 410-337-0747
               E-mail: sidran@sidran.org
                             www.sidran.org

Richard Moskovitz

Dr. Moskovitz considers BPD to be part of the dissociative continuum, as it has many causes, symptoms and behaviors in common with Dissociative Disorder. This book is intended for people diagnosed with BPD, their families and therapists. Outlines the features of BPD, including abuse histories, dissociation, mood swings, self harm, impulse control problems and many more. Includes an extensive resource section. *$12.95*

190 pages

846 Multiple Personality and Dissociation, 1791-1992: Complete Bibliography

200 E Joppa Road
Suite 207
Baltimore, MD 21286   410-825-8888
                             888-825-8249
                    Fax: 410-337-0747
               E-mail: sidran@sidran.org
                             www.sidran.org

This second edition is expanded, revised, updated and reorganized. It serves as an ideal resource for anyone interested in the history of trauma studies. *$9.95*

156 pages

847 Rebuilding Shattered Lives: Responsible Treatment of Complex Post-Traumatic and Dissociative Disorders

John Wiley & Sons
605 3rd Avenue
New York, NY 10058-0180   212-850-6000
                         Fax: 212-850-6008

Essential for anyone working in the field of trauma therapy. Part I discusses recent findings about child abuse, the changes in attitudes toward child abuse over the last two decades and the nature of traumatic memory. Part II is an overview of principles of trauma treatment, including symptom control, establishment of boundaries and therapist self-care. Part III covers special topics, such as dissociative identity disorder, controversies, hospitalization and acute care. *$47.50*

271 pages ISBN 0-471247-32-4

848 Trauma, Memory, and Dissociation

American Psychiatric Publishing
1000 Wilson Boulevard
Suite 1825
Arlington, VA 22209-3901   703-907-7322
                                  800-368-5777
                         Fax: 703-907-1091
                    E-mail: appi@psych.org
                                  www.appi.org

Katie Duffy, Marketing Assistant

Comprehensive text on dissociation and memory alterations in trauma. Presents empirical data on dissociative symptoms associated with exposure to psychological trauma, including combat, childhood abuse, as well as the important relationships dissociative disorder has with other conditions associated with extreme stress such as post traumatic stress disorder. *$54.00*

439 pages ISBN 0-880487-53-4

849 Treatment of Multiple Personality Disorder

American Psychiatric Publishing
1000 Wilson Boulevard
Suite 1825
Arlington, VA 22209-3901　　　**703-907-7322**
　　　　　　　　　　　　　　800-368-5777
　　　　　　　　　Fax: 703-907-1091
　　　　E-mail: appi@psych.org
　　　　　　　　　www.appi.org

Katie Duffy, Marketing Assistant

Authorities in the Multiple Personality Disorder field merge clinical understanding and research into therapeutic approaches that can be employed in clinical practice. *$22.50*

258 pages ISBN 0-880480-96-3

850 Understanding Dissociative Disorders and Addiction

200 E Joppa Road
Suite 207
Townson, MD 21286　　　**410-825-8888**
　　　　　　　　　　　　　　888-825-8249
　　　　　　　　Fax: 410-337-0747
　　　E-mail: sidran@sidran.org
　　　　　　　　www.sidran.org

Esther Giller, Presidnet and Director
Sheila Giller, Secretary/Treasurer
J.G. Goellner, Diector Emertius
Stanly Platman M.D., Medical Advisor

This booklet discusses the origins and symptoms of dissociation, explains the links between dissociative disorder and chemical dependency. Addresses treatment options available to help in your recovery. The work book includes exercises and activities that help you acknowledge, accept and manage both your chemical dependency and your disociative disorder. *$9.00*

Web Sites

851 www.alt.support.dissociation

Dissociative disorders.

852 www.cyberpsych.org
CyberPsych

Hosts the American Psychoanalyists Foundation, American Association of Suicideology, Society for the Exploration of Psychotherapy Intergration, and Anxiety Disorders Association of America. Also subcategories of the anxiety disorders, as well as general information, including panic disorder, phobias, obsessive compulsive disorder (OCD), social phobia, generalized anxiety disorder, post traumatic stress disorder, and phobias of childhood. Book reviews and links to web pages sharing the topics.

853 www.fmsf.com
False Memory Syndrome Facts

Access to literature.

854 www.issd.org
International Society for the Study of Dissociation

A nonprofit, professional society that promotes research and training in the identification and treatment of dissociative disorders, provides professional and public education about dissociative states, and serves as a catalyst for international communication and cooperation among clinicians and researchers working in this field.

855 www.planetpsych.com
Planetpsych.com

Learn about disorders, their treatments and other topics in psychology. Articles are listed under the related topic areas. Ask a therapist a question for free, or view the directory of professionals in your area. If you are a therapist sign up for the directory. Current features, self-help, interactive, and newsletter archives.

856 www.psychcentral.com
Psych Central

Personalized one-stop index for psychology, support, and mental health issues, resources, and people on the Internet.

857 www.sidran.org/trauma.html
Trauma Resource Area

Resources and Articles on Dissociative Experiences Scale and Dissociative Identity Disorder, PsychTrauma Glossary and Traumatic Memories.

Introduction

Eating is integral to human health, and for many people food is a pleasure that can be enjoyed without giving it too much thought. But an increasing number of people (mostly, but not exclusively, women) have eating disorders, which cause them to use food and dieting in ways that are extremely unhealthy, even life-threatening. The two principal eating disorders are Anorexia Nervosa and Bulimia Nervosa; though different in the symptoms they manifest, the two disorders are quite similar in their underlying pathology: an obsessive concern with food, body image, and body weight.

Many people believe that eating disorders are, in part, culturally determined: in the Western world, and particularly the US, a pervasive cultural preference for slimness causes many people to spend extraordinary amounts of time, money and energy dieting and exercise to stay slim. Cultural preference is likely to exert pressure on people, especially young women, who may be genetically or psychologically predisposed to the illness. It is important to be wary of some forms of media, including the internet, which can offer exposure to counterproductive influence. There is some tendency to include overeating as a type of Eating Disorder, as it reflects the paradox that, as society values thinness more and more, more and more people are obese. Eating Disorders may do serious and lasting physical damage; because of this, treatment first restores a patient to a safe and healthy body weight. But treatment of the disorder is liable to be a long-term process, involving both anti-depressant medication and psychotherapy. Fortunately, most people who are appropriately treated can and do recover.

SYMPTOMS

Anorexia Nervosa:
•Refusal to maintain body weight at or above eighty-five percent of a minimally normal weight for age and height;
•Intense fear of gaining weight or becoming fat, even though underweight;
•Disturbance in the way one's body weight or shape is experienced, undue influence of body weight or shape on self-evaluation, or denial of the seriousness of the current low body weight;
•In menstruating females, the absence of at least three consecutive menstrual cycles;
•Physical damage often occurs, such as imbalances in body chemicals, which if severe can cause cardiac arrest; purging often erodes tooth enamel, in which case a dentist might make the diagnosis. A gynecologist may also diagnose Anorexia Nervosa, as it is associated with amenorrhea and often results in infertility.

Bulimia Nervosa:
•Recurrent episodes of binge eating characterized by eating more food than most people would eat during a similar period of time and under similar circumstances;
•A sense of loss of control over eating;
•Recurrent inappropriate behavior in order to prevent weight gain, such as self-induced vomiting or misuse of laxatives, and excessive fasting or exercise;
•The binge-eating and inappropriate behaviors both occur, on average, at least twice a week for three months;
•Self-evaluation is unduly influenced by body shape and weight;
•The disturbance does not occur exclusively during episodes of Anorexia Nervosa.

ASSOCIATED FEATURES

Patients with Anorexia Nervosa may be severely depressed, and may experience insomnia, irritability, and diminished interest in sex. These features may be exacerbated if the patient is severely underweight. People with Eating Disorders also share many of the features of Obsessive Compulsive Disorder. For instance, someone with an Eating Disorder may have an excessive interest in food; they may hoard food, or spend unusual amounts of time reading and researching about foods, recipes and nutrition. People with Anorexia Nervosa may also exhibit a strong need to control their environment, and may be socially and emotinally withdrawn.

Individuals with Bulimia Nervosa are often within the normal weight range, but prior to the development of the disorder they may frequently be overweight. Depression and Mood Disorders are common among people with bulimia, and patients often ascribe their bulimia to the Mood Disorders. In other cases, however, it appears that the Mood Disorders precede the Eating Disorders. Substance abuse occurs in about one-third of individuals with bulimia.

Anxiety Disorders are common, and fear of social situations can be a precipitating factor in binging episodes.

PREVALENCE

Prevalence studies in females have found rates of 0.5 to one percent for Anorexia Nervosa. There is only limited data for the prevalence of Anorexia Nervosa in males. The prevalence of Bulimia Nervosa among adolescent females is approximately one to three percent. The rate of the disorder among males is approximately one-tenth of that in females.

TREATMENT OPTIONS

Medications, especially the newest SSRIs (Selective Serotonin Reuptake Inhibitors, which were originally developed as antidepressants), have been found to be very effective in the treatment of Eating Disorders. They can help restore and build self-esteem, and thereby help the patient maintain a positive attitude as well as a safe and healthy body image and body weight.

Because of the physical damage that an Eating Disorder can do to a patient, nutritional counseling and monitoring is often vital to restore and maintain proper body weight.

It is critical to recognize that Eating Disorders are, in addition to being life-threatening, extremely complex: simply restoring the patient to an acceptable body weight is not enough. Many patients have complex and conflicting psychological issues that trigger the compulsion to binge, or the morbid fear of gaining weight. These issues need to be addressed by psychotherapy. Forms of psychotherapy that may be useful in treating Eating Disorders include psychodynamic psychotherapy (in which longstanding and sometimes unconscious emotional issues related to the eating disorders are explored) and cognitive behavior therapy, which aims to identify the thought patterns that trigger the Eating Disorder and to establish healthy eating habits. Recent literature suggests that psychotherapeutic approaches are often more effective than medications in the treatment of Anorexia. Family involvement in treatment is critical, and peer pressure can be utilized to compel patients to maintain adequate nutrition. Eating Disorders are serious and treatment may be required over a course of many years.

Associations & Agencies

859 American Anorexia/Bulimia Association
293 Central Park W
Suite 1R
New York, NY 10024　　　　212-891-8686

Organization dedicated to increasing the awareness of eating disorders and offering information on prevention and treatment.

860 Anorexia Bulimia Treatment and Education Center
615 S New Ballas Road
Saint Louis, MO 63141-8221　　314-569-6000
　　　　　　　　　　　　Fax: 314-569-6910

Offers education on the prevention of eating disorders and information on various treatment options.

861 Anorexia Nervosa and Associated Disorders National Association (ANAD)
PO Box 7
Highland Park, IL 60035-0007　　847-831-3438

Vivian Hanson Meehan, President

Sponsors national and local programs to prevent eating disorders and assist people with eating disorders and their families. Provides a national clearinghouse of information and is a grassroots association for laypeople and professionals. It operates a national network of free support groups for people with eating disorders and their families, and provides prevention information and education to students and lecturers.

862 Anorexia Nervosa and Related Eating Disorders
PO Box 5102
Eugene, OR 97405-0102　　　541-344-1144
　　　　　　　　E-mail: jarinor@rio.com
　　　　　　　　　　　www.anred.com

We are a nonprofit organization that provides information about anorexia nervosa, bulimia nervosa, binge eating diorder, and other less-well-known food and weight disorders.

863 Center for Family Support (CFS)
333 7th Avenue
New York, NY 10001-5004　　　212-629-7939
　　　　　　　　　　Fax: 212-239-2211
　　　　　　　　　　　www.cfsny.org

Steven Vernickofs, Executive Director

Service agency devoted to the physical well-being and development of the retarded child and the sound mental health of the parents. Helps families with retarded children with all aspects of home care including counseling, referrals, home aide service and consultation. Offers intervention for parents at the birth of a retarded child with in-home support, guidance and infant stimulation. Pioneered training of nonprofessional women as home aides to provide supportive services in homes.

864 Center for Mental Health Services Knowledge Exchange Network
US Department of Health and Human Services
PO Box 42490
Washington, DC 20015-4800
　　　　　　　　　　　800-789-2647
　　　　　　　　　Fax: 301-984-8796
　　　　　E-mail: ken@mentalhealth.org
　　　　　　　　www.mentalhealth.org

Information about resources, technical assistance, research, training, networks, and other federal clearing houses, and fact sheets and materials. Information specialists refer callers to mental health resources in their communities as well as state, federal and non-profit contacts. Staff available Monday through Friday, 8:30 AM - 5:00 PM, EST, excluding federal holidays. After hours, callers may leave messages and an information specialist will return their call.

865 Change for Good Coaching and Counseling
3801 Connecticut Avenue NW
Washington, DC 20008-4530　　202-362-3009
　　　　　　　　　　Fax: 443-654-2420
　　　E-mail: brockhansenlcsw@aol.com
　　　　　　　　www.shamebusters.com

866 Council on Size and Weight Discrimination (CSWD)
PO Box 305
Mount Marion, NY 12456-0305　　845-679-1209
　　　　　　　　　　Fax: 845-679-1206
　　　　　　　　E-mail: info@cswd.org
　　　　　　　　　　www.cswd.org

Miriam Berg, President
Lynn McAfee, Director of Medical Advocacy
William J. Fabrey, Media Project
Nancy Summer, Fund Raising

The Council on Size and Weight Discrimination is a not-for-profit group which works to change people's attitudes about weight. We act as consumer advocated for larger people, especially in the areas of medical treatment, job discrimination, and media images.

867 Eating Disorders Awareness and Prevention
603 Stewart Street
Suite 803
Seattle, WA 98101-1263　　　　206-382-3587
　　　　　　　　　　Fax: 206-829-8501
　　　　　　　　　　　www.edap.org

NEDA is dedicated to expanding public understanding of eating disorders and promoting access to quality treatment for those affected along with support for their families through education, advocacy and research.

868 International Association of Eating Disorders Professionals

PO Box 1295
Pekin, IL 61555-1295   309-346-3341
                              800-800-8126
                         Fax: 775-239-1597
        E-mail: iaedpmembers@earthlink.net
                         www.iaedp.com

Bonnie Harken, Managing Director
Vicki Berkus MD CEDS, President

Offers professional counseling and assistance to the medical community, courts, law enforcement officials, and social welfare agencies.

869 Largesse, The Network for Size Esteem

PO Box 9404
New Haven, CT 06534-0404   203-787-1624
                         Fax: 203-787-1624
           E-mail: largesse@eskimo.com
                www.eskimo.com/~largesse

Karen W Stimson, Co-Director

Our mission is to create personal awareness and social change which promotes a positive image, health and equal rights for people of size.

870 NADD: Association for Persons with Developmental Disabilities and Mental Health Needs

132 Fair Street
Kingston, NY 12401-4802   845-334-4336
                              800-331-5362
                         Fax: 845-331-4569
                E-mail: nadd@mhv.net
                     www.thenadd.org

Dr. Robert Fletcher, Executive Director

Nonprofit organization designed to promote interest of professional and parent development with resources for individuals who have the coexistence of mental illness and mental retardation. Provides conference, educational services and training materials to professionals, parents, concerned citizens and service organizations. Formerly known as the National Association for the Dually Diagnosed.

871 National Alliance for the Mentally Ill

2107 Wilson Boulevard
Suite 300
Arlington, VA 22201-3042   703-524-7600
                              800-950-6264
                         Fax: 703-524-9094
                         TDD: 703-516-7227
             E-mail: helpline@nami.org
                         www.nami.org

Laurie Flynn, Executive Director

Nation's leading self-help organization for all those affected by severe brain disorders. Mission is to bring consumers and families with similar experiences together to share information about services, care providers, and ways to cope with the challenges of schizophrenia, manic depression, and other serious mental illnesses.

872 National Association of Anorexia Nervosa and Associated Disorders (ANAD)

PO Box 7
Highland Park, IL 60035-0007   847-831-3438
                             Fax: 847-433-4632
                E-mail: anad20@aol.com
                             www.anad.org

Dawn Rics, Administrator

National education/advocacy organization that assists sufferers of eating disorders, their families, and works to prevent eating disorders. Some of the services provided include the national hotline, self help groups for victims and families, educational and prevention programs, referrals to health care professionals, as well as referrals to inpatient/outpatient programs, promotes research and works on a variety of advocacy issues.

873 National Association to Advance Fat Acceptance (NAAFA)

PO Box 431
Oscoda, MI 48750   866-623-5223
                         Fax: 886-623-5224
             E-mail: naafa@charter.net
                         www.naafa.org

Maryanne Bodoky, Executive Director

Nonprofit organization dedicated to improving the quality of life for fat people. Opposes discrimination against fat people including discrimination in advertising, employment, fashion, medicine, insurance, social acceptance, the media, schooling and public accomodations. Monitors legislative activity and litigation affecting fat people. Publications: NAAFA Newsletter, bimonthly. Annual conference and symposium, always mid-August.

874 National Eating Disorders Association

603 Stewart Street
Suite 803
Seattle, WA 98101   206-382-3587
                              800-931-2237
      E-mail: info@NationalEatingDisorders.org
                www.NationalEatingDisorders.org

Dr. Laura Hill, Director

Offers a national information phone line, an international treatment referral directory, and a support group directory. The organization sponsors an annual conference and offers a speakers' bureau with a wide range of eating disorder professionals and volunteers for the general public as well as professionals.

875 National Institute of Mental Health Eating Disorders Program

Building 10 Room 35231
Bethesda, MD 20892-0001   301-496-1891
                         Fax: 301-402-1561

876 National Mental Health Consumer's Self-Help Clearinghouse

1211 Chestnut Street
Suite 1207
Philadelphia, PA 19107   215-751-1810
                                800-553-4539
                       Fax: 215-636-6312
              E-mail: info@mhselfhelp.org
                       www.mhselfhelp.org

Alex Morrsey, Information/Referral

Funded by the National Institute of Mental Health Community Support Program, the purpose of the Clearinghouse is to encourage the development and growth of consumer self-help groups.

Year Founded: 1992

877 O-Anon General Service Office (OGSO)

PO Box 1314
North Folk, CA 93643   597-877-3615
                       Fax: 559-877-3015

Jack Finley, Chairman

For families and friends of compulsive overeaters. Provides support groups that offer opportunities for the sharing of experiences and viewpoints to offer comfort, hope and friendship. Also to grow spiritually by working with the Twelve Steps and to give understanding and encouragement to the compulsive overeater. Works in cooperation with Overeaters Anonymous. Publications: Newsletter, three to four times a year. Offers periodic retreats and workshops.

878 TOPS Club

4575 S 5th Street
PO Box 07360
Milwaukee, WI 53207-0360   414-482-4620
                                800-932-8677
                       Fax: 414-482-3955
              E-mail: comm@globaldialog.com
                       www.tops.org

Betty Domenoe, President

TOPS is an international family of all ages, sizes, and shapes from all walk of life. Dedicated to helping each other Take Off and Keep Off Pounds Sensibly. We offer fellowship while you change to a healthier, new lifestyle andlearn to maintain it.

879 We Insist on Natural Shapes

PO Box 19938
Sacramento, CA 95819
                                800-600-9467
                       www.winsnews.org

A nonprofit organization educates about normal, healthy shapes.

Books

880 American Psychiatric Association Practice Guideline for Eating Disorders

American Psychiatric Publishing
1000 Wilson Boulevard
Suite 1825
Arlington, VA 22209-3901   703-907-7322
                                800-368-5777
                       Fax: 703-907-1091
              E-mail: appi@psych.org
                       www.appi.org

James Scully MD, President
Katie Duffy, Marketing

Includes information on all aspects of anorexia nervosa and bulimia nervosa, including self induced vomiting, laxative or diuretic use, strict diesting or fasting, and vigorous exercise to prevent weight gain. $22.50

48 pages ISBN 0-890423-00-8

881 Anorexia Nervosa & Recovery: a Hunger for Meaning

Haworth Press
10 Alice Street
Binghamton, NY 13904-1503   607-722-5857
                                800-429-6784
                       Fax: 607-722-1424
              E-mail: getinfo@haworthpress.com
                       www.haworthpress.com

Presents the most objective, complete, and compassionate picture of what anorexia nervosa is about. $14.95

146 pages ISBN 0-918393-95-7

882 Beyond Anorexia

Cambridge University Press
40 W 20th Street
New York, NY 10011-4211   212-924-3900
                                800-872-7423
                       Fax: 212-691-3239
              E-mail: marketing@cup.org
                       www.cup.org

Beyond Anorexia is a sociological exploration of how people recover from what medicine lables 'eating disorders'. $59.95

248 pages

883 Binge Eating: Nature, Assessment and Treatment

Guilford Publications
72 Spring Street
New York, NY 10012   212-431-9800
                                800-365-7006
                       Fax: 212-966-6708
              E-mail: info@guilford.com
                       www.guilford.com

Informative and practical text brings together original and significant contributions from leading experts from a wide variety of fields. Detailed manual covers all those who binge eat, including those who are overweight. *$21.95*

419 pages ISBN 0-898628-58-X

884 Body Betrayed

American Psychiatric Publishing
1000 Wilson Boulevard
Suite 1825
Arlington, VA 22209-3901
703-907-7322
800-368-5777
Fax: 703-907-1091
E-mail: appi@psych.org
www.appi.org

Katie Duffy, Marketing Assistant

Concentrating on women, eating disorders and treatments. *$20.00*

440 pages ISBN 0-880485-22-1

885 Body Image Workbook: An 8 Step Program for Learning to Like Your Looks

New Harbinger Publications
5674 Shattuck Avenue
Oakland, CA 94609-1662
510-652-2002
800-748-6273
Fax: 510-652-5472
E-mail: customerservice@newharbinger.com
www.newharbinger.com

Workbook offering a program to help transform your relationship with your body. *$17.95*

224 pages ISBN 1-572240-62-8

886 Body Image, Eating Disorders, and Obesity in Youth

APA Books
750 First Street NE
Washington, DC 20090
202-336-5500
800-374-2721
Fax: 202-336-5500
TDD: 202-336-6123
E-mail: order@apa.org
www.apa.org/books

Provides for clinicians including research, assessment and treatment suggestions on body image disturbances and eating disorders in children and adolescents. *$49.95*

517 pages ISBN 1-557987-58-0

887 Brief Therapy and Eating Disorders

Jossey-Bass Publishers
989 Market Street
San Francisco, CA 94103
415-433-1740
Fax: 415-433-0499
www.josseybass.com

Demonstrates how solution-focused brief therapy is on of the more eefficient approaches in treating eating disorders. *$36.95*

284 pages ISBN 0-787900-53-2

888 Bulimia

Jossey-Bass Publishers
989 Martket Street
San Francisco, CA 94103
415-433-1740
Fax: 415-433-0499
www.josseybass.com

A step-by-step guide to this complex disease. Filled with practical information and advice, this essential resource offers hope to millions of bulimics and their loved ones. *$17.95*

167 pages ISBN 0-787903-61-2

889 Bulimia Nervosa

University of Minnesota Press
111 3rd Avenue S
Suite 290
Minneapolis, MN 55401
612-627-1970
Fax: 612-627-1980
E-mail: ump@tc.umn.edu
www.upress.umn.edu

A practical guide for health-care professionals to the diagnosis, treatment and management of bulimia by a leading expert in the field of eating disorders. Hardcover.

188 pages ISBN 0-816616-26-4

890 Bulimia Nervosa & Binge Eating: A Guide To Recovery

New York University Press
838 Broadway
3rd Floor
New York, NY 10003
212-998-2575
Fax: 212-995-3833
www.nyupress.nyu.edu

A self-help book designed to guide bilimics and binge-eaters to recovery. *$35.00*

160 pages ISBN 0-814715-22-2

891 Bulimia: a Guide to Recovery

Gurze Books
PO Box 2238
Carlsbad, CA 92018-2238
760-434-7533
800-756-7533
Fax: 760-434-5476
E-mail: gzcatl@aol.com
www.gurze.net

Lindsey Cohn, Co-Owner Gurze Books

Guidebook offers a complete understanding of bulimia and a plan for recovery. Includes a two-week program to stop binging, things-to-do instead of binging, a two-week guide for support groups, specific advice for loved ones, and Eating Without Fear - Hall's story of self-cure which has inspired thousands of other bulimics. *$14.95*

285 pages ISBN 0-936077-31-X

892 Consumer's Guide to Psychiatric Drugs

New Harbinger Publications
5674 Shattuck Avenue
Oakland, CA 94609-1662
510-652-2002
800-748-6273
Fax: 510-652-5472
E-mail: customerservice@newharbinger.com
www.newharbinger.com

Helps consumers understand what treatment options are available and what side effects to expect. Covers possible interactions with other drugs, medical conditions, and other concerns. Explains how each drug works, and offers detailed information about treatments for depression, bipolar disorder, anxiety, and sleep disorders, as well as other conditions. *$16.95*

340 pages ISBN 1-572241-11-X

893 Controlling Eating Disorders with Facts, Advice and Resources

Oryx Press
88 Post Road W
Westport, CT 06881
203-226-3571
Fax: 603-431-2214
E-mail: info@oryxpress.com
www.oryxpress.com

894 Conversations with Anorexics: A Compassionate & Hopeful Journey

Jason Aronson
230 Livingston Street
Northvale, NJ 07647
800-782-0015
Fax: 201-767-1576
www.aronson.com

A compassionate and hopeful journey through the theraputic process. In this book Bruch presents some of her most challenging cases, offering deeply moving accounts of the cource and cure. *$30.00*

238 pages ISBN 1-568212-61-5

895 Coping with Eating Disorders

Rosen Publishing Group
29 E 21st Street
New York, NY 10010-6209
800-237-9932
Fax: 888-436-4643
E-mail: info@rosenpub.com
www.rosenpublishing.com

Offers practical suggestions on coping with eating disorders. *$16.95*

ISBN 0-823921-33-6

896 Cult of Thinness

Boston University Press
14 Mayflower Road
Chestnut Hill, MA 02467
617-552-3350
www.bc.edu/bc_org/rvp/pubaf/chronicle

$25.00

256 pages ISBN 0-195082-41-9

897 Deadly Diet

New Harbinger Publications
5674 Shattuck Avenue
Oakland, CA 94609-1662
510-652-2002
800-748-6273
Fax: 510-652-5472
E-mail: customerservice@newharbinger.com
www.newharbinger.com

Offering proven cognitive behavioral techniques, this book's self help program teaches effective coping strategies in three areas: stress reduction, behavior change, and cognitive change. It provides essential techniques for confronting the inner voice that's responsible for the shame, guilt, and low self worth that fuels eating disorders. *$14.95*

256 pages ISBN 1-879237-42-3

898 Developmental Psychopathology of Eating Disorders: Implications for Research, Prevention and Treatment

Lawrence Erlbaum Associates
10 Industrial Avenue
Mahwah, NJ 07430-2262
201-825-3200
800-926-6577
Fax: 201-236-0072
E-mail: orders@erlbaum.com
www.erlbaum.com

This text provides backround material from developmental psychology and psychopathology - following the theory that eating problems and disorders are typically rooted in childhood. Applications are then outlined, including research, treatment, protective factors and primary prevention. *$79.95*

456 pages ISBN 0-805817-46-8

899 Eating Disorders & Obesity: a Comprehensive Handbook

Guilford Publications
72 Spring Street
New York, NY 10012
212-431-9800
800-365-7006
Fax: 212-966-6708
E-mail: info@guilford.com
www.guilford.com

Presents and integrates virtually all that is currently known about eating disorders and obesity in one authorative, accessible and eminently practical volume. *$57.95*

583 pages ISBN 0-898628-50-4

900 Eating Disorders Sourcebook

Omnigraphics
PO Box 625
Holmes, PA 19043
800-234-1340
Fax: 800-875-1340
E-mail: info@omnigraphics.com
www.omnigraphics.com

Omnigraphics is the publisher of the Health Reference Series, a growing consumer health information resource with more than 100 volumes in print. Each title in the series features an easy to understand format, nontechnical language, comprehensive indexing and resources for further information. Material in each book has been collected from a wide range of government agencies, professional associations, periodicals and other sources. *$78.00*

322 pages ISBN 0-780803-35-3

901 Eating Disorders: Reference Sourcebook

Oryx Press
88 Post Road W
Westport, CT 06881   **203-226-3571**
                                Fax: 603-431-2214
                    E-mail: info@oryxpress.com
                            www.oryxpress.com

Listings of 200 centers and groups for care and treatment of eating disorders, such as anorexia nervosa, bulimia nervosa, and compulsive overeating. *$49.95*

902 Eating Disorders: When Food Turns Against You

Franklin Watts
90 Old Sherman Turnpike
Danbury, CT 06816-0001
                                800-621-1115
                            Fax: 203-797-3657
                                www.grolier.com

$14.50

96 pages ISBN 0-531111-75-0

903 Emotional Eating: A Practical Guide to Taking Control

Lexington Books
4501 Forbes Boulevard
Suite 200
Lanham, MD 20706   **717-794-3800**
                                800-426-6420
                            Fax: 717-794-3803
                    www.lexingtonbook.com

Using case histories he explores some of the cuases of emotional eating (childhoos programing, family life, sexual abuse) and the manifestos of emotional eating ("sneaky snaking",gazing, and binging). Of particulat intrest in the last chaper, which helps the reader determine whether or not it is a good or bad time to diet. While not a diet book or a 12-step primer, this is a tool for developing healthier ways of handling emotions and food. *$19.95*

200 pages ISBN 0-029002-15-0

904 Encyclopedia of Obesity and Eating Disorders

Facts on File
11 Penn Plaza
New York, NY 10001-2006   **212-290-8090**
                                800-322-8755
                            Fax: 212-678-3633

From abdominoplasty to Zung Rating Scale, this volume defines and explains these disorders, along with medical and other problems associated with them. *$50.00*

272 pages

905 Etiology and Treatment of Bulimia Nervosa

Jason Aronson
506 Clement Street
Dunmore, PA 18512-1523   **415-387-2272**
                            Fax: 415-387-2377
                    E-mail: info@greepapplebooks.com
                            www.aronson.com

$35.00

352 pages ISBN 1-568213-39-5

906 Feminist Perspectives on Eating Disorders

Guilford Publications
72 Spring Street
New York, NY 10012   **212-431-9800**
                                800-365-7006
                            Fax: 212-966-6708
                    E-mail: info@guilford.com
                            www.guilford.com

Explores the relationship between the anguish of eating disorder sufferers and the problems of ordinary women. Examines the sociocultural pressure on women to conform to culturally ideal body types and how this affects individual self concept. Controversial topics include the relationship between sexual abuse and eating disorders, the use of medications and the role of hospitalization and 12-step programs. *$25.95*

465 pages ISBN 1-572301-82-1

907 Food for Recovery: The Next Step

Crown Publishing Group
201 E 50th Street
New York, NY 10022-7703   **212-572-6117**
                            Fax: 212-572-6192

A very practicle guide on every aspect needed by the patient and councelor to utilize nutrtion as a therapeutic tool. *$14.00*

ISBN 0-517586-94-0

908 Golden Cage, The Enigma of Anorexia Nervosa

Random House
1745 Broadway 15-3
New York, NY 10019   **212-782-9000**
                            Fax: 212-572-6066
                    www.randomhouse.com

One of the world's leading authorities offers a vivid and moving account of the causes, effects and treatment of this devastating disease. *$9.00*

ISBN 0-394726-88-X

909 Group Psychotherapy for Eating Disorders

American Psychiatric Publishing
1000 Wilson Boulevard
Suite 1825
Arlington, VA 22209-3901
703-907-7322
800-368-5777
Fax: 703-907-1091
E-mail: appi@psych.org
www.appi.org

Katie Duffy, Marketing Assistant

The first book to fully explore the use of group therapy in the treatment of eating disorders. *$46.00*

353 pages ISBN 0-880484-19-5

910 Helping Athletes with Eating Disorders

Human Kinetics Publishers
PO Box 5076
Champaign, IL 61825-5076
800-747-4457
Fax: 217-351-1549
E-mail: orders@hkusa.com

Gives readers the information they need to identify and address major eating disorders such as: anorexia, bulimia nervosa, and eating disorders not otherwise specified. *$25.00*

208 pages ISBN 0-873223-83-7

911 Hunger So Wide and Deep

University of Minnesota Press
111 3rd Avenue S
Suite 290
Minneapolis, MN 55401
612-627-1970
Fax: 612-627-1980
E-mail: um@tc.umn.edu
www.upress.um.edu

ISBN 0-816624-35-6

912 Hungry Self; Women, Eating and Identity

Harper Collins
10 E 53rd Street
New York, NY 10022
212-207-7000
Fax: 212-207-6978
www.harpercollins.com

Answers the need for help among the five million American women who suffer from eating disorders. Paperback. *$13.00*

256 pages ISBN 0-060925-04-3

913 Insights in the Dynamic Psychotherapy of Anorexia and Bulimia

Jason Aronson
506 Clemant Street
San Francisco, CA 94118
415-387-2272
Fax: 415-387-2377
www.greenapplebooks.com

The clinical insights that guide the dynamic psychotheraoy of anorexic and bulimic patients. *$45.00*

288 pages ISBN 0-876685-68-8

914 Lifetime Weight Control

New Harbinger Publications
5674 Shattuck Avenue
Oakland, CA 94609-1662
510-652-2002
800-748-6273
Fax: 510-652-5472
E-mail: customerservice@newharbinger.com
www.newharbinger.com

Program of lifetime weight management in seven steps: 1. Eat spontaneously to settle into your 'setpoint' weight. 2. Accept yourself as okay, regardless of your weight. 3. Determine how and why you eat, learning all the reasons besides hunger. 4. Satisfy emotional needs directly, saving food for satisfying real hunger. 5. Improve nutrition. 6. Increase activity. 7. Stick to it. *$13.95*

208 pages ISBN 0-934986-83-5

915 Making Peace with Food

Harper Collins
10 E 53rd Street
New York, NY 10022-5244
212-207-7000
800-242-7737
Fax: 212-207-7617
www.harpercollins.com

For millions of diet-conscious Americans, the scientifically proven, step-by-step guide to overcoming repeated weight loss and gain, binge eating, guilt and anxieties about food and body image. *$15.00*

224 pages ISBN 0-060963-28-X

916 Obesity: Theory and Therapy

Raven Press
I 185 Avenue of the Americas
New York, NY 10036
212-930-9500
800-638-3030
Fax: 212-869-3495
www.lww.com

A classic reference for clinicians dealing with obesity, this volume provides the most up-to-date research, preclinical and clinical information.

500 pages ISBN 0-881678-84-8

917 Overeaters Anonymous

Metro Intergroup of Overeaters Anonymous
350 Third Avenue
PO Box 759
New York, NY 10001
212-946-4599
E-mail: NYOAMentroOffice@yahoo.com

Personal stories demonstrating the struggles overcome and accomplishments made. *$7.50*

204 pages

918 Practice Guidelines for Eating Disorders

American Psychiatric Publishing
1000 Wilson Boulevard
Suite 1825
Arlington, VA 22209-3901
703-907-7322
800-368-5777
Fax: 703-907-1091
E-mail: appi@psych.org
www.appi.org

Katie Duffy, Marketing Assistant

Designed for health care professionals, this guideline includes information on all aspects of anorexia nervosa and bulimia nervosa, including self-induced vomiting, use of laxatives and vigorous exercise to prevent weight gain. *$22.50*

38 pages ISBN 0-890423-00-8

919 Psychobiology and Treatment of Anorexia Nervosa and Bulimia Nervosa

American Psychiatric Publishing
1000 Wilson Boulevard
Suite 1825
Arlington, VA 22209-3901   **703-907-7322**
                                       800-368-5777
                               Fax: 703-907-1091
                   E-mail: appi@psych.org
                                    www.appi.org

Katie Duffy, Marketing Assistant

Combines clinical research concerning these distinct disorders and provides an overview of the psychobiology and treatment. *$48.50*

356 pages ISBN 0-880485-06-X

920 Psychodynamic Technique in the Treatment of the Eating Disorders

Jason Aronson
400 Keystone Industrial Park
Dunmore, PA 18512-1523   **570-342-1320**
                                      800-782-0015
                               Fax: 201-767-1576
                                    www.aronson.com

Provides a blueprint for the treatment of the eating disorders. *$50.00*

440 pages ISBN 0-876686-22-6

921 Psychosomatic Families: Anorexia Nervosa in Context

Harvard University Press
79 Garden Street
Cambridge, MA 02138   **800-405-1619**
                          Fax: 800-406-9145
      E-mail: CONTACT_HUP@harvard.edu
                        www.hup.harvard.edu

Hardcover. *$38.50*

351 pages ISBN 0-674722-20-5

922 Self-Starvation

Jason Aronson
400 Keystone Industrial Park
Dunmore, PA 18512-1523   **570-342-1320**
                                      800-782-0015
                               Fax: 201-767-1576
                                    www.aronson.com

Argues that anorexia nervoso is a social disease reflecting unbearable conflicts within the family. *$30.00*

312 pages ISBN 1-568218-22-2

923 Sexual Abuse and Eating Disorders

200 E Joppa Road
Suite 207
Baltimore, MD 21286   **410-825-8888**
                                   888-825-8249
                            Fax: 410-337-0747
           E-mail: sidran@sidran.org
                                 www.sidran.org

Explores the complex relationship between sexual abuse and eating disorders. Sexual abuse is both an extreme boundary violation and a disruption of attachment and bonding; victims of such abuse are likely to exhibit symptoms of self injury, including eating disorders. This volume is a discussion of the many ways that sexual abuse and eating disorders are related, also has accounts by a survivor of both. Investigates the prevalence of sexual abuse among individuals with eating disorders. Also examines how a history of sexual violence can serve as a predictor of subsequent problems with food. *$34.95*

228 pages

924 Starving to Death in a Sea of Objects

Jason Aronson
400 Keystone Industrial Park
Dunmore, PA 18512-1523   **570-342-1320**
                                      800-782-0015
                               Fax: 201-840-7242
                                    www.aronson.com

Makes the central dilemma clear: how emancipation can come to mean secutiry and pleasure for the anorectic. *$30.00*

464 pages ISBN 0-876684-35-5

925 Surviving an Eating Disorder: Perspectives and Strategies

Harper Collins
10 E 53rd Street
New York, NY 10022-5244   **212-207-7132**
                              Fax: 212-207-7946
                          www.harpercollins.com

Addresses the cutting-edge advances made in the field of eating disorders, discusses how the changes in health care have affected treatment and provides additional strategies for dealing with anorexia, bulimia and binge eating disorder. It also includes updated readings and a list of support organizations. A terrrific resource for those suffering from eating disorders, their families and professionals. Paperback. *$13.00*

256 pages ISBN 0-060952-33-4

926 Treating Eating Disorders

Jossey-Bass Publishers
10475 Crosspoint Boulevard
Indianapolis, IN 46256   **877-762-2974**
                              Fax: 800-597-3299
          E-mail: consumers@wiley.com
                               www.josseybass.com

Details how some of the most eminent clinicians in the field combine and intergrate a wide varitey of contemporary therapies — rainging from psychodynamic to systematic to cognitive behavioral—to successfully treat clients with anorexia nervosa, bulimia nervosa, and bringe eating diorders. Filled with up to date information and important approaches to assessment and treatment, the book offers a hands-on approach that cogently illustrates both theory and technique. *$29.95*

416 pages ISBN 0-787903-30-2

927 Understanding Anorexia Nervosa

Charles C Thomas Publisher
2600 S 1st Street
Springfield, IL 62704-4730   217-789-8980
                                        800-258-8980
                                   Fax: 217-789-9130
                         E-mail: books@ccthomas.com
                                   www.ccthomas.com

Contents: Course of Illness; Social Influences; Adolescence; At the Hospital; Techniques for Weight Gain; Psychotherapy; After the Hospital. *$30.95*

116 pages ISBN 0-398051-91-7

928 Weight Loss Through Persistence

New Harbinger Publications
5674 Shattuck Avenue
Oakland, CA 94609-1662   510-652-2002
                                       800-748-6273
                                  Fax: 510-652-5472
          E-mail: customerservice@newharbinger.com
                              www.newharbinger.com

This book distills current scientific findings about losing weight into a step by step program that shows you how you can achieve a long term commitment to effective weight control. Includes five healthy eating plans and a wealth of other ideas about how to exercise, cope, and persist. *$13.95*

281 pages ISBN 1-879237-64-4

929 When Food Is Love

Geneen Roth and Associates
PO Box 2852
Santa Cruz, CA 95063

                                       877-243-6336
                                  Fax: 831-685-8602
          E-mail: GeneenRoth@GeneenRoth.com
                              www.geneenroth.com

Lindsey Cohn, Bookseller

Shows how dieting and compulsive eating often become a subsititue for intimacy. Drwaing on painful personal experiece as well as the candid stories of thoes she has helped in her seminars, Roth ecamins the crucial issues that surrounf compilsive eating: need for control, dependency on melodrama, desire for what is fobidden, and the belief that the wrong move can mean catastrophe. She shows why many people overeat in an attempt to satisfy their emotional hunger, and why weightloss frequently just uncovers a new set of problems. But her welcome message is that the cycle of compulsive behavior. This book will help readers break destructive, self-pertetuating patterns and learn to satisfy all the hungers - physical and emoitional - thak makes us human. *$10.00*

205 pages

Periodicals & Pamphlets

930 American Anorexia/Bulimia Association News

293 Central Park West
Suite 1R
New York, NY 10002-4   212-501-8351
                                  Fax: 212-501-0342

Offers information on the latest treatments, medications, books, conferences, support groups, and workshops for persons with eating disorders.

931 Anorexia: Am I at Risk?

ETR Associates
4 Carbonero Way
Scotts Valley, CA 95066   831-438-4060
                                       800-321-4407
                                  Fax: 800-435-8433
                    E-mail: customerservice@etr.org
                                   www.etr.org

Offers a clear overview of anorexia; Lists symptoms; Explains helath problems.

932 Body Image

ETR Associates
4 Carbonero Way
Scotts Valley, CA 95066   831-438-4060
                                       800-321-4407
                                  Fax: 800-435-8433
                    E-mail: customerservice@etr.org
                                   www.etr.org

Discusses the difference between healthy and disorted body image; the link between poor body image and low self esteem; five point list to help people check out their own body image.

933 Bulimia

ETR Associates
4 Carbonero Way
Scotts Valley, CA 95066   831-438-4060
                                       800-321-4407
                                  Fax: 800-435-8433
                    E-mail: customerservice@etr.org
                                   www.etr.org

Includes warning signs that someone's bulimic, health consequesnces of bulimia, and how to help a friend.

934 Eating Disorder Sourcebook

Gurze Books
PO Box 2238
Carlsbad, CA 92018-2238   760-434-7533
                                 800-756-7533
                         Fax: 760-434-5476
                E-mail: gzcatl@aol.com
                         www.bulimia.com

Leigh Cohn, Co-Owner

Includes 125 books and tapes on eating disorders and related subjects for both lay and professional audiences, basic facts about eating disorders, a list of national organizations and treatment facilities. Also publishes a bimonthly newsletter for clinicians and are executive editors of Eating Disorders the Journal of Treatment and Prevention.

28 pages 1 per year

935 Eating Disorders

ETR Associates
4 Carbonero Way
Scotts Valley, CA 95066   831-438-4060
                                 800-321-4407
                         Fax: 800-435-8433
                E-mail: customerservice@etr.org
                                 www.etr.org

Includes anorexia and bulimia, eating patterns versus eating disorders, treatment and getting help.

936 Eating Disorders Factsheet

Center for Mental Health Services: Knowledge Exchange Network
PO Box 42490
Washington, DC 20015
                                 800-789-2647
                         Fax: 301-984-8796
                         TDD: 866-889-2647
                E-mail: ken@mentalhealth.org
                         www.mentalhealth.org

This fact sheet provides basic information on the symptoms, medical complications, formal diagnosis, and treatment for anorexia nervousa and bulimia nervousa.

2 pages

937 Eating Disorders: Facts About Eating Disorders and the Search for Solutions

National Institute of Mental Health
6001 Executive Boulevard
Room 8184
Bethesda, MD 20892-9663
                                 866-615-6464
                         Fax: 301-443-4279
                         TTY: 301-443-8431
                E-mail: nimhinfo@nih.gov
                         www.nimh.nih.gov

Eating is controlled by many factors, including appetite, food availability, family, peer, and cultural practices, and attempts at voluntary control. Dieting to a body weight leaner than needed for health is highly promoted by current fashion trends, sales campaigns for special foods, and in some activities and professions. Eating disorders involve serious disturbances in eating behavior, such as extreme and unhealthy reduction of food intake or severe overeating, as well as feelings of distress or extreme concern about body shape or weight. There is help, and there is every hope for recovery.

8 pages

938 Fats of Life

ETR Associates
4 Carbonero Way
Scotts Valley, CA 95066   831-438-4060
                                 800-321-4407
                         Fax: 800-435-8433
                E-mail: customerservice@etr.org
                                 www.etr.org

Stresses that health, not body weight, is what's important; dispels myths about dieting; includes chart to help people determine their body mass index.

939 Food and Feelings

ETR Associates
4 Carbonero Way
Scotts Valley, CA 95066   831-438-4060
                                 800-321-4407
                         Fax: 800-435-8433
                E-mail: customerservice@etr.org
                                 www.etr.org

Helps students recognize eating disorders; emphasizes the seriousness of eating disorders; encourages the sufferers to seek treatment.

940 Getting What You Want from Your Body Image

ETR Associates
4 Carbonero Way
Scotts Valley, CA 95066   831-438-4060
                                 800-321-4407
                         Fax: 800-435-8433
                E-mail: customerservice@etr.org
                                 www.etr.org

Discusses topics such as the influence of the media, the truth about dieting, and body image survival tips.

941 Restrictive Eating

ETR Associates
4 Carbonero Way
Scotts Valley, CA 95066   831-438-4060
                                 800-321-4407
                         Fax: 800-435-8433
                E-mail: customerservice@etr.org
                                 www.etr.org

Discusses the spectrum of eating patterns, signs of restrictive eating and why it is a problem, how to help a friend, and where to go for help.

942 Teen Image

ETR Associates
4 Carbonero Way
Scotts Valley, CA 95066   831-438-4060
                                 800-321-4407
                            Fax: 800-435-8433
        E-mail: customerservice@etr.org
                                 www.etr.org

Dispels unrealistic media images; offers ways to boost
body image and self esteem; includes tips to maintain
a good body image.

943 Working Together

National Association of Anorexia Nervosa and Asso-
ciated Disorders
PO Box 7
Highland Park, IL 60035-0007   847-831-3438
                            Fax: 847-433-4632
              E-mail: anad20@aol.com
                                 www.anad.org

Dawn Ries, Administrator

Designed for individuals, families, group leaders and
professionals concerned with eating disorders. Provides updates on treatments, resources, conferences,
programs, articles by therapists, recovered victims,
group members and leaders.

2 pages 4 per year

Research Centers

944 Center for the Study of Adolescence

Michael Reese Hospital and Medical Center
2929 S. Ellis Avenue
Chicago, IL 60616   312-791-2000
        www.michaelreesehospital.com

**945 Center for the Study of Anorexia and
Bulimia**

1841 Broadway 4th Floor
New York, NY 10023   212-333-3444
                            Fax: 212-333-5444

Jill M. Pollack, Executive Director
Jaclyn Kodosky, Program Administrator

Established as a division of the Institute for Contemporary Psychotherapy in 1979 and is the oldest
non-profit eating disorders clinic in New York City.
Using an ecelctic apporaoch, the professional staff
and affiliats are on the cutting edge of treatment in
their field. The treatment staff includes social workers, psychologists, registered nurses and nutrionists,
all with special training in the treatment of eating disorders.

**946 Eating Disorders Research and
Treatment Program**

Michael Reese Hospital and Medical Center
2929 S Ellis Avenue
Chicago, IL 60616   312-791-2000

Regina Casper, Director

947 Obesity Research Center

St. Luke's-Roosevelt Hospital
1090 Amsterdam Avenue 14th Floor
New York, NY 10025-1710   212-523-4196
                            Fax: 212-523-3416
              E-mail: dg108@columbia.edu

Dr. Xavier Pi-Sunyer, Director

Helps reduce the the incidence of obesity and realted
diseases through leadership in basic research, clinical
reserch, epidemiology and public health, patient care,
and public education.

**948 University of Pennsylvania Weight and
Eating Disorders Program**

3535 Market Street
Suite 3108
Philadelphia, PA 19104   215-898-7314
                            Fax: 215-898-2878
        E-mail: weight@upsnet.med.upenn.edu

Dr. Tom Wadden, Director

Conducts a wide variety of studies on the causes and
treatment of weight-related disorders.

Support Groups & Hot Lines

949 Compulsive Eaters Anonymous

5500 E Atherton Street, Suite 227-B
Long Beach, CA 90815-4017   562-342-9344
                            Fax: 562-342-9346
              E-mail: admin@ceahow.org
                                 www.ceahow.org

Our purpose is to stop eating compulsively... and we
welcome in fellowship and friendly understanding all
those who share our common problem.

950 Food Addicts Anonymous

4623 Forest Hill Boulevard
Suite 109-4
W Palm Beach, FL 33415-9120   561-967-3871
                  www.foodadictsanonymous.org

951 MEDA

92 Pearl Street
Newton, MA 02458   617-558-1881
                            Fax: 617-558-1771
              E-mail: meda@medainc.org
                                 www.medainc.org

Claudia Eaton, Product Manager
John W Hird, Career Development Manager
Rebecka Manley, Founder

MEDA ia a nonprofit organization dedicated to the prevention, education and treatment of eating disorders based on a model of full recovery. MEDA instills hope by providing innovative services and critical resources to clients, professionals, and educators. MEDA wasfounded in 1994 by Rebecca Manley who had the vision to provide services to the underserved individual, family and firends to prevent and treat eating disorders. MEDA is a group of mental healht professionals and revocered individuals, on staff memebers of our referral network, working to achieve that goal. MEDA is not funded by the state of Massachusetts and relies solely on contributions and income from servicest to opperate.

952   National Anorexic Aid Society

Harding Hospital
1670 Upham Drive
Columbus, OH 43229-3517   614-293-9600

953   National Center for Overcoming Overeating

PO Box 1257
Old Chelsea Station
New York, NY 10113-0920   212-875-0442
www.OvercomingOvereating.com

954   Overeaters Anonymous

World Service Office
6075 Zenith Court NE
PO Box 44020
Rio Rancho, NM 87124-6424   505-891-2664
Fax: 505-891-4320
E-mail: overeater@technet.nm.org
www.overeatersanonymous.org

Twelve step program for compulsive eaters.

Video & Audio

955   Eating Disorder Video

Active Parenting Publishers
1955 Vaughn Road NW
Suite 108
Kennesaw, GA 30144-7808   770-429-0565
800-825-0060
Fax: 770-429-0334
E-mail: cservice@activeparenting.com
www.activeparenting.com

Features compelling interviews with several young people who have suffered from anorexia nervosa, bulimia and compulsive eating. Discusses the treatments, causes and techniques for prevention with field experts. *$39.95*

ISSN Q6456

956   Eating Disorders: When Food Hurts

Fanlight Productions
4196 Washington Street
Suite 2
Boston, MA 01231   617-524-0980
800-937-4113
Fax: 617-469-3379
E-mail: fanlight@fanlight.com
www.fanlight.com

Kelli English, Publicity Coordinator

People recovering from anorexia and bulimia, together with a therapist specializing in eating disorders, discuss their experiences of confronting these dangerous conditions. Encourages people with eating disorders to get help, as well as educating teachers, counselors, and others who work with young women. *$195.00*

Web Sites

957   www.alt.support.eating.disord

Alternative Support for Eating Disorder

Information for anorexics, also a bulletin board.

958   www.anred.com

Anorexia Nervosa and Related Eating Disorders

The factual materials are detailed and organized.

959   www.closetoyou.org/eatingdisorders

Close to You

Information on nutrition, normal eating, diet drugs.

960   www.closetoyou.org/eatingdisorders/disth ink htm

15 Styles of Distorted Thinking

Reference useful for cognitive therapy.

961   www.closetoyou.org/eatingdisorders/road. html

Road to an Eating Disorder is Paved with Diet Rules

962   www.closetoyou.org/eatingdisorders/sitem ap. htm

Eating Disorders

Offers information on eating disorders - treatment, therapy, medical, and articles.

Eating Disorders/Web Sites

963 www.cyberpsych.org
CyberPsych

Hosts the American Psychoanalyists Foundation, American Association of Suicideology, Society for the Exploration of Psychotherapy Intergration, and Anxiety Disorders Association of America. Also subcategories of the anxiety disorders, as well as general information, including panic disorder, phobias, obsessive compulsive disorder (OCD), social phobia, generalized anxiety disorder, post traumatic stress disorder, and phobias of childhood. Book reviews and links to web pages sharing the topics.

964 www.edap.org
Eating Disorders Awareness and Prevention

A source of educational brochures and curriculum materials.

965 www.gurze.com/titlecat.htm
Gurze Bookstore

Hundreds of books on eating disorders.

966 www.healthyplace.com/Communities/Eating_ Disorders/peacelovehope
Peace, Love, and Hope

Click on Body Views for information on body dysmorphic disorder.

967 www.hedc.org/about.html
Harvard Eating Disorders Center

Help in identifying an eating distorder.

968 www.kidsource.com/nedo/
National Eating Disorders Organization

Educational materials on dynamics, causative factors and evaluating treatment options.

969 www.mentalhelp.net/factsfam/anorexia.htm
Anorexia Nervosa General Information

Introductory text on Anorexia Nervosa.

970 www.mentalhelp.net/guide/eating.htm
Mental Health Net, Eating Disorders

971 www.mirror-mirror.org/eatdis.htm
Mirror, Mirror

Relapse prevention for eating disorders.

972 www.noah-health.org/english/illness/ mentalhealth/mental.hmtl
Eating Disorders Articles

973 www.planetpsych.com
Planetpsych.com

Learn about disorders, their treatments and other topics in psychology. Articles are listed under the related topic areas. Ask a therapist a question for free, or view the directory of professionals in your area. If you are a therapist sign up for the directory. Current features, self-help, interactive, and newsletter archives.

974 www.psychcentral.com
Psych Central

Personalized one-stop index for psychology, support, and mental health issues, resources, and people on the Internet.

975 www.rcpsych.ac.uk/public/help/anor/anor _ frame.htm
Anorexia and Bulimia

Describes causes, symptoms, and treatment.

976 www.something-fishy.com
Something Fishy Music and Publishing

Eating disorder website concentrating on the creative.

977 www.something-fishy.org
Something Fishy

Site for therapists and clients on eating disorders.

978 www.something-fishy.org/doctors/tips.php
Tips for Doctors

Sensitizes heatlh care providers to the fears of patients.

979 **www.utexas.edu/student/cmhc.eating.html**
Is Food a Problem?

Three factual brochures.

Gender Identification Disorder/

Introduction

With a wide scope of questions and confusion surrounding human sexuality and gender-explicit roles in the modern era, many children, adolescents and adults have been perplexed by the concepts of homosexuality and cross-gender identification. Homosexuality is a matter of sexual orientation: whether one is sexually attracted to men or women. Gender identity is a matter of what gender one feels oneself to be; people with Gender Identity Disorder, therefore, feel that their psychological experience conflicts with the physical body with which they were born. The American Psychiatric Association ceased to classify homosexuality as an illness in 1973. While a homosexual orientation does not stem from a mental affliction or emotional conflict, Gender Identification Disorder can have serious social and occupational repercussions.

Diagnosis of Gender Identification Disorder requires two sets of criteria: (1) a heavy and persistent insistence that the individual is, or has a strong desire to be, of the opposite sex, and (2) a constant discomfort about his/her designated sex, a feeling of inappropriateness towards his/her biological designation. Typically, boys conceding to the disorder are predisposed to dressing as girls, drawing explicit pictures of females, playing with pre-designated feminine toys, fantasizing and role playing as females and interacting primarily with the opposite sex. Girls with the condition have tendencies towards participating in contact sports, have an aversion to wearing dresses, are often mistaken for boys due to attire and hair style, and may assert that they will develop to be a man. For adolescents and adults, ostracism in school and the workplace is likely to occur, as is a profound inability to associate with others and poor relationships with family members and members of either sex.

SYMPTOMS

In boys
•A marked preoccupation with traditionally femi-
nine activites;
•A preference for dressing as a girl;
•Attraction to stereotypical female games and toys;
•Portraying female characters in role playing;
•Assertion he is a girl;
•Insistence on sitting to urinate;
•Displaying disgust for his genitals, wishing to remove them.

In girls
•Aversion to traditional female attire;
•Shared interest in contact games;
•A preference for associating with boys;
•Refusing to urinate sitting down;
•Show little interest in playing with stereotypical female toys such as dolls;
•Assertion that she will grow a penis, not breasts;
•Identification with strong male figures.

In adolescents
•Ostracism in school and social situations;
•Social isolation, peer rejection and peer teasing;
•Significant cross-gender identification and mannerisms;
•Similar symptoms as children.

In adults
•Adoption of social roles, physical appearance, and mannerisms of opposite sex;
•Surgical and/or hormonal manipulation of biological state;
•Discomfort in being regarded by others, or functioning, as his/her designated sex;
•Cross-dressing;
•Transvestic Fetishism.

ASSOCIATED FEATURES

Those who have Gender Identification Disorder are at risk of mental and physical harm resulting from the reactions of other people to their condition. In children, a manifestation of Separation Anxiety Disorder, Generalized Anxiety Disorder and symptoms of Depression may result from Gender Identification Disorder. For adolescents, depression and suicidal thoughts or ideas, as well as actual suicide attempts can result from prolonged feelings of ostracism by peers. Relationships with either one or both parents may weaken from resentment, lack of communication and misunderstanding; many with this disorder may drop out of or avoid school due to peer teasing. For many, lives are built around decreasing gender distress. They are often preoccupied with appearance. In extreme cases, males with the disorder perform their own castration. Prostitution has been linked with the disorder because young people who are rejected by their families and ostracized by others may resort to prostitution as the only way to support themselves, a practice which increases the risk of acquiring sexually transmitted diseases. Some people with Gender Identitification Disorder resort to substance abuse and other forms of abuse in an attempt to deal with the stress.

TREATMENT OPTIONS

With the exception of individuals who seek to change their sex, therapists who attempt to pathologize sexual orientation have been generally unsuccessful. Conversion therapy can instigate more harm than good. Some people with Gender Identification Disorder decide to live as a member of the opposite sex; some choose to undergo sex-change surgery. Psychological assistance can help individuals to gain acceptance of themselves, and can teach methods of dealing with discrimination, prejudice and violence.

Associations & Agencies

981 **Center for Family Support (CFS)**
333 7th Avenue
New York, NY 10001-5004   212-629-7939
Fax: 212-239-2211
www.cfsny.org

Steven Vernickofs, Executive Director

Service agency devoted to the physical well-being and development of the retarded child and the sound mental health of the parents. Helps families with retarded children with all aspects of home care including counseling, referrals, home aide service and consultation. Offers intervention for parents at the birth of a retarded child with in-home support, guidance and infant stimulation. Pioneered training of nonprofessional women as home aides to provide supportive services in homes.

982 **Center for Mental Health Services Knowledge Exchange Network**
US Department of Health and Human Services
PO Box 42557
Washington, DC 20015-4800
800-789-2647
Fax: 301-984-8796
TDD: 866-889-2647
E-mail: ken@mentalhealth.org
www.mentalhealth.org

Information about resources, technical assistance, research, training, networks, and other federal clearing houses, and fact sheets and materials. Information specialists refer callers to mental health resources in their communities as well as state, federal and nonprofit contacts. Staff available Monday through Friday, 8:30 AM - 5:00 PM, EST, excluding federal holidays. After hours, callers may leave messages and an information specialist will return their call.

983 **NADD: Association for Persons with Developmental Disabilities and Mental Health Needs**
132 Fair Street
Kingston, NY 12401-4802   845-334-4336
800-331-5362
Fax: 845-331-4569
E-mail: nadd@mhv.net
www.thenadd.org

Dr. Robert Fletcher, Executive Director

Nonprofit organization designed to promote interest of professional and parent development with resources for individuals who have the coexistence of mental illness and mental retardation. Provides conference, educational services and training materials to professionals, parents, concerned citizens and service organizations. Formerly known as the National Association for the Dually Diagnosed.

984 **National Gay and Lesbian Task Force**
1325 Massachusetts Avenue NW
Suite 600
Washington, DC 20005   202-393-5177
Fax: 202-393-2241
TTY: 202-393-2284
E-mail: ngltf@ngltf.com
www.ngltf.org

Matt Foreman, Executive Director

Offers community support for gay and lesbian individuals.

985 **National Institute of Mental Health**
6001 Executive Blvd
Room 8184
Bethesda, MD 20892-9663   301-443-4513
Fax: 301-443-4279
TTY: 301-443-8431
E-mail: nimhinfo@nih.gov
www.nimh.nih.gov

Thomas R Insel MD, Director
Richard K Nakamura, Deputy Director

The mission of the National Institute of Mental Health is to reduce the burden of mental illness and behavioral disorders through research on mind, brain, and behavior.

986 **National Mental Health Consumer's Self-Help Clearinghouse**
1211 Chestnut Street
Suite 1207
Philadelphia, PA 19107   215-751-1810
800-553-4539
Fax: 215-636-6312
E-mail: info@mhselfhelp.org
www.mhselfhelp.org

Alex Morrsey, Information/Referral

Funded by the National Institute of Mental Health Community Support Program, the purpose of the Clearinghouse is to encourage the development and growth of consumer self-help groups.

Year Founded: 1992

987 **Parents and Friends of Lesbians and Gays**
1726 M Street NW
Suite 400
Washington, DC 20036   202-467-8180
Fax: 202-467-8194
E-mail: info@pflag.org
www.pflag.org

David Tseng, Executive Director
Jeanne Bourgeois, Chief of Staff

Organization of families and friends of lesbian and gay individuals, dedicated to offer support and understanding.

Books

988 Gender Identify Disorder and Psychosexual Problems in Children and Adolescents

Book News
5739 NE Summer Street
Portland, OR 97218   503-281-9230
                           Fax: 503-287-4485
          E-mail: booknews@booknews.com
                           www.booknews.com

An in-depth resource on the diagnosis, assessment, etiology, and treatment of gender identity disorder in children and adolescents, reviewing recent clinical work and research in the field. *$55.00*

989 Identity Without Selfhood

Cambridge University Press
40 W 20th Street
New York, NY 10011-4211   212-924-3900
                                 800-872-7423
                            Fax: 212-691-3239
             E-mail: marketing@cup.org
                                 www.cup.org

Mariam Fraser

Situated at the crossroads of feminism, queer theory, and poststructuralist debates around identity, this is a book that shows how key Western concepts such as individuality constrain attempts to deconstruct the self and prevent bisexuality being understood as an identity. *$75.00*

226 pages ISBN 0-521623-57-x

Web Sites

990 www.cyberpsych.org

CyberPsych

Hosts the American Psychoanalyists Foundation, American Association of Suicideology, Society for the Exploration of Psychotherapy Intergration, and Anxiety Disorders Association of America. Also subcategories of the anxiety disorders, as well as general information, including panic disorder, phobias, obsessive compulsive disorder (OCD), social phobia, generalized anxiety disorder, post traumatic stress disorder, and phobias of childhood. Book reviews and links to web pages sharing the topics.

991 www.healthfinder.gov Healthfinder

Healthfinder is a key source for finding the best government and nonprofit health and human services information on the internet.

992 www.intelihealth.com

Aetna US Healthcare & Johns Hopkins University Health System

Aetna InteliHealth is to empower people with trusted solutions for healthier lives. We accomplish this by providing credible information from the most trusted sources.

993 www.kidspeace.org

KidsPeace

KidsPeace is a private, not-for-profit charity dedicated to serving the critical behavioral and mental health needs of children, preadolescents, and teens. KidsPeace provides specialized residential treatment services and comprehensive range of treatment programs and educational services to help families help kids anticipate and avoid crisis whenever possible.

994 www.mayohealth.org

Mayo Clinic Health Oasis

To empower people to manage their health. We accomplish this by providing useful and up-to-date information and tools that reflect the expertise and standard of excellence of Mayo Clinic.

995 www.nih.gov/health

National Institutes of Health

The National Institutes of Health is the steward of medical and behavioral research for the Nation. It is the Agency under the U.S. Department of Health and Human Services.

996 www.nlm.nih.gov

National Library of Medicine

The National Library of Medicine provides many of its products and services on the Web, including the highly used PubMed database, a collection of millions of citations for biomedical articles back to the 1950's, and Medline Plus, an extensive source of health information from the National Institute of Health and other trusted sources.

997 www.planetpsych.com

Planetpsych.com

Learn about disorders, their treatments and other topics in psychology. Articles are listed under the related topic areas. Ask a therapist a question for free, or view the directory of professionals in your area. If you are a therapist sign up for the directory. Current features, self-help, interactive, and newsletter archives.

998   **www.psychcentral.com**

Psych Central

Personalized one-stop index for psychology, support,
and mental health issues, resources, and people on the
Internet.

Introduction

Almost everyone has experienced a situation where they are tempted to do something that is not good for them but they do it anyway. This kind of behavior only becomes a disorder when a person is repeatedly and persistently unable to resist a temptation which is always harmful to them or to others. Usually the person feels a rising tension before acting on the need, feels pleasure and relief when giving in to the impulse and, sometimes, feels remorse and guilt afterwards. Four different disorders are included in this category.

KLEPTOMANIA

Symptoms
•Recurrent failure to resist the impulse to steal objects; often they are objects the individual could have paid for or doesn't particularly want;
•Increased sense of tension immediately before the theft;
•Pleasure and relief during the stealing;
•The theft is not due to anger, delusions or hallucinations.
•Awareness that stealing is senseless and wrong;
•Feelings of depression and guilt after stealing.

Associated Features
Kleptomania should not be confused with shoplifting or other thefts which are deliberate and for personal gain, or those that are sometimes done by adolescents on a dare or as a rite of passage. Kleptomania is strongly associated with Depression, Anxiety Disorders, and Eating Disorders.

Prevalence
Kleptomania appears to be very rare, less than five percent of shoplifters have the disorder. However, Kleptomania is usually kept secret by the person, so this estimate may be low. It is much more common among females than males and may continue in spite of convictions for shoplifting.

Treatment Options
Behavior therapy, which is psychotherapy focusing on changing the behavior, has had some success, as has anti-depressant medication. A combination of these is most likely to help the person curb the impulse to steal while treating some of the underlying problems.

PYROMANIA

Symptoms
• Purposefully setting fires more than once;
•Increased tension before the deed;
•Fascination with and curiosity about fire and its paraphernalia;
•Pleasure or relief when setting or watching fires;
•The fire is not set for financial gain, revenge, or political reasons.

Associated Features
Many with this disorder make complicated preparations for setting a fire, and seem not to care about the serious consequences. They may get pleasure from the destruction. Most juveniles who set fires also have symptoms of Attention-Deficit/Hyperactivity Disorder or Adjustment Disorder.

Prevalence
Over forty percent of people arrested for arson in the US are under 18, but among children, the disorder is rare. Fire setting occurs mostly among males, and is more common for males with alcohol problems, learning problems and poor social skills.

Treatment Options
There is no agreed-upon best treatment. Pyromania is difficult to treat because the person usually does not take responsibility for the fire setting, and is in denial. Some therapies focused directly on the psychotherapy with the individual and with the family have been helpful. There is some indication that antidepressants may be effective.

PATHOLOGICAL GAMBLING

Symptoms
 Recurrent gambling;
 Gambling distrupts family, personal and work activities;
 Preoccupation with gambling, thinking about

past plays, planning future gambling and how to get money for more gambling;

Seeks excitement more than money. Bets become bigger and risks greater to produce the needed excitement;

Gambling continues despite repeated efforts to stop with accompanying restlessness and irritability;

Person may gamble to escape depression, anxiety, guilt;

Chasing losses may become a pattern;

May lie to family, therapists, and others to conceal gambling;

May turn to criminal behavior (forgery, fraud, theft) to get money for gambling;

May lose job, relationships, career opportunities;

Bailout behavior, that is turning to family and others when in desperate financial straits.

Associated Features

Compulsive gamblers are distorted in their thinking. They are superstitious, deny they have a problem, and may be overconfident. They believe that money is the cause of, and solution to, all their problems. They are often competitive and easily bored. They may be extravagantly generous and very concerned with other people's approval. Compulsive gamblers are prone to medical problems connected with stress, such as hypertension and migraine. They also have a higher rate of Attention-Deficit/Hyperactivity Disorder; up to seventy-five percent suffer from Major Depressive Disorder, one third from Bipolar Disorder, and more than fifty percent abuse alcohol. Twenty percent are reported to have attempted suicide.

Prevalence

Gambling takes different forms in different cultures, e.g. cock-fights, horse racing, the stock market. Both males and females are compulsive gamblers. Men usually begin gambling in adolescence, women somewhat later.

Women are more likely to use gambling as an escape from Depression. The prevalence of pathological gambling is high and rising between one percent and three percent of the adult US population.

It is estimated that half of pathological gamblers are women, though women only make up from two percent to four percent of Gamblers Anonymous. Women may not go to treatment programs because of greater stigma attached to women gamblers.

Treatment Options

It is a difficult disorder to treat, but psychotherapy that concretely targets the behavior had limited success. Gamblers Anonymous, a 12-step program, may enable some to stop gambling. Treatment of the underlying disorders and involving family members may be helpful.

TRICHOTILLOMANIA

Symptoms

Repeated hair pulling so that hair loss is noticeable;

Increasing tension just before the behavior or when trying to resist it;

Pleasure or relief when pulling;

Causes clear distress and problems in personal work, or social functioning.

Associated Features

Examining the hair root, pulling the hair between the teeth, or eating hairs (Trichophagia) may accompany Trichotillomania. Hair pulling is usually done in private or in the presence of close family members. Pain is not usually reported. The hair pulling is mostly denied and concealed by wigs, hairstyling and cosmetics. People with this disorder may also have Major Depressive Disorder, General Anxiety Disorder, Eating Disorder or Mental Retardation.

Prevalence

Among children, both males and females can have the disorder, but among adults, it is far more frequent in females. There are no recent prevalence figures for the general population, but in studies of college students, one percent to two percent have experienced Trichotillomania.

Treatment Options

There is no agreement about the cause of this disorder, making treatment more difficult. Professionals are often not consulted. Variable treatments that have been proposed include behavior therapy, hypnosis, and stress reduction. Medication has sometimes been helpful.

Associations & Agencies

1000 Career Assessment & Planning Services

Goodwill Industries-Suncoast
10596 Gandy Boulevard
St. Petersburg, FL 33733   727-523-1512
          Fax: 727-563-9300
E-mail: gw.marketing@goodwill-suncoast.com
          www.goodwill-suncoast.org

R Lee Waits, President / CEO
Dan R Johnson, Secretary

We provide diagnostic services aimed at determining the readiness of individuals for community resources that could improve the quality of life for those who are unprepared for immediate placement in employment.

1001 Center for Family Support (CFS)

333 7th Avenue
New York, NY 10001-5004   212-629-7939
          Fax: 212-239-2211
          www.cfsny.org

Steven Vernickofs, Executive Director

Service agency devoted to the physical well-being and development of the retarded child and the sound mental health of the parents. Helps families with retarded children with all aspects of home care including counseling, referrals, home aide service and consultation. Offers intervention for parents at the birth of a retarded child with in-home support, guidance and infant stimulation. Pioneered training of nonprofessional women as home aides to provide supportive services in homes.

1002 Center for Mental Health Services Knowledge Exchange Network

US Department of Health and Human Services
PO Box 42557
Washington, DC 20015-4800
          800-789-2647
          Fax: 301-984-8796
          TDD: 866-889-2647
E-mail: ken@mentalhealth.org
          www.mentalhealth.org

A Kathryn Power M Ed, Director

Information about resources, technical assistance, research, training, networks, and other federal clearing houses, and fact sheets and materials. Information specialists refer callers to mental health resources in their communities as well as state, federal and non-profit contacts. Staff available Monday through Friday, 8:30 AM - 5:00 PM, EST, excluding federal holidays. After hours, callers may leave messages and an information specialist will return their call.

1003 NADD: Association for Persons with Developmental Disabilities and Mental Health Needs

132 Fair Street
Kingston, NY 12401-4802   845-334-4336
          800-331-5362
          Fax: 845-331-4569
          E-mail: nadd@mhv.net
          www.thenadd.org

Dr. Robert Fletcher, Executive Director

Nonprofit organization designed to promote interest of professional and parent development with resources for individuals who have the coexistence of mental illness and mental retardation. Provides conference, educational services and training materials to professionals, parents, concerned citizens and service organizations. Formerly known as the National Association for the Dually Diagnosed.

1004 National Mental Health Consumer's Self-Help Clearinghouse

1211 Chestnut Street
Suite 1207
Philadelphia, PA 19107   215-751-1810
          800-553-4539
          Fax: 215-636-6312
          E-mail: info@mhselfhelp.org
          www.mhselfhelp.org

Alex Morrsey, Information/Referral

Funded by the National Institute of Mental Health Community Support Program, the purpose of the Clearinghouse is to encourage the development and growth of consumer self-help groups.

Year Founded: 1992

1005 Suncoast Residential Training Center/Developmental Services Program

Goodwill Industries-Suncoast
10596 Gandy Boulevard
St. Petersburg, FL 33733   727-523-1512
          Fax: 727-563-9300
E-mail: gw.marketing@goodwill-suncoast.com
          www.goodwill-suncoast.org

R Lee Waits, President / CEO
Dan R Johnson, Secretary

A large group home which serves individuals diagnosed as mentally retarded with a secondary diagnosed of psychiatric difficulties as evidenced by problem behavior. Providing residential, behavioral and instructional support and services that will promote the development of adaptive, socially appropriate behavior, each individual is assessed to determine, socialization, basic academics and recreation. The primary intervention strategy is applied behavior analysis. Professional consultants are utilized to address the medical, dental, psychiatric and pharmacological needs of each individual. One of the most popular features is the active community integration component of SRTC. Program customers attend an average of 15 monthly outings to various community events.

Books

1006 104 Activities That Build: Self Esteem, Teamwork, Communication, Anger Management, Self Discovery & Coping Games

Childs Work/Childs Play
135 Dupont Street
PO Box 760
Plainville, NY 11803-0760

800-962-1141
Fax: 800-262-1886
E-mail: info@Childswork.com
www.Childswork.com

Full of interactive and fun games and activities that can be used with small or large groups, or even one on one. *$23.95*

271 pages

1007 Angry All the Time

Courage to Change
PO Box 1268
Newburgh, NY 12551

800-440-4003
Fax: 800-772-6499

Help for those who lose control too often. Identify the causes of anger, avoid problems steming as a result of unmanged anger and learn how to change with eight steps of anger management. *$12.95*

136 pages

1008 Check Up from the Neck Up, Ensuring your Mental Health in the New Millennium

Hope Press
PO Box 188
Duarte, CA 91009-0188

818-303-0644
800-321-4039
Fax: 818-358-3520
www.hopepress.com

Provides concise coping techniques for adults who have difficulties due to anxiety, depression, short temper, irritability, rage-attacks, compulsions, obbsession and attention deficit hyperactivity disorder. *$19.95*

550 pages ISBN 1-878267-09-4

1009 Dysinhibition Syndrome How to Handle Anger and Rage in Your Child or Spouse

Hope Press
PO Box 188
Duarte, CA 91009-0188

818-303-0644
800-321-4039
Fax: 818-358-3520
www.hopepress.com

How to understand and handle rage and anger in your children or spouse. The book presents behavioral approaches that can be very effective and an understanding that can be family saving. *$24.95*

271 pages ISBN 1-878267-08-6

1010 Impulsivity and Compulsivity

American Psychiatric Publishing
1000 Wilson Boulevard
Suite 1825
Arlington, VA 22209-3901

703-907-7322
800-368-5777
Fax: 703-907-1091
E-mail: appi@psych.org
www.appi.org

Katie Duffy, Marketing Assistant

Leading researchers and clinicians share their expertise on the phenomenological, biological, psychodynamic, and treatment aspects of these disorders. *$40.00*

294 pages ISBN 0-880486-76-7

1011 Trichotillomania

American Psychiatric Publishing
1000 Wilson Boulevard
Suite 1825
Arlington, VA 22209-3901

703-907-7322
800-368-5777
Fax: 703-907-1091
E-mail: appi@psych.org
www.appi.org

Katie Duffy, Marketing Assistant

Study of hair pulling from both a clinical and a research perspective. Documenting the clinical phenomenology, morbidity and management of trichotillomania. The use of medication, the value of behavioral interventions and the role of hypnotherapy are also thoroughy discussed. *$45.00*

368 pages ISBN 0-880487-59-3

Support Groups & Hot Lines

1012 Gam-Anon Family Groups

PO Box 157
Whitestone, NY 11357

718-352-1671

Twelve-step program for relatives and friends of compulsive gamblers.

1013 Gamblers Anonymous

PO Box 17173
Los Angeles, CA 90017

213-386-8789
Fax: 213-386-0030
E-mail: isomain@gamblersanonymous.org
www.gamblersanonymous.org

Web Sites

1014 www.alzwell.com/Clues.html

When Anger Hurts: Quieting the Storm Within

Recognizing trigger behavior that usually precedes and precipitates a violent outburst.

1015 www.apa.org/pubinfo/anger.html

Controlling Anger-Before It Controls You

From the American Psychological Association.

1016 www.cyberpsych.org

CyberPsych

Hosts the American Psychoanalyists Foundation, American Association of Suicideology, Society for the Exploration of Psychotherapy Intergration, and Anxiety Disorders Association of America. Also sub-categories of the anxiety disorders, as well as general information, including panic disorder, phobias, obsessive compulsive disorder (OCD), social phobia, generalized anxiety disorder, post traumatic stress disorder, and phobias of childhood. Book reviews and links to web pages sharing the topics.

1017 www.drkoop.com/wellness/mental_health/

Compulsive Gambling

1018 www.incestabuse.about.com/library/

Anger-Part II: Using Anger's Power Safely

Excellent overview.

1019 www.incestabuse.about.com/library/weekly/

Anger-Part I: Identifying Anger

Excellent overview.

1020 www.members.aol.com/AngriesOut

Get Your Angries Out

Guidelines for kids, teachers, and parents.

1021 www.mentalhelp.net/psyhelp/chap7

Anger and Aggression

Therapeutic approaches.

1022 www.npin.org/library/pre1998/n00216/n00216. html

Plain Talk About...Dealing with the Angry Child

From US Department of Health and Human Services.

1023 www.npin.org/pnews/pnews997/pnew997g .html

Temper Tantrums: What Causes Them and How Can You Respond?

Parent's News publication.

1024 www.planetpsych.com

Planetpsych.com

Learn about disorders, their treatments and other topics in psychology. Articles are listed under the related topic areas. Ask a therapist a question for free, or view the directory of professionals in your area. If you are a therapist sign up for the directory. Current features, self-help, interactive, and newsletter archives.

1025 www.psychcentral.com

Psych Central

Personalized one-stop index for psychology, support, and mental health issues, resources, and people on the Internet.

1026 www.queendom.com/articles/arguing_intro.html

Arguing and Relationships: Introduction

Constructive arguing and communication skills.

1027 www.topchoice.com/~psyche/love/misc communicate.html

Communication When Anger is Involved

Clear on how disagreements are normal, but escalation is not.

Introduction

Movement Disorders, though widely believed to be mental disorders, are actually classified as diseases which affect an individual's ability to move normally. Medication-induced Movement Disorders include Parkinson's Disease, Neuroleptic Malignant Syndrome, Acute Dystonia, Acute Akathisia, and Tardive Dyskinesia. Typical symptoms include tremors, tics, and other involuntary movements. Here we will focus on Tardive Dyskinesia, which is a serious side effect, or complication, of treatment with some antipsychotic medications, though some newer medications carry a much reduced risk of the condition.

SYMPTOMS

•Involuntary movement of the tongue, jaw, torso, or limbs developed in association with the use of neuroleptic (antipsychotic) medication;
•The involuntary movements are present over at least four weeks, in the following patterns:
Choreiform (rapid, jerky non-repetitive);
Athetoid (slow, sinous, continual);
Rhythmic (sterotyped);
•These symptoms develop during exposure to an antipsychotic medication or within four weeks of withdrawal from an oral form of the medication;
•There has been at least a three-month exposure to antipsychotic medication (one month for those 60 years or older);
•Symptoms are not due to a neurological or a general medical condition, ill-fitting dentures, or other medications that cause acute reversible dyskinesia (e.g., L-dopa).

ASSOCIATED FEATURES

The involuntary movements of Tardive Dyskinesia are often facial, such as chewing, sucking, and grimacing, but may include arms, legs, and respiratory muscles. Although it is more common in people who have been taking antipsychotic drugs for years, neither the amount taken nor the length of time on the drug seems to be the main determinant. Thus, the precise cause is not clear.

More than seventy-five percent of those with the disorder have abnormal facial movements; about fifty percent have abnormal limb movements; and up to twenty-five percent show abnormal movements of the torso. About ten percent are affected in all these regions. Facial movements are more common among the elderly; limb and trunk movement are more often found among younger people. The movements can be made worse by stimulants and other medications, and may also be temporarily intensified by emotional stress. Relaxation and voluntary movement in the affected parts can reduce them, and they generally do not appear during sleep.

Tardive Dyskinesia can begin at any age and usually starts with very slight involuntary movements which may not even be noticed. When the movements are severe, they may be associated with other serious conditions: ulcers in cheek or tongue, enlargement of the tongue, difficulty in swallowing, breathing, walking, weight loss and depression. The disorder is sometimes associated with people who have some form of brain pathology or emotional disorders.

PREVALENCE

Prevalence of Tardive Dyskinesia in those who have had long-term treatment with antipsychotic medication is between twenty percent and thirty percent. It appears to develop in twenty percent to forty percent of schizophrenic patients who receive long-term antipsychotic drug treatment. In general, the disorder is more common among the elderly, with prevalence up to fifty percent among elderly people receiving antipsychotic drugs over long periods.

Among young people, there are no gender differences, but among elderly, women are more often affected than men. The disorder is more common in the chronically institutionalized.

TREATMENT OPTIONS

No treatment is completely effective. Paradoxically, neuroleptic medication can mask the condition. When the neuroleptic medication is stopped, five percent to forty percent of all cases cease to have abnormal involuntary movements and, if the movement disorder is mild, fifty percent ot ninety percent go into remission. In general, younger people are more likely to show improvement, and among the elderly the disorder is more likely to become more severe.

Patients on neuroleptic medications should be regularly assessed for signs of Tardive Dyskinesia. The risks of this disorder must be carefully weighed against the risks of untreated psychotic illness.

Associations & Agencies

1029 American Parkinson's Disease Association

60 Bay Street
Staten Island, NY 10301

802-223-2732
Fax: 718-981-4399

National organization dedicated to support and serve those individuals striken with Parkinson's disease by providing information on treatment, education, referrals. Also supports victim's caregivers.

1030 Center for Family Support (CFS)

333 7th Avenue
New York, NY 10001-5004

212-629-7939
Fax: 212-239-2211
www.cfsny.org

Steven Vernickofs, Executive Director

Service agency devoted to the physical well-being and development of the retarded child and the sound mental health of the parents. Helps families with retarded children with all aspects of home care including counseling, referrals, home aide service and consultation. Offers intervention for parents at the birth of a retarded child with in-home support, guidance and infant stimulation. Pioneered training of nonprofessional women as home aides to provide supportive services in homes.

1031 Center for Mental Health Services Knowledge Exchange Network

US Department of Health and Human Services
PO Box 42490
Washington, DC 20015-4800

800-789-2647
Fax: 301-984-8796
E-mail: ken@mentalhealth.org
www.mentalhealth.org

Information about resources, technical assistance, research, training, networks, and other federal clearing houses, and fact sheets and materials. Information specialists refer callers to mental health resources in their communities as well as state, federal and nonprofit contacts. Staff available Monday through Friday, 8:30 AM-5:00 PM, EST, excluding federal holidays. After hours, callers may leave messages and an information specialist will return their call.

1032 NADD: Association for Persons with Developmental Disabilities and Mental Health Needs

132 Fair Street
Kingston, NY 12401-4802

845-334-4336
800-331-5362
Fax: 845-331-4569
E-mail: nadd@mhv.net
www.thenadd.org

Dr. Robert Fletcher, Executive Director

Nonprofit organization designed to promote interest of professional and parent development with resources for individuals who have the coexistence of mental illness and mental retardation. Provides conference, educational services and training materials to professionals, parents, concerned citizens and service organizations. Formerly known as the National Association for the Dually Diagnosed.

1033 National Mental Health Consumer's Self-Help Clearinghouse

1211 Chestnut Street
Suite 1207
Philadelphia, PA 19107

215-751-1810
800-553-4539
Fax: 215-636-6312
E-mail: info@mhselfhelp.org
www.mhselfhelp.org

Alex Morrsey, Information/Referral

Funded by the National Institute of Mental Health Community Support Program, the purpose of the Clearinghouse is to encourage the development and growth of consumer self-help groups.

Year Founded: 1992

1034 National Parkinson Foundation

1501 NW 9th Avenue
Bob Hope Road
Miami, FL 33136-1494

305-547-6666
800-327-4545
Fax: 305-243-4403
E-mail: mailbox@parkinson.org
www.parkinson.org

Daniel Arty, President
Paul F Oreffice, Co-Chairman

1035 Tardive Dyskinesia: Tardive Dystonia National Association

PO Box 45732
Seattle, WA 98145-0732

206-522-3166
Fax: 206-528-2117
E-mail: skjaer@halcyon.com
www.icomm.ca/geninfo/dystoria.htm

Sonja Kjaer, Director

A voluntary nonprofit self help organization dedicated to providing information and support to individuals with Tardive Dyskinesia or Tardive Dystonia, family members, health care professionals and the general public. Committed to encouraging research on Tardive Dyskinesia & Dystonia. Enabling affected individuals to exchange information, support and resources through its networking program. Advocates on behalf of affected individuals. Offers a variety of educational materials including reports, journal article reprints, and brochures.

Books

1036 Adverse Effects of Psychotropic Drugs

Gilford Press
72 Spring Street
New York, NY 10012   212-431-9800

$63.00

1037 Management of Tardive Dyskinesia

American Psychiatric Publishing
1000 Wilson Boulevard
Suite 1825
Arlington, VA 22209-3901   703-907-7322
                                 800-368-5777
                            Fax: 703-907-1091
                     E-mail: appi@psych.org
                                 www.appi.org

Katie Duffy, Marketing Assistant

$7.50

ISBN 0-890420-04-1

1038 Tardive Dyskinesia: Biological Mechanisms & Clinical Aspects, Progress in Psychiatry

American Psychiatric Publishing
1000 Wilson Boulevard
Suite 1825
Arlington, VA 22209-3901   703-907-7322
                                 800-368-5777
                            Fax: 703-907-1091
                     E-mail: appi@psych.org
                                 www.appi.org

$13.50

290 pages ISBN 0-880481-76-5

1039 Understanding & Treating Tardive Dyskinesia

Guilford Publications
72 Spring Street
New York, NY 10012   212-431-9800
                                 800-365-7006
                            Fax: 212-966-6708
                   E-mail: info@guilford.com
                                 www.guilford.com

$52.50

363 pages ISBN 0-898621-75-5

Video & Audio

1040 Questions & Answers About Tardive Dyskinesia

Duvall Media

Neva Duyndam, Editor

Discusses tardive dyskinesia, a possible side effect of anit-spychotic drugs. Audio cassette. *$9.95*

Year Founded: 1989 ISBN 1-878159-07-0

Web Sites

1041 www.apdaparkinson.com

American Parkinson Disease Association

Basic Parkinson's information.

1042 www.michaeljfox.org

Michael J Fox Foundation

A user-friendly information source.

1043 www.ninds.nih.gov/health_and_medical/ disorder_index.htm

National Institute of Neurological Disorders and Stroke

High quality information.

1044 www.parkinson.org

National Parkinson Foundation

The information is well presented and covers all the issues related to Parkinson's.

1045 www.parkinsonsinstitute.org

Parkinson's Institute

Consumer friendly information on Parkinson's and other movement disorders.

1046 www.pdf.org

Parkinson's Disease Foundation

A well organized and comprehensive site.

1047 www.pharmacology.about.com/health/ pharmacology/library/weekly/aa970710.h tm

About.com on Parkinson's Disease Drugs and Treatments

About Parkinson's Disease drugs.

1048 www.planetpsych.com

Planetpsych.com

Learn about disorders, their treatments and other topics in psychology. Articles are listed under the related topic areas. Ask a therapist a question for free, or view the directory of professionals in your area. If you are a therapist sign up for the directory. Current features, self-help, interactive, and newsletter archives.

1049 www.psychcentral.com

Psych Central

Personalized one-stop index for psychology, support, and mental health issues, resources, and people on the Internet.

1050 www.wemove.org

We Move: Worldwide Education and Awareness for Movement Disorders

Deals with movement disorders and offers information, chat room, webcast presentations, and links.

1051 www.wpda.org

World Parkinson Disease Association

Articles that cover treatment and research.

Obsessive Compulsive Disorder/Introduction

Introduction

Obsessive Compulsive Disorder (OCD) is a diagnosis given to individuals who have overwhelming obsessions and/or compulsions. Obsessions are repeated, intrusive, unwanted thoughts that cause distressing emotions such as anxiety or disgust. A person may worry constantly about infection and contamination, for instance. Or a person may fear that he will embarrass himself in public. A compulsion, which often accompanies an obsession, is a ceaseless urge to do something to lessen the anxiety and discomfort caused by the obession. People who have obsessions and compulsions often engage in rituals (a highly systematized set of repetitious actions).

Obsessive Compulsive Disorder may be mild or severe: an indvidual may engage in a private ritual that may be out of the ordinary, but which does not significantly impede the individual from doing other activites. In more severe cases, the rituals may consume an entire day making normal functioning impossible. But because obsessions and compulsions often make the individual feel powerless, even mild cases can cause significant distress.

A remarkable amount of research activity is being conducted on OCD, and treatments (including medication and behavior therapy) are frequently successful. The vast majority of patients who are properly treated can live normal lives.

SYMPTOMS

Recurrent and persistent thoughts, impulses or images that are experienced as intrusive and inappropriate and that cause marked anxiety or distress:
•The thoughts or images are not simply excessive worries about real-life problems;
•Repetitive behaviors that the person feels driven to perform in response to an obsession, or according to rules that must be applied rigidly;
•The person recognizes that the obession or compulsions are unreasonable;

•The obsessions or compulsions cause marked distress, are time consuming, or significantly interfere with the person's normal routine, occupational or academic functioning, or usual social activities.

ASSOCIATED FEATURES

The most common obsessions in people with OCD are repeated thoughts about contamination, repeated doubts (for instance about whether one has hurt someone in a traffic accident or left a door unlocked or the stove on) and a need to have things in a particular order. Other common obsessions include concern about aggressive impulses, such as a fear that one will hurt one's child or shout obscenities in a public place. Also common are unreasonable fears about one's health, with repeated visits to the doctor.

The individual with OCD knows that these concerns are unreasonable, but feels powerless to stop them. And the individual usually undertakes some kind of ritualistic action to quell the anxieties caused by his or her obsession.

Because of the distress caused by the condition, people with OCD will often avoid situations that trigger the obsession. For instance, a person with a fear of contamination and a compulsion to wash hands may avoid shaking hands with strangers or eating in public restaurants. Performing compulsions can become virtually a full-time task, severely disrupting relationships and impeding the individual's ability to participate in normal life.

PREVALENCE

Although OCD usually begins in adolescence or early adulthood, it may begin in childhood. Age at onset is earlier in males than in females: between the ages of six and 15 years for males and 20 and 29 for females. Symptoms of OCD in children are generally similar to those in adults. Washing, checking, and ordering rituals are particularly common in children. The disorder is equally common in men as in women. Although OCD was once thought to be relatively rare, recent studies have estimated that two and one-half percent of the population may have the disorder.

TREATMENT OPTIONS

Patients with OCD may benefit from behavioral therapy and/or a variety of medications. Currently, one of the most effective therapies is a kind of behavior therapy called exposure and response prevention. Using this therapy, a patient, with a therapist, is carefully exposed to situations that generally cause anxiety and provoke the obsessive compulsive behavior. Slowly, the patient learns to decrease and later stop the ritualistic behavior altogether. In behavior therapy, a patient must sometimes agree to abide by certain guidelines established by the therapist. For instance, a patient who is a compulsive handwasher might agree to spend no more than ten minutes a day washing. People who are compulsive checkers might agree to check door locks and gas stoves only once a day. Some patients may use medication. Medications often used for depression have been found to be successful for OCD; these drugs include fluoxetine, fluvoxamine, paroxeatine, sertraline, and clomipramine. In very severe cases, in which the OCD is disabling, brain surgery is an option.

Associations & Agencies

1053 Career Assessment & Planning Services

Goodwill Industries-Suncoast
10596 Gandy Boulevard
St. Petersburg, FL 33733   727-523-1512
                              Fax: 727-563-9300
E-mail: gw.marketing@goodwill-suncoast.com
                    www.goodwill-suncoast.org

R Lee Waits, President / CEO
Loreen M Spencer, Chairman

Provides diagnostic services aimed at determining the
readiness of individuals for employment and training.
In addition to making employment and training recommendations, Goodwill identifies community resources that could improve the quality of life for those
who are unprepared for immmediate placement in employment.

1054 Center for Family Support (CFS)

333 7th Avenue
New York, NY 10001-5004   212-629-7939
                              Fax: 212-239-2211
                                  www.cfsny.org

Steven Vernickofs, Executive Director

Service agency devoted to the physical well-being and
development of the retarded child and the sound mental health of the parents. Helps families with retarded
children with all aspects of home care including counseling, referrals, home aide service and consultation.
Offers intervention for parents at the birth of a retarded child with in-home support, guidance and infant stimulation. Pioneered training of
nonprofessional women as home aides to provide supportive services in homes.

1055 Center for Mental Health Services Knowledge Exchange Network

US Department of Health and Human Services
PO Box 42490
Washington, DC 20015-4800
                                  800-789-2647
                              Fax: 301-984-8796
              E-mail: ken@mentalhealth.org
                    www.mentalhealth.org

Information about resources, technical assistance, research, training, networks, and other federal clearing
houses, and fact sheets and materials. Information
specialists refer callers to mental health resources in
their communities as well as state, federal and nonprofit contacts. Staff available Monday through Friday, 8:30 AM - 5:00 PM, EST, excluding federal
holidays. After hours, callers may leave messages and
an information specialist will return their call.

1056 NADD: Association for Persons with Developmental Disabilities and Mental Health Needs

132 Fair Street
Kingston, NY 12401-4802   845-334-4336
                                  800-331-5362
                              Fax: 845-331-4569
                    E-mail: nadd@mhv.net
                          www.thenadd.org

Dr. Robert Fletcher, Executive Director

Nonprofit organization designed to promote interest
of professional and parent development with resources for individuals who have the coexistence of
mental illness and mental retardation. Provides conference, educational services and training materials to
professionals, parents, concerned citizens and service
organizations. Formerly known as the National Association for the Dually Diagnosed.

1057 National Mental Health Consumer's Self-Help Clearinghouse

1211 Chestnut Street
Suite 1207
Philadelphia, PA 19107   215-751-1810
                                  800-553-4539
                              Fax: 215-636-6312
              E-mail: info@mhselfhelp.org
                    www.mhselfhelp.org

Alex Morrsey, Information/Referral

Funded by the National Institute of Mental Health
Community Support Program, the purpose of the
Clearinghouse is to encourage the development and
growth of consumer self-help groups.

Year Founded: 1992

1058 Obsessive Compulsive Anonymous

PO Box 215
New Hyde Park, NY 11040   516-741-4901

National, nonprofit, self help organization consisting
of a fellowship of individuals dedicated to sharing
their experience, strength and hope with one another
to enable them to solve their common problems and
help others recover from OCD. Established in 1988,
OCA is a fellowship of people who use the Twelve
Steps, adapted for OCA, to help obtain relief from obsessions and compulsions. Consisting of approximately 1,000 members and 50 chapters, OCA is not
allied with any sect, denomination, organization or institution. Provides informational pamphlets and meeting contact lists with contacts throughout the United
States and Canada.

1059 Obsessive Compulsive Foundation

676 State Street
New Haven, CT 06511   203-401-2070
                              Fax: 203-401-2076
              E-mail: info@ocfoundation.org
                    www.ocfoundation.org

Janet S Emmerman, President
Joy Kant, Treasurer

For sufferers of obsessive-compulsive disorder and their families and friends. To educate the public and professional communities about OCD and related disorders; to provide assistance to individuals with OCD and related disorders, their family and friends, and to support research into the causes and effective treatments.

1060 Obsessive Compulsive Information Center

Madison Institute of Medicine
7617 Mineral Point Road
Suite 300
Madison, WI 53717-1623   608-827-2470
                               Fax: 608-827-2479
                          E-mail: mim@miminc.org
                               www.miminc.org

Provides information packets, booklets, patient guides, and telephone information services.

1061 Suncoast Residential Training Center/Developmental Services Program

Goodwill Industries-Suncoast
10596 Gandy Boulevard
St. Petersburg, FL 33733   727-523-1512
                                 Fax: 727-563-9300
E-mail: gw.marketing @goodwill-suncoast.com
                          www.goodwill-suncoast.org

R Lee Waits, President/CEO
Loreen M Spencer CPA, Chairman

A large group home which serves individuals diagnosed as mentally retarded with a secondary diagnosed of psychiatric difficulties as evidenced by problem behavior. Providing residential, behavioral and instructional support and services that will promote the development of adaptive, socially appropriate behavior, each individual is assessed to determine, socialization, basic academics and recreation. The primary intervention strategy is applied behavior analysis. Professional consultants are utilized to address the medical, dental, psychiatric and pharmacological needs of ech individual. One of the most popular features is the active community integration component of SRTC. Program customers attend an average of 15 monthly outings to various community events.

Books

1062 A Thousand Frightening Fantasies: Understanding and Healing Scrupulosity and Obsessive Compulsive Disorder

National Book Network
PO Box 190
Blue Ridge Summit, PA 17214
                               800-462-6420

$19.95

228 pages ISBN 0-824516-05-2

1063 Boy Who Couldn't Stop Washing: Experience and Treatment of Obsessive-Compulsive Disorder

Penguin Group
375 Hudson Street
New York, NY 10014   212-366-2000
                           800-631-8571
                      Fax: 201-366-2679
          E-mail: online@penguinputnam.com
                    www.penguinputnam.com

A comprehensive treatment of obsessive-compulsive disorder that summarizes evidence that the disorder is neurobiological. It also describes the effect of medication combined with behavioral therapy. *$6.99*

304 pages Year Founded: 1991 ISBN 0-451172-02-7

1064 Brain Lock: Free Yourself from Obsessive Compulsive Behavior

Harper Collins
10 E 53rd Street
New York, NY 10022-5244   212-207-7000
                                 800-242-7737
                            Fax: 800-822-4090
                            www.harpercollins.com

A simple four-step method for overcoming OCD that is so effective, it's now used in academic treatment centers throughout the world. Proved by brain-imaging tests to actually alter the brain's chemistry, this method dosen't rely on psychopharmaceuticals but cognitive self-therapy and behavior modification to develop new patterns of response. Offers real-life stories of actual patients. Paperback. *$ 13.00*

219 pages ISBN 0-060987-11-1

1065 Brief Strategic Solution-Oriented Therapy of Phobic and Obsessive Disorders

Jason Aronson
400 Keystone Industrial Park
Dunmore, PA 18512-1523   570-342-1320
                                800-782-0015
                           Fax: 201-767-1576
                           www.aronson.com

Using a strategic framework, the therapist focuses on reframing the patient's representations of self and other. *$45.00*

216 pages ISBN 1-568218-04-4

1066 Check Up from the Neck Up, Ensuring your Mental Health in the New Millennium

Hope Press
PO Box 188
Duarte, CA 91009-0188   818-303-0644
                               800-321-4039
                          Fax: 818-358-3520
                          www.hopepress.com

Provides concise coping techniques for adults who have difficulties due to anxiety, depression, short temper, irritability, rage-attacks, compulsions, obbsession and attention defect hyperactivity disorder. *$19.95*

550 pages ISBN 1-878267-09-4

1067 Childhood Obsessive Compulsive Disorder (Developmental Clinical Psychology and Psychiatry)

Sage Publications
2455 Teller Road
Thousand Oaks, CA 91320   **805-499-9774**
                                     800-818-7243
                         Fax: 800-583-2665
                    E-mail: info@sagepub.com
                         www.sagepub.com

$21.95

ISBN 0-803959-22-2

1068 Freeing Your Child from Obsessive-Compulsive Disorder

Crown Publishing Group
201 E 50th Street
New York, NY 10022-7703   **212-572-6117**
                         Fax: 212-572-6192

ISBN 0-812931-16-5

1069 Funny, You Don't Look Crazy: Life With Obsessive Compulsive Disorder

Dilligaf Publishing
64 Court Street
Ellsworth, ME 04605   **207-667-5031**

A honest look at people who live with Obsessive Compulsive Disorder and those who love them.

128 pages Year Founded: 1994 ISBN 0-963907-00-X

1070 Getting Control: Overcoming Your Obsessions and Compulsions

Penguin Putnam
375 Hudson Street
New York, NY 10014-3658   **212-366-2000**
                                     800-227-9604
                         Fax: 201-896-8569
                    www.pengumputnam.com

Updated guide to treating OCD based on clinically proven techniques of behavior therapy. Offers a step-by-step program including assessing symptoms, setting realistic goals and creating specific therapeutic exercises.

ISBN 0-452281-77-6

1071 Imp of the Mind: Exploring the Silent Epidemic of Obsessive Bad Thoughts

Penguin Putnam
375 Hudson Street
New York, NY 10014-3658   **212-366-2000**
                                     800-227-9604
                         Fax: 201-896-8569
                    www.pengumputnam.com

Draws on new advances to explore the causes of obsessive thoughts, and the difference between harmless and dangerous bad thoughts.

ISBN 0-525945-62-8

1072 Let's Talk Facts About Obsessive Compulsive Disorder

American Psychiatric Publishing
1000 Wilson Boulevard
Suite 1825
Arlington, VA 22209-3901   **703-907-7322**
                                      800-368-5777
                         Fax: 703-907-1091
                    E-mail: appi@psych.org
                         www.appi.org

Katie Duffy, Marketing Assistant

$12.50

8 pages ISBN 0-890423-58-X

1073 OCD Workbook: Your Guide to Breaking Free From Obsessive-Compulsive Disorder

New Harbinger Publications
5674 Shattuck Avenue
Oakland, CA 94609-1662   **510-652-2002**
                                    800-748-6273
                         Fax: 510-652-5472
        E-mail: customerservice@newharbinger.com
                    www.newharbinger.com

ISBN 1-572241-69-1

1074 OCD in Children and Adolescents: a Cognitive-Behavioral Treatment Manual

Guilford Publications
72 Spring Street
New York, NY 10012   **212-431-9800**
                                800-365-7006
                         Fax: 212-966-6708
                    E-mail: info@guilford.com
                         www.guilford.com

Written for clinicians, the book includes tips for parents, and treatment guidelines. The cognitive - behavioral approach to OCD has been problematic for many to understand because patients with symptoms of increased anxiety are told that their treatment initially involves further increases in their anxiety levels. The authors provide this in a modified and developmentally appropriate approach. *$32.00*

298 pages

1075 Obsessive-Compulsive Disorder

American Psychiatric Publishing
1000 Wilson Boulevard
Suite 1825
Arlington, VA 22209-3901   703-907-7322
                                 800-368-5777
                        Fax: 703-907-1091
                  E-mail: appi@psych.org
                              www.appi.org

Katie Duffy, Marketing Assistant

Contents include an introduction to OCD, epidemiology, clinical picture, OCD with comorbid conditions, spectrum disorder, biological substrates, drug treatment, psychological approaches to treatment, treatment resistant OCD, and management of OCD. $14.95

64 pages ISBN 1-853173-87-8

1076 Obsessive-Compulsive Disorder Across the Life Cycle

American Psychiatric Publishing
1000 Wilson Boulevard
Suite 1825
Arlington, VA 22209-3901   703-907-7322
                                 800-368-5777
                        Fax: 703-907-1091
                  E-mail: appi@psych.org
                              www.appi.org

Katie Duffy, Marketing Assistant

Obsessive - compulsive disorder in children, adolescents, adults, during pregnancy and in later life. $25.00

144 pages ISBN 0-880484-47-0

1077 Obsessive-Compulsive Disorder Casebook

American Psychiatric Publishing
1000 Wilson Boulevard
Suite 1825
Arlington, VA 22209-3901   703-907-7322
                                 800-368-5777
                        Fax: 703-907-1091
                  E-mail: appi@psych.org
                              www.appi.org

Katie Duffy, Marketing Assistant

Presents 60 case histories of OCD with a discussion by the author and editors regarding their opinion on each diagnosis. $39.95

336 pages ISBN 0-880487-29-1

1078 Obsessive-Compulsive Disorder Spectrum

American Psychiatric Publishing
1000 Wilson Boulevard
Suite 1825
Arlington, VA 22209-3901   703-907-7322
                                 800-368-5777
                        Fax: 703-907-1091
                  E-mail: appi@psych.org
                              www.appi.org

Katie Duffy, Marketing Assistant

Comprehensive examination of OCD, related disorders and treatment regimens. $68.50

338 pages ISBN 0-880487-07-0

1079 Obsessive-Compulsive Disorder in Children and Adolescents: A Guide

Madison Institute of Medicine
7617 Mineral Point Road
Suite 300
Madison, WI 53717-1623   608-827-2470
                        Fax: 608-827-2479
                  E-mail: mim@miminc.org
                              www.miminc.org

The guide is a comprehensive introduction to obsessive-compulsive disorder for parents who are learning about the illness. Discusses treating symptoms by a combination of behavioral therapy and medication and describes various drugs that can be used with children and adolescents in terms of their effects on brain functioning, symptom control, and side-effects. The book is attuned to the difficulties families of OCD children face. $5.95

66 pages ISBN 1-890802-28-X

1080 Obsessive-Compulsive Disorder in Children and Adolescents

American Psychiatric Publishing
1000 Wilson Boulevard
Suite 1825
Arlington, VA 22209-3901   703-907-7322
                                 800-368-5777
                        Fax: 703-907-1091
                  E-mail: appi@psych.org
                              www.appi.org

Katie Duffy, Marketing Assistant

Examines the early development of obsessive - compulsive disorder and describes to effective treatments. $47.50

360 pages ISBN 0-880482-82-6

1081 Obsessive-Compulsive Disorder: Theory, Research and Treatment

Guilford Publications
72 Spring Street
New York, NY 10012   212-431-9800
                                 800-365-7006
                        Fax: 212-966-6708
                  E-mail: info@guilford.com
                              www.guilford.com

Part I: Psychopathology and Theoretical Perspectives; Part II: Assessment and Treatment; Part III: Obsessive Compulsive Spectrum Disorders; Appendix: List of Resources. $50.00

478 pages ISBN 1-572303-35-2

1082 Obsessive-Compulsive Disorders: A Complete Guide to Getting Well and Staying Well

Oxford University Press
198 Madison Avenue
New York, NY 10016   212-726-6000
                                 800-451-7556
                        Fax: 919-677-1303
                              www.oup-usa.org

ISBN 0-195140-92-3

1083 Obsessive-Compulsive Disorders: Practical Management

Mosby
11830 Westline Industrial Drive
Saint Louis, MO 63146   314-872-8370
800-325-4177
Fax: 314-432-1380

Topics include the clinical picture, illnesses relation to obsessive-compulsive disorder, spectrum disorders, patient and clinical management and pathophysiology and assessment. *$117.50*

885 pages ISBN 0-815138-40-7

1084 Obsessive-Compulsive Related Disorders

American Psychiatric Publishing
1000 Wilson Boulevard
Suite 1825
Arlington, VA 22209-3901   703-907-7322
800-368-5777
Fax: 703-907-1091
E-mail: appi@psych.org
www.appi.org

Katie Duffy, Marketing Assistant

Discusses the way compulsivity and impulsivity are understood, diagnosed and treated. *$22.50*

286 pages ISBN 0-880484-02-0

1085 Over and Over Again: Understanding Obsessive-Compulsive Disorder

Jossey-Bass/Wiley
111 River Street
Hoboken, NJ 07030-5774   201-748-6000
Fax: 201-748-6088
E-mail: custserv@wiley.com
www.wiley.com

This sensitive and insightful book, the result of the author's years of research and experimentation, is a much needed survival manual for OCD sufferers and the families and friends who share their pain. *$25.00*

240 pages Year Founded: 1997 ISBN 0-787908-76-2

1086 Phobic and Obsessive-Compulsive Disorders: Theory, Research, and Practice

Kluwer Academic/Plenum Publishers
233 Spring Street
New York, NY 10013   212-620-8000
Fax: 212-463-0742
www.kluweronline.com

$80.00

Year Founded: 1990 ISBN 0-306410-44-3

1087 Real Illness: Obsessive-Compulsive Disorder

National Institute of Mental Health
6001 Executive Boulevard
Room 8184
Bethesda, MD 20892-9663   866-615-6464
Fax: 301-443-4279
TTY: 301-443-8431
E-mail: nimhinfo@nih.gov
www.nimh.nih.gov

Do you have disturbing thoughts and behaviors you know don't make sense but that you can't seem to control? This easy brochure explains how to get help.

9 pages

1088 School Personnel: A Critical Link in the Identification, Treatment and Management of OCD in Children and Adolescents

Obsessive-Compulsive Foundation
PO Box 9593
New Haven, CT 06535-9573   203-315-2190

Recognizing OCD in the school setting, current treatments, the role of school personnel in identification, assessment, and educational interventions, are thoroughly covered in this brief, but informative booklet especially targeted to educators and guidance counselors. *$4.00*

24 pages

1089 Teaching the Tiger, a Handbook for Individuals Involved in the Education of Students with Attention Deficit Disorders, Tourette Syndrome, or Obsessive - Compulsive Disorder

Hope Press
PO Box 188
Duarte, CA 91009-0188   818-303-0644
800-321-4039
Fax: 818-358-3520
www.hopepress.com

Innovative methods of teaching children with ADD, Tourette Syndrome, Obsessive-Compulsive Disorders *$35.00*

ISBN 1-878267-34-5

1090 Tormenting Thoughts and Secret Rituals: The Hidden Epidemic of Obsessive-Compulsive Disorder

Random House
1745 Broadway
3rd Floor
New York, NY 10019   212-782-9000
Fax: 212-572-6066
www.randomhouse.com

Discusses the various forms Obsessive-Compulsive Disorder (OCD) takes and, using the most common focuses of obsession, presents detailed cases whose objects are filth, harm, lust, and blasphemy. He explains how the disorder is currently diagnosed and how it differs from addiction, worrying, and preoccupation. He summarizes the recent findings in the areas of brain biology, neuroimaging and genetics that show OCD to be a distinct chemical disorder of the brain. *$14.95*

336 pages Year Founded: 1999 ISBN 0-440508-47-9

1091 When Once Is Not Enough: Help for Obsessive Compulsives

New Harbinger Publications
5674 Shattuck Avenue
Oakland, CA 94609-1662   510-652-2002
                                 800-748-6273
                              Fax: 510-652-5472
E-mail: customerservice@newharbinger.com
                              www.newharbinger.com

Kerrin White MD

How to recognize and confront fears, using simple rituals, positive coping strategies and handling complications. *$14.95*

229 pages ISBN 0-934986-87-8

1092 When Perfect Isn't Good Enough: Strategies for Coping with Perfectionism

New Harbinger Publications
5674 Shattuck Avenue
Oakland, CA 94609-1662   510-652-2002
                                 800-748-6273
                              Fax: 510-652-5472
E-mail: customerservice@newharbinger.com
                              www.newharbinger.com

This step by step guide explores the nature of perfectionism and offers a series of exercises to help you challenge unrealistic expectations and work on the specific situations in your life where perfectionism is a problem. *$13.95*

252 pages ISBN 1-572241-24-1

Periodicals & Pamphlets

1093 OCD Newsletter

676 State Street
New Haven, CT 06511   203-401-2070
                          Fax: 203-401-2076
         E-mail: info@ocfoundation.org
                  www.ocfoundation.org

For sufferers of obsessive-compulsive disorder and their families and friends.

8-12 pages Year Founded: 1986

Support Groups & Hot Lines

1094 Obsessive-Compulsive Anonymous

PO Box 215
New Hyde Park, NY 11040-0910   516-739-0662
                              Fax: 212-768-4679
              www.hometown.aol.com/west 24th

Self-help program for obsessive compulsive disorder. Provides meetings, fellowship, literature and audio tapes.

ISBN 0-962806-62-5

1095 Obsessive-Compulsive Foundation

676 State Street
New Haven, CT 06511   203-401-2070
                          Fax: 203-401-2076
         E-mail: info@ocfoundation.org
                  www.ocfoundation.org

For sufferers of obsessive-compulsive disorders and their families and friends. To educate the public and professional communities about OCD and related disorders; to provide assistance to individuals with OCD and related disorders, their family and friends, and to support research into the causes and effective treatments.

Video & Audio

1096 Hope & Solutions for Obsessive Compulsive Disorder: Part III

Awareness Foundation for OCD
3N374 Limberi Lane
Afocd c/o Gail Adams
Saint Charles, IL 60175-7655   630-513-9234
                              www.ocawareness.com

An educational psychologist offers educators effective classroom strategies that school personnel may implement with students who have obsessive compulsive disorder and addresses federal law as it pertains to students with disabilities. *$19.95*

1097 Hope and Solutions for OCD

ADD WareHouse
300 NW 70th Avenue
Suite 102
Plantation, FL 33317   954-792-8100
                                 800-233-9273
                              Fax: 954-792-8545
         E-mail: sales@addwarehouse.com
                  www.addwarehouse.com

Finally, a video series about obsessive compulsive disorder with some straight forward solutions and advice for individuals with OCD, their families, doctors, and school personnel. Viewers will learn what OCD is and how to treat it. Discusses how OCD can affect students in school and the impact on the family life. 85 minutes. *$89.95*

1098 Touching Tree

Obsessive-Compulsive Foundation
676 State Street
New Haven, CT 06511   **203-401-2070**
                          Fax: 203-401-2076
                E-mail: info@ocfoundation.org
                      www.ocfoundation.org

This video will foster awareness of early onset obsessive-compulsive disorder (OCD) and demonstrate the symptoms and current therapies that are most successful. Typical ritualistic compulsions of children and adolescents such as touching, hand washing, counting, etc. are explained. *$49.95*

Year Founded: 1993

1099 Understanding and Treating the Hereditary Psychiatric Spectrum Disorders

Hope Press
PO Box 188
Duarte, CA 91009-0188   **818-303-0644**
                               800-321-4039
                          Fax: 818-358-3520
                          www.hopepress.com

David E Comings MD, Presenter

Learn with ten hours of audio tapes from a two day seminar given in May 1997 by David E Comings MD. Tapes cover: ADHD, Tourette Syndrome, Obsessive-Compulsive Disorder, Conduct Disorder, Oppositional Defiant Disorder, Autism and other Hereditary Psychiatric Spectrum Disorders. Eight audio tapes. *$75.00*

Year Founded: 1997

Web Sites

1100 www.cyberpsych.org

CyberPsych

Hosts the American Psychoanalyists Foundation, American Association of Suicideology, Society for the Exploration of Psychotherapy Intergration, and Anxiety Disorders Association of America. Also subcategories of the anxiety disorders, as well as general information, including panic disorder, phobias, obsessive compulsive disorder (OCD), social phobia, generalized anxiety disorder, post traumatic stress disorder, and phobias of childhood. Book reviews and links to web pages sharing the topics.

1101 www.fairlite.com/ocd/

OCD Web Server

Abstracts found from the University of Kentucky's Medical Library. Information on medications taken directly from the manufacturers' brochures.

1102 www.interlog.com/~calex/ocd

Obsessive-Compulsive Disorder Web Sites

List of links.

1103 www.lexington-on-line.com/naf.ocd.2.html

Obsessive-Compulsive Disorder

A five page explanation.

1104 www.mayohealth.org/mayo/9809/htm/ocd.htm

Obsessive-Compulsive Disorder

Mayo Clinic 5 page publication.

1105 www.nimh.nih.gov/anxiety/anxiety/ocd/index.htm

National Institute of Health

Information on anxiety disorders and OCD.

1106 www.nimh.nih.gov/publicat/ocdmenu.cfm

Obsessive-Compulsive Disorder

Introductory handout with treatment recommendations.

1107 www.nursece.com/OCD.htm

Obsessive Compulsive Disorder

Features and treatments.

1108 www.ocdhope.com/gdlines.htm

Guidelines for Families Coping with OCD

1109 www.ocfoundation.org

Obsessive-Compulsive Foundation

Chat, newsletters, research, book reviews, and conferences

1110 www.planetpsych.com

Planetpsych.com

Learn about disorders, their treatments and other topics in psychology. Articles are listed under the related topic areas. Ask a therapist a question for free, or view the directory of professionals in your area. If you are a therapist sign up for the directory. Current features, self-help, interactive, and newsletter archives.

1111 www.psychcentral.com

Psych Central

Personalized one-stop index for psychology, support, and mental health issues, resources, and people on the Internet.

1112 www.psychguides.com/eks_oche.htm

Expert Consensus Treatment Guidelines for Obsessive-Compulsive Disorder: A Guide for Patients and Families.

Introduction

Paraphilias are sexual disorders or perversions in which intercourse is not the desired goal. Instead, the desire is to use non-human objects or non-sexual body parts for sexual activities sometimes involving the suffering of, or inflicting pain onto, non-consenting partners.

SYMPTOMS

•Recurrent, intense, sexually arousing fantasies, urges, or behavior involving the particular perversion for at least six months;
•The fantasies, urges, or behavior cause distress and/or disruption in the person's functioning in social, work, and interpersonal areas.

There are eight Paraphilias, described below, categorized as either victimless, or as victimizing someone who has not consented to be subjected to the sexual activity, with relevant associated features.

Exhibitionism
The exposure of the genitals to a stranger or group of strangers. Sometimes the paraphiliac masturbates during exposure. The onset of this disorder usually occurs before age 18 and becomes less severe after age 40.

Fetishism
Using non-living objects i.e. the fetish for sexual gratification. Objects commonly used include women's underwear, shoes or other articles of women's clothes. The person often masturbates while holding, rubbing, or smelling the fetish object. This disorder usually begins in adolescence; it is chronic and often lifelong.

Frotteurism
Sexual arousal, and sometimes masturbation to orgasm, while rubbing against a non-consenting person. The behavior is usually planned to occur in a crowded place, such as on a bus, subway, or in a swimming pool, where detection is less likely. Frotteurism usually begins in adolescence, is most frequent between the ages of 15 and 25, then gradually declines.

Pedophilia
Sexual Activity with a prepubertal child, generally 13 years or younger. The pedophiliac must be at least 16 and at least five years older than his victim. Pedophiliacs are usually attracted to children in a certain age range.
The frequency of the behavior may be associated with the degree of stress in the person's life. It usually begins in adolescence and is chronic. Pedophiles usually report a higher incidence of severe marital discord.

Sexual Masochism
Acts of being bound, beaten, humiliated, or made to suffer in some other way in order to become sexually aroused. The behaviors can be self-inflicted or performed with a partner, and include physical bondage, blindfolding and humiliation. Masochistic sexual fantasies are likely to have been present since childhood. The activities themselves begin at different times but are common by early adulthood; they are usually chronic. The severity of the behaviors may increase over time.

Sexual Sadism
Acts in which the person becomes sexually excited through the physical or psychological suffering of someone else. Some Sexual Sadists may conjure up the sadistic fantasies during sexual activity without acting on them. Others act on their sadistic urges with a consenting partner (who may be a Sexual Masochist), or act on their urges with a non-consenting partner. The behavior may involve forcing the other person to crawl, be caged or tortured. Sadistic sexual fantasies are likely to have been present inchildhood. The onset of the behavior varies but is common by early adulthood. The disorder is usually chronic. The severity of the sadistic acts tends to increase over time. When the disorder is severe or coupled with Antisocial Personality Disorder, the person will likely seriously injure or kill his victim.

Transvestic Fetishism
Heterosexual males either dressing in women's clothes and then masturbating, or dressing com-

pletely as females including wearing makeup. When not cross dressed, the man looks like an ordinary masculine man. It is important to note that there is considerable controversy over this diagnosis; some people who cross dress seem to have little distress and function normally. This condition typically begins in childhood or adolescence. Often the cross dressing is not done publicly until adulthood.

Voyeurism

Peeping Tom disorder, involving the act of observing one or more unsuspecting persons (usually strangers) who are naked, in the process of undressing, or engaged in sexual activity, to become sexually excited. Sexual activity with the people being observed is not usually sought. The Voyeur may masturbate during the observation or later. The onset of this disorder is usually before age 15. It tends to be chronic.

PREVALENCE

Paraphiliacs are almost exclusively male. Very few volunteer to disclose their activities or to seek treatment. It is estimated that most have deficits in interpersonal or sexual relationships. In one study, two thirds were diagnosed with Mood Disorders and fifty percent had alcohol or drug abuse problems.

Recent studies provide evidence that the great majority of Paraphiliacs are active in more than one form of sexually perverse behavior; less than ten percent have only one form; and thirty-eight percent engage in five or more different sexually deviant behaviors. In a survey of college students, it was found that young males often fantasize about forced sex, and almost half have engaged in some form of sexual misconduct or sexual behavior with someone younger than age 14.

At the same time, the incidence and prevalence of some sexual perversions are hard to estimate, or unknown, because they are rarely reported or the people involved do not come into contact with the authorities or the health care system.

TREATMENT OPTIONS

All the Paraphilias are difficult to treat. It is important for the professional making the diagnosis to take a very careful history, and to be sensitive to the presence of other, e.g., personality, disorders. Relapse is common.

Diagnostic techniques are used, such as penile plethysmography, in which the degree of penile erection is measured while the individual is exposed to visual sexual stimuli. Some people are treated in a formal Sex Offenders Program, developed for individuals arrested for and convicted of paraphilias that are crimes. Sometimes treatment occurs within the context of individual therapy where trust can be established. Others have been treated by means of conditioning techniques, e.g., where a fetish object is paired with an aversive stimulus such as mild electric shock. Medication is also used. Pedophilia is sometimes treated through so-called chemocastration which, through the use of female hormones or other medications, diminishes sexual appetite.

Treatment can be difficult because many individuals do not wish to be punished and do not necessarily have any real interest in being treated: they may deliberately deceive the professional, or deny the problem. Sex offenders are also more likely to exaggerate treatment gains, resist treatment, or end treatment prematurely.

The fact that these conditions are classified as mental disorders does not relieve individuals who violate laws of criminal responsibility.

Associations & Agencies

1114 Center for Family Support (CFS)

333 7th Avenue
New York, NY 10001-5004   212-629-7939
                                 Fax: 212-239-2211
                                 www.cfsny.org

Steven Vernickofs, Executive Director

Service agency devoted to the physical well-being and development of the retarded child and the sound mental health of the parents. Helps families with retarded children with all aspects of home care including counseling, referrals, home aide service and consultation. Offers intervention for parents at the birth of a retarded child with in-home support, guidance and infant stimulation. Pioneered training of nonprofessional women as home aides to provide supportive services in homes.

1115 Center for Mental Health Services Knowledge Exchange Network

US Department of Health and Human Services
PO Box 42490
Washington, DC 20015-4800

                                 800-789-2647
                                 Fax: 301-984-8796
                                 E-mail: ken@mentalhealth.org
                                 www.mentalhealth.org

Information about resources, technical assistance, research, training, networks, and other federal clearing houses, and fact sheets and materials. Information specialists refer callers to mental health resources in their communities as well as state, federal and non-profit contacts. Staff available Monday through Friday, 8:30 AM - 5:00 PM, EST, excluding federal holidays. After hours, callers may leave messages and an information specialist will return their call.

1116 NADD: Association for Persons with Developmental Disabilities and Mental Health Needs

132 Fair Street
Kingston, NY 12401-4802   845-334-4336
                                    800-331-5362
                                    Fax: 845-331-4569
                                    E-mail: nadd@mhv.net
                                    www.thenadd.org

Dr. Robert Fletcher, Executive Director

Nonprofit organization designed to promote interest of professional and parent development with resources for individuals who have the coexistence of mental illness and mental retardation. Provides conference, educational services and training materials to professionals, parents, concerned citizens and service organizations. Formerly known as the National Association for the Dually Diagnosed.

1117 National Mental Health Consumer's Self-Help Clearinghouse

1211 Chestnut Street
Suite 1207
Philadelphia, PA 19107   215-751-1810
                                    800-553-4539
                                    Fax: 215-636-6312
                                    E-mail: info@mhselfhelp.org
                                    www.mhselfhelp.org

Alex Morrsey, Information/Referral

Funded by the National Institute of Mental Health Community Support Program, the purpose of the Clearinghouse is to encourage the development and growth of consumer self-help groups.

Year Founded: 1992

Web Sites

1118 www.mentalhealth.com

Internet Mental Health

On-line information and a virtual encyclopedia related to mental disorders, possible causes and treatments. News, articles, on-line diagnostic programs and related links. Designed to improve understanding, diagnosis and treatment of mental illness throughout the world. Awarded the Top Site Award and the NetPsych Cutting Edge Site Award.

1119 www.planetpsych.com

Planetpsych.com

Learn about disorders, their treatments and other topics in psychology. Articles are listed under the related topic areas. Ask a therapist a question for free, or view the directory of professionals in your area. If you are a therapist sign up for the directory. Current features, self-help, interactive, and newsletter archives.

1120 www.psychcentral.com

Psych Central

Personalized one-stop index for psychology, support, and mental health issues, resources, and people on the Internet.

Introduction

Everyone has personality characteristics that are likable and unlikable, attractive and unattractive. Our personality is deeply rooted in our sense of ourselves and how others see us; it is formed from a complex intermingling of genetic factors and life experience. By adulthood, most of us have personality traits that are exceedingly difficult to change. Sometimes, these deeply rooted personality traits can get in the way of our happiness, hinder relationships, and even cause harm to ourselves or others.

A person may have a tendency to be deeply suspicious of other people with no good reason. Another person may assume a haughty, arrogant manner that is difficult to be around. Personality Disorders, by definition, do not cause symptoms; they are defined as a whole set of traits and behaviors and inner experiences that pervade every or nearly every aspect of a person's life.

A diagnosis of a Personality Disorder should be distinguished from labeling someone a bad or disagreeable person, and not be used to label or stigmatize people who are simply unpopular, rebellious or otherwise unorthodox. Rather, a Personality Disorder refers to an enduring pattern of experience and behavior that is inflexible, long lasting (often beginning in adolescence or early adulthood) and which leads to distress and impairment. Ten distinct personality disorders have been identified:
•Paranoid Personality Disorder;
•Schizoid Personality Disorder;
•Schizotypal Personality Disorder;
•Antisocial Personality Disorder;
•Borderline Personality Disorder;
•Histrionic Personality Disorder;
•Narcissistic Personality Disorder;
•Avoidant Personality Disorder;
•Dependent Personality Disorder;
•Obsessive-Compulsive Personality Disorder.

SYMPTOMS

An enduring pattern of inner experience and behavior that deviates markedly from the expectations of the individual's culture:
•This pattern is manifested in two or more of the following areas: cognition, affectivity, interpersonal functioning, and impulse control;
•The enduring pattern is inflexible and pervasive across a broad range of personal and social situations;
•The enduring pattern leads to clinically significant distress or impairment in social, occupational, or other important areas of functioning;
•The pattern is stable and of long duration and its onset can be traced back at least to adolescence or early adulthood;
•The enduring pattern is not better accounted for as a manifestation or consequence of another mental disorder;
•The enduring pattern is not due to the direct physiological effects of a substance or a general medical condition;
•Feelings that the problem is with other people: others do not respect or take care of him or her; others are out to trick and cheat him or her; others are too intrusive or too sloppy.

TREATMENT OPTIONS

Most people who suffer from a Personality Disorder do not see themselves as having a problem, and therefore do not seek treatment. For those who do, the most effective treatment is long-term (at least one year) psychotherapy. People with Personality Disorders may seek treatment only because they are distressed that others do not behave as patients think they should, or because the patients' behaviors cause them to have significant problems with employment and relationships. It is important for a patient to find a mental health professional with expert knowledge and experience in treating personality disorders. Some therapists specialize in treating Borderline Personality Disorder and use a treatment called Dialectal Behavioral Therapy. Antisocial Personality Disorder is notably difficult to treat, especially in extreme cases, when the affected individual lacks all concern for harming others.

Psychotherapy encourages patients to talk about their suspicions, doubts and other personality traits that have a negative impact on their lives, and therefore helps to improve social interactions.

Psychotherapeutic treatment should include attention to family members, stressing the importance of emotional support, reassurance, explanation of the disorder, and advice on how to manage and respond to the patient. Group therapy is helpful in many situations.

Antipsychotic medication can be useful in patients with certain Personality Disorders, specifically Schizotypal and Borderline Disorders.

Associations & Agencies

1122 Career Assessment & Planning Services

Goodwill Industries-Suncoast
10596 Gandy Boulevard
St. Petersburg, FL 33702   727-523-1512
                             888-279-1988
                        Fax: 727-563-9300
E-mail: gw.marketing@goodwill-suncoast.org
              www.goodwill-suncoast.org

Chris Ward, Marketing Media Manager
R Lee Waits, President/CEO

Provides a comprehensive assessment, which can predict current and future employment and potential adjustment factors for physically, emotionally, or developmentally disabled persons who may be unemployed or underemployed. Assessments evaluate interests, aptitudes, academic achievements, and physical abilities (including dexterity and coordination) through coordinated testing, interviewing and behavioral observations.

1123 Center for Family Support (CFS)

333 7th Avenue
New York, NY 10001-5004   212-629-7939
                        Fax: 212-239-2211
                             www.cfsny.org

Steven Vernickofs, Executive Director

Service agency devoted to the physical well-being and development of the retarded child and the sound mental health of the parents. Helps families with retarded children with all aspects of home care including counseling, referrals, home aide service and consultation. Offers intervention for parents at the birth of a retarded child with in-home support, guidance and infant stimulation. Pioneered training of nonprofessional women as home aides to provide supportive services in homes.

1124 Center for Mental Health Services Knowledge Exchange Network

US Department of Health and Human Services
PO Box 42490
Washington, DC 20015-4800
                             800-789-2647
                        Fax: 301-984-8796
              E-mail: ken@mentalhealth.org
                   www.mentalhealth.org

Information about resources, technical assistance, research, training, networks, and other federal clearing houses, and fact sheets and materials. Information specialists refer callers to mental health resources in their communities as well as state, federal and nonprofit contacts. Staff available Monday through Friday, 8:30 AM - 5:00 PM, EST, excluding federal holidays. After hours, callers may leave messages and an information specialist will return their call.

1125 NADD: Association for Persons with Developmental Disabilities and Mental Health Needs

132 Fair Street
Kingston, NY 12401-4802   845-334-4336
                             800-331-5362
                        Fax: 845-331-4569
              E-mail: nadd@mhv.net
                   www.thenadd.org

Dr. Robert Fletcher, Executive Director

Nonprofit organization designed to promote interest of professional and parent development with resources for individuals who have the coexistence of mental illness and mental retardation. Provides conference, educational services and training materials to professionals, parents, concerned citizens and service organizations. Formerly known as the National Association for the Dually Diagnosed.

1126 National Alliance for the Mentally Ill

2107 Wilson Boulevard
Suite 300
Arlington, VA 22201-3042   703-524-7600
                             800-950-6264
                        Fax: 703-524-9094
                        TDD: 703-516-7227
              E-mail: helpline@nami.org
                   www.nami.org

Laurie Flynn, Executive Director

Nation's leading self-help organization for all those affected by severe brain disorders. Mission is to bring consumers and families with similar experiences together to share information about services, care providers, and ways to cope with the challenges of schizophrenia, manic depression, and other serious mental illnesses.

1127 National Mental Health Consumer's Self-Help Clearinghouse

1211 Chestnut Street
Suite 1207
Philadelphia, PA 19107   215-751-1810
                             800-553-4539
                        Fax: 215-636-6312
              E-mail: info@mhselfhelp.org
                   www.mhselfhelp.org

Alex Morrsey, Information/Referral

Funded by the National Institute of Mental Health Community Support Program, the purpose of the Clearinghouse is to encourage the development and growth of consumer self-help groups.

Year Founded: 1992

1128 Suncoast Residential Training Center/Developmental Services Program

Goodwill Industries-Suncoast
10596 Gandy Boulevard
PO Box 14456
St. Petersburg, FL 33702   727-523-1512
                        Fax: 727-563-9300
                   www.goodwill-suncoast.org

Personality Disorders/Books

Jay McCloe, Director Resource Development

A large group home which serves individuals diagnosed as mentally retarded with a secondary diagnosed of psychiatric difficulties as evidenced by problem behavior. Providing residential, behavioral and instructional support and services that will promote the development of adaptive, socially appropriate behavior, each individual is assessed to determine, socialization, basic academics and recreation. The primary intervention strategy is applied behavior analysis. Professional consultants are utilized to address the medical, dental, psychiatric and pharmacological needs of ech individual. One of the most popular features is the active community integration component of SRTC. Program customers attend an average of 15 monthly outings to various community events.

Books

1129 Angry Heart: Overcoming Borderline and Addictive Disorders

New Harbinger Publications
5674 Shattuck Avenue
Oakland, CA 94609-1662   **510-652-2002**
                                    800-748-6273
                              Fax: 510-652-5472
E-mail: customerservice@newharbinger.com
                        www.newharbinger.com

This self help guide uses a variety of exercises and step by step techniques to help individuals with borderline and addictive disorders come to terms with their destructive lifestyle and take steps to break out of its dysfunctional cycle of self defeating thoughts and behavior. *$14.95*

272 pages ISBN 1-572240-80-6

1130 Assess Dialogue Personality Disorders

Cambridge University Press
40 W 20th Street
New York, NY 10011-4221   **212-924-3900**
                              Fax: 212-691-3239
                  E-mail: information@cup.org
                              www.cup.org

Cambridge University Press is the printing and publishing house of the University of Cambridge. It is an integral part of the University and is devoted constitutionally to printing and publishing for "the acquisition, advancement, conservation, and dissemination of knowledge in all subjects". As such, it is a charitable, not-for-profit organization, free from tax worldwide.

1131 Biological and Neurobehavioral Studies of Borderline Personality Disorder

American Psychiatric Publishing
1000 Wilson Boulevard
Suite 1825
Arlington, VA 22209-3901   **703-907-7322**
                                    800-368-5777
                              Fax: 703-907-1091
                  E-mail: appi@psych.org
                              www.appi.org

Katie Duffy, Marketing Assistant

Provides a review of a broad series of biological and neurobehavioral studies of patients with borderline personality disorder. *$35.00*

288 pages ISBN 0-880484-80-2

1132 Biology of Personality Disorders, Review of Psychiatry

American Psychiatric Publishing
1000 Wilson Boulevard
Suite 1825
Arlington, VA 22209-3901   **703-907-7322**
                                    800-368-5777
                              Fax: 703-907-1091
                  E-mail: appi@psych.org
                              www.appi.org

Katie Duffy, Marketing Assistant

Contents include neurotransmitter function in personality disorders, new biological research strategies for personality disorders, genetics and psychobiology of s e v e n - f a c t o r m o d e l o f p e r s o n a l i t y, psychopharmacological management, and significance of biological research for a biopsychosocial model of personality disorders. *$25.00*

166 pages ISBN 0-880488-35-2

1133 Borderline Personality Disorder

American Psychiatric Publishing
1000 Wilson Boulevard
Suite 1825
Arlington, VA 22209-3901   **703-907-7322**
                                    800-368-5777
                              Fax: 703-907-1091
                  E-mail: appi@psych.org
                              www.appi.org

Katie Duffy, Marketing Assistant

Guide to the diagnosis and treatment of borderline personality disorder. *$34.00*

256 pages ISBN 0-880486-89-9

1134 Borderline Personality Disorder: Multidimensional Approach

American Psychiatric Publishing
1000 Wilson Boulevard
Suite 1825
Arlington, VA 22209-3901   **703-907-7322**
                                    800-368-5777
                              Fax: 703-907-1091
                  E-mail: appi@psych.org
                              www.appi.org

Katie Duffy, Marketing Assistant

Practical approach to the management of patients with BPD. *$33.00*

288 pages ISBN 0-880486-55-4

1135 Borderline Personality Disorder: Etilogy and Treatment

American Psychiatric Publishing
1000 Wilson Boulevard
Suite 1825
Arlington, VA 22209-3901   703-907-7322
                                  800-368-5777
                              Fax: 703-907-1091
                         E-mail: appi@psych.org
                                   www.appi.org

Katie Duffy, Marketing Assistant

Provides empirical data as the basis for progress in understanding and treating the borderline patient. $50.00

420 pages ISBN 0-880484-08-X

1136 Borderline Personality Disorder: Tailoring the Psychotherapy to the Patient

American Psychiatric Publishing
1000 Wilson Boulevard
Suite 1825
Arlington, VA 22209-3901   703-907-7322
                                  800-368-5777
                              Fax: 703-907-1091
                         E-mail: appi@psych.org
                                   www.appi.org

Katie Duffy, Marketing Assistant

Emphasizes how the clinician should decide between the use of supportive as opposed to expressive techniques, depending upon the characteristics of the patient. $34.00

256 pages ISBN 0-880486-89-9

1137 Challenging Behavior

Cambridge University Press
40 W 20th Street
New York, NY 10011-4221   212-924-3900
                             Fax: 212-691-3239
                      E-mail: marketing@cup.org
                                   www.cup.org

1138 Childhood Antecedents of Multiple Personality Disorder

American Psychiatric Publishing
1000 Wilson Boulevard
Suite 1825
Arlington, VA 22209-3901   703-907-7322
                                  800-368-5777
                              Fax: 703-907-1091
                         E-mail: appi@psych.org
                                   www.appi.org

Katie Duffy, Marketing Assistant

Professional discussion of early causes of this condition. $22.50

258 pages ISBN 0-880480-82-3

1139 Clinical Assessment and Management of Severe Personality Disorders

American Psychiatric Publishing
1000 Wilson Boulevard
Suite 1825
Arlington, VA 22209-3901   703-907-7322
                                  800-368-5777
                              Fax: 703-907-1091
                         E-mail: appi@psych.org
                                   www.appi.org

Katie Duffy, Marketing Assistant

Focuses on issues relevant to the clinician in private practice, including the diagnosis of a wide range of personality disorders and alternative management approaches. $33.00

260 pages ISBN 0-880484-88-8

1140 Clinical Perspectives on Multiple Personality Disorder

American Psychiatric Publishing
1000 Wilson Boulevard
Suite 1825
Arlington, VA 22209-3901   703-907-7322
                                  800-368-5777
                              Fax: 703-907-1091
                         E-mail: appi@psych.org
                                   www.appi.org

Katie Duffy, Marketing Assistant

Discusses psychotherapy of Multiple Personality Disorder, post traumatic and dissociative phenomena in transference and countertransference, treament as a posttraumatic condition, and provides case studies that exhibits the application of techniques, approaches and insights important when treating MPD. $52.00

398 pages ISBN 0-880483-65-2

1141 Cognitive Analytic Therapy & Borderline Personality Disorder: Model and the Method

John Wiley & Sons
605 3rd Avenue
New York, NY 10058-0180   212-850-6000
                             Fax: 212-850-6008
                       E-mail: info@wiley.com
                                  www.wiley.com

Amy Bazarnik, Conventions Coordinator

1142 Consumer's Guide to Psychiatric Drugs

New Harbinger Publications
5674 Shattuck Avenue
Oakland, CA 94609-1662   510-652-2002
                                800-748-6273
                            Fax: 510-652-5472
       E-mail: customerservice@newharbinger.com
                             www.newharbinger.com

Helps consumers understand what treatment options are available and what side effects to expect. Covers possible interactions with other drugs, medical conditions and other concerns. Explains how each drug works, and offers detailed information about treatments for depression, bipolar disorder, anxiety and sleep disorders, as well as other conditions. $16.95

340 pages ISBN 1-572241-11-X

1143 Developmental Model of Borderline Personality Disorder: Understanding Variations in Course and Outcome

American Psychiatric Publishing
1000 Wilson Boulevard
Suite 1825
Arlington, VA 22209-3901   703-907-7322
                                  800-368-5777
                             Fax: 703-907-1091
                        E-mail: appi@psych.org
                                  www.appi.org

Landmark work on this difficult condition. Emphasizes a developmental approach to BPD based on treatment of inpatients at Chestnut Lodge in Rockville, Maryland, during the years through 1975. Using information gleaned from the original clinical notes and follow-up studies, the authors present four intriguing case studies to chart the etiology, long-term course, and clinical manifestations of BPD. *$34.95*

256 pages Year Founded: 2002 ISBN 0-880485-15-9

1144 Disordered Personalities

Rapid Psychler Press
3560 Pine Grove Avenue
Suite 374
Port Huron, MI 48060   519-433-7642
                              888-779-2453
                         Fax: 888-779-2457
                  E-mail: rapid@psychler.com
                            www.psychler.com

David Robinson, Publisher

$34.95

406 pages ISBN 0-968209-44-0

1145 Disorders of Narcissism: Diagnostic, Clinical, and Empirical Implications

American Psychiatric Publishing
1000 Wilson Boulevard
Suite 1825
Arlington, VA 22209-3901   703-907-7322
                                  800-368-5777
                             Fax: 703-907-1091
                        E-mail: appi@psych.org
                                  www.appi.org

Katie Duffy, Marketing Assistant

Addresses important subjects at the forefront of the study of narcissism, including cognitive treatment, normal narcissism, pathological narcissism and suicide, and the connection between pathological narcissism, trauma, and alexithymia. *$42.50*

304 pages ISBN 0-880487-01-1

1146 Field Guide to Personality Disorders

Rapid Psychler Press
3560 Pine Grove Avenue
Suite 374
Port Huron, MI 48060   519-433-7642
                              888-779-2453
                         Fax: 888-779-2457
                  E-mail: rapid@psychler.com
                            www.psychler.com

David Robinson, Publisher

$14.95

186 pages ISBN 0-968032-46-X

1147 Lost in the Mirror: An Inside Look at Borderline Personality Disorder

200 E Joppa Road
Suite 207
Baltimore, MD 21286   410-825-8888
                             888-825-8249
                        Fax: 410-337-0747
                   E-mail: sidran@sidran.org
                             www.sidran.org

Richard Moskovitz

Dr. Moskovitz considers BPD to be part of the dissociative continuum, as it has many causes, symptoms and behaviors in common with Dissociative Disorder. This book is intended for people diagnosed with BPD, their families and therapists. Outlines the features of BPD, including abuse histories, dissociation, mood swings, self harm, impulse control problems and many more. Includes an extensive resource section. *$12.95*

190 pages

1148 Management of Countertransference with Borderline Patients

American Psychiatric Publishing
1000 Wilson Boulevard
Suite 1825
Arlington, VA 22209-3901   703-907-7322
                                  800-368-5777
                             Fax: 703-907-1091
                        E-mail: appi@psych.org
                                  www.appi.org

Katie Duffy, Marketing Assistant

Open and detailed discussion of the emotional reactions that clinicians experience when treating borderline patients. *$34.50*

254 pages ISBN 0-880785-63-9

1149 Personality and Psychopathology

American Psychiatric Publishing
1000 Wilson Boulevard
Suite 1825
Arlington, VA 22093-901   703-907-7322
                                 800-368-5777
                            Fax: 703-907-1091
                       E-mail: appi@psych.org
                                 www.appi.org

Katie Duffy, Marketing Assistant

Compiles the most recent findings from more than 30 internationally recognized experts. Analyzes the association between personality and psychopathology from several interlocking perspective, descriptive, developmental, etiological, and therapeutic. *$58.50*

496 pages ISBN 0-880489-23-5

1150 Role of Sexual Abuse in the Etiology of Borderline Personality Disorder

200 E Joppa Road
Suite 207
Baltimore, MD 21286   410-825-8888
888-825-8249
Fax: 410-337-0747
E-mail: sidran@sidran.org
www.sidran.org

Presenting the latest generation of research findings about the impact of traumatic abuse on the development of BPD. This book focuses on the theoretical basis of BPD, including topics such as childhood factors associated with the development, the relationship of child sexual abuse to dissociation and self-mutilation, severity of childhood abuse, borderline symptoms and family environment. Twenty six contributors cover every aspect of BPD as it relates to childhood sexual abuse. *$42.00*

248 pages

1151 Shorter Term Treatments for Borderline Personality Disorders

New Harbinger Publications
5674 Shattuck Avenue
Oakland, CA 94609-1662   510-652-2002
800-748-6273
Fax: 510-652-5472
E-mail: customerservice@newharbinger.com
www.newharbinger.com

This much needed guide offers approaches designed to help clients stabilize emotions, decrease vulnerability and work toward more adaptive day-to-day functioning. Covers diagnostic issues and details treatment strategies drawn from a variety of models and approaches. *$ 49.95*

184 pages ISBN 1-572240-92-X

1152 Stop Walking on Eggshells: Taking Back Your Life Back When Someone You Care About Has Borderline Personality Disorder

New Harbinger Publications
5674 Shattuck Avenue
Oakland, CA 94609-1662   510-652-2002
800-748-6273
Fax: 510-652-5472
E-mail: customerservice@newharbinger.com
www.newharbinger.com

This guide for the family and friends of those who have BPD is designed to help them understand how the disorder affects their loved ones and recognize what they can do to establish personal limits and enforce boundaries, communicate more effectively, cope with self destructive behavior, and take care of themselves. *$14.95*

272 pages ISBN 1-572241-08-X

1153 Structured Interview for DSM-IV Personality (SIDP-IV)

American Psychiatric Publishing
1000 Wilson Boulevard
Suite 1825
Arlington, VA 22209-3901   703-907-7322
800-368-5777
Fax: 703-907-1091
E-mail: appi@psych.org
www.appi.org

Katie Duffy, Marketing Assistant

Semistructured interview uses nonpejorative questions to examine behavior and personality traits from the patient's perspective. *$21.95*

48 pages ISBN 0-880489-37-5

1154 Type A Behavior

Sage Publications
2455 Teller Road
Thousand Oaks, CA 91320   805-499-9774
800-818-7243
Fax: 800-583-2665
E-mail: info@sagepub.com
www.sagepub.com

This important book brings together leading scholars to answer questions about environmental and genetic factors role in the development of Type A behavior, whether or not gender has an effect and if Type A parents raise Type A children. Presents current Type A reserch and discusses issues including theoretical advances, hostility, special populations, measurement and prediction refinements, work settings, medical and psychological refinements and extensions and interventions. *$48.00*

436 pages

Support Groups & Hot Lines

1155 SAFE Alternatives

7115 W North Avenue
PMB 319
Oak Park, IL 60302
800-366-8288
www.selfinjury.com

Karen Conterio, Contact

At SAFE, we try to create a culture of safety in which the injurer comes to realize that self-injury destroys relationships, but safety brings people closer to them. We also do not employ infantilizing, restrictive methods of behavior control, which reinforce the individual's sense of helplessness and powerlessness.

Web Sites

1156 www.cyberpsych.org

CyberPsych

Hosts the American Psychoanalyists Foundation, American Association of Suicideology, Society for the Exploration of Psychotherapy Intergration, and Anxiety Disorders Association of America. Also subcategories of the anxiety disorders, as well as general information, including panic disorder, phobias, obsessive compulsive disorder (OCD), social phobia, generalized anxiety disorder, post traumatic stress disorder, and phobias of childhood. Book reviews and links to web pages sharing the topics.

1157 www.mentalhealth.com

Internet Mental Health

On-line information and a virtual encyclopedia related to mental disorders, possible causes and treatments. News, articles, on-line diagnostic programs and related links. Designed to improve understanding, diagnosis and treatment of mental illness throughout the world. Awarded the Top Site Award and the NetPsych Cutting Edge Site Award.

1158 www.navicom.com/patty/

Borderline Personality Disorder Sanctuary

Recovery information for people with the borderline personality disorder. Latest research regarding etiology and treatment of the borderline personality disorder, with suicide information.

1159 www.nimh.nih.gov/publicat/ocdmenu.cfm

Obsessive-Compulsive Disorder

Introductory handout with treatment recommendations.

1160 www.ocdhope.com/gdlines.htm

Guidelines for Families Coping with OCD

1161 www.planetpsych.com

Planetpsych.com

Learn about disorders, their treatments and other topics in psychology. Articles are listed under the related topic areas. Ask a therapist a question for free, or view the directory of professionals in your area. If you are a therapist sign up for the directory. Current features, self-help, interactive, and newsletter archives.

1162 www.psychcentral.com

Psych Central

Personalized one-stop index for psychology, support, and mental health issues, resources, and people on the Internet.

Introduction

Traumatic events can stay with us for a long time. Such events can range from the rare and horrific, such as severe torture, to more common events such as an automobile accident or a violent crime. Veterans of war often spend years reliving, or trying to forget, the experience of combat. Effects of some childhood experiences can last well into adulthood. When the after-effects of a traumatic event are so severe and so persistent that they impair functioning, professional help is necessary. Post-Traumatic Stress Disorder, or PTSD, is a diagnosis made to describe the psychological and physiological symptoms that arise from experiencing, witnessing or participating in a traumatic event.

SYMPTOMS

Exposure to a traumatic event in which the person experienced, witnessed, or was confronted by death or serious injury, or a threat to the physical integrity of self or others, and the person's response involved intense fear, helplessness, or horror, can result in three basic types of symptoms: re-experiencing, numbing, and/or increased emotional arousal. Re-experiencing includes:
•Recurrent and intrusive distressing recollections of the event, including images, thoughts or perceptions;
•Recurrent distressing flashbacks, nightmares and/or dreams of the event;
•Acting or feeling as if the traumatic event were recurring.
Increased arousal includes:
•Intense psychological distress at exposure to internal or external cues that symbolize or resemble an aspect of the traumatic event;
•Physiological reactivity on exposure to internal or external cues that symbolize or resemble an aspect of the traumatic event;
•Persistent avoidance of stimuli associated with the trauma.
Numbing includes:
•Diminished general responsiveness;
•Desensitization of emotional reactiveness.

Duration of the disturbance is usually more than one month, and the disturbance causes clinically significant distress or impairment in social, occupational, or other important settings.

ASSOCIATED FEATURES

Response to traumatic events can vary from person to person. Some characteristics, however, are common among individuals with PTSD. If a person has survived a life-threatening event, there may be a profound sense of guilt, particularly if others did not survive the event. These guilt feelings may be exacerbated if the individual perceives that his or her survival occurred at the expense of others' safety.

People with PTSD often avoid situations that remind them of the traumatic event, and this can be disruptive to normal life. They may also experience dissociative symptoms, meaning that in certain situations that are threatening they may revert to a state that they will be unable to recall later. In other cases, a person with PTSD may complain of physical symptoms that have no discernible anatomic or physiological explanation, but which are manifestations of psychic distress; these are known as somatic complaints. The patient with PTSD is also liable to experience a range of feelings that make it difficult or impossible for him or her to carry on with life in a normal fashion. They may feel that the trauma they experienced damaged them permanently and irreparably, or give up on previously strongly-held beliefs; in some cases people with PTSD undergo a profound change of personality. Patients with PTSD may also have any number of other distinctive mental illnesses at the same time: Depression, Obsessive-Compulsive Disorder, Social Phobia, or Substance-Abuse Related Disorders.

PREVALENCE

Anyone who experiences a traumatic event can have Post Traumatic Stress Disorder. PTSD was first diagnosed in war veterans, and many people associate it with soliders, but women and children are actually more vulnerable to PTSD than are men, and account for more than half the cases. Studies in the community reveal a prevalence ranging from one percent to fourteen percent. However, men and women, on average, suffer different kinds of trauma; women are more likely to experience sexual assault than men, and sexual assault is more likely to result in PTSD than some other types of trauma. Yet when men are sexually assaulted, they are even more likely to develop PTSD than women are. When the study population is made up of combat veterans who have experienced a traumatic event, or victims of criminal violence, the prevalence ranges from three percent to fifty-eight percent.

TREATMENT OPTIONS

Therapies include medication and/or psychotherapy. As with many psychiatric disorders, treatment often involves some combination of therapy and medicine. SSRI (Selective Seratonin Reuptake Inhibitor) medications can be especially helpful, and sertraline and paroxetine have specific FDA indications for PTSD. Also useful in some situations are benzodiazepines, which are tranquillizers that can be used to block the symptoms of anxiety at the time they occur. Beta-blocker medications block the physical signs and symptoms of anxiety, such as fast heart rate. SSRIs, on the other hand, are used on an everyday basis rather than just when symptoms occur. Eye Movement Desensitization treatment has been used to help patients with PTSD, though the results are not consistent.

Behavior therapy is a kind of psychotherapy that focuses on helping the patient recognize the thought processes that result in traumatic stress reactions. By working with a professional and learning methods for relaxing and countering the stress reactions, the individual can master the reactions triggered by the traumatic event, or reminders of it. Behavior therapy may involve exposing the patient in a safe and controlled environment to stimuli that prompt a stress reaction; through repeated exposures, the patient slowly is desensitized and in time will be able to experience the stimuli without having a stress reaction. Traditional

psychodynamic psychotherapy may also be useful to help the patient examine conscind unconscious psychological conflicts surrounding the traumatic event. It can also be useful to rebuild self-confidence and self-esteem. Participation in a support group can also be extremely beneficial to individuals with PTSD. Groups have formed around particular issues and particular traumatic experiences; for instance, there are support groups for survivors of rape, incest, or the sudden loss of a loved one. Support groups also exist for combat veterans and other trauma victims.

Associations & Agencies

1164 Association of Traumatic Stress Specialists

PO Box 2747
Georgetown, TX 78627   512-868-3677
Fax: 512-868-3678
E-mail: admin@ATSS-HQ.com
www.ATSS-HQ.com

Jo Halligan, Executive Director

ATSS is an international multidisciplinary membership organization offering certification to qualified individuals who provide services, intervention and treatment in the field of traumatic stress. Available services include referrals, annual international conferences, newsletters, certification recognition, and other services.

4 per year

1165 Career Assessment & Planning Services

Goodwill Industries-Suncoast
10596 Gandy Boulevard
PO Box 14456
St. Petersburg, FL 33702   727-523-1512
Fax: 727-577-2749
www.goodwill-suncoast.org

Jay McCloe, Director Resource Development

Provides a comprehensive assessment, which can predict current and future employment and potential adjustment factors for physically, emotionally, or developmentally disabled persons who may be unemployed or underemployed. Assessments evaluate interests, aptitudes, academic achievements, and physical abilities (including dexterity and coordination) through coordinated testing, interviewing and behavioral observations.

1166 Center for Family Support (CFS)

333 7th Avenue
New York, NY 10001-5004   212-629-7939
Fax: 212-239-2211
www.cfsny.org

Steven Vernickofs, Executive Director

Service agency devoted to the physical well-being and development of the retarded child and the sound mental health of the parents. Helps families with retarded children with all aspects of home care including counseling, referrals, home aide service and consultation. Offers intervention for parents at the birth of a retarded child with in-home support, guidance and infant stimulation. Pioneered training of nonprofessional women as home aides to provide supportive services in homes.

1167 Center for Mental Health Services Knowledge Exchange Network

US Department of Health and Human Services
PO Box 42490
Washington, DC 20015-4800
800-789-2647
Fax: 301-984-8796
E-mail: ken@mentalhealth.org
www.mentalhealth.org

Information about resources, technical assistance, research, training, networks, and other federal clearing houses, and fact sheets and materials. Information specialists refer callers to mental health resources in their communities as well as state, federal and non-profit contacts. Staff available Monday through Friday, 8:30 AM - 5:00 PM, EST, excluding federal holidays. After hours, callers may leave messages and an information specialist will return their call.

1168 International Society for Traumatic Stress Studies

60 Revere Drive
Suite 500
Northbrook, IL 60062   847-480-9028
Fax: 847-480-9282
E-mail: istss@istss.org
www.istss.org

Provides a forum for sharing research, clinical strategies, public policy concerns and theoretical formulation on trauma in the US and worldwide. Dedicated to discovery and dissemination of knowledge and to the stimulation of policy, program and service initiatives that seek to reduce traumatic stressors and their permanent and long-term consequences. Members include psychiatrists, psychologists, social workers, nurses, counselors, researchers, adminsitrators, advocates, and others.

1169 NADD: Association for Persons with Developmental Disabilities and Mental Health Needs

132 Fair Street
Kingston, NY 12401-4802   845-334-4336
800-331-5362
Fax: 845-331-4569
E-mail: nadd@mhv.net
www.thenadd.org

Dr. Robert Fletcher, Executive Director

Nonprofit organization designed to promote interest of professional and parent development with resources for individuals who have the coexistence of mental illness and mental retardation. Provides conference, educational services and training materials to professionals, parents, concerned citizens and service organizations. Formerly known as the National Association for the Dually Diagnosed.

1170 National Alliance for the Mentally Ill

2107 Wilson Boulevard
Suite 300
Arlington, VA 22201-3042   703-524-7600
800-950-6264
Fax: 703-524-9094
TDD: 703-516-7227
E-mail: helpline@nami.org
www.nami.org

Laurie Flynn, Executive Director

Nation's leading self-help organization for all those affected by severe brain disorders. Mission is to bring consumers and families with similar experiences together to share information about services, care providers, and ways to cope with the challenges of schizophrenia, manic depression, and other serious mental illnesses.

1171 National Mental Health Consumer's Self-Help Clearinghouse

1211 Chestnut Street
Suite 1207
Philadelphia, PA 19107   215-751-1810
800-553-4539
Fax: 215-636-6312
E-mail: info@mhselfhelp.org
www.mhselfhelp.org

Alex Morrsey, Information/Referral

Funded by the National Institute of Mental Health Community Support Program, the purpose of the Clearinghouse is to encourage the development and growth of consumer self-help groups.

Year Founded: 1992

1172 Suncoast Residential Training Center/Developmental Services Program

Goodwill Industries-Suncoast
10596 Gandy Boulevard
PO Box 14456
St. Petersburg, FL 33702   727-523-1512
Fax: 727-577-2749
www.goodwill-suncoast.org

Jay McCloe, Director Resource Development

A large group home which serves individuals diagnosed as mentally retarded with a secondary diagnosed of psychiatric difficulties as evidenced by problem behavior. Providing residential, behavioral and instructional support and services that will promote the development of adaptive, socially appropriate behavior, each individual is assessed to determine, socialization, basic academics and recreation. The primary intervention strategy is applied behavior analysis. Professional consultants are utilized to address the medical, dental, psychiatric and pharmacological needs of ech individual. One of the most popular features is the active community integration component of SRTC. Program customers attend an average of 15 monthly outings to various community events.

1173 Traumatic Incident Reduction Association

13 NW Barry Road, PMB 214
Kansas City, MO 64155-2728   816-468-4945
800-499-2751
Fax: 816-468-6656
E-mail: info@tira.org
www.tira.org

Devoted to reducing the affects of traumatic incidents and providing education on how to deal with traumatic events.

Books

1174 After the Crash: Assessment and Treatment of Motor Vehicle Accident Survivors

American Psychological Publishing
750 1st Street NE
Washington, DC 20002-4241   202-336-5500
Fax: 202-216-7610
www.apa.org

Katie Duffy, Marketing Assistant

$39.95

1175 Aging and Post Traumatic Stress Disorder

American Psychiatric Publishing
1000 Wilson Boulevard
Suite 1825
Arlington, VA 22209-3901   703-907-7322
800-368-5777
Fax: 703-907-1091
E-mail: appi@psych.org
www.appi.org

Katie Duffy, Marketing Assistant

Provides both literature reviews and data about animal and clinical studies and training for important current concepts of aging, the stress response and the interaction between them. *$37.50*

268 pages ISBN 0-880485-13-2

1176 Children and Trauma: Guide for Parents and Professionals

Courage to Change
PO Box 1268
Newburgh, NY 12551-1268   800-440-4003
Fax: 800-772-6499

Comprehensive guide to the emotional aftermath of children's crises. Discusses warning signs that a child may need professional help, and explores how parents and professionals can help children heal, reviving a sense of well being and safety. *$19.95*

240 pages

1177 Coping with Post-Traumatic Stress Disorder

Rosen Publishing Group
29 E 21st Street
New York, NY 10010   800-237-9932
Fax: 888-436-4643
E-mail: info@rosenpub.com
www.rosenpublishing.com

$26.50

Year Founded: 2002 ISBN 0-823934-56-X

1178 Coping with Trauma: a Guide to Self-Understa nding

American Psychiatric Publishing
1000 Wilson Boulevard
Suite 1825
Arlington, VA 22209-3901   703-907-7322
                                  800-368-5777
                             Fax: 703-907-1091
                        E-mail: appi@psych.org
                                  www.appi.org

Katie Duffy, Marketing Assistant

$16.00

385 pages ISBN 0-880489-96-0

1179 EMDR: Breakthrough Therapy for Overcoming Anxiety, Stress and Trauma

200 E Joppa Road
Suite 207
Baltimore, MD 21286   410-825-8888
                                 888-825-8249
                            Fax: 410-337-0747
                       E-mail: sidran@sidran.org
                                 www.sidran.org

EMDR - Eye Movement Desensitization and Reprocessing, has successfully relieved symptoms like depression, phobias and nightmares of PTSD survivors, with a rapidity that almost defies belief. In this book for general audiences, Shapiro, the originator of EMDR, explains how she created the groundbreaking therapy, how it works and how it can help people who feel stuck in negative reactions and behaviors. Included with the text are a variety of compelling case studies. *$16.00*

284 pages

1180 Effective Treatments for PTSD

Guilford Publications
72 Spring Street
New York, NY 10012   212-431-9800
                                 800-365-7006
                            Fax: 212-966-6708
                       E-mail: info@guilford.com
                                 www.guilford.com

Represents the collaborative work of experts across a range of theoretical orientations and professional backgrounds. Addresses general treatment considerations and methodological issues, reviews and evaluates the salient literature on treatment approaches for children, adolescents and adults. *$44.00*

379 pages ISBN 1-572305-84-3

1181 Herbs for the Mind: What Science Tells Us about Nature's Remedies for Depression, Stress, Memory Loss and Insomnia

Guilford Publications
72 Spring Street
New York, NY 10012   212-431-9800
                                 800-365-7006
                            Fax: 212-966-6708
                       E-mail: info@guilford.com
                                 www.guilford.com

Offers an authoritive guide to the most popular herbs for the mind: St. John's wort, kava, valerian and ginkgo. Clear guidelines are provided for developing an herbal self - help regimen, evaluating its ongoing effectiveness and recognizing when professional intervention may be necessary. A reliable scientific source for answers to frequently asked questions about herbal remedies. *$14.95*

265 pages ISBN 1-572304-76-6

1182 I Can't Get Over It: Handbook for Trauma Survivors

Courage To Change
PO Box 1268
Newburgh, NY 12551
                                 800-440-4003
                            Fax: 800-772-6499

Guides readers through the healing process of recovering from Post Traumatic Stress Disorder. From the emotional experience to the process of healing, this book is written for survivors of all types of trauma including war, sexual abuse, crime, family violence, rape and natural catastrophes. *$16.95*

374 pages ISBN 1-572240-58-

1183 Post-Traumatic Stress Disorder: Additional Perspectives

Charles C Thomas Publisher
2600 S 1st Street
Springfield, IL 62704-4730   217-789-8980
                                 800-258-8980
                            Fax: 217-789-9130
                      E-mail: books@ccthomas.com
                                 www.ccthomas.com

Comprehensive review of symptoms and treatment of PTSD. Tips on making diagnosis consistent. Treatment of each symptom is thoroughly reviewed. Prevention of PTSD is considered in detail with clear and logical innovative recommendations. Discusses special considerations in treating combat veterans, legal considerations, and recommendations for dealing with disasters. All without technical terminology. *$55.95*

258 pages ISSN 0-398-06242-0ISBN 0-398058-99-7

1184 Post-Traumatic Stress Disorder: Assessment, Differential Diagnosis, and Forensic Evaluation

Professional Resource Press
PO Box 15560
Sarasota, FL 34277-1560   941-343-9601
                                 800-443-3364
                            Fax: 941-343-9201
                      E-mail: orders@prpress.com
                                 www.prpress.com

Debra Fink, Managing Editor

A concise yet thorough examination of PTSD. An excellent resource for psychologists, psychiatrists, and lawyers involved in litigation concerning PTSD. *$26.95*

264 pages ISBN 0-943158-35-4

1185 Post-Traumatic Stress Disorder: Complete Treatment Guide

200 E Joppa Road
Suite 207
Baltimore, MD 21286   410-825-8888
                            888-825-8249
                       Fax: 410-337-0747
              E-mail: sidran@sidran.org
                       www.sidran.org

Excellent for clinicians who want to work more effectively with trauma survivors, this textbook provides a step by step description of PTSD treatment strategies. Includes chapters on definitions, diagnostic criteria and the biochemistry of PTSD. Reflects a generalized ideal structure of the healing process. Includes cognitive and behavioral techniques for managing flashbacks, anxiety attacks, sleep disturbances and dissociation; a comprehensive program for working through deeper layers of pain; plus PTSD related problems such as survivor guilt, secondary wounding, low self esteem, victim thinking, anger and depression. Presents trauma issues clearly for both general audiences and trauma professionals. *$49.95*

345 pages

1186 Posttraumatic Stress Disorder in Litigation: Guidelines for Forensic Assessment

American Psychiatric Publishing
1000 Wilson Boulevard
Suite 1825
Arlington, VA 22209-3901   703-907-7322
                                  800-368-5777
                             Fax: 703-907-1091
                    E-mail: appi@psych.org
                             www.appi.org

This essential collection by 13 leading US experts sheds important new light on forensic guidelines for effective assessment and diagnosis and determination of disability, serving both plaintiffs and defendants in litigation involving PTSD claims. Mental health and legal professionals, third-party payers, and interested laypersons will welcome this balanced approach to a complex and difficult field. *$44.95*

272 pages Year Founded: 2003 ISBN 1-585620-66-1

1187 Psychological Trauma

American Psychiatric Publishing
1000 Wilson Boulevard
Suite 1825
Arlington, VA 22209-3901   703-907-7322
                                  800-368-5777
                             Fax: 703-907-1091
                    E-mail: appi@psych.org
                             www.appi.org

Katie Duffy, Marketing Assistant

Epidemiology of trauma and post-traumatic stress disorder. Evaluation, neuroimaging, neuroendocrinology and pharmacology. *$29.00*

206 pages ISBN 0-880488-37-9

1188 Rebuilding Shattered Lives: Responsible Treatment of Complex Post-Traumatic and Dissociative Disorders

John Wiley & Sons
605 3rd Avenue
New York, NY 10058-0180   212-850-6000
                             Fax: 212-850-6008
                    E-mail: info@wiley.com
                             www.wiley.com

Essential for anyone working in the field of trauma therapy. Part I discusses recent findings about child abuse, the changes in attitudes toward child abuse over the last two decades and the nature of traumatic memory. Part II is an overview of principles of trauma treatment, including symptom control, establishment of boundaries and therapist self - care. Part III covers special topics, such as dissociative identity disorder, controversies, hospitalization and acute care. *$47.50*

271 pages ISBN 0-471247-32-4

1189 Risk Factors for Posttraumatic Stress Disorder

American Psychiatric Publishing
1000 Wilson Boulevard
Suite 1825
Arlington, VA 22209-3901   703-907-7322
                                  800-368-5777
                             Fax: 703-907-1091
                    E-mail: appi@psych.org
                             www.appi.org

Katie Duffy, Marketing Assistant

Strategies to study risk for the development of PTSD including epidemiological risk factors for trauma and PTSD, genetic risk factors for a twin study, family studies, parental PTSD as a risk factor, neurocognitive risk factors and risk factors for the acute biological and psychological response to trauma. *$42.50*

320 pages ISBN 0-880488-16-6

1190 Take Charge: Handling a Crisis and Moving Forward

American Institute for Preventive Medicine
30445 Northwestern Highway
Suite 350
Farmington Hills, MI 48334-3102   248-539-1800
                             Fax: 248-539-1808
                    E-mail: aipm@healthy.net
                             www.HealthyLife.com

Sue Jackson, VP

Take Charge helps people effectively live their lives after September 11th. This full color booklet provides just the right amount of information to effectively address the many concerns people have today. It will help people to be prepared for any kind of disaster, be it a terrorist attack, fire or flood.

32 pages

1191 Traumatic Stress: Effects of Overwhelming Experience on Mind, Body and Society

Guilford Publications
72 Spring Street
New York, NY 10012   212-431-9800
                            800-365-7006
                       Fax: 212-966-6708
                  E-mail: info@guilford.com
                          www.guilford.com

The current state of research and clinical knowledge on traumatic stress and its treatment. Contributions from leading authorities summarize knowledge emerging. Addresses the uncertainties and controversies that confront the field of traumatic stress, including the complexity of posttraumatic adaptations and the unproven effectiveness of some approaches to prevention and treatment. *$62.00*

596 pages ISBN 1-572300-88-4

1192 Trust After Trauma: a Guide to Relationships for Survivors and Those Who Love Them

New Harbinger Publications
5674 Shattuck Avenue
Oakland, CA 94609-1662   510-652-2002
                                800-748-6273
                           Fax: 510-652-5472
      E-mail: customerservice@newharbinger.com
                           www.newharbinger.com

Survivors guided through process of strengthening existing bonds, building new ones, and ending cycles of withdrawal and isolation. *$15.95*

344 pages ISBN 1-572241-01-2

1193 Understanding Post Traumatic Stress Disorder and Addiction

200 E Joppa Road
Suite 207
Baltimore, MD 21286   410-825-8888
                             888-825-8249
                        Fax: 410-337-0747
                  E-mail: sidran@sidran.org
                          www.sidran.org

This booklet discusses PTSD, how to recognize it and how to begin a dual recovery program from chemical dependency and PTSD. The workbook includes information to enhance your understanding of PTSD, activities to help identify the symptoms of dual disorders, a self evaulation of your recovery process and ways to handle situations that may trigger PTSD. *$9.00*

Post Traumatic Stress Disorder

1194 Posttraumatic Stress Disorder: A Guide

Madison Institute of Medicine
7617 Mineral Point Road
Suite 300
Madison, WI 53717-1623   608-827-2470
                           Fax: 608-827-2479
                  E-mail: mim@miminc.org
                          www.miminc.org

This informative guide provides a comprehensive overview of the causes and effective treatments of posttraumatic stress disorder (PTSD). *$5.95*

69 pages

Periodicals & Pamphlets

1195 Anxiety Disorders

Center for Mental Health Services: Knowledge Exchange Network
PO Box 42490
Washington, DC 20015   800-789-2647
                          Fax: 301-984-8796
                          TDD: 866-889-2647
              E-mail: ken@mentalhealth.org
                          www.mentalhealth.org

This fact sheet presents basic information on the symptoms, formal diagnosis, and treatment for generalized anxiety disorder, panic disorders, phobias, and posttraumatic stress disorder.

3 pages

1196 Helping Children and Adolescents Cope with Violence and Disasters

National Institute of Mental Health
6001 Executive Boulevard
Room 8184
Bethesda, MD 20892-9663   866-615-6464
                             Fax: 301-443-4279
                             TTY: 301-443-8431
                  E-mail: nimhinfo@nih.gov
                          www.nimh.nih.gov

Fact sheets that discuss children and adolescents' reactions to violence and disasters, emphasizing the wide range of responses and the role that parents, teachers and therapists can play in the healing process.

1197 Let's Talk Facts About Post-Traumatic Stress Disorder

American Psychiatric Publishing
1000 Wilson Boulevard
Suite 1825
Arlington, VA 22209-3901   703-907-7322
                                  800-368-5777
                             Fax: 703-907-1091
                  E-mail: appi@psych.org
                          www.appi.org

Katie Duffy, Marketing Assistant

$12.50

8 pages ISBN 0-890423-63-6

1198 Real Illness: Post-Traumatic Stress Disorder

National Institute of Mental Health
6001 Executive Boulevard
Room 8184
Bethesda, MD 20892-9663

866-615-6464
Fax: 301-443-4279
TTY: 301-443-8431
E-mail: nimhinfo@nih.gov
www.nimh.nih.gov

Do you avoid reminders of a bad accident, war or another traumatic event? Do you have nightmares, fear, emotional numbness? Read this pamphlet of simple information about how to get help.

9 pages

Video & Audio

1199 Treating Trauma Disorders Effectively

Colin A Ross Institute for Psychological Trauma
1701 Gateway
Suite 349
Richardson, TX 75080

972-918-9588
Fax: 972-918-9069
www.rossinst.com

This video illustrates two fundamental treatment principles: attachment to the perpetrator and locus of control shift. For clinicians, the program provides immediately usable techniques for their practices; for the layperson it provides a clear explanation for two consequences of childhood trauma. *$85.00*

Web Sites

1200 www.apa.org/practice/traumaticstress.html

Managing Traumatic Stress

American Psychological Association five page publication.

1201 www.bcm.tmc.edu/civitas/caregivers.htm

Caregivers Series

Sophisticated articles describing the effects of childhood trauma on brain development and relationships.

1202 www.cyberpsych.org

CyberPsych

Hosts the American Psychoanalyists Foundation, American Association of Suicideology, Society for the Exploration of Psychotherapy Intergration, and Anxiety Disorders Association of America. Also subcategories of the anxiety disorders, as well as general information, including panic disorder, phobias, obsessive compulsive disorder (OCD), social phobia, generalized anxiety disorder, post traumatic stress disorder, and phobias of childhood. Book reviews and links to web pages sharing the topics.

1203 www.factsforhealth.org

Madison Institute of Medicine

Resource to help identify, understand and treat a number of medical conditions, including social anxiety disorder and posttraumatic stress disorder.

1204 www.icisf.org

International Critical Incident Stress Foundation

A nonprofit, open membership foundation dedicated to the prevention and mitigation of disabling stress by education, training and support services for all emergency service professionals. Continuing education and training in emergency mental health services for psychologists, psychiatrists, social workers and licensed professional counselors.

1205 www.mentalhealth.com

Internet Mental Health

On-line information and a virtual encyclopedia related to mental disorders, possible causes and treatments. News, articles, on-line diagnostic programs and related links. Designed to improve understanding, diagnosis and treatment of mental illness throughout the world. Awarded the Top Site Award and the NetPsych Cutting Edge Site Award.

1206 www.ncptsd.org

National Center for PTSD

Clinical and research information on post-traumatic stress disorder (PTSD); includes over 21,000 article titles and abstracts on trauma-related literature.

1207 www.planetpsych.com

Planetpsych.com

Learn about disorders, their treatments and other topics in psychology. Articles are listed under the related topic areas. Ask a therapist a question for free, or view the directory of professionals in your area. If you are a therapist sign up for the directory. Current features, self-help, interactive, and newsletter archives.

1208 www.psychcentral.com

Psych Central

Personalized one-stop index for psychology, support, and mental health issues, resources, and people on the Internet.

1209 www.ptsdalliance.org

Website of the Post Traumatic Stress Disorder Alliance.

1210 www.sidran.org
Sidran Foundation

Focuses on dissociation and traumatic memories.

1211 www.sidran.org/trauma.html
Trauma Resource Area

Resources and Articles on Dissociative Experiences Scale and Dissociative Identity Disorder, PsychTrauma Glossary and Traumatic Memories.

1212 www.sni.net/trips/links.html
Post Traumatic Stress Resources

Links to major pages and metasites.

1213 www.trauma-pages.com

Information on post-traumatic stress disorder.

1214 www.trauma-pages.com/index.html
David Baldwin's Trauma Information Pages

Articles, resources and support.

1215 www.trauma-pages.com/t-facts.htm
Trauma Response

Listing of symptoms, ways to cope.

Introduction

Officially known as Somatizing Disorders, the disorders in this category are characterized by multiple physical symptoms or the conviction that one is ill or that there is something physically wrong despite negative medical examinations and laboratory tests. Those who have a Somatizing Disorder persist in believing they are ill or experience physical symptoms over long periods, regardless of evidence to the contrary, and their beliefs negatively affect all areas of their functioning.

Two main types of Somatizing Disorders are Hypochondriasis, which consists of one being convinced that he or she is ill despite all evidence to the contrary, and Somatization Disorder, consisting of one's experiencing physical symptoms without a discernible basis.

HYPOCHONDRIASIS SYMPTOMS

•Preoccupation with fears of having a serious illness based on a misinterpretation of bodily symptoms or sensations;
•A patient is more concerned about the symptoms than about being seriously ill;
•The preoccupation persists in spite of medical reassurance;
•The preoccupation is a source of distress and difficulty in social, work, and other areas;
•The duration of the preoccupation is at least six months.

SOMATIZATION DISORDER SYMPTOMS

•A history of physical complaints beginning before age 30 and continuing over years, resulting in a search for treatment or clear difficulties in social, work, or interpersonal areas;
•Four pain symptoms related to at least four places or functions;
•Two gastrointestinal problems other than pain, e.g., nausea, diarrhea;
•One sexual symptom other than pain, e.g., irregular menstruation, sexual disinterest, erectile dys-

function;
•One pseudoneurological symptom other than pain, e.g., weakness, double vision;
•Post-exam, symptoms cannot be explained by a medical condition;
•When a medical condition exists, physical complaints and social difficulties are greater than normal.

ASSOCIATED FEATURES

The person with either of these Somatizing Disorders visits many doctors, but neither physical examinations nor lab testing confirm their belief of illness; the individual often believes they are not getting proper care but lab findings and medical examinations consistently find nothing. The person with these disorders often suffers from anxiety and depression, and sufferers can have general medical disorders at the same time as Somatizing Disorders. Physical symptoms appearing after the somatization diagnosis is made, however, should not be dismissed completely out of hand.

The person may be treated by several doctors at once, which can lead to unwitting and possibly dangerous combinations of treatments. There may be suicide threats and attempts, and deteriorating personal relationships. Individuals with these disorders often have associated Personality Disorders, such as Histrionic, Borderline, or Antisocial Personality Disorder.

PREVALENCE

Hypochondriasis is equally common in both sexes. Its prevalence in the general population is not known. In general medical practice, four percent to nine percent of patients have the disorder. It is usually chronic.

Somatization Disorder is slightly more rare among men in the US than in other countries, but not uncommon in general medical practice. It is more common among Puerto Rican and Greek men, which suggests that cultural factors influence the sex ratios.

TREATMENT OPTIONS

These disorders are chronic by definition, and are difficult to manage. Repeated reassurance is not successful. The aim is to limit the extent to which the physical concerns and symptoms preoccupy an individual's thoughts and activities, and drain family emotional and financial resources. Individuals suffering from these disorders often resist mental health referral because they interpret it, sometimes correctly, as an indication that their symptoms are not being taken seriously. Treatment, whether by the primary care or mental health professional or both, should focus on maintaining function despite the symptoms. It is important that the psychological management and treatment is coordinated with medical treatment if possible by one physician only; one person should oversee all the medical treatment, including the psychological, so that care does not become fragmented and/or repetitive as the patient sees many different clinicians. Some individuals with Hypochondriasis respond to treatment which combines medication with intensive behavioral and cognitive techniques to manage anxiety and modify beliefs about the origin and course of physical symptoms.

Associations & Agencies

1217 Career Assessment & Planning Services

Goodwill Industries-Suncoast
10596 Gandy Boulevard
St. Petersburg, FL 33733   727-523-1512
                    Fax: 727-563-9300
E-mail: gw.marketing@goodwill-suncoast.com
                    www.goodwill-suncoast.org

R Lee Waits, President/CEO
Loreen M Spencer, Chair Person

Provides a comprehensive assessment, which can predict current and future employment and potential adjustment factors for physically, emotionally, or developmentally disabled persons who may be unemployed or underemployed. Assessments evaluate interests, aptitudes, academic achievements, and physical abilities (including dexterity and coordination) through coordinated testing, interviewing and behavioral observations.

1218 Center for Family Support (CFS)

333 7th Avenue
New York, NY 10001-5004   212-629-7939
                    Fax: 212-239-2211
                    www.cfsny.org

Steven Vernickofs, Executive Director

Service agency devoted to the physical well-being and development of the retarded child and the sound mental health of the parents. Helps families with retarded children with all aspects of home care including counseling, referrals, home aide service and consultation. Offers intervention for parents at the birth of a retarded child with in-home support, guidance and infant stimulation. Pioneered training of nonprofessional women as home aides to provide supportive services in homes.

1219 Center for Mental Health Services

SAMSHA
PO Box 42557
Washington, DC 20015
                    800-789-2647
                    Fax: 301-984-8796
                    TDD: 866-889-2647
                    www.mentalhealth.samhsa.com

Kathryn A Power M.Ed, Director

CMHS leads federal efforts to treat mental illnesses by promoting mental health and by preventing the development or worsening of mental health when possible.

1220 Center for Mental Health Services Knowledge Exchange Network

US Department of Health and Human Services
PO Box 42490
Washington, DC 20015-4800
                    800-789-2647
                    Fax: 301-984-8796
E-mail: ken@mentalhealth.org
                    www.mentalhealth.org

Information about resources, technical assistance, research, training, networks, and other federal clearing houses, and fact sheets and materials. Information specialists refer callers to mental health resources in their communities as well as state, federal and nonprofit contacts. Staff available Monday through Friday, 8:30 AM - 5:00 PM, EST, excluding federal holidays. After hours, callers may leave messages and an information specialist will return their call.

1221 Deborah MacWilliams

548 SW 13th Street
Suite B-3
Bend, OR 97702   541-617-0351
                    Fax: 541-617-0351

Deborah MacWilliams PhD PMHNP

Providing individual psychiatric evaluation, psychotherapy, and medical management for adults and teens. Specializing in thorough assessments and personalized treatment planning.

1222 Institute for Contemproary Psychotherapy

1841 Broadway 60th Street Fourth Floor
New York, NY 10023-7603   212-333-3444
                    Fax: 212-333-5444
                    www.icpnyc.org

Leslie Goldstein C.S.W, Vice Chairman
Fred Lipschitz, Treasurer
Sydney Ratner C.S.W, Secretry
Ronald Taffel PhD, Chairman

ICP is dedicated to providing high quality therapy at low to moderate cost, offering post-graduate training for therapists and educatiing the public about mental health issues.

1223 NADD: Association for Persons with Developmental Disabilities and Mental Health Needs

132 Fair Street
Kingston, NY 12401-4802   845-334-4336
                    800-331-5362
                    Fax: 845-331-4569
                    E-mail: nadd@mhv.net
                    www.thenadd.org

Dr. Robert Fletcher, Executive Director

Nonprofit organization designed to promote interest of professional and parent development with resources for individuals who have the coexistence of mental illness and mental retardation. Provides conference, educational services and training materials to professionals, parents, concerned citizens and service organizations. Formerly known as the National Association for the Dually Diagnosed.

1224 National Mental Health Consumer's Self-Help Clearinghouse

1211 Chestnut Street
Suite 1207
Philadelphia, PA 19107   215-751-1810
                    800-553-4539
                    Fax: 215-636-6312
                    E-mail: info@mhselfhelp.org
                    www.mhselfhelp.org

Alex Morrsey, Information/Referral

Funded by the National Institute of Mental Health Community Support Program, the purpose of the Clearinghouse is to encourage the development and growth of consumer self-help groups.

Year Founded: 1992

1225 Suncoast Residential Training Center/Developmental Services Program

Goodwill Industries-Suncoast
10596 Gandy Boulevard
St. Petersburg, FL 33733-4456   727-523-1512
                                           888-279-1988
                              Fax: 727-563-9300
E-mail: gw.marketing@goodwill-suncoast.com
                www.goodwill-suncoast.org

R Lee Waits, President/CEO
Loreen M Spencer, Chair Person

A large group home which serves individuals diagnosed as mentally retarded with a secondary diagnosed of psychiatric difficulties as evidenced by problem behavior. Providing residential, behavioral and instructional support and services that will promote the development of adaptive, socially appropriate behavior, each individual is assessed to determine, socialization, basic academics and recreation. The primary intervention strategy is applied behavior analysis. Professional consultants are utilized to address the medical, dental, psychiatric and pharmacological needs of ech individual. One of the most popular features is the active community integration component of SRTC. Program customers attend an average of 15 monthly outings to various community events.

Books

1226 Hypochondria: Woeful Imaginings

University of California Press
2120 Berkeley Way
Berkeley, CA 94720-5804   501-642-4247
                              Fax: 510-643-7127
E-mail: askucp@ucpress.edu
                www.ucpress.edu

Susan Baur illuminates the process by which hypochondriacs come to adopt and maintain illness as a way of life. *$25.00*

260 pages Year Founded: 1989 ISBN 0-520067-51-7

1227 Journal of Psychosomatic Research

Elsevier Science
655 Avenue of the Americas
New York, NY 10010   212-633-3730
                              Fax: 212-633-3680

The Journal of Psychosomatic Research is a multidisciplinary research jounral covering all aspects of the relationships between psychology and medicine. The scope is broad and ranges from basic biological and psychological research to evaluations of treatment and services. Papers will normally be concerned with illness or patients rather than studies of healthy populations. Studies concerning special populations, such as the elderly and children and adolescents, are welcome. In addition to peer-reviewed original papers, the journal publishes editoirals, reviews, and other papers related to the journal's aims.

1228 Mind-Body Problems: Psychotherapy with Psychosomatic Disorders

Jason Aronson
230 Livingston Street
Northvale, NJ 07647   570-342-1320
                                 800-782-0015
                              Fax: 201-767-1576
                www.aronson.com

Shows us the causes and treatments of the major pychosomatic sympstons. *$70.00*

376 pages ISBN 1-568216-54-8

1229 Phantom Illness: Recognizing, Understanding, and Overcoming Hypochondria

Houghton Mifflin Company
222 Berkeley Street
Boston, MA 02116   617-351-5000
                E-mail: inquiries@hmco.com
                              www.hmco.com

Offers hope to those who suffer from the debilitating disorder of hypochondria. Carla Cantor's long, dark road to hypochondria began when she crashed a car, killing a friend of hers. She couldn't forgive herself, and a few years later began imagining that she was suffering from lupis. Many years and two hospitalizations later, she wrote this book not only about her experiences, but about hypochondria in general, now more politely referred to as a 'somatoform disorder'. Paperback. *$15.00*

351 pages ISBN 0-395859-92-1

Video & Audio

1230 Effective Learning Systems

3451 Bonita Bay Boulevard
Suite 205
Bonita Springs, FL 34134   239-948-1660
                                       800-966-5683
                              Fax: 239-948-1664
                E-mail: info@efflearn.com
                              www.efflearn.com

Robert E Griswold, President
Deirdre M Griswold, VP

Audio tapes for stress management, deep relaxation, anger control, peace of mind, insomnia, weight and smoking, self-image and self-esteem, positive thinking, health and healing. Since 1972, Effective Learning Systems has helped millions of people take charge of their lives and make positive changes. Over 75 titles available, each with a money-back guarantee. Price range $12-$14.

Web Sites

1231 www.mentalhealth.com

Internet Mental Health

On-line information and a virtual encyclopedia related to mental disorders, possible causes and treatments. News, articles, on-line diagnostic programs and related links. Designed to improve understanding, diagnosis and treatment of mental illness throughout the world. Awarded the Top Site Award and the NetPsych Cutting Edge Site Award.

1232 www.planetpsych.com

Planetpsych.com

Learn about disorders, their treatments and other topics in psychology. Articles are listed under the related topic areas. Ask a therapist a question for free, or view the directory of professionals in your area. If you are a therapist sign up for the directory. Current features, self-help, interactive, and newsletter archives.

1233 www.psychcentral.com

Psych Central

Personalized one-stop index for psychology, support, and mental health issues, resources, and people on the Internet.

1234 www.users.lanminds.com/~eds/manual.html

Trauma Treatment Manual

On-line treatment manual gives professionals an overview of trauma treatment from one psychologist's viewpoint, treatment guidelines and examples.

Introduction

Schizophrenia is a devastating disease of the brain that severely impairs an individual's ability to think, feel and function normally. Though not a common disorder, it is one of the most destructive, disrupting the lives of sufferers, as well as of family members and loved ones. Long misunderstood, people with Schizophrenia and their families have also borne a stigma in addition to the burden of their illness.

Fortunately, much has been learned about the disease in recent years and treatments have improved markedly. If properly treated, many people with Schizophrenia can live stable, happy, and productive lives without relapse.

Today, Schizophrenia is understood to be a genetically determined disorder of the brain, and older theories of poor parenting or unhappy families have been discredited. Many theories exist to explain the neurological origin and cause of Schizophrenia; one theory is that it is a disorder of information processing resulting from a defect in the prefrontal cortex of the brain. Because this system is defective, an individual with Schizophrenia is easily overwhelmed by the amount of information and stimuli coming from the environment. Typically, a person with Schizophrenia may hear voices. He or she may also have strange thoughts and ideas triggered by hallucinations and/or delusions, e.g., believing that he or she is God or a famous historical figure. Schizophrenia is a chronic disease, and once diagnosed, a person is liable to need treatment for the rest of his or her life. However, great strides have been made in treating the disease.

SYMPTOMS

Positive symptoms:
•Delusions or false and bizarre beliefs;
•Hallucinations;

Negative symptoms:

•Withdrawing from social contact;
• Speaking less;
•Losing interest in things and the ability to enjoy them;
•Disorganized speech;
•Grossly disorganized or catatonic behavior (extremely agitated or zombie-like);
•The symptoms cause social and occupational dysfunction;
•Signs of the disturbance persist for at least six months;
•The symptoms are not related to mood or depressive disorders, substance abuse or general medical conditions.

ASSOCIATED FEATURES

People with Schizophrenia, because their disease causes difficulty in perceiving their environment and responding to it normally, will often act strange, and have odd beliefs. They sometimes react to stimuli (voices or images originating inside their brains) as though they were originating in their environment; hallucinations and delusions can make a person's behavior appear bizarre to others. A person with the disease may act socially inappropriately for instance, by smiling, laughing or being silly for no reason. Anhedonia, the inability to enjoy pleasurable activities is common in Schizophrenia, as are sleep disturbances and abnormalities of psychomotor activity. The latter may take the form of pacing, rocking, or immobility. Negative symptoms can be more disabling than positive ones, and can cause family members to think the individual is just lazy. Schizophrenia takes many forms, and there are a number of subtypes of the illness, including paranoid schizophrenia.

Individuals with untreated Schizophrenia, under the influence of hallucinations and delusions, have a slightly greater propensity for violence than the general population, especially when there is co-existing alcohol or substance abuse, which is quite common. However, it is important to emphasize that this is not always the case; Schizophrenia is known as a heterogenous disease, meaning that the illness takes many forms, depending on a variety of individual characteristics and circumstances.

It has been established that patients who receive appropriate treatment are not more violent than the general population.

The life expectancy of people with Schizophrenia is shorter then the general population for a variety of resons: suicide is common among people with the disease and people with Schizophrenia often have poorer overall health, and are often too ill to take care of themselves.

PREVALENCE

The first episode of Schizophrenia usually occurs in teenage years, although some cases may occur in the late thirties or forties. Onset prior to puberty is rare, though cases as early as five year olds have been reported. Women are more likely to have a later onset and a better prognosis. Estimates of the prevalence of Schizophrenia vary widely around the world, but probably about one percent of the population has the disease.

TREATMENT OPTIONS

Because Schizophrenia is known to be a disease of the brain, medications used to treat the disease are designed to correct chemical imbalances in the brain. Two drugs, Clozapine and Risperidal, have been remarkably successful in correcting the positive symptoms of Schizophrenia, those symptoms that cause hallucinations, voices, and other overt behavioral abnormalities. However, Clozapine causes a low incidence of a life-threatening blood disorder; therefore people who take it must have blood tests at regular intervals. There are several new medications, all of which seem to be more effective in treating the negative, as well as the positive, symptoms. They are Seroquel, Zyprexa, and Geodon.

Antipsychotic medications can have serious side effects, the most prominent being Tardive Dyskinesia which causes involuntary muscular movements (see Movement Disorders). Often, patients report that antipsychotic medications make them feel foggy, or lethargic. The newer antipsychotic medications are less sedating and have a decreased risk of causing Tardive Dyskinesia, but are associated with significant weight gain and increased risk of diabetes.

Having Schizophrenia interferes with taking care of oneself and getting proper medical care in several ways; Schizophrenia often depletes financial resources so that patients cannot afford medication, nutrition, and medical care. Schizophrenia can also interfere with an individual's ability to understand signs and symptoms of medical diorders. Compliance with medication is often a problem, and failure to continue taking medication is a major cause of relapse. For this reason, treatment should include supportive therapy, in which a psychiatrist or other mental health professional provides counseling aimed at helping the patient maintain a positive and optimistic attitude focused on staying healthy. Other forms of therapy, such as social skills training, have also found some success and may be useful in helping a person with Schizophrenia learn appropriate social and interpersonal behavior.

Associations & Agencies

1236 Career Assessment & Planning Services

Goodwill Industries-Suncoast
10596 Gandy Boulevard
St. Petersburg, FL 33733   727-523-1512
Fax: 727-563-9300
E-mail: gw.marketing@goodwill-suncoast.org
www.goodwill-suncoast.org

R Lee Waits, President/CEO
Loreen M Spencer, Chair Person

Provides a comprehensive assessment, which can predict current and future employment and potential adjustment factors for physically, emotionally, or developmentally disabled persons who may be unemployed or underemployed. Assessments evaluate interests, aptitudes, academic achievements, and physical abilities (including dexterity and coordination) through coordinated testing, interviewing and behavioral observations.

1237 Center for Family Support (CFS)

333 7th Avenue
New York, NY 10001-5004   212-629-7939
Fax: 212-239-2211
www.cfsny.org

Steven Vernickofs, Executive Director

Service agency devoted to the physical well-being and development of the retarded child and the sound mental health of the parents. Helps families with retarded children with all aspects of home care including counseling, referrals, home aide service and consultation. Offers intervention for parents at the birth of a retarded child with in-home support, guidance and infant stimulation. Pioneered training of nonprofessional women as home aides to provide supportive services in homes.

1238 Center for Mental Health Services

SAMSHA
PO Box 42557
Washington, DC 20015
800-789-2647
Fax: 301-984-8796
TDD: 866-889-2647
www.mentalhealth.org

Edward B Searle MBA, Acting Deputy Director
Jeffrey A Buck MD, Associate Director

Develops national mental health policies, that promote Federal/State coordination and benefit from input from consumers, family members and providers. Ensures that high quality mental health services programs are implemented to benefit seriously mentally ill populations, disasters or those involved in the criminal justice system.

1239 Center for Mental Health Services Knowledge Exchange Network

US Department of Health and Human Services
PO Box 42490
Washington, DC 20015-4800
800-789-2647
Fax: 301-984-8796
E-mail: ken@mentalhealth.org
www.mentalhealth.org

Information about resources, technical assistance, research, training, networks, and other federal clearing houses, and fact sheets and materials. Information specialists refer callers to mental health resources in their communities as well as state, federal and non-profit contacts. Staff available Monday through Friday, 8:30 AM - 5:00 PM, EST, excluding federal holidays. After hours, callers may leave messages and an information specialist will return their call.

1240 NADD: Association for Persons with Developmental Disabilities and Mental Health Needs

132 Fair Street
Kingston, NY 12401-4802   845-334-4336
800-331-5362
Fax: 845-331-4569
E-mail: nadd@mhv.net
www.thenadd.org

Dr. Robert Fletcher, Executive Director

Nonprofit organization designed to promote interest of professional and parent development with resources for individuals who have the coexistence of mental illness and mental retardation. Provides conference, educational services and training materials to professionals, parents, concerned citizens and service organizations. Formerly known as the National Association for the Dually Diagnosed.

1241 National Alliance for Research on Schizophrenia and Depression

60 Cutter Mill Road
Suite 404
Great Neck, NY 11021-3104   516-829-0091
800-829-8289
Fax: 516-487-6930
E-mail: info@narsad.org
www.narsad.org

Constance E Lieber, President

NARSAD is a private, not-for-profit public charity 501 (C) (3) organized for the purpose of raising and distributing funds for scientific research into the causes, cures, treatments and prevention of severe psychiatric brain disorders, such as schizophrenia and depression.

1242 National Alliance for the Mentally Ill

2107 Wilson Boulevard
Suite 300
Arlington, VA 22201-3042   703-524-7600
800-950-6264
Fax: 703-524-9094
TDD: 703-516-7227
E-mail: helpline@nami.org
www.nami.org

Laurie Flynn, Executive Director

Nation's leading self-help organization for all those affected by severe brain disorders. Mission is to bring consumers and families with similar experiences together to share information about services, care providers, and ways to cope with the challenges of schizophrenia, manic depression, and other serious mental illnesses.

1243 National Mental Health Association

2001 N Beauregard Street
12th Floor
Alexandria, VA 22311   703-684-7722
        800-969-6642
    Fax: 703-684-5968
    TTY: 800-433-5959
    E-mail: infoctr@nmha.org
    www.nmha.org

Mike Fienza, Executive Director
Chris Condayn, Communications

Dedicated to improving treatments, understanding and services for adults and children with mental health needs. Working to win political support for funding for school mental health programs. Provides information about a wide range of disorders.

1244 National Mental Health Consumer's Self-Help Clearinghouse

1211 Chestnut Street
Suite 1207
Philadelphia, PA 19107   215-751-1810
      800-553-4539
    Fax: 215-735-0275
    E-mail: info@mhselfhelp.org
    www.mhselfhelp.org

Alex Morrsey, Information/Referral

Funded by the National Institute of Mental Health Community Support Program, the purpose of the Clearinghouse is to encourage the development and growth of consumer self-help groups.

Year Founded: 1992

1245 Suncoast Residential Training Center/Developmental Services Program

Goodwill Industries-Suncoast
10596 Gandy Boulevard
St. Petersburg, FL 33733   727-523-1512
    Fax: 727-563-9300
    E-mail: gw.marketing@goodwill-suncoast.org
    www.goodwill-suncoast.org

R Lee Waits, President/CEO
Loreen M Spencer, Chair Person

A large group home which serves individuals diagnosed as mentally retarded with a secondary diagnosed of psychiatric difficulties as evidenced by problem behavior. Providing residential, behavioral and instructional support and services that will promote the development of adaptive, socially appropriate behavior, each individual is assessed to determine, socialization, basic academics and recreation. The primary intervention strategy is applied behavior analysis. Professional consultants are utilized to address the medical, dental, psychiatric and pharmacological needs of ech individual. One of the most popular features is the active community integration component of SRTC. Program customers attend an average of 15 monthly outings to various community events.

Books

1246 Biology of Schizophrenia and Affective Disease

American Psychiatric Publishing
1000 Wilson Boulevard
Suite 1825
Arlington, VA 22209-3901   703-907-7322
    800-368-5777
    Fax: 703-907-1091
    E-mail: appi@psych.org
    www.appi.org

Katie Duffy, Marketing Assistant

Provides a state-of-the-art look at the biological bases of several mental illness from the perspective of the researchers making these discoveries. *$58.50*

464 pages ISBN 0-880487-46-1

1247 Breakthroughs in Antipsychotic Medications: a Guide for Consumers, Families, and Clinicians

National Alliance for the Mentally Ill
Colonial Place Three
2107 Wilson Boulevard Suite 300
Arlington, VA 22201-3042   703-524-7600
    800-950-6264
    Fax: 703-524-9094
    TDD: 703-516-7227
    E-mail: campaign@nami.org
    www.nami.org

Helps consumers and their families weigh the pros and cons of switching from older antipsychotics to newer ones. Answers frequently asked questions about antipsychotics and guides readers through the process of switching. Includes fact sheets on the new medications and their side effects. *$22.95*

207 pages Year Founded: 1999 ISBN 0-393703-03-7

1248 Concept of Schizophrenia: Historical Perspectives

American Psychiatric Publishing
1000 Wilson Boulevard
Suite 1825
Arlington, VA 22209-3901   703-907-7322
                                  800-368-5777
                              Fax: 703-907-1091
                        E-mail: appi@psych.org
                                    www.appi.org

Katie Duffy, Marketing Assistant

$65.00

211 pages

1249 Contemporary Issues in the Treatment of Schizophrenia

American Psychiatric Publishing
1000 Wilson Boulevard
Suite 1825
Arlington, VA 22209-3901   703-907-7322
                                  800-368-5777
                              Fax: 703-907-1091
                        E-mail: appi@psych.org
                                    www.appi.org

Covers approaches to the patient by investigating biological, pharmacological and psychosocial treatments. *$99.95*

960 pages ISBN 0-880486-81-3

1250 Coping with Schizophrenia: a Guide for Families

New Harbinger Publications
5674 Shattuck Avenue
Oakland, CA 94609-1662   510-652-2002
                                  800-748-6273
                              Fax: 510-652-5472
         E-mail: customerservice@newharbinger.com
                            www.newharbinger.com

Provides detailed, step by step strategies for preventing relapses, regulating medications, establishing household rules, dealing with depression and anxiety, overcoming alcohol and drug abuse, responding to crises, improving quality of life, and planning for the patient's future. *$15.95*

368 pages ISBN 1-879237-78-4

1251 Encyclopedia of Schizophrenia and the Psychotic Disorders

Facts on File
132 W 31st Street
17th Floor
New York, NY 10001-2006
                                  800-322-8755
                              Fax: 800-678-3633
            E-mail: custserv@factsonfile.com
                            www.factsonfile.com

Details recent theories and research findings on schizophrenia and psychotic disorders, together with a complete overview of the field's history. *$65.00*

368 pages Year Founded: 2000 ISBN 0-816040-70-2

1252 Family Care of Schizophrenia: a Problem-Solving Approach...

Guilford Publications
72 Spring Street
New York, NY 10012   212-431-9800
                                  800-365-7006
                              Fax: 212-966-6708
                    E-mail: info@guilford.com
                                www.guilford.com

Falloon and his colleagues have developed a model for the broad-based community treatment of schizophrenia and other severe forms of mental illness that taps this underutilized potential. The goal of their program is not merely the reduction of stress that can trigger florid episodes, but also the restoration of the patient to a level of social functioning that permits employment and socialization with people outside the family. As the author demonstrates, families can, with proper guidance, be taught to modulate intrafamilial stress, whether it derives from family tensions or external life events. *$27.95*

451 pages ISBN 0-898629-23-3

1253 Family Work for Schizophrenia: a Practical Guide

American Psychiatric Publishing
1000 Wilson Boulevard
Suite 1825
Arlington, VA 22209-3901   703-907-7322
                                  800-368-5777
                              Fax: 703-907-1091
                        E-mail: appi@psych.org
                                    www.appi.org

Katie Duffy, Marketing Assistant

1254 First Episode Psychosis

American Psychiatric Publishing
1000 Wilson Boulevard
Suite 1825
Arlington, VA 22209-3901   703-907-7322
                                  800-368-5777
                              Fax: 703-907-1091
                        E-mail: appi@psych.org
                                    www.appi.org

Katie Duffy, Marketing Assistant

Professional discussion of early Psychosis presentation. *$39.95*

160 pages ISBN 1-853174-35-1

1255 Group Therapy for Schizophrenic Patients

American Psychiatric Publishing
1000 Wilson Boulevard
Suite 1825
Arlington, VA 22209-3901   703-907-7322
                                  800-368-5777
                              Fax: 703-907-1091
                        E-mail: appi@psych.org
                                    www.appi.org

Katie Duffy, Marketing Assistant

Acquaints mental health practitioners with this cost-effective method of treatment. *$29.00*

192 pages ISBN 0-880481-72-2

1256 Guidelines for the Treatment of Patients with Schizophrenia

American Psychiatric Publishing
1000 Wilson Boulevard
Suite 1825
Arlington, VA 22209-3901   703-907-7322
                                  800-368-5777
                          Fax: 703-907-1091
                          E-mail: appi@psych.org
                                  www.appi.org

Katie Duffy, Marketing Assistant

Provides therapists with a set of patient care strategies that will aid their clinical decison making. Describes the best and most appropriate treatments available to patients. *$22.50*

160 pages ISBN 0-890423-09-1

1257 How to Cope with Mental Illness In Your Family: a Guide for Siblings and Offspring

Health Source
1404 K Street, NW
Washington, DC 20005-2401   202-789-7303
                                   800-713-7122
                           Fax: 202-789-7899
                   E-mail: healthsourcebooks@psych.org
                           www.healthsourcebooks.org

This book explores the nature of illnesses such as schizophrenia, major depression, while providing the tools to overcome the devasting effects of growing up or living in a family where they exist. Readers are led through the essential stages of recovery, from revisiting their childhood to revising their family legacy, and ultimately, to reclaiming their life. *$14.00*

240 pages ISBN 0-874779-23-5

1258 Innovations in the Psychological Management of Schizophrenia: Assessment, Treatment & Services

John Wiley & Sons
605 3rd Avenue
New York, NY 10058-0180   212-850-6000
                         Fax: 212-850-6008
                         E-mail: info@wiley.com
                                 www.wiley.com

$80.00

338 pages ISBN 0-471929-35-2

1259 Innovative Approaches for Difficult to Treat Populations

American Psychiatric Publishing
1000 Wilson Boulevard
Suite 1825
Arlington, VA 22209-3901   703-907-7322
                                  800-368-5777
                          Fax: 703-907-1091
                          E-mail: appi@psych.org
                                  www.appi.org

Firsthand look at the future direction of clinical services. Focuses on services for individuals who use the highest proportion of mental health resources and for whom traditional services have not been effective. *$65.00*

512 pages ISBN 0-880486-80-5

1260 Natural History of Mania, Depression and Schizophrenia

American Psychiatric Publishing
1000 Wilson Boulevard
Suite 1825
Arlington, VA 22209-3901   703-907-7322
                                  800-368-5777
                          Fax: 703-907-1091
                          E-mail: appi@psych.org
                                  www.appi.org

Katie Duffy, Yarketing Assistant

An unusual look at the course of mental illness, based on data from the Iowa 500 Research Project. *$42.50*

336 pages ISBN 0-880487-26-7

1261 New Pharmacotherapy of Schizophrenia

American Psychiatric Publishing
1000 Wilson Boulevard
Suite 1825
Arlington, VA 22209-3901   703-907-7322
                                  800-368-5777
                          Fax: 703-907-1091
                          E-mail: appi@psych.org
                                  www.appi.org

Discusses the new class of antipsychotic agents that promise superior efficacy and more favorable side-effects; offers an improved understanding of how to employ existing pharmachotherapeutic agents. *$32.50*

272 pages ISBN 0-880484-91-8

1262 Office Treatment of Schizophrenia

American Psychiatric Publishing
1000 Wilson Boulevard
Suite 1825
Arlington, VA 22209-3901   703-907-7322
                                  800-368-5777
                          Fax: 703-907-1091
                          E-mail: appi@psych.org
                                  www.appi.org

Katie Duffy, Marketing Director

Examines options in outpatient treatment of schizophrenic patients. *$31.00*

208 pages

1263 Outcome & Innovation in Psychological Treatment of Schizophrenia

John Wiley & Sons
605 3rd Avenue
New York, NY 10058-0180   212-850-6000
                         Fax: 212-850-6008
                         E-mail: info@wiley.com
                                 www.wiley.com

$65.00

65 pages ISBN 0-471976-59-8

1264 Plasma Homovanillic Acid in Schizophrenia: Implications for Presynaptic Dopamine Dysfunction

American Psychiatric Publishing
1000 Wilson Boulevard
Suite 1825
Arlington, VA 22209-3901   703-907-7322
                                  800-368-5777
                            Fax: 703-907-1091
                       E-mail: appi@psych.org
                                  www.appi.org

Katie Duffy, Marketing Assistant

Provides the most comprehensive and current collection of information on plasma HVA levels. Provides a concise synthesis and critique of current data. *$33.00*

216 pages ISBN 0-880484-89-6

1265 Practicing Psychiatry in the Community: a Manual

American Psychiatric Publishing
1000 Wilson Boulevard
Suite 1825
Arlington, VA 22209-3901   703-907-7322
                                  800-368-5777
                            Fax: 703-907-1091
                       E-mail: appi@psych.org
                                  www.appi.org

Katie Duffy, Marketing Assistant

Addresses the major issues currently facing community psychiatrists. *$67.50*

560 pages ISBN 0-880486-63-5

1266 Prenatal Exposures in Schizophrenia

American Psychiatric Publishing
1000 Wilson Boulevard
Suite 1825
Arlington, VA 22209-3901   703-907-7322
                                  800-368-5777
                            Fax: 703-907-1091
                       E-mail: appi@psych.org
                                  www.appi.org

Considers a range of epigenetic elements thought to interact with abnormal genes to produce the onset of illness. Attention to the evidence implicating obstetric complications, prenatal infection, autoimmunity and prenatal malnutrition in brain disorders. *$36.50*

352 pages ISBN 0-880484-99-3

1267 Psychiatric Rehabilitation of Chronic Mental Patients

American Psychiatric Publishing
1000 Wilson Boulevard
Suite 1825
Arlington, VA 22209-3901   703-907-7322
                                  800-368-5777
                            Fax: 703-907-1091
                       E-mail: appi@psych.org
                                  www.appi.org

Katie Duffy, Marketing Assistant

Provides highly detained prescriptions for assesment and treatment techniques with case examples and learning exercises. *$28.00*

320 pages ISBN 0-880482-01-X

1268 Psychoeducational Groups for Patients with Schizophrenia: Guide for Practitioners

Aspen Publishers
1185 Avenue of the Americas
New York, NY 10036   212-597-0200
                      Fax: 212-597-0338
                      www.aspenpublishers.com

This unique resource provides a comprehensive, step-by-step intervention program designed to assist the therapist who conducts psychoeducation groups for patients with schizophrenia, on an inpatient or outpatient basis. Special features include assessment questionnaires specifically designed to measure pre-and-post-intervention change, samples of questions frequently asked by patients, easy-to-read worksheets, handouts and group evaluation forms. *$161.90*

292 pages ISBN 0-834201-97-6

1269 Psychoses and Pervasive Development Disorders in Childhood and Adolescence

American Psychiatric Publishing
1000 Wilson Boulevard
Suite 1825
Arlington, VA 22209-3901   703-907-7322
                                  800-368-5777
                            Fax: 703-907-1091
                       E-mail: appi@psych.org
                                  www.appi.org

Katie Duffy, Marketing Assistant

Provides a concise summary of currently knowledge of psychoses and pervasive developmental disorders of childhood and adolescence. Discusses recent changes in aspects of diagnosis and definition of these disorders, advances in knowledge, and aspects of treatment. *$46.50*

368 pages ISBN 1-882103-01-7

1270 Return From Madness

Jason Aronson
200 Livingston Street
Northvale, NJ 07647   201-767-4093
                             800-782-1005
                        Fax: 201-767-1576
                             www.aronson.com

This book offers a new approach to helping people who have emerged from madness. *$50.00*

256 pages ISBN 1-568216-25-4

1271 Schizophrenia

American Psychiatric Publishing
1000 Wilson Boulevard
Suite 1825
Arlington, VA 22209-3901 703-907-7322
800-368-5777
Fax: 703-907-1091
E-mail: appi@psych.org
www.appi.org

Katie Duffy, Marketing Assistant

Ideas in treating the disease, and how many patients can lead productive lives without relapse. *$165.00*

760 pages ISBN 0-632032-76-6

1272 Schizophrenia Revealed: From Nuerons to Social Interactions

WW Norton & Company
500 5th Avenue
New York, NY 10110 212-790-9456
Fax: 212-869-0856
E-mail: admalmud@wwnorton.com
www.wwnorton.com

Helps explain some of the former mysteries of Schizophrenia that are now possible to study through advances in neuroscience. *$ 28.00*

272 pages ISSN 70326-6

1273 Schizophrenia and Genetic Risks

National Alliance for the Mentally Ill
Colonial Place Three
2107 Wilson Boulevard
Arlington, VA 22201 703-524-7600
800-950-6264
Fax: 703-524-9094
TDD: 703-516-7227
E-mail: info@nami.org
www.nami.org

Provides basic facts about schizophrenia and its familial distribution so consumers and mental health workers can become informed enough to initiate appropriate actions. Includes suggested resources.

1274 Schizophrenia and Manic Depressive Disorder

National Alliance for the Mentally Ill
Colonial Place Three
2107 Wilson Boulevard Suite 300
Arlington, VA 22201 703-524-7600
800-950-6264
Fax: 703-524-9094
TDD: 703-516-7227
E-mail: info@nami.org
www.nami.org

Explores the biological roots of mental illness with a primary focus on schizophrenia. *$27.00*

274 pages ISBN 0-465072-85-2

1275 Schizophrenia and Primitive Mental States

Jason Aronson Publishing
276 Livingston Street
Northvale, NJ 07647 570-342-1320
800-782-0015
Fax: 201-767-1576
www.aronson.com

In this volume, reowned therapist Peter Giovacchini shows readers how to do more psychotic patients than rely on medication to reduce their florid symptoms. Instead, he demonstrates how schizophrenic patients can be offered true cure and the possibility of living a full and related life through intensive psychotherapeutic treatment. *$50.00*

288 pages ISBN 0-765700-27-1

1276 Schizophrenia in a Molecular Age

American Psychiatric Publishing
1000 Wilson Boulevard
Suite 1825
Arlington, VA 22209-3901 703-907-7322
800-368-5777
Fax: 703-907-1091
E-mail: appi@psych.org
www.appi.org

Katie Duffy, Marketing Assistant

Explores the multidimensional phenotype of schizophrenia, and use of molecular biology and anti-psychotic medications. Reviews the implications of early sensory procesing and subcortical involvement of cognitive dysfuntion inschizophrenia. Functional neuroimaging applied to the syndrome of schizophrenia. *$26.50*

224 pages ISBN 0-880489-61-8

1277 Schizophrenia: From Mind to Molecule

American Psychiatric Publishing
1000 Wilson Boulevard
Suite 1825
Arlington, VA 22209-3901 703-907-7322
800-368-5777
Fax: 703-907-1091
E-mail: appi@psych.org
www.appi.org

Katie Duffy, Marketing Assistant

Provides a thorough look at schizophrenia that includes neurobehavioral studies, traditional and emerging technologies, psychosocial and medical treatments, and future research opportunities. *$34.00*

278 pages ISBN 0-800489-50-2

1278 Schizophrenia: Straight Talk for Family and Friends

William Morrow & Company
10 East 53rd Street
New York, NY 10022 212-261-6500
Fax: 212-261-6549
www.williammorrow.com

Lists more than 150 local chapters of the National Alliance for the Mentally Ill. *$17.95*

Year Founded: 1985

1279 Stigma and Mental Illness

American Psychiatric Publishing
1000 Wilson Boulevard
Suite 1825
Arlington, VA 22209-3901   703-907-7322
                                  800-368-5777
                             Fax: 703-907-1091
                        E-mail: appi@psych.org
                                  www.appi.org

Katie Duffy, Marketing Assistant

Collection of firsthand accounts on how society has stigmatized mentally ill individuals, their families and their caregivers. *$36.00*

236 pages ISBN 0-880484-05-5

1280 Surviving Schizophrenia: A Manual for Families, Consumers and Providers

Harper Collins
10 E 53rd Street
New York, NY 10022-5244   212-207-7000
                                 800-242-7737
                            Fax: 212-207-2271
                          www.harpercollins.com

Since its first publication nearly twenty years ago, this has become the standard reference book on this disease, helping thousands of patients, families and mental health professionals to better deal with the condition. Dr. Fuller Torrey explains the nature causes, symptoms, and treatment of this often misunderstood illness. This fully revised 4th edition of Surviving Schizophrenia is a must-have for the multitude of people affected both directly and indirectly by this serious, yet treatable, disorder. *$15.00*

544 pages ISBN 0-060959-19-3

1281 Treating Schizophrenia

Jossey-Bass / John Wiley & Sons
111 River Street
Hokoken, NJ 07030-5774   201-748-6000
                           Fax: 201-748-6088
                       E-mail: custserv@wiley.com
                                 www.wiley.com

Using case studies from their own practices, the contributors describe how to conduct a successful assessment of schizophrenia. They then explore in detail the major treatment methods, including inpatient treatment, individual therapy, family therapy, group therapy, and the crucial role of medication. Th authors also address the timely issue of treating schizophrenia in the era of managed care. *$ 121.60*

372 pages Year Founded: 1995

1282 Understanding Schizophrenia: Guide to the New Research on Causes & Treatment

Free Press
1120 Avenue of the Americas
New York, NY 10036-6700   800-456-6798
                            Fax: 800-943-9831
                               E-mail: con-
sumer.customerservice@simonandschuster.com
                             www.simonsays.com

Two noted researchers provide an accessible, timely guide to schizophrenia, discussing the nature of the disease, recent advances in understanding brain structure and function, and the latest psychological and drug treatments. *$25.95*

283 pages Year Founded: 1994 ISBN 0-029172-47-0

1283 Water Balance in Schizophrenia

American Psychiatric Publishing
1000 Wilson Boulevard
Suite 1825
Arlington, VA 22209-3901   703-907-7322
                                  800-368-5777
                             Fax: 703-907-1091
                        E-mail: appi@psych.org
                                  www.appi.org

Katie Duffy, Marketing Assistant

Provides clinicians with a consolidated guide to polydipsia - hyponatramia, associated with schizophrenia. *$54.95*

304 pages ISBN 0-880484-85-3

Periodicals & Pamphlets

1284 Schizophrenia

National Institute of Mental Health
6001 Executive Boulevard
Room 8184
Bethesda, MD 20892-9663
                                  866-615-6464
                             Fax: 301-443-4279
                             TTY: 301-443-8431
                        E-mail: nimhinfo@nih.gov
                                  www.nimh.nih.gov

This booklet answers many common questions about schizophrenia, one of the most chronic, severe and disabling mental disorders. Current research-based information is provided for people with schizophrenia, their family members, friends and the general public about the symptoms and diagnosis of schizophrenia, possible causes, treatments and treatment resources.

28 pages Year Founded: 1999

1285 Schizophrenia Bulletin: Superintendent of Documents

Government Printing Office
732 N Capital Street NW
Washington, DC 20401   202-698-3277

ISBN 0-160105-89-7

1286 Schizophrenia Fact Sheet

Center for Mental Health Services: Knowledge Exchange Network
PO Box 42490
Washington, DC 20015

800-789-2647
Fax: 301-984-8796
TDD: 866-889-2647
E-mail: ken@mentalhealth.org
www.mentalhealth.org

This fact sheet provides information on the symptoms, diagnosis, and treatment for schizophrenia.

2 pages

1287 Schizophrenia Research

11830 Westline Industrial Drive
St Louis, MO 63146

212-633-3730
800-545-2522
Fax: 800-535-9935
E-mail: usbkinfo@elsevier.com
www.elsevier.nl/locate/schres

A publication of new international research that contributes to the understanding of schizophrenia disorders. It is hoped that this journal will aid in bringing together previously separated biological, clinic and psychological research on this disorder, and stimulate the synthesis of these data into cohesive hypotheses.

ISSN 0920-9964

Research Centers

1288 National Alliance for Research on Schizophrenia and Depression

60 Cutter Mill Road
Suite 404
Great Neck, NY 11021-3104

800-829-8289
Fax: 516-487-6930
E-mail: info@narsad.org
www.narsad.org

Raises funds for research on schizophrenia, depression and other mental illnesses. Affiliated with National Alliance for the Mentally Ill, National Depressive and Manic Depressive Association and National Mental Health Association.

1289 Schizophrenia Research Branch: Division of Clinical and Treatment Research

6001 Executive Boulevard
Room 18 MSC 9663
Bethesda, MD 20892-9663

301-443-4513
866-615-6464
Fax: 301-443-5158
TTY: 301-443-8431
E-mail: nimhinfo@nih.gov
www.nimh.nih.gov

Plans, supports, and conducts programs of research, research training, and resource development of schizophrenia and related disorders. Reviews and evaluates research developments in the field and recommends new program directors. Collaborates with organizations in and outside of the National Institute of Mental Health (NIMH) to stimulate work in the field through conferences and workshops.

1290 Schizophrenic Biologic Research Center

VA Medical Center
130 W Kingsbridge Road
Bronx, NY 10468-3992

718-579-1630
Fax: 718-933-2121

Michael Davidson MD, Director

Focuses on mental illness and schizophrenia.

Support Groups & Hot Lines

1291 Family-to-Family: National Alliance for the Mentally Ill

200 N Glebe Road
Suite 1015
Arlington, VA 22203-3728

703-524-7600
800-950-6264
Fax: 703-524-9094
TDD: 703-516-7227
E-mail: lynn@nami.org
www.nami.org

Lynn Saunders, Program Coordinator

Twelve-week course for families of individuals with severe brain disorders, curriculum focuses on schizophrenia, bipolar disorder, clinical depression, panic disorder and obsessive compulsive disorder; discusses the clinical treatment of these illnesses and teaches the knowledge and skills that family members need to cope more effectively. Available across the country.

1292 Recovery

802 N Dearborn Street
Chicago, IL 60610-3364

312-337-5661
Fax: 312-337-5756
E-mail: inquiries@recovery-inc.com
www.recovery-inc.com

Kelly Garcia, Executive Director
Maurine Pyle, Assistant Director

Techniques for controlling behavior, changing attitudes for recovering mental patients. Systematic method of self-help offered.

1293 Schizophrenics Anonymous Forum

Mental Health Association in Michigan
30233 Southfield Road
Suite 220
Southfield, MI 48076

248-647-1711
Fax: 248-647-1732
E-mail: inquiries@nsfoundation.org
www.mha-mi.org

Elizabeth A Plant, Director

Self-help organization sponsored by American Schizophrenia Association. Groups are comprised of dignosed schizophrenics who meet to share experiences, strengths and hopes in an effort to help each other cope with common problems and recover from the disease, rehabilitation program follows the 12 principles of Alcoholics Anonymous. Publications: Newsletter, semi-annual. Monthly support group meeting.

Video & Audio

1294 Bonnie Tapes

Mental Illness Education Project
PO Box 470813
Brookline Village, MA 02447-0813   617-562-1111
800-343-5540
Fax: 617-779-0061
E-mail: info@miepvideos.org
www.miepvideos.org

Christine Ledoux, Executive Director
Jack Churchill, President
Lucia Miller, Marketing Director

Bonnie's account of coping with schizophrenia will be a revelation to people whose view of mental illness has been shaped by the popular media. She and her family provide an intimate view of a frequently feared, often misrepresented, and much stigmatized illness-and the human side of learning to live with a psychiatric disability. Set of three tapes $143.88 or $59.95 per tape.

Year Founded: 1997

1295 Families Coping with Mental Illness

Mental Illness Education Project
PO Box 470813
Brookline Village, MA 02247-0244   617-562-1111
800-343-5540
Fax: 617-779-0061
E-mail: info@miepvideos.org
www.miepvideos.org

Christine Ledoux, Executive Director

10 family members share their experiences of having a family member with schizophrenia or bipolar disorder. Designed to provide insights and support to other families, the tape also profoundly conveys to professionals the needs of families when mental illness strikes. In two versions: a twenty two minute version ideal for short classes and workshops, and a richer forty three minute version with more examples and details. Discounted price for families/consumers. *$68.95*

Year Founded: 1997

Web Sites

1296 www.cyberpsych.org

CyberPsych

Hosts the American Psychoanalyists Foundation, American Association of Suicideology, Society for the Exploration of Psychotherapy Intergration, and Anxiety Disorders Association of America. Also subcategories of the anxiety disorders, as well as general information, including panic disorder, phobias, obsessive compulsive disorder (OCD), social phobia, generalized anxiety disorder, post traumatic stress disorder, and phobias of childhood. Book reviews and links to web pages sharing the topics.

1297 www.health-center.com/mentalhealth/schizophrenia/default.htm

Schizophrenia

Basic information for beginners.

1298 www.med.jhu.edu/schizophrenia

Department of Psychiatry and Behavioral Sciences

Learn more about research and how you can sign up for various studies.

E pages

1299 www.members.aol.com/leonardjk/USA.htm

Schizophrenia Support Organizations

1300 www.mentalhealth.com/book/p40-sc01.html

Schizophrenia: Handbook for Families

Mostly unique information.

1301 www.mentalhealth.com/book/p40-sc02.html

Schizophrenia: Youth's Greatest Disabler

Comprehensive and realistic coverage of schizophrenia.

1302 www.mentalhelp.net/guide/schizo.htm

Mentalhelp

Collection of articles and links.

1303 www.mgl.ca/~chovil

Experience of Schizophrenia

Home page containing a biography, advice, resources, and diagrams for teaching.

1304 www.mhsource.com/
advocacy/narsad/order.html

Brochures, books, and videos.

1305 www.mhsource.com/advocacy/
narsad/newsletter.html

Public service announcements.

1306 www.mhsource.com/advocacy/narsad
/narsadfaqs.html

Medical questions and answers.

1307 www.mhsource.com/advocacy/narsad/
studyops.html

Research studies.

1308 www.mhsource.com/narsad.html

National Alliance for Research on Schizophrenia and Depression

Raises funds for research on schizophrenia, depression and other mental illnesses. Affiliated with National Alliance for the Mentally Ill, National Depressive and Manic Depressive Association and National Mental Health Association.

1309 www.nami-nyc-metro.org

New York National Alliance for the Mentally Ill

Hundreds of articles.

1310 www.nimh.nih.gov/publicat/schizoph.htm

Schizophrenia

National Institute of Mental Health.

1311 www.planetpsych.com

Planetpsych.com

Learn about disorders, their treatments and other topics in psychology. Articles are listed under the related topic areas. Ask a therapist a question for free, or view the directory of professionals in your area. If you are a therapist sign up for the directory. Current features, self-help, interactive, and newsletter archives.

1312 www.psychcentral.com

Psych Central

Personalized one-stop index for psychology, support, and mental health issues, resources, and people on the Internet.

1313 www.recovery-inc.com

Recovery

Describes the organizations approach.

1314 www.schizophrenia.com

Schizophrenia.com

Offers basic and in-depth information, discussion and chat.

1315 www.schizophrenia.com/discuss/Disc3.html

Schizophrenia.com Home Page

On-line support for patients and families.

1316 www.schizophrenia.com/newsletter

Schizophrenia.com

Comprehensive psychoeducational site on schizophrenia.

1317 www.schizophrenia.com/newsletter/buckets/ success.html

Schizophrenia.com

Success stories including biographical accounts, links to stories of famous people who have schizophrenia, and personal web pages.

Introduction

It is common, of course, not to feel sexual desire or be sexually aroused sometimes, and not always to be able to achieve orgasm. A Sexual Disorder is diagnosed when such events are repeated and persist over time and when they interfere with the person's functioning in important areas of life.

Sexual Disorders are divided into four groups: Disorders of Sexual Desire; Disorders of Sexual Arousal; Orgasmic Disorders, and Disorders involving Sexual Pain.

SEXUAL DESIRE DISORDERS SYMPTOMS

Hypoactive Sexual Desire Disorder (HSDD)

•Persistent or repeated lack of sexual fantasies and desire for sexual activities;
•The lack of sexual fantasies and desire cause marked distress or interpersonal problems.

Sexual Aversion Disorder (SAD)

•Persistent or repeated extreme aversion to, and avoidance of, all or almost all genital sexual contact with a sexual partner;
•The aversion causes marked distress or interpersonal problems.

Associated Features
The person with a Sexual Desire Disorder commonly has a poor body image and avoids nudity. In HSDD, a person does not initiate sexual activity, or respond to the partner's initiation attempts. The disorder is often associated with the inability to achieve orgasm in women, and the inability to achieve an erection in men. It can also be connected to other psychiatric and medical problems, including a history of sexual trauma and abuse.

Prevalence
HADD is common in both men and women but twice as many women as men report it. It is estimated at twenty percent overall, and as high as sixty-five-percent among those seeking treatment for sexual disorders. The prevalence of SAD is unknown.

SEXUAL AROUSAL DISORDER SYMPTOMS

Female Sexual Arousal Disorder (FSAD)

•Persistent or repeated inability to attain or maintain adequate lubrication-swelling (sexual excitement) response throughout sexual activity;
•The disorder causes clear distress or interpersonal problems.

Male Erectile Disorder (MED)

•Persistent or repeated inability to maintain an adequate erection throughout sexual activity;
•The difficulty causes clear distress or interpersonal problems.

Associated Features
While both these disorders are common, men are often more emotionally affected than women. Issues interacting with the disorder include performance anxiety (especially in men), fear of failure, inadequate stimulation, and relationship conflicts. Other problems are also associated with FSAD and MED, such as childhood sexual trauma, sexual identity concerns, religious orthodoxy, depression, lack of intimacy or trust, and power conflicts. MED is frequently associated with diabetes, peripheral nerve disorders, and hypertension, and is a side effect of a variety of medications; men with MED must be evaluated for these conditions. In addition, the medications used to treat MED are contraindicated in some medical conditions, such as heart conditions.

Prevalence
Prevalence information varies for FSAD. In one study, 13.6 percent of women reported a lack of lubrication during most or all sexual activity; twenty-three percent had such problems occasionally; and 44.2 percent of post-menopausal women reported having lubrication problems. In a study of happily married couples, about one third of women complained of difficulty in achieving or maintaining sexual excitement.

Erectile difficulties in men are estimated to be very common, affecting 20-30 million men in the US. The frequency of erectile problems increases steeply with age. In one survey, fifty-two percent of men aged 40-70 reported erectile problems, with three times as many older men reporting difficulties. The disorder is common among married, single, heterosexual and homosexual men.

Treatment Options

In FSAD, a cognitive-behavioral psychotherapy is often recommended, including practical help such as the use of water-soluble lubricating products. Hormone treatment, such as testosterone-estrogen compounds, is sometimes helpful.

An array of treatments is available for Male Erectile Dysfunction, including prosthetic devices for physiological penile problems. In cases of hormonal problems, testosterone treatments have had some results. However, the use of testosterone to treat sexual disorders in menopausal women can have serious side effects. Viagra, a relatively new drug therapy, is producing success, as are two newer medications for MED, vardenafil (Levitra) and tadalafil (Cialis).

ORGASMIC DISORDER SYMPTOMS

Female and Male Orgasmic Disorders

Persistent or repeated delay in, or absence of, orgasm despite a normal sexual excitement phase;
The disorder causes clear distress of interpersonal problems.

Premature Ejaculation

Persistent or recurring ejaculation with minimal sexual stimulation before, upon, or shortly after penetration and earlier than desired;
The disorder causes clear distress of interpersonal problems.

Associated Features

When FOD or MOD occur only in certain situations, difficulty with desire and arousal are often also present.

All of these disorders are associated with poor body image, self-esteem or relationship problems. In FOD or MOD, medical or surgical conditions can also play a role, such as multiple sclerosis, spinal cord injury, surgical prostatectomy (males), and some medications. PE is likely to be very distruptive. Some males may have had the disorder all their lives, for others it may be situational. Few illnesses or drugs are associated with PE.

Prevalence

FOD is probably the most frequent sexual disorder among females. Among those who have sought sex therapy twenty-four percent to thirty-seven percent report the problem. In general population samples, 15.4 percent of premenopausal women report the disorder, and 34.7 percent of postmenopausal women do so. More single than married women report that they have never had an orgasm. There is no association between FOD and race, socioeconomic status, education, or religion. MOD is relatively rare; only three percent to eight percent of men seeking treatment report having the disorder, though there is a higher prevalence among homosexual males (ten percent to fifteen percent).

PE is very common: twenty-five percent to forty percent of adult males report having, or having had, this problem.

Treatment Options

Psychotherapeutic treatments are similar to those for Sexual Desire and Sexual Arousal Disorders. In both males and females with Orgasmic Disorders there may be a lack of desire, performance anxiety, and fear of impregnation or disease. Therapy should take into account contextual and historical information concerning the onset and course of the problem. Cognitive-behavioral methods to help change the assumptions and thinking of the person have sometimes been helpful.

SEXUAL PAIN DISORDER SYMPTOMS

Dyspareunia

Recurring or persistent pain with sexual intercourse in a male or female;
The disorder causes clear distress or interpersonal problems.

Vaginismus

Persistent or recurrent involunatry spasm of the vagina that interferes with sexual intercourse;
The disorder causes clear distress or interpersonal problems.

Associated Features

Both Dyspareunia and Vaginismus may be associated with lack of desire or arousal. Women with Vaginismus tend to avoid gynecological exams, and the disorder is most often associated with psychological and interpersonal issues. Various physical factors are associated with Dyspareunia, such as pelvic inflammatory disease, hymenal scarring, and vulvar vestibulitis. Dyspareunia is not a clear symptom of any physical condition. In women it is often combined with Depression and interpersonal conflicts. Other associated psychosocial factors include religious orthodoxy, low self-esteem, poor body image, poor couple communication, and history of sexual trauma.

Prevalence

Dyspareunia is frequent in females but occurs infrequently in males. Vaginismus is seen quite often in sex therapy clinics - in fifteen percent to seventeen percent of women coming for treatment.

Treatment Options

Probably the most successful treatment for women with these disorders is the reinsertion of a graduated sequence of dilaters in the vagina. The woman's partner should be present, and a participant in this treatment. This treatment should be done in conjunction with relaxation training, sensate focusing exercises, (which help people focus on the pleasures of sex rather than the performance) and sex therapy.

General Treatment Options

The professional making the diagnosis of a Sexual Disorder should be trained and experienced in Sexual Disorders and sex therapy. It is important to know whether or not a medical or medication issue is present. However, many with these disorders do not seek treatment. Their lack of desire for sex is often combined with a lack of desire for sex therapy. Even with therapy, relapse is commonly reported. Treatments that have had some success are ones that challenge the cognitive assumptions and distortions of client(s), e.g., that sex should be perfect, that without intercourse and without both partners having an orgasm it isn't real sex. Therapy often also includes sensate focusing in which the person is encouraged and trained to give up the role of agitated spectator to love-making in favor of participating in it.

Associations & Agencies

1319 Center for Family Support (CFS)
333 7th Avenue
New York, NY 10001-5004   212-629-7939
Fax: 212-239-2211
www.cfsny.org

Steven Vernickofs, Executive Director

Service agency devoted to the physical well-being and development of the retarded child and the sound mental health of the parents. Helps families with retarded children with all aspects of home care including counseling, referrals, home aide service and consultation. Offers intervention for parents at the birth of a retarded child with in-home support, guidance and infant stimulation. Pioneered training of nonprofessional women as home aides to provide supportive services in homes.

1320 Center for Mental Health Services
SAMSHA
PO Box 42557
Washington, DC 20015
800-789-2647
Fax: 301-984-8796
TDD: 866-889-2647
www.mentalhealth.org

Irene S Levine PhD, Deputy Director

Develops national mental health policies, that promote Federal/State coordination and benefit from input from consumers, family members and providers. Ensures that high quality mental health services programs are implemented to benefit seriously mentally ill populations, disasters or those involved in the criminal justice system.

1321 Center for Mental Health Services Knowledge Exchange Network
US Department of Health and Human Services
PO Box 42490
Washington, DC 20015-4800
800-789-2647
Fax: 301-984-8796
E-mail: ken@mentalhealth.org
www.mentalhealth.org

Information about resources, technical assistance, research, training, networks, and other federal clearing houses, and fact sheets and materials. Information specialists refer callers to mental health resources in their communities as well as state, federal and nonprofit contacts. Staff available Monday through Friday, 8:30 AM - 5:00 PM, EST, excluding federal holidays. After hours, callers may leave messages and an information specialist will return their call.

1322 NADD: Association for Persons with Developmental Disabilities and Mental Health Needs
132 Fair Street
Kingston, NY 12401-4802   845-334-4336
800-331-5362
Fax: 845-331-4569
E-mail: nadd@mhv.net
www.add.org

Dr. Robert Fletcher, Executive Director

Nonprofit organization designed to promote interest of professional and parent development with resources for individuals who have the coexistence of mental illness and mental retardation. Provides conference, educational services and training materials to professionals, parents, concerned citizens and service organizations. Formerly known as the National Association for the Dually Diagnosed.

1323 National Mental Health Consumer's Self-Help Clearinghouse
1211 Chestnut Street
Suite 1207
Philadelphia, PA 19107   215-751-1810
800-553-4539
Fax: 215-636-6312
E-mail: info@mhselfhelp.org
www.mhselfhelp.org

Alex Morrsey, Information/Referral

Funded by the National Institute of Mental Health Community Support Program, the purpose of the Clearinghouse is to encourage the development and growth of consumer self-help groups.

Year Founded: 1992

Books

1324 Back on Track: Boys Dealing with Sexual Abuse
200 E Joppa Road
Suite 207
Baltimore, MD 21286   410-825-8888
888-825-8249
Fax: 410-337-0747
E-mail: sidran@sidran.org
www.sidran.org

Leslie Bailey Wright
Mindy B Loiselle

Written for boys age ten and up, this wookbook addresses adolescent boys directly, answering commonly asked questions, offering concrete suggestions for getting help and dealing with unspoken concerns such as homosexuality. Contains descriptions of what therapy may be like and brief explanations of social services and courts, as well as sections on family and friends. Exercises and interesting graphics break up the text. The book's important message is TELL: Just keep telling until someone listens who STOPS the abuse. *$14.00*

144 pages

1325 Dangerous Sex Offenders: a Task Force Report of the American Psychiatric Association

American Psychiatric Publishing
1000 Wilson Boulevard
Suite 1825
Arlington, VA 22209-3901   703-907-7322
                                  800-368-5777
                              Fax: 703-907-1091
                         E-mail: appi@psych.org
                                  www.appi.org

Katie Duffy, Marketing Assistant

$40.95

224 pages ISBN 0-890422-80-X

1326 Interviewing the Sexually Abused Child

American Psychiatric Publishing
1000 Wilson Boulevard
Suite 1825
Arlington, VA 22209-3901   703-907-7322
                                  800-368-5777
                              Fax: 703-907-1091
                         E-mail: appi@psych.org
                                  www.appi.org

Katie Duffy, Marketing Assistant

Guide for mental health professionals who need to know if a child has been sexually abused. Presents guidelines on the structure of the interview and covers the use of free play, toys, and play materials by focusing on the investigate interview of the suspected victim. *$27.95*

80 pages ISBN 0-880486-12-0

1327 Masculinity and Sexuality: Selected Topics in the Psychology of Men

American Psychiatric Publishing
1000 Wilson Boulevard
Suite 1825
Arlington, VA 22209-3901   703-907-7322
                                  800-368-5777
                              Fax: 703-907-1091
                         E-mail: appi@psych.org
                                  www.appi.org

Katie Duffy, Marketing Assistant

$37.50

200 pages ISBN 0-880489-62-6

1328 Physician Sexual Misconduct

American Psychiatric Publishing
1000 Wilson Boulevard
Suite 1825
Arlington, VA 22209-3901   703-907-7322
                                  800-368-5777
                              Fax: 703-907-1091
                         E-mail: appi@psych.org
                                  www.appi.org

Katie Duffy, Marketing Assistant

Warning signs and appropriate actions are discussed. *$66.50*

304 pages ISBN 0-880487-60-2

1329 Sexual Abuse and Eating Disorders

200 E Joppa Road
Suite 207
Baltimore, MD 21286   410-825-8888
                                  888-825-8249
                              Fax: 410-337-0747
                        E-mail: sidran@sidran.org
                                  www.sidran.org

Explores the complex relationship between sexual abuse and eating disorders. This volume is a discussion of the many ways that sexual abuse and eating disorders are related, also has accounts by a survivor of both. Investigates the prevalence of sexual abuse amoung individuals with eating disorders. Also examines how a history of sexual violence can serve as a predictor of subsequent problems with food. Looks at related social factors, reviews trauma based theories, more controversial territory and discusses delayed memory versus false memory. *$34.95*

228 pages

1330 Sexual Aggression

American Psychiatric Publishing
1000 Wilson Boulevard
Suite 1825
Arlington, VA 22209-3901   703-907-7322
                                  800-368-5777
                              Fax: 703-907-1091
                         E-mail: appi@psych.org
                                  www.appi.org

Katie Duffy, Marketing Assistant

Appropriate diagnosis and treatment options are presented. *$64.00*

364 pages ISBN 0-880487-57-7

1331 Sexuality and People with Disabilities

Indiana Institute on Disability and Community
Indiana University
2853 E Tenth Street
Bloomington, IN 47408-2696   812-855-6508
                                  800-280-7010
                              Fax: 812-855-9630
                              TTY: 812-855-9396
                       E-mail: uap@indiana.edu
                                www.iidc.indiana.edu

Sexuality information for people with disabilities is available but difficult to find. This publication discusses the importance of having sexuality information available and provides numerous sexuality-related resources. *$5.00*

16 pages

1332 Therapy for Adults Molested as Children: Beyond Survival

200 E Joppa Road
Suite 207
Baltimore, MD 21286   410-825-8888
                                  888-825-8249
                              Fax: 410-337-0747
                        E-mail: sidran@sidran.org
                                  www.sidran.org

Substantially expanded and revised, this new edition includes detailed information on how to treat sexual abuse survivors more effectively. Chapters cover topics such as client dissociation during therapy, the false/recovered memory controversy, gender differences in abuse treatment. The appendix analyzes the Trauma Symptom Inventory, a 100 item test of post traumatic stress and other psycological sequelae of traumatic events. *$36.95*

256 pages

1333 Treating Intellectually Disabled Sex Offenders: a Model Residential Program

Safer Society Foundation
PO Box 340
Brandon, VT 05733-0340   **802-247-3132**
                          Fax: 802-247-4233
               E-mail: gina@safersociety.org
                     www.safersociety.org

Gina Brown, Sales/Marketing Manager

Describes how the intensive residential specialized Social Skills Program at Oregon State Hospital combines the principles of respect, self-help, and experiential learning with traditional sex-offender treatment methods. *$24.00*

152 pages ISBN 1-884444-30-X

Periodicals & Pamphlets

1334 Family Violence & Sexual Assault Bulletin

Family Violence & Sexual Assault Institute
6160 Cornerstone Court E
San Diego, CA 92121   **858-623-2777**
                     Fax: 858-646-0761
                          www.fvsai.org

David Westgate, Director

Book club, research and quarterly newsletter. *$35.00*

60-70 pages

Web Sites

1335 www.cs.uu.nl/wais/html/na-bng/alt.support.ab use-partners.html

Partners of sexual abuse survivors.

1336 www.emdr.com
EMDR Institute

EMDR is an acronym for Eye Movement Desensitization and Reprocessing. It is an innovative clinical treatment that has successfully helped over a million indiviguals who have survived trauma, including sexual abuse, domestic violence, combat, crime and thouse suffering from a number of other disorders including depressions, addictions, phobias and a variety of self-esteem issues.

1337 www.firelily.com/gender/sstgfaq

Transgendered and intersexed persons.

1338 www.mentalhealth.com
Internet Mental Health

On-line information and a virtual encyclopedia related to mental disorders, possible causes and treatments. News, articles, on-line diagnostic programs and related links. Designed to improve understanding, diagnosis and treatment of mental illness throughout the world. Awarded the Top Site Award and the NetPsych Cutting Edge Site Award.

1339 www.planetpsych.com
Planetpsych.com

Learn about disorders, their treatments and other topics in psychology. Articles are listed under the related topic areas. Ask a therapist a question for free, or view the directory of professionals in your area. If you are a therapist sign up for the directory. Current features, self-help, interactive, and newsletter archives.

1340 www.priory.com/sex.htm
Sexual Disorders

Diagnoses and treatments.

1341 www.psychcentral.com
Psych Central

Personalized one-stop index for psychology, support, and mental health issues, resources, and people on the Internet.

1342 www.shrinktank.com
Shrinktank

Psychology-related programs, shareware and freeware.

1343 www.xs4all.nl/~rosalind/cha-assr.html

For people going through sex reassignment surgery or procedures.

Introduction

Sleep Disorders are a group of disorders characterized by extreme disruptions in normal sleeping patterns. These include Primary Insomnia, Primary Hypersomnia, Narcolepsy, Breathing-related Sleep Disorder, Circadian Rhythm Sleep Disorder, and Substance Abuse Induced Sleep Disorder. There are also Nightmare Disorder and Sleep Terror Disorder. Primary Insomnia entails the inability to sleep, and causes excessive sleepiness for at least one month, as evidenced by either prolonged sleep episodes or daytime sleep episodes that occur almost daily. Narcolepsy is characterized by chronic, involuntary and irresistible sleep attacks; typically a person with the disorder will fall asleep at any time of the day.

Breathing-related Sleep Disorder is diagnosed when sleep is distrupted by an obstruction of the breathing apparatus. Circadian Rhythm Sleep Disorder is a disruption of normal sleep patterns leading to a mismatch between the schedule required by a person's environment and his or her sleeping patterns; i.e., the individual is irresistibly sleepy when he or she is required to be awake, and awake at those times that he or she should be sleeping. Nightmare Disorder is diagnosed when there is a repeated occurrence of frightening dreams that lead to waking. Sleep Terror Disorder is the repeated occurrence of sleep terrors, or abrupt awakenings from sleeping with a shriek or a cry.

SYMPTOMS

Because of the variety of Sleep Disorders, we will address here only the disorder with the greatest prevalence: Primary Insomnia. A diagnosis of Primary Insomnia is made if the following criteria are met:
•Difficulty initiating or maintaining sleep or nonrestorative sleep for at least one month;
•The impairment causes clinically significant distress or impairment in social, occupational or other important areas of functioning;
•The disturbance does not occur exclusively during the course of other sleep-related disorders;
•The disturbance is not due to the direct physiological effects of a substance.

ASSOCIATED FEATURES

Individuals with primary insomnia have a history of light sleeping, and interpersonal or work-related problems typically arise because of lack of sleep. Accidents and injuries may result from lack of attentiveness during waking hours, and medications are liable to be misused or abused by people with primary insomnia.

PREVALENCE

Surveys indicate a one-year prevalence of insomnia complaints in thirty percent to forty percent of adults, though the percentage of those who would have a diagnosis of Primary Insomnia is unknown. In clinics specializing in Sleep Disorders, about fifteen percent to twenty-five percent of individuals with chronic insomnia are diagnosed with Primary Insomnia.

TREATMENT OPTIONS

Treatment for Sleep Disorders should combine an examination by a primary care physician to determine physical condition and sleeping habits, and a discussion with a somologist, a professional trained in Sleep Disorders, or other mental health professional to determine the individual's emotional state.

Referrals may be made to sleep clinics, which are usually situated in hospitals, or sleep disorder centers, which could be part of hospitals, universities or psychiatric institutions. To determine the cause of sleep disturbances, an individual in a sleep clinic or sleep disorder center may undergo interviews, psychological tests and laboratory observation. Medications that may be part of treatment for Sleep Disorders include drugs known as Hypnotics, or sleeping tablets, including temazepam, Ambien, and Sonata. There is also a new drug, Provigil, which helps people with Narcoleopsy to stay awake. Many cases will resolve with improved sleep hygiene, treatment of pain and other remediable causes, once diagnosed and treated.

Associations & Agencies

1345 American Academy of Sleep Medicine

One Westbrook Corporate Center
Suite 920
Westchester, IL 60154
708-492-0930
Fax: 708-492-0943
E-mail: info@aasmnet.org
www.aasmnet.org

Jerome A Barrett, Executive Director
Rebecca Chipman, Public Relations Coordinator
Jennifer Markkanen, Dir. Professional Development

National not-for-profit professional membership organization dedicated to the advancement of sleep medicine. The Academy's mission is to assure quality care for patients with sleep disorders, promote the advancement of sleep research and provide public and professional education. The AASM delivers programs, information and services to and through its members and advocates sleep medicine supportive policies in the medical community and the public sector.

1346 Center for Family Support (CFS)

333 7th Avenue
New York, NY 10001-5004
212-629-7939
Fax: 212-239-2211
www.cfsny.org

Steven Vernickofs, Executive Director

Service agency devoted to the physical well-being and development of the retarded child and the sound mental health of the parents. Helps families with retarded children with all aspects of home care including counseling, referrals, home aide service and consultation. Offers intervention for parents at the birth of a retarded child with in-home support, guidance and infant stimulation. Pioneered training of nonprofessional women as home aides to provide supportive services in homes.

1347 Center for Mental Health Services

SAMSHA
PO Box 42557
Washington, DC 20015
800-789-2647
Fax: 301-984-8796
TDD: 866-889-2647
www.mentalhealth.org

Irene S Levine PhD, Deputy Director

Develops national mental health policies, that promote Federal/State coordination and benefit from input from consumers, family members and providers. Ensures that high quality mental health services programs are implemented to benefit seriously mentally ill populations, disasters or those involved in the criminal justice system.

1348 Center for Mental Health Services Knowledge Exchange Network

US Department of Health and Human Services
PO Box 42490
Washington, DC 20015-4800
800-789-2647
Fax: 301-984-8796
E-mail: ken@mentalhealth.org
www.mentalhealth.org

Information about resources, technical assistance, research, training, networks, and other federal clearing houses, and fact sheets and materials. Information specialists refer callers to mental health resources in their communities as well as state, federal and non-profit contacts. Staff available Monday through Friday, 8:30 AM - 5:00 PM, EST, excluding federal holidays. After hours, callers may leave messages and an information specialist will return their call.

1349 NADD: Association for Persons with Developmental Disabilities and Mental Health Needs

132 Fair Street
Kingston, NY 12401-4802
845-334-4336
800-331-5362
Fax: 845-331-4569
E-mail: nadd@mhv.net
www.thenadd.org

Dr. Robert Fletcher, Executive Director

Nonprofit organization designed to promote interest of professional and parent development with resources for individuals who have the coexistence of mental illness and mental retardation. Provides conference, educational services and training materials to professionals, parents, concerned citizens and service organizations. Formerly known as the National Association for the Dually Diagnosed.

1350 National Alliance for the Mentally Ill

2107 Wilson Boulevard
Suite 300
Arlington, VA 22201-3042
703-524-7600
800-950-6264
Fax: 703-524-9094
TDD: 703-516-7227
E-mail: helpline@nami.org
www.nami.org

Laurie Flynn, Executive Director

Nation's leading self-help organization for all those affected by severe brain disorders. Mission is to bring consumers and families with similar experiences together to share information about services, care providers, and ways to cope with the challenges of schizophrenia, manic depression, and other serious mental illnesses.

1351 National Mental Health Consumer's Self-Help Clearinghouse

1211 Chestnut Street
Suite 1207
Philadelphia, PA 19107
215-751-1810
800-553-4539
Fax: 215-636-6312
E-mail: info@mhselfhelp.org
www.mhselfhelp.org

Alex Morrsey, Information/Referral

Funded by the National Institute of Mental Health Community Support Program, the purpose of the Clearinghouse is to encourage the development and growth of consumer self-help groups.

Year Founded: 1992

1352 Sleep Disorders Unit of Beth Israel Hospital

330 Brookline Avenue
Boston, MA 02215   **617-667-7000**
www.bidmc.harvard.edu/home.asp

Jean K Matheson MD, Contact

Provides testing and treatment for those with sleep disorders and offers educational workshops, plus support for their families.

Books

1353 Concise Guide to Evaluation and Management of Sleep Disorders

American Psychiatric Publishing
1000 Wilson Boulevard
Suite 1825
Arlington, VA 22209-3901   **703-907-7322**
                                      800-368-5777
                                  Fax: 703-907-1091
                          E-mail: appi@psych.org
                                         www.appi.org

Katie Duffy, Marketing Assistant

Overview of sleep disorders medicine, sleep physiology and pathology, insomnia complaints, excessive sleepiness disorders, parasomnias, medical and psychiatric disorders and sleep, medications with sedative-hypnotic properties, special problems and populations. *$29.95*

304 pages ISBN 0-880489-06-5

1354 Consumer's Guide to Psychiatric Drugs

New Harbinger Publications
5674 Shattuck Avenue
Oakland, CA 94609-1662   **510-652-2002**
                                       800-748-6273
                                  Fax: 510-652-5472
        E-mail: customerservice@newharbinger.com
                               www.newharbinger.com

Helps consumers understand what treatment options are available and what side effects to expect. Covers possible interactions with other drugs, medical conditions and other concerns. Explains how each drug works, and offers detailed information about treatments for depression, bipolar disorder, anxiety and sleep disorders, as well as other conditions. *$16.95*

340 pages ISBN 1-572241-11-X

1355 Dream Encyclopedia

Visible Ink Press
43311 Joy Road #414
Canton, MI 48187-2075   **734-667-3211**
                                  Fax: 734-667-4311
                                     www.visibleink.com

Organizations involved in the study of dreams, including sleep research centers and laboratories. Principal content is 250 dream topics, along with possible symbol interpretations. *$19.95*

454 pages Year Founded: 1995 ISBN 0-787601-56-X

1356 Getting to Sleep

New Harbinger Publications
5674 Shattuck Avenue
Oakland, CA 94609-1662   **510-652-2002**
                                       800-748-6273
                                  Fax: 510-652-5472
        E-mail: customerservice@newharbinger.com
                               www.newharbinger.com

Outlines effective methods for falling and staying asleep. *$12.95*

224 pages ISBN 0-934986-93-2

1357 Principles and Practice of Sleep Medicine

Elsevier/WB Saunders Company
Curtis Center, Suite 300E
170 S Independence Mall W
Philadelphia, PA 19106-3399   **215-238-7800**
                                       800-523-1649
                                  Fax: 800-238-7883
                              www.us.elsevierhealth.com

Covers the recent advances in basic sciences as well as sleep pathology in adults. Encompasses developments in this rapidly advancing field and also includes topics related to psychiatry, circadian rhythms, cardiovascualr diseases and sleep apnea diagnosis and treatment. Hardcover. *$159.00*

1336 pages Year Founded: 2000 ISBN 0-721676-70-7

1358 Sleep Disorders Sourcebook

Omnigraphics
PO Box 625
Holmes, PA 19043
                                       800-234-1340
                                  Fax: 800-875-1340
                        E-mail: info@omnigraphics.com
                                    www.omnigraphics.com

Omnigrahphics is the publisher of the Health Reference Series, a growing consumer health information resource with more than 100 volumes in print. Each title in the series features an easy to understand format, nontechnical language, comprehensive indexing and resources for further information. Material in each book has been collected from a wide range of government agencies, professional associations, periodicals and other sources. *$78.00*

439 pages ISBN 1-780802-34-9

1359 Snoring from A to Zzzz

Spencer Press
2525 NW Lovejoy Street
Suite 402
Portland, OR 97210-2865

503-223-4959
Fax: 503-223-1608

Covers organizations, associations, support groups, and manufacturers of sleep-related medical products relevant to sleep disorders. Discusses every aspect of snoring and sleep apnea from causes to cures. *$14.95*

248 pages ISBN 0-965070-81-6

Web Sites

1360 www.asda.org

American Academy of Sleep Medicine

Valuable information on troubles with sleep and links.

1361 www.cyberpsych.org

CyberPsych

Hosts the American Psychoanalyists Foundation, American Association of Suicideology, Society for the Exploration of Psychotherapy Intergration, and Anxiety Disorders Association of America. Also subcategories of the anxiety disorders, as well as general information, including panic disorder, phobias, obsessive compulsive disorder (OCD), social phobia, generalized anxiety disorder, post traumatic stress disorder, and phobias of childhood. Book reviews and links to web pages sharing the topics.

1362 www.mentalhealth.com

Internet Mental Health

On-line information and a virtual encyclopedia related to mental disorders, possible causes and treatments. News, articles, on-line diagnostic programs and related links. Designed to improve understanding, diagnosis and treatment of mental illness throughout the world. Awarded the Top Site Award and the NetPsych Cutting Edge Site Award.

1363 www.nhlbi.nih.gov/about/ncsdr

National Institute of Health National Center on Sleep Disorders

Requires Adobe Acrobat Reader.

1364 www.nlm.nih.gov/medlineplus/sleepdisorders. html

MEDLINEplus on Sleep Disorders

Compilation of links directs you to information on sleep disorders.

1365 www.planetpsych.com

Planetpsych.com

Learn about disorders, their treatments and other topics in psychology. Articles are listed under the related topic areas. Ask a therapist a question for free, or view the directory of professionals in your area. If you are a therapist sign up for the directory. Current features, self-help, interactive, and newsletter archives.

1366 www.psychcentral.com

Psych Central

Personalized one-stop index for psychology, support, and mental health issues, resources, and people on the Internet.

1367 www.sleepdisorders.about.com

About.com on Sleep Disorders

Well-organized information including new developments and a chat room.

1368 www.sleepdisorders.com

SleepDisorders.com

Updated monthly and organized by sleep disorders with quality links.

1369 www.sleepfoundation.org

National Sleep Foundation

Frequently updated credible site, with free newsletter.

1370 www.sleepnet.com

Sleepnet.com

Categorizes sleep disorders for research, forums are up-dated frequently and posts are thoughtful and insightful.

1371 www.talhost.net/sleep/links.htm

For those who have sleep disorders and have a problem sleeping.

Introduction

The substances referred to in this section include: amphetamines; marijuana; cocaine (and its purer derivative, crack); hallucinogens, such as LSD; inhalants, such as butane gas or cleaning fluid; opioids, such as morphine, heroin, or codeine; and benzodiazepines like Valium and Xanax. Caffeine and nicotine are not included.

SYMPTOMS

Substance Abuse Symptoms

•Repeated substance use resulting in inability to fulfill fundamental obligations at work, school, or home, e.g., repeated absences, poor work performance, family neglect;
•Repeated substance use, resulting in dangerous situations, e.g., driving or operating a machine while impaired;
•Repeated substance-related legal problems e.g., arrests for disorderly conduct;
•Continued substance use despite persistent social or interpersonal problems worsened by the effects of substance abuse.

Substance Dependence Symptoms

•Tolerance:

(a) need for increased amounts of the substance to achieve desired effect;
(b) clear diminished effect with continued use of the same amount of substance.

•Withdrawl:

(a) characteristic withdrawal syndrome, prolonged taking and then stopping/reducing substance causing clear difficulties in social, work, and other areas;
(b) the same or a related substance is taken to avoid/alleviate the withdrawal symptoms;

•Substance is often taken in greater amounts or for a longer period than intended;
•Repeated wish or unsuccessful attempts to control substance use;
•A great deal of time is taken to get and use substance or to recover from its effects;
•Important social, work, or recreational activities are missed because of substance use;
•Substance use continues in spite of the person knowing about the persistent psychological or physical problems it causes (e.g., depression induced by cocaine or continued drinking).

ASSOCIATED FEATURES

Genetics has a considerable influence on a person's propensity for substance abuse disorders, and such disorders are associated with significant changes in the brain.

Many individuals with drug-use disorders take more than one substance, a person who suffers from anxiety when coming down from cocaine may drink alcohol to deal with the anxiety. Many with drug-related disorders complain of anxiety, insomnia, and depression. Other mental disorders are also associated with substance use: for example, the use may often represent one aspect of a mental disorder. Individuals with Depression, Post Traumatic Stress Disorder, or Bipolar Disorder sometimes abuse drugs in an attempt to medicate themselves. Forty-seven percent of people with Schizophrenia have drug abuse disorders. Furthermore, people with Antisocial Personality Disorder may abuse substances, including amphetamines such as cocaine. Substance-related disorders can also lead to other mental disorders. Use of the synthetic hallucinogen Ecstasy is associated with acute and paranoid psychoses, and the prolonged use of cocaine (a stimulant) can lead to paranoid psychosis with violent behavior.

Childhood sexual abuse is strongly associated with substance dependence. Chronic drug and alcohol abuse can lead to difficulty in memory and problem solving, and impaired sexual functioning.

Substance Abuse & Dependence/Introduction

PREVALENCE

There are large cultural differences in attitudes to substances. In some cultures, mood altering drugs, including alcohol, are well accepted; in others they are strictly forbidden.

Those between the ages of 18 and 24 have a high prevalence for abuse of all substances. Early adolescent drug and alcohol use is associated with a slight but important decline in intellectual abilities. Substance related disorders are more common among males than females. The lifetime prevalence of all drugs (except alcohol) is 11.9 percent in the US; in males it is twice as high as in females. About thirteen percent of the general population is estimated to use cannabis (marijuana); about ten percent have used benzodiazepines (e.g., Valium, Xanax); about seven percent to nine percent of 18-25 year-olds have used amphetamines at least once; eight percent to 15.5 percent of 26-34 year-olds have used hallucinogens like LSD at least once. Even inhalants have been used at least once by five percent of the population. Inhalants are used mainly by boys between eight and 19 years old (and especially by 13-15 year-olds).

TREATMENT OPTIONS

Treatment can be very difficult for several reasons, among them a patient's denial that there is a problem, and his or her highly unstable motivation for continuing treatment. Treatment is also difficult because a patient's cravings can be overwhelmingly intense, and the individual's social circle is often composed of other substance abusers, making it hard for the individual to maintain relationships while becoming or remaining abstinent. The goal in treatment is to achieve and maintain abstinence. A wide range of interventions may be needed. There should be a general assessment, including a history of the drug abuse, and evaluation of medical, social, and psychological problems. It is best to involve the partner/family/friends of the person in order to help the person gain new understanding of the problem and to add information to the general assessment. An explicit treatment plan should be

worked out with the person (and partner/family/friends if appropriate) with concrete goals for which the person takes responsibility. The goals should include not only stopping substance use, but dealing with associated problems concerning health, personal relationships, and work. If the withdrawal symptoms are severe, the person may have to be hospitalized. Group therapy has been most widely used for problem drinkers through such organizations as Alcoholics Anonymous (AA), and has had some success with abuse and dependence of other drugs, e.g., cocaine. The goal is for the person to identify destructive patterns and to assume responsibility for decisions. AA and other 12-step programs involve recognizing that one has a lifelong problem, acknowledging the damage done to others, and taking responsibility for one's future behavior. Intensive psychotherapy is often desirable to deal with associated problems.

Another option is maintenance therapy, in which a drug is prescribed that has a slower action and is less addictive than the street drug, e.g., methadone instead of heroin. This is combined with therapy to help the person with withdrawal and with problems associated with drug use.

Cognitive-behavioral therapy can help increase the substance user's personal skills so that there is less dependency on drugs and the drug culture as a source of satisfaction. Identifying triggers for drug use and drug relapse is important as a basis for planning ways of avoiding them. Prescription drugs and relaxation techniques associated with withdrawal symptoms can help alleviate depression.

Rehabilitation in a therapeutic community is a further option for treatment. This is often peer directed and provides confrontation as well as high levels of support. Ethnic and cultural similarity of client and therapist is often helpful.

It is important to note that most people who successfully achieve abstinence have experienced several previous episodes of treatment relapse. One relapse is not an indication that treatment has failed.

Associations & Agencies

1373 American Academy of Addiction Psychiatry (AAAP)

7301 Mission Road
Suite 252
Prairie Village, KS 66208-3075   913-262-6161
Fax: 913-262-4311
E-mail: info@aaap.org
www.aaap.org

Jeanne G Trumble, Executive Director
Becky Stien, Deputy Executive Director

Professional membership organization with approximately 1,000 members in the United States and around the world. The membership consists of psychiatrists who work with addiction in their practices, faculty at various academic institutions, nonpsychiatrist professionals who are making a contribution to the field of addiction psychiatry, residents and medical students. The Academy offers various educational opportunities including addiction psychiatry review courses, annual meetings, and buprenorphine training. Annual meetings held in December.

1374 Career Assessment & Planning Services

Goodwill Industries-Suncoast
10596 Gandy Boulevard
PO Box 14456
St. Petersburg, FL 33702   727-523-1512
Fax: 727-577-2749
www.goodwill-suncoast.org

Jay McCloe, Director of Resource Development

Provides a comprehensive assessment, which can predict current and future employment and potential adjustment factors for physically, emotionally, or developmentally disabled persons who may be unemployed or underemployed. Assessments evaluate interests, aptitudes, academic achievements, and physical abilities (including dexterity and coordination) through coordinated testing, interviewing and behavioral observations.

1375 Center for Family Support (CFS)

333 7th Avenue
New York, NY 10001-5004   212-629-7939
Fax: 212-239-2211
www.cfsny.org

Steven Vernickofs, Executive Director

Service agency devoted to the physical well-being and development of the retarded child and the sound mental health of the parents. Helps families with retarded children with all aspects of home care including counseling, referrals, home aide service and consultation. Offers intervention for parents at the birth of a retarded child with in-home support, guidance and infant stimulation. Pioneered training of nonprofessional women as home aides to provide supportive services in homes.

1376 Center for Mental Health Services

SAMSHA
PO Box 42557
Washington, DC 20015
800-789-2647
Fax: 301-984-8796
TDD: 866-889-2647
www.mentalhealth.org

Irene S Levine PhD, Deputy Director

Develops national mental health policies, that promote Federal/State coordination and benefit from input from consumers, family members and providers. Ensures that high quality mental health services programs are implemented to benefit seriously mentally ill populations, disasters or those involved in the criminal justice system.

1377 Center for Mental Health Services Knowledge Exchange Network

US Department of Health and Human Services
PO Box 42490
Washington, DC 20015-4800
800-789-2647
Fax: 301-984-8796
E-mail: ken@mentalhealth.org
www.mentalhealth.org

Information about resources, technical assistance, research, training, networks, and other federal clearing houses, and fact sheets and materials. Information specialists refer callers to mental health resources in their communities as well as state, federal and nonprofit contacts. Staff available Monday through Friday, 8:30 AM - 5:00 PM, EST, excluding federal holidays. After hours, callers may leave messages and an information specialist will return their call.

1378 NADD: Association for Persons with Developmental Disabilities and Mental Health Needs

132 Fair Street
Kingston, NY 12401-4802   845-334-4336
800-331-5362
Fax: 845-331-4569
E-mail: nadd@mhv.net
www.thenadd.org

Dr. Robert Fletcher, Executive Director

Nonprofit organization designed to promote interest of professional and parent development with resources for individuals who have the coexistence of mental illness and mental retardation. Provides conference, educational services and training materials to professionals, parents, concerned citizens and service organizations. Formerly known as the National Association for the Dually Diagnosed.

1379 National Alliance for the Mentally Ill

2107 Wilson Boulevard
Suite 300
Arlington, VA 22201-3042   703-524-7600
800-950-6264
Fax: 703-524-9094
TDD: 703-516-7227
E-mail: helpline@nami.org
www.nami.org

Laurie Flynn, Executive Director

Nation's leading self-help organization for all those affected by severe brain disorders. Mission is to bring consumers and families with similar experiences together to share information about services, care providers, and ways to cope with the challenges of schizophrenia, manic depression, and other serious mental illnesses.

1380 National Association of State Alcohol and Drug Abuse Directors

808 17th Street NW
Suite 410
Washington, DC 20006-3910   202-293-0090
                              Fax: 202-293-1250
                         E-mail: dcoffice@nasadad.org
                              www.nasadad.org

Lewis Gallant PhD, Executive Director
Vannera So, Prevention Director

A private, nonprofit educational, scientific and informational organization that serves all state alcoholism and drug agency directors. NASADADs basic purpose is to foster and support the development of effective alcohol and other drug abuse prevention and treatment programs throughout each state. NASADAD serves as a focal point for the examination of alcohol and other drug-related issues of common interest to both national organizations and federal agencies.

Year Founded: 1971

1381 National Clearinghouse for Alcohol and Drug Information

Substance Abuse and Mental Services
5600 Fishers Lane
Rm 12-105 Parklawn Building
Rockville, MD 20847-2345   301-443-4795
                              Fax: 301-443-0284
                              www.health.org

Service of the US Substance Abuse and Mental Health Services Administration (SAMHSA). Collects, prepares, classifies and distributes information concerning alcohol, tobacco and other drugs, prevention strategies and materials, research, treatment approaches and resources, and training programs for professionals, community education programs, parents, children, and all interested persons. Provides a variety of free printed material including pamphlets, booklets, posters, resource guides and directories.

1382 National Council on Alcoholism and Drug Dependence

20 Exchange Place, Suite 2902
New York, NY 10005   212-269-7797
                              Fax: 212-269-7510
                         E-mail: national@ncadd.org
                              www.ncadd.org

Fights the stigma and the disease of alcoholism and other drug addictions. Founded by Marty Mann, the first woman to find long-term sobriety in Alcoholics Anonymous, NCADD provides education, information, intervetion and treatment through offices in New York and Washington, and a nationwide network of Affiliates.

Year Founded: 1944

1383 National Mental Health Consumer's Self-Help Clearinghouse

1211 Chestnut Street
Suite 1207
Philadelphia, PA 19107   215-751-1810
                              800-553-4539
                         Fax: 215-636-6312
                    E-mail: info@mhselfhelp.org
                              www.mhselfhelp.org

Alex Morrsey, Information/Referral

Funded by the National Institute of Mental Health Community Support Program, the purpose of the Clearinghouse is to encourage the development and growth of consumer self-help groups.

Year Founded: 1992

1384 Section for Psychiatric and Substance Abuse Services (SPSPAS)

1 N Franklin Street
Chicago, IL 60606-3421   312-422-3000
                              Fax: 312-422-4796
                              www.aha.org

Dick Davidson, President
Richard J Pollack, Executive VP

Institutional members of the American Hospital Association who provide psychiatric substance abuse, clinical psychology and other behavorial health services and assists the AHA in development and implementation of policies and programs to promote psychiatric substance abuse, clinical psychiatry and other behavioral health services. Active in formulating and commenting on federal legislation and regulations relating to psychiatric and substance abuse services.

1385 Suncoast Residential Training Center/Developmental Services Program

Goodwill Industries-Suncoast
10596 Gandy Boulevard
PO Box 14456
St. Petersburg, FL 33702   727-523-1512
                              Fax: 727-577-2749
                         www.goodwill-suncoast.org

Jay McCloe, Director Resource Development

A large group home which serves individuals diagnosed as mentally retarded with a secondary diagnosed of psychiatric difficulties as evidenced by problem behavior. Providing residential, behavioral and instructional support and services that will promote the development of adaptive, socially appropriate behavior, each individual is assessed to determine, socialization, basic academics and recreation. The primary intervention strategy is applied behavior analysis. Professional consultants are utilized to address the medical, dental, psychiatric and pharmacological needs of ech individual. One of the most popular features is the active community integration component of SRTC. Program customers attend an average of 15 monthly outings to various community events.

Books

1386 Addiction Workbook: a Step by Step Guide to Quitting Alcohol and Drugs

New Harbinger Publications
5674 Shattuck Avenue
Oakland, CA 94609-1662
510-652-2002
800-748-6273
Fax: 510-652-5472
E-mail: customerservice@newharbinger.com
www.newharbinger.com

This comprehensive workbook explains the facts about addiction and provides simple, step by step directions for working through the stages of the quitting process. *$17.95*

160 pages ISBN 1-572240-43-1

1387 Addictive Behaviors: Readings on Etiology, Prevention & Treatment

American Psychological Publishing
750 1st Street NE
Washington, DC 20002
202-336-5500
Fax: 202-216-7610
E-mail: appi@psych.org
www.appi.org

1388 American Psychiatric Association Practice Guideline for the Treatment of Patients With Substance Use Disorders : Alcohol, Cocaine, Opioids

American Psychiatric Publishing
1000 Wilson Boulevard
Suite 1825
Arlington, VA 22209-3901
703-907-7322
800-368-5777
Fax: 703-907-1091
E-mail: appi@psych.org
www.appi.org

James Scully MD, President
Katie Duffy, Marketing Assistant

Offers guidance to psychiatrists caring for patients with substance use disorders. *$29.50*

126 pages ISBN 0-890423-03-2

1389 Clinical Supervision in Alcohol and Drug Abuse Counseling

Jossey-Bass / Wiley & Sons
111 River Street
Hoboken, NJ 07030-5774
201-748-6000
Fax: 201-748-6088
E-mail: custserv@wiley.com
www.josseybass.com

This is the throughly revised edition of the groundbreaking, definitive text for supervisors in substance abuse counseling. *$25.95*

400 pages ISBN 0-787973-77-7

1390 Concerned Intervention: When Your Loved One Won't Quit Alcohol or Drugs

New Harbinger Publications
5674 Shattuck Avenue
Oakland, CA 94609-1662
510-652-2002
800-748-6273
Fax: 510-652-5472
E-mail: customerservice@newharbinger.com
www.newharbinger.com

John O'Neill
Pat O'Neill

Practical guide to group intervention techniques with lessons from experiences of families seeking counseling and treatment. *$13.95*

208 pages ISBN 1-879237-36-9

1391 Concise Guide to Treatment of Alcoholism and Addictions

American Psychiatric Publishing
1000 Wilson Boulevard
Suite 1825
Arlington, VA 22209-3901
703-907-7322
800-368-5777
Fax: 703-907-1091
E-mail: appi@psych.org
www.appi.org

Katie Duffy, Marketing Assistant

Presents information on available treatment options for alcoholism and addictions, substance abuse in the workplace and laboratory testing. *$29.95*

172 pages ISBN 0-880483-26-1

1392 Critical Incidents: Ethical Issues in Substance Abuse Prevention and Treatment

Hazelden
15251 Pleasant Valley Road
PO Box 176
Center City, MN 55012-0176
651-213-4000
800-328-9000
Fax: 651-213-4590
E-mail: info@hazelden.org
www.hazelden.org

An excellent resource for ethical questions, this book by William White, is a hands-on situational guide with approximately 200 examples of ethical problems, which are useful in clarifying ethical issues and providing questions for discussion. *$25.00*

276 pages ISBN 0-938475-03-7

1393 Drug Abuse Sourcebook

Omnigraphics
PO Box 625
Holmes, PA 19043
800-234-1340
Fax: 800-875-1340
E-mail: info@omnigraphics.com
www.omnigraphics.com

Omnigraphics is the publisher of the Health Reference Series, a growing consumer health information resource with more than 100 volumes in print. Each title in the series features an easy to understand format, nontechnical language, comprehensive indexing and resources for further information. Material in each book has been collected from a wide range of governmental agencies, professional associations, periodicals and other sources. *$78.00*

629 pages ISBN 0-780802-42-x

1394 Drug Abuse and Addiction Information/Treatment Directory

American Business Directories
5711 S 86th Circle
PO Box 27347
Omaha, NE 68127-0347
402-593-4600
800-555-6124
Fax: 402-331-5481
E-mail: directory@abii.com
www.abbi.com

1 per year

1395 Drug Facts and Comparisons

Facts and Comparisons
111 Westport Plaza
Suite 300
Saint Louis, MO 63146-3098
800-223-0554
Fax: 314-878-1574
www.drugfacts.com

Laura Hartel, Marketing Manager

Health care professionals choice for authoritative, comprehensive, and timely drug information. Contains information about more than 22,000 prescription and OTC products; divides drugs into logical, related therapeutic groups, categorizing them so that similar drugs may be easily compared.

ISBN 1-574391-10-0

1396 Drug Interaction Facts

Facts and Comparisons
111 Westport Plaza
Suite 300
Saint Louis, MO 63146-3014
314-216-2100
800-223-0554
Fax: 314-878-5563
www.drugfacts.com

Drug Interaction Facts loose-leaf edition provides drug-drug and drug food interaction information in a quick reference format. Drug Facts covers more than 20,000 brand and generic drugs and more 70 therapeutic classes. Available as bound edition, CD-ROM, or loose-leaf. *$209.00*

ISBN 1-574390-15-5

1397 Drug, Alcohol, and Other Addictions: A Directory of Treatment Centers and Prevention Programs Nationwide

Oryx Press
88 Post Road W
Westport, CT 06881
203-226-3571
Fax: 603-431-2214
E-mail: info@oryxpress.com
www.oryxpress.com

Covers nearly 12,000 federal, state, and local addiction treatment programs including public and private centers. *$195.00*

656 pages

1398 Dynamics of Addiction

Hazelden
15251 Pleasant Valley Road
PO Box 176
Center City, MN 55012-0176
651-213-2400
800-257-7810
Fax: 651-213-4411
E-mail: info@hazelden.org
www.hazelden.org

Pamphlet about addictions.

12 pages ISBN 0-935908-38-2

1399 Getting Beyond Sobriety

Jossey-Bass / Wiley & Sons
111 River Street
Hoboken, NJ 07030-5774
201-748-5774
Fax: 201-748-6088
E-mail: custserv@wiley.com
www.wiley.com

This method will lead to a change in behavior within the individual, while developing and expanding connection with others. *$ 42.50*

198 pages Year Founded: 1997 ISBN 0-787908-40-1

1400 Helping Women Recover: Special Edition for Use in the Criminal Justice System

Jossey-Bass / Wiley & Sons
111 River Street
Hoboken, NJ 07030-5774
201-748-6000
Fax: 201-748-6088
E-mail: custserv@wiley.com
www.wiley.com

Designed to meet the unique needs of substance-abusing women. Created for use with women's groups in a variety of correctional settings. Offers mental health professionals, corrections personnel, and program administrators the tools they need to implement this highly effective program.

384 pages ISBN 0-787946-10-5

1401 How Drugs Can Affect Your Life: The Effects of Drugs on Safety and Well Being: With Special Emphasis on Prevention of Drug Use

Charles C Thomas Publisher
2600 S First Street
Springfield, IL 62704-4730   217-789-8980
                                    800-258-8980
                              Fax: 217-789-9130
                    E-mail: books@ccthomas.com
                                www.ccthomas.com

$41.95

294 pages Year Founded: 1992 ISBN 0-398057-62-1

1402 Kicking Addictive Habits Once & For All

Jossey-Bass / Wiley & Sons
111 River Street
Hoboken, NJ 07030
                                    800-956-7739
                              Fax: 800-605-2665
                      E-mail: custserv@wiley.com
                                  www.wiley.com

All aspects of changing bad habits and developing a balance lifestyle are addressed in the book. *$22.50*

224 pages ISBN 0-787940-68-2

1403 LSD: Still With Us After All These Years

Jossey-Bass / Wiley & Sons
111 River Street
Hoboken, NJ 07030   201-748-6000
                      Fax: 201-748-6088
              E-mail: custserv@wiley.com
                          www.wiley.com

Facts about LSD. *$21.50*

176 pages ISBN 0-787943-79-7

1404 Let's Talk Facts About Substance Abuse & Addiction

American Psychiatric Publishing
1000 Wilson Boulevard
Suite 1825
Arlington, VA 22209-3901   703-907-7322
                                  800-368-5777
                            Fax: 703-907-1091
                     E-mail: appi@psych.org
                                www.appi.org

Katie Duffy, Marketing Assistant

Straight talk about a difficult subject. *$26.95*

1405 Lives At Risk: Understanding and Treating Young People with Dual Diagnosis

Free Press
1120 Avenue of the Americas
New York, NY 10036-6700   212-698-7000
                            Fax: 212-632-4989
                          www.simonsays.com

Lives at Risk addresses a population of concern: young men and women in early adulthood who are stalled and endangered by problems of mental illness and/or personality disorders combined with substance abuse. Through four vividly presented cases, the authors trace the complexities of the problems, define subgroups of the population, and discuss what can be done in contemporary treatment. *$30.00*

272 pages ISBN 0-684828-07-3

1406 Living Skills Recovery Workbook

Elsevier Science
11830 Westline Industrial Drive
St. Louis, MO 63146   314-453-7010
                             800-325-4177
                       Fax: 314-453-7095
           E-mail: custserv.ehs@elsevier.com
                          www.elsevier.com

Provides clinicians with the tools necessary to help patients with dual diagnoses acquire basic living skills. Focusing on stress management, time management, activities of daily living, and social skills training, each living skill is taught in relation to how it aids in recovery and relapse prevention for each patient's individual lifestyle and pattern of addiction. *$36.95*

197 pages Year Founded: 1999 ISBN 0-750671-18-1

1407 Living Sober I

Jossey-Bass / Wiley & Sons
111 River Street
Hoboken, NJ 07030   201-748-8677
                      Fax: 201-748-2665
                          www.wiley.com

Emphasizes the specific coping skills essential to a client's recovery. *$495.00*

87 pages Year Founded: 1999

1408 Living Sober II

Jossey-Bass / Wiley & Sons
111 River Street
Hoboken, NJ 07030   201-748-6000
                      Fax: 201-748-6088
                          www.wiley.com

Emphasizes the specific coping skills essential to a client's recovery. *$395.00*

1409 Meaning of Addiction

Jossey-Bass / Wiley & Sons
111 River Street
Hoboken, NJ 07030   201-748-6000
                      Fax: 201-748-6088
                          www.wiley.com

A controversial and persuasive analysis of addiction. *$30.50*

224 pages Year Founded: 1998 ISBN 0-787943-82-7

Substance Abuse & Dependence/Books

1410 Medical Aspects of Chemical Dependency Active Parenting Publishers

Hazelden
15251 Pleasant Valley Road
PO Box 176
Center City, MN 55012-0176   651-213-4000
800-328-9000
Fax: 651-213-4590
E-mail: info@hazelden.org
www.hazelden.org

This curriculum helps professionals educate clients in treatment and other settings about medical effects of chemical use and abuse. The program includes a video that explains body and brain changes that can occur when using alcohol or other drugs, a workbook that helps clients apply the information from the video to their own situations, a handbook that provides in-depth information on addiction, brain chemistry and the physiological effects of chemical dependency and a pamphlet that answers critical questions clients have about the medical effects of chemical dependency. Available to purchase separately. Program value packages available. $244.70

1411 Mother's Survival Guide to Recovery: All About Alcohol, Drugs & Babies

New Harbinger Publications
5674 Shattuck Avenue
Oakland, CA 94609-1662   510-652-2002
800-748-6273
Fax: 510-652-5472
E-mail: customerservice@newharbinger.com
www.newharbinger.com

Offers a strong message of hope to help women cope with the challenges of recovering, deal with prenatal care and parenting issues, and take steps toward creating the healthy, happy families they want to have. $12.95

160 pages ISBN 1-572240-49-0

1412 Motivating Behavior Changes Among Illicit-Drug Abusers

American Psychological Association
750 First Street NE
Washington, DC 20002-4241   202-336-5500
800-374-2721
Fax: 202-216-7610
www.apa.org

Scientifically based method focused on the use of incentives to change behavior. Research in multiple applications of contingency management techniques. Test case of effective utilization of the method in treating illicit-drug abusers. $39.95

547 pages Year Founded: 1999 ISBN 1-557985-70-7

1413 Narcotics and Drug Abuse: A-Z

Croner Publications
10951 Sorrento Valley Road
Suite 1D
San Diego, CA 92121-1613   800-441-4033
Fax: 800-809-0334
E-mail: paul@croner.com
www.croner.com

Covers agencies, organizations, facilities, companies and persons actively opposed to the use and/or abuse of narcotics and drugs. $100.00

900 pages 1 per year

1414 National Directory of Drug and Alcohol Abuse Treatment Programs

Substance Abuse & Mental Health Services
Adminsitration
5600 Fishers Lane
Room 16-105, Office of Applied Studies
Rockville, MD 20857   301-443-6239
Fax: 301-443-9847
E-mail: findtreatment@samhsa.gov
www.findtreatment.samhsa.gov

Geraldine Scott Pinkney, Statistician

Directory of substance abuse treatment programs for use by persons seeking treatment and by professionals. Lists facility name, address, telephone number and services offered. Updated annually. Available in paperback. Searchable on-line version on web site.

596 pages 1 per year

1415 New Treaments for Chemical Addictions

American Psychiatric Publishing
1000 Wilson Boulevard
Suite 1825
Arlington, VA 22209-3901   703-907-7322
800-368-5777
Fax: 703-907-1091
E-mail: appi@psych.org
www.appi.org

Katie Duffy, Marketing Assistant

Examines new approaches for an old problem. $37.50

248 pages ISBN 0-880488-38-7

1416 Points for Parents Perplexed about Drugs

Hazelden
15251 Pleasant Valley Road
PO Box 176
Center City, MN 55012-0176   651-213-4000
800-257-7810
Fax: 651-213-4411
E-mail: info@hazelden.org
www.hazelden.org

Clear guidelines help teachers, parents, family members and others recognize, evaluate, and deal with adolescent drug abuse. Excellent support for family counseling programs. $3.25

16 pages Year Founded: 1996 ISBN 0-894861-40-9

1417 Principles of Addiction Medicine

American Society of Addiction Medicine
4601 N Park Avenue
Suite 101, Upper Arcade
Chevy Chase, MD 20815   301-987-9278
800-844-8948
E-mail: email@asa.com
www.asam.org

James F Callahan DPA, Executive VP/CEO

Textbook on the basic and clinical science of prevention and treatment of alcohol, nicotine, and other drug dependencies and addictions. *$155.00*

1338 pages ISBN 1-880425-04-0

1418 Research Society on Alcoholism: Directory

7801 N Lamar Boulevard, Suite D-89
Austin, TX 78752-1038   512-454-0022
                               Fax: 512-454-0812
          E-mail: debbyrsa@bga.com
                    www.rsoa.org

Covers about 1,200 member researchers concerned with alcoholism and other related problems. *$5.00*

50 pages 1 per year

1419 Science of Prevention: Methodological Advances from Alcohol and Substance Research

American Psychological Association
750 First Street NE
Washington, DC 20002-4241   202-336-5500
                               800-374-2721
                    Fax: 202-216-7610
          E-mail: executiveoffice@apa.org
                    www.apa.org

Carolyn Valliere, Marketing Specialist

This book explores ways for bringing greater methodological rigor to prevention research, gathering together the analyses and insights of prominent researchers who present examples of the problems and the solutions they have encountered in their own work. *$39.95*

458 pages Year Founded: 1997 ISBN 1-557984-39-5

1420 Selfish Brain: Learning from Addiction

Hazelden
15251 Pleasant Valley Road
PO Box 176
Center City, MN 55012-0176   651-213-4000
                               800-328-9000
                    Fax: 651-213-4590
          E-mail: customerservice@hazelden.org
                    www.hazelden.org

Helps clients or loved ones face addiction and recovery by exploring the biological, historical and cultural aspects of addiction and its destructiveness. *$18.95*

544 pages ISBN 1-568383-63-0

1421 Sex, Drugs, Gambling and Chocolate: Workbook for Overcoming Addictions

Impact Publishers
PO Box 6016
Atascadero, CA 93423-6016   805-466-5917
                               800-246-7228
                    Fax: 805-466-5919
          E-mail: info@impactpublishers.com
                    www.impactpublishers.com

There is an alternative to 12-step. You can reduce almost any type of addictive behavior from drinking to sex, eating, and the Internet... with this practical and effective workbook. Teaches general principles of addictive behavior change, so readers can apply them as often as they need. *$15.95*

240 pages ISBN 1-886230-55-2

1422 Substance Abuse Directory and Related Services

Department of Public Health
321 E 12th Street
Des Moines, IA 50319-0075   515-281-7689
                               800-247-0614
                    Fax: 515-281-4535
          www.idph.state.ia.us/do/default

Mary Mincer Hansen, Director

Covers about 190 alcohol and drug abuse treatment and prevention programs, parent and community support groups and national substance abuse organizations and agencies.

1 per year

1423 Substance Abuse Librarians and Information Specialists Directory

PO Box 9513
Berkeley, CA 94709-0513   510-642-5208
                               Fax: 510-642-7175
          E-mail: salis@arg.org
                    www.salis.org

Covers approximately 200 libraries, clearinghouses, and information centers worldwide that offer resource information about substance abuse; and approximately 300 other organizations. *$45.00*

148 pages 3 per year

1424 Talking Back to Prozac

Center for the Study of Psychiatry and Psychology
101 East State Street
Ithaca, NY 14850   607-272-5328
                               Fax: 607-272-5329
          E-mail: breggin@tmn.com
                    www.breggin.com

Discusses the principles of drug withdrawl from many psychiatric drugs. Patients can develop serious and even life-threatening emotional and physical reactions. *$6.99*

Year Founded: 1995 ISBN 0-312956-06-1

1425 Treating Substance Abuse: Part 1

American Counseling Association
5999 Stevenson Avenue
Alexandria, VA 22304-3300   800-422-2648
                               Fax: 703-823-0252
                               TDD: 703-823-6862
          E-mail: webmaster@counseling.org
                    www.counseling.org

The first of a two-volume set presents up-to-date findings on the treatment of alcoholism and addiction to cocaine, caffeine, hallucinogens, and marijuana. Techniques and case examples are offered from a variety of approaches, including motivational enhancement therapy, marriage and family therapy as well as cognitive-behavioral. *$26.95*

280 pages ISBN 1-886330-48-4

1426 Treating Substance Abuse: Part 2

American Counseling Association
5999 Stevenson Avenue
Alexandria, VA 22304-3300

800-422-2648
Fax: 703-823-0252
E-mail: webmaster@counseling.org
www.counseling.org

For treating select populations of substance-abusing clients, including those with disabilities, psychiatric disorders, schizophernia and major depression. Also serves adolescents, older adults, pregnant women and clients whose addictions affect their ability to function in the workplace. *$29.95*

311 pages ISBN 1-886330-49-2

1427 Twelve-Step Facilitation Handbook

Hazelden Publishing
15251 Pleasant Valley Road
PO Box 176
Center City, MN 55012-0176

651-213-4000
800-328-9000
Fax: 651-213-4590
E-mail: customersupport@hazelden.org
www.hazelden.com

This book provides clinicians with the tools they need to encourage chemically dependent clients to take advantage of the healing power of twelve-step programs. Learn how to integrate these time-tested principles into your practice. *$24.95*

214 pages Year Founded: 2003 ISBN
1-592850-96-0

1428 Twenty-Four Hours a Day

Hazelden
15251 Pleasant Valley Road
PO Box 176
Center City, MN 55012-0176

651-213-2121
800-328-9000
Fax: 651-213-4590
www.hazelden.org

Daily meditation in this classic book helps clients develop a solid foundation in a spiritual program, learn to relate the Twelve Steps to their everyday lives and accomplish their treatment and aftercare goals. Includes 366 daily meditations with special consideration and extra encouragement given during holidays. Helps clients find the power to stay sober each day and not to take that first drink. Hardcover - $12.00, Softcover - $10.00. *$12.00*

400 pages ISBN 0-894860-12-7

1429 Understanding Dissociative Disorders and Addiction

Hazelden Publishing
15251 Pleasant Valley Road
Center City, MN 55012-0176

410-825-8888
800-328-9000
Fax: 651-213-4577
E-mail: customersupport@hazelden.org
www.hazelden.org

A Scott Winter, MD

This booklet discusses the origins and symptoms of dissociation, explains the links between dissociative disorder and chemical dependency. Addresses treatment options available to help in your recovery. The work book includes exercises and activities that help you acknowledge, accept and manage both your chemical dependency and your disociative disorder. *$2.95*

1430 Understanding Post-Traumatic Stress Disorder and Addiction

200 E Joppa Road
Suite 207
Baltimore, MD 21286

410-825-8888
888-825-8249
Fax: 410-337-0747
E-mail: sidran@sidran.org
www.sidran.org

This booklet discusses PTSD, how to recognize it and how to begin a dual recovery program from chemical dependency and PTSD. The workbook includes information to enhance your understanding of PTSD, activities to help identify the symptoms of dual disorders, a self evaulation of your recovery process and ways to handle situations that may trigger PTSD. *$9.00*

1431 Woman's Journal, Special Edition for Use in the Criminal Justice System

Jossey-Bass / Wiley & Sons
111 River Street
Hoboken, NJ 07030

201-748-6000
Fax: 201-748-6088
E-mail: customer@wiley.com
www.wiley.com

Designed to meet the unique needs of substance-abusing women. Created for use with women's groups in a variety of correctional settings. Offers mental health professionals, corrections personnel, and program administrators the tools they need to implement this highly effective program. *$23.50*

144 pages Year Founded: 1999 ISBN
0-787946-10-9

1432 You Can Free Yourself From Alcohol & Drugs: Work a Program That Keeps You in Charge

New Harbinger Publications
5674 Shattuck Avenue
Oakland, CA 94609-1662

510-652-2002
800-748-6273
Fax: 510-652-5472
E-mail: customerservice@newharbinger.com
www.newharbinger.com

Reworking of the Twelve Steps approach into a program that helps addicts and alcoholics make needed changes in their lifestyle. *$13.95*

214 pages ISBN 1-572241-18-7

1433 Your Brain on Drugs

Hazelden
15251 Pleasant Valley Road
PO Box 176
Center City, MN 55012-0176   **651-213-4000**
800-328-9000
Fax: 651-213-4590
E-mail: info@hazelden.org
www.hazelden.org

This pamphlet explains the effects of alcohol and other drugs on the brain through illustrations, activities and exercise that help to reinforce the easy-to-read text. *$4.00*

36 pages

Periodicals & Pamphlets

1434 About Crack Cocaine

ETR Associates
4 Carbonero Way
Scotts Valley, CA 95066   **831-438-4060**
800-321-4407
Fax: 800-435-8433
E-mail: customerservice@etr.org
www.etr.org

Describes what crack cocaine is and why it's dangerous and lists the effects on the body. *$16.00*

1435 Addiction

ETR Associates
4 Carbonero Way
Scotts Valley, CA 95066   **831-438-4060**
800-321-4407
Fax: 800-435-8433
E-mail: customerservice@etr.org
www.etr.org

Includes answers to commonly asked questions about drug addiction, a 13'x 17' wall chart presents the stages of addiction and recovery, covers denial, withdrawal and relapse. *$18.00*

1436 Alcoholism and Drug Abuse Weekly

Manisses Communications Group
208 Governor Street
Providence, RI 02906   **401-831-6020**
800-333-7771
Fax: 401-861-6370
E-mail: manisssescs@manisses.com
www.manisses.com

Reports on state and private agencies on issues of importance to professionals in the field of alcohol and drug abuse treatment and prevention. *$499.00*

48 per year ISSN 1042-1394

1437 American Journal on Addictions

American Academy of Addiction Psychiatry
7301 Mission Road
Suite 252
Prairie Village, KS 66208-3075   **913-262-6161**
Fax: 913-262-4311
E-mail: info@aaap.org
www.aaap.org

Jeanne G Trumble, Executive Director

1438 Brown University: Digest of Addiction Theory and Application

Manisses Communications Group
208 Governor Street
Providence, RI 02906   **401-831-6020**
800-333-7771
Fax: 401-861-6370
E-mail: manissescs@manisseses.com
www.manisses.com

Karienne Stovell, Sr Managing Editor

Digests and abstracts articles from more than 80 international scholarly journals. Presents articles in summarized formats with comments on their applications. *$189.00*

12 pages 12 per year ISSN 1040-6328

1439 Designer Drugs

ETR Associates
4 Carbonero Way
Scotts Valley, CA 95066   **831-438-4060**
800-321-4407
Fax: 800-435-8433
E-mail: customerservice@etr.org
www.etr.org

Traces the evolution of designer drugs like China White and MDMA, explains how addiction works and suggests why designer drugs are so addicted. *$16.00*

1440 Drug ABC's

ETR Associates
4 Carbonero Way
Scotts Valley, CA 95066   **831-438-4060**
800-321-4407
Fax: 800-435-8433
E-mail: customerservice@etr.org
www.etr.org

26 good reasons to stay away from drugs, facts of different drugs, and motivation for being drug-free. *$16.00*

1441 Drug Dependence, Alcohol Abuse and Alcoholism

Elsevier Publishing
11830 Westline Industrial Drive
St Louis, MO 63146
800-542-2522
Fax: 800-535-9938
E-mail: usbkinfo@elsevier.com
www.elsevier.com

This journal aims to provide its readers with a swift, yet complete, current awareness service. This is achieved both by the scope and structure of the journal.

ISSN 0925-5958

1442 Drug Facts Pamphlet

ETR Associates
4 Carbonero Way
Scotts Valley, CA 95066   **831-438-4060**
                                     800-321-4407
               Fax: 800-435-8433
        E-mail: customerservice@etr.org
                       www.etr.org

Overview of 11 of the most commonly abused drugs includes: Description of drug, short-term effects and long-term effects.

1443 DrugLink

Facts and Comparisons
111 Westport Plaza
Suite 300
Saint Louis, MO 63146-3014   **314-216-2100**
                                        800-223-0554
               Fax: 314-878-5563
               www.drugsfacts.com

DrugLink is an eight-page newsletter that provides abstracts of drug-related articles from various journals. DrugLink allows health care professionals to stay up-to-date on hot topics without having to subscribe to multiple publications. *$52.95*

8 pages ISBN 1-089559-0 -

1444 Drugs: Talking With Your Teen

ETR Associates
4 Carbonero Way
Scotts Valley, CA 95066   **831-438-4060**
                                     800-321-4407
               Fax: 800-435-8433
        E-mail: customerservice@etr.org
                       www.etr.org

Suggestions for effective communication include: avoid scare tatics, clarify family rules, other alternative for drug use. *$ 16.00*

1445 Hazelden Voice

Hazelden Foundation
PO Box 11
Center City, MN 55012-0011   **612-213-4000**
                                        800-257-7810
               Fax: 651-213-4411
        E-mail: info@hazelden.org
                       www.hazelden.org

Marty Duda, Editor

Reports on Hazelden activities and programs, and discusses developments and issues in chemical dependency treatment and prevention. Carries notices of professional education opportunities, reviews of resources in the field, and a calendar of events.

1446 ICPA Reporter

ICPADD
12501 Old Columbia Pike
Silver Spring, MD 20904-6601   **301-680-6719**
               Fax: 301-680-6707
        E-mail: The ICPA@hotmail.com
                       www.icpa-dd.org

Reports on activities of the Commission worldwide, which seeks to prevent alcoholism and drug dependency. Recurring features include a calendar of events and notices of publications available.

4 pages 4 per year

1447 Journal of Substance Abuse Treatment

Elsevier Publishing
11830 Westline Industrial Drive
St Louis, MO 63146
                                        800-545-2522
               Fax: 800-535-9935
        E-mail: usbkinfo@elsevier.com
                       www.elsevier.com

The Journal of Substance Abuse Treatment features original reviews, training and educational articles, special commentary, and especially research articles that are meaningful to the treatment of nicotine, alcohol, and other drugs of dependence.

ISSN 0740-5472

1448 Marijuana ABC's

ETR Associates
4 Carbonero Way
Scotts Valley, CA 95066   **831-438-4060**
                                     800-321-4407
               Fax: 800-435-8433
        E-mail: customerservice@etr.org
                       www.etr.org

Discusses the effects of marijuana, legal consequences, and strategies for saying no.

1449 National Institute of Drug Abuse: NIDA

6001 Executive Boulevard
Room 5213
Bethesda, MD 20892-9561   **301-443-1124**
               Fax: 301-443-7397
        E-mail: information@lists.nida.nih.gov
                       www.nida.nih.gov

Beverly Jackson, Public Information

Covers the areas of drug abuse treatment and prevention research, epidemiology, neuroscience and behavioral research, health services research and AIDS. Seeks to report on advances in the field, identify resources, promote an exchange of information, and improve communications among clinicians, researchers, administrators, and policymakers. Recurring features include synopses of research advances and projects, NIDA news, news of legislative and regulatory developments, and announcements.

16 pages 24 per year

1450 Prevention Researcher

Integrated Research Services
66 Club Road
Suite 370
Eugene, OR 97401-2463   541-683-9278
                               800-929-2955
                    E-mail: info@tpronline.org
                          www.tpronline.org

Provides information on behavioral research to health
and human services professionals, with a primary emphasis on adolescent substance abuse issues. *$20.00*

12-16 pages 4 per year ISSN 1086-4385

1451 Save Our Sons and Daughters Newsletter (SOSAD)

2441 W Grand Boulevard
Detroit, MI 48208   313-361-5200
                    E-mail: sosadb@aol.com

Serves as a forum for the organization, parents and
supporters of children killed in street violence who began working together to create positive alternatives
for young people. Provides commentaries, news of
neighborhood coalitions, rallies, other social activities. Crisis Intervention and Violence Prevention
News.

8 pages 12 per year

1452 Substance Abuse Report: Warren, Gorham & Lamont

White Pond Colony
Carmel, NY 10512   845-225-2935
                         Fax: 845-225-5395

Alison Knopf, Editor

Concentrates on regulatory news, trends, and developments in the field of drug and alcohol abuse including managed care and funding. Discusses treatment
methods and community facilities for handling substance abuse. Recurring features include news of upcoming conferences. *$275.00*

8 pages

1453 When Someone You Care About Abuses Drugs and Alcohol: When to Act, What to Say

Hazelden
15251 Pleasant Valley Road
PO Box 176
Center City, MN 55012-0176   651-213-4000
                               800-257-7810
                         Fax: 651-213-4411
                  E-mail: info@hazelden.org
                          www.hazelden.org

This pamphlet shows family, friends, and co-workers
how to confront someone who may be abusing alcohol
or other drugs. *$2.25*

16 pages Year Founded: 1993

Research Centers

1454 National Clearinghouse for Alcohol and Drug Information

PO Box 2345
Rockville, MD 20847-2345   301-468-2600
                               800-729-6686
                        Fax: 301-468-7394
                             www.health.org

One-stop resource for information about substance
abuse prevention and addiction treatment.

Support Groups & Hot Lines

1455 Alateen

1600 Corporate Landing Parkway
Virginia Beach, VA 23454-5617   757-563-1600
                                 888-425-2666
                          Fax: 757-563-1655
                   E-mail: wso@al-anon.org
                       www.alanon.alateen.org

Mary Ann Keller, Director Members Services

Support program for teenagers who are the relatives
or friends of problem drinkers. Meetings are
facilitable by Alateen members. An Adult- Al-Anon
member provides guidance as the Alateen Sponsor.

1456 Chemically Dependent Anonymous

PO Box 423
Severna Park, MD 21146   410-647-7060

Twelve-step program for friends and relatives of
chemically dependent people.

1457 Cocaine Anonymous

3740 Overland Avenue
Suite C
Los Angeles, CA 90034-6337   310-559-5833
                               800-347-8998
                         Fax: 310-559-2554
                     E-mail: cawso@ca.org
                               www.ca.org

1458 Infoline

Connecticut United Way
1344 Silas Deane Highway
Rocky Hill, CT 06067   860-571-7500
                         Fax: 860-571-7525
          E-mail: unitedwayservices@ctunitedway.org
                             www.211.org

Melanie Loewenstein, Senior VP
Debi Colacrai, CEO/CFO

Infoline is a free, confidential, help-by-telephone service for information, referral, and crisis intervention. Trained professionals help callers find information, discover options or deal with a crisis by locating hundreds of services in their area on many different issues, from substance abuse to elder needs to suicide to volunteering in your community. Infoline is certified by the American Association of Suicidology. Operates 24 hours a day, everyday. Multilingual caseworkers are available. For Child Care Infoline, call 1-800-505-1000.

1459 Marijuana Anonymous

PO Box 2912
Van Nuys, CA 91404

800-766-6779

Twelve-step program for marijuana addiction.

1460 Nar-Anon World Wide Service

PO Box 2562
Palos Verde, CA 90274-0119   310-547-5800

Twelve-step program for families and friends of addicts.

1461 Narcotics Anonymous

PO Box 9999
Van Nuys, CA 91409   818-773-9999
Fax: 818-700-0700
E-mail: info@na.org
www.na.org

For narcotic addicts: Peer support for recovered addicts.

1462 National Mental Health Association

2001 N Beauregard Street
12th Floor
Alexandria, VA 22311   703-684-7722
800-969-6642
Fax: 703-684-5968
TTY: 800-433-5959
E-mail: infoctr@nmha.org
www.nmha.org

Michael Faenza, President/CEO

NMHA is America's oldest and only nonprofit organization that addresses all the aspects of mental health and mental illness.

1463 Pathways to Promise

5400 Arsenal Street
Saint Louis, MO 63139-1300   314-644-8400
Fax: 314-644-8834
E-mail: pathways@mimh.edu
www.pathways2promise.org

Pathways to Promise is an interfaith technical assistance and resource center which offers liturgical and educational materials, program models, and networking information to promote a caring ministry with people with mental illness and their families.

1464 Self Management and Recovery Training

24000 Mercantile Road
Suite 11
Beachwood, OH 44122   216-292-0220
www.smartrecovery.org

Cognitive behavioral abstinence-based approach.

Video & Audio

1465 Cocaine & Crack: Back from the Abyss

Hazelden
15251 Pleasant Valley Road
PO Box 176
Center City, MN 55012-0176   651-213-4000
800-257-7810
Fax: 651-213-4411
E-mail: info@hazelden.org
www.hazelden.org

Provides clients in correctional, educational, and treatment settings an understanding of the history, pharamacology, and medical impact of cocaine/crack use through personal stories of addiction and recovery. Reveals proven methods for overcoming addiction and discusses the best ways to maintain recovery. 46 minutes. *$225.00*

Year Founded: 1998

1466 Cross Addiction: Back Door to Relapse

Hazelden
15251 Pleasant Valley Road
PO Box 176
Center City, MN 55012-0176   651-213-2121
800-328-9000
Fax: 651-213-4590
www.hazelden.org

Presents a overview of the nature of cross-addiction. What it looks like, how it happens and why the addict is so susceptible to it. Explains to clients understanding the impact of different drugs and multiple drugs on the mind and body. *$195.00*

1467 Heroin: What Am I Going To Do?

Hazelden
15251 Pleasant Valley Road
PO Box 176
Center City, MN 55012-0176   651-213-4000
800-328-9000
Fax: 651-213-4590
E-mail: info@hazelden.org
www.hazelden.org

Shares powerful stories and keen insights from recovering heroin addicts and the rewards of clean living. Teaches clients how to use honesty, surrender and responsibility as the power tools for a successful recovery. Deglamorizes heroin use, with an portrait of drug's inevitable degration of the mind, body and spirit. 30 minutes. *$225.00*

Year Founded: 1997

1468 Inhalant Abuse: Kids in Danger/Adults in the Dark

Hazelden
15251 Pleasant Valley Road
PO Box 176
Center City, MN 55012-0176

651-213-2121
800-328-9000
Fax: 651-213-4590
E-mail: info@hazelden.org
www.hazelden.org

Allen Mondell, Director
Cynthia Salzman, Director

An excellent video to help professionals recognize inhalant abuse amoung young people and implement proper prevention and intervention techniques. Not recommended for viewing by children. 18 minute. *$ 150.00*

Year Founded: 1990

1469 Intervention, How to Help Someone Who Doesn't Want Help

Hazelden
15251 Pleasant Valley Road
PO Box 176
Center City, MN 55012-0176

651-213-4000
800-328-9000
Fax: 651-213-4590
E-mail: info@hazelden.org
www.hazelden.org

This video describes how chemical dependence affects those around the dependent person, including a spouse, children, neighbors, and co-workers. A 30-point of assessment questionaire teaches those concerned how they can intervene by effectively confronting the dependent person with reality. A 48 minute video. *$495.00*

Year Founded: 1986

1470 Marijuana: Escape to Nowhere

Hazelden
15251 Pleasant Valley Road
PO Box 176
Center City, MN 55012-0176

651-213-4000
800-328-9000
Fax: 651-213-4590
E-mail: info@hazelden.org
www.hazelden.org

Challenges myths about marijuana by clearly stating that marijuana is addictive and use results in physical, emotional and spiritual consequences. Explains to clients in simple language the pharmacology of today's more potent marijuana and shares the hope and healing of recovery. 30 minutes. *$225.00*

Year Founded: 1999

1471 Medical Aspects of Chemical Dependency Active Parenting Publishers

Hazelden
15251 Pleasant Valley Road
PO Box 176
Center City, MN 55012-0176

651-213-2121
800-328-9000
Fax: 651-213-4590
www.hazelden.org

This curriculum helps professionals educate clients in treatment and other settings about medical effects of chemical use and abuse. The program includes a video that explains body and brain changes that can occur when using alcohol or other drugs, a workbook that helps clients apply the information from the video to their own situations, a handbook that provides in-depth information on addiction, brain chemistry and the physiological effects of chemical dependency and a pamphlet that answers critical questions clients have about the medical effects of chemical dependency. Available to purchase separately. Program value packages available. *$244.70*

1472 Methamphetamine: Decide to Live

Hazelden
15251 Pleasant Valley Road
PO Box 176
Center City, MN 55012-0176

651-213-4000
800-328-9000
Fax: 651-213-4590
E-mail: info@hazelden.org
www.hazelden.org

Methamphetamine: Decide to Live presents the latest information on the devasting consequences of meth addiction and the struggles and rewards of recovery. Facts, medical aspects, personal stories, and insights on the recovery process illuminate the path to healing. The video is divided into two parts and is 38 minutes long. *$225.00*

Year Founded: 1998

1473 Methamphetamine: a Methamphetamine Prevention Video

Hazelden
15251 Pleasant Valley Road
PO Box 176
Center City, MN 55012-0176

651-213-4000
800-328-9000
Fax: 651-213-4590
E-mail: info@hazelden.org
www.hazelden.org

This video appeals to young people to provide information about the pharmacology of methamphetamines and the physical and social consequences of its use. Testimonials, animation, graphics and a musical soundtrack deliver a strong message suitable for high school prevention and youth treatment settings. 20 minute. *$225.00*

Year Founded: 1999

1474 Prescription Drugs: Recovery from the Hidden Addiction

Hazelden
15251 Pleasant Valley Road
PO Box 176
Center City, MN 55012-0176

651-213-4000
800-328-9000
Fax: 651-213-4590
E-mail: info@hazelden.org
www.hazelden.org

Combines essential facts about prescription drugs with vivid personal stories of addiction and recovery. Classifies prescription medications and gives the corresponding street forms. Offers solutions to problems unique to presciption drugs, addresses the particular needs of older adults and elaborates on the dangers of cross-addiction. 31 minutes. *$225.00*

Year Founded: 1998

1475 Reality Check: Marijuana Prevention Video

Hazelden
15251 Pleasant Valley Road
PO Box 176
Center City, MN 55012-0176   **651-213-4000**
                                        800-328-9000
                          Fax: 651-213-4590
            E-mail: info@hazelden.org
                      www.hazelden.org

This video creates a strong message for kids about the dangers of marijuana use. A combination of humor, animated graphics, testimonials and music deliver the facts on the pharmacology of marijuana and both it's short and long use consequences. Suitable for kids grades 7-12.   15 minute video. *$225.00*

Year Founded: 1999

1476 SmokeFree TV: a Nicotine Prevention Video

Hazelden
15251 Pleasant Valley Road
PO Box 176
Center City, MN 55012-0176   **651-213-4000**
                                        800-328-9000
                          Fax: 651-213-4590
            E-mail: info@hazelden.org
                      www.hazelden.org

Key facts, consequences of use and refusal skills guide children in understanding why they should avoid nicotine. Animated graphics, stories, humor, and music appeal to young people. Pharmacology of nicotine, its consequences and ways to refuse it are also explored. 15 minute video. *$225.00*

Year Founded: 1999

1477 Straight Talk About Substance Use and Violence

ADD WareHouse
300 NW 70th Avenue
Suite 102
Plantation, FL 33317   **954-792-8100**
                                  800-233-9273
                     Fax: 954-792-8545
        E-mail: sales@addwarehouse.com
                www.addwarehouse.com

Substance abuse and violence prevention begins with this three video program featuring the frank testimonials of 19 teens with significant chemical deppendency issues who range in age from 13 to 22. In the starkest terms they discuss their most personal issues: substance abuse, sexual abuse, physical abuse, suicide attempts, violent acting out, depression, and abusive relationships. Includes 95 page discussion guide and three 30 minute videos. *$259.00*

1478 Twenty-Four Hours a Day Audio

Hazelden
15251 Pleasant Valley Road
PO Box 176
Center City, MN 55012-0176   **651-213-4000**
                                        800-328-9000
                          Fax: 651-213-4590
            E-mail: info@hazelden.org
                      www.hazelden.org

Twenty-Four Hours a Day is intended as a help for A.A. members in our program of living one day at a time, but can also be of help to anyone who wishes to begin each day with a few minutes of thought, meditation, and prayer. This audio tape is 3 hours long. *$17.95*

Year Founded: 1998 ISBN 1-574532-65-0

1479 Vernon Johnson's Complete Guide to Intervention

Hazelden
15251 Pleasant Valley Road
PO Box 176
Center City, MN 55012-0176   **651-213-4000**
                                        800-328-9000
                          Fax: 651-213-4590
            E-mail: info@hazelden.org
                      www.hazelden.org

A detailed synthesis of all aspects of intervention from the founder of the process that has helped many chemically dependent people and their families. Album of twelve audios. *$77.00*

Web Sites

1480 www.addictionresourceguide.com
Addiction Resource Guide

Descriptions of inpatient, outpatient programs.

1481 www.alcoholism.about.com/library/weekly/
Alcohol and the Elderly

Links to other pages relevant to overuse of alcohol and drugs in the elderly.

1482 www.doitnow.org/pages/pubhub.hmtl
The Do It Now Foundation

Copies of brochures on drugs, alcohol, smoking, drugs and kids, and street drugs.

1483 www.erols.com/ksciacca/
Dual Diagnosis Website, Kathleen Sciacca

Articles about the treatment of dually diagnosed patients, a bibliography, links to other on-line resources, a discussion forum, and an interactive chat area.

1484 www.health.org

Preveline - Prevention Online

Designed for access by drug name or publication series.

1485 www.health.org/

PrevLine: National Clearinghouse for Alcohol and Drug Information

Substance abuse resources directed toward professionals, fact sheets, research news and updates.

1486 www.jacsweb.org

JACS

Ten articles dealing with denial and ignorance.

1487 www.jointogether.org/

Join Together

Alcohol and substance abuse information, legislative alerts, new and updates.

1488 www.mentalhealth.com

Internet Mental Health

On-line information and a virtual encyclopedia related to mental disorders, possible causes and treatments. News, articles, on-line diagnostic programs and related links. Designed to improve understanding, diagnosis and treatment of mental illness throughout the world. Awarded the Top Site Award and the NetPsych Cutting Edge Site Award.

1489 www.mhsource.com/pt/p950536.html

Public and Research Views of Dual-Diagnosis Explored

Explains interactions of mental illness and substance abuse.

1490 www.naadac.org

National Association of Alcohol and Drug Abuse Counselors

Its mission is to lead, unify, and empower global addiction focused professionals to achieve excellence through education, advocacy, knowledge, standards of practice, ethics, professional development, and research. Advocates on behalf of addiction professionals and the people they serve. Establishes and promotes the highest possible standards of practice and qualifications for addiction professionals.

1491 www.nida.nih.gov

National Institute on Drug Abuse

Many publications useful for patients. Research Reports, summaries about chemicals and treatments.

1492 www.nida.nih.gov/DrugsofAbuse.html

Commonly Abused Drugs: Street Names for Drugs of Abuse

Current names, periods of detection, medical uses.

1493 www.nida.nih.gov/researchreports/cocaine

Cocaine Abuse and Addiction

From the National Institute on Drug Abuse.

1494 www.psychcentral.com

Psych Central

Personalized one-stop index for psychology, support, and mental health issues, resources, and people on the Internet.

1495 www.pta.org/commonsense

Common Sense: Strategies for Raising Alcoholic/Drug-/Free Children

Drug facts, warning signs, and guidance.

1496 www.samhsa.gov/

Substance Abuse and Mental Health Services Administration

Provides links to government resources related to substance abuse and mental health.

1497 www.uiuc.edu/departments/mckinley/

Drug/Alcohol Brochures

Single page handouts with basic information.

1498 www.well.com/user/woa/
Web of Addictions

Links to fact sheets from trustworthy sources.

Introduction

Suicide used to be considered both a sin and a crime. Today, suicide is viewed primarily as a psychiatric problem. It is not in itself a mental disorder but the risk of suicide is considerably raised in the presence of certain mental disorders. Suicide often involves a complex interaction of problems in which psychological, neurological, medical, social, and family factors may all play a part.

Most professionals distinguish at least two suicide groups: those who actually kill themselves, i.e., completed suicides; and those who attempt it, usually harming themselves, but survive. Those who succeed in killing themselves are nearly always suffering from one or more psychiatric disorders. They plan the suicide very carefully, including making discovery unlikely, and they use lethal means (shooting themselves, or jumping from a high place). Among those who make the attempt but survive, most are acting impulsively, in a way that makes discovery probable, and their means are not likely to be lethal (e.g. taking insufficient pills). Nevertheless, there is an overlap: plenty of people commit suicide impulsively, and others have their careful plans interrupted by circumstance or ambivalence. Each unsuccessful attempt increases the likelihood of a completed suicide in the future.

ASSOCIATED FEATURES

Nine of 10 suicides are associated with some form of mental disorder, especially Depression, Schizophrenia, Alcohol Abuse, Bipolar Disorder, and Panic Disorder. In addition, Personality Disorders have been diagnosed in one-third to one-half of people who kill themselves. These are often seen in younger people who live in an environment where drug and alcohol abuse, as well as violence, are common. The most common personality disorders associated with suicide are Borderline Personality Disorder, Antisocial Personality Disorder, and Narcissistic Personality Disorder. Among people with Schizophrenia, suicide is the main reason for premature death; they have a lifetime risk of ten percent, especially those suffering from Paranoid Schizophrenia.

Drug and alcohol abuse is also a risk factor for suicide: among 113 young people who killed themselves in California, fifty-five percent had some kind of substance abuse problems, usually long standing and including different drugs.

Another associated factor is severe, debilitating, or terminal physical illness. The pain, restricted function, and dread of dependence can all contribute to suicidal behavior, especially in illnesses such as Huntington's Disease, cancer, multiple sclerosis, spinal cord injuries, and AIDS. Some or many of these risk factors are present in most completed suicides. But it's inaccurate to conclude that most people with one or more of these risk factors are likely to kill themselves. Quite the opposite is true, making it very difficult to predict suicide for any given individual.

PREVALENCE

Suicide is the ninth leading cause of death in the US and the third leading cause among 15-24 year-olds. It is estimated that over five million people have suicidal thoughts each year, though there are only 30,000 deaths from suicide each year. This may be a serious underestimate, however, since suicide is still considered a stigma and often goes unreported. In the general population there are 11.2 reported suicides for every 100,000 people. It is reported even less in children: among 5-14 year-olds, 0.7 percent per 100,000. Among 15-19 year-olds, 13.2 percent per 100,000, and has recently increased sharply. Boys are more likely to commit suicide than girls and more likely to use firearms. Compared to other countries, guns are particularly common in the US as a means of suicide. Children who kill themselves often have a history of antisocial behavior, and depression and suicide is more common in their families than in families in general.

More males than females commit suicide, both among adults and adolescents. Among adults, the most likely suicides will be men who are widowed, divorced, or single, who lack social support, who are unemployed, who have a diagnosis of mental disorder (especially Depression), who have a physical illness, a family history of suicide, who are in psychological turmoil, who have made previous suicide attempts, who use or abuse alcohol, and who have easy access to firearms. Among adolescents, the most likely suicides are married males (or unwed and pregnant females), who have suffered from parental absence or abuse, who have academic problems, affective disorders (especially Bioplar Disorder), who are substance abusers, suffer from Attention-Deficit/Hyperactivity Disorder or epilepsy, who have Conduct Disorder, problems with impulse control, a family history of suicide, and/or access to firearms. Keeping guns in the home is a suicide risk for both males and females.

Elderly people (those over age 65) are more likely than any other age group to commit suicide. While only twelve percent of the population is elderly, twenty percent of all those who kill themselves are elderly. As in other population groups, elderly men are more likely to kill themselves than elderly women but the difference between the sexes is much bigger in this age group than in other age groups. Among all ages, the rate of suicide for men is about 20 per 100,000 and for women five per 100,000. Among the elderly, the rate for men is about 42 per 100,000 and for women about six and one-half per 100,000. Thus the great overall gender differences become even bigger among the elderly and more so as the elderly get older. The highest rate of suicide is among white elderly men, probably because their economic and social status drops severely with age, because they usually do not have a good support system and because they are highly unlikely to ask for help.

Although all the factors discussed here are risk factors, it should be kept in mind that 99.9 percent of those at risk do not commit suicide.

TREATMENT OPTIONS

Considering the risk factors, a professional must first make a careful assessment, taking all the risk factors into account, including the availability of weapons, pills and other lethal means, as well as suicidal ideation and whether or not the person has conveyed the intention to commit suicide, and whether the method the patient plans to use is available (one can only jump off a bridge if there is a bridge, or drive into a wall if one has access to a vehicle). Someone who has no thought of death or has thoughts of death that are not connected with suicide is at a lower risk than someone who is thinking of suicide. Among those who are thinking of it, those who have not worked out the means of committing suicide are at a lower risk than those who think of suicide and a specific method of carrying it out. Treatment is partly based on the level of intervention that is believed to be required. If the person is seriously depressed and is also anxious, tense, and angry, and in overwhelming psychological anguish, the risk is more acute and the person is less able to take charge. This means that the professional must do so. The first priority is to ensure the safety of the client. Sometimes hospitalization is necessary.

After safety is assured, treatment is aimed at the underlying disorder. It may include psychological support, medication and other therapies: group; art; dance/movement. Professional treatment should involve working with the family if possible and other medical staff, e.g., a physician. Regular reassessments should take place.

In cases where there are Personality Disorders, there may be anger and aggression, and the suicidal thoughts and ideas may be chronic or repetitive. This is a particular strain on professionals, patients, and family. The patient, family, and clinician must work together to understand the chronicity of the condition, and the fact that suicide cannot always be prevented. It is essential to develop a working alliance between therapist and client, based on trust, mutual respect, and on the client's belief that the therapist genuinely cares about him/her. Reassessments include getting information from other professionals involved in treating the person, including reassessment of medication with the prescribing physician, and from family members or others significant in the life of the client who should participate in planning and following up. Assessment must also include assessment of the client's ability to understand and participate in the treatment, information about his/her psychological state (hopeless, despairing, depressed) and cognitive competence.

Associations & Agencies

1500 American Association of Suicidology

4201 Connecticut Avenue NW
Suite 408
Washington, DC 20008-1158   202-237-2280
Fax: 202-237-2282
E-mail: info@suicidology.org
www.suicidology.org

Dr. Alan Berman, Executive Director

A nonprofit organization devoted to understanding and preventing suicide. Promotes public awareness, research, public education, and training for professionals and volunteers.

1501 American Foundation for Suicide Prevention

120 Wall Street
22 Floor
New York, NY 10005-4023   212-363-3500
888-333-2377
Fax: 212-363-6237
E-mail: lteegarden@afsp.org
www.afsp.org

Lance Teegarden, Communications Manager

The American Foundation for Suicide Prevention (AFSP) is the only national not-for-profit exclusively dedicated to funding suicide prevention research, initiating treatment projects and offering educational programs and conferences for survivors, mental health professionals, physicians, and the public.

1502 American Suicide Foundation

1045 Park Avenue
Suite 3C
New York, NY 10028   212-210-1111
800-273-4042

Referrals to support groups for survivors.

1503 Center for Mental Health Services

SAMSHA
PO Box 42557
Washington, DC 20015

800-789-2647
Fax: 301-984-8796
TDD: 866-889-2647
www.mentalhealth.org

Irene S Levine PhD, Deputy Director

Develops national mental health policies, that promote Federal/State coordination and benefit from input from consumers, family members and providers. Ensures that high quality mental health services programs are implemented to benefit seriously mentally ill populations, disasters or those involved in the criminal justice system.

1504 Center for Mental Health Services Knowledge Exchange Network

US Department of Health and Human Services
PO Box 42490
Washington, DC 20015-4800

800-789-2647
Fax: 301-984-8796
E-mail: ken@mentalhealth.org
www.mentalhealth.org

Information about resources, technical assistance, research, training, networks, and other federal clearing houses, and fact sheets and materials. Information specialists refer callers to mental health resources in their communities as well as state, federal and non-profit contacts. Staff available Monday through Friday, 8:30 AM - 5:00 PM, EST, excluding federal holidays. After hours, callers may leave messages and an information specialist will return their call.

1505 National Alliance for the Mentally Ill

2107 Wilson Boulevard
Suite 300
Arlington, VA 22201-3042   703-524-7600
800-950-6264
Fax: 703-524-9094
TDD: 703-516-7227
E-mail: helpline@nami.org
www.nami.org

Laurie Flynn, Executive Director

Nation's leading self-help organization for all those affected by severe brain disorders. Mission is to bring consumers and families with similar experiences together to share information about services, care providers, and ways to cope with the challenges of schizophrenia, manic depression, and other serious mental illnesses.

1506 National Mental Health Consumer's Self-Help Clearinghouse

1211 Chestnut Street
Suite 1207
Philadelphia, PA 19107   215-751-1810
800-553-4539
Fax: 215-636-6312
E-mail: info@mhselfhelp.org
www.mhselfhelp.org

Alex Morrsey, Information/Referral

Funded by the National Institute of Mental Health Community Support Program, the purpose of the Clearinghouse is to encourage the development and growth of consumer self-help groups.

Year Founded: 1992

1507 Suicide Prevention Advocacy Network (SPAN)

1025 Vermont Avenue NW
Suite 1200
Washington, DC 20005   202-449-3600
Fax: 202-449-3601
E-mail: info@spanusa.org
www.spanusa.org

Gerald H Weyrauch, Chairman
Sandy Martin, Lifekeeper Foundation Founder
Elise P Weyrauch, Administrator

SPAN USA is dedicated to the creation and implementation of effective national suicide prevention stratagies.

Books

1508 Adolescent Suicide

American Psychiatric Publishing
1000 Wilson Boulevard
Suite 1825
Arlington, VA 22209-3901   **703-907-7322**
                                       800-368-5777
                                 Fax: 703-907-1091
                        E-mail: appi@psych.org
                                   www.appi.org

Katie Duffy, Marketing Assistant

Presents techniques that allow psychiatrists and other professionals to respond to signs of distress with timely therapeutic intervention. *$38.95*

212 pages ISBN 0-873182-08-1

1509 Adolescent Suicide: A School-Based Approach to Assessment and Intervention

Research Press
Dept 24 W
PO Box 9177
Champaign, IL 61826   **217-352-3273**
                                 800-519-2707
                           Fax: 217-352-1221
                  E-mail: rp@researchpress.com
                        www.researchpress.com

Russell Pense, VP Marketing

Presents the information required to accurately identify potentially suicidal adolescents and provides the skills necessary for effective intervention. The book includes many case examples derived from information provided by parents, mental health professionals and educators, as well as adolescents who have considered suicide or survived suicide attempts. An essential resource for school counseling staff, psychologists, teachers and administrators. *$14.95*

190 pages ISBN 0-878223-36-3

1510 Anatomy of Suicide: Silence of the Heart

Charles C Thomas Publisher
2600 S First Street
Springfield, IL 62704-4730   **217-789-8980**
                                         800-258-8980
                                   Fax: 217-789-9130
                     E-mail: books@ccthomas.com
                                www.ccthomas.com

The author explores the scope of this problem which involves clinical and ethical issues; the myth of depression; the path to suicide; unfinished business; staying alive; early warnings; first interventions; the self-contract; cases in point; and the future of suicide. Written for psychologists, counselors, and mental health professionals, this book is an excellent resource that will further our understanding of suicide and seek new ways for prevention. *$42.95*

170 pages Year Founded: 1998 ISSN 0-398-06803-8ISBN 0-398068-02-X

1511 Choosing to Live: How to Defeat Suicide through Cognitive Therapy

New Harbinger Publications
5674 Shattuck Avenue
Oakland, CA 94609-1662   **510-652-2002**
                                     800-748-6273
                               Fax: 510-652-5472
       E-mail: customerservice@newharbinger.com
                           www.newharbinger.com

Thomas E Ellis, PsyD
Cory F Newman, PhD

Self help guide to those considering suicide with step by step program for change. *$12.95*

192 pages ISBN 1-572240-56-3

1512 Consumer's Guide to Psychiatric Drugs

New Harbinger Publications
5674 Shattuck Avenue
Oakland, CA 94609-1662   **510-652-2002**
                                     800-748-6273
                               Fax: 510-652-5472
       E-mail: customerservice@newharbinger.com
                           www.newharbinger.com

Helps consumers understand what treatment options are available and what side effects to expect. Covers possible interactions with other drugs, medical conditions and other concerns. Explains how each drug works, and offers detailed information about treatments for depression, bipolar disorder, anxiety and sleep disorders, as well as other conditions. *$16.95*

340 pages ISBN 1-572241-11-X

1513 Harvard Medical School Guide to Suicide Assessment and Intervention

Jossey-Bass / Wiley & Sons
111 River Street
Hoboken, NJ 07030-5774   **201-748-6000**
                               Fax: 201-748-6088
                E-mail: consumers@wiley.com
                                 www.wiley.com

Presents a multidimensional model of suicide assessment by offering clear techniques for intervention in both inpatient and outpatient settings. Also describes the use of psychopharmacology and prevention in the context of managed care. *$59.95*

736 pages Year Founded: 1998 ISBN 0-787943-03-7

1514 In the Wake of Suicide

Jossey-Bass / Wiley & Sons
111 River Street
Hoboken, NJ 07030-5774   **201-748-6000**
                      Fax: 201-748-6088
           E-mail: consumers@wiley.com
                      www.wiley.com

Breathtaking stories of incredible power for anyone struggling to find the meaning in the suicide death of a loved one and for all readers seeking writing that moves and inspires. *$27.00*

256 pages Year Founded: 1998 ISBN 0-787940-52-6

1515 Left Alive: After a Suicide Death in the Family

Charles C Thomas Publisher
2600 S 1st Street
Springfield, IL 62704-4730   **217-789-8980**
                      800-258-8980
                 Fax: 217-789-9130
         E-mail: books@ccthomas.com
                 www.ccthomas.com

Contents: Richard Killed Himself Today; The Fragmented Family; 'If Only I Had...'; If Only 'They' Had; My Child Chose Death; Ruptures in the Relationship; Dad—We're Half a Family Now; My Brother, My Friend; Reaching and Recovering. Epilogue. *$21.95*

120 pages ISBN 0-398066-50-7

1516 Suicidal Adolescents

Charles C Thomas Publisher
2600 S First Street
Springfield, IL 62704-4730   **217-789-8980**
                      800-258-8980
                 Fax: 217-789-9130
         E-mail: books@ccthomas.com
                 www.ccthomas.com

Contents: The History of Social Attitudes Toward Suicide; Adolescence and Suicide; An Overview; The Motivation Underlying Suicidal Behavior; The Etiology of Suicidal Behavior; Prodromal Clues; Treatment; Prevention; Intervention; Postvention; Summary; Recommendations for Those in Contact With Adolescents. References, Glossary. *$32.95*

108 pages ISBN 0-398048-66-5

1517 Suicidal Patient: Principles of Assesment, Treatment, and Case Management

American Psychiatric Publishing
1000 Wilson Boulevard
Suite 1825
Arlington, VA 22209-3901   **703-907-7322**
                      800-368-5777
                 Fax: 703-907-1091
         E-mail: appi@psych.org
                 www.appi.org

Katie Duffy, Marketing Assistant

Presents a clinical approach and valuable assessment strategies and techniques. Demonstrates an easy to use innovative clinical model with specific stages of treatment and associated interventions outlined for inpatient and outpatient settings. *$45.50*

282 pages ISBN 0-800485-54-X

1518 Suicide Over the Life Cycle

American Psychiatric Publishing
1000 Wilson Boulevard
Suite 1825
Arlington, VA 22209-3901   **703-907-7322**
                      800-368-5777
                 Fax: 703-907-1091
         E-mail: appi@psych.org
                 www.appi.org

Katie Duffy, Marketing Assistant

Helps readers understand risk factors and treatment of suicidal patients. *$82.50*

836 pages ISBN 0-880483-07-5

1519 Understanding and Preventing Suicide: New Perspectives

Charles C Thomas Publisher
2600 S 1st Street
Springfield, IL 62704-4730   **217-789-8980**
                      800-258-8980
                 Fax: 217-789-9130
         E-mail: books@ccthomas.com
                 www.ccthomas.com

Seven perspectives for understanding and preventing suicidal behavior, illustrating their implications for prevention. This book discusses suicide from a crimnological perspective, and whether the theories in it have any applicability to suicidal behavior, both in furthering our understanding of suicide and in seeing new ways to prevent suicide. Armed with this information, we may move far toward understanding and preventing suicide in the twenty-first century. *$35.95*

137 pages Year Founded: 1990 ISSN 0-398-06235-8ISBN 0-398057-09-5

1520 Youth Suicide: Issues, Assesment and Intervention

Charles C Thomas Publisher
2600 S 1st Street
Springfield, IL 62704-4730   **217-789-8980**
                      800-258-8980
                 Fax: 217-789-9130
         E-mail: books@ccthomas.com
                 www.ccthomas.com

$33.95

138 pages ISBN 0-398057-06-0

Periodicals & Pamphlets

1521 Suicide (Fast Fact 3)

Center for Mental Health Services: Knowledge Exchange Network
PO Box 42490
Washington, DC 20015

800-789-2647
Fax: 301-984-8796
TDD: 866-889-2647
E-mail: ken@mentalhealth.org
www.mentalhealth.org

This fact card provides statistics and a list of resources on suicide.

1 pages Year Founded: 2000

1522 Suicide Talk: What To Do If You Hear It

ETR Associates
4 Carbonero Way
Scotts Valley, CA 95066

831-438-4060
800-321-4407
Fax: 800-435-8433
E-mail: customerservice@etr.org
www.etr.org

Includes suicide warning signs, how to help a friend, and ways to relieve stress. *$16.00*

1523 Suicide: Who Is at Risk?

ETR Associates
4 Carbonero Way
Scotts Valley, CA 95066

831-438-4060
800-321-4407
Fax: 800-435-8433
E-mail: customerservice@etr.org
www.etr.org

Includes warning signs, symptoms, and what to do. *$16.00*

Support Groups & Hot Lines

1524 Friends for Survival

PO Box 214463
Sacramento, CA 95821

916-392-0664
800-646-7322

Assists family, friends, and professionals following a suicide death.

1525 NineLine

460 W 41st Street
New York, NY 10036

800-999-9999
www.covenanthouse.org/nineline/kid.html

Nationwide crisis/suicide hotline.

1526 Survivors of Loved Ones' Suicides (SOLOS)

PO Box 1716
Springfield, VA 22151-0716

www.1000deaths.com

Web Sites

1527 www.alt.suicide.holiday

Suicide discussion.

1528 www.cyberpsych.org

CyberPsych

Hosts the American Psychoanalyists Foundation, American Association of Suicideology, Society for the Exploration of Psychotherapy Intergration, and Anxiety Disorders Association of America. Also subcategories of the anxiety disorders, as well as general information, including panic disorder, phobias, obsessive compulsive disorder (OCD), social phobia, generalized anxiety disorder, post traumatic stress disorder, and phobias of childhood. Book reviews and links to web pages sharing the topics.

1529 www.lollie.com/suicide.html

Comprehensive Approach to Suicide Prevention

Readings for anyone contemplating suicide.

1530 www.members.aol.com/dswgriff/suicide.html

Now Is Not Forever: A Survival Guide

Print out a no-suicide contract, do problem solving, and other exercises.

1531 www.members.tripod.com/~suicideprevention/ index

Suicide Prevention Help

Coping with suicidal thoughts and friends.

1532 www.mentalhealth.com

Internet Mental Health

On-line information and a virtual encyclopedia related to mental disorders, possible causes and treatments. News, articles, on-line diagnostic programs and related links. Designed to improve understanding, diagnosis and treatment of mental illness throughout the world. Awarded the Top Site Award and the NetPsych Cutting Edge Site Award.

1533 www.metanoia.org/suicide/

If You Are Thinking about Suicide...Read This First

Excellent suggestions, information and links for the suicidal.

1534 www.planetpsych.com

Planetpsych.com

Learn about disorders, their treatments and other topics in psychology. Articles are listed under the related topic areas. Ask a therapist a question for free, or view the directory of professionals in your area. If you are a therapist sign up for the directory. Current features, self-help, interactive, and newsletter archives.

1535 www.psychcentral.com

Psych Central

Personalized one-stop index for psychology, support, and mental health issues, resources, and people on the Internet.

1536 www.psycom.net/depression.central.suicid e. html

Suicide and Suicide Prevention

List of links to material on suicide.

1537 www.save.org

SA/VE - Suicide Awareness/Voices of Education

1538 www.vcc.mit.edu/comm/samaritans/broch ure. html

How to Help Someone You Care About

Guidelines for family.

1539 www.vvc.mit.edu/comm/samaritans/warni ng. html

Signs of Suicide Risk

Introduction

A tic is described as a sudden, rapid, recurrent, non-rhythmic motor movement or vocalization. Four disorders are associated with tics: Chronic Motor or Vocal Tick Disorder, Transient Tic Disorder, Tic Disorder Not Otherwise Specified, and Tourette's Syndrome. Both motor and vocal tics can be classified as either simple or complex. Tourette's Syndrome is the most extreme case displaying multiple motor tics and one or more vocal tics, and will be the focus of this chapter.

SYMPTOMS

•Multiple motor, as well as one or more vocal tics have been present during the illness, not necessarily at the same time;
•The tics occur many times during a day (often in bouts) nearly every day or intermittently throughout for more than one year, and during this period there was never a tic-free period of more three consecutive months;
•The disturbance causes clear distress or difficulties in social, work, or other areas;
•The onset is before age 18;
•The involuntary movements or vocalizations are not due to the direct effects of a substance (e.g., stimulants) or a general medication condition.

ASSOCIATED FEATURES

Between ten percent and forty percent of people with Tourette's Syndrome also have echolalia (repeating words spoken by others) or echopraxia (imitating someone else's movements). Relatively few (less than ten percent) have coprolalia (the involuntary uterance of obscenities).
There seems to be a clear association between tic disorders, such as Tourette's Syndrome and Obsessive Compulsive Disorder (OCD). As many as twenty percent to thirty percent of people with OCD report having or having had tics, and between five percent and seven percent of those with OCD also have Tourette's Syndrome. In studies of patients with Tourette's Syndrome it was found that thirty-six percent to fifty-two percent also meet the criteria for OCD. This is evidence that Tourette's Syndrome and Obsessive Compulsive Disorder share a genetic basis or some underlying pathological/physiological condition. The genetic evidence is further strengthened by the concordance rate in twins (i.e., the likelihood that if one member of the pair has the disorder, the other will also develop it): in identical twins the concordance is fifty-three percent, whereas in fraternal twins it is eight percent.

Other conditions commonly associated with Tourette's Syndrome are hyperactivity, distractibility, impulsivity, difficulty in learning, emotional disturbances, and social problems. The nature of the disorder is often accompanied by social uneasiness, shame, self-consciousness, and depression. The person may be rejected by others and may develop anxiety about the tics, negatively affecting social, school, and work functioning. In severe cases, the disorder may interfere with everyday activities like reading and writing.

PREVALENCE

Tourette's Syndrome is reported in a variety of ethnic and cultural groups. It is one and one-half to three times more common in males than females and about 10 times more prevalent in children and adolescents than in adults. Overall prevalence is estimated at between four and five people in 10,000.

While the age of onset can be as early as two years, it commonly begins during childhood or early adolescence. The median age for the development of tics is seven years. The disorder usually lasts for the life of the person, but there may be periods of remission of weeks, months, or years. The severity, frequency, and variability of the tics often diminish during adolescence and adulthood. In some cases, tics can disappear entirely by early adulthood.

TREATMENT OPTIONS

Many treatments have been tried. Haloperidol, an antipsychotic drug, is the most effective; it acts directly on the brain source of the tic, counteracting the overactivity, and can have a calming effect, but also can have unfortunate side effects. In very severe, disabling cases of OCD, brain surgery is an option. SSRIs (Selective Serotonin Reuptake Inhibitors) have also been effective in some cases of Tic Disorders. Symptoms of the disorder usually diminish with increasing age, and many people learn to live with them.

Associations & Agencies

1541 Center for Family Support (CFS)

333 7th Avenue
New York, NY 10001-5004   212-629-7939
                                  Fax: 212-239-2211
                                  www.cfsny.org

Steven Vernickofs, Executive Director

Service agency devoted to the physical well-being and development of the retarded child and the sound mental health of the parents. Helps families with retarded children with all aspects of home care including counseling, referrals, home aide service and consultation. Offers intervention for parents at the birth of a retarded child with in-home support, guidance and infant stimulation. Pioneered training of nonprofessional women as home aides to provide supportive services in homes.

1542 Center for Mental Health Services Knowledge Exchange Network

US Department of Health and Human Services
PO Box 42490
Washington, DC 20015-4800

                                  800-789-2647
                                  Fax: 301-984-8796
                                  E-mail: ken@mentalhealth.org
                                  www.mentalhealth.org

Information about resources, technical assistance, research, training, networks, and other federal clearing houses, and fact sheets and materials. Information specialists refer callers to mental health resources in their communities as well as state, federal and nonprofit contacts. Staff available Monday through Friday, 8:30 AM - 5:00 PM, EST, excluding federal holidays. After hours, callers may leave messages and an information specialist will return their call.

1543 NADD: Association for Persons with Developmental Disabilities and Mental Health Needs

132 Fair Street
Kingston, NY 12401-4802   845-334-4336
                                  800-331-5362
                                  Fax: 845-331-4569
                                  E-mail: nadd@mhv.net
                                  www.thenadd.org

Dr. Robert Fletcher, Executive Director

Nonprofit organization designed to promote interest of professional and parent development with resources for individuals who have the coexistence of mental illness and mental retardation. Provides conference, educational services and training materials to professionals, parents, concerned citizens and service organizations. Formerly known as the National Association for the Dually Diagnosed.

1544 National Alliance for the Mentally Ill

2107 Wilson Boulevard
Suite 300
Arlington, VA 22201-3042   703-524-7600
                                  800-950-6264
                                  Fax: 703-524-9094
                                  TDD: 703-516-7227
                                  E-mail: helpline@nami.org
                                  www.nami.org

Laurie Flynn, Executive Director

Nation's leading self-help organization for all those affected by severe brain disorders. Mission is to bring consumers and families with similar experiences together to share information about services, care providers, and ways to cope with the challenges of schizophrenia, manic depression, and other serious mental illnesses.

1545 National Mental Health Consumer's Self-Help Clearinghouse

1211 Chestnut Street
Suite 1207
Philadelphia, PA 19107   215-751-1810
                                  800-553-4539
                                  Fax: 215-636-6312
                                  E-mail: info@mhselfhelp.org
                                  www.mhselfhelp.org

Alex Morrsey, Information/Referral

Funded by the National Institute of Mental Health Community Support Program, the purpose of the Clearinghouse is to encourage the development and growth of consumer self-help groups.

Year Founded: 1992

1546 Tourette Syndrome Association

42-40 Bell Boulevard
Suite 205
Bayside, NY 11361-2820   718-224-2999
                                  888-486-8738
                                  Fax: 718-279-9596
                                  E-mail: ts@tsa-usa.org
                                  www.tsa-usa.org

Tracy Flynn, Public Information

National, nonprofit voluntary health organization with 50 chapters in the US and over 45 contacts in other countries. Members include people with TS, their relatives and other interested, concerned supporters. Maintains a crisis hotline, physician referral listings by state, and medical referrals in other countries. Publishes a brochure titled Questions and Answers about Tourette Syndrome.

Books

1547 Adam and the Magic Marble

Hope Press
PO Box 188
Duarte, CA 91009-0188

                                  800-321-4039
                                  Fax: 818-358-3520
                                  E-mail: dcomings@mail.earthlink.net
                                  www.hopepress.com

Exciting reading for all ages, and a must for those who have been diagnosed with Tourette syndrome or other disabilities. An up-beat story of three heros, two with Tourette syndrome, one with cerebal palsy. Constantly taunted by bullies, the boys find a marble full of magic power, they aim a spell at the bullies and the adventure begins. *$6.95*

1548 Children with Tourette Syndrome: A Parent's Guide

ADD WareHouse
300 NW 70th Avenue
Suite 102
Plantation, FL 33317　　　　**954-792-8100**
800-233-9273
Fax: 954-792-8545
E-mail: sales@addwarehouse.com
www.addwarehouse.com

The first guide written specifically for parents and other family members is a collaboration by a team of medical specialists, therapists, people with TS, and parents. It provides a complete introduction to TS and how it's diagnosed and treated. Also, chapters on family life, emotions, education and legal rights. *$17.00*

340 pages

1549 Don't Think About Monkeys: Extraordinary Stories Written by People with Tourette Syndrome

Hope Press
PO Box 188
Duarte, CA 91009-0188
800-321-4039
Fax: 626-358-3520
www.hopepress.com

Collection of fourteen stories written by teenager and adults with Tourette syndrome, describing how they have managed to cope and live with disorder. Especially inspiring to others with this and similar disorders. *$12.95*

200 pages ISBN 1-878267-33-7

1550 Echolalia: an Adult's Story of Tourette Syndrome

Hope Press
PO Box 188
Duarte, CA 91009-0188　　　　**818-303-0644**
800-321-4039
Fax: 818-358-3520
www.hopepress.com

Story of best selling writer Jackson Evans, who was diagnosed at age 35 as having Tourette syndrome and obsessive-compulsive disorder. At first he is grateful for the answers it brings him, but Jackson soon realizes that the real problems are just beginning. Story is told in a poetic style that captures the rhythms that smooth the Tourette. It ends with the ultimate truth, the answer isn't in being diagnosed, the answer is in living. *$11.95*

165 pages ISBN 1-878267-31-0

1551 Hi, I'm Adam: a Child's Story of Tourette Syndrome

Hope Press
PO Box 188
Duarte, CA 91009-0188　　　　**818-303-0644**
800-321-4039
Fax: 818-358-3520
www.hopepress.com

Adam Buehrens is ten years old and has Tourette syndrome. Adam wrote and illustrated this book because he wants everyone to know he and other children with Tourette syndrome are not crazy. They just hava a common neurological disorder. If you know a child that has tics, temper tantrums, unreasonable fears, or problems dealing with school, you will find this a reassuring story. *$4.95*

35 pages ISBN 1-878267-29-9

1552 Mind of its Own, Tourette's Syndrome: Story and a Guide

Oxford University Press
198 Madison Avenue
New York, NY 10016　　　　**212-726-6000**
800-451-7556
Fax: 919-677-1303
www.oup-usa.org/orbs/

Composed of two parts which interdigitate with each other. One part is an on-going story about Michael, a boy with TS, and his family and friends. Michael is a fictional composite character drawn from experience with many patients. Portrays a relatively mild case because the majority of the cases are mild. The second part consists of factural information which we have tried to present in a clear and readable manner. Includes illustration, some tables and other materials that may be of interest.

174 pages ISBN 0-195065-87-5

1553 RYAN: a Mother's Story of Her Hyperactive/Tourette Syndrome Child

Hope Press
PO Box 188
Duarte, CA 91009-0188　　　　**818-303-0644**
800-321-4039
Fax: 818-358-3520
E-mail: dcomings@mail.earthlink.net
www.hopepress.com

A moving and informative story of how a mother struggled with the many behavioral problems presented by her son with Tourette syndrome, ADHD and oppositional defiant disorder. *$9.95*

302 pages ISBN 1-878267-25-6

1554 Raising Joshua

Hope Press
PO Box 188
Duarte, CA 91009-0188　　　　**818-303-0644**
800-321-4039
Fax: 818-358-3520
E-mail: dcomings@mail.earthlink.net
www.hopepress.com

A mothers story of Josh, a boy with Tourette Syndrome and Attention Deficit Hyperactivity Disorder. *$14.95*

ISBN 0-965750-17-

1555 Teaching the Tiger, a Handbook for Individuals Involved in the Education of Students with Attention Deficit Disorders, Tourette Syndrome, or Obsessive - Compulsive Disorder

Hope Press
PO Box 188
Duarte, CA 91009-0188   **818-303-0644**
                                   800-321-4039
                        Fax: 818-358-3520
     E-mail: dcomings@mail.earthlink.net
                        www.hopepress.com

Innovative methods of teaching children with ADD, Tourette Syndrome, Obsessive-Compulsive Disorders. *$35.00*

ISBN 1-878267-34-5

1556 Tourette Syndrome

Dilligaf Publishing for Awareness Project
64 Court Street
Ellsworth, ME 04605   **207-667-5031**
          E-mail: awareness@acadia.net

Includes an overview of the syndrome and tips of how to recognize traditional tics in the classroom; evaulation and referral are the basic components of this easy-to-read, basic book for the classroom teacher.

20 pages

1557 Tourette Syndrome and Human Behavior

Hope Press
PO Box 188
Duarte, CA 91009-0188   **818-303-0644**
                                   800-321-4039
                        Fax: 818-358-3520
     E-mail: dcomings@mail.earthlink.net
                        www.hopepress.com

How Tourette syndrome, a common hereditary disorder, provides insights into the cause and treatment of a wide range of human behavioral problems. It covers diagnosis, associated behaviors including ADHD, learning disorders, dyslexia, conduct disorder, obsessive-compulsive behaviors, alcoholism, drug abuse, obesity, depression, panic attacks, phobias, night terrors, bed wetting, sleep disturbances, lying, steeling, inappropiate sexual behavior, and others, brain structure and chemistry and implications for society. *$39.95*

850 pages ISBN 1-878267-28-0

1558 Tourette's Syndrome, Tics, Obsession, Compulsions: Developmental Psychopathology & Clinical Care

John Wiley & Sons
605 3rd Avenue
New York, NY 10058-0180   **212-850-6000**
                        Fax: 212-850-6008
          E-mail: info@wiley.com
                        www.wiley.com

Once thought to be rare, Tourette's Syndeome is now seen as a relatively common childhood disorder either in its complete or partial incarnations. Drawing on the work of contributors hailing from the Yale Unversity Child Psychiatry Department, this edited volume explores the disorder from many perspectives, mapping out the diagnosis, genetics, phenomenology, natural history, and treatment of Tourette's Syndrome. *$189.00*

584 pages ISBN 0-471160-37-7

1559 Tourette's Syndrome: The Facts

Oxford University Press
198 Madison Avenue
New York, NY 10016   **212-726-6000**
                                800-451-7556
                        Fax: 919-677-1303
                www.oup-usa.org/orbs/

Paperback. *$16.95*

128 pages ISBN 0-198523-98-X

1560 Tourette's Syndrome: Tics, Obsessions, Compulsions

ADD WareHouse
300 NW 70th Avenue
Suite 102
Plantation, FL 33317   **954-792-8100**
                                   800-233-9273
                        Fax: 954-792-8545
     E-mail: sales@addwarehouse.com
                        www.addwarehouse.com

Drawing on the work of contributors hailing from the prestigious Yale University Child Psychiatry Department, this edited volume explores the disorder from many perspectives, mapping out the diagnosis, genetics, phenomenology, natural history and treatment of Tourette's Syndrome. *$89.95*

584 pages

1561 What Makes Ryan Tic?: a Family's Triunph Over Tourette's Syndrome and Attention Deficit Hyperactivity Disorder

Hope Press
PO Box 188
Duarte, CA 91009-0188   **818-303-0644**
                                   800-321-4039
                        Fax: 818-358-3520
     E-mail: dcomings@mail.earthlink.net
                        www.hopepress.com

A moving and informative story of how a mother struggled with the many behavioral problems presented by her son with Tourette syndrome, ADHD and oppostional defiant disorder. *$15.95*

303 pages ISBN 1-878267-35-3

Support Groups & Hot Lines

1562 Tourette Syndrome Association

42-40 Bell Boulevard
Bayside, NY 11361-2820

718-224-2999
Fax: 718-224-9596
E-mail: ts@tsa-usa.org
www.tsa-usa.org

Tracy Flynn, Public Information

National voluntary, nonprofit organization working to identify the cause of, find the cure for and control the effects of this disorder. Today, TSA has grown into a major organization with 50 US chapters and 300 support groups, plus international contacts around the world.

Year Founded: 1972

Video & Audio

1563 After the Diagnosis...The Next Steps

Tourette Syndrome Association
42-40 Bell Boulevard
Suite 205
Bayside, NY 11361-2874

718-224-2999
888-486-8738
Fax: 718-279-9596
E-mail: ts@tsa-usa.org
www.tsa-usa.org

When the diagnosis is Tourette Syndrome, what do you do first? How do you sort out the complexities of the disorder? Whose advice do you follow? What steps do you take to lead a normal life? Six people with TS—as different as any six people can be—relate the sometimes difficult, but finally triumphant path each took to lead the rich, fulfilling life they now enjoy. Narrated by Academy Award-winning actor, Richard Dreyfuss, the stories are refreshing blends of poignancy, fact, and inspiration illustrating that a diagnosis of TS can be approached with confidence and hope. Includes comments by family and friends, teachers, counselors and leading medical authorities on Tourette Syndrome. A must-see for the newly diagnosed child, teen or adult.

1564 Clinical Counseling: Toward a Better Understanding of TS

Tourette Syndrome Association
42-40 Bell Boulevard
Suite 205
Bayside, NY 11361-2874

718-224-2999
888-486-8738
Fax: 718-279-9596
E-mail: ts@tsa-usa.org
www.tsa-usa.org

Certain key issues often surface during the counseling sessions of people wwith TS and their families. These important areas of concern are explored for counselors, social workers, educators, psychologists and other allied professionals. Expert clinical practitioners offer invaluable insights for those working with people affected by Tourette Syndrome.

1565 Complexities of TS Treatment: Physician's Roundtable

Tourette Syndrome Association
42-40 Bell Boulevard
Suite 205
Bayside, NY 11361-2874

718-224-2999
888-486-8738
Fax: 718-279-9596
E-mail: ts@tsa-usa.org
www.tsa-usa.org

Three of the most highly regarded experts in the diagnosis and treatment of Tourette Syndrome offer insight, advice and treatment strategies to fellow physicians and other healthcare professionals.

1566 Family Life with Tourette Syndrome... Personal Stories

Tourette Syndrome Association
42-40 Bell Boulevard
Suite 205
Bayside, NY 11361-2874

718-224-2999
888-486-8738
Fax: 718-279-9596
E-mail: ts@tsa-usa.org
www.tsa-usa.org

In extended, in-depth interviews, all the people engagingly profiled in After the Diagnosis...The Next Steps, reveal the individual ways they developed to deal with TS. Each shows us that the key to leading a successful life in spite of having TS, is having a loving, supportive network of family and friends. Available in its entirety or as separate vignettes.

1567 Understanding and Treating the Hereditary Psychiatric Spectrum Disorders

Hope Press
PO Box 188
Duarte, CA 91009-0188

818-303-0644
800-321-4039
Fax: 818-358-3520
www.hopepress.com

David E Comings MD, Presenter

Learn with ten hours of audio tapes from a two day seminar given in May 1997 by David E Comings, MD. Tapes cover: ADHD, Tourette Syndrome, Obsessive-Compulsive Disorder, Conduct Disorder, Oppositional Defiant Disorder, Autism and other Hereditary Psychiatric Spectrum Disorders. Eight Audio tapes. *$75.00*

Year Founded: 1997

Web Sites

Web site of the association dedicated to identifying the cause, finding the cure and controlling the effects of TS.

1568 www.mentalhealth.com
Internet Mental Health

On-line information and a virtual encyclopedia related to mental disorders, possible causes and treatments. News, articles, on-line diagnostic programs and related links. Designed to improve understanding, diagnosis and treatment of mental illness throughout the world. Awarded the Top Site Award and the NetPsych Cutting Edge Site Award.

1569 www.planetpsych.com
Planetpsych.com

Learn about disorders, their treatments and other topics in psychology. Articles are listed under the related topic areas. Ask a therapist a question for free, or view the directory of professionals in your area. If you are a therapist sign up for the directory. Current features, self-help, interactive, and newsletter archives.

1570 www.psychcentral.com
Psych Central

Personalized one-stop index for psychology, support, and mental health issues, resources, and people on the Internet.

1571 www.tourette-syndrome.com

Online community devoted to children and adults with Tourette Syndrome disorder and their families, friends, teachers, and medical professionals. Provides an interactive meeting place for those interested in TS.

1572 www.tourettesyndrome.net
Tourette Syndrome Plus

Parent and teacher friendly site on Tourette Syndrome, Attention Deficit Disorder, Executive Dysfunction, Obessive Compulsive Disorder, and related conditions.

1573 www.tsa-usa.com
Tourette Syndrome Association

Educational information for patients, caregivers and physicians.

1574 www.tsa-usa.org
Tourette Syndrome Association

Associations & Agencies

1575 American Academy of Child and Adolescent Psychiatry

3615 Wisconsin Avenue NW
Washington, DC 20016-3007   202-966-7300
                                Fax: 202-966-2891
                                www.aacap.org

Professional medical organization comprised of child and adolescent psychiatrist trained to promote healthy development and to evaluate, diagnose, and treat children and adolescents and their families who are affected by disorders of feeling, thinking and behavior. Child and adolescent psychiatrists are physicians who are uniquely qualified to integrate knowledge about human behavior, social, and cultural perspectives with scientific, humanistic, and collaborative approaches to diagnosis, treatment and the promotion of mental health.

1576 American Academy of Pediatrics

141 NW Point Boulevard
Elk Grove Village, IL 60007   847-434-4000
                                 Fax: 847-434-8000
                                 E-mail: cme@aap.org
                                 www.aap.org

Provides information on diagnosis and treatment of physical and mental pediatric conditions by offering programs, training, and resources.

1577 American Association for Geriatric Psychiatry

7910 Woodmont Avenue
Suite 1050
Bethesda, MD 20814-3084   301-654-7850
                                 Fax: 301-654-4137
                                 E-mail: main@aagponline.org
                                 www.aagpgpa.org

Christine deVries, Executive Director
Marjerie Vanderbilt, Dir Government Affairs
Jeannine Rowe, Director of Education

American Association for Geriatric Psychiatry (AAGP) is a national association representing and serving its members and the field of geriatric psychiatry. It is dedicated to promoting the mental health and well-being of older people and improving the care of those with late life mental disorders. AAGP enhances the knowledge base and standards of practice in geriatric psychiatry through education and research and by advocating for meeting the mental health needs of older Americans.

1578 American Pediatrics Society

3400 Research Forest Drive
Suite B-7
The Woodlands, TX 77381   281-419-0052
                                 Fax: 281-419-0082
                                 E-mail: info@aps-spr.org
                                 www.aps-spr.org

Society of professionals working with pediatric health care issues; offers seminars and a variety of publications.

1579 Association for the Help of Retarded Children

200 Park Avenue S
Suite 1201
New York, NY 10003-1503   212-780-2500
                                 Fax: 212-777-5893
                                 E-mail: ahrcnyc@dti.net
                                 www.ahrcnyc.org

Shirley Berenstein, Director
Jennifer Rossiter, Contact

Developmentally disabled children and adults, their families, and interested individuals. Provides support services, training programs, clinics, schools and residential facilities to the developmentally disabled. Publications: The Chronicle, quarterly newsletter.

1580 Center for Family Support (CFS)

333 7th Avenue
New York, NY 10001-5004   212-629-7939
                                 Fax: 212-239-2211
                                 www.cfsny.org

Steven Vernickofs, Executive Director

Service agency devoted to the physical well-being and development of the retarded child and the sound mental health of the parents. Helps families with retarded children with all aspects of home care including counseling, referrals, home aide service and consultation. Offers intervention for parents at the birth of a retarded child with in-home support, guidance and infant stimulation. Pioneered training of nonprofessional women as home aides to provide supportive services in homes.

1581 Federation for Children with Special Needs (FCSN)

1135 Tremont Street
Suite 420
Boston, MA 02120   617-236-7210
                                 800-331-0688
                                 Fax: 617-572-2094
                                 E-mail: fcsninfo@fcsn.org
                                 www.fcsn.org

Rich Robison, Executive Director

The federation provides information, support, and assistance to parents of children with disabilities, their professional partners and their communities.

1582 Federation of Families for Children's Mental Health

1101 King Street
Suite 420
Alexandria, VA 22314   703-684-7710
                                 Fax: 703-836-1040
                                 E-mail: ffcmh@ffcmh.org
                                 www.ffcmh.org

Barbara Huff, Executive Director

National family-run organization dedicated exclusively to children and adolesents with mental health needs and their families. Our voice speaks through our work in policy, training and technical assistance programs. Publishes a quarterly newsletter and sponsors an annual conference and exhibits.

1583 Lifespire

345 Hudson Street
3rd Floor
New York, NY 10014   212-741-0100
Fax: 212-463-9814
E-mail: info@lifespire.org
www.lifespire.com

Professionals, parents, sibilings, and others interested in mentally retarded and developmentally disabled adults. Offers professionally supervised programs for mentally retarded and developmentally disabled adults including vocational rehabilitation, dual diagnosis programs, job placement, rehabilitation workshops, activities for daily living, day treatment, day training, supported work, and family support programs.

1584 Mentally Ill Kids in Distress

755 E Willetta Street, Suite 128
Phoenix, AZ 85006   602-253-1240
Fax: 602-523-1250
E-mail: mikidaz@qwest.net
www.mikid.org

1585 Michigan Association for Children's Mental Health

941 Abbott Road
Suite P
East Lansing, MI 48823-3104   517-336-7222
Fax: 517-336-8884
E-mail: acmhlori@acd.net
www.acmh-mi.org

Sara Way, Director

Promotes development of a system of care for families of children with emotional, behavioral or mental health disorders through community education and awareness, family support and involvement and the persistent pursuit of advocacy to improve the quality of life.

1586 National Child Support Network

PO Box 1018
Fayetteville, AR 72702-1018
800-729-5437
www.childsupport.org

1587 National Information Center for Children and Youth with Disabilities

PO Box 1492
Washington, DC 20013
800-695-0285

1588 National Technical Assistance Center for Children's Mental Health

Georgetown University Child Development Center
3307 M Street NW
Washington, DC 20007   202-687-5000
Fax: 202-687-1954
TTY: 202-687-5503
E-mail: gucdc@georgetown.edu
www.dml.georgetown.edu/research/gucdc/cassp.html

Integral part of the Georgetown University Center for Child and Human Development at the Georgetown University Medical Center. Nationally recognized for its work in assisting states and communities build systems of care for mental health concerns.

Year Founded: 1984

1589 Parents Helping Parents

3041 Olcott Street
Santa Clara, CA 95054   408-727-5775
Fax: 408-727-0182
E-mail: general@php.com
www.php.com

Lois Jones, Executive Director

Nonprofit family resource center offering culturally sensitve information and peer counseling, provides a forum for parents and professionals to get information. PHP does not promote or recommend any treatment, therapy, institution or professional.

1590 Parents Information Network FFCMH

1101 King Street
Suite 420
Alexandria, VA 22314   703-684-7710
Fax: 703-836-1040
E-mail: ffcmh@ffcmh.org
www.ffcmh.org/local.htm

Bridget Schneider, Facilitator

National parent run organization focused on the needs of children and youth with emotional, behavioral or mental disorders and their families.

1591 Pilot Parents: PP

Ollie Webb Center
1941 S 42nd Street
Suite 122
Omaha, NE 68105-2942   402-346-5220
Fax: 402-346-5253
E-mail: jvarner@olliewebb.org
www.olliebebb.org

Jennifer Varner, Coordinator

Parents, professionals and others concerned with providing emotional and peer support to new parents of children with special needs. Sponsors a parent-matching program which allows parents who have had sufficient experience and training in the care of their own children to share their knowledge and expertise with parents of children recently diagnosed as disabled. Publications: The Gazette, newsletter, published 6 times a year. Also available in Arizona and limited other states.

1592 Research and Training Center for Children's Mental Health

Univerity of South Florida
13303 Bruce B Downs Boulevard
Department of Child and Family
Tampa, FL 33612 813-974-4661
Fax: 813-974-6257
www.rtckids.fmhi.usf.edu

Bob Frieman PhD, Department Chairman

State initiative for clinical studies of pediatric mental health issues.

1593 Research and Training Center on Family Support and Children's Mental Health

Portland State University/Regional Research Institute
PO Box 751
Portland State University
Portland, OR 97207-0751 503-725-4040
Fax: 503-725-4180
E-mail: gordon@pdx.edu
www.rtc.pdx.edu

Lynwood Gordon, Public Information/Outreach
Janet Walker, Editor

Dedicated to promoting effective community based, culturally competent, family centered services for families and their children who are or may be affected by mental, emotional or behavioral disorders. This goal is accomplished through collaborative research partnerships with family members, service providers, policy makers, and other concerned persons. Major efforts in dissemination and training include: An annual conference, an award winning web site to share information about child and family mental services and policy issues which includes Focal Point, a national bulletin regarding family support and children's mental health.

1594 Resources for Children with Special Needs

116 E 16th Street
5th Floor
New York, NY 10003 212-677-4650
Fax: 212-254-4070
E-mail: info@resourcesnyc.org
www.resourcenyc.org

Karen T Schlesinger, Executive Director
Dianne Littwin, Director Publications

Information, referral, advocacy, training, publications for New York City parents of youth with disabilities or special needs and the professionals who work with them.

1595 United Families for Children's Mental Health

13301 Bruce B Downs Boulevard
FMHI Box 2, Room 2514
Tampa, FL 33612 813-974-7930
Fax: 813-974-7712
E-mail: ffcmh@earthlink.net

Carol Baier

1596 Young Adult Institute and Workshop (YAI)

460 W 34th Street
New York, NY 10001-2382 212-273-6100
www.yai.org

Joel M Levy, Executive Director/CEO
Phil Levy, President/COO

Serves more than 15,000 people of all ages and levels of mental retardation, developmental and learning disabilities. Provides a full range of early intervention, preschool, family supports, employment training and placement, clinical and residential services, as well as recreation and camping services. YAI/National Intitute for People with Disabilities is also a professional organization, nationally renowned for its publications, conferences, training seminars, video training tapes and innovative television programs.

1597 Youth Services International

1819 Main Street
Suite 1000
Sarasota, FL 34236 941-953-9199
Fax: 941-953-9198
E-mail: YSIWEB@youthservices.com
www.youthservices.com

1598 Zero to Three

2000 M Street NW
Suite 200
Washington, DC 20036 202-638-1144
800-899-4301
Fax: 202-638-0851
E-mail: oto3@presswarehouse.com
www.zerotothree.org

Matthew E Melmed JD, Executive Director
Emily Fanichel, Associate Director

Professionals and researchers in the health care industry, policymakers and parents working to improve the healthy physical, cognitive and social development of infants, toddlers and their families. Sponsors training and technical assistance activities. Publications: Clinical Infant Reports, book series. Public Policy Pamphlets, 1 to 3 times per year. Zero to Three, 6 times per year, Annual National Training Institute conference and exhibits, usually in December.

Books

1599 13 Steps to Help Families Stop Fighting and Solve Problems Peacefully

Childs Work/Childs Play
135 Dupont Street
PO Box 760
Plainville, NY 11803-0760
800-962-1141
Fax: 800-262-1886
E-mail: info@Childswork.com
www.Childswork.com

Candid views on why families fight, and solutions to conflict. *$15.95*

1600 Aggression Replacement Training: A Comprehensive Intervention for Aggressive Youth

Research Press
Dept 24 W
PO Box 9177
Champaign, IL 61826

217-352-3273
800-519-2707
Fax: 217-352-1221
E-mail: rp@researchpress.com
www.researchpress.com

Russell Pense, VP Marketing

Aggression Replacement Training (ART) offers a comprehensive intervention program designed to teach adolescents to understand and replace aggression and antisocial behavior with positive alternatives. The book is designed to be user-friendly and teacher-oriented. It contains summaries of ART's outcome evaluations and it discusses recent applications in schools and other settings. *$24.95*

366 pages ISBN 0-878223-79-7

1601 Bibliotherapy Starter Set

Childs Work/Childs Play
135 Dupont Street
PO Box 760
Plainville, NY 11803-0760

800-962-1141
Fax: 800-262-1886
E-mail: info@Childswork.com
www.Childswork.com

Eight popular books for helping children ages four - twelve. Titles include Self Esteem, Divorce, ADHD, Feelings, and Anger. *$89.95*

1602 Book of Psychotheraputic Homework

Childs Work/Childs Play
135 Dupont Street
PO Box 760
Plainville, NY 11803-0760

800-962-1141
Fax: 800-262-1886
E-mail: info@Childswork.com
www.Childswork.com

More than 80 home activities to guarantee your therapy won't lose momentum. Appropriate for ages five - ten. *$20.95*

1603 Breaking the Silence: Teaching the Next Generation About Mental Illness

NAMI Queens/Nassau
1983 Marcus Avenue
Lake Success, NY 11042

516-326-0797
Fax: 576-437-5785
E-mail: btslessonplans@aol.com
www.btslessonplans.org

Amy Lax, Director PR/Educational Outreach
Janet Susin, Project Director
Lorraine Kaplan, Director Educational Training

Breaking the Silence (BTS) is an innovative teaching package which includes lesson plans, games and posters on serious mental illness for three grade levels: upper elementary, middle and high school. It is designed to fight stigma by putting a human face on mental illness, replacing fear and ridicule with compassion. BTS meets national health standards.

1604 CARE Child and Adolescent Risk Evaluation: A Measure of the Risk for Violent Behavior

Research Press
Dept 24 W
PO Box 9177
Champaign, IL 61826

217-352-3273
800-519-2707
Fax: 217-352-1221
E-mail: rp@researchpress.com
www.researchpress.com

Russell Pense, VP Marketing

The CARE was developed as a prevention tool to identify youth, as early as possible, who are at risk for committing acts of violence. Unlike other evaluation programs, CARE includes a case management planning form that provides the information needed to develop a risk management intervention plan. The CARE Kit includes 25 assessment forms, 25 case management planning forms and manual. *$75.00*

1605 Children and Trauma: Guide for Parents and Professionals

Courage to Change
PO Box 1268
Newburgh, NY 12551-1268

800-440-4003
Fax: 800-772-6499

Comprehensive guide to the emotional aftermath of children's crises. Discusses warning signs that a child may need professional help, and explores how parents and professionals can help children heal, reviving a sense of well being and safety. *$19.95*

240 pages

1606 Childs Work/Childs Play

135 Dupont Street
PO Box 760
Plainview, NY 11803-0760

800-962-1141
Fax: 800-262-1886
E-mail: info@Childswork.com
www.Childswork.com

Catalog of books, games, toys and workbooks relating to child development issues such as recognizing emotions, handling uncertainty, bullies, ADD, shyness, conflicts and other things that children may need some help navigating.

Pediatric & Adolescent Issues/Books

1607 Creative Therapy with Children and Adolesent s

Impact Publishers
PO Box 6016
Atascadero, CA 93423-6016
805-466-5917
800-246-7228
Fax: 805-466-5919
E-mail: info@impactpublishers.com
www.impactpublishers.com

Over 100 activities to be used in working with children, adolesents and families. Encourages creativity in therapy and helps therapists facilitate change by gaining rapport with children and other clients who find it difficult to talk about feelings and experiences. $21.95

192 pages ISBN 1-886230-19-6

1608 Forms Book Set

Childs Work/Childs Play
135 Dupont Street
PO Box 760
Plainville, NY 11803-0760
800-962-1141
Fax: 800-262-1886
E-mail: info@Childswork.com
www.Childswork.com

Five-book pack with reproducible forms titled: Oppositional Child, Children with OCD, Counseling Children, ADHD Child and Socially Fearful Child.

1609 Forms for Behavior Analysis with Children

Research Press
Dept 24 W
PO Box 9177
Champaign, IL 61826
217-352-3273
800-519-2707
Fax: 217-352-1221
E-mail: rp@researchpress.com
www.researchpress.com

Russell Pense, VP Marketing

A unique collection of 42 reproducible assessment forms designed to aid counselors and therapists in making proper diagnoses and in developing treatment plans for children and adolescents. Different assessment formats are included, ranging from direct observations and interviews to informant ratings and self-reports. Certain forms are to be filled out by children and adolescents, while others are to be completed by parents, school personnel, significant others or the therapist. $ 39.95

208 pages ISBN 0-878222-67-7

1610 Gangs in Schools: Signs, Symbols and Solutions

Research Press
Dept 24 W
PO Box 9177
Champaign, IL 61826
217-352-3273
800-519-2707
Fax: 217-352-1221
E-mail: rp@researchpress.com
www.researchpress.com

Russell Pense, VP Marketing

Written by noted authority Arnold Goldstein and gang expert Donald Kodluboy, this book is an essential resource for educators and administrators who are concerned about gang presence or the possibility of gang presence in their schools. The book describes effective gang prevention and intervention strategies. It includes a helpful checklist on how to recognize early gang presence in schools. And it presents a comprehensive plan for maximizing school safety. $19.95

256 pages ISBN 0-878223-82-7

1611 Gender Respect Workbook

Childs Work/Childs Play
135 Dupont Street
PO Box 760
Plainville, NY 11803-0760
800-962-1141
Fax: 800-262-1886
E-mail: info@Childswork.com
www.Childswork.com

Over 100 activities appropriate for ages 8 and up, to help teachers and counselors raise conciousness of sexisim and sexist practices. $18.95

1612 I Wish Daddy Didn't Drink So Much

Childs Work/Childs Play
135 Dupont Street
PO Box 760
Plainville, NY 11803-0760
800-962-1141
Fax: 800-262-1886
E-mail: info@Childswork.com
www.Childswork.com

Realistic and sensitive book about how a girl handles disappointment in her father's problems. Ages 6 - 12. $6.95

1613 Kid Power Tactics for Dealing with Depression & Parent's Survival Guide to Childhood Depression

Childs Work/Childs Play
135 Dupont Street
PO Box 760
Plainville, NY 11803-0760
800-962-1141
Fax: 800-262-1886
E-mail: info@Childswork.com
www.Childswork.com

Two-volume set was wriiten by a child who suffered from depression and his mother. Plain language and a wealth of information for children ages 8 and over, plus their parents and teachers. $30.95

1614 My Body is Mine, My Feelings are Mine

Childs Work/Childs Play
135 Dupont Street
PO Box 760
Plainville, NY 11803-0760
800-962-1141
Fax: 800-262-1886
E-mail: info@Childswork.com
www.Childswork.com

248

For ages 3 - 8. First part to be read to children, the second part teaches adults how to educate children about body safety. Sexual victimization can be prevented through explanation of how to identify inappropriate touching and what to do about it. *$18.95*

1615 My Listening Friend

Childs Work/Childs Play
135 Dupont Street
PO Box 760
Plainview, NY 11803-0760

800-962-1141
Fax: 800-262-1886
E-mail: info@Childswork.com
www.Childswork.com

For ages five - twelve, explores the feelings a child has the first time they see a counselor. Written from the point of view of the child. *$13.50*

60 pages

1616 Saddest Time

Childs Work/Childs Play
135 Dupont Street
PO Box 760
Plainville, NY 11803-0760

800-962-1141
Fax: 800-262-1886
E-mail: info@Childswork.com
www.Childswork.com

Helps children ages 6 - 12 understand that death is sad and sometimes tragic, but it is also part of life. *$13.95*

1617 Teen Relationship Workbook

Childs Work/Childs Play
135 Dupont Street
PO Box 760
Plainville, NY 11803-0760

516-349-5520
800-962-1141
Fax: 800-262-1886
E-mail: info@childswork.com
www.childswork.com

A reproducible workbook, this hands-on tool helps teens develop healthy relationships and prevent dating abuse and domestic violence. *$44.95*

135 pages

1618 What Works When with Children and Adolescents: A Handbook of Individual Counseling Techniques

Research Press
Dept 24 W
PO Box 9177
Champaign, IL 61826

217-352-3273
800-519-2707
Fax: 217-352-1221
E-mail: rp@researchpress.com
www.researchpress.com

Russell Pense, VP Marketing

This practical handbook is designed for counselors, social workers and psychologists in schools and mental health settings. It offers over 100 creative activities and effective interventions for individual counseling with children and adolescents (ages 6-18). Dr. Vernon provides strategies for establishing a therapeutic relationship with students who are sometimes apprehensive or opposed to counseling. Several case studies are included to help illustrate the counseling techniques and interventions. The book also includes a chapter on working with parents and teachers. *$39.95*

344 pages ISBN 0-878224-38-6

Periodicals & Pamphlets

1619 Anxiety Disorders in Children and Adolescents

Center for Mental Health Services: Knowledge Exchange Network
PO Box 42490
Washington, DC 20015

800-789-2647
Fax: 301-984-8796
TDD: 866-889-2647
E-mail: ken@mentalhealth.org
www.mentalhealth.org

This fact sheet defines anxiety disorders, identifies warning signs, discusses risk factors, describes types of help available, and suggests what parents or other caregivers can do.

3 pages

1620 Attention-Deficit/Hyperactivity Disorder in Children and Adolescents

Center for Mental Health Services: Knowledge Exchange Network
PO Box 42490
Washington, DC 20015

800-789-2647
Fax: 301-984-8796
TDD: 866-889-2647
E-mail: ken@mentalhealth.org
www.mentalhealth.org

This fact sheet defines attention-deficit/hyperactivity disorder, describes the warning signs, discusses types of help available, and suggests what parents or other caregivers can do.

3 pages

1621 Autism Spectrum Disorders in Children and Adolescents

Center for Mental Health Services: Knowledge Exchange Network
PO Box 42490
Washington, DC 20015

800-789-2647
Fax: 301-984-8796
TDD: 866-889-2647
E-mail: ken@mentalhealth.org
www.mentalhealth.org

This fact sheet defines autism, describes the signs and causes, discusses types of help available, and suggests what parents or other caregivers can do.

2 pages

1622 Conduct Disorder in Children and Adolescents

Center for Mental Health Services: Knowledge Exchange Network
PO Box 42490
Washington, DC 20015

800-789-2647
Fax: 301-984-8796
TDD: 866-889-2647
E-mail: ken@mentalhealth.org
www.mentalhealth.org

This fact sheet defines conduct disorder, identifies risk factors, discusses types of help available, and suggests what parents or other caregivers can do.

2 pages

1623 Families Can Help Children Cope with Fear, Anxiety

Center for Mental Health Services: Knowledge Exchange Network
PO Box 42490
Washington, DC 20015

800-789-2647
Fax: 301-984-8796
TDD: 866-889-2647
E-mail: ken@mentalhealth.org
www.mentalhealth.org

This fact sheet defines conduct disorder, identifies risk factors, discusses types of help available, and suggests what parents or other caregivers to common signs of fear and anxiety.

1624 Helping Hand

Performance Resource Press
1270 Rankin Drive
Suite F
Troy, MI 48083-2843

248-588-7733
800-453-7733
Fax: 800-499-5718
www.prponline.com

Educates teachers and parents about child and adolescents behavioral health.

4 pages 9 per year

1625 Major Depression in Children and Adolescents

Center for Mental Health Services: Knowledge Exchange Network
PO Box 42490
Washington, DC 20015

800-789-2647
Fax: 301-984-8796
TDD: 866-889-2647
E-mail: ken@mentalhealth.org
www.mentalhealth.org

This fact sheet defines depression and its signs, identifies types of help available, and suggests what parents or other caregivers can do.

2 pages

1626 Mental, Emotional, and Behavior Disorders in Children and Adolescents

Center for Mental Health Services: Knowledge Exchange Network
PO Box 42490
Washington, DC 20015

800-789-2647
Fax: 301-984-8796
TDD: 866-889-2647
E-mail: ken@mentalhealth.org
www.mentalhealth.org

This fact sheet describes mental, emotional, and behavioral problems that can occur during childhood and adolescence and discusses related treatment, support services, and research.

4 pages

Support Groups & Hot Lines

1627 Alateen and Al-Anon Family Groups

1600 Corporate Landing Parkway
Virginia Beach, VA 23454-5617

757-563-1600
888-425-2666
Fax: 757-563-1655
E-mail: wso@al-anon.org
www.al-anon.org

Mary Ann Keller, Director Members Services

A fellowship of youth affected by another persons drinking.

1628 Boys Town National Hotline

1 Hansen Place
Suuite 1301
Brooklyn, NY 11243

718-622-1667
800-448-3000

Crisis intervention and referrals.

1629 CANDU Parent Group

24W681 Woodcrest Road
Naperville, IL 60540-3624

630-983-9027
www.ffcmh.org/local.htm

Cathy Bozett, Facilitator

Support group for parents. Sub-group of the Federation of Families for Children's Mental Health.

1630 CHADD: Children and Adults with AD/HD

8181 Professional Place
Suite 150
Landover, MD 20785

301-306-7070
800-233-4050
Fax: 301-306-7090
www.chadd.org

1631 International Youth Council

401 N Michigan Avenue
Chicago, IL 60611-4212

800-637-7974

Brings together teens living in a single parent homes.

1632 Just Say No International

2101 Webster Street
Oakland, CA 94612-3027

800-258-2766

Provides assistance in avoiding destructive behavior.

1633 Kid Save

3438 Route 309
Orefield, PA 18069

800-999-9999
E-mail: kidsave@kidspeace.org
www.kidspeace.org

Offers information and referrals to children and adolescents.

1634 National Youth Crisis Hotline

5331 Mount Alifan Drive
San Diego, CA 92111-2622

800-448-4663

Information and referral for runaways, and for youth and parents with problems.

1635 NineLine

460 W 41st Street
New York, NY 10036

800-999-9999
www.covenanthouse.org/nineline/kid.html

Nationwide crisis/suicide hotline.

1636 Rainbows

1111 Tower Road
Schaumburg, IL 60173   708-310-1880

Peer support groups for adults and children who are grieving.

1637 SADD: Students Against Drunk Drivers

PO Box 800
Marlboro, MA 01752   508-481-3568

Video & Audio

1638 Aggression Replacement Training Video: A Comprehensive Intervention for Aggressive Youth

Research Press
Dept 24 W
PO Box 9177
Champaign, IL 61826   217-352-3273
800-519-2707
Fax: 217-352-1221
E-mail: rp@researchpress.com
www.researchpress.com

Russell Pense, VP Marketing

For staff training-illustrates the training procedures in the Aggression Replacement Training (ART) book. A free copy of the book accompanies the video program. *$125.00*

1639 Children: Experts on Divorce

Courage to Change
PO Box 1268
Newburgh, NY 1268

800-440-4003
Fax: 800-772-6499

Children of divorced parents are interviewed about their feelings and views of how adults can relate to their children during and after a separation and divorce. The information on this video can help to prevent some of the long-term harm that they may feel. Ages of these children are four to fifteen. 38 minutes. *$34.95*

1640 Chill: Straight Talk About Stress

Childs Work/Childs Play
135 Dupont Street
PO Box 760
Plainview, NY 11803-0760

800-962-1141
Fax: 800-262-1886
E-mail: info@Childswork.com
www.Childswork.com

Encourages youth to recognize, analyze and handle the stresses in their lives. 22 minutes. *$96.95*

1641 Legacy of Childhood Trauma: Not Always Who They Seem

Research Press
Dept 24 W
PO Box 9177
Champaign, IL 61826   217-352-3273
800-519-2707
Fax: 217-352-1221
E-mail: rp@researchpress.com
www.researchpress.com

Russell Pense, VP Marketing

This powerful video focuses on the connection between so-called "delinquent youth" and the experience of childhood trauma such as emotional, sexual, or physical abuse. It inspires viewers to comprehend the emotional betrayal felt by abused children and encourages caregivers to identify strategies for healing and transformation. *$195.00*

Web Sites

1642 www.Al-Anon-Alateen.org

Al-Anon and Alateen

AA literature may serve as an introduction.

1643 www.CHADD.org

CHADD: Children/Adults with Attention Deficit/Hyperactivity Disorder

1644 www.TheAtlantic.com/politics/family/divorce

Divorce and the Family in America

Historical perspective on the family and divorce.

1645 www.abcparenting.com

ABCs of Parenting

1646 www.aboutteensnow.com/dramas

Teen Dramas

Realistic conflicts played out and discussed by a therapist.

1647 www.adhdnews.com.ssi.htm

Social Security

Applying for disability benefits for children with ADHD.

1648 www.adhdnews.com/Advocate.htm

Advocating for Your Child

1649 www.adhdnews.com/sped.htm

Special Education Rights and Responsibilities

Writing IEP's and TIEPS. Pursuing special education services.

1650 www.cfc-efc.ca/docs/00000095.htm

Helping Your Child Cope with Separation and Divorce

1651 www.couns.uiuc.edu

Self-Help Brochures

Address issues teens deal with.

1652 www.divorcedfather.com

Still a Dad

For divorced fathers.

1653 www.duanev/family/dads.html

So What are Dads Good For

1654 www.education.indiana.edu/cas/adol/adol.html

Adolescence Directory On-Line

A collection of documents on the growth and development of adolescents.

1655 www.ericps.crc.uiuc.edu/npin/index.html

NPIN: National Parent Information Network

Information on education.

1656 www.ericps.crc.uiuc.edu/npin/library/texts.html

NPIN Resources for Parents: Full Texts of Parenting-Related Material

1657 www.fathermag.com

Fathering Magazine

Hundreds of articles online.

1658 www.fathers.com

Fatherhood Project

1659 www.flyingsolo.com

Flying Solo

Site on single parenting.

1660 www.fsbassociates.com/fsg/whydivorce.html

Breaking the News

Clear rules on how not to tell kids about divorce.

1661 www.geocities.com/EnchatedForest/1068

Bipolar Kids Homepage

Set of links.

1662 www.home.clara.net/spig/guidline.htm

Guidelines for Separating Parents

1663 www.hometown.aol.com/DrgnKprl/BPCAT.html

Bipolar Children and Teens Homepage

1664 www.ianr.unl.edu/pubs/NebFacts/nf223.htm

Supporting Stepfamilies: What Do the Children Feel

Deals with emotions of children in blended families.

1665 www.kidshealth.org/kid/feeling/index.html

Dealing with Feelings

Ten readings. Examples are: Why Am I So Sad; Are You Shy; Am I Too Fat or Too Thin; and A Kid's Guide to Divorce.

1666 www.kidsource.com/kidsource/pages/parenting

Parenting: General Parenting Articles

1667 www.klis.com/chandler/pamphlet/bipolar/bipolarpamphlet.html

Bipolar Affective Disorder in Children and Adolescents

An introduction for families.

1668 www.klis.com/chandler/pamphlet/dep/depressionpamphlet.htm

Depression in Children and Adolescents

1669 www.klis.com/chandler/pamphlet/panic/

Panic Disorder, Separation, Anxiety Disorder, and Agoraphobia

1670 www.magicnet.net/~hedyyumi/child.html

Learning to Get Along for the Best Interest of the Child

1671 www.mentalhealth.org/publications/allpubs/

Attention-Deficit/Hyperactiviy Disorder in Children and Adolescents

Lists symptoms very fully.

1672 www.muextension.missouri.edu/xpor/hesguide/

Focus on Kids: The Effects of Divorce on Children

Discusses stresses on kids.

1673 www.naturalchild.com/home

Natural Child Project

Articles by experts.

1674 www.nichcy.org

National Information Center for Children and Youth with Disabilities

Excellent information in English and Spanish.

1675 www.nnfr.org/curriculum/topics/sep_div.html

Coping with Separation and Divorce: A Parenting Seminar

1676 www.nospank.org/toc.htm

Project NoSpank

Site for those against paddling in schools.

1677 www.npin.org/library/pre1998/n00216/n00216. html

Plain Talk About...Dealing with the Angry Child

From US Department of Health and Human Services.

Pediatric & Adolescent Issues/Web Sites

1678 www.npin.org/pnews/pnews997/pnew997g
.html
**Temper Tantrums: What Causes Them and How
Can You Respond?**

Parents News publication.

1679 www.oznet.ksu.edu/library/famlf2/
Family Life Library

1680 www.parentcity.com/read/library
Parent City Library

Many articles on parenting.

1681 www.parenthoodweb.com
ParenthoodWeb

Focusing on early childhood.

1682 www.parenthoodweb.com/parent_cfmfiles
/pros. cfm/155
Blended Families

Resolving conflicts.

1683 www.personal.psu.edu/faculty/n/x/nxd10/
Family Relations

Information parenting and family problems.

1684 www.positive-way.com/step.htm
Stepfamily Information

Introduction and tips for stepfathers, stepmothers and
remarried parents.

1685 www.pta.org/commonsense
**Common Sense: Strategies for Raising Alco-
holic/Drug-/Free Children**

Drug facts, warning signs, and guidence.

1686 www.snowcrest.net/skiing/stepmom.htm
Wicked Stepmothers, Fact or Fiction

Details the harm done by stereotyping stepmothers.

1687 www.stepfamily.org/tensteps.htm
Ten Steps for Steps

Guidelines for stepfamilies.

1688 www.stepfamilyinfo.org/sitemap.htm
Stepfamily in Formation

1689 www.teenwire.com/index.asp
Teenwire

Information on relationships and sexuality.

1690 www.todaysparent.com
Today's Parent Online

1691 www.users.aol.com:80/jimams/answers1.h
tml
Questions from Younger Children about ADD

Responses to children's questions.

1692 www.users.aol.com:80/jimams/answers2.h
tml
Questions from Adolescents about ADD

Responses to children's questions.

1693 www.wholefamily.com/kidteencenter/inde
x.html
About Teens Now

Addresses important issues in teens lives.

1694 www.worldcollegehealth.org
World Health College

Dedicated to adolescent health issues including learning disabilities and grief. Written by experts.

1695 www1.tpgi.com.au/users/revolve/ncprepo
rt/ furstenberg
**Parenting Apart: Patterns of Childrearing after
Marital Disruption**

National survey of family relations.

1696 www2.mc.duke.edu/pcaad

**Duke University's Program in Child and Adolescent
Anxiety Disorder**

National

1697 AAMR: American Association on Mental Retardation

444 N Capitol Street NW
Suite 846
Washington, DC 20001-1512
202-387-1968
800-424-3688
Fax: 202-387-2193
E-mail: dcroser@aamr.org
www.aamr.org

Ann P Turnbull, President
Doreen Croser, Executive Director

Promotes progressive policies, sound research, effective practices, and universal human rights for people with intellectual disabilities.

1698 Advocates for Human Potential

323 Boston Post Road
Sudbury, MA 01776-3022
978-443-0055
Fax: 978-443-4722
E-mail: nshifman@ahpnet.com

Neal Shifman, President/CEO

Under contract with the Center for Mental Health Services (CMHS), Advocates for Human Potential (AHP) provides technical assistance to states and local providers regarding the Projects for Assistance in Transition from Homelessness (PATH) Program.

1699 Aleppos Foundation

39 Fairway E
Colts Neck, NJ 07722-1418
732-946-4489
Fax: 732-946-3344
E-mail: ilynch@monmouth.com
www.aleppos.org

Focuses on self-education: to learn about our inner and outer selves; to face up to our past; and to learn to communicate our true selves to others.

1700 Alliance of Genetic Support Groups

4301 Connecticut Avenue NW
Suite 404
Washington, DC 20008-2369
202-966-5557
800-336-4363
Fax: 202-966-8553
E-mail: info@geneticalliance.org
www.geneticalliance.org

A non-profit coalition of voluntary genetic support groups, consumers and professionals addressing the needs of individuals and families affected by genetic disorders from a national perspective. Specializes in linking people intrested in generic conditions with organization which can provide support and information.

1701 American Academy of Child and Adolescent Psychiatry

3615 Wisconsin Avenue NW
Washington, DC 20016-3007
202-966-7300
Fax: 202-966-2891
www.aacap.org

Marilyn Benoit, MD, President

Information is provided as a public service to aid in the understanding and treatment of the developmental, behavioral, and mental disorders which affect an estimated 7 to 12 million children and adolescents at any given time in the United States.

1702 American Academy of Pediatrics

141 NW Point Boulevard
Elk Grove Village, IL 60007
847-434-4000
Fax: 847-434-8000
E-mail: cme@aap.org
www.aap.org

Provides information on diagnosis and treatment of physical and mental pediatric conditions by offering programs, training, and resources.

1703 American Association for Geriatric Psychiatry

7910 Woodmont Avenue
Suite 1050
Bethesda, MD 20814-3084
301-654-7850
Fax: 301-654-4137
E-mail: main@aagponline.org
www.aagpgpa.org

American Association for Geriatric Psychiatry (AAGP) is a national association representing and serving its members and the field of geriatric psychiatry. It is dedicated to promoting the mental health and well-being of older people and improving the care of those with late life mental disorders. AAGP enhances the knowledge base and standards of practice in geriatric psychiatry through education and research and by advocating for meeting the mental health needs of older Americans.

1704 American Association of Psychiatric Services for Children (AAPSC)

440 1st Street NW
3rd Floor
Washington, DC 20001-2085
202-638-2952

Dr. Sydney Koret, Executive Director

Fosters prevention and treatment of mental and emotional disorders of the child, adolescent and family and furthers the development and application of clinical knowledge. Researches and supports projects dealing with child and adolescent mental health. Sponsors educational programs and compiles statistics. Publications: AAPSC Membership Directory, annual. AAPSC Newsletter, bimonthly. Child Psychiatry and Human Development, quarterly. Annual conference and exhibit usually in February or March.

1705 American Holistic Health Association

PO Box 17400
Anaheim, CA 92817-7400
714-779-6152
E-mail: mail@ahha.org
www.ahha.org

Michael Morton, PhD., President
Suzan Walter, Secretary/Treasurer

Promotes holistic principles honoring the whole person and encouraging people to actively participate in their own health and healthcare.

1706 American Managed Behavioral Healthcare Association

1101 Pennsylvania Avenue NW
6th Floor
Washington, DC 20004
Fax: 202-756-7308
www.ambha.org

Pamela Greenberg MPP, Executive Director

Represents and promotes the interests of specialty managed behavioral health care organizations.

1707 American Network of Community Options and Resources (ANCOR)

1101 King Street
Suite 380
Alexandria, VA 22314
703-532-7850
Fax: 703-535-7860
E-mail: ancor@ancor.org
www.ancor.org

Represents providers of case to persons with disabilities (including MR/NH). Promotes high standard of ethics. Conducts educational programs.

1708 American Pediatrics Society

3400 Research Forest Drive
Suite B-7
The Woodlands, TX 77381
281-419-0052
Fax: 281-419-0082
E-mail: info@aps-spr.org
www.aps-spr.org

Larry Shapiro, M.D., President
Elizabeth McAnarney, M.D., Vice President

Society of professionals working with pediatric health care issues; offers seminars and a variety of publications.

1709 American Psychiatric Association

1000 Wilston Boulevard
Suite 1825
Arlington, VA 22209-3901
703-907-7300
E-mail: apa@psych.org
www.psych.org

Marcia Kraft Goin, MD, President

Medical specialty society recognized world-wide. Both U.S. and international member physicians work together to ensure humane care and effective treatment for all persons with mental disorder, including mental retardation and substance-related disorders.

1710 American Psychological Association

750 1st Street NE
Washington, DC 20002-4242
202-336-5500
800-374-2721
Fax: 202-336-6063
TDD: 202-336-6123
TTY: 202-336-6123
www.apa.org

Largest scienctific and professional organziation representing psychology in the United States and is the world's largest association of psychologists. Works to advance psychology as a science, as a profession, and as a means of promoting human welfare.

1711 Association for the Care of Children's Health

19 Mantua Road
Mount Royal, NJ 08061-1006
609-224-1742
Fax: 609-224-1742

1712 Association for the Help of Retarded Children

200 Park Avenue S
Suite 1201
New York, NY 10003-1503
212-780-2500
Fax: 212-777-5893
E-mail: ahrcnyc@dti.net
www.ahrcnyc.org

Shirley Berenstein, Director

Offer disabled individuals day to day living that is as rich, absorbing and worthwhile as possible, with an emphasis on helping clients live up to their maximum potential in the community.

1713 Association of Mental Health Librarians (AMHL)

13301 Bruce B Downs Blvd
Tampa, FL 33612-3899
813-974-4471
Fax: 813-974-7242
E-mail: hanson@fmhi.usf.edu
www.fmhi.usf.edu/amhl

Ardis Hanson, President

An organization that is working in the field of mental health information delivery. Its members come from a variety of settings. AMHL provides opportunities for its members to enhance their professional skills; encourage research activities in mental health librarianship; and strengthens the role of the librarian within the mental health community.

1714 Bazelon Center for Mental Health Law

1101 15th Street NW
Suite 1212
Washington, DC 20005
202-467-5730
Fax: 202-223-0409
TDD: 202-467-4232
E-mail: webmaster@bazelon.org
www.bazelon.org

Robert Bernstein, Executive Director
Ira Burnim, Director

National legal advocate for people with mental disabilities. Through precedent-setting litigation and in the public policy arena, the Bazelon Center works to advance and preserve the rights of people with mental illnesses and development disabilities.

1715 Best Buddies International (BBI)

100 SE 2nd Street
#1990
Miami, FL 33131   305-374-2233
800-892-8339
Fax: 305-374-5305
E-mail: LaverneLewis@BestBuddies.org
www.bestbuddies.org

Anthony Shriver, Founder
J.R. Fry, Director

A nonprofit organization dedicated to enhancing the lives of people with intellectual disabilities by providing opportunities for one-to-one friendships and integrated employment.

1716 Bethesda Lutheran Homes and Services

700 Hoffman Drive
Watertown, WI 53094   920-261-3050
800-369-4636
Fax: 920-261-8441

Matthew Becker

Provides religious education, habilitation services, therapeutic services, vocational training and residential care for persons with mental retardation. Paid summer co-op positions in nursing, social work, psychology, special education, recreation, Christian education. Provides free information and referral services nationwide for parents, pastors, teachers, and mental retardation professionals.

1717 Black Mental Health Alliance (BMHA)

733 W 40th Street
Suite 10
Baltimore, MD 21211-2107   410-338-2642
Fax: 410-338-1771

Seeks to increase clinicians, clergy, educators and social service professionals awareness of African-Americans mental health needs and concerns on issues including stress, violence, racism, substance abuse and parenting. Provides consultation, public information and resource referrals. Publications: Visions, quarterly. Annual meeting and dinner-dance. Annual Optimal Mental Health for African American Families Conference.

1718 Center for Attitudinal Healing (CAH)

33 Buchanan Drive
Sausalito, CA 94965-1650   415-331-6161
Fax: 415-331-4545
E-mail: home123@aol.com
www.attitudinalhealing.org

Don Gowewy, Executive Director

Nonsectarian organization established to supplement traditional health care by offering free attitudinal healing services for children and adults with life-threatening illnesses or other crisis. Offers support groups and arranges home and hospital visits for children, youth and adults. Publications: Advice to Doctors and Other Big People, book. Another Look at the Rainbow, book. Rainbow Connection, newsletter, three times a year. There is a Rainbow Behind Every Dark Cloud, book. Workshops, five times a year.

1719 Center for Family Support (CFS)

333 7th Avenue
New York, NY 10001-5004   212-629-7939
Fax: 212-239-2211
www.cfsny.org

Steven Vernickofs, Executive Director

Service agency devoted to the physical well-being and development of the retarded child and the sound mental health of the parents. Helps families with retarded children with all aspects of home care including counseling, referrals, home aide service and consultation. Offers intervention for parents at the birth of a retarded child with in-home support, guidance and infant stimulation. Pioneered training of nonprofessional women as home aides to provide supportive services in homes.

1720 Center for Mental Health Services

SAMSHA
PO Box 42557
Washington, DC 20015

800-789-2647
Fax: 301-984-8796
TDD: 866-889-2647
www.mentalhealth.org

Irene S Levine PhD, Deputy Director

Develops national mental health policies, that promote Federal/State coordination and benefit from input from consumers, family members and providers. Ensures that high quality mental health services programs are implemented to benefit seriously mentally ill populations, disasters or those involved in the criminal justice system.

1721 Center for the Study of Issues in Public Mental Health

Nathan S Kline Institute for Psychiatric Research
140 Old Orangeburg Road
Orangeburg, NY 10962-1157   845-398-6594
Fax: 845-398-6592
E-mail: penney@nki.rfmh.org
www.rfmh.org

Carole Siegel, PhD, Director
Kim Hopper, PhD, Co-Director
Dixianne Penney, Administrator Director

The Center is committed to developing and conducting research within the contents of a rigorous research program that is strongly influenced by the requirements of a public mental health system and, in turn, influences the development of policy and practice in this arena.

1722 Child Welfare League of America

440 1st Street NW
Third Floor
Washington, DC 20001-2085   202-638-2952
Fax: 202-638-4004
www.cwla.org

1723 Christian Horizons

PO Box 3381
Grand Rapids, MI 49501   616-956-7063
Fax: 616-956-7063
E-mail: info@christianhorizonsinc.org
www.christianhorizonsinc.org

A Christian organization dedicated to enriching the lives of people with mental impairments. Provides day programs, camping ministries, and Bible studies. Assists churches in identifying persons with special needs and supports parents of those with special needs.

1724 Coalition of Voluntary Mental Health Agencies

90 Broad Street
8th Floor
New York, NY 10004   212-742-1600
Fax: 212-742-2080
E-mail: mailbox@cvmha.org
www.cvmha.org/

An umbrella advocacy organization of New York City's mental health community, representing over 100 non-profit community based mental health agencies that serve more than 500,000 clients in the five boroughs of New York City. Founded in 1972, the Coalition is entirely membership supported with limited foundation and government funding for special purpose advocacy and assistance projects.

1725 Community Access

666 Broadway
3rd Floor
New York, NY 10012-2317   212-780-1400
Fax: 212-780-1412
www.communityaccess.net

Donald Starcke, Director of Development

A nonprofit agency providing housing and advocacy for people with psychiatric disabilities. Provides 430 affordable housing units for people with psychiatric disabilities, families with disabilities, and low income people from local neighborhoods.

1726 Community Service Options

7575 S Kostner Avenueue
Chicago, IL 60652   773-884-1000
Fax: 773-838-9362
www.ffcmh.org/local.htm

1727 Council for Learning Disabilities

PO Box 4014
Leesburg, VA 20177   571-258-1010
Fax: 571-258-1011
www.cldinternational.org

Kirsten McBride, Executive Secretary

Professional membership association for professionals working with individuals who have learning disabilities. Committed to enhancing the educational and life span development of the learning disabled. Sponsors conferences and publishes journals in the field of learning disabilities.

1728 Council on Quality and Leadership

100 W Road
Suite 406
Towson, MD 21204   410-583-0060
Fax: 410-583-0063
E-mail: info@thecouncil.org
www.thecouncil.org

James F Gardner PhD, President/CEO
Michael Chapman, VP

An international nonprofit organization dedicated to advancing the quality of services and supports to people with disabilities. This is accomplished through its accreditation services, training programs and research division. The Council is currently providing support to organizations and providers thoughout the United States, Canada, England, Ireland and Australia.

1729 Eye Movement Desensitization and Reprocessing International Association (EMDRIA)

PO Box 141925
Austin, TX 78714-9125   512-451-5200
Fax: 512-451-5256
E-mail: info@emdria.org
www.emdria.org

Carol York, Executive Director
Rosalie Thomas, President

The primary objective of EMDRIA is to establish, maintain and promote the highest standards of excellence and integrity in Eye Movement Desensitization and Reprocessing practice, research and education.

1730 Families Anonymous

PO Box 3475
Culver City, CA 90231-3475
Fax: 310-815-9682
E-mail: famanon@familiesanonymous.org
www.familiesanonymous.org

For concerned relatives and friends of youth with drug abuse or related behavior problems.

1731 Family Advocacy & Support Association

PO Box 73367
Washington, DC 20056-3367   202-526-5436
Fax: 202-326-3039

Phyllis Morgan, President

Self-help, nonprofit, support, education and advocacy organization comprised of parents/family members and service providers dedicated to improving the quality of life for children and youth with emotional, behavioral and learning disabilities.

1732 Family Violence & Sexual Assault Institute

6160 Cornerstone Court E
San Diego, CA 92121   858-623-2777
Fax: 858-646-0761
www.fvsai.org

David Westgate, Director

Book club, research, and quarterly newsletter.

1733 Federation for Children with Special Needs (FCSN)

1135 Tremont Street
Suite 420
Boston, MA 02120

617-236-7210
800-331-0688
Fax: 617-572-2094
E-mail: fcsninfo@fcsn.org
www.fcsn.org

Rich Robison, Executive Director

The federation provides information, support, and assistance to parents of children with disabilities, their professional partners and their communities.

1734 Federation of Families for Children's Mental Health

1101 King Street
Suite 420
Alexandria, VA 22314

703-684-7710
Fax: 703-836-1040
E-mail: ffcmh@ffcmh.org
www.ffcmh.org

Barbara Huff, Executive Director

National family-run organization dedicated exclusively to children and adolesents with mental health needs and their families. Our voice speaks through our work in policy, training and technical assistance programs. Publishes a quarterly newsletter and sponsors an annual conference and exhibits.

1735 Healing for Survivors

PO Box 4698
Fresno, CA 93744-4698

559-442-3600
Fax: 559-442-3600
E-mail: hfshope@email.com
www.hfshope.org

Jan Kister, Director
Tammie Wineland, Administrative Assistant

Support center for adults who were physically, emotionally, or sexually abused as children. Provides weekly support groups, weekend workshops, individual counseling, partners groups and couples groups.

1736 Human Services Research Institute

2336 Massachusetts Avenue
Cambridge, MA 02140-1813

617-876-0426
Fax: 617-492-7401
www.hsri.org

Valerie Bradley, President
H Stephen Leff PhD, Senior VP

Assists state and federal government to enhance services and support people with mental illness and people with mental retardation.

1737 Information Centers for Lithium, Bipolar Disorders Treatment & Obsessive Compulsive Disorder

Madison Institute of Medicine
7617 Mineral Point Road
Suite 300
Madison, WI 53717-1623

608-827-2470
Fax: 608-827-2479
E-mail: mim@miminc.org
www.miminc.org

The Information Centers publish information booklets. Authored by experts on each disorder, these patient guides offer information about various psychiatric disorders and their treatments, and address the questions most frequently asked by patients and their families.

1738 Institute of Living Anxiety Disorders Center

Hartford Hospital
200 Retreat Avenue
Hartford, CT 06106

800-673-2411
Fax: 860-545-7068
www.instituteofliving.org/ADC

David Tolin, PhD, Director

Provides evaluation and treatment for individuals suffering from anxiety disorders as well as training and education for clinicians.

1739 International Society of Psychiatric-Mental Health Nurses

1211 Locust Street
Philadelphia, PA 19107-5409

215-545-2843
800-826-2950
Fax: 215-545-8107
E-mail: info@ispn-psych.org
www.ispn-psych.org

Lynette Jack PhD, RN, CARN, President
Geraldine S Pearson PhD, RN, CS, Secratary
Mary Jo Regan-Kubinski PhD, RN, Treasurer

To unite and enhance the presence and the voice of specialty psychiatric mental health nurses while influencing heatlhcare policy to promote equitable, evidence-based and effective treatment and care for individuals, families and communities.

1740 Judge Baker Children's Center

3 Blackfan Circle
Boston, MA 02115-5794

617-232-8390
Fax: 617-232-8399
E-mail: info@jbcc.harvard.edu
www.jbcc.harvard.edu

Stewart Hauser, MD, PhD, President
Kevin Lee Hepner, VP

A nonprofit organization dedicated to improving the lives of children whose emotional and behavioral problems threaten to limit their potential.

1741 Langley Porter Psychiatric Institute

University of California
401 Parnassus Avenue
San Francisco, CA 94143-9911

415-476-7000

Samuel Barnodes MD, Director

Conducts clinical studies of psychiatric disorders.

1742 Learning Disability Association of America

4156 Library Road
Pittsburgh, PA 15234-1349

412-341-1515
Fax: 412-344-0224
E-mail: info@ldaamerica.org
www.ldanatl.org

John E Muench, National Executive Director

Offers information and referral services to the learning disabled. Free pamphlets, fact sheets and bibliography regarding learning disabilities.

1743 Life Development Institute

18001 N 79th Avenue, Suite E71
Phoenix, AZ 85308   623-773-2774
Fax: 623-773-2788
E-mail: LDIinARIZ@aol.com
www.life-development-inst.org

Robert Crawford, President

Serves older adolescents and adults with learning disabilities and related disorders. Conducts programs to assist individuals to achieve careers/employment commensurate with capabilities and independent status.

1744 Lifespire

345 Hudson Street
3rd Floor
New York, NY 10014   212-741-0100
Fax: 212-463-9814
E-mail: info@lifespire.org
www.lifespire.com

Professionals, parents, sibilings, and others interested in mentally retarded and developmentally disabled adults. Offers professionally supervised programs for mentally retarded and developmentally disabled adults including vocational rehabilitation, dual diagnosis programs, job placement, rehabilitation workshops, activities for daily living, day treatment, day training, supported work, and family support programs.

1745 Menninger Clinic

2801 Gessner
PO Box 809045
Houston, TX 77280-9045   713-275-5000
800-351-9058
Fax: 713-275-5107
www.menninger.edu

Dr. Herbert Spohn, Director

A national specialty psychiatric care facility offering diagnostic and treatment programs for adoloscents and adults.

1746 Mental Health and Aging Network (MHAN) of the American Society on Aging (ASA)

Ameican Society on Aging
833 Market Street
Suite 511
San Francisco, CA 94103-1824   415-974-9600
800-537-9728
Fax: 415-974-0300
E-mail: info@asaging.org
www.asaging.org

Rodney Jackson, Registration

Dedicated to improving the supportive interventions for older adults with mental health problems and their caregivers by: Creating a cadre of professionals with expertise in geriatric mental health, Assuring that service professionals are multi capable, Improving the systems of care, Providing a voice for the underserved and Advocating for the services that advance quality of life for our clients.

1747 Mental Illness Education Project

PO Box 470813
Brookline Village, MA 02447-0813   617-562-1111
800-343-5540
Fax: 617-779-0061
E-mail: info@miepvideos.org
www.miepvideos.org

Christine Ledoux, Executive Director

Engaged in the production of video-based educational and support materials for the following specific populations: people with psychiatric disabilities; families, mental health professionals, special audiences, and the general public. The Project's videos are designed to be used in hospital, clinical and educational settings, and at home by individuals and families.

1748 Mentally Ill Kids in Distress

755 E Willetta Street
Phoenix, AZ 85006   602-253-1240
Fax: 602-523-1250
E-mail: mikidaz@qwest.net
www.mikid.org

1749 NADD: Association for Persons with Developmental Disabilities and Mental Health Needs

132 Fair Street
Kingston, NY 12401-4802   845-334-4336
800-331-5362
Fax: 845-331-4569
E-mail: nadd@mhv.net
www.thenadd.org

Dr. Robert Fletcher, Executive Director

Nonprofit organization designed to promote interest of professional and parent development with resources for individuals who have the coexistence of mental illness and mental retardation. Provides conference, educational services and training materials to professionals, parents, concerned citizens and service organizations. Formerly known as the National Association for the Dually Diagnosed.

1750 Nathan S Kline Institute for Psychiatric Research

140 Old Orangeburg Road
Orangeburg, NY 10962   845-398-5500
Fax: 845-398-5510
E-mail: webmaster@nki.rfmh.org
www.rfmh.org/nki

Robert Cancro MD, Director
Jerome Levine Md, Deputy Director

Research programs in Alzheimers disease, analytical psychopharmacology, basic and clinical neuroimaging, cellular and molecular neurobiology, clinical trail data management, co-occuring disorders and many other mental health studies.

1751 National Alliance for the Mentally Ill

2107 Wilson Boulevard
Suite 300
Arlington, VA 22201-3042   **703-524-7600**
800-950-6264
Fax: 703-524-9094
TDD: 703-516-7227
E-mail: elizabetha@nami.org
www.nami.org

Deborah White, Membership
Elizabeth Adams, Public Relations

Alliance of self help and advocacy groups concerned with severe and chronic mentally ill individuals and provides emotional support and practical guidance to families. Educates and informs the public about mental illnesses. Conducts consumer advocacy activities to enact legislation and promotes funding for the seriously mentally ill. Operates a speakers' bureau. Publications: Media Watch Kit. NAMI Advocate, bimonthly. Brochures, handbooks and newsletters. Annual meeting and exhibit.

1752 National Association for Rural Mental Health

3700 W Division Street
Suite 105
Saint Cloud, MN 56301-3728   **320-202-1820**
Fax: 320-202-1833
E-mail: NARMH@facts.ksu.edu
www.narmh.org

Rick Peterson, President
LuAnn Rice, Manager

Provides a forum for rural mental health professionals and advocates to identify problems, find solutions, and work cooperatively toward improving the delivery of rural mental health services, promote the unique needs and concerns of rural mental health policy and practice issues, sponsor an annual conference where rural mental health professionals benefit from the sharing of knowledge and resources. NARMH was founded to develop, enhance and support mental health services and providers in rural America.

Year Founded: 1977

1753 National Association of Protection and Advocacy Systems

900 2nd Street NE
Suite 211
Washington, DC 20002-3557   **202-408-9514**
Fax: 202-408-9520
TDD: 202-408-9521
E-mail: info@napas.org
www.protectionandadvocacy.com

Curtis L Decker, Executive Director

NAPAS was established under the Protection and Advocacy for Individuals with Mental Illness (PAIMI) Act. PAIMI programs protect and advocate for the legal rights of persons with mental illness. The programs investigate reports of abuse or neglect and provide technical assistance, information, and legal counseling. Publishes a free, quarterly newsletter, P&A News.

1754 National Association of State Mental Health Program Directors

66 Canal Center Plaza
Suite 302
Alexandria, VA 22314   **703-739-9333**
Fax: 703-548-9517
E-mail: roy.praschil@nasmhpd.org
www.nasmhpd.org

Robert W Glover PhD, Executive Director
Roy Praschil, Director Operations
Jackee Williams, Meeting Manager

Nonprofit membership organization that adovacates at the national level for the collective interests of state mental health agency commissioners and staff. Operates under a cooperative agreement with the National Governor's Association. NASMHPD is committed to working with other stakeholders to improve public mental health systems and the lives of persons with serious mental illnesses who access these and other systems. Its core services focus on legislative advocacy, technical assistance and information dissemination.

Year Founded: 1959

1755 National Association of Therapeutic Wilderness Camps

698 Dinner Bell-Ohiopyle Road
Ohiopyle, PA 15470
E-mail: info@natwc.org
www.natwc.org

Represents nearly fifty therapeutic wilderness camps located all over the US. We believe therapeutic wilderness camps represent the most effective method to help troubled young people change the way they deal with their parents, school, and other authorities.

1756 National Center for Learning Disabilities

381 Park Avenue S
Room 1401
New York, NY 10016   **212-545-7510**
888-575-7373
Fax: 212-545-9665
www.CD.org

National, non profit organization dedicated to improving the lives of those affected by learning didabilities (LD). Services include national information and referral, public outreach and communications, legislative advocacy and public policy. Its mission is to promote public awareness and understanding of learning disabilities and to provide national leadership on behalf of children and adults with LD so they may achieve thier potential and enjoy full participation in society. Our website offers a free monthly e mail newsletter, and much more information for contacts and referrals.

1757 National Center on Addiction and Substance Abuse at Columbia University

633 3rd Avenue
19th Floor
New York, NY 10017-6706   212-841-5200
                         Fax: 212-956-8020
          E-mail: info@casacolumbia.org
                    www.casacolumbia.org

William H Foster PhD, COO
Richard Mulieri, Communications

Unique think/action tank that engages all disiplines to study every form of substance abuse as it affects our society.

1758 National Child Support Network

PO Box 1018
Fayetteville, AR 72702-1018
                              800-729-5437
                    www.childsupport.org

1759 National Council for Community Behavioral Healthcare

12300 Twinbrook Parkway
Suite 320
Rockville, MD 20852-1606   301-984-6200
                         Fax: 301-881-7159
          E-mail: administration@nccbh.org
                    www.nccbh.org

Jeannie Campbell, CEO
David Schuerholz, Marketing/Communications

Behavioral healthcare administrators. Publishes the Journal of Behavioral Health Sciences and Research, ABHM Leader. Annual training conferences. See web for additional information.

1760 National Empowerment Center

National Empowerment Center
599 Canal Street
Lawrence, MA 01840   978-685-1518
                              800-769-3728
                         Fax: 978-681-6426
                    www.power2u.org

Daniel B Fisher MD, PhD, Executive Director
Laurie Ahern, Educator

Technical assistance center, providing information and education to consumer/survivor/ex-patients, family members and professionals. Carries a message of recovery, empowerment, hope and healing to people who have been diagnosed with mental illness.

1761 National GAINS Center for People with Co-Occurring Disorders in the Justice System

345 Delaware Avenue
Delmar, NY 12054-1123   518-439-7415
                              800-311-4246
                         Fax: 518-439-7612
          E-mail: sdavidson@prainc.com
                    www.gainsctr.com

Joseph J Cocozza PhD, Co-Director
Henry Steadman PhD, Co-Director
Susan Davidson, Division Manager

Center is a national focus for the collection and dissemination of information about effective, integrated mental health and substance abuse services for people with co-ocurring disorders who come in contact with the criminal justice system, including law enforcement, jails, prisons, and community corrections. The center is operated by Policy Research, inc. of Delmar, NY and is supported by the National Institute of Corrections, the Center for Substance Abuse Treatment and the Center for Mental Health Services.

1762 National Institute of Drug Abuse: NIDA

6001 Executive Boulevard
Room 5213
Bethesda, MD 20892-9561   301-443-1124
                         Fax: 301-443-7397
          E-mail: information@lists.nida.nih.gov
                    www.nida.nih.gov

Beverly Jackson, Public Information

Covers the areas of drug abuse treatment and prevention research, epidemiology, neuroscience and behavioral research, health services research and AIDS. Seeks to report on advances in the field, identify resources, promote an exchange of information, and improve communications among clinicians, researchers, administrators, and policymakers. Recurring features include synopses of research advances and projects, NIDA news, news of legislative and regulatory developments, and announcements.

1763 National Institute of Mental Health Information Resources and Inquiries Branch

6001 Executive Boulevard
Room 8184
Bethesda, MD 20892-9663
                              866-615-6464
                         Fax: 301-443-4279
                         TTY: 301-443-8431
          E-mail: nimhinfo@nih.gov
                    www.nimh.nih.gov

1764 National Mental Health Association

2001 N Beauregard Street
12th Floor
Alexandria, VA 22311   703-684-7722
                              800-969-6642
                         Fax: 703-684-5968
                         TTY: 800-433-5959
          E-mail: infoctr@nmha.org
                    www.nmha.org

Mike Fienza, Executive Director
Chris Condayn, Communications

Dedicated to improving treatments, understanding and services for adults and children with mental health needs. Working to win political support for funding for school mental health programs. Provides information about a wide range of disorders, such as panic disorder, obsessive-compulsive disorder, post traumatic stress, generalized anxiety disorder and phobias. Also advocates for programs to diagnose and treat children in juvenille justice systems.

1765 National Mental Health Consumer's Self-Help Clearinghouse

1211 Chestnut Street
Suite 1207
Philadelphia, PA 19107   **215-751-1810**
800-553-4539
Fax: 215-636-6312
E-mail: info@mhselfhelp.org
www.mhselfhelp.org

Alex Morrsey, Information/Referral

Funded by the National Institute of Mental Health Community Support Program, the purpose of the Clearinghouse is to encourage the development and growth of consumer self-help groups.

Year Founded: 1992

1766 National Organization on Disability

910 16th Street NW
Suite 600
Washington, DC 20006   **202-293-5960**
Fax: 202-293-7999
TTY: 202-293-5968
E-mail: ability@nod.org
www.nod.org

Elizabeth A Davis, VP/Director
Charles Dey, VP/Director
Glynnis Breen, Development

Nonprofit organization dedicated to promoting the full and equal participation of America's 49 million women, men and children with disabilities in all aspects of life. Consisting of 4,500 members and 250 chapters, NOD produces educational materials including fact sheets, brochures, a directory and various booklets including From Barriers To Bridges and Loving Justice. Offers many groups, partnerships and programs all orientated around expanding, promoting and advocating for people affected with disabilities.

Year Founded: 1982

1767 National Rehabilitation Association

633 S Washington Street
Alexandria, VA 22314   **703-836-0850**
Fax: 703-836-0848
TDD: 703-836-0849
E-mail: info@nationalrehab.org
www.nationalrehab.org

Anne Marie Hohman, Executive Director
John D'Angelo, Director Operations

Concerned with the rights of people with disabilities, our mission is to provide advocacy, awareness and career advancement for professionals in the fields of rehabilitation. Our members include rehab counselors, physical, speech and occupational therapists, job trainers, consultants, independent living instructors and other professionals involved in the advocacy of programs and services for people with disabilities.

1768 National Resource Center on Homelessness & Mental Illness

345 Delaware Avenue
Delmar, NY 12054

    800-444-7415
Fax: 518-439-7612
E-mail: nrc@prainc.com
www.nrchmi.samsa.gov

Francine Williams, Director
Deborah Dennis, VP/Project Director

Focused on the effective organization and delivery of services for people who are homeless and have serious mental illnesses. The Resource Center's activites enable the Center for Mental Health Services to facilitate service systems change through field-based knowledge development, synthesis, exchange and adoption of effective practices. Our staff provides a vital link between emerging knowledge and everyday practice by offering workshops and training opportunities on promising trends and practices, providing targeted technical assistance, developing referral lists, fact sheets and publications on homelessness, housing and mental health, maintaining a resource library and responding to information requests.

1769 National Self-Help Clearinghouse Graduate School and University Center

365 5th Avenue
Suite 3300
New York, NY 10016   **212-817-1822**
E-mail: info@selfhelpweb.org
www.selfhelpweb.org

Audrey Gardner, Co Director
Frank Riessman, Co Director

Facilitates access to self-help groups and increases the awareness of the importance of mutual support. The clearinghouse provides services by: assisting human service agencies on self-help principles, conducting training for self-help group leaders and group facilitators, researches the effectiveness of self-help and relationships with formal caregiving systems and provides media outreach.

Year Founded: 1976

1770 National Technical Assistance Center for Children's Mental Health

Georgetown University Child Development Center
3307 M Street NW
Washington, DC 20007   **202-687-5000**
Fax: 202-687-1954
TTY: 202-687-5503
E-mail: gucdc@georgetown.edu
www.dml.georgetown.edu/re-
search/gucdc/cassp.html

Integral part of the Georgetown University Center for Child and Human Development at the Georgetown University Medical Center. Nationally recognized for its work in assisting states and communities build systems of care for mental health concerns.

Year Founded: 1984

1771 New Hope Foundation

PO Box 201
Kensington, MD 20895-0201   **301-946-6395**
Fax: 301-946-1402
E-mail: newhope@nhfi.org
www.newhopfoundationinc.org

Daphne Stegmaier, Volunteer

Nonprofit organization integrates the many techniques proven effective in dealing with serious mental problems. Presents an innovative, replicable program designed to maximize the ability of chronically ill mental patients to achieve stable, self supporting lives in the community.

1772 PRO Behavioral Health

7600 E Eastman Avenue, Building #3
Suite 500
Denver, CO 80231   303-695-6007
                                888-687-6755
                                Fax: 303-695-0100
                                www.probh.com

Mari Teitelman LCSW, Business Development

PRO Behavioral Health is one of the nation's leading mental health and substance abuse managed care firms. Founded and directed by behavioral health clinicians and managers, PRO brings a clinically driven behavioral health service model to the market. Client organizations enjoy the benefits of PRO's client-specific customized programs, highly responsible customer service, behavioral health care coordinated with medical care, continuous quality improvement and reduced costs.

1773 Parents Helping Parents

3041 Olcott Street
Santa Clara, CA 95054   408-727-5775
                                Fax: 408-727-0182
                                E-mail: general@php.com
                                www.php.com

Lois Jones, Executive Director

Nonprofit family resource center offering culturally sensitive information, peer counseling and provides a forum for parents and professionals to get information. PHP does not promote or recommend any treatment, therapy, institution or professional.

1774 Parents Information Network

1101 King Street
Suite 420
Alexandria, VA 22314   703-684-7710
                                Fax: 703-836-1040
                                E-mail: ffcmh@ffcmh.org
                                www.ffcmh.org/local.htm

Bridget Schneider, Facilitator

National parent run organization focused on the needs of children and youth with emotional, behavioral or mental disorders and their families.

1775 People First of Oregon

PO Box 12642
Salem, OR 97309-0642   503-362-0336
                                Fax: 503-587-8459
                                E-mail: people1@open.org
                                www.open.org/people1

Develpmentally disabled people joining together to learn how to speak for themselves. Offers support, a united voice, advocacy to its members, information to communities, developing service projects to communities you live in, assistance in starting new People First groups, information to countries around the world, and participation on DD Council and A.R.C. Boards, Transit Boards.

1776 Professional Assistance Center for Education (PACE)

National-Louis University
2840 Sheridan Road
Evanston, IL 60201-1730   847-475-2670
                                Fax: 847-256-1057
                                E-mail: cburns@nl.edu
                                www.2.nl.edu/pace

Carol Burns, Director

Non-credit, non degree, two-year postsecondary program for students with learning disabilities. The program prepares young adults for careers as aides in preschools or human service agencies. In addition to professional preparation coursework, the curriculum also focuses on social skills and independent living skills. Students receive a certificate of completion at the conclusion of the program. College residential life is an integral part of the program. Transitional program where appropriate.

1777 Psychiatric Clinical Research Center

University of Illinois at Chicago
1740 W Taylor Street
Medical Center
Chicago, IL 60612-7232   312-996-0443
                                800-842-1002
                                www.uillinoismedcenter.org

Ramon Gomez, Director

The Center offers those whose quality of life is affected by severe mental disorders the opportunity to receive an accurate diagnosis and treatment for their condition using the latest methods of care. Those who participate in the clinical research give our staff the opportunity to learn more about these serious mental disorders.

1778 Reasearch Center for Severe Mental Illnesses

11301 Wilshire Boulevard #116
W LA VA Medical Center, Building 208 R
Los Angeles, CA 90073-1003   310-477-7927
                                E-mail: rpl@ucla.edu
                                www.npi.ucla.edu/crc/products/products

Robert Paul Liberman MD, Director
Jim Mintz PhD, Associate Director

For more than 20 years the center has given priority to the design, validation and dissemination of the practical, user-friendly assesment, treatment and rehabilitation techniques for practitioners.

1779 Reclamation

2502 Waterford Drive
San Antonio, TX 78217-5037   210-822-3569
                                www.community-2.webtv/stigmanet/POSITIVEVISIBILITY

Don H Culwell, Director

Former mental patients and interested others. Seeks to eliminate the stigma of mental illness and reclaim members' dignity. Serves as a voice for mental health patients in consumer, social and political affairs. Helps members to live outside a hospital setting by providing assistance in the areas of resocialization, employment and housing. Monitors the media and encourages positive media coverage. Publications: Positive Visibility, quarterly newsletter. Annual Reclamation conference.

1780 Recovery

802 N Dearborn Street
Chicago, IL 60610-3364   312-337-5661
Fax: 312-337-5756
E-mail: inquiries@recovery-inc.com
www.recovery-inc.com

Kelly Garcia, Executive Director
Maurine Pyle

Recovery method is to help prevent relapses in former mental patients and to forestall chronicity in nervous patients. Recovery provides training in a systematic method of self-help aftercare for these patients, based on the system of self-help principles described in Low's book, Mental Health Through Will Training.

1781 Refuah

PO Box 1212
Randolph, MA 02368   781-961-2815
Fax: 781-986-5070
E-mail: nblrefuah@aol.com
www.refuahboston.org

Nancy Blake Lewis, Executive Director

Expanding network of concerned Jewish family members and friends with loved ones of any race or creed suffering from chronic mental illness.

1782 Research and Training Center on Family Support and Children's Mental Health

Portland State University/Regional Research Institute
PO Box 751
Portland State University
Portland, OR 97207-0751   503-725-4040
Fax: 503-725-4180
E-mail: gordon@pdx.edu
www.rtc.pdx.edu

Lynwood Gordon, Public Information/Outreach
Janet Walker, Editor

Dedicated to promoting effective community based, culturally competent, family centered services for families and their children who are or may be affected by mental, emotional or behavioral disorders. This goal is accomplished through collaborative research partnerships with family members, service providers, policy makers, and other concerned persons. Major efforts in dissemination and training include: An annual conference, an award winning web site to share information about child and family mental services and policy issues which includes Focal Point, a national bulletin regarding family support and children's mental health.

1783 Resources for Children with Special Needs

116 E 16th Street
5th Floor
New York, NY 10003   212-677-4650
Fax: 212-254-4070
E-mail: info@resourcesnyc.org
www.resourcesnyc.org

Karen T Schlesinger, Executive Director
Dianne Littwin, Director Publications

Information, referral, advocacy, training, publications for New York City parents of youth with disabilities or special needs and the professionals who work with them.

1784 Sidran Traumatic Stress Institute

200 E Joppa Road
Suite 207
Baltimore, MD 21286   410-825-8888
888-825-8249
Fax: 410-337-0747
E-mail: sidran@sidran.org
www.sidran.org

Esther Giller, Executive Director

A nonprofit charitable organization devoted to education, advocacy and research to benefit people who are suffering from injuries of traumatic stress. Whether caused by family violence, crime, disaster, war or any other overwhelming experience, the disabling effects of trauma can be overcome with understanding, support and appropriate treatment. To support people with traumatic stress conditions and to educate mental health professionals and the public. Sidran has developed many service, training and bookself information sources.

1785 Systems Advocacy

National Mental Health Consumers' Self-Help
Clearinghouse
1211 Chestnut Street
Suite 1000
Philadelphia, PA 19107-4103   215-751-1810
800-553-4539
Fax: 212-636-6312
E-mail: THEKEY@delphi.com
www.mhselfhelp.org

1786 Thresholds Psychiatric Rehabilitation

4101 N Ravenswood Avenue
Chicago, IL 60613   773-880-6260
888-997-3422
Fax: 773-880-9050
E-mail: thresholds@thresholds.org
www.thresholds.org

Mary Jo Herseth, President
Tony M Zipple, CEO

Psychosocial rehabilitation agency serving persons with severe and persistent mental illness.

1787 United Families for Children's Mental Health

13301 Bruce B Downs Boulevard
FMHI Box 2, Room 2514
Tampa, FL 33612   813-974-7930
Fax: 813-974-7712
E-mail: ffcmh@earthlink.net

Carol Baier

1788 Voice of the Retarded

5005 Newport Drive
Suite 108
Rolling Meadows, IL 60008-3837   847-253-6020
Fax: 847-253-6054
E-mail: vor@compuserve.com
www.vor.net

Tamie Hopp, Executive Director
Nancy Ward, President

VOR is a national advocacy organization. Its mission
is to ensure quality care and choice in services and
supports received by people with mental retardation.
Through a weekly e-mail update, a quarterly newsletter and frequent action alerts, we empower our members and coordinate grass roots advocacy.
Membership is $25 per year.

1789 Warren Grant Magnuson Clinical Center

9000 Rockville Pike
Building 10, Room 1C255
Bethesda, MD 20892-0001   301-496-2563
E-mail: occc@cc.nih.gov
www.cc.nih.gov

Established as the research hospital of the National Institutes of Health. Designed with patient care facilities close to research laboratories so new findings of
basic and clinical scientists can be quickly applied to
the treatment of patients. Upon referral by physicians,
patients are admitted to NIH clinical studies.

Year Founded: 1953

1790 Washington Institute for Mental Illness Research and Training

Washington State University, Spokane
310 N Riverpoint Blv
PO Box 1495
Spokane, WA 99210-1495   509-358-7500
Fax: 509-358-7619
E-mail: 20contacts
www.spokane.wsu.edu/research&ser-
vice/WIMIRT/#key%

Gary G Galbraith, Director

Governmental organization focusing on mental illness research.

1791 Windhorse Associates

211 North Street
Suite 1
Northampton, MA 01060   413-586-0207
877-844-8181
Fax: 413-585-1521
E-mail: admissions@windhorseassociates.org
www.windhorseassociates.org

Jeff Fortuna, Executive Director

Promoting recovery from serious mental disturbances. Programs of care are individually tailored and
based in the client's home: a therapeutic household
created in partnership with the client and his or her
family and one or two housemates. Clinical staff are
highly qualified and form a close-knit team for each
client. Compassion, belief in recovery, mindfulness,
and attention to the whole person are basic principles
of treatment.

1792 World Federation for Mental Health

Secretariat
PO Box 16810
Alexandria, VA 22302-0810   703-838-7525
Fax: 703-519-7648
E-mail: info@wfmh.com
www.wfmh.com

Gwen Dixon, Office Administrator

Education and advocacy organization. Our primary
goal is to educate the public on mental health and to
advocate for those who deal with mental health issues.
Working to protect the human rights of those defined
as mentally ill.

1793 Young Adult Institute and Workshop (YAI)

460 W 34th Street
New York, NY 10001-2382   212-273-6100
www.yai.org

Joel M Levy, Executive Director/CEO
Phil Levy, President/COO

Serves more than 15,000 people of all ages and levels
of mental retardation, developmental and learning
disabilities. Provides a full range of early intervention, preschool, family supports, employment training and placement, clinical and residential services,
as well as recreation and camping services. YAI/Na-
tional Intitute for People with Disabilities is also a
professional organization, nationally renowned for its
publications, conferences, training seminars, video
training tapes and innovative television programs.

1794 Youth Services International

1819 Main Street
Suite 1000
Sarasota, FL 34236   941-953-9199
Fax: 941-953-9198
E-mail: YSIWEB@youthservices.com
www.youthservices.com

1795 Zero to Three

2000 M Street NW
Suite 200
Washington, DC 20036   202-638-1144
800-899-4301
Fax: 202-638-0851
E-mail: oto3@presswarehouse.com
www.zerotothree.org

Matthew E Melmed JD, Executive Director
Emily Fenichel, Associate Director

Professionals and researchers in the health care industry, policymakers and parents working to improve the healthy physical, cognitive and social development of infants, toddlers and their families. Sponsors training and technical assistance activities. Publications: Clinical Infant Reports, book series. Public Policy Pamphlets, 1 to 3 times per year. Zero to Three, 6 times per year, Annual National Training Institute conference and exhibits, usually in December.

By State
Alabama

1796 Alabama Alliance for the Mentally Ill

6900 6th Avenue S
Suite B
Birmingham, AL 35212-1902   205-833-8336
                                   800-626-4199
                            Fax: 205-833-8309
                    E-mail: alaami@aol.com

Ann Denbo, President

Advocacy, education and support for and about the Alabama mental health community.

1797 Birmingham Psychiatry

1 Independence Plaza
Homewood, AL   205-879-7953
                            Fax: 205-870-7987

1798 Horizons School

2111 University Boulevard
Birmingham, AL 35233   205-322-6606
                                   800-822-6242
                            Fax: 205-322-6605
                    www.horizonsschool.org

Marie McElheny, Admissions Coordinator
Jade Carter, Director

College based, non degree program for students with specific learning disabilities and other mild learning problems. This specially-designed, two-year program prepares individuals for successful transitions to the community. Classes teach life skills, social skills and career training.

1799 Mental Health Board of North Central Alabama

4110 Highway 31 South
PO Box 2479
Decatur, AL 35603   256-355-5904
                                   800-365-6008
                    E-mail: mentalhealth@mhcnca.org
                            www.mhcnca.org

1800 Mental Health Center of North Central Alabama

4110 Highway 31 S
Decatur, AL 35603   256-335-6091
                                   800-337-3162
                            Fax: 256-355-6091
                    E-mail: mentalhealth@mhcna.org
                            www.mhcnca.org

We support all people with mental health disorders to achieve respect and dignity, to reach their full potential and to be free from stigma and prejudice.

Alaska

1801 Alaska Alliance for the Mentally Ill

144 W 15th Avenue
Suite B
Anchorage, AK 99501   907-277-1300
                    E-mail: info@nami-alaska.org
                            www.nami-alaska.org

Beth LaCross, Board President
Yvonne Evans, Support Group Facilitator

Mission is to bring consumers and families with similar experiences together to share information about services, care providers, and ways to cope with the challenges of schizophrenia, manic depression, and other serious mental illnesses.

1802 Alaska Mental Health Association

4050 Lake Otis Parkway
Suite 209
Anchorage, AK 99508-5221   907-563-0880
                            Fax: 907-563-0881
                    www.alaska.net/~mhaa

Arizona

1803 Arizona Alliance for the Mentally Ill

2210 N 7th Street
Phoenix, AZ 85006-1604   602-244-8166
                                   800-626-5022
                            Fax: 602-244-9264
                    E-mail: azami@azami.org
                            www.az.nami.org

Sue Davis, Executive Director
Joan Abbot, Membership

Advocacy, education and support groups for families in Arizona who have loved ones dealing with mental health concerns.

1804 Community Partnership of Southern Arizona

4575 E Broadway
Tucson, AZ 85711   520-318-6900
                            Fax: 520-325-1441
                    E-mail: nogra@cpsa-rhba.org
                            www.cpsa-rhba.org

Neal Cash, CEO
Judy Johnson PhD, Deputy Director

Administrative organization responsible for the coordination of behavioral health treatment and preventitive services in southern and southeastern Arizona. We are a local community based nonprofit organization that is dedicated to ensuring the provision of accessible high quality and cost effective behavioral health services for adults and children.

1805 Devereux Arizona Treatment Network

11000 N Scottsdale Road
Suite 260
Scottsdale, AZ 85254-4581   480-998-2920
                                   800-345-1292
                                   Fax: 480-443-5587
                                   www.devereux.org

Jim Cole, Executive Director

National non-profit treatment centers for emotional disorders.

1806 Healthcare Southwest

2016 S 4th Avenue
Tucson, AZ 85713-3509   520-458-8767
                               Fax: 520-458-8767

1807 Mental Health Association of Arizona

6411 E Thomas Road
Scottsdale, AZ 85251-6005   480-994-4407
                                   800-642-4407
                                   www.mhaaz.com

Tiffany Bock, Executive Director
Julie Clark, Community Education

Allfiliate of the National Mental Health Association, we support all people with mental disorders to achieve respect and dignity, to reach their full potential and to be free from stigma and prejudice.

Year Founded: 1954

1808 Navajo Nation K'E Project: Children & Families Advocacy Corporation

PO Box 3390
200 Parkway Administration Building 1
Window Rock, AZ 86515   928-871-7160
                               Fax: 928-871-7255

Janet Hillis

1809 Navajo Nation K'E Project: Chinle Children & Families Advocacy Corporation

PO Box 3390
Chinle, AZ 86515   928-871-7160
                          Fax: 928-871-7255

Shirley Etsitty

1810 Navajo Nation K'E Project: Tuba City Children & Families Advocacy Corporation

PO Box 3390
200 Parkway Administration Building 1
Window Rock, AZ 86515   928-871-7160
                               Fax: 928-871-7255

Rueben McCabe

1811 Navajo Nation K'E Project: Winslow Children & Families Advocacy Corporation

PO Box 3390
200 Parkway Administration Building 1
Window Rock, AZ 86515   928-871-7160
                               Fax: 928-871-7255

Jayne Clark

Arkansas

1812 Arkansas Alliance for the Mentally Ill

4313 W Markham Street
Hendrix Hall, Room 203
Little Rock, AR 72205-4096   501-661-1548
                                    800-844-0381
                       E-mail: tenewman@aol.com
                                    www.nami.org

Laurie Flynn, Executive Director

Bringing consumers and families with similar experiences together to share information about services, care providers, and ways to cope with the challenges of schizophrenia, manic depression, and other serious mental illnesses.

California

1813 Assistance League of Southern California

1360 North Street
Andrews Plaza
Hollywood, CA 90028   323-469-1973
                             Fax: 323-469-3533
          E-mail: email@assistanceleague.net
                       www.assistanceleague.net

Sandy Doerschlag, Chief Executive Director
Janet Harrison, Public Relations

Provides mental health services to childeren over 5 years of age, individuals and families. Parent education and domestic violence classes are available. Services in English, Spanish and Armenian.

Year Founded: 1919

1814 California Alliance for the Mentally Ill

National Alliance for the Mentally Ill
1111 Howe Avenue
Suite 475
Sacramento, CA 95825-8541   916-567-0163
                                   Fax: 916-567-1757
     E-mail: grace. mcandrews@namicalifornia.org
                       www.namicalifornia.org

Laurie Flynn, Executive Director

Nation's leading self-help organization for all those affected by severe brain disorders. Mission is to bring consumers and families with similar experiences together to share information about services, care providers, and ways to cope with the challenges of schizophrenia, manic depression, and other serious mental illnesses. The California office answers questions from hundreds of individuals and groups outside NAMI who turn to us for accurate information about mental illness, NAMI affiliates near them, and where to turn for help.

Year Founded: 1977

1815 California Association of Marriage and Family Therapists

7901 Raytheon Road
San Diego, CA 92111-1606   858-292-2638
                                  Fax: 858-292-2666
                                  www.camft.org

Mary Riemersma, Executive Director

Independent professional organization representing the interests of licensed marriage and family therapists. Dedicated to advancing the profession as an art and a science, to maintaining high standards of professional ethics, to upholding the qualifications for the profession and to expanding the recognition and awareness of the profession.

1816 California Association of Social Rehabilitation Agencies

815 Marina Vista, Suite D
PO Box 388
Martinez, CA 94553   925-229-2300
                               Fax: 925-229-9088
                    E-mail: casra@casra.org
                            www.casra.org

Betty Dahlquist, Executive Director
Peggy Harris, Executive Assistant
Dave Hosseini, Public Policy
Sheryle Stafford, Public Policy

Dedicated to improving services and social conditions for people with psychiatric disabilities by promoting their recovery, rehabilitation and rights. A diagnosis is not a destiny.

1817 California Health Information Association

1915 N Fine Avenue
Suite 104
Fresno, CA 93727-1510   559-251-5038
                               Fax: 559-251-5836
                E-mail: info@californiahia.org
                         www.californiahia.org

LaVonne LaLamoreaux, Executive Director
Marilyn R Taylor, Operations Manager

Nonprofit association that provides leadership, education, resources and advocacy for California's health information management professionals. Contributes to the delivery of quality patient care through excellence in health information management practice.

1818 California Institute for Mental Health

2030 J Street
Sacramento, CA 95814-3904   916-556-3480
                               Fax: 916-446-4519
                    E-mail: sgoodwin@cimh.org
                            www.cimh.org

Sandra Naylor-Goodwin, Executive Director
Bill Carter, Deputy Director
Ed Diksa, Director Training

Promoting excellence in mental health services through training, technical asistances, research and policy development.

1819 California Psychiatric Association: CPA

1400 K Street
Suite 302
Sacramento, CA 95814   916-442-5196
                               Fax: 916-442-6515
                E-mail: calpsych@worldnet.att.net
                            www.calpsych.org

Barbara Gard, Executive Director
Randall Hagar, Director Government Relations

Represents psychiatrists and the interests of their patients as those interests are affected by state government. CPA is area six of the American Psychiatric Association, and is composed of members of APA's five district branches in California.

1820 California Psychological Association

1022 G Street
Sacramento, CA 95814-0817   916-325-9786
                               Fax: 916-325-9790
           E-mail: calpsychlink@calpsychlink.org
                         www.calpsychlink.org

Claudia Foutz, Executive Director
Patricia VanWoerkom, Deputy Director
Annie Norris, Member Services

Nonprofit professional association for licensed psychologists and others affiliated with the delivery of psychological services. Sponsors many legislative proposals dealing with access to mental health care services, managed care, hospital practice, prescription privilege authority and other issues. Regularly provides free public service through programs such as the well respected disaster response service.

Year Founded: 1948

1821 Calnet

1916 Creston Road
Paso Robles, CA 93446-4465   805-239-3332
                               Fax: 805-239-4545
                E-mail: blandis@calnetcare.com
                            www.calnetcare.com

Brent Lamb, President
Barbara Orlando, Marketing/Communications

Nonprofit membership association of mental health facilities networking mental health and chemical dependency treatment providers throughout the state of California.

1822 Community Resource Council

1945 Palo Verde Avenue
Suite 202
Long Beach, CA 90815-3445   562-430-3099
                               Fax: 562-749-3355

Barry Leedy, Executive Director

Agency provides groups and classes to all ages. Sliding fee scale.

1823 Five Acres: Boys and Girls Aid Society of Los Angeles County

760 W Mountain View Street
Altadena, CA 91001-4925   626-798-6793
                               Fax: 626-797-7722
                               TTY: 626-204-1375
                E-mail: for5acres@earthlink.com
                            www.5acres.org

Robert A Ketch, Executive Director
Sandi Zaslow, Assistant Executive Director
Cathy Clement, Director Development

Works to: prevent child abuse and neglect, care for, treat and educate emotionally disturbed, abused and neglected children and their families in residential and outreach programs, advance the welfare of children and families by research, advocacy and collaboration, strive for the highest standards of excellence by professionals and volunteers, and provide research and educational resources to families, the community and professionals for the prevention and treatment of child abuse and neglect.

Year Founded: 1888

1824 Gold Coast Alliance for the Mentally Ill

520 N Main Street, Room 203
PO Box 1088
Angels Camp, CA 95222   **209-736-4264**
E-mail: gcami@goldrush.com
www.nami.org

Laurie Flynn, Executive Director

Local chapter of the national self-help organization (NAMI) for all those affected by severe brain disorders. Mission is to bring consumers and families with similar experiences together to share information about services, care providers, and ways to cope with the challenges of schizophrenia, manic depression, and other serious mental illnesses.

1825 Health Services Agency: Mental Health

1080 Emeline Avenue
Santa Cruz, CA 95060-1966   **831-454-4000**
Fax: 831-454-4770
TDD: 831-454-2123
E-mail: info@santacruzhealth.org
www.santacruzhealth.org

Rama Khalsa PhD, Health Services Administrator
David McNutt MD, County Health Officer

Exists to protect and improve the health of the people in Santa Cruz County. Provides programs in environmental health, public health, medical care, substance abuse prevention and treatment, and mental health. Clients are entitled to information on the costs of care and their options for getting health insurance coverage through a variety of programs.

1826 National Association of Mental Illness: California

1111 Howe Avenue
Suite 475
Sacramento, CA 95825-8541   **916-567-0163**
Fax: 916-567-1757
E-mail: grace.mcandrews@namicalifornia.org
www.namicalifornia.org

Grace McAndrews, Executive Director

Provides support, information and education for families of seriously mentally ill individuals. NAMI California's efforts focus on support, referral, advocacy, research and education. Available are the Journal Magazine, videos, educational classes, and support groups.

1827 National Health Foundation

Hospital Association of Southern California
6633 Telephone Road
Suite 210
Ventura, CA 93003-5569   **805-650-1243**
Fax: 805-650-6456
E-mail: mclark@hasc.org
www.hasc.org

Monty Clark, Regional Vice President

Charitable affiliate whose mission is to improve and enhance the health of the underserved by developing and supporting inovative programs that can become independently viable, systemic solutions to gaps in healthcare access and delivery and have potential to be replicated nationally.

1828 Northern California Psychiatric Society

1631 Ocean Avenue
San Francisco, CA 94112-1796   **415-334-2418**
Fax: 415-239-2533
E-mail: info@ncps.org
www.ncps.org

Marvin Firestone, President
Byron Whittlin, VP
Janice Tagart, Executive Director

A district branch of the American Psychiatric Association. A nonprofit organization that tries to improve the treatment, rehabilitation, and care of the mentally ill, the developmentally disabled, and the emotionally disturbed.

1829 Orange County Psychiatric Society

300 S Flower Street
Orange, CA 92868-3417   **949-978-3016**
Fax: 949-978-6039

Works to improve public awareness of mental illness and increase financial support.

1830 UCLA Department of Psychiatry & Biobehavioral Sciences

C8-871 Neuropsychiatry Institute
Box 951759
Los Angeles, CA 90095-1759   **310-825-0511**
www.psychiatry.ucla.edu

Programs for clinical research treatment for adults and children suffering from psychiatric illness.

1831 United Advocates for Children of California

1401 El Camino Avenue
Suite 340
Sacramento, CA 95815   **916-643-1530**
Fax: 916-643-1592
TTY: 916-643-1532
E-mail: information@uacc4families.org
www.uacc4families.org

A nonprofit organization that works on behalf of children and youth with serious emotional disturbances and their families.

Colorado

1832 Adolescent and Family Institute of Colorado

10001 W 32nd Avenue
Wheat Ridge, CO 80033-5601   303-238-1231
                                   Fax: 303-238-0500
                                   www.aficonline.com

Eric Meyer, MD, Executive Director

A licensed and accredited adolescent psychiatric and substance abuse 24 hour facility.

1833 CHINS UP Youth and Family Services

25 Farragut Avenue
Colorado Springs, CO 80909-5601   719-475-0562
                                     Fax: 719-634-0562
                        E-mail: shinsupinc@aol.com
                                     www.chinsup.org

Gerard H Heneman, Executive Director

Chins Up is a nonprofit multi-service agency serving children and families in the child welfare and juvenile justice systems. Chins Up strives to heal the broken lives of children and families.

1834 Colorado Health Networks-Value Options

7150 Campus Drive
Suite 300
Colorado Springs, CO 80919
                                     800-804-5040
                              www.valueoptions.com

CHN is comprised of partnerships between ValueOptions and seven community mental health centers.

1835 Craig Counseling & Biofeedback Services

611 Breeze Street
Craig, CO 81625-2503   970-824-7475
                                     Fax: 970-824-7475
                        E-mail: drhadlee@hotmail.com

Frank Hadley MA, DAPA, Director
Bert Dech MD, Medical Director

Full-service mental health and biofeedback center with two male and one female therapist and a board certified adult, adolescent and child psychiatrist.

1836 Federation of Families for Children's Mental Health

Colorado Chapter
901 W 14th Avenue
Suite 1
Denver, CO 80204   303-572-0302
                                     Fax: 303-572-0304
                        www.coloradofederation.org

To promote mental health for all children, youth and families.

1837 Mental Health Association of Colorado

6795 E Tennessee Avenue
Suite 425
Denver, CO 80224-1614   303-377-3040
                                     800-456-3249
                                Fax: 303-377-4920
                                www.mhacolorado.org

Jeanne Mueller Rohner, Executive Director
Michelle Hoffer, Director Development
Kristen Gravatt, Director Community Relations

A nonprofit association providing leadership to address the full range of mental health issues in Colorado. The association is a catalyst for improving diagnosis, care and treatment for people of all ages with mental health problems.

Connecticut

1838 Connecticut Families United for Children's Mental Health

PO Box 151
New London, CT 06320   860-439-0710
                                     866-439-0788
                                Fax: 860-439-0711
              E-mail: ctfamiliesunited@sbcglobal.net
                  www.ctfamiliesunited.homestead.com

A nonprofit organization providing statewide emotional support, family and systems advocacy and information and referrals.

1839 Connecticut National Association of Mentally Ill

30 Jordan Lane
Wethersfield, CT 06109   860-882-0236
                                     800-215-3021
                                Fax: 860-586-7477
                                     www.namict.org

Marilyn Ricci, President
Debra Anderson, Executive Director

Dedicated to improving the lives of people with serious mental illnesses and their families.

1840 Family & Community Alliance Project

110 Washington Street
Hartford, CT 06106-4405   860-566-6810
                                     Fax: 860-246-8778

Support group for families who have children with a mental illness.

1841 Mental Health Association: Connecticut

1480 Bedford Street
Stamford, CT 06905-5309   203-323-0124
                                     Fax: 203-323-0383
                                     www.mhct.org

To advocate and work for everyone's mental health.

1842 Thames Valley Programs

1 Ohio Avenue
Norwich, CT 06360-1536
                                     866-445-2616
                                     Fax: 860-886-6567

Marek Kukulka, LMFT, Program Manager

The Thames Valley Programs offer a continuum of care services with the goal of stabilization for children and adolescents who suffer from a broad range of behavioral and emotional problems. Programs utilize a positive, goal oriented approach to treatment that emphasizes patients' strength and success in the effort to maintain recovery and desired outcomes. Individualized, highly structured treatment programs offered at Thames Valley include: Partial Hospital Program, Intensive Outpatient Program, and Extended Day Program.

1843 Women's Support Services

PO Box 341
Sharon, CT 06069   860-364-1080
E-mail: wssdv@snet.net

Linda Everett, President

Support and advocacy for those affected by domestic violence and abuse in the towns of Cannan, Cornwall, Kent, North Cannan, Salisbury, and Sharon.

Delaware

1844 Delaware Alliance for the Mentally Ill

2400 W 4th Street
Wilmington, DE 19805   302-427-0787
888-427-2643
Fax: 302-427-2075
E-mail: namide@namide.org
www.namide.org

John P Smoots, President
Richard Taylor, Vice President
Rita A Marocco, Executive Director

A statewide organization of families, mental health consumers, friends and professionals dedicated to improving the quality of life for those affected by life changing brain diseases such as schizophrenia, bipolar disorder and major depression.

1845 Delaware Guidance Services for Children and Youth

1156 Walker Road
Dover, DE 19904-6540   302-678-9316
Fax: 302-678-9317
www.delawareguidance.com

To provide quality mental health services for children , youth and their families.

1846 Mental Health Association of Delaware

100 W 10th Street
Wilmington, DE 19810   302-654-6833
Fax: 302-654-6838
www.mhinde.org

Marjorie Mudrick

To deliver mental health education, advocacy and support, and to collaborate to provide mental health leadership in Delaware

1847 National Association of Social Workers: Delaware Chapter

3301 Green Street
Claymont, DE 19703-2052   302-792-0356
Fax: 302-792-0678
E-mail: naswae@aol.com
www.naswdc.org

Works to enhance the professional growth and development of its members, to create and maintain professional standards, and to advance sound social policies.

District of Columbia

1848 DC Alliance for the Mentally Ill

422 8th Street SE
Washington, DC 20003-2832   202-546-0646
Fax: 202-546-6817
E-mail: namidc@aol.com
www.nami.org/about/namidc

Joan Bowser, President
Nancy Head, Executive Director

Nation's leading self-help organization for all those affected by severe brain disorders. Mission is to bring consumers and families with similar experiences together to share information about services, care providers, and ways to cope with the challenges of schizophrenia, manic depression, and other serious mental illnesses.

1849 Family Advocacy & Support Association

1289 Brentwood Road NE
Washington, DC 20002   202-526-5436
Fax: 202-265-7877
www.mentalhealth.org

Comprehensive community mental health services program for children and their families.

Florida

1850 Department of Human Services For Youth & Families

2929 NW 17th Avenue
Miami, FL 33125-1118   305-633-6481
Fax: 305-633-5632

1851 Family Network on Disabilities of Florida

2735 Whitney Road
Clearwater, FL 33760-1610   727-523-1130
800-825-5736
Fax: 727-523-8687
E-mail: fnd@fndfl.org
www.fndfl.org

Jan LaBelle, Executive Director
Laura Mataluni, Executive Assistant

A statewide network of families and individuals who may be at risk, have disabilities, or have special needs.

1852 Florida Alcohol and Drug Abuse Association

1030 E Lafayette Street
Suite 100
Tallahassee, FL 32301-4559   850-878-2196
                                    Fax: 850-878-6584
                                    E-mail: fadaa@fadaa.org
                                    www.fadaa.org

John Daigle, Executive Director

Statewide membership organization that represents more than ninety community-based substance abuse treatment and prevention agencies throughout Florida. FADAA has provided advocacy for substance abuse programs and the clients they serve for the past twenty seven years, as well as quality training programs for substance abuse professionals and up-to-date information on substance abuse to the general public.

1853 Florida Federation of Families for Children's Mental Health

734 Shadeville Highway
Crawfordville, FL 32327   850-926-3514
                                 877-926-3514
                                 Fax: 413-480-2947
                                 E-mail: ejwells@sprynet.com
                                 www.fifionline.org

Conni Wells

A nationally affiliated parent-run organization focused on the needs of children and youth with emotional, behavioral or mental disorders and their families.

1854 Florida Health Care Association

307 W Park Avenue
Tallahassee, FL 32301   850-224-3907
                               Fax: 850-681-2075
                               www.fhca.org

Kelley Rice-Schild, President

FHCA is dedicated to providing the highest quality care for elderly, chronically ill, and disabled individuals.

1855 Florida National Alliance for the Mentally Ill

911 E Park Avenue
Tallahassee, FL 32301-2646   850-671-4445
                                    Fax: 850-671-5272
                                    E-mail: lynne@namifl.org
                                    www.namifl.org

Lynn Montgomery, Executive Director

Nation's leading self-help organization for all those affected by severe brain disorders. Mission is to bring consumers and families with similar experiences together to share information about services, care providers, and ways to cope with the challenges of schizophrenia, manic depression, and other serious mental illnesses.

1856 Mental Health Association of West Florida

840 W Lakeview Avenue
Pensacola, FL 32501   850-438-9879
                             Fax: 850-438-5901

Offers special information and referrals for families of mental health.

1857 National Association of Social Workers Florida Chapter

1931 Dellwood Drive
Tallahassee, FL 32303   850-224-2400
                               800-352-6279
                               Fax: 850-561-6279
                               E-mail: naswfl@naswfl.org
                               www.naswfl.org

Jim Akin, Executive Director

NASW is a membership organization for professional social workers in Florida. NASWFL provides: continuing education, information center, advocacy for employment and legislation.

Georgia

1858 Georgia Association of Homes and Services for Children

34 Peachtree Street NW
Suite 710
Atlanta, GA 30303-2301   404-572-6170
                                Fax: 404-572-6171
                                E-mail: norman@gahsc.org
                                www.gahsc.org

GAHSC is an association that is dedicated to supporting those who care for children who are at risk of abuse and neglect. Member agencies of GAHSC include family foster care, community group homes, education programs and others.

1859 Georgia National Alliance for the Mentally Ill

3050 Presidential Drive
Suite 202
Atlanta, GA 30340-3916   770-234-0855
                                800-728-1052
                                Fax: 770-234-0237
                                E-mail: nami-ga@nami.orgcom
                                www.nami.org

Sally Montgomery, President
Mary Sloan, Executive Director

NAMI is nonprofit, grassroots, self-help, support and advocacy organization of consumers, families and friends of people with severe mental illnesses such as schizophrenia, bipolar disorder, major despressive disorder, and other severe and persistent mental illnesses that affect the brain.

1860 Georgia Parent Support Network

1381 Metropolitan Parkway
Atlanta, GA 30310   404-758-4500
                           800-832-8645
                           Fax: 404-758-6833
                           E-mail: slsmith2@ix.netcom.com
                           www.gspn.org

Cynthia Wainscott, Chairperson
Kathy Dennis, Vice President
Linda Seay, Secretary/Treasurer

The Georgia Parent Support Network is dedicated to providing support, education and advocacy for children and youth with mental illness, emotional disturbances and behavioral difference and their families.

1861 Grady Health Systems: Central Fulton CMHC

80 Jesse Hill Jr Drive S.E.
Atlanta, GA 30303-3050   404-616-4307
Fax: 404-616-5998

Robert L Brown, FAIA Chairman
Clayton Sheptherd, Treasurer

Grady Health System improves the health of the community by providing quality, comprehensive health care in a compassionate, culturally competent, ethical and fiscally responsible manner. Grady maintains its commitment to the underserved of Fulton and DeKalb counties, while also providing care for residents of metro Atlanta and Georgia. Grady leads through its clinical exellence, innovative research and progressive medical education and training.

Hawaii

1862 Hawaii Alliance for the Mentally Ill

1126 12th Avenue
Suite 205
Honolulu, HI 96816-3714   808-737-2778
www.nami.org

Laurie Flynn, Executive Director

Nation's leading self-help organization for all those affected by severe brain disorders. Mission is to bring consumers and families with similar experiences together to share information about services, care providers, and ways to cope with the challenges of schizophrenia, manic depression, and other serious mental illnesses.

1863 Hawaii Families As Allies

PO Box 700310
Kapolei, HI 96709-0310   808-487-8785
866-361-8825
Fax: 808-487-0514
www.mentalhealth.org

Sharon Nobriga, Co Executive Director

Parent Advocacy group for those with children who have mental disorders.

1864 National Alliance for the Mentally Ill in Hawaii

770 Kapiolani Boulevard
Suite 613
Honolulu, HI 96813-5240   808-591-1297
Fax: 808-591-2058

Marion Poirier, Exective Director

The National Alliance for the Mentally Ill maintains a helpline for informaiton on mental illness and referalls to local groups.

Idaho

1865 Idaho Alliance for the Mentally Ill

PO Box 68
Albion, ID 83311   208-673-6672
800-572-9940
Fax: 208-673-6685
www.nami.org

Laurie Flynn, Executive Director

NAMI Idaho is a non-profit, tax exempt family organization for people with brain disorders.

Illinois

1866 Allendale Association

PO Box 1088
Lake Villa, IL 60046-1088   847-356-2351
888-255-3631
Fax: 847-356-0289
www.allendale4kids.org

Mary Shahbazian, President
Ronald Howard, VP Reisdential Programs
Dr. Pat Taglione, VP Clinical/Community Services

The Allendale Association is a private, non-profit organization dedicated to the excellence and innovation in the care, education, treatment and advocacy for troubled children, youth and their families.

1867 Baby Fold

108 E Wilow Street
PO Box 327
Normal, IL 61761-0327   309-452-1170
Fax: 309-452-0115
E-mail: info@thebabyfold.org

The Baby Fold is a multi-service agency that provides Residential, Special Education, Child Welfare, and Family Support Services to children and families in central Illinois.

1868 Chaddock

205 S 24th Street
Quincy, IL 62301-4492   217-222-0034
888-242-3625
Fax: 217-222-3865
E-mail: dreer@chaddock.org
www.chaddock.org

Gene Simon, President
Reg Ankrom, Director of Support Services
Jerry Douglas, Director of Education
Conran Dvorak, Director of Residential Services

Chaddock's mission is to empower children and families to become self-reliant, contributing members of their communities by providing quality programs and services in caring settings.

1869 Chicago Child Care Society

5467 S University Avenue
Chicago, IL 60615-5193   773-643-0452
Fax: 773-643-0620

Mrs. Hugo Sonnenschein, President
Robert L Rinder, Vice President
Mary O'Brian Pearlman, Vice President
Judith Lavender, Secretary

Chicago Child Care Society exist to protect vulnerable children and strengthen their families. We strive to be among the permier providers of high quality and effective child welfare services. We believe the quality of life for future generations depends upon the quality of care provided for children today. We believe children should be provided with services and opportunities tha will enable them to reach their optimism physical, mental and social development. We believe all the children are entitled to the protection and nurturing care of adults, preferably within their birth families. However, if family can't fulfill these basic functions, we believe society, by either public or private means should provide the best alternative care.

1870 Children's Home Association of Illinois

2130 N Knoxville Avenue
Peoria, IL 61603-2460   309-685-1047
                        Fax: 309-687-7299
                        www.chail.org

James G , Sherman

Nonprofit, non-sectarian multiple program and social service organization. Giving children a childhood and future by protecting them, teaching them, healing them and by building strong communities and loving families.

1871 Coalition of Illinois Counselors Organization

PO Box 1086
Norhtbrook, IL 60065   847-205-4432
                        Fax: 847-205-4423

We collaberate with other mental health disciplines; human services organizations, industries and business as well as representatives of the government, to promote emotional health care interests. We are commited to upholding high standards for clients in Illinois.

1872 Family Service Association of Greater Elgin Area

22 S Spring Street
Elgin, IL 60120-6412   847-695-3680
                        Fax: 847-695-4552
                        E-mail: JZahm@fsaelgin.org
                        www.fsaelgin.org

Lisa A La Forge, Executive Director
Dr. Sandra Angelo, Dir. Consumer Credit Counseling
Jon A Zahm, Developmental/Community Rel.

A non-profit agancy, Family service Associaition has served the Greater Elgin Area since 1931. Supported both publicly and privately, most of the funding is recieved from such local sources as United Ways, corporate and individual contributions and client fees.

1873 Human Resources Development Institute

222 S Jefferson Street
Chicago, IL 60661   312-441-9009
                        Fax: 312-441-9019
                        www.hrdi.org

Martina Jones, Executive Director
Kimberly Sutton PhD, Sr VP Clinical/Program Support

Community based behavioral health and human services organization. This nonprofit agency on the south side of Chicago, is concerned with mental health and substance abuse solutuions. Offering more than 40 programs at 20 sites.

Year Founded: 1974

1874 Illinois Alcoholism and Drug Dependency Association

937 S 2nd Street
Springfield, IL 62704-2701   217-528-7335
                            Fax: 217-528-7340
                            www.iadda.org

Angela M Bowman, CEO
Sara Moscato, Associate Director
Pel Thomas, Business Manage
May Jo Pevey, Prevention Coordinator

IADDA is a statewide organization established in 1967 respresenting more than 100 prevention and treatment agencies, as well as individuals who are interested in the substance abuse field. The Association advocates for sound public policy that will create healthier families and safer communites. IADDA members educate government officials in Springfield and Washington, and work to increase the public understanding of substance abuse and addiction.

1875 Illinois Alliance for the Mentally Ill

730 E Vine Street
Suite 209
Springfield, IL 62703-2553   217-522-1403
                            800-346-4572
                            Fax: 217-522-3598
                            E-mail: namiill@sbcglobal.net
                            www.il.namil.org

Tom Lambert, President

We are committed to a future where recovery is the expected outcome and when mental illness can be prevented or cured. We envision a nation where everyone with a mental illness will have access to early detection and the effective treatment and support essential to live, work, learn and participate fully in their community.

1876 Illinois Federation of Families for Children's Mental Health

PO Box 1357
Vienna, IL 62995   618-658-2059
                    800-871-8400
                    Fax: 618-658-2720
                    E-mail: iffcmh@msn.com
                    www.iffcmh.ner/contact.htm

Dian Ledbetter, Executive Director
Beth Berndt, Family Resource Director
Lejeune Burdine, Vienna Office Manager
Beverly Hartig, Austim Project Management

Goal is to create a statewide network for individuals and groups throughout Illinois so: Families are not alone in caring for their children with difficult behavior; Parents are better informed on social services, legal, educational and medica resources; research prevention, and early intervenion.

1877 Larkin Center

1212 Larkin Avenue
Elgin, IL 60123-6098   847-695-5656
                                    Fax: 847-695-0897
                                    www.larkincenter.org

Dennis L Graf MS, Executive Director
Richard Peterson MSW, Executive Director
Martine Lyle, Admissions And QA Director
Michelle Potter MS LCPC, Clinical Director

Our mission is achieved through the efforts of Larkins Center's team of skilled professionals in creative co-operation with the community.

1878 Little City Foundation (LCF)

1760 W Algonquin Road
Palatine, IL 60067-4799   847-358-5510
                                    Fax: 847-358-3291
                            E-mail: people@littlecity.org
                                    www.LittleCity.org

Alex Alexandrou, Pesident
Alex Gianaras, Vice President
Fred G Lebed, Secretary
Quentin Johnson, Treasurer

The mission of Little City Foundation is to provide state of the art services to help children and adults with mental retardation or other developmental emotional and behavioral challenges to lead meaningful, productive, and dignified lives.

1879 Metropolitan Family Services

14 E Jackson Boulevard
Chicago, IL 60604-2259   312-986-4340
                                    Fax: 312-986-4187
                    E-mail: contactus@metrofamily.org
                                    www.metrofamily.org

Richard L Jones PhD, President and CEO
Nancy Kim Philips, Chief Operating Officer
Denis Hurley, Chife Financial Offcer
Evelyn Engler, Vice President, Human ResourcesS

Our mission is to help Chicago - area families become strong, stable and self-sufficient.

1880 West Central Federation of Families for Children's Mental Health

PO Box 813
Jacksonville, IL 62651-0813   217-785-5787
                                    Fax: 217-243-5299
                                    www.ffcmh.org/local.htm

Robert Dennis

Non-profit organization focused on the needs of children and youth, with emotional, behavioral or mental disorders and their families.

Indiana

1881 Indiana Alliance for the Mentally Ill

PO Box 22697
Indianapolis, IN 46222-0697   317-925-9399
                                        800-677-6442
                                    Fax: 317-925-9398
                                    www.nami.org

Laurie Flynn, Executive Director

NAMI Indiana is dedicated to improving the quality of life for those persons who are affected by mental illness.

1882 Indiana University Psychiatric Management

PO Box 2087
Indianapolis, IN 46224-3784   317-278-9100
                                        800-230-4876
                                    Fax: 317-278-9142
                            E-mail: iupm@iupui.edu

IUPM is a managed mental health program development within Indiana University which links quality mental health and substance abuse providers in the community with a superior academic psychiatric program.

1883 Mental Health Association in Marion County Consumer Services

2506 Willowbrook Parkway
Suite 100
Indianapolis, IN 46205-1542   317-251-0005
                                    Fax: 317-254-2800
                                    www.mcmha.org

Shary Johnson, President
Dan Collins, Vice President
Mike Simmons, Secretary
David Vonnegut-Gabovitch, Treasurer

The mission of the Association is to provide education, advocacy and service through programs designed to promote health; positively affect public attiudes and perceptions of mental illness through support and knowledge; and improve care and treatment of persons with mental ilness.

1884 Villages, Program Administration

85-175 Farrington Highway
Apt. A418
Waianae, HI 96792-2171   808-524-5900
                                    Fax: 808-585-9459
                        E-mail: nami-hi@hawaii.rr.com
                                    www.nami.org

Mike Durant, President

NAMI is dedicated to the eradication of mental illnesses and to the improvement of the quality of life of all whose lives are affected by these diseases.

Iowa

1885 Iowa Alliance for the Mentally Ill

5911 Meredith Drive
Suite E
Des Moines, IA 50322-1903   515-254-0417
                                        800-417-0417
                                    Fax: 515-254-1103
                            E-mail: amiiowa@aol.com
                                    www.nami.org

Kathy Trotter, President
Margret Stout, Executive Director

NAMI is dedicated to the education of mental illnesses and to the improvement of the quality of life of all whose lives are affected by these diseases.

1886 Iowa Federation of Families for Children's Mental Health

112 S Williams
PO Box 362
Anamosa, IA 52205-7321   319-462-2187
888-400-6302
Fax: 319-462-6789
E-mail: help@iffcmh.org
www.ffcmh.org/local.htm

Lori Reynolds

Our mission is to link families to community, county and state partners for needed support and services; and to promote system change that will enable families to live in a safe, stable and respectful environment.

1887 University of Iowa, Mental Health: Clinical Research Center

University of Iowa Hospitals & Clinics
200 Hawkins Drive
Iowa City, IA 52242-1009   319-356-4720
877-575-2864
Fax: 319-356-2587

Dr. Nancy C Andreassen, Director

We seek to improve the precision with which specific disease categories are defines and to increase our understanding of their underlying mechanisms and causes. Our primary emphasis is on schizophrenia spectrum disorders, including schizophrenia, schizoaffective disorder, schizopherniform disorder and schizotypal personality.

Kansas

1888 Kansas Alliance for the Mentally Ill

112 SW 6th
PO Box 675
Topeka, KS 66601   913-233-4804
800-539-2660
www.nami.org

Laurie Flynn, Executive Director

Nation's leading self-help organization for all those affected by severe brain disorders. Mission is to bring consumers and families with similar experiences together to share information about services, care providers, and ways to cope with the challenges of schizophrenia, manic depression, and other serious mental illnesses.

1889 Kansas Schizophernia Anonymous

112 SW 6th
PO Box 675
Topeka, KS 66601   913-233-1730

Laurie Flynn, Executive Director

Self-help organization for all those coping with the challenges of schizophrenia.

1890 Keys for Networking: Federation Families for Children's Mental Health

1301 S Topeka
Topeka, KS 66612   785-233-8732
800-499-8732
Fax: 785-235-6659
E-mail: jadams@keys.org
www.keys.org

Jane Adams

State family organization serving families whose children have serious emotional disabilities.

Kentucky

1891 Children's Alliance

420 Capitol Avenue
Frankfort, KY 40601   502-875-3399
Fax: 502-223-4200
E-mail: melissa.lawson@childrensallianceky.org
www.childrensallianceky.org

Bart Baldwin, President
Melissa Lawson, Member Services
Nannette Lenington, Business Manager

Our mission is to shape public policy, inform constituencies and provide leadership in advocacy for Kentucky's children and families.

1892 Clearsprings/Options

4010 Dupont Circle
Suite 283
Louisville, KY 40207-4847   502-899-3999
Fax: 502-894-4445

1893 FACES of the Blue Grass

570 E Main Street
Lexington, KY 40508-2342   606-254-3106
www.ffcmh.org/local.htm

Jim Powell

Support group for families who have children diagnosed with mental illness.

1894 KY-SPIN

10301-B Deering Road
Louisville, KY 40272   502-937-6894
800-525-7746
Fax: 502-937-6464
E-mail: spininc@aol.com
www.kyspin.com

Non-profit organization dedicated to promoting programs which will enable persons with disabilities and their families to enhance their quality of life.

1895 Kentucky Alliance for the Mentally Ill

10510 LeGrange Road
Building 103
Louisville, KY 40223-1228   502-245-5284
800-257-5081
Fax: 502-245-6390
E-mail: namiky@mindspring.com
www.nami.org

Harry Mills, Executive Director
Lois Anderson, President

Nation's leading self-help organization for all those affected by severe brain disorders. Mission is to bring consumers and families with similar experiences together to share information about services, care providers, and ways to cope with the challenges of schizophrenia, manic depression, and other serious mental illnesses.

1896 Kentucky IMPACT

275 E Main Street
Frankfort, KY 40621-0001   **502-564-7610**
                    E-mail: kyimpact@krccnet.com
                    www.mhmr.chs.ky.gov

Kentucky IMPACT is a statewide program which coordinates services for children with severe emotional disabilities and their families.

1897 Kentucky Psychiatric Association

PO Box 198
Frankfort, KY 40602-0198   **502-695-4843**
                              877-597-7924
                    Fax: 502-695-4441
                    E-mail: waltonkpa@aol.com
                    www.icypsych.org

Theresa Walton, Executive Director

A non-profit association of medical doctors who have completed a psychiatry residency.

1898 National Association of Social Workers: Kentucky Chapter

304 West Liberty Street
Suite 201
Louisville, KY 40202
                    800-526-8098
                    Fax: 502-589-3602
                    E-mail: naswky@aol.com
                    www.naswky.org

Professional membership organization, for state social workers.

1899 Project Vision

2210 Goldsmith Lane
Suite 118
Louisville, KY 40218-1038   **502-456-0923**
                              800-525-7746
                    Fax: 502-456-0893
                    www.ffcmh.org/local.htm

Laurie Cottrell

1900 SPOKES Federation of Families for Children's Mental Health

275 E Main Street
Frankfort, KY 40621-0001   **502-564-7610**
                              Fax: 502-564-9010
          E-mail: danderson@mhrdmc.chr.state.ky.us
                    www.ffcmh.org/local.htm

Debbie Anderson

Non-profit organization focused on the need of children and youth with emotional, behavioral or mental disorders and their families.

Louisiana

1901 Louisiana Alliance for the Mentally Ill

PO Box 64585
Baton Rouge, LA 70896   **504-343-6928**
                              www.la.nami.org

Diane Pitts, President

Nation's leading self-help organization for all those affected by severe brain disorders. Mission is to bring consumers and families with similar experiences together to share information about services, care providers, and ways to cope with the challenges of schizophrenia, manic depression, and other serious mental illnesses.

1902 Louisiana Federation of Families for Children's Mental Health

200 Lafayette Street
Suite 420
Baton Rouge, LA 70801   **225-346-4020**
                              Fax: 225-346-0770
                              www.laffcmh.com

The purpose of the FFCMH is to serve the needs of children with serious emotional, behavioral and mental disorders and their families.

Maine

1903 Familes United for Children's Mental Health

PO Box 2107
Augusta, ME 04338-2107   **207-622-3309**
                              Fax: 207-622-1661
                              www.ffcmh.org/local.htm

Pat Hunt

Non-profit organization providing statewide individual emotional suuport, information and referrals, help in locating services, news regarding children's mental health issues and current events, support groups, newsletter, family and professional collaborations, family and systems advocacy, family member participation in policy and system development.

1904 Maine Alliance for the Mentally Ill

1 Bangor Street
Augusta, ME 04330   **207-622-5767**
                              800-464-5767
                    Fax: 207-621-8430
                    E-mail: NAMI-ME@nami.org
                    www.me.nami.org

David Sturtevant, Executive Director

Nation's leading self-help organization for all those affected by severe brain disorders. Mission is to bring consumers and families with similar experiences together to share information about services, care providers, and ways to cope with the challenges of schizophrenia, manic depression, and other serious mental illnesses.

1905 Maine Psychiatric Association

PO Box 190
Manchester, ME 04351-0190   207-622-7743
                                   Fax: 207-622-3332
          E-mail: weldridge@mainemed.com

Warene Chase Eldridge, Executive Secretary

To provide treatment for all persons with mental disorder, including mental retardation and substance-related disorders.

Maryland

1906 Community Behavioral Health Association of Maryland: CBH

18 Egges Lane
Cantonsville, MD 21228-4511   410-788-1865
                                     Fax: 410-788-1768
          E-mail: mdcbh@aol.com
               www.cbh.bluestep.net

Carol Veater, Administration

Professional association for Maryland's network of community behavioral health programs operating in the public and private sectors.

1907 Department of Health and Human Services/OAS

200 Independence Avenue SW
Washington, DC 20201   202-619-0257
                              877-696-6775
                              www.dhhs.gov

The DHHS is the United States government's principal agency for protecting the health of all Americans and providing essential human services, especially for those who are least able to help themselves.

1908 Families Involved Together

2219 Maryland Avenue
Baltimore, MD 21218   410-235-5222
                             Fax: 410-235-4222
          E-mail: diane@familiesinvolved.org

Diane Sakwa

Parents of children with special needs.

1909 Health Resources and Services Administration

Parklawn Building
5600 Fishers Lane
Rockville, MD 20857   301-594-4060
                             Fax: 301-594-4984
                             www.hrsa.gov

Elizabeth Duke PhD, Administrator
Stephen Smith, Senior Advisor

The Health Resources and Services Administration's mission is to improve and expand access to quality health care for all.

1910 Institute of Psychiatry and Human Behavior: University of Maryland

701 West Pratt Street
Suite 388
Baltimore, MD 21201-1542   410-328-6736
          E-mail: VPorter@psych.umaryland.edu
               www.medschool.umaryland.edu

John Talbot MD, Director

conducts studies of psychiatric disorders.

1911 Maryland Alliance for the Mentally Ill

711 W 40th Street
Suite 451
Baltimore, MD 21211   410-467-7100
                             800-467-0075
                             Fax: 410-467-7195
          E-mail: amimd@aol.com
               www.nami.org

Barbara Bellack, Executive Director

Nation's leading self-help organization for all those affected by severe brain disorders. Mission is to bring consumers and families with similar experiences together to share information about services, care providers, and ways to cope with the challenges of schizophrenia, manic depression, and other serious mental illnesses.

1912 Maryland Psychiatric Research Center

PO Box 21247
Baltimore, MD 21228-0747   410-402-7666
                             www.mprc.umaryland.edu

Dr. William Carpenter Jr, Director

To study the manifestations, causes, and innovative treatment of zchizophrenia.

1913 Mental Health Association of Maryland

711 W 40th Street
Suite 460
Baltimore, MD 21211-2110   410-235-1178
                                  800-572-6426
                                  Fax: 410-235-1180
          E-mail: info@mhamd.org
               www.mhamd.org

Christine McKee, Public Education Director
Diane Cabot, Regional Director
Linda Raines, Executive Director

The Mental Health Association of Maryland is dedicated to promoting mental health, preventing mental disorders and achieving victory over mental illness through advocacy, education, research and service.

1914 National Association of Social Workers: Maryland Chapter

5740 Executive Drive
Suite 208
Baltimore, MD 21228-1759   410-788-1066
                                  800-867-6776
                                  Fax: 410-747-0635
          E-mail: nasw.md@verizon.net
               www.nasw-md.org

The mission of the NASW-MD chapter is to support, promote and advocate for the social work profession and its clients, promote just and equitable social policies and for the health and welfare of the people of Maryland.

1915 Sheppard Pratt Health System

6501 N Charles Street
Baltimore, MD 21285   410-938-3000
                            888-938-4207
                        Fax: 410-938-3159
            E-mail: info@sheppardpratt.org
                    www.sheppardpratt.org

Dr Steven S Sharfstein, President/CEO
Dr Robert Roca, VP & Medical Director

Private, nonprofit behavioral health system with inpatients, partial outpatient, residential, crisis, contract management.

1916 Survey & Analysis Branch

5600 Fishers Lane
Rockwall II Suite 15C
Rockville, MD 20857-0002   301-443-3343
                            Fax: 301-443-7926
                            www.samhsa.gov

Dr. Ronald Manderscheid, Branch Chief

Federally funded agency studying mental health issues.

Massachusetts

1917 Concord-Assabet Family and Adolescent Services

380 Massachusetts Avenue
Acton, MA 07120-3745   978-369-4909
                        Fax: 978-263-3088
                            www.cafas.org

Kathi Geisler, Director Public Relations

Provides individual, couples, family, group counseling, education/preventive programs, outreach/advocacy, services for older adults, young parents and youths.

1918 Depressive and Manic-Depressive Association of Boston

115 Mill Street
PO Box 102
Belmont, MA 02478-0001   617-855-2795
                        Fax: 617-855-3666
            E-mail: info@mddaboston.org
                    www.mddaboston.org/

MDDA-BOSTON is resource for people with affective disorders and their families and friends.

1919 Greater Lynn Mental Health & Retardation Association

37 Friend Street
PO Box 408
Lynn, MA 01903-0508   781-593-1088
                        Fax: 781-593-5731
                            www.glmh.org

Robert Stearns, CEO
Elaine White, Director of Facilities

Private, non-profit corporation that provides residential, clinical, recreation, day and employment, work training, affordable housing, and multi-cultural and community education services for people with disabilities, their families, and advocates in Northeastern Massachusetts.

1920 Jewish Family and Children's Services

31 New Chardon Street
Boston, MA 02114-4701   617-227-6641
                        Fax: 617-227-3220

Jewish Family and Children's Services is here to help individuals and families of all ages through human service and health care programs that reflect Jewish values of social responsibility and concern for all members of the community.

1921 Massachusetts Alliance for the Mentally Ill

400 W Cummings Park
Suite 6650
Woburn, MA 01801-6528   781-938-4048
                            800-370-9085
                        Fax: 781-938-4069
            E-mail: namimass@aol.com
                    www.namimass.org

Toby Fisher, Executive Director
Philip Hadley, President

Nation's leading self-help organization for all those affected by severe brain disorders. Mission is to bring consumers and families with similar experiences together to share information about services, care providers, and ways to cope with the challenges of schizophrenia, manic depression, and other serious mental illnesses.

1922 Massachusetts Behavioral Health Partnership

120 Front Street
Suite 315
Worcester, MA 01608   508-890-6400
                        Fax: 508-890-6410

The Massachusetts Behavioral Behavioral Health Partnership manages the mental health and substance abuse services for MassHealth Members who select the Division's Primary Care Clinician Plan.

1923 Mental Health and Substance Abuse Corporations of Massachusetts

251 W Central Street
Natick, MA 01760   508-647-8385
                        Fax: 508-647-8311

To promote community-based mental health and substance abuse services as the most appropriate, clinically effective, and cost-sensitive method for providing care to individuals in need.

1924 Parent Professional Advocacy League

59 Temple Place
Suite 664
Boston, MA 02111   617-542-7860
                                      800-537-0446
                              Fax: 617-542-7832
                          E-mail: info@ppal.net
                          www.http://ppal.net

Provides support, education, and advocacy around issues related to children's mental health

Michigan

1925 Ann Arbor Consultation Services Performance & Health Solutions

5331 Plymouth Road
Ann Arbor, MI 48105-9520   313-996-9111
                              Fax: 313-996-1950

Outpatient services for mental health and chemical dependency issues.

1926 Borgess Behavioral Medicine Services

1521 Gull Road
Kalamazoo, MI 49048   269-226-7000
                              Fax: 269-324-8665
                                  www.borgess.com

Alan O Kogan MD, Medical Director
Denise Crawford MSW, Referal Development Division

Offers patients and families a wide array of services to address their mental health concerns.

1927 Boysville of Michigan

8759 Clinton Macon Road
Clinton, MI 49236-9572   517-423-7451
                              Fax: 517-423-5442
                    E-mail: djablons@boysville.org
                              www.boysville.org

David Jablonski, Director of Communications
Francis Boylan, President/CEO

Boysville of Michigan works with one thousand plus boys and girls and their families on a daily basis in both residential and community based programs throughout Michigan and northwestern Ohio.

1928 Justice in Mental Health Organizations

421 Seymour Avenue
Lansing, MI 48933-1116   517-371-2794
                                      800-831-8035
                              Fax: 517-371-5770
                      E-mail: jimhojim@aol.com

Lisa Howell, Executive Director

The JMHO is a non-profit 501 (c) (3) organization in Lansing, Michigan. It is an advocacy group, as well as a mutual self-help organization that offers a network of support to thousands of individuals living in the community.

1929 Lapeer County Community Mental Health Center

1570 Suncrest Drive
Lapeer, MI 48446-1154   810-667-0500
                              Fax: 810-664-8728
                          E-mail: iccmhc@tir.com
                              www.countylapeer.org

Michael K Vizena, Executive Director
Lauren J Emmons, Associate Director

Comprehensive community mental health services to children and adults of all ages. Services are limited to Lapeer County residents. Most insurance plans are honored. A sliding fee schedule is applied for those without insurance benefits. The center is licensed by the state of Michigan and is fully accredited by JCAHO.

1930 Macomb County Community Mental Health

10 N Main
5th Floor
Mt Clemens, MI 48043   586-948-0222
                              Fax: 586-469-7674

Provides a wide variety of mental health treatment and support services to adults and children with mental illness, developmental disabilities, and substance abuse treatment needs.

1931 Manic Depressive and Depressive Association of Metropolitan Detroit

PO Box 32531
Detroit, MI 48232-0531   734-284-5563
                          www.mdda-metro-detroit.org

Educates patients, families, and professionals, and the public concerning the nature of depressive and manic-depressive illness as treatable medical diseases; to foster self-help for patients and families; to eliminate discrimination and stigma; to improve access to care; and to advocate for research toward the elimination of these illnesses.

1932 Metropolitan Area Chapter of Federation of Families for Children's Mental Health

5504 Kreger
Sterling Heights, MI 48310   810-978-1221
                              www.ffcmh.org/local.htm

Pat Boyer

Dedicated to children and adolescents with mental health needs and their families.

1933 Michigan Alliance for the Mentally Ill

921 N Washington Avenue
Lansing, MI 48906   517-485-4049
                                      800-331-4264
                              Fax: 517-485-2333
                    E-mail: namimichigan@acd.net
                              www.mi.nami.org

Hubert Huebl, President

Nation's leading self-help organization for all those affected by severe brain disorders. Mission is to bring consumers and families with similar experiences together to share information about services, care providers, and ways to cope with the challenges of schizophrenia, manic depression, and other serious mental illnesses.

1934 Michigan Association for Children with Emotional Disorders: MACED

230233 Southfield Road
Suite 219
Southfield, MI 48076-0000　　　248-433-2200
Fax: 248-433-2299
E-mail: info@michkids.org
www.michkids.org

Samuel L Davis, Clinical Director

Ensures that children with serious emotional disorders receive appropriate mental health and educational services so that they reach their full potential. To provide support to families and to encourage community understanding of the need for specialized programs for their children.

1935 Michigan Association for Children's Mental Health

941 Abbott Road
Suite P
East Lansing, MI 48823-3104　　517-336-7222
800-782-0883
Fax: 517-336-8884
E-mail: acmhlori@acd.net
www.ffcmh.org

Robin Laurain, Family Advocacy Consultant

Provides advocacy, resources and educational training to parents of emotionally impaired children.

1936 Northpointe Behavioral Healthcare Systems

715 Pyle Drive
Kingsford, MI 49802-4456　　　906-774-9522
Fax: 906-774-1570
E-mail: info@nbhs.org
www.nbhs.org

Michigan Community Mental Health agency serving Dickinson, Menominee and Iron counties. Provides a full spectrum of managed behavioral healthcare services to the chronically mentally ill and developmentally disabled. A corporate services division provides employee assistance programs both in Michigan and outside the state.

1937 Southwest Counseling & Development Services

1700 Waterman Street
Detroit, MI 48209-3317　　　　313-841-8905
Fax: 313-841-4470
www.comnet.org

John Van Camp, President/CEO
Graciela Villalobos, Program Director of Outpatient

A mental health agency working to promote community well being. The mission is to enhance the well being of individuals, families and the community by providing effective leadership and innovative, quality mental health services.

1938 Woodlands Behavioral Healthcare Network

960 M-60 East
Cassopolis, MI 49031　　　　　269-445-2451
Fax: 269-445-3216
www.woodlandsbhn.org

Provides community mental health services.

Minnesota

1939 Centre for Mental Health Solutions: Minnesota Bio Brain Association

2000 South Plymouth Road
Suite 220
Minnetonka, MN 55305　　　　952-922-6916
877-853-6916
Fax: 952-922-3412
E-mail: info@mentalhealthsolutions.org
www.tcfmhs.org

Tamera Shumaker, Executive Director
Nicole Zivalich, CEO

Our goal and primary focus is to investigate the underlying core causes in the body's biochemistry that allows illness to present itself and to provide information and education about healthy lifestyles, exercise, nutritious foods, proper nutritional supplements, clean air and water, sunshine and right thinking and attitudes that will ultimately manifest into vibrant health.

1940 Minnesota Association for Children's Mental Health

165 Western Avenue
Suite 2
Saint Paul, MN 55102　　　　　651-644-7333
800-528-4511
Fax: 651-644-7391
E-mail: dsaxhaug@macmh.org
www.macmh.org

Deborah Saxhaug

The mission of the Minnesota Association for Children's Mental Health is to enhance the quality of life for children with emotional or behavioral disorders and their families.

1941 Minnesota National Alliance for the Mentally Ill

970 Raymond Avenue S
Suite 105
Saint Paul, MN 55114-1164　　　651-645-2948
888-473-0237
Fax: 651-645-7379
E-mail: nami-mn@nami.org
www.nami.org/namimn

Sue Abderholden, Executive Director

Advocates for justice, dignity and respect for all people affected by mental illness and biological brain disorders. Through education, advocacy and support we strive to eliminate the pervasive stigma of mental illness, effect positive changes in the mental health system as well as increasing public and professional understanding of mental illness.

1942 Minnesota Psychiatric Society

4707 Highway 61
#232
Saint Paul, MN 55110-3227   651-407-1873
Fax: 651-407-1754
www.mnpsychoc.org

Laura Vukelich, Executive Director

The Minnesota Psychiatric Society is a professional association of psychiatrics. Our vision is accessible, quality mental health care for the patients that we service.

1943 Minnesota Psychological Association

1711 W County Road B
Suite 310N
Roseville, MN 55113-4036   651-697-0440
Fax: 651-697-0439
www.mnpsych.org

Enhances public and psychological interests by promoting the science of psychology and its applications.

1944 NASW Minnesota Chapter

Iris Park Place, Suite 340
1885 University Avenue W
Saint Paul, MN 55104   651-293-1935
Fax: 651-293-0952
E-mail: email@naswmn.org
www.naswmn.org

To promote the profession of Social Work by establishing and maintaining professional standards and by advancing the authority and credibility of Social Work; to provide services to its members by supplying opportunities for professional development and leadership and by enhancing communication among its members; to advocate for clients by promoting political action and community education.

1945 North American Training Institute: Division of the Minnesota Council on Compulsive Gambling

314 W Superior Street
Suite 702
Duluth, MN 55802-1805   218-722-1503
888-989-9234
Fax: 218-722-0346
E-mail: info@nati.org
www.nati.org

Elizabeth M George, Chief Executive Director

The NATI conducts web based clinical courses to provide specific knowledge and advanced training leading to national certification for professionals in the prevention, treatment, and rehabilitation of patholgical gamblers.

1946 Pacer Center

8161 Normandale Boulevard
Minneapolis, MN 55437   952-838-9000
800-537-2237
Fax: 952-838-0199
TTY: 952-838-0190
E-mail: pacer@pacer.org
www.pacer.org

To expand opportunities and anhance the quality of life of children and young adults with disabilities and their families, based on the concept of parents helping parents.

Mississippi

1947 Mississippi Alliance for the Mentally Ill

411 Briarwood Drive
Suite 401
Jackson, MI 39206   601-899-9058
800-357-0388
Fax: 601-956-6380
E-mail: namimiss1@aol.com
www.nami.org

Teri Brister, Executive Director
Annette Giessner, President

Nation's leading self-help organization for all those affected by severe brain disorders. Mission is to bring consumers and families with similar experiences together to share information about services, care providers, and ways to cope with the challenges of schizophrenia, manic depression, and other serious mental illnesses.

1948 Mississippi Families as Allies

5166 Keele Street
Suite B100
Jackson, MS 39206-4319   601-981-1618
800-833-9671
Fax: 601-981-1696
E-mail: msfam@netdoor.com
www.cecp.air.org

Tressa Eide, Family Support Coordinator

To provide information and emotional support to families, provide education and training for families and professionals and advocate for improvements in the System of Care for Mississippi's children.

Missouri

1949 Depressive and Manic-Depressive Association of St. Louis

1905 S Grand Boulevard
Saint Louis, MO 63104-1542   314-776-3969
Fax: 314-776-7071
E-mail: dmdastl@aol.com
www.ndmda.org

A consumer drop-in center, friendship line, peer support and self-help group.

1950 Mental Health Association of Greater St. Louis

1905 S Grand Boulevard
Saint Louis, MO 63104-1542　　314-773-1399
Fax: 314-773-5930
E-mail: mhagstleaol.com
www.mhagstl.org

The Mental Health Association (MHA) of Greater St. Louis serves St. Louis City and the counties of St. Louis, St. Charles, Lincoln, Warren, Franklin and Jefferson. Services include educational literature/reference library, referrals to mental health professionals and self-help groups, representative payee services, educational course (BRIDGES), speakers bureau and more.

1951 Missouri Alliance for the Mentally Ill

1001 SW Boulevard
Suite E
Jefferson City, MO 65109-2501　　314-634-7727
800-374-2138
Fax: 573-761-5636
E-mail: mocami@aol.com

Steven R Wilhelm, President
Cindi Keele, Executive Director

The Missouri Coalition of Alliance for the Mentally Ill is a family organization for persons with brain disorders. It has 15 active chapters throughout Missouri.

1952 Missouri Institute of Mental Health

University of Missouri
5400 Arsenal Street
Saint Louis, MO 63139-1300　　314-644-8787
Fax: 314-644-8834
www.mimh.edu

1953 Missouri Statewide Parent Advisory Network: MO-SPAN

440 A Rue Street Francois
Florissant, MO 63031　　314-972-0600
Fax: 314-972-0606
www.mo.span.org

Donna Dittrich, Executive Director
Tina Var Vera, Administrative Assistant

The mission of MO-SPAN is to improve the lives of children and youth with serious emotional disorders and their families by supporting and mobilizing families through training, education, advocacy and systems change. MO-SPAN is a statewide, nonprofit organization which is directed by a Board of Directors, the majority of who are parents of children with severe emotional disabilities.

Montana

1954 Family Support Network

3302 4th Avenue
Suite 103
Billings, MT 59104-1366　　406-256-7783
Fax: 406-256-9879
www.ffcmh.org/local.htm

Barbara Sample, Executive Director

Dedicated to children and adolescents with mental health needs and their families.

1955 Mental Health Association of Montana

25 S Ewing
Suite 206
Helena, MT 59601　　406-442-4276
Fax: 406-442-4986
E-mail: mmha@in-tch.com
www.mhamontana.org

Charles McCarthy, Executive Director
Betty DeYoung, Administrative Assistant

Providing public education and advocacy for mental health services in Montana for over fifty years. Provides a hot line, conferences, libraries and has five local affiliates. Over twelve hundred individual and organization memberships.

1956 Montana Alliance for the Mentally Ill

554 Toole Court
Helena, MT 59602-6946　　406-443-7871
888-280-6264
Fax: 406-862-6357
E-mail: namimt@ixi.net
www.mt.nami.org

Gary Mihelish, President

Nebraska

1957 Department of Health and Human Services Regulation and Licensure

Credentialing Division
301 Centennial Mall South 3rd Floor
Lincoln, NE 68509-5007　　402-471-2155
Fax: 402-471-3577
E-mail: marie.mcclatchey@hhss.state.ne.us
www.hhs.state.ne.us/crl/crlindex.htm

Dick Nelson, Director
Helen Meeks, Division Administrator

The Credentialing Division's mission is to assure the public that health-related practices provided by individuals, facilities and programs are safe, of acceptable quality, and that the cost of expanded services is justified by the need.

1958 Mutual of Omaha Companies: Integrated Behavioral Services and Psychiatric Programs

Mutual of Omaha Plaza
Omaha, NE 68175-0001　　402-351-8364
Fax: 402-351-2880

1959 National Association of Social Workers: Nebraska Chapter

PO Box 83732
Lincoln, NE 68501-3732　　402-477-7344
877-816-6279
Fax: 402-476-6547
E-mail: naswne@assocoffice.net
www.naswne.org

June Remington, Executive Director

Nebraska chapter is an affiliate of the National Association of Social Workers with a membership of six hundred plus.

1960 Nebraska Alliance for the Mentally Ill

1941 S 42nd Street
Suite 517
Omaha, NE 68105

402-345-8101
877-463-6264
Fax: 402-346-4070
E-mail: cwuebben@nami.org
www.ne.nami.org

Colleen M Wuebben, Executive Director
Carole Denton, President

The office of NAMI Nebraska, a non-profit organization dedicated to providing support, education and advocacy to and for anyone whose life has been touched by a mental illness.

1961 Nebraska Family Support Network

3801 Harney Street
2nd Floor
Omaha, NE 68131

402-505-4608
800-245-6081
Fax: 402-444-7722

1962 Pilot Parents: PP

Ollie Webb Center
1941 S 42nd Street
Suite 122
Omaha, NE 68105-2942

402-346-5220
Fax: 402-346-5253
E-mail: jvarner@olliewebb.org
www.olliewebb.org

Jennifer Varner, Coordinator

Parents, professionals and others concerned with providing emotional and peer support to new parents of children with special needs. Sponsors a parent-matching program which allows parents who have had sufficient experience and training in the care of their own children to share their knowledge and expertise with parents of children recently diagnosed as disabled. Publications: The Gazette, newsletter, published 6 times a year. Also has chapters in Arizona and limited other states.

Nevada

1963 Carson City Alliance for the Mentally Ill Share & Care Group

Carson City, NV 89701-6122

775-882-9749
Fax: 775-665-1639
www.nami.org

Ruth Paxton

Part of the nation's leading self-help organization for all those affected by severe brain disorders. Mission is to bring consumers and families with similar experiences together to share information about services, care providers, and ways to cope with the challenges of schizophrenia, manic depression, and other serious mental illnesses.

1964 Nevada Alliance for the Mentally Ill

6150 Transverse Drive #104
Las Vegas, NV 89146

702-258-1618
Fax: 702-258-6931
www.nami-nevada.org

Rosetta Johnson, President

Organization composed of families, friends, and professionals who are dedicated to helping people with mental illness and their families in coping with the devastation of the illness.

1965 Nevada Principals' Executive Program

2355 Red Rock Street
Suite 106
Las Vegas, NV 89146

702-388-8899
800-216-5188
Fax: 702-388-2966
E-mail: pepinfo@nvpep.org
www.nvpep.org

Karen Taycher

To strengthen and renew th knowledge, skills, and beliefs of public school leaders so that they might help improve the conditions for teaching and learning in schools and school districts.

New Hampshire

1966 Monadnock Family Services

64 Main Street
Suite 301
Keene, NH 03431-3701

603-357-6878
Fax: 603-357-6896
E-mail: rboyd@mfs.org
www.mfs.org

Ken Jue, CEO
Gary Barnes, COO
Peter Skalahan, CFO

A nonprofit community mental health center serving the mental health needs of families, buisness and other public and private organizations with comprehensive continuum of education, prevention and treatment services.

1967 New Hampshire Alliance for the Mentally Ill

15 Green Street
Concord, NH 03301-4020

603-225-5359
800-242-6264
Fax: 603-228-8848
E-mail: naminh@naminh.org
www.naminh.org

Michael Cohen, Executive Director
Sam Adams, President

Nation's leading self-help organization for all those affected by severe brain disorders. Mission is to bring consumers and families with similar experiences together to share information about services, care providers, and ways to cope with the challenges of schizophrenia, manic depression, and other serious mental illnesses.

New Jersey

1968 Association for Advancement of Mental Health

819 Alexander Road
Princeton, NJ 08540-6303

609-452-2088
Fax: 609-452-0627
E-mail: info@aamh.org

Richard McDonnell, Executive Director
Bruce Moehler, Director of Development

A private, non-profit community-based mental health agency licensed by the NJ State Division of Mental Health and Hospitals, that provides comprehensive services to Mercer County individuals and their families who lives are adversely affected by emotional distress, psychiatric illness and development disability. Fees are based on ability to pay.

1969 Association for Children of New Jersey

35 Halsey Street
2nd Floor
Newark, NJ 07102-3000   **973-643-3876**
                                Fax: 973-643-9153
                                www.acnj.org

Suzanne Poole, Office Manager

The organization primarily works through community education, research and public policy analysis to improve opportunities for all of New Jersey's children and their families.

1970 Eating Disorders Association of New Jersey

10 Station Place
Metuchen, NJ 08840
                                800-522-2230
                                Fax: 609-688-1544
                                E-mail: njaaba@aol.com
                                www.njaaba.org

Leigh Garfield, President

Self-help organization which offers information and referrals, and professionally-run support groups at 12 locations state-wide for people with eating disorders, their families, friends and interested professionals.

1971 Jewish Family Service of Atlantic County and Cape

3 S Weymouth Avenue
Ventnor City, NJ 08406-2948   **609-822-1108**
                                    Fax: 609-882-1106
                                    www.jfsatlantic.org

Multi-service familty counseling agency dedicated to promoting, strengthening and preserving individual, family, and community weel-being in a manner consistent with Jewish philosophy and values.

1972 Mental Health Association of New Jersey

1562 US Highway 130
North Brunswick, NJ 08902   **732-940-0991**
                                  Fax: 732-940-0355
                                  E-mail: naminj@optonline.net
                                  www.naminj.org

Sylvia Axelrod, Executive Director
Mark Perrin, President

Nation's leading self-help organization for all those affected by severe brain disorders. Mission is to bring consumers and families with similar experiences together to share information about services, care providers, and ways to cope with the challenges of schizophrenia, manic depression, and other serious mental illnesses.

1973 National Association for the Mentally Ill of New Jersey

1562 Route 130
N Brunswick, NJ 08902   **732-940-0991**
                              Fax: 732-940-0355
                              E-mail: naminj@optonline.net
                              www.naminj.org

Mark Perrin MD, President
Sylvia Axelrod, Executive Director

NAMI New Jersey is a statewide non profit organization dedicated to improving the lives of individuals and families who are affected by mental illness.

1974 New Jersey Association of Mental Health Agencies

The Neuman Building
3575 Quakerbridge Road, Suite 102
Mercerville, NJ 08619   **609-838-5488**
                              Fax: 609-838-5489
                              www.njamha.org

Debra L Wentz

To champion opprotunities that advance its members' ability to deliver accessible, quality, efficient and effective integrated behavioral health care services to mental health consumers and their families.

1975 New Jersey Protection and Advocacy

210 S Broad Street
3rd Floor
Trenton, NJ 08608-2404   **609-292-9742**
                               800-922-7233
                               Fax: 609-777-0187
                               TDD: 609-633-7106
                               E-mail: advocate@njpanda.org
                               www.njpanda.org

Richard West, Secretary
Marilyn Goldstein, Vice-Chair

Legal and non legal advocacy, information and referral, technical assistance and training, outreach and education in support of the human, civil, and legal rights of people with disabilities in New Jersey.

1976 New Jersey Psychiatric Association

PO Box 8008
Bridgewater, NJ 08807-8008   **908-685-0650**
                                   Fax: 908-725-8610
                                   E-mail: psychnj@optonline.net

Carla A Ross, Executive Director

The New Jersey Psychiatric Association is a professional organization of about 900 physicians qualified by training and experience in the treatment of mental illness. NJPA is a District Branch of the American Psychiatric Association and is the official voice of organized psychiatry in New Jersey.

1977 New Jersey Support Groups

Anorexia/Bulimia Association of New Jersey
10 Station Place
Metuchen, NJ 08840   **609-252-0202**

Offers various support groups across the state for anorexics and bulimics.

New Mexico

1978 Navajo Nation K'E Project-Shiprock Children & Families Advocacy Corp

PO Box 1240
Shiprock, NM 87420-1240   505-368-4479
                                 Fax: 505-368-5582

Evelyn Balwin

Provides community-based behavioral and/or mental health and related services to children and familieswith serious emotional difficulties.

1979 New Mexico Alliance for the Mentally Ill

6001 Marble NE Suite 8
PO Box 3086
Albuquerque, NM 87190-3086   505-260-0154
                                Fax: 505-260-0342
                                E-mail: naminm@aol.com
                                www.naminm.org

Elaine Jones, Executive Director
Elaine Miller, Administrator Assistant

Nation's leading self-help organization for all those affected by severe brain disorders. Mission is to bring consumers and families with similar experiences together to share information about services, care providers, and ways to cope with the challenges of schizophrenia, manic depression, and other serious mental illnesses.

New York

1980 Alliance for the Mentally Ill: Friends & Advocates of the Mentally Ill

New York, NY 10018-6505   212-684-3264
                                E-mail: helpline@naminyc.org
                                www.nami-nyc-metro.org

Evelyn Roberts, Executive Director

The AMI/FAMI is an affiliate of the National Alliance for the Mentally Ill. Offers a wide range of support groups, educational lectures, a newsletter and public access cable television program, Resource Center, Help Line and advocacy efforts.

1981 Babylon Consultation Center

206 Deer Park Avenue
Babylon, NY 11702-1929   631-587-1924
                                www.kindesigns.com

Michael J Beck PhD, Founder
Dr Jacob Kesten PhD, Consulting Psychologist

The Babylon Consultation Center is a community based provider of full gamut of mental health services for over 20 years, and consists of a multi-disciplinary group of professional independent contractors representing the fields of psychology, social work, marriage and family counseling, mediation also education and business consulting.

1982 Compeer

259 Monroe Avenue
Suite B1
Rochester, NY 14607-3632   585-546-8280
                                800-836-0475
                                Fax: 585-325-2558
                                E-mail: compeerp@rochester.rr.com
                                www.compeer.org

Bernice Skirboll, Executive Director
Andrea Miller, VP

National nonprofit organization which matches community volunteers in supportive friendship relationships with children and adults recieving mental health treatment.

1983 Eating Disorder Council of Long Island

50 Charles Lindbergh Boulevard
Suite 400
Uniondale, NY 11553   516-229-2393

The EDCLI is a non-profit organization devoted to prevention, education and support prevention of eating disorders, and support to sufferers of eating disorders, their families and their friends.

1984 Families Together in New York State

15 Elk Street
Albany, NY 12207   518-432-0333
                                888-326-8644
                                Fax: 518-434-6478
                                E-mail: info@ftnys.org
                                www.ftnys.org

Non-profit, parent-run organization that strives to establish a unified voice for children with emotional, behavioral, and social challenges.

1985 Finger Lakes Parent Network

25 W Steuben Street
Bath, NY 14810   585-928-9894
                                Fax: 585-928-9894

Patti DiNardo

Parent-governed, non-profit organization focused on the needs of children and youth with emotional, behavioral or mental disorders and their families.

1986 Healthcare Association of New York State

1 Empire Drive
Rensselaer, NY 12144   518-431-7600
                                Fax: 518-431-7915
                                E-mail: info@hanys.org
                                www.hanys.org

Cindy Levernois, Director Behavioral Health

Serves as the primary advocate for more than 550 non-profit and public hospitals, health systems, long-term care, home care, hospice, and other health care organizations throughout New York State.

1987 Mental Health Association in Albany County

260 S Pearl Street
Albany, NY 12202   518-447-4555
                                Fax: 518-447-4661

To ensure that persons with mental illness are provided a full range of services that promote stabilization, rehabilitation and recovery for the purpose of enhancing or improving their lives.

1988 Mental Health Association in Dutchess County

510 Haight Avenue
Poughkeepsie, NY 12603-2434   845-473-2500
Fax: 845-473-4870
E-mail: mhadc@hvc.rr.com
www.mhadc.com

The Mental Health Association in Dutchess County is a voluntary, not-for-profit dedicated to the promotion of mental health, the prevention of mental illness and the improved care and treatment of persons with mental illnesses.

1989 Metro Intergroup of Overeaters Anonymous

350 Third Avenue
PO Box 759
New York, NY 10010   212-946-4599
E-mail: NYOAMetroOffice@yahoo.com

Offers various support groups and meetings.

1990 National Association of Social Workers New York State Chapter

188 Washington Avenue
Albany, NY 12210-2394   518-463-4741
Fax: 518-463-6446
E-mail: info@naswnys.com
www.naswnys.org

The National Association of Social Workers is the largest membership organization of professional social workers in the world, with more than 155,000 members. NASW works to enhance the professional growth and development of its members, to create and maintain professional standards, and to advance sound social policies.

1991 New York Association of Psychiatric Rehabilitation Services

1 Columbia Place
2nd Floor
Albany, NY 12207-1006   518-436-0008
Fax: 518-436-0044
E-mail: nyaprs@aol.com
www.nyaprs.org

Harvey Rosenthal, Executive Director
Kelly Adams, Administrative Coordinator

New York Association of Psychiatric Services (NYAPRS) is a statewide coalition of New Yorkers, who are in recovery from mental illness and the professionals who work alongside them in rehabilitation and peer support services located throughout New York State. NYAPRS' mission is to promote the partnership of consumers, providers and families seeking to increase opportunities for community integration and independence for persons who have experienced a mental illness.

1992 New York Business Group on Health

386 Park Avenue S
Suite 703
New York, NY 10016   212-252-7440
Fax: 212-252-7448
E-mail: nybgh@nybgh.org
www.nybgh.org

Laurel Pickering, Executive Director
Janaera J Gaston MPA, Programs Director

NYBGH is a not-for-profit coalition of 150 businesses and is the only organization in the New York Metropolitan area exclusively devoted to employer health benefit issues. The mission is to provide leadership and knowledge to employers to promote a value-based, market-driven healthcare system.

1993 New York State Alliance for the Mentally Ill

260 Washington Avenue
Albany, NY 12210-1336   518-462-2000
800-950-3228
Fax: 518-462-3811
E-mail: info@naminys.org
www.naminys.org

Sean C Moran, Program/Outreach Manager
J David Seay, Executive Director
Jeff Keller, Deputy Director

Organization comprised of families of individuals with mental illness. Members work to improve the quality of life for all people with mental illness and to eradicate the stigma associated with mental illness.

1994 Orange County Mental Health Association

20 Walker Street
Goshen, NY 10924   845-294-7411
Fax: 845-294-7348
www.mhaorangeny.com

Rosalyn Goldman

Promotes th epositive mental health and emotional well-being of Orange County residents, working towards reducing the stigma of mental illness, developmental disabilities, and providing support to victims of sexual assault and other crimes.

1995 Parents United Network: Parsons Child Family Center

60 Academy Road
Albany, NY 12208   518-426-2600
Fax: 518-447-5234

Joan Valery

County wide peer support organization providing support and advocacy for the special needs of families caring for children suffering from emotional, social and behavioral disorders. Is a local chapter of the national organization Federation of Families united Network, and is affiliated with state chapter.

1996 Project LINK

Ibero-American Action League
817 E Main Street
Rochester, NY 14605-2722   **585-256-8900**
                                          Fax: 585-256-0120
                              E-mail: eamarlin@iaal.org
                                          www.iaal.org

Julio Vasquez, Executive Director

As well as our other activities in the Hispanic community, we continue to be committed to the betterment and quality of life of the mentally ill. We advocate for the severely and persistently mentally ill individual who is at risk of becoming involved or is involved with the criminal justice system. Projeck LINK operates in partnership with the University of Rochester, Strong-Memorial Department of Psychiatry, Action for a Better Community, Monroe County Mental Health Clinic for Socio-Legal Services, St. Mary's Hospital, the Urban League of Rochester and the Ibero-American Action League.

1997 State University of New York at Stony Brook: Mental Health Research

450 Clarkson Avenue
PO Box 1195
Brooklyn, NY 11203-2056   **718-270-1270**

Oliver David, Director

1998 Westchester Alliance for the Mentally Ill

101 Executive Boulevard
Suite 2
Elmsford, NY 10523   **914-592-5458**
                                          www.nami.org

Provides support and education for families who are feeling alone and in pain with a member of their family suffering from mental illness; no meeting fee.

1999 Westchester Task Force on Eating Disorders

3 Mount Joy Avenue
Scarsdale, NY 10583-2632   **914-472-3701**

Karen Cohen

A professionally-led support group for people with eating disorders including anorexia, bulimia and compulsive overeating; families and professionals interested in learning about the disorder are welcome to the meetings.

2000 Yeshiva University: Soundview-Throgs Neck Community Mental Health Center

2527 Glebe Avenue
Bronx, NY 10461-3109   **718-904-4400**
                                          Fax: 718-931-7307

Dr. Itamar Salamon, Director

Mental health counseling for adults and children. Accepts Medicaid and private insurance. Sliding scale fee.

North Carolina

2001 National Association of Social Workers: North Carolina Chapter

412 Morson Street
PO Box 27582
Raleigh, NC 27611-7582   **919-828-9650**
                                          800-280-6207
                              Fax: 919-828-1341
                      E-mail: naswnc@naswnc.org
                                          www.naswnc.org

Katherine Boyd, Executive Director

NASW is a membership organization that promotes, develops, and protects the practice of social work and social workers. NASW also seeks to enhance the effective functioning and well-being of individuals, families, and communities through its work and through advocacy.

2002 North Carolina Alliance for the Mentally Ill

309 W Millbrook Road
Suite 121
Raleigh, NC 27609   **919-788-0801**
                                          800-451-9682
                              Fax: 919-788-0906
                      E-mail: mail@naminc.org
                                          www.nami.nc.org

Gloria Harrison, Helpline Director

Nation's leading self-help organization for all those affected by severe brain disorders. Mission is to bring consumers and families with similar experiences together to share information about services, care providers, and ways to cope with the challenges of schizophrenia, manic depression, and other serious mental illnesses.

2003 North Carolina Mental Health Consumers Organization

PO Box 27042
Raleigh, NC 27611-7042   **919-832-2286**
                                          800-326-3842
                              Fax: 919-828-6999

NC MHCO is a private non-profit organization not affilated with NAMI NC. This organization has been providing advocacy and support to adults with mental illness since 1989.

2004 Western North Carolina Families CAN (Children and Adolescents Network)

PO Box 665
Arden, NC 28704   **828-687-1157**
                      E-mail: wncfamilies@bellsouth.net

Ann May

Mutual support and community collaboration, provides resources, referrals, education, and advocacy for families who have children with challenging behaviors and serious emotional disorders.

North Dakota

2005 National Association of Social Workers: North Dakota Chapter

PO Box 1775
Bismarck, ND 58502-1775   701-223-4161
Fax: 701-224-9824

Tom Tupa, Executive Director

NASW Dakotas, serves the critical and diverse needs of the entire social work profession.

2006 North Dakota Federation of Families for Children's Mental Health: Region II

PO Box 3061
Bismarck, ND 58502-3061   701-222-1223
Fax: 701-250-8835
E-mail: ndffrg19@idt.net

Valorie Keeney

To provide support and information to families of children and adolescents with serious emotional, behavioral, or mental disorders.

2007 North Dakota Alliance for the Mentally Ill

Minot, ND 58702-6016   701-852-8202
E-mail: jsabol@ndak.net
www.nami.org

Janet Sabol

Nation's leading self-help organization for all those affected by severe brain disorders. Mission is to bring consumers and families with similar experiences together to share information about services, care providers, and ways to cope with the challenges of schizophrenia, manic depression, and other serious mental illnesses.

2008 North Dakota Federation of Families for Children's Mental Health: Region V

214 2nd Avenue
W Fargo, ND 58078   701-235-9923

Pat Harles

To provide support and information to families fo children and adolescents with serious emotional, behavioral, or mental disorders.

2009 North Dakota Federation of Families for Children's Mental Health: Region VII

PO Box 3061
Bismarck, ND 58502-3061   701-222-1223
Fax: 701-250-8835
E-mail: ndffrg19@idt.net

Carlotta McCleary

To rpovide support and information to families of children and adolescents with serious emotional, behavioral, or mental disorders.

2010 North Dakota Federation of Families for Children's Mental Health

PO Box 3061
Bismarck, ND 58502-3061   701-222-1223
Fax: 701-250-8835
E-mail: ndffrg19@idt.net

Liz Sweet

To provide support and informatin to families of children and adolescents with serious emotional, behavioral, or mental disorders.

2011 South Valley Mental Health Association

1 North 2nd Street
Suite 314
Fargo, ND 58102-4915   701-293-3384
E-mail: mkaspari@aol.com
www.nmha.org

Susan Rae Halgeland, Regional Director

Advocacy, education and referrals.

Ohio

2012 Concerned Advocates Serving Children & Families

9195 2nd Street
Canton, OH 44704-1132   330-454-7917
Fax: 330-455-2026

Connie Truman

Support group for families of children diagnosed with mental illness.

2013 Mental Health Association of Summit

405 Tallmadge Road
PO Box 639
Cuyahoga Falls, OH 44222   330-923-0688
Fax: 330-923-7573
E-mail: info@mhasc.net
www.mentalhealthassociationofsummitcounty.org

Rudy Libertini, Executive Director
Sandy Soful, Associate Director

The Mental Health Association of Summit is part of a network of professionals and volunteers committed to improving America's mental health seeking victory over mental illness. To help achieve this national goal we are working to improve mental health services, to initiate services where none exist and to monitor the use of mental health tax dollars in the community.

2014 Mount Carmel Behavioral Healthcare

1808 E Broad Street
Columbus, OH 43203-2003   614-251-8242
800-227-3256
E-mail: mcbhinfo@mchs.com
www.mcbh.com

Mark Ridenour, Executive Director
Marc Clemente MD, MBA, Medical Director

Mount Carmel Behavioral Healthcare is a behavioral healthcare management organization offering a cost-effective, comprehensive continuum of behavioral healthcare services.

2015 National Association of Social Workers: Ohio Chapter

33 N Third Street
Suite 530
Columbus, OH 43215   614-461-4484
                           Fax: 614-461-9793
                  E-mail: ohnasw@ameritech.net
                           www.naswoh.org

Elaine C Schiwy, Executive Director
Sarah E Hamilton, Membership Coordinator

The mission of NASW is to strengthen, support, and unify the social work profession, to promote the development of social work standards and practice, and to advocate for social policies that advance social justice and diversity.

2016 Ohio Alliance for the Mentally Ill

747 E Broad Street
Columbus, OH 43205   614-224-2700
                           800-686-2646
                           Fax: 614-224-5400
                  E-mail: amiohio@amiohio.org
                           www.namiohio.org

Terry L Russell, Executive Director
Stacey Smith, Operations Director

Nation's leading self-help organization for all those affected by severe brain disorders. Mission is to bring consumers and families with similar experiences together to share information about services, care providers, and ways to cope with the challenges of schizophrenia, manic depression, and other serious mental illnesses.

2017 Ohio Association of Child Caring Agencies

400 E Town Street
Suite G-10
Columbus, OH 43215-4700   614-461-0014
                                 Fax: 614-228-7004
                        E-mail: PWyman@oacca.org
                                 www.oacca.org

Penny M Wyman, Executive Director
George E Biggs, Assistant Executive Director

The Ohio Association of Child Caring Agencies is to promote and strengthen a fully-integrated, private/public network of high-quality services for Ohio's children and their families through advocacy, education, and support of member agencies.

2018 Ohio Council of Behavioral Healthcare Providers

35 E Gay Street
Suite 401
Columbus, OH 43215-3138   614-228-0747
                                 Fax: 614-228-0740
                E-mail: staff@ohiocouncil-bhp.org
                        www.ohiocouncil-bhp.org

Pat Bridgman, Associate Director
Brenda Cornett, Membership Services

A trade association representing provider organizations throughout Ohio which provide behavioral healthcare services to their communities.

2019 Ohio Department of Mental Health

30 E Broad Street
Room 1180
Columbus, OH 43215-3414   614-466-2596
                                 877-275-6364
                           Fax: 614-752-9453
                           TDD: 614-752-9696
                           TTY: 888-636-4889
                           www.mh.state.oh.us

State agency responsible for oversight and funding of public mental health programs and services.

2020 Planned Lifetime Assistance Network of Northeast Ohio

2490 Lee Boulevard
Suite 204
Cleveland Heights, OH 44118-1269   216-321-3611
                                 Fax: 216-321-0021
                  E-mail: info@planNEohio.org
                           www.planneohio.org

Provides individualized home-based social services and advocacy to assist families who have a neurobiologically disabled family member to function at their maximum. LISW staff provides therapy and works with existing service providers to ensure quality of care. Offers a wide range of community-based, social, and recreational activities for its participants.

2021 Positive Education Program

3100 Euclid Avenue
Cleveland, OH 44115-2508   216-361-4400
                                 Fax: 216-361-8600
                  E-mail: pepgen@pepcleve.org
                           www.pepcleve.org

Frank A Fecser Ph D, Executive Director
Tom Valore Ph D, Program Director

The Positive Education Program (PEP) is to help troubled and troubling children and their families build skills to grow and learn successfully.

2022 Six County

2845 Bell Street
Zanesville, OH 43701-1794   740-454-9766
                                 Fax: 740-588-6452
                  E-mail: info@sixcounty.org
                           www.sixcounty.org

Helping community mental health needs in Coshocton, Guernsey, Morgan, Muskingum, Noble and Perry counties. In addition to the traditional treatment services, specialized services have been developed to reach people with ever changing needs. Employee assistance, sheltered employment, intensive outpatient, and residential services.

Oklahoma

2023 Child & Adolescent Network

5131 N Classen Boulevard
Suite 110
Oklahoma City, OK 73118-4433   405-848-4330
                                      800-645-5437
                                 Fax: 405-840-4746
                           www.ffcmh.org/local.htm

Palma Bucher

Dedicated to children and adolescents with mental health needs and their families.

2024 Oklahoma Alliance for the Mentally Ill

500 N Broadway Avenue
Suite 100
Oklamhoma City, OK 73102-6200   405-230-1900
800-583-1264
Fax: 405-230-1903
E-mail: nami-OK@swbell.net
www.ok.nami.org

Jeff Tallent, Executive Director
Hope Ingle, President

Nation's leading self-help organization for all those affected by severe brain disorders. Mission is to bring consumers and families with similar experiences together to share information about services, care providers, and ways to cope with the challenges of schizophrenia, manic depression, and other serious mental illnesses.

2025 Oklahoma Mental Health Consumer Council

5131 N Classen Boulevard, Suite 200
Oklahoma City, OK 73118   405-840-0607
Fax: 405-840-4177

OMHCC is the statewide advocacy organization of and for mental health consumers. Offers support groups, speakers' bureau and advocacy consultations on all issues affecting consumers.

2026 Oklahoma Psychiatric Physicians Association

PO Box 1328
Norman, OK 73070-1328   405-360-5066
Fax: 405-447-1053
E-mail: oklapsychiatry@yahoo.com
www.oklahomapsychiatry.org

District branch of the American Psychiatric Association, is a medical specialty society recognized world-wide. Pysicians specialize in the diagnosis and treatment of mental and emotional illnesses and substance abuse disorders.

Oregon

2027 Anorexia Nervosa & Related Eating Disorders

PO Box 5102
Eugene, OR 97405-0102   503-344-1144
www.anred.com

Works with the Sacred Heart General Hospital in Eugene, Oregon, to provide information, assessments, support groups and treatment for anorexics and bulimics.

2028 Oregon Alliance for the Mentally Ill

2620 Greenway Drive NE
Suite 17
Salem, OR 97301-4538   503-370-7774
800-343-6264
Fax: 503-370-9452
E-mail: namior@comcast.net
www.namioregon.org

Monica Kosman, President
Stephen Loaiza, Executive Director

Dedicated to the eradication of mental illnesses and to the improvement of the quality of life of all whose lives are affected by these diseases. A self-help, support and advocacy organization of consumers, families, and friends of people with severe mental illnesses.

2029 Oregon Family Support Network

15544 S Clackamas River Drive
Oregon City, OR 97045   503-656-5440
Fax: 503-581-4841
E-mail: ofsn@open.org
www.ofsn.org

Maureen H Breckenridge, JD, Executive Director

Families throughout Oregon supporting other families who have children and adolescents with mental, emotional and behavioral disorders.

2030 Oregon Psychiatric Association

PO Box 2042
Salem, OR 97308-2042   503-370-7019
Fax: 503-587-8063
E-mail: assoc@wvi.com

John McCulley, Executive Secretary

To ensure human care and effective treatment for all persons with mental disorder, including mental retardation and substance-related disorders.

Pennsylvania

2031 Health Federation of Philadelphia

1211 Chestnut Street
Suite 801
Philadelphia, PA 19107-4120   215-567-8001
Fax: 215-567-7743

Natalie Levkovich, Executive Director

A private, non-profit membership organization which provides shared services to a consortium of community and federally qualified health centers in Philadelphia.

2032 Mental Health Association of South East Pennsylvania

1211 Chestnut Street
Philadelphia, PA 19401-4931   215-751-1800
800-688-4226
E-mail: mcps@mhasp.org
www.mhasp.org

Joseph A Rogers, President/CEO
Jack Boyle, Senior VP/COO

The Mental Health Association of Southeastern Pennsylvania is a nonprofit citizen's organization that develops, supports and promotes innovative education and advocacy programs.

2033 Montgomery County Project SHARE

538 Dekalb Street
Norristown, PA 19401-4931 610-272-7997
E-mail: mcps@mhasp.org

Jeffrey Siemsen, Director

2034 Parents Involved Network

1211 Chestnut Street
Philadelphia, PA 19107-4103 215-751-1800
800-688-4226
E-mail: pin@pinofpa.org

Parents Involved Network of Pennsylvania is an organization that assists parents or caregivers of children and adolescents with emotional and behavioral disorders. PIN provides information, helps parents find services and will advocate on their behalf with any of the public systems that serve children.

2035 Pennsylvania Alliance for the Mentally Ill

2149 N 2nd Street
Harrisburg, PA 17110-1005 717-238-1514
800-223-0500
Fax: 717-238-4390
E-mail: nami-pa@nami.org
www.namipa.org

James W Jordan Jr, Executive Director
Carol Caruso, President

The largest statewide non-profit organization dedicated to helping mental health consumers and their families rebuild their lives and conquer the challenges posed by severe and persistent mental illness.

2036 Pennsylvania Chapter of the American Anorexia Bulimia Association

PO Box 1287
Langhorne, PA 19047 215-221-1864
Fax: 215-702-8944
www.aabaphila.org

The American Anorexia Bulimia Association of Philidelphia is a non-profit, providing services and programs for anyone interested in or affected by, Anorexia, Bulimia and/or related disorders.

2037 Pennsylvania Society for Services to Children

415 S 15th Street
Philadelphia, PA 19146-1637 215-875-3400
Fax: 215-875-3411
www.pssckids.org

Helen B Dennis, Executive Director
Carla Thompson Neal, Program Director

Philadelphia Society for Services to Children is a recognized leader in child abuse prevention in the Delaware Valley. Provides and advocate for services that will help each child to grow up in a safe, stable and supportive family environment.

2038 Southwestern Pennsylvania Alliance for the Mentally Ill

4721 McKnight Road
Suite 216
Pittsburgh, PA 15237-3415 412-366-3788
888-264-7972
Fax: 412-366-3935
E-mail: www.info@namiswpa.org
www.swpa.nami.org

NAMI Southwestern Pennsylvania is a non-profit organization that serves a ten-county region in Southwestern Pennsylvania. We address the increasing need for families and consumers to have a stronger voice in the mental health system.

2039 University of Pittsburgh Medical Center

200 Lothrop Street
Pittsburgh, PA 15213-2585 412-647-8762
800-533-8762
E-mail: upmcweb@upmc.edu
www.upmc.com

The University of Pittsburgh Medical Center is the leading health care system in western Pennsylvania and one of the largest nonprofit integrated health care systems in the United States.

Rhode Island

2040 Central Falls Alliance for the Mentally Ill

Community Support Service
101 Bacon Street
Pawtucket, RI 02888 401-724-7946
www.nami.org

Laurie Flynn, Executive Director

Nation's leading self-help organization for all those affected by severe brain disorders. Mission is to bring consumers and families with similar experiences together to share information about services, care providers, and ways to cope with the challenges of schizophrenia, manic depression, and other serious mental illnesses.

2041 Davis Park Alliance for the Mentally Ill

VA Hospital
Room 384
Providence, RI 02904 401-821-1577
www.nami.org

Laurie Flynn, Executive Director

Nation's leading self-help organization for all those affected by severe brain disorders. Mission is to bring consumers and families with similar experiences together to share information about services, care providers, and ways to cope with the challenges of schizophrenia, manic depression, and other serious mental illnesses.

2042 East Bay Alliance for the Mentally Ill

St. Jean Baptiste
328 Main Street
Warren, RI 02885 401-245-2386
www.nami.org

Laurie Flynn, Executive Director

Nation's leading self-help organization for all those affected by severe brain disorders. Mission is to bring consumers and families with similar experiences together to share information about services, care providers, and ways to cope with the challenges of schizophrenia, manic depression, and other serious mental illnesses.

2043 Kent County Alliance for the Mentally Ill

Hillsgrove House
70 Minnesota Avenue
Warwick, RI 02818   **401-821-5601**
                              www.nami.org

Laurie Flynn, Executive Director

Nation's leading self-help organization for all those affected by severe brain disorders. Mission is to bring consumers and families with similar experiences together to share information about services, care providers, and ways to cope with the challenges of schizophrenia, manic depression, and other serious mental illnesses.

2044 New Avenues Alliance for the Mentally Ill

Johnston Mental Health Services
1516 Atwood Avenue
Johnston, RI 02919   **401-351-4309**
                              www.nami.org

Laurie Flynn, Executive Director

Nation's leading self-help organization for all those affected by severe brain disorders. Mission is to bring consumers and families with similar experiences together to share information about services, care providers, and ways to cope with the challenges of schizophrenia, manic depression, and other serious mental illnesses.

2045 Newport County Alliance for the Mentally Ill

Channing Memorial
Pelham Street
Newport, RI 02840   **401-423-2951**
                              www.nami.org

Laurie Flynn, Executive Director

Nation's leading self-help organization for all those affected by severe brain disorders. Mission is to bring consumers and families with similar experiences together to share information about services, care providers, and ways to cope with the challenges of schizophrenia, manic depression, and other serious mental illnesses.

2046 Northern Rhode Island Alliance for the Mentally Ill

Landmark Medical Center
Cass Avenue
Newport, RI 02840   **401-334-2434**
                              www.nami.org

Laurie Flynn, Executive Director

Nation's leading self-help organization for all those affected by severe brain disorders. Mission is to bring consumers and families with similar experiences together to share information about services, care providers, and ways to cope with the challenges of schizophrenia, manic depression, and other serious mental illnesses.

2047 Parent Support Network of Rhode Island

400 Warwick Avenue
Suite 12
Warwick, RI 02888   **401-467-6855**
                              800-483-8844
                         Fax: 401-467-6903

Cathy Ciano, Executive Director

Organization of families supporting families with children and youth who are at risk for or have serious behavioral, emotional, and/or mental health challenges, having consideration for their backround and values. The goals of PSN are to: strengthen and preserve families; enable families in advocacy; extend social networks, reduce family isolation and develop social policy systems of care. Parent Support Network accomplishes these goals through providing advocacy, education and training, promoting outreach and public awareness, facilitating social events for families, participating on committees responsible for developing, implementing and evaluating policies and systems of care.

2048 Rhode Island Alliance for the Mentally Ill

1255 N Main Street
Providence, RI 02904   **401-331-3060**
                       E-mail: AMIofRI@aol.com
                              www.nami.org

Laurie Flynn, Executive Director

Nation's leading self-help organization for all those affected by severe brain disorders. Mission is to bring consumers and families with similar experiences together to share information about services, care providers, and ways to cope with the challenges of schizophrenia, manic depression, and other serious mental illnesses.

2049 Siblings & Offspring Group Alliance for the Mentally Ill

1255 N Main Street
Providence, RI 02904   **401-331-3060**
                              www.nami.org

Laurie Flynn, Executive Director

Nation's leading self-help organization for all those affected by severe brain disorders. Mission is to bring consumers and families with similar experiences together to share information about services, care providers, and ways to cope with the challenges of schizophrenia, manic depression, and other serious mental illnesses.

2050 Spouses & Partners' Group Alliance for the Mentally Ill

Butler Hospital
345 Blackstone Boulevard
Providence, RI 02904   **401-331-3060**
                              www.nami.org

Laurie Flynn, Executive Director

Nation's leading self-help organization for all those affected by severe brain disorders. Mission is to bring consumers and families with similar experiences together to share information about services, care providers, and ways to cope with the challenges of schizophrenia, manic depression, and other serious mental illnesses.

2051 Washington County Alliance for the Mentally Ill

South Shore Mental Health
33 Cherry Lane
Wakefield, RI 02879   **401-295-1956**
www.nami.org

Laurie Flynn, Executive Director

Nation's leading self-help organization for all those affected by severe brain disorders. Mission is to bring consumers and families with similar experiences together to share information about services, care providers, and ways to cope with the challenges of schizophrenia, manic depression, and other serious mental illnesses.

South Carolina

2052 Federation of Families of South Carolina

PO Box 1266
Columbia, SC 29202   **803-779-0402**
866-779-0402
Fax: 803-779-0017
www.ffcmh.org

Diane Revels-Flashnick, Executive Director

Nonprofit organization established to serve the families of children with any degree of emotional, behavioral or psychiatric disorder. The services and programs by the Federation are designed to meet the individual needs of families around the state. Through support networks, educational materials, publications, conferences, workshops and other activities, the Federation provides many avenues of support for families of children with emotional, behavioral or psychiatric disorders.

2053 National Mental Health Association: Georgetown County

PO Box 2097
Georgetown, SC 29442-2097   **843-546-8101**
Fax: 843-527-8101

Advocates for people with mental illness including referrals to counseling and provides education about mental illness.

2054 South Carolina Alliance for the Mentally Ill

PO Box 1267
5000 Thurmond Mall Boulevard, Suite 338
Columbia, SC 29202-1267   **803-733-9592**
800-788-5131
Fax: 803-733-9593
E-mail: namiofsc@logicsouth.com
www.namisc.org

Ken Howell, President
David Almeida, Executive Director

Non-profit with 17 local groups throughout the state. Provide support, education and advocacy for families and friends of people with serious mental illness.

2055 South Carolina Alliance for the Mentally Ill

PO Box 2538
Columbia, SC 29202-2538   **803-779-7849**
800-788-5131
www.nami.org

Laurie Flynn, Executive Director

Nation's leading self-help organization for all those affected by severe brain disorders. Mission is to bring consumers and families with similar experiences together to share information about services, care providers, and ways to cope with the challenges of schizophrenia, manic depression, and other serious mental illnesses.

2056 South Carolina Family Support Network

PO Box 2538
Columbia, SC 29202-2538   **803-779-7849**
800-788-5131
www.ffcmh.org/local.htm

Diane Flashnick

Focused on the needs of children and youth with emotional, behavioral or mental disorders and their families.

2057 Village Program

1 Carriage Lane
#G
Charleston, SC 29407-6060   **843-852-4130**
Fax: 843-852-4125
www.ffcmh.org/local.htm

Donna Steinhilber

South Dakota

2058 Brookings Alliance for the Mentally Ill

211 4th Street
PO Box 221
Brookings, SD 57006   **605-697-2850**
E-mail: SDAMIdonna@aol.com
www.nami.org

Laurie Flynn, Executive Director

Nation's leading self-help organization for all those affected by severe brain disorders. Mission is to bring consumers and families with similar experiences together to share information about services, care providers, and ways to cope with the challenges of schizophrenia, manic depression, and other serious mental illnesses.

2059 Huron Alliance for the Mentally Ill

79 Second Street SW
Huron, SD 57350-1204   **605-352-4499**
800-551-2531
Fax: 605-352-5573
E-mail: namisd@santel.net
www.sd.nami.org

Dedicated to the eradication of mental illness and the improvement of the quality of life of all whose lives are affected by these diseases.

Tennessee

2060 Bridges

PO Box 90
Paris, TN 38242-0090

800-590-0901

Based on the belief that those with mental illness 'can and do recover a new and valued sense of self and purpose' in accepting and overcoming the challenges of a disability that has affected every aspect of life: physical, intellectual, emotional, and spiritual.

2061 Geriatric Care Centers of America

415 Highway 135
Waverly, TN 37185

931-296-0106
Fax: 931-296-1013

2062 Memphis Business Group on Health

5100 Poplar Avenue
Suite 600
Memphis, TN 38137-0600

901-323-1808
Fax: 901-767-6592

To facilitate the purchase of efficient and effective health care services for the Memphis community.

2063 Tennessee Alliance for the Mentally Ill

5410 Homberg Drive
Suite 4
Knoxville, TN 37919

423-602-7900
www.nami.org

Laurie Flynn, Executive Director

Nation's leading self-help organization for all those affected by severe brain disorders. Mission is to bring consumers and families with similar experiences together to share information about services, care providers, and ways to cope with the challenges of schizophrenia, manic depression, and other serious mental illnesses.

2064 Tennessee Association of Mental Health Organization

42 Rutledge Street
Nashville, TN 37210-2043

615-244-2220
Fax: 615-254-8331
www.tamho.org

State wide trade association representing primarily community mental health centers, community-owned corporation that have historically served the needs of the mentally ill and chemically dependent citizens of Tennessee regardless of their ability to pay.

2065 Tennessee Mental Health Consumers' Association

116 Dalton Street
Kingsport, TN 37665

800-459-2925
Fax: 423-245-6100
E-mail: tnmhca@aol.com

Irene Russell, Executive Director

Not-for-profit organization whose members are mental health consumers and other individuals and groups who support the mission of TMHCA.

2066 Tennessee Voices for Children

1315 8th Avenue S
Nashville, TN 37203

800-670-9882
Fax: 615-269-8914
E-mail: tnvoices.org
www.ffcmh.org/local.htm

Charlotte Bryson, Executive Director

Non-profit, non-partisan organization of families, professionals, business and community leaders, and government representatives committed to improving and expanding services related to the emotional and behavioral well-being of children.

2067 Vanderbilt University: John F Kennedy Center for Research on Human Development

PO Box 40
Peabody College
Nashville, TN 37203-5701

615-322-8240
Fax: 615-322-8236
TDD: 615-343-2958
E-mail: kc@vanderbilt.edu
www.kc.vanderbilt.edu

Pat Leavitt PhD, Center Acting Director
Jan Rosemergy PhD, Director Communications

Research and research training related to disorders of thinking, learning, perception, communication, mood and emotion caused by disruption of typical development. Available services include behavior analysis clinic, referrals, lectures and conferences, and a free quarterly newsletter.

Texas

2068 Children's Mental Health Partnership

1430 Collier Street
Austin, TX 78704

512-445-7780
Fax: 512-445-7701
www.mhatexas.org

A coalition of human services providers, parents, educators and juvenile court professionals who care about the special mental health needs of Austin area youth and families.

2069 Dallas Federation of Families for Children's Mental Health

2629 Sharpview Lane
Dallas, TX 75228-6047

214-320-3750
Fax: 214-320-1825
www.ffcmh.org/local.htm

Susan Rogers

2070 Depression and Bipolar Support Alliance of Houston and Harris County

PO Box 270341
Houston, TX 77277-0341

713-528-1546
Fax: 281-933-3299
www.dbsahouston.org

Self-help, nonprofit organization for those who have been diagnosed or have symptoms of mood disorder. Families and friens of people with mood disorders are also involved. Provides personal support and direct services to its members, educates the public about the nature and management of these treatable disorders, and promotes related research.

2071 Fox Counseling Service

1900 Pease Street
Suite 310
Vernon, TX 76384-4625   940-553-3783
800-687-9439
Fax: 940-553-3783

Fred Fox, Sole Proprietor

Marital counseling using PREP, family counseling, ADHD diagnosis and management. Couseling for mental health issues... depression, anxiety, stress, etc.

2072 Jewish Family Service

13140 Coit Road
Suite 400
Dallas, TX 75240-5725   214-437-9950
Fax: 214-437-1988

2073 Jewish Family Service of San Antonio

12500 NW Military Hwy
#250
San Antonio, TX 78231-1871   210-302-6920
Fax: 210-349-6952
E-mail: johnsonb@jfs-sa.org

2074 Mental Health Association

670 N 7th Street
Beaumont, TX 77702-1741   409-833-9657

Non-profit agency offering free information, referral services, educational programs, and advocay to all of Jefferson County.

2075 Parent Connection

1020 Riverwood Center
Conroe, TX 77304-2811   409-756-8321
800-839-8876
Fax: 409-756-8326

2076 Texas Alliance for the Mentally Ill

10 E 7th Street
Suite 208
Austin, TX 78702-3257   512-474-2225
800-633-3760
www.nami.org

Laurie Flynn, Executive Director

Nation's leading self-help organization for all those affected by severe brain disorders. Mission is to bring consumers and families with similar experiences together to share information about services, care providers, and ways to cope with the challenges of schizophrenia, manic depression, and other serious mental illnesses.

2077 Texas Counseling Association

316 W 12th Street
Suite 402
Austin, TX 78701-1840   512-472-3403
800-580-8144
Fax: 512-472-3756

Darlene Stevens, Office Manager

The Texas Counseling Association is the state association for professional couselors. The 1999 Professional Growth Conference will be held in Corpus Christi on November 10 - 13.

2078 Texas Federation of Families for Children's Mental Health

1020 Tiverwood Center
Conroe, TX 77304   409-756-8319
Fax: 409-525-2746
www.ffcmh.org/local.htm

Patti Derr

2079 Texas Psychological Association

6633 E Highway 290
Suite 305
Austin, TX 78723-1158   512-454-2449

2080 Texas Society of Psychiatric Physicians

401 W 15th Street
Suite 675
Austin, TX 78701-1665   512-478-0605

2081 University of Texas Southwestern Medical Center

5323 Harry Hines Boulevard
Dallas, TX 75390   214-648-3111
Fax: 214-648-8955

Utah

2082 Allies for Youth & Families

2900 S State Street
Suite 260
S Salt Lake City, UT 84115   801-467-1500
Fax: 801-467-0328

Cheran Zullo

2083 DMDA Southern Utah and Nevada

PO Box 2187
Saint George, UT 84771-2187
800-385-2877
Fax: 801-652-9333

2084 Healthwise of Utah

2505 Parleys Way
Suite 30804
Salt Lake City, UT 84109   801-481-6176

2085 Utah Alliance for the Mentally Ill

PO Box 58047
Salt Lake City, UT 84158-0047   801-584-2023
www.nami.org

Laurie Flynn, Executive Director

Nation's leading self-help organization for all those affected by severe brain disorders. Mission is to bring consumers and families with similar experiences together to share information about services, care providers, and ways to cope with the challenges of schizophrenia, manic depression, and other serious mental illnesses.

2086 Utah Parent Center

2290 E 4500 Street
Suite 110
Salt Lake City, UT 84117-4428   **801-272-1051**
800-468-1160
Fax: 801-272-8907
E-mail: upc@inconnect.com
www.utahparentcenter.org

The Utah Parent Center is a statewide nonprofit organization founded in 1984 to provide training, information, referral and assistance to parents of children and youth with all disabilities: physical, mental, learning and emotional. Staff at the center are primarily parents of children and youth with disabilities who carry out the philosophy of Parents Helping Parents.

2087 Utah Psychiatric Association

2885 Swiss Drive
Santa Clara, UT 84765-5101   **801-674-5600**
Fax: 801-674-7149

Vermont

2088 Brattleboro Retreat

75 Linden Street
PO Box 803
Brattleboro, VT 05302-0803   **802-257-1207**
800-738-7328
Fax: 802-258-3796

2089 Fletcher Allen Health Care

111 Colchester Avenue
Burlington, VT 05401-1416   **802-656-3270**
Fax: 802-656-2733

2090 Spruce Mountain Inn

PO Box 153
Plainfield, VT 05667-0153   **802-454-8353**
Fax: 802-454-1008
E-mail: smi@together.net
www.s-m-i.com

2091 Vermont Alliance for the Mentally Ill

230 Main Street
Room 203
Brattleboro, VT 05301-2840   **802-257-5546**
800-639-6480
www.nami.org

Laurie Flynn, Executive Director

Nation's leading self-help organization for all those affected by severe brain disorders. Mission is to bring consumers and families with similar experiences together to share information about services, care providers, and ways to cope with the challenges of schizophrenia, manic depression, and other serious mental illnesses.

2092 Vermont Employers Health Alliance

104 Church Street
Burlington, VT 05401-4449   **802-865-0525**
Fax: 805-862-5443

2093 Vermont Federation of Families for Children's Mental Health

28 Barre Street
PO Box 607
Montpelier, VT 05601-0607   **802-223-4917**
800-639-6071
Fax: 802-828-2159
E-mail: VFFCMH@together.net

Pamela Dow, Executive Director

Virginia

2094 First Hospital Corporation

240 Corporate Boulevard
Norfolk, VA 23502-4948   **751-451-5100**
Fax: 757-412-6604

2095 Garnett Day Treatment Center

1 Garnet Center Drive
Charlottesville, VA 22911-8572   **434-977-3425**
Fax: 434-977-8529

2096 NAMI

Colonial Place Three
2107 Wilson Blvd. Ste 300
Arlington, VA 22201-3042   **703-524-7600**
800-950-6264
Fax: 703-524-9094
TDD: 703-516-7227
www.nami.org

Margaret Stout, President
Edward Foulks, 1st VP
Betsy Smith, 2nd VP

Nonprofit self help support and advocacy organization of consumers, families, and friends of people with mental illnesses, such as schizophrenia, bipolar disorder, major depressive disorder, and other severe and persistent mental illnesses that affect the brain.

2097 Newport News Support Group

PO Box 6644
Newport News, VA 23606-0644   **757-875-1307**

2098 Parent Resource Center

PO Box 26691
Richmond, VA 23261-6691   **804-559-6833**
800-477-0946
Fax: 804-559-6835
www.ffcmh.org

Beverly Bell

2099 Parents & Children Coping Together: PACCT

PO Box 26691
Richmond, VA 23261-6691   **804-559-6833**
Fax: 804-559-6835
E-mail: pacct@infionline.net
www.pacct.net

Joyce B Kube, Executive Director
Randy Del Rossi, Family Support Coordinataor

Support and education for parents and family members of children and adolescents with mental, emotional and behavioral disorders.

2100 Parents & Children Coping Together: Roanoke Valley

PO Box 21112
Roanoke, VA 24018-0113   540-989-5042
                    E-mail: kellyd@airmail.net
                    www.ffcmh.org/local.htm

Sue Scheibe

2101 Parents and Children Coping Together

PO Box 26691
Richmond, VA 23261-6691   804-559-6833
                              800-477-0946
                    E-mail: pacct@infionline.net
                              www.pacct.net

Joyce Kube

2102 Piedmont Behavioral Health Center

42009 Victory Lane
Leesburg, VA 20176-6269   703-777-0800
                              800-777-8855
                         Fax: 703-777-6970

Elizabeth Thomas, Admissions
Mari Jo Banner, Director Community Relations

Offers fifteen acute psychiatric/chemical dependency beds for adolescents and adults, fifty two beds for adolescent residential treatment patients, and six beds for sexual offenders. Has a campus academy and a partial hospitalization program for all populations including senior adults.

2103 Richmond Support Group

Warwick Medical & Professional Center
Richmond, VA   804-320-7881

2104 Trigon BC/BS of Virginia

2221 Edward Holland Drive
Richmond, VA 23230-2518   804-354-2007
                         Fax: 804-354-2536

2105 Virginia Alliance for the Mentally Ill

PO Box 1903
Richmond, VA 23218   804-255-8264
                              800-484-7753
                    E-mail: va ami@aol.com
                              www.nami.org

Laurie Flynn, Executive Director

Nation's leading self-help organization for all those affected by severe brain disorders. Mission is to bring consumers and families with similar experiences together to share information about services, care providers, and ways to cope with the challenges of schizophrenia, manic depression, and other serious mental illnesses.

2106 Virginia Beach Community Service Board

Pembroke 6
Suite 208
Virginia Beach, VA 23462   757-437-5770
                         Fax: 804-490-5736

2107 Virginia Federation of Families for Children's Mental Health

1101 King Street
Suite 420
Alexandria, VA 22314   703-684-7710
                         Fax: 703-836-1040
                    E-mail: ffcmh@ffcmh.org
                              www.ffcmh.org

Barbara Huff, Executive Director
Cynthia Warger, Claiming Children Editor
Linda Donahue, Administrative Assistant
Trina Osher, Coordinator Policy/Research

Family-run organization dedicated exclusively to children and adolesents with mental health needs and their families. Our work speaks through our work in policy, training and technical assistance programs. Publishes a quarterly newsletter and sponsors an annual conference and exhibits.

Washington

2108 Bellevue Alliance for the Mentally Ill

Overlake Hospital
Bellevue, WA 98004   206-747-1262
                              www.nami.org

Laurie Flynn, Executive Director

Nation's leading self-help organization for all those affected by severe brain disorders. Mission is to bring consumers and families with similar experiences together to share information about services, care providers, and ways to cope with the challenges of schizophrenia, manic depression, and other serious mental illnesses.

2109 Children's Alliance

2017 E Spruce
Seattle, WA 98122   206-324-0340
                         Fax: 206-325-6291
          E-mail: seattle@childrensalliance.org
                    www.childrensalliance.org

Paola Maranan, Executive Director
Deborah Bowler, Administration
Ruth Schubert, Communications

Washington's statewide child advocacy organization. We champion public policies and practices that deliver the essentials that kids need to thrive — confidence, stability, health and safety.

2110 Common Voice for Pierce County Parents

801 141st Street E
Tacoma, WA 98445-2768   253-537-2145
                         Fax: 253-537-2162

Marge Critchlow

Family support group.

2111 Family Support Group Alliance for the Mentally Ill

Fairfax Hospital
10200 NE 132nd
Kirkland, WA 98033   206-821-2000
                                www.nami.org

Laurie Flynn, Executive Director

Nation's leading self-help organization for all those affected by severe brain disorders. Mission is to bring consumers and families with similar experiences together to share information about services, care providers, and ways to cope with the challenges of schizophrenia, manic depression, and other serious mental illnesses.

2112 Good Sam-W/Alliance for the Mentally Ill Family Support Group

325 Pioneer Avenue E
Puyallup, WA 98371   206-848-5571
                                www.nami.org

Laurie Flynn, Executive Director

Nation's leading self-help organization for all those affected by severe brain disorders. Mission is to bring consumers and families with similar experiences together to share information about services, care providers, and ways to cope with the challenges of schizophrenia, manic depression, and other serious mental illnesses.

2113 Gray's Harbour Alliance for the Mentally Ill

Elma City Hall
Elma City, WA 98541   206-482-2981
                                 www.nami.org

Laurie Flynn, Executive Director

Nation's leading self-help organization for all those affected by severe brain disorders. Mission is to bring consumers and families with similar experiences together to share information about services, care providers, and ways to cope with the challenges of schizophrenia, manic depression, and other serious mental illnesses.

2114 King County Federation of Families for Children's Mental Health

2211 NE 12th Street
Renton, WA 98056-2915   425-277-0426
                          E-mail: kellyd@airmail.net
                          www.ffcmh.org/local.htm

Marilyn Williams

2115 Kitsap County Alliance for the Mentally Ill

Health Center
109 Austin Drive NE
Bremerton, WA 98310   206-377-2910
                                 www.nami.org

Laurie Flynn, Executive Director

Nation's leading self-help organization for all those affected by severe brain disorders. Mission is to bring consumers and families with similar experiences together to share information about services, care providers, and ways to cope with the challenges of schizophrenia, manic depression, and other serious mental illnesses.

2116 Managed Care Washington

4319 Stone Way N
Seattle, WA 98103-7420   206-441-1722
                                Fax: 206-441-4823

2117 North Sound Regional Alliance for the Mentally Ill

1401 Cleveland
Senior Center
Moutn Vernon, WA 98273   206-387-0981
                                 www.nami.org

Laurie Flynn, Executive Director

Nation's leading self-help organization for all those affected by severe brain disorders. Mission is to bring consumers and families with similar experiences together to share information about services, care providers, and ways to cope with the challenges of schizophrenia, manic depression, and other serious mental illnesses.

2118 North Sound Regional Support Network

117 N 1st Street
Suite 8
Mount Vernon, WA 98273-2858   360-416-7013
                                         800-684-3555
                                   Fax: 360-416-7017
                                   TTY: 360-419-9008
                          E-mail: nsrsn@nsrsn.org
                          www.http://nsrsn.org

Charles Benjamin, Executive Director
Greg Long, Assistant Director/Planner

2119 Nueva Esperanza Counseling Center

720 W Court Street
Suite 8
Pasco, WA 99301-4178   509-545-6506

2120 Pierce County Alliance for the Mentally Ill

1201 S Proctor
Tacoma, WA 98498   206-272-3070
                              www.nami.org

Laurie Flynn, Executive Director

Nation's leading self-help organization for all those affected by severe brain disorders. Mission is to bring consumers and families with similar experiences together to share information about services, care providers, and ways to cope with the challenges of schizophrenia, manic depression, and other serious mental illnesses.

2121 Seattle University District Alliance for the Mentally Ill

PO Box 45732
Seattle, WA 98060-9814   206-522-3166
                                www.nami.org

Laurie Flynn, Executive Director

Nation's leading self-help organization for all those affected by severe brain disorders. Mission is to bring consumers and families with similar experiences together to share information about services, care providers, and ways to cope with the challenges of schizophrenia, manic depression, and other serious mental illnesses.

2122 Sharing & Caring for Consumers, Families Alliance for the Mentally Ill

N of Tacoma General Hospital
Tacoma, WA 98498   206-383-3056
                                www.nami.org

Laurie Flynn, Executive Director

Nation's leading self-help organization for all those affected by severe brain disorders. Mission is to bring consumers and families with similar experiences together to share information about services, care providers, and ways to cope with the challenges of schizophrenia, manic depression, and other serious mental illnesses.

2123 South King County Alliance for the Mentally Ill

600 E Smith
Kent Senior Center
Kent, WA 98031   206-852-0731
                                www.nami.org

Laurie Flynn, Executive Director

Nation's leading self-help organization for all those affected by severe brain disorders. Mission is to bring consumers and families with similar experiences together to share information about services, care providers, and ways to cope with the challenges of schizophrenia, manic depression, and other serious mental illnesses.

2124 Southwest Alliance for the Mentally Ill

2600 SW Holden
Seattle, WA 98060   206-848-5571
                                www.nami.org

Laurie Flynn, Executive Director

Nation's leading self-help organization for all those affected by severe brain disorders. Mission is to bring consumers and families with similar experiences together to share information about services, care providers, and ways to cope with the challenges of schizophrenia, manic depression, and other serious mental illnesses.

2125 Spanish Support Group Alliance for the Mentally Ill

2601 Elliott Avenue
Suite 4143
Seattle, WA 98060   206-441-9965
                                www.nami.org

Laurie Flynn, Executive Director

Nation's leading self-help organization for all those affected by severe brain disorders. Mission is to bring consumers and families with similar experiences together to share information about services, care providers, and ways to cope with the challenges of schizophrenia, manic depression, and other serious mental illnesses.

2126 Spokane Mental Health

107 S Division Street
Spokane, WA 99202-1586   509-838-4651
                                Fax: 509-458-7449

David Panken, CEO
Marilyn Wilson, Clinical Director
Susan Legel, CFO

County provider of mental health services.

2127 Washington Alliance for the Mentally Ill

802 NW 70th Street
Seattle, WA 98117   206-789-7722
                                800-782-9264
                                www.nami.org

Laurie Flynn, Executive Director

Nation's leading self-help organization for all those affected by severe brain disorders. Mission is to bring consumers and families with similar experiences together to share information about services, care providers, and ways to cope with the challenges of schizophrenia, manic depression, and other serious mental illnesses.

2128 Washington State Psychological Association

711 N 35th Street
Suite 206
Seattle, WA 98103   206-547-4220
                                Fax: 206-547-6366
                                E-mail: wspa@wapsych.org
                                www.wapsych.org

To support, promote and advance the science, education and practice of psychology in the public interest.

2129 Western State Hospital Alliance for the Mentally Ill

S Hall Activity Center
Tacoma, WA 98498   206-756-2650
                                800-782-9264
                                www.nami.org

Laurie Flynn, Executive Director

Nation's leading self-help organization for all those affected by severe brain disorders. Mission is to bring consumers and families with similar experiences together to share information about services, care providers, and ways to cope with the challenges of schizophrenia, manic depression, and other serious mental illnesses.

2130 Whidbey Island Alliance for the Mentally Ill

Whidbey Island, WA 98498   360-383-3056
                                www.nami.org

Laurie Flynn, Executive Director

Nation's leading self-help organization for all those affected by severe brain disorders. Mission is to bring consumers and families with similar experiences together to share information about services, care providers, and ways to cope with the challenges of schizophrenia, manic depression, and other serious mental illnesses.

West Virginia

2131 Mountain State Parents Children Adolescent Network

PO Box 6658
Wheeling, WV 26003-0906   304-232-4881
800-244-5385
Fax: 304-233-3847
E-mail: toothman@mspcan.org
www.mspcan.org

Teri Toothman, Executive Director

Support, education and training for families who have a child with serious emotional disturbance.

2132 West Virginia Alliance for the Mentally Ill

PO Box 2706
Charleston, WV 25330-2706   304-342-0497
800-598-5653
E-mail: WVAMAIL@aol.com
www.nami.org

Laurie Flynn, Executive Director

Nation's leading self-help organization for all those affected by severe brain disorders. Mission is to bring consumers and families with similar experiences together to share information about services, care providers, and ways to cope with the challenges of schizophrenia, manic depression, and other serious mental illnesses.

2133 West Virginia University Department Family Medicine

WVU HSC Family Practice Center
Morgantown, WV 26505   304-293-5204

Wisconsin

2134 Charter BHS of Wisconsin/Brown Deer

4600 W Schroeder Drive
Brown Deer, WI 53223-1469   414-355-2273
Fax: 414-355-6726

2135 Child and Adolescent Psychopharmacology Information

Wisconsin Psychiatric Institute and Clinic
6001 Research Park Boulevard
#1568
Madison, WI 53719-1176   608-263-6171

2136 Stoughton Family Counseling

1520 Vernon Street
Stoughton, WI 53589-2260   608-873-6422
Fax: 608-873-6014

2137 We Are the Children's Hope

2943 N 9th Street
Milwaukee, WI 53206-3217   414-263-3375
E-mail: kelly@airmail.net
www.ffcmh.org/local.htm

Zelodius Brown

2138 Wisconsin Alliance for the Mentally Ill

1410 Northport Drive
Madison, WI 53704-2041   608-242-7223
800-236-2988
Fax: 608-242-7225
E-mail: amiwisc@aol.com
www.nami.org

Robert Beliman MD, President

Self-help organization for all those affected by severe brain disorders. Mission is to bring consumers and families with similar experiences together to share information about services, care providers, and ways to cope with the challanges of schizophrenia, manic depression, and other serious mental illnesses.

2139 Wisconsin Association of Family and Child Agency

131 W Wilson Street
Suite 901
Madison, WI 53703-3245   608-257-5939
Fax: 608-257-6067

2140 Wisconsin Family Ties

16 N Carroll Street
Suite 830
Madison, WI 53703-2726   608-267-6888
800-422-7145
Fax: 608-267-6801
E-mail: kellyd@airmail.net
www.ffcmh.org/local.htm

JoAnn Stormer

Wyoming

2141 Concerned Parent Coalition

1125 Sioux Ave
Gillette, WY 82718-6529   307-682-6684
E-mail: kellyd@airmail.net
www.ffcmh.org/local.htm

Michelle Gerlosky

2142 Pineridge at Lander Valley

1320 Bishop Randall Drive
Lander, WY 82520-3939   307-332-5700
Fax: 307-335-6465

2143 Uplift

PO Box 664
Cheyenne, WY 82003-0664   307-778-8686
888-875-4383
Fax: 307-778-8681
E-mail: uplift@wyoming.com
www.uplift-wyoming.com

Peggy Nikkel, Executive Director

Wyoming Chapter of the Federation of Familes for Children's Mental Health. Providing support, education, advocacy, information and referral for parents and professionals focusing on emotional, behavioral and learning needs of children and youth.

2144 Wyoming Alliance for the Mentally Ill

656 Granite Drive
Rock Springs, WY 82901   **307-362-3333**
                               www.nami.org

Laurie Flynn, Executive Director

Nation's leading self-help organization for all those affected by severe brain disorders. Mission is to bring consumers and families with similar experiences together to share information about services, care providers, and ways to cope with the challenges of schizophrenia, manic depression, and other serious mental illnesses.

Federal

2145 Administration for Children and Families

370 Lenfant SW
Washington, DC 20447-0001   202-690-7027
                                 Fax: 202-401-6400

Responsible for federal programs that promotes the economic and social well-being of families, children, individuals, and communities.

2146 Administration for Children, Youth and Families

US Department of Health & Human Services
400 6th Street SW
Washington, DC 20024-2706   202-619-0257
                                         888-877-696
                                 Fax: 202-690-7203
                                 www.os.dhhs.gov

Dodie Truman, Commissioner

Advises Health and Human Services department on plans and programs related to early childhood development; operates the Head Start day care and other related child service programs; provides leadership, advice, and services that affect the general well-being of children and youths.

2147 Administration on Aging

1 Massachusetts Avenue
Suites 4100 & 5100
Washington, DC 20201   202-619-0724
                               www.aoa.gov

One of the nation's largest providers of home and community-based care for older persons and their caregivers. The mission is to promote the dignity and independence of older people, and help society prepare for an aging population.

2148 Administration on Developmental Disabilities US Department of Health & Human Services

Washington, DC 20201   202-690-6590
                             Fax: 202-690-6904
                             TTY: 202-690-6415
                        www.acf.dhs.gov/programs/ada

Develops and administers programs protecting rights and promoting independence, productivity and inclusion; funds state grants, protection and advocacy programs, University Affiliated Programs and other national projects.

2149 Agency for Healthcare Research and Quality: Office of Communications and Knowledge Transfer

540 Gaither Road
Suite 200
Rockville, MD 20852-4908   301-427-1200
                              E-mail: info@ahrq.org
                                      www.ahrq.org

Provides policymakers and other health care leaders with information needed to make critical health care decisions.

2150 Association of Maternal and Child Health Programs (AMCHP)

1220 19th Street NW
Suite 801
Washington, DC 20036   202-775-0436
                             Fax: 202-775-0061
                        E-mail: info@amchp.org
                                www.amchp.org

National non-profit organization representing state public health workers. Provides leadership to assure the health and well-being of women of reproductive age, children, youth, including those with special health care needs and their families.

2151 Center for Mental Health Services Homeless Programs Branch

Substance Abuse and Mental Health Services Administration
5600 Fishers Lane
Room 11C-05
Rockville, MD 20857-0002   301-443-3706
                             Fax: 301-443-0256
                             TDD: 301-443-9006
                             www.mentalhealth.org

Walter Leginski PhD, Chief

Federal agency concerned with the prevention and treatment of mental illness and the promotion of mental health. Homeless Programs Branch administers a variety of programs and activities. Provides professional leadership for collaborative intergovernmental initiatives designed to assist persons with mental illnesses who are homeless. Also supports a contract for the National Resource Center on Homelessness and Mental Illness.

2152 Center for Substance Abuse Treatment

5600 Fishers Lane
Rockwall II Suite 880
Rockville, MD 20857-0002   301-443-7747
                             Fax: 301-443-8345

2153 Centers for Disease Control & Prevention

1600 Clifton Road NE
Mail Stop D51
Atlanta, GA 30329-4018   404-639-3311
                                      800-311-3435
                             TTY: 404-639-3312

Protecting the health and safety of people — at home and abroad, providing credible information to enhance health decisions, and promoting health through strong partnership. Serves as the national focus for developing and applying disease prevention and control, environmental health, and health promotion in education activities designed to improve the health of the people of the United States.

2154 Centers for Medicare & Medicaid Services: Health Policy

200 Independence Avenue SW
Room 325-H
Washington, DC 20201-0004   202-690-7941
                             Fax: 202-690-6262

2155 Commission on Mental Health Services: Department of Human Services

2700 Martin Luther King Jr Avenue SE
Building A-5
Washington, DC 20032-2601   800-368-1019
                             Fax: 757-363-1460

To provide the treatment and support services needed by adults with mental disorders and children with serious emotional problems.

2156 Committee for Truth in Psychiatry: CTIP

PO Box 1214
New York, NY 10003   212-665-6587
                      E-mail: ctip@erols.com
        www.harborside.com/~equinox/ect.htm

Linda Andre, Director

Former psychiatric patients who have had electroconvulsive therapy (ECT's), working toward informed consent to shock treatment. Works to retain ECT's current FDA classification as a high-risk procedure. Publications: Synopsis of the Conflict Over ECT at the FDA, pamphlet. FDA's Regulatory Proceedings Concerning ECT, pamphlet. Shockwaves, quarterly. Future patients should be informed before they give their consent to such treatment.

2157 Equal Employment Opportunity Commission

1801 L Street NW
Room 6407
Washington, DC 20507-0001   202-663-4264

To eradicate employment discrimination at workplace.

2158 Health and Human Services Office of Assistant Secretary for Planning & Evaluation

200 Independence Avenue SW
Room 438F
Washington, DC 20201-0004   202-690-6141
                             Fax: 202-690-6518

2159 Information Resources and Inquiries Branch

National Institute of Mental Health
6001 Executive Boulevard
Room 8184
Bethesda, MD 20892-9663

                      866-615-6464
                 Fax: 301-443-4279
                 TTY: 301-443-8431
        E-mail: nimhinfo@nih.gov
               www.nimh.nih.gov

A component of the National Institute of Health, the NIMH conducts and supports research that seeks to understand, treat and prevent mental illness. The Institute's Information Resources and Inquiries Branch (IRIB) responds to information requests from the lay public, clinicians and the scientific community with a variety of publications on subjects such as basic behavioral research, neuroscience of mental health, rural mental, children's mental disorders, schizophrenia, paranoia, depression, bipolar disorder, learning disabilities, Alzheimer's disease, panic, obsessive compulsive and other anxiety disorders. A publication list is available upon request.

2160 National Institutes of Mental Health Division of Extramural Activities

6001 Executive Boulevard
Room # 8184 MSC 9663
Bethesda, MD 20892-9663   301-443-4513
                           866-615-6464
                      Fax: 301-443-4279
                      TTY: 301-443-4513

2161 National Center of HIV, STD and TB Prevention

1600 Clifton Road
Mail E-07
Atlanta, GA 30333   404-639-8011

2162 National Clearinghouse for Drug & Alcohol

11426-28 Rockville Pike
Suite 200
Rockville, MD 20852   301-770-5800
                       Fax: 301-468-6433

2163 National Institute of Alcohol Abuse and Alcoholism: Treatment Research Branch

6001 Executive Boulevard
Room #8184 MSC 9663
Bethesda, MD 20892-9663   301-443-4513
                           866-615-6464
                      Fax: 301-446-8431
                      TTY: 301-443-8431
        E-mail: nimhinfo@nih.gov
               www.nimh.nih.gov

2164 National Institute of Alcohol Abuse and Alcoholism: Homeless Demonstration and Evaluation Branch

5600 Fishers Lane
Room 13C-06
Rockville, MD 20857-0002   301-443-3885

2165 National Institute of Alcohol Abuse and Alcoholism: Office of Policy Analysis

5600 Fishers Lane
Room 16-95
Rockville, MD 20857-0002   301-443-3864

2166 National Institute of Drug Abuse: NIDA

6001 Executive Boulevard
Room 5213
Bethesda, MD 20892-9561   301-594-6145
Fax: 301-443-7397
E-mail: information@lists.nida.nih.gov
www.nida.nih.gov

Beverly Jackson, Public Information

Covers the areas of drug abuse treatment and prevention research, epidemiology, neuroscience and behavioral research, health services research and AIDS. Seeks to report on advances in the field, identify resources, promote an exchange of information, and improve communications among clinicians, researchers, administrators, and policymakers. Recurring features include synopses of research advances and projects, NIDA news, news of legislative and regulatory developments, and announcements.

2167 National Institute of Health (NIH): Division Research

PO Box 5180
Baltimore, MD 21224-0180   410-550-1427
Fax: 410-550-1528

2168 National Institute of Mental Health: Schizophrenia Research Branch

5600 Fishers Lane
Room 18C-14
Rockville, MD 20857-0002   301-443-4707

2169 National Institute of Mental Health: Office of Science Policy and Program Planning

5600 Fishers Lane
Room 17C-27
Rockville, MD 20857-0002   301-443-1639
Fax: 301-443-4045

2170 National Institute on Drug Abuse Science: Policy and Analysis Division

5600 Fishers Lane
Room 10A-55
Rockville, MD 20857-0002   301-443-6071

2171 National Institute on Drug Abuse: Division of Clinical Research

5600 Fishers Lane
#10A-30
Rockville, MD 20857-0002   301-443-011
Fax: 301-443-2317

2172 National Institutes of Mental Health: Office on AIDS

5600 Fishers Lane
#10-95
Rockville, MD 20857-0002   301-443-7281
Fax: 301-443-9719

2173 National Institutes of Mental Health: Mental Disorders of the Aging

5600 Fishers Lane
#18-105
Rockville, MD 20857-0002   301-443-1185
Fax: 301-594-6784

2174 National Library of Medicine

8600 Rockville Pike
Bethesda, MD 20894-0001

2175 Office of Applied Studies, SA & Mental Health Services

5600 Fishers Lane
OAS/SAMHSA
Rockville, MD 20857-0002   301-443-6239
Fax: 301-443-9847

2176 Office of Disease Prevention & Health Promotion

12132 330 C Street SW
Washington, DC 20201-0001   202-205-8611

2177 Office of Health Care Financing

2100 Martin Luther King Jr Avenue SE
Washington, DC 20020-5719   202-939-1860

2178 Office of Mental Health System Development

2700 Martin Luther King Jr Avenue SE
Washington, DC 20032-2601   202-373-7847

2179 Office of National Drug Control Policy

Executive Office of the President
Washington, DC 20013   301-794-4827

2180 Office of Prepaid Health Care, HCFA

330 Independence Avenue SW
Suite 4406
Washington, DC 20201-0001   202-619-1063

2181 Office of Program and Policy Development

4350 EW Highway
Floor 7
Bethesda, MD 20814-4410   301-594-4060
Fax: 301-594-4984

2182 Office of Science Policy

9000 Rockville Pike
Suite 218
Bethesda, MD 20892-0001   301-496-1454
Fax: 301-402-0280

2183 President's Committee on Mental Retardation

US DHHS, Administration for Children & Families, PCMR
370 L'Enfatne Promenade SW
Aerospace Center, Room 701
Washington, DC 20447
202-619-0634
Fax: 202-205-9519
www.acf.dhhs.gov/programs/pcmr

The PCMR acts in an advisory capacity to the President and the Secretary of Health and Human Services on matters relating to programs and services for persons with mental retardation. It has adopted several national goals in order to better recognize and uphold the right of all people with mental retardation to enjoy a quality of life that promotes independence, self-determination and participation as productive members of society.

2184 Presidential Commission on Employment of the Disabled

1331 F Street NW
Washington, DC 20004-1107
202-376-6200

2185 Presidents Committee on Mental Retardation: Administration for Children & Families

330 C Street SW
Room 3086
Washington, DC 20201-0001
202-619-0634
Fax: 202-205-9519
E-mail: gblumenthal@acf.dhhs.gov
www.acf.dhhs.gov/programs/pcmr

Gary Blumenthal, Executive Director
Olivia Golden, Asst. Sec. for Children/Families

Administers the Education of the Handicapped Act and related programs for the education of handicapped children, including grants to institutions of higher learning and fellowships to train educational personnel. Grants to states for the education of handicapped children, research and demonstration.

2186 Protection and Advocacy Program for the Mentally Ill

US Department of Health and Human Services
5600 Fishers Lane
Room C-22
Rockville, MD 20857-0002
301-443-3667
Fax: 301-443-4868

Natalie Reatia, Chief
Norma Hatot, Director

Federal formula grant program to protect and advocate the rights of people with mental illnesses who are in residential facilities and to investigate abuse and neglect in such facilities.

2187 Public Health Foundation

1220 L Street NW
Washington, DC 20005-4018
202-898-5600
Fax: 202-898-5609

2188 Substance Abuse & Mental Health Services Adminstration (SAMHSA)

5600 Fishers Lane
Rockville, MD 20857-0002
301-443-3343
Fax: 301-443-7926

Agency within the United States Department of health and human services that works to improve the quality and availability of substance abuse prevention, addiction treatment and mental health services.

2189 Substance Abuse and Mental Health Services Administration

SAMSHA
500 Fishers Lane
Room 12C-05
Rockville, MD 20857-0001
301-443-2403
Fax: 301-443-1726
www.samsha.org

Agency charged with improving the quality and availability of prevention, treatment, and rehabilitative services in order to reduce illness, death, disability, and cost to society resulting from substance abuse and mental illnesses.

2190 Substance Abuse and Mental Health Services Administration: Homeless Program

SAMHSA
5600 Fishers Lane
Room 11C-05
Rockville, MD 20857-0002
301-443-3706
Fax: 301-443-0256

2191 Substance Abuse and Mental Health Services Administration: Center for Mental Health Services

SAMHSA
PO Box 42557
Washington, DC 20015
800-789-2647
Fax: 301-984-8796
TDD: 866-889-2647
www.mentalhealth.org

2192 US Department of Health and Human Services Planning and Evaluation

200 Independence Ave SW
Room 442E
Washington, DC 20201-0004
888-644-6226
866-464-3616
Fax: 866-464-3616

2193 US Department of Health and Human Services Bureau of Primary Health

4350 EW Highway
Room 3
Bethesda, MD 20814-4410
301-594-4491
Fax: 301-594-0089

2194 US Department of Health and Human Services: Office of Women's Health

200 Independence Avenue SW
Hurbert H Humphrey Building, Room 728E
Washington, DC 20201-0004   202-690-7650
                                   Fax: 202-690-7172

2195 US Department of Public Health: Indian Services

5600 Fishers Lane
Room 5A-20
Rockville, MD 20857-0002   301-443-4297
                                  Fax: 301-443-7623

2196 US Veterans Administration: Mental Health and Behavioral Sciences Services

810 Vermont Avenue
Room 900
Washington, DC 20410-0001   202-273-8434

By State

Alabama

2197 Alabama Department of Human Resources

50 N Ripley Street
Montgomery, AL 36130-0624   334-242-1310
                                   Fax: 334-353-1115

Member of the National Leadership Council

2198 Alabama Department of Mental Health and Mental Retardation

100 N Union Street
PO Box 301410
Montgomery, AL 36130-1410   334-242-3417
                                   800-367-0955
                             Fax: 334-353-3894
          E-mail: bsievers@mh.state.al.us
                        www.mh.state.al.us

Kathy E Sawyer, Commissioner
Amy Hinton, Spokesperson
John Houston, Executive Asst. to Commissioner

State agency charged with providing services to citizens with mental illness, mental retardation and substance abuse disorders.

2199 Alabama Department of Public Health

PO Box 303017
Montgomery, AL 36130-3017   334-261-5052

Claude Fox, State Health Officer

2200 Alabama Disabilities Advocacy Program

PO Box 870395
Tuscaloosa, AL 35487-0395   205-348-4928
                             Fax: 205-348-3909
                             TDD: 205-348-9484
                             TTY: 205-348-4928
                E-mail: ADAP@law.ua.edu
                              www.adap.net

Ann Marshall, Coordinator Outreach/Training

Federally mandated, statewide, Protection and Advocacy system serving eligible individuals with disabilities in Alabama. ADAP's five programs are: Protection and Advocacy for Persons with Developmental Disabilities, Protection and Advocacy for Individuals with Mental Illness, Protection and Advocacy of Individual Rights, Protection and Advocacy for Assistive Technology and Protection and Advocacy for Beneficiaries of Social Security.

2201 Alabama State Department of Mental Health

200 Interstate Park Drive
Montgomery, AL 36109-5404   334-240-6833

Richard E Hanan, Commissioner

Alaska

2202 Alaska Department of Health & Social Services

Pouch H-04
Juneau, AK 99811   907-465-3370
                          800-465-4828
                     Fax: 907-465-2668
          www.hss.state.ak.us/dmhdd/

2203 Alaska Division of Medical Assistance/DHSS

4501 Business Park Boulevard, Suite 24
Building M
Anchorage, AK 99503-7117   907-561-2171
                                  Fax: 907-561-1684

2204 Alaska Division of Mental Health and Developmental Disabilities

PO Box 110620
Juneau, AK 99811-0620   907-465-3370
                               Fax: 907-465-2668

Karl R Brimner, Director
Constance E Anderson, DD Program Administrator
Leonard Abel PhD, CMHS Prgram Administrator

2205 Alaska Division of Mental Health and Developmental Disabilities

701 E Tudor Road
Suite 260
Anchorage, AK 99503-7457   907-269-3600
                                  Fax: 907-269-3623

2206 Alaska Mental Health Association

4045 Lake Otis Parkway
Suite 209
Anchorage, AK 99508-5227   907-563-0880
                                  Fax: 907-563-0881

2207 Alaska Mental Health Board

431 N Franklin Street
Suite 200
Juneau, AK 99801-1186   907-465-3071
                               Fax: 907-465-3079
                E-mail: amhb@alaska.net
                       www.alaska.net/~amhb

Walter Majoros, Executive Director

Planning and advocacy body for public mental health services. The board works to ensure that Alaska's mental health program is integrated and comprehensive. It recommends operating and capital budgets for the program. The Governor appoints twelve - sixteen members to the board. At least half the members must be consumers of mental health services or family members. Two members are mental health service providers and one an attorney.

Arizona

2208 Arizona Department of Health Services

150 North 18th Avenue
Phoenix, AZ 85007   602-542-1001
Fax: 602-154-0883
www.webmaster@hs.state.az.us

2209 Arizona Department of Health Services: Behavioral Services

2122 E Highland Avenue
Suite 100
Phoenix, AZ 85016-4740   602-381-8995
Fax: 602-553-9140

2210 Arizona Department of Health Services: Child Fatality Review

1740 W Adams Street
Suite 308
Phoenix, AZ 85007-2670   602-542-1875
Fax: 602-542-1265

2211 Arizona Department of Health: Substance Abuse

150 N 18th Avenue
#200
Phoenix, AZ 85007   602-542-1001
Fax: 602-542-0883
www.http://www.hs.state.az.us/bhs/bsagmh.htm

2212 Governor's Division for Children

1700 W Washington Street
Suite 404
Phoenix, AZ 85007-2812   602-542-3191
Fax: 602-542-4644

2213 Northern Arizona Regional Behavioral Health Authority

1300 S Yale Street
Flagstaff, AZ 86001   928-774-7128

Arkansas

2214 Arkansas Department of Health

4815 W Markham
Little Rock, AR 72205   501-661-2000
Fax: 501-280-4999

2215 Arkansas Department of Human Services

4313 W Markham Street
Little Rock, AR 72205-4023   501-686-9164
877-227-0007
Fax: 501-686-9182

2216 Arkansas Division of Children & Family Service

PO Box 1437
Slot 808
Little Rock, AR 7220   501-682-8462
Fax: 501-682-8094

Member of the National Leadership Council

2217 Arkansas Division on Youth Services

PO Box 1437
Slot 450
Little Rock, AR 72203-1437   502-682-8654
Fax: 501-682-1339

2218 Arkansas State Mental Hospital

4313 W Markham
Little Rock, AR 72205   501-686-9000
Fax: 501-686-9655

2219 Mental Health Council of Arkansas

501 Woodlane Drive
Suite 200
Little Rock, AR 72201-1025   501-372-7062
Fax: 501-372-8039

California

2220 California Department of Alcohol and Drug Programs

1700 K Street
Suite 5
Sacramento, CA 95814-4022   916-654-5326
800-879-2772
Fax: 916-323-1270

2221 California Department of Alcohol and Drug Programs: Mentor Resource Center

1700 K Street
Floor 1
Sacramento, CA 95814-4022   916-445-0834
800-444-3066
Fax: 916-323-1270

2222 California Department of Corrections: Health Care Services

1515 S Street
Sacramento, CA 95814-7243   916-324-4755

2223 California Department of Education: Healthy Kids, Healthy California

PO Box 944272
Sacramento, CA 94244-2720   510-670-4581
Fax: 510-670-4582
www.californiahealthykids.org

2224 California Department of Health Services: Medicaid

714 P Street
Room 1253
Sacramento, CA 95814-6401   916-657-1496
Fax: 916-657-1156
www.dhs.ca.gov

2225 California Department of Health Services: Medi-Cal Drug Discount

714 P Street
Room 213
Sacramento, CA 95814-6401   916-654-0532

2226 California Department of Health and Human Services

200 Independence Avenue SW
Washington, DC 20201   202-619-0257
                              877-696-6775
                         Fax: 202-690-7203

2227 California Department of Mental Health

1600 9th Street
Suite 120
Sacramento, CA 95814-6414   916-654-2487
                              Fax: 916-654-2804

2228 California Health & Welfare Agency

1600 9th Street
Suite 151
Sacramento, CA 95814-6414   916-654-2309
                              Fax: 916-654-3198
                              www.dmh.cahwnet.gov

2229 California Health and Welfare Agency

1600 9th Street
Suite 460
Sacramento, CA 95814-6414   916-654-3454
                              Fax: 916-654-3343

2230 California Hispanic Commission on Alcohol Drug Abuse

2921 P Street
Sacramento, CA 95814   916-443-5473
                         Fax: 916-443-1732

2231 California Institute for Mental Health

2030 J Street
Sacramento, CA 95814-3904   916-556-3480
                              Fax: 916-446-4519
                    E-mail: sgoodwin@cimh.org
                              www.cimh.org

Sandra Naylor-Goodwin, Executive Director
Bill Carter, Deputy Director
Ed Diksa, Director Training

Promoting excellence in mental health services through training, technical asistances, research and policy development.

2232 California Mental Health Directors Association

2030 J Street
Sacramento, CA 95814-3932   916-556-3477
                              Fax: 916-446-4519
                              www.cmhda.org

Patricia Ryan, Executive Director

2233 California Women's Commission on Addictions

14622 Victory Boulevard
Suite 100
Van Nuys, CA 91411-1621   818-376-0470
                            Fax: 818-376-1307

Colorado

2234 Colorado Department of Health Care Policy and Finance

1575 Sherman Street
4th Floor
Denver, CO 80203-1702   303-866-2859
                          Fax: 303-866-2803

2235 Colorado Department of Human Services: Alcohol and Drug Abuse Division

4300 Cherry Creek Drive S
Denver, CO 80220-1530   303-692-2930
                          Fax: 303-853-9775

2236 Colorado Department of Institions

3520 W Oxford Avenue
Denver, CO 80236-3108   303-866-7500

2237 Colorado Department of Social Services

1575 Sherman Street
10th Floor
Denver, CO 80203-1702   303-866-5800

2238 Colorado Division of Medical Assistance

1575 Sherman Street
Suite 5
Denver, CO 80203-1702   303-866-2445

2239 Colorado Division of Mental Health

3520 W Oxford Avenue
Denver, CO 80236-3108   719-546-4000
                          Fax: 719-546-4627

George Kawamura, Director

2240 Denver County Department of Social Services

1200 Federal Boulevard
Denver, CO 80204-3221   720-944-3666
                          Fax: 720-944-3096
          E-mail: roxane.white@dhs.co.denver.co.us

2241 El Paso County Human Services

105 N Spruce Street
Colorado Springs, CO 80905-1409   719-444-5531
                              Fax: 719-444-5598

Connecticut

2242 Connecticut Department of Mental Health and Addiction Services

PO Box 341431
Hartford, CT 06134-1431   860-418-7000
                            Fax: 860-418-6697

2243 Connecticut Department of Children and Families

505 Hudson Street
Hartford, CT 06106-7107   860-550-6352

Member of the National Leadership Council

2244 Connecticut Department of Mental Health

410 Capitol Avenue
Hartford, CT 06106-1308   860-418-6827
                                 800-446-7348
                                 Fax: 860-418-6786
                                 www.state.ct.us/

Delaware

2245 Delaware Department of Health & Social Services

1901 N Dupont Highway
Main Building
New Castle, DE 19720-1100   302-255-9040
                                 302-744-4700
                                 Fax: 302-255-4429

2246 Delaware Division of Child Mental Health Services

Excelsior Building
Wilmington, DE 19801   302-633-2600
                                 Fax: 302-633-2614

Julian Taplin, Executive Director

2247 Delaware Division of Family Services

1825 Faulkland Road
Wilmington, DE 19805-1121   302-663-2665

District of Columbia

2248 DC Commission on Mental Health Services

1536 U Street NW
Washington, DC 20009-3912   202-373-7297
                                 Fax: 202-373-5384

2249 DC Department of Human Services

801 East Building
2700 Martin Luther King Jr Avenue SE
Washington, DC 20032-2601   202-279-6002
                                 Fax: 202-279-6014

2250 Health and Medicine Council of Washington

506 Capital Court NE
Suite 200
Washington, DC 20002-4339   202-544-7499
                                 Fax: 202-546-7105

Dale P Dirks, President

Florida

2251 Florida Department of Alcohol, Drug Abuse & Mental Health

1317 Winewood Boulevard
Tallahassee, FL 32301   850-488-9800
                                 Fax: 850-414-7474

2252 Florida Department of Children and Families

1317 Winewood Boulevard
Building 6
Tallahassee, FL 32399-0700   850-488-8304
                                 Fax: 850-487-2239
                                 E-mail: johnbryant@dcf.state.fl.us

Provides rules, regulations, monitoring of fifteen district mental health program offices and mental health providers throughout the state.

2253 Florida Department of Health and Human Services

1317 Winewood Boulevard
Building 6
Tallahassee, FL 32399-6570   850-487-4441

2254 Florida Department of Health and Rehab Services: Substance Abuse Program

1317 Winewood Boulevard
Building 3ROM
Tallahassee, FL 32399-6570   850-487-2920
                                 Fax: 850-487-2239

2255 Florida Department of Mental Health and Rehabilitative Services

1317 Winewood Boulevard
Tallahassee, FL 32399-6570   850-487-2920
                                 Fax: 850-487-2239

Dr. Ira Rose, Director

2256 Florida Medicaid

2727 Fort Knox Boulevard
Tallahassee, FL 32308-6261   850-488-9525
                                 Fax: 850-922-7303

Georgia

2257 Georgia Department Human Resources: Behavioral Health Plan

1256 Briarcliff Road NE
Atlanta, GA 30306-2636   404-657-2174
                                 Fax: 404-657-2187

2258 Georgia Department of Human Resources

12 Peachtree Street
Suite 3-130
Atlanta, GA 30303   404-657-2164
                                 Fax: 717-654-2187

2259 Georgia Department of Health and Human Services

101 Marietta Street NW
Suite 701
Atlanta, GA 30323-0001   404-331-2329
                                800-633-4277
                                www.hcfa.gov

2260 Georgia Department of Human Resources

2 Peachtree Street NW
4th Floor
Atlanta, GA 30303   404-657-2252
                          Fax: 404-657-1137
                    www.dmh.dhr.state.ga.us

2261 Georgia Department of Medical Assistance

2 Martin Luther King Jr Drive SW
Suite 1220
Atlanta, GA 30334-9000   404-656-4479

2262 Georgia Division of Mental Health and Mental Retardation

2 Peachtree Street NW
Suite 4-152
Atlanta, GA 30303-3181   404-657-2346
                          Fax: 404-657-2359

2263 Georgia Division of Mental Health: Mental Retardation and Substance Abuse

2 Peachtree Street NW
Suite 4, 130
Atlanta, GA 30303   404-657-2252
                          Fax: 404-657-1137

Carl E Roland Jr, Director

Hawaii

2264 Hawaii Department of Adult Mental Health

PO Box 3378
Honolulu, HI 96801-3378   808-334-0800
                          Fax: 208-334-0828

Dr. Nalene Andratti, Director

2265 Hawaii Department of Health

1250 Punchbowl Street
Honolulu, HI 96801-3378   808-586-4416
                          Fax: 808-586-4444
        E-mail: alswanso@mail.health.state.hi.us

Anita Swanson, Director Behavioral Health

Idaho

2266 Department of Health and Welfare: Medicaid Division

3380 American Terrace
PO Box 83720
Boise, ID 83720   208-334-5795
                          Fax: 208-364-1846

2267 Department of Health and Welfare: Community Rehab

450 W State Street
Boise, ID 83702-6005   208-334-5531
                          Fax: 208-334-5694

2268 Idaho Department of Health & Welfare

450 W State
#7
Boise, ID 83720-0001   208-334-5528
                          Fax: 208-334-6699

2269 Idaho Bureau of Maternal and Child Health

PO Box 83720
Boise, ID 83720-3720   208-334-5967
                          Fax: 208-334-6581

2270 Idaho Bureau of Mental Health and Substance Abuse, Division of Family & Community Service

450 W State Street, 5th Floor
PO Box 83720
Boise, ID 83720-0001   208-334-5528
                          Fax: 208-334-6699

2271 Idaho Department of Health and Welfare: Family and Child Services

1720 Westgate Drive
Boise, ID 83704-7164   208-334-6728
                          Fax: 208-334-6738

2272 Idaho Mental Health Center

1720 Westgate Drive
Boise, ID 83704-7164   208-334-0800
                          Fax: 208-334-0828

Dr. Gary Payne, Director

Illinois

2273 Illinois Alcoholism and Drug Dependency Association

937 S 2nd Street
Springfield, IL 62704-2701   217-528-7335
                          Fax: 217-528-7340

2274 Illinois Department of Alcoholism and Substance Abuse

100 W Randolph Street
Suite 5-600
Chicago, IL 60601-3224   312-814-2291
                          Fax: 312-814-2419

2275 Illinois Department of Children and Family Services

100 W Randolph Street
Suite 6-100
Chicago, IL 60601-3225   312-814-8744
                          Fax: 312-814-1905

2276 Illinois Department of Health and Human Services

233 N Michigan Avenue
Suite 060
Chicago, IL 60601   312-886-6432
                          Fax: 312-353-0252

2277 Illinois Department of Human Services

1580 E Knox Street
Galesburg, IL 61401   309-342-8144
                          Fax: 309-342-4518

2278 Illinois Department of Human Services: Office of Mental Health

100 S Grand Avenue E
Harris II, 2nd Floor
Springfield, IL 62762   217-782-3731
                          Fax: 217-782-2406
          E-mail: dhsmhyb@dhs.state.il.us

Leigh Steiner PhD, Associate Director

Works to improve the lives of persons with mental illness by integrating state operated services, community based programs, and other support services to create an effective and responsive treatment and care network. Management office which plans, organizes, and controls the activities of the organization, but does not offer services to the public.

2279 Illinois Department of Mental Health and Drug Dependence

160 N La Salle Street
Chicago, IL 60601-3103   312-814-4963
                          Fax: 312-814-4832

2280 Illinois Department of Mental Health and Developmental Disabilities

Springfield, IL 62765-0001   217-782-2753
                          Fax: 217-524-0835

Jess McDonald, Director

2281 Illinois Department of Public Aid

201 S Grand Avenue E
Springfield, IL 62763   217-782-2570
                          Fax: 217-782-5672

2282 Illinois Department of Public Health: Division of FDD

525 W Jefferson Street
Springfield, IL 62761-0001   217-782-7532
                          Fax: 217-524-0802

2283 Illinois State Psychiatric Institute

1601 W Taylor Street
Chicago, IL 60612-4397   312-433-8568
                          Fax: 312-433-8570

James T Barter MD, Director

2284 Mental Health Association in Illinois

188 W Randolph Street
Suite 2225
Chicago, IL 60601-2901   312-368-9070
                          Fax: 312-368-0283
                E-mail: mhai@mhai.org
                        www.mhai.org

Jan Halcomb, Chief Executive Director

The Mental Health Association in Illinois works to promote mental health, prevent mental and emotional disorders, and improve the care and treatment of persons suffering from mental and emotional problems.

Indiana

2285 Indiana Bureau of Family Protection

402 W Washington Street
Room W-364
Indianapolis, IN 46204-2739   765-741-0200

2286 Indiana Consortium for Mental Health Services

1122 N Oxford Street
Indianapolis, IN 46201-1323   317-274-8589
                          Fax: 317-278-3654

2287 Indiana Department of Family & Social Services

402 W Washington Street
Room W-353
Indianapolis, IN 46204-2739   317-232-7844
                          Fax: 317-233-3472

2288 Indiana Department of Public Welfare

402 W Washington Street
Room W-364
Indianapolis, IN 46204-2739   317-232-7116

2289 Indiana Family and Social Services Administration: Division of Mental Health

402 W Washington Street
Suite W-353
Indianapolis, IN 46204-2739   317-233-4319
                          Fax: 317-233-3472

2290 Indiana Family and Social Services Administration

402 W Washington Street
Indianapolis, IN 46204-2739   317-233-4452
                          Fax: 317-233-4693

2291 Indiana Medicaid

100 N Senate Avenue
Indianapolis, IN 46204-2207   317-232-4966

Iowa

2292 Iowa Department Human Services

1200 University Avenue
Des Moines, IA 50314-2330   515-281-7737
                          Fax: 515-242-6316

2293 Iowa Department of Public Health

Lucas State Office Building
Des Moines, IA 50319-0001
515-281-4417
Fax: 515-281-4535

2294 Iowa Department of Public Health: Division of Substance Abuse

321 12th Street
Des Moines, IA 50309-3402
515-242-6514
Fax: 515-281-4535

2295 Iowa Deptartment of Social Services

Hoover State Office Building
Des Moines, IA 50319-0001
515-281-5723
Fax: 515-281-4597

2296 Iowa Division of Mental Health & Developmental Disabilities: Department of Human Services

Hoover State Office Building
1305 E Walnut St
Des Moines, IA 50319-0114
515-281-5874
Fax: 515-281-8512

Kansas

2297 Comcare of Sedgwick County

635 N Main Street
Wichita, KS 67203
316-832-0318
Fax: 316-383-7925

2298 Division of Health Care Policy

915 SW Harrison
10th Floor N
Topeka, KS 66612
785-296-7272
Fax: 785-296-6142

Donna Doolin, Assistant Director SATR
Karene Suddeth, Director

The Substance Abuse Treatment and Recovery Unit licenses all substance abuse treatment facilities in Kansas, oversees the credentialing of substance abuse counselors, and provides substance abuse treatment to low-income Kansans through a statewide network of funded providers.

2299 Kansas Department of Mental Health and Retardation and Social Services

10th & Topeka Street
Topeka, KS 66612
785-296-3773
888-888-582
Fax: 785-296-6142
www.ink.org

Darvin Hirsch, Director MR/DD Services

2300 Kansas Department of Social and Rehabilitation Services

915 SW Harrison Street
5th Floor N
Topeka, KS 66612-1505
785-296-2608
Fax: 785-296-2861

Kentucky

2301 Kentucky Cabinet for Human Resources

275 E Main Street
Frankfort, KY 40604
502-564-4527
Fax: 502-564-5478

2302 Kentucky Department for Medicaid Services

275 E Main Street
Frankfort, KY 40624
502-564-4321
Fax: 502-564-0509

2303 Kentucky Department for Social Services

275 E Main Street
Frankfort, KY 40621
502-564-2147
Fax: 502-564-5995

2304 Kentucky Department of Mental Health and Mental Retardation

275 E Main Street
Frankfort, KY 40621-0001
205-564-2880
Fax: 502-564-3844

2305 Kentucky Justice Cabinet: Department of Juvenile Justice

1025 Capital Center Drive
Frankfort, KY 40601-1851
502-564-2738
Fax: 502-564-4308

Louisiana

2306 Louisiana Commission on Law Enforcement and Administration

1885 Wooddale Boulevard
Suite 708
Baton Rouge, LA 70806-1550
225-925-4418
Fax: 225-925-1998

2307 Louisiana Department of Health and Hospitals: Office of Mental Health

PO Box 4049
Bin #12
Baton Rouge, LA 70821-4049
255-342-2540
Fax: 255-342-5066

2308 Louisiana Department of Health and Hospitals: Division of Programs

PO Box 871
Bin #15
Baton Rouge, LA 70821-0871
504-342-3800
Fax: 504-342-4497

2309 Louisiana Department of Health

PO Box 629
Baton Rouge, LA 70821-0629
225-642-4707
Fax: 504-342-9508

2310 Louisiana Department of Health & Hospitals

PO Box 4049
Bin #12
Baton Rouge, LA 70821-4049   225-342-9238
                              Fax: 225-342-5066

2311 Louisiana Department of Health & Human Services

PO Box 3318
Baton Rouge, LA 70821-3318   504-342-4086

2312 Louisiana Department of Health and Hospitals: Office of Alcohol and Drug Abuse

PO Box 2790
Bin #18
Baton Rouge, LA 70821-2790   225-342-6717
                              Fax: 255-342-3875

2313 Louisiana Division of Mental Health

PO Box 4049
Baton Rouge, LA 70821-4049   504-342-2540
                              Fax: 504-342-5066

Jerry Vincent, Director

2314 Louisiana Office for Prevention and Recovery

PO Box 53129
Baton Rouge, LA 70892-3129   504-922-0730

Maine

2315 Maine Department Mental Health and Bureau of Children

State House Station
Augusta, ME 04333-0001   207-287-4250
                              Fax: 207-287-4268

2316 Maine Department Services for Children with Special Needs

State House Station
Augusta, ME 04333-0001   207-287-4251
                              Fax: 207-287-4291

2317 Maine Department of Behavioral and Developmental Services

State House Station 40
Augusta, ME 04333-0040   207-287-4223
                              Fax: 207-287-4268
                              TDD: 207-287-2000
E-mail: gary.r.sawyer@state.me.us.web
        www.STATE.ME.US/dmhmrsa/

Lynn F Duby, Commissioner

Provides community services to idividuals with mental illnesses, mental retardation, substance abuse issues and children with special needs. Provides psychiatric inpatient services at two mental health facilities.

2318 Maine Department of Human Services: Children's Emergency Services

State House Station
Augusta, ME 04333-0001   207-287-2983
                              Fax: 207-287-5065

2319 Maine Division of Mental Health

State House Station
#1
Augusta, ME 04333-0001   207-287-4260
                              Fax: 207-287-7286

2320 Maine Office of Substance Abuse: Information and Resource Center

159 State House Station
Augusta, ME 04333-0159   207-287-2595
                              800-499-0027
                              Fax: 207-287-8910
E-mail: osa.ircosa@maine.gov
        www.maine.gov/bds/osa

Provides Maine's citizens with alcohol, tobacco and other drug information, resources and research for prevention, education and treatment.

Maryland

2321 Centers for Medicare & Medicaid Services: Office of Research/Demonstration

6325 Security Boulevard
Suite 2302
Baltimore, MD 21207   410-966-6676

2322 Centers for Medicare & Medicaid Services

7500 Security Boulevard
Baltimore, MD 21244   410-786-0727
                              866-226-1819
                              Fax: 410-966-3252
                              www.cms.hhs.gov

2323 Centers for Medicare & Medicaid Services: Division of Payment Policy

6325 Security Boulevard
Room 200
Baltimore, MD 21207   641-966-3236
                              Fax: 410-966-3252

2324 Maryland Health Care Financing Administration: Divison of Coverage Policy

6235 Security Boulevard
Room 200
Baltimore, MD 21207   410-966-5648
                              Fax: 410-966-3252

2325 Maryland Alcohol and Drug Abuse Administration

201 W Preston Street
Baltimore, MD 21201-2323   410-225-6925
                              Fax: 410-333-7206

2326 Maryland Department of Health and Mental Hygiene

201 W Preston Street
Room 405
Baltimore, MD 21201-2399   410-767-6860
                                  877-461-3464
                             Fax: 410-767-6489
E-mail: healthmd@dhmh.state.md.us
                    www.dhmh.state.md.us/

2327 Maryland Department of Human Resources

311 W Saratoga Street
Baltimore, MD 21201-3500   410-767-7713
                             Fax: 410-333-6556
                        www.dhr.state.mdus

2328 Maryland Division of Mental Health

2301 Argonne Drive
Baltimore, MD 21218-1628   410-767-6860
                             Fax: 410-333-7482

2329 Maryland Health Care Financing Administration: Division of Eligiblity Policy

6325 Security Boulevard
Room 200
Baltimore, MD 21207   410-966-4451
                             Fax: 410-966-3252

2330 Maryland Health Care Financing Administration

7500 Security Boulevard
Baltimore, MD 21244-1850   410-786-7614
                             Fax: 410-786-5010

2331 Maryland Health Systems Financing Administration

300 W Preston Street
Baltimore, MD 21201-2308   410-225-1459

2332 Maryland Office of State Healthcare Reform

6325 Security Boulevard
Room 2306
Baltimore, MD 21207   710-966-2671
                             Fax: 717-783-1116

Massachusetts

2333 Massachusetts Bureau of Substance Abuse Services

250 Washington Street
#3
Boston, MA 02108-4603   617-624-5111
                             Fax: 617-624-5185

2334 Massachusetts Department of Mental Health

25 Staniford Street
Boston, MA 02114-2503   617-626-8075
                             Fax: 617-626-8077

Eileen Elias, Commissioner

2335 Massachusetts Department of Public Health

250 Washington Street
Boston, MA 02108-4603   617-624-5111
                             Fax: 617-624-5185

2336 Massachusetts Department of Public Welfare

600 Washington Street
Boston, MA 02111   617-348-8500
                             Fax: 617-348-8575
                        www.spat.ma.us/dta

2337 Massachusetts Department of Social Services

24 Farnsworth Street
Boston, MA 02210-1264   617-727-3171
                             Fax: 617-261-7435

2338 Massachusetts Division of Medical Assistance

600 Washington Street
Floor 5
Boston, MA 02111-1704   617-348-5617
                             Fax: 617-348-8590

2339 Massachusetts Executive Office of Public Safety

1 Ashburton Place
Room 2110
Boston, MA 02108-1518   617-727-6300
                             Fax: 617-727-5356

Michigan

2340 Michigan Department of Community Health: Treatment Policy Section

320 S Walnut Street
Lewis Cass Building, Floor 5
Lansing, MI 48913   517-335-0161
                             Fax: 517-241-2611

2341 Michigan Department of Community Health: System Development and Monitoring

320 S Walnut Street
Lewis Cass Building, Floor 6
Lansing, MI 48913   517-335-0178
                             Fax: 517-241-4729

James K Habbem Jr, Director

2342 Michigan Department of Community Health

320 S Walnut Street
Lewis Cass Building
Lansing, MI 48913   517-373-3500
                             Fax: 517-335-3090

2343 Michigan Department of Community Health: Prevention Policy

320 S Walnut Street
Lewis Cass Building, Floor 5
Lansing, MI 48913-0001   517-241-2599

2344 Michigan Department of Mental Health

320 Walnut Boulevard
6
Lansing, MI 48913-0001   517-373-3500
                                Fax: 517-373-4288

**2345 Michigan Department of Mental Health
Bureau of Community Mental Health
Services**

320 S Walnut Street
Lewis Cass Bldg
Lansing, MI 48913-0001   000-151-7373
                                Fax: 517-335-6775

2346 Michigan Department of Public Health

3423 N Martin Luther King Jr Boulevard
Lansing, MI 48906-2934   517-335-8088
                                Fax: 517-335-8837

2347 Michigan Department of Social Services

400 S Pine Street
PO Box 30037
Lansing, MI 48909-7537   517-335-5001
                                Fax: 517-335-5007

**2348 Michigan Division of Substance Abuse
Quality & Planning**

3423 N Martin Luther King Boulevard
Lansing, MI 48909   517-335-0278
                              Fax: 517-241-2611

Deborah Hollis, Director

**2349 Michigan State Representative: Co-Chair
Public Health**

State Capitol
Lansing, MI 48913-0001   517-373-1705
                                Fax: 517-373-5968

**2350 National Council on Alcoholism and Drug
Dependence of Michigan**

913 W Holmes Road
Suite 111
Lansing, MI 48910   517-394-1252
                              Fax: 517-394-1518

Minnesota

**2351 Department of Human Services:
Chemical Health Division**

444 Lafayette Road N
Saint Paul, MN 55155-3823   651-582-1832
                                Fax: 651-582-1865
                                www.dhs.state.mn.us

Don Eubanks, Director

**2352 Minnesota Department of Human
Services**

444 Lafayette Road N
Saint Paul, MN 55155-3828   651-296-6117
                                Fax: 651-296-6244

**2353 Minnesota Department of Mental Health
and Human Services**

444 Lafayette Road N
Saint Paul, MN 55155-3828   651-296-4497
                                Fax: 651-582-1831

2354 Minnesota Youth Services Bureau

244 North Lake Street
Forest Lake, MN 55025-2647   651-464-3685
                                Fax: 651-464-3687

Mississippi

**2355 Department of Rehabilitation Services:
Vocational Rehab**

PO Box 1698
Jackson, MS 39215-1698   601-853-5100
                                Fax: 601-853-5205

**2356 Mississippi Alcohol Safety Education
Program**

103 Mississippi Research Park
PO Box 5287
Mississippi State, MS 39762-5287   662-325-3423
                                    800-678-2534
                                Fax: 662-325-9439
                                www.ssrc.misstate.edu/

MASEP is the statewide program for first-time offenders convicted of driving under the influence of alcohol or another substance which has impaired one's
ability to operate a motor vehicle.

2357 Mississippi Bureau of Mental Retardation

1101 Robert E Lee Building
Jackson, MS 39201-1311   601-664-6000
                                Fax: 601-354-6945

Roger McMurtry, Chief

**2358 Mississippi Department of Human
Services**

PO Box 352
Jackson, MS 39205-0352   601-359-4981
                                Fax: 601-359-4226

**2359 Mississippi Department of Mental Health:
Division of Alcohol and Drug Abuse**

239 N Lamar Street
1101 Robert F Lee Building
Jackson, MS 39201-1309   601-359-1288
                                Fax: 601-359-6295

Dr. Albert Randel Hendrix, Executive Director
Herb Loving, Director Alcohol/Drug Abuse
Roger McMurtry, Chief of Bureau of Mental Health

State authority on mental health, mental retardation,
alcohol and substance abuse and Alzheimer's disease.

2360 Mississippi Department of Mental Health

1101 Robert E Lee Building
Jackson, MS 39201-1311   601-359-1288
                                Fax: 601-359-6295

Albert Hendricks PhD, Director

2361 Mississippi Department of Mental Health: Division of Medicaid

239 N Lamar Street
Suite 1101
Jackson, MS 39201   601-359-1288
Fax: 601-359-6295

Missouri

2362 Missouri Department of Mental Health

1706 E Elm
Jefferson City, MO 65101   573-751-4122
800-364-9687
Fax: 573-751-8224
E-mail:
royc.wilsonmd.web.www.state.mo.us/dmh
www.modhmg.state.mo.us

Keith Schafer, Director

2363 Missouri Department of Public Safety

Truman Office Building, Room 870
PO Box 749
Jefferson City, MO 65102-0749   573-751-4905
Fax: 573-751-5399

2364 Missouri Department of Social Services: Aging Division

PO Box 1527
Jefferson City, MO 65102-1527   573-751-2270

2365 Missouri Department of Social Services

PO Box 1527
Jefferson City, MO 65102-1527   314-751-4815
800-735-2966
Fax: 314-751-3203

2366 Missouri Department of Social Services: Medical Services Division

PO Box 6500
Jefferson City, MO 65102-6500   573-751-4905
Fax: 573-751-5399

2367 Missouri Division of Alcohol and Drug Abuse

1706 E Elm Street
Jefferson City, MO 65101-4130   573-751-4942
Fax: 573-751-7814

2368 Missouri Division of Comprehensive Psychiatric Service

PO Box 687
1706 E Elm Street
Jefferson City, MO 65102-0687   573-751-5212
Fax: 573-751-7815

2369 Missouri Division of Medical Services

615 Howerton Court
PO Box 6500
Jefferson City, MO 65109-6806   573-751-6922
Fax: 573-751-6564

2370 Missouri Division of Mental Retardation and Developmental Disabilities

1706 E Elm Street
PO Box 687
Jefferson City, MO 65102-0687   573-751-4054
Fax: 573-751-9207

Montana

2371 Monatana Department of Mental Health and Human Services

1359 11th Avenue
Helena, MT 59601-3919   406-444-3969
Fax: 406-444-4920

2372 Montana Department of Health and Human Services: Child & Family Services Division

PO Box 8005
Helena, MT 59604-8005   406-444-5991

2373 Montana Department of Institutions

1539 11th Avenue
Helena, MT 59601-4526   406-444-3969
Fax: 460-444-4435

2374 Montana Department of Public Health & Human Services: Addictive and Mental Disorders

PO Box 202951
Helena, MT 56902   406-444-3964
Fax: 406-444-4435

2375 Montana Department of Social & Rehabilitation Services

111 Sander Street
PO Box 4210
Helena, MT 59604-4210   406-444-1710

Nebraska

2376 Nebraska Department of Health and Human Services

PO Box 95044
Lincoln, NE 68509-5044   402-471-2306
Fax: 402-471-4619

2377 Nebraska Department of Public Institutions

PO Box 94728
Lincoln, NE 68509-4728   402-471-2850
Fax: 402-479-5162

2378 Nebraska Department of Public Institutions: Office of Community Mental Health

PO Box 94728
Lincoln, NE 68509-4728   402-471-2851
Fax: 402-479-5145

2379 Nebraska Department of Social Services

PO Box 95044
Lincoln, NE 68509-5044   402-471-9331
                                TDD: 402-471-2306

**2380 Nebraska Department of Social Services:
Medical Services Division**

301 Centennial Mall S
Lincoln, NE 68509   402-471-9379
                                Fax: 402-471-9092

Bob Seifert, Director

2381 Nebraska Mental Health Centers

7160 S 29th
Lincoln, NE 68516   402-423-6990
                                Fax: 402-423-7045
          E-mail: nmhc@nmhc-clinics.com
                  www.mmhc-clinics.com

Dr. Matthew Nessetti, Director

Nevada

2382 Nevada Department of Human Resources

505 E King Street
Building 603
Carson City, NV 89710-0001   702-486-6000
                                Fax: 702-486-6248

**2383 Nevada Department of Human
Resources: Medicaid & Welfare Division**

2527 N Carson Street
Carson City, NV 89706-0147   702-687-4378

**2384 Nevada Department of Human
Resources: Bureau of Alcohol & Drug
Abuse**

1830 E Sahara Avenue
Suite 314
Las Vegas, NV 89104-3737   702-486-8250
                                Fax: 702-486-8253

2385 Nevada Department of Human Services

6171 W Charleston Boulevard
Building 15
Las Vegas, NV 89146-1126   702-486-7650
                                Fax: 702-486-7626

**2386 Nevada Division of Mental Health &
Developme ntal Services**

505 E King Street
Suite 602
Carson City, NV 89701   775-684-5943
                                Fax: 775-684-5964
          www.mhds@dhr.state.nv.us

Dr. Kevin Crowe, Chief Planning/Evaluation

The Nevada Division of Mental Health provides a full
array of clinical services to over 24,000 consumers
each year. Services include: crisis intervention, hospital care, medication clinic, outpatient counseling, residential support and other mental health services
targeted to individuals with serious mental illness.

**2387 Nevada Division of Mental Health and
Mental Retardation**

1330 S Curry Street
Carson City, NV 89703   775-687-4195
                                Fax: 775-687-4103

**2388 Nevada Employment Training &
Rehabilitation Department**

505 E King Street
Suite 500
Carson City, NV 89701-3703   775-684-4190
                                Fax: 775-684-4185

**2389 Southern Nevada Adult Mental Health
Services**

6161 W Charleston Boulevard
Las Vegas, NV 89146-1148   702-486-6000
                                Fax: 702-486-6248

State operated community mental health center. Provides inpatient and outpatient psychiatric services.

**2390 State of Nevada: Nevada Mental Health
Institute**

480 Galletti Way
Sparks, NV 89431-5573   702-688-2193
                                Fax: 702-688-2192

New Hampshire

**2391 Division of Human Services: Office of
Medical Service**

6 Hazel Drive
Concord, NH 03301-3431   603-271-4353

**2392 Division of Mental Health and
Developmental Services**

105 Pleasant Street
Concord, NH 03301-3852   603-271-5064

**2393 Division of Mental Health: Community
Mental**

105 Pleasant Street
#2
Concord, NH 03301-3852   603-271-5031
                                Fax: 603-271-5040

**2394 New Hampshire Department of Health &
Human Services: Behavioral Health**

105 Pleasant Street
State Office Park
Concord, NH 03301-3852   603-271-5007
                                Fax: 603-271-5058

**2395 New Hampshire Department of Health &
Welfare**

65 Beacon Street W
PO Box 634
Laconia, NH 03247-0634   603-524-4485

Government Agencies/By State/New Jersey

2396 New Hampshire Department of Mental Health

State Office Park S
Concord, NH 03301   603-271-5000
                          Fax: 603-271-5058

Donald Shumway, Director
Paul Garmon

New Jersey

2397 Juvenile Justice Commission

840 Bear Tavern Road
CN 107
Trenton, NJ 08628-1019   609-530-5203
                               Fax: 609-530-3465

2398 New Jersey Department of Social Services

50 E State, 3rd Floor, Capitol Center
PO Box 727
Trenton, NJ 08625-0727
                          Fax: 609-777-0662
          E-mail: webmaster@dhs.state.nj.us
          www.state.nj.us/humanservices/dhsmahl.html

Alan G Kaufman, Director

2399 New Jersey Division Of Mental Health Services

Capital Center
PO Box 727
Trenton, NJ 08625   609-777-0700
                          800-382-6717
                          Fax: 609-777-0662
          E-mail: dmhsmail@dhs.state.nj.us
          www.state.nj.us/humanservices/dmhs

Allan Kaufman, Director

State mental health authority

2400 New Jersey Division of Mental Health Services

CN 727
Trenton, NJ 08625   609-777-0810
                          Fax: 609-777-0835

2401 New Jersey Division of Youth & Family Services

50 E State Street
Suite 5
Trenton, NJ 08608-1715   609-984-2380

2402 New Jersey Office of Managed Care

Department of Health
CN-367
Trenton, NJ 18625   609-588-2510
                          Fax: 609-588-7823

New Mexico

2403 New Mexico Behavioral Health Services Division

1190 S St. Francis Drive
Santa Fe, NM 87502   505-827-2658
                           Fax: 505-827-0097
                           www.health.state.nm.us

Mary Schumacher, Director
Elizabeth Mendoza, Acting Administrative Assistant

2404 New Mexico Children: Youth and Families Department

PO Box 5160
Santa Fe, NM 87502-5160   505-827-7623
                                Fax: 505-827-5883

2405 New Mexico Department of Health

1190 S St. Francis Drive
PO Box 26110
Santa Fe, NM 87502-0110   505-827-2613
                                Fax: 505-827-0097
                                www.health.state.nm.us

2406 New Mexico Department of Human Services

PO Box 2348
Santa Fe, NM 87504-2348   505-827-4315
                                Fax: 505-827-3185

2407 New Mexico Department of Human Services: Medical Assistance Programs

PO Box 2348
Santa Fe, NM 87504-2348   505-827-9454
                                Fax: 505-827-4402

2408 New Mexico Health & Environment Department

1190 St. Francis Drive
Room 3150N
Santa Fe, NM 87503-0001   505-827-2651
                                Fax: 505-827-2695

New York

2409 New York County Department of Social Services

40 Howard Street
Albany, NY 12207-1684   518-447-7300

2410 New York Department of Mental Health

44 Holland Avenue
Albany, NY 12208-3411   518-474-2568

Richard Surles PhD, Director
James Stone

2411 New York Department of Social Services

40 N Pearl Street
Albany, NY 12207-2729   518-463-4829

2412 New York Office of Alcohol & Substance Abuse Services

1450 Western Avenue
Albany, NY 12203-3536   646-728-4513
                              Fax: 646-728-4690

Frank McCorry PhD

State agency responsible for funding, licensing and monitering substance abuse prevention and treatment services in New York State.

North Carolina

2413 North Carolina Department of Human Resources: Mental Health Developmental Disabilities & Substance Abuse Division
325 N Salisbury Street
Raleigh, NC 27603-1388   919-733-7011
                                Fax: 919-733-9455

2414 North Carolina Department of Human Resources
PO Box 29529
Raleigh, NC 27626-0529   919-733-2833
                                Fax: 919-733-2796

2415 North Carolina Department of Mental Health
325 N Salisbury Street
Raleigh, NC 27603-1388   919-733-7011
                                Fax: 919-733-1221

Mike Pedneau, Director
Dr. John S Baggatt

2416 North Carolina Division of Mental Health: Drug Dependency and Substance Abuse Services
325 N Salisbury Street
Suite 679
Raleigh, NC 27603-1388   919-733-4460
                                Fax: 919-715-3604

2417 North Carolina Division of Social Services
325 N Salisbury Street
Raleigh, NC 27603-1388   919-733-7011

2418 North Carolina Governor's Office of Substance Abuse Policy
301 W Jones Street, Suite 250
3021 Mail Service
Raleigh, NC 27603-1300   919-715-5989
                                Fax: 919-715-2360
                                www.dhhs.state.nc.us

2419 North Carolina Mental Health Services
325 N Salisbury Street
Raleigh, NC 27603-1388   919-733-4660
                                Fax: 919-715-3604

2420 North Carolina Substance Abuse Profession Certification Board
PO Box 10126
Raleigh, NC 27605-0126   919-832-0975

North Dakota

2421 North Dakota Department of Human Services: Medicaid Program
600 E Boulevard Avenue
Judicial Wing
Bismarck, ND 58505-0250   701-328-2321
                                 Fax: 701-328-1544
                       E-mail: dhsmed@state.nd.us
                    www.state.dd.us/humanservices

David J Zentner, Director Medical Services

Pays for a wide array of medical services including mental health services for certain low-income residents of North Dakota. Anyone interested in applying for services should contact their local County Social Service Board office.

2422 North Dakota Department of Human Services: Mental Health Services Division
600 E Boulevard Avenue
Bismarck, ND 58505-0660   701-328-8940
                                 Fax: 701-328-8969

2423 North Dakota Department of Human Services: Division of Mental Health and Substance Abuse
600 S 2nd Street
Bismarck, ND 58504   701-328-8940
                                 Fax: 701-328-8969

2424 North Dakota Department of Mental Health
600 S 2nd Street, Suite 1 D
State Capitol Bldg
Bismarck, ND 58505-0660   328-894-0090
                                 Fax: 701-328-8969

Sam Ismir, Director

Ohio

2425 Ohio Community Drug Board
725 E Market Street
Akron, OH 44305-2421   330-434-4141
                                 Fax: 330-434-7125

2426 Ohio Department of Mental Health
30 E Broad Street
8th Floor
Columbus, OH 43215-3414   614-466-2337
                                 Fax: 614-752-9453

Oklahoma

2427 Oklahoma Department of Human Services
PO Box 26768
Oklahoma City, OK 73125-0352   405-522-5818
                                 Fax: 405-521-6684

2428 Oklahoma Department of Mental Health and Substance Abuse Service

1200 NE 13th Street
PO Box 53277
Oklahoma City, OK 73152-3277   405-522-3908
Fax: 405-522-3650
TDD: 405-522-3851
www.odmhsas.org

Terry Cline PhD, Commissioner
Dave Statton, COO
Jeffrey Dismukes, Director Public Information

State agency responsible for mental health, substance abuse, and domestic violence and sexual assault services.

2429 Oklahoma Healthcare Authority

4545 N Lincoln Boulevard
Suite 124
Oklahoma City, OK 73105-3400   405-271-4200
Fax: 405-271-3431

2430 Oklahoma Office of Juvenile Affairs

PO Box 268812
Oklahoma City, OK 73126-8812   918-246-8000
Fax: 918-241-0647
E-mail: stegri@oja.state.ok.us
www.oja.state.ok.us

Richard DeLaughter, Executive Director
James Johnson, Deputy Director
Stephen Grissom PhD, Chief Psychologist

State agency charged with delivery of programs and services to delinquent youth. Services include delinquency prevention, diversion, counseling in both community and secure residential programs. OJA provides counseling services with counselors, social workers and psychologists, as well as contracted service providers.

2431 Oklahoma's Mental Health Consumer Council

5131 N Classen Boulevard
Suite 200
Oklahoma City, OK 73118-4433   405-840-0607
888-424-1305
Fax: 405-840-4177
E-mail: omhcc@sbcglobal.net
www.okmentalhealth.org

Consumer run statewide advocacy organization for education, empowerment, quality of life, encouragement and rights protection of persons with mental illness. Services include empowerment training, systems advocacy, peer support and jail diversion programs.

Oregon

2432 Marion County Health Department

3180 Center Street NE
Suite 2100
Salem, OR 97310-0001   503-588-5357
Fax: 503-364-6552

2433 Mental Health and Developmental Disability Division: Department of Human Services

2575 Bittern Street NE
Salem, OR 97310-0520   503-945-9700
Fax: 503-373-7327

2434 Office of Mental Health and Addiction Services Training & Resource Center

2575 Bittern Street NE, Room 119A
PO Box 14250
Salem, OR 97309-0740   503-945-9701
800-822-6772
Fax: 503-373-7327
E-mail: oprc@open.org
www.open.org/~oprc/

Wendy Hausotter, Coordinator
Sandi Lacher, Resource Specialist
Dixie Montague, Webmaster

We are a library and clearinghouse, your connection to resources for prevention and treatment of disorders related to the use of alcohol, tobacco, other drugs and problem gambling. Our goal is to provide current, accurate and timely information to professionals and the public. We also seek to promote use of research based practices and promising approaches to prevention and treatment.

2435 Oregon Commission on Children and Families

530 Center Street NE
Suite 300
Salem, OR 97310-0001   503-373-1570
Fax: 503-378-8395

2436 Oregon Department of Human Resources: Medical Assistance Program

500 Summer Street NE
Salem, OR 97310-1002   503-945-5769
Fax: 503-373-7689

2437 Oregon Department of Human Resources: Health Service Section

318 Public Service Building
Salem, OR 97310-0001   503-945-6492

2438 Oregon Department of Mental Health

2600 Center Street NE
Salem, OR 97310-1319   503-954-9499
Fax: 503-378-3796

Stan Mazurhart, Director

2439 Oregon Health Plan Unit

2575 Bittern Street NE
Salem, OR 97310-1312   503-945-9827
Fax: 503-947-1023

Pennsylvania

2440 Dauphin County Drug and Alcohol

25 S Front Street
Floor 8
Harrisburg, PA 17101-2025   717-780-7030
Fax: 717-635-2266

2441 Pennsylvania Bureau of Community Program Standards

PO Box 90
Harrisburg, PA 17108-0090   717-783-8665

2442 Pennsylvania Department of Health: Office of Drug and Alcohol Programs

PO Box 90
Harrisburg, PA 17108-0090   717-783-8200
                                 Fax: 717-787-6285

2443 Pennsylvania Department of Mental Health

120 South Street
Harrisburg, PA 17101-1210   717-787-6443
                                 Fax: 717-787-5394

Susan Reider, Director

2444 Pennsylvania Department of Public Welfare

PO Box 8021
Harrisburg, PA 17105-8021   717-772-6198
                                 Fax: 717-772-6328

2445 Pennsylvania Department of Public Welfare: Office of Mental Health

PO Box 2675
Harrisburg, PA 17105-2675   717-787-6443
                                 Fax: 717-787-5394

2446 Pennsylvania Deputy Secretary for Public Health Programs

PO Box 90
Harrisburg, PA 17108-0090   717-783-1457
                                 Fax: 717-772-0608
                E-mail: kmagaro@state.pa.us

Gary L Gurian, Deputy Secretary

2447 Pennsylvania Division of Drug and Alcohol Training: Information

PO Box 90
Harrisburg, PA 17108-0090   717-787-2606

2448 Pennsylvania Division of Drug and Alcohol Program: Monitoring

PO Box 90
Harrisburg, PA 17108-0090   717-783-8307

2449 Pennsylvania Division of Drug and Alcohol Prevention: Intervention and Treatment

PO Box 90
Harrisburg, PA 17108-0090   717-787-2712

2450 Pennsylvania Medical Assistance Programs

PO Box 8043
Harrisburg, PA 17105-8043   717-782-6142

Rhode Island

2451 Rhode Island Council on Alcoholism and Other Drug Dependence

500 Prospect Street
Pawtucket, RI 02860-6260   401-728-7800
                                 800-622-7422

2452 Rhode Island Department of Human Services

600 New London Avenue
Cranston, RI 02920-3041   401-464-2183

2453 Rhode Island Department of Mental Health

Cottage 405 Ct B
Cranston, RI 02920   401-462-3201
                                 Fax: 401-462-3204
                                 TDD: 401-462-6087

Reed Cosper, Director

2454 Rhode Island Department of Mental Health: Mental Retardation and Hospital

14 Harrington Road
Cranston, RI 02920   401-462-3201
                                 Fax: 401-462-3204
                                 www.hrh.state.ri.us

2455 Rhode Island Division of Mental Health

600 New London Avenue
Cranston, RI 02920-3024   401-462-3201
                                 Fax: 401-462-3204

2456 Rhode Island Division of Substance Abuse

25 Howard Avenue
Building 057
Cranston, RI 02920-3001   401-464-2091
                                 Fax: 401-464-2089

South Carolina

2457 Lexington/Richland Drug and Alcohol Abuse Council

PO Box 50597
Columbia, SC 29250-0597   803-733-1376
                                 Fax: 803-733-1377

2458 Mental Health Association in South Carolina

1823 Gadsden Street
Columbia, SC 29201-2344   803-779-5363

2459 South Carolina Bureau of Drug Control

2600 Bull Street
Columbia, SC 29201-1708   803-935-7817
                                 Fax: 803-935-7820

2460 South Carolina Department of Alcohol and Other Drug Abuse Services
101 Business Park Boulevard
Columbia, SC 29203-9498   803-896-5555
Fax: 803-896-5557
www.daodas.state.sc.us

Rick C Wade, Director

DAODAS is the cabinet-level department responsible for ensuring the availability of comprehensive alcohol and other drug abuse services for the citizens of South Carolina.

2461 South Carolina Department of Mental Health and Mental Retardation
PO Box 485
Columbia, SC 29202-0485   803-898-8581
Fax: 803-898-8316

Maureen Donnelly, Director

2462 South Carolina Department of Social Services
PO Box 1520
Columbia, SC 29202-1520   803-734-5670

2463 South Carolina Health and Human Services Finance Commission
PO Box 8206
Columbia, SC 29202-8206   803-253-4137

South Dakota

2464 South Dakota Department of Human Services: Division of Mental Health
E Highway 34, Hillsview Plaza
500 E Capitol Avenue
Pierre, SD 57501   605-773-5991
800-265-9684
Fax: 605-773-7076
E-mail: infoMH@dhs.state.sd.us
www.state.sd.us/dhs/dmh/

Kim Malsam-Rysdon, Director
Amy Iversen-Pollreisz, Community Based Mental Health

Serves as the point of contact for state funded services, support and treatment for adults with severe and persistent mental illness (SPMI), and children with serious emotional disturbance (SED).

2465 South Dakota Department of Social Services
700 Governors Drive
Pierre, SD 57501-2291   605-773-3165
Fax: 605-773-4855

2466 South Dakota Department of Social and Medical Services
700 Governors Drive
Pierre, SD 57501-2291   605-773-5246

2467 South Dakota Division of Mental Health
500 E Capitol
Pierre, SD 57501-5070   605-773-7172
Fax: 605-773-7076
E-mail: infoMH@dhs.state.sd.us

2468 South Dakota Human Services Center
3515 Broadway Avenue
PO Box 76
Yankton, SD 57078-0076   605-668-3100
Fax: 605-668-3460

Cory Nelson, Interim Administrator

Tennessee

2469 Alcohol and Drug Council of Middle Tennessee
2612 Westwood Drive
PO Box 40387
Nashville, TN 37204-2710   615-269-0029
800-427-4188
Fax: 615-269-0299
TDD: 615-269-0344
E-mail: office@adcmt.org
www.adcmt.org

Robert G Currie, Executive VP

2470 Bureau of TennCare: State of Tennessee
729 Church Street
Nashville, TN 37203-3503   615-532-6706
800-669-1851
Fax: 615-532-1383

2471 Chattanooga/Plateau Council for Alcohol and Drug Abuse
207 Spears Avenue
Chattanooga, TN 37405-3840   423-756-7644
877-282-2327
Fax: 432-756-7646

2472 Memphis Alcohol and Drug Council
1450 Poplar Avenue
Memphis, TN 38104-2901   901-274-0056
Fax: 901-274-0086

2473 Tennessee Commission on Children and Youth
710 James Robertson Parkway
9th Floor
Nashville, TN 37243-0800   615-741-2633
Fax: 615-741-5956
www.state.tn.us/teey

Linda O'Neal, Executive Director
Pat Wade, Program Director

2474 Tennessee Department of Health
425 5th Avenue N
Nashville, TN 37247   651-741-7305
Fax: 615-532-2286

2475 Tennessee Department of Health: Alcohol and Drug Abuse

425 5th Avenue N
3rd Fl
Nashville, TN 37247   615-741-1921
Fax: 615-532-2419

2476 Tennessee Department of Human Services

1000 2nd Avenue N
Nashville, TN 37243-1403   615-532-4000

2477 Tennessee Department of Mental Health and Mental Retardation

706 Church Street
Doctors Building, Suite 600
Nashville, TN 37203-3586   615-532-6564
Fax: 615-741-0770

2478 Tennessee Department of Mental Health and Mental Disabilities

425 5th Avenue
Nashville, TN 37243   615-532-6610
Fax: 615-741-4557
E-mail: martha.robinson@state.tn.us
www.state.tn.us/mental

Elisabeth Rukeyser, Commissioner
Martha Robinson, Public Information/Education

Tennessee's mental health and developmental disabilities authority. It has responsibility for system planning, setting policy and quality standards, system monitering and evaluation, disseminating public information and advocating for persons of all ages who have mental illness, serious emotional disturbance or developmental disabilities.

2479 Tennessee Neuropsychiatric Institute

Middle Tennessee Mental Health Institute
1501 Murfreesboro Pike
Nashville, TN 37217-2800   615-399-3238

Michael Ebert MD, Director

2480 Williamson County Council on Alcohol and Drug Prevention

1320 W Main Street
Suite 418
Franklin, TN 37064-3737   615-790-5783
Fax: 615-790-5783

Texas

2481 Austin Travis County Mental Health: Mental Retardation Center

1430 Collier Street
Austin, TX 78704-2911   512-447-4141
Fax: 512-440-4081
E-mail: help@atcmhmr.com
www.atcmhmr.com

Abraham Minjarez, Acting Dir, Adult Mental Health
David Evans, Executive Director

Provides mental health, mental retardation and substance services to the Austin-Travis County community.

2482 Dallas County Mental Health: Mental Retardation Center

1341 W Mockingbird Lane
Suite 1000
Dallas, TX 75247-6913   214-634-4550
Fax: 214-630-3469

2483 Harris County Mental Health: Mental Retardation Authority

2850 Fannin Street
Suite 200
Houston, TX 77002-9220   281-863-7000
Fax: 281-863-7767

2484 Tarrant County Mental Health: Mental Retardation Services

3840 Hulen Street
Fort Worth, TX 76107-7277   817-569-4300
Fax: 817-569-4499

2485 Texas Commission on Alcohol and Drug Abuse

9001 NIH 35
Suite 105
Austin, TX 78753-5233   866-214-0547
866-373-1253

2486 Texas Department of Human Services

PO Box 149030
Austin, TX 78714-9030   512-438-3045

2487 Texas Department of Mental Health: Retardation

PO Box 12668
Capitol Station
Austin, TX 78711-2668   512-206-4588
Fax: 512-206-4560
www.mhmr.state.tx.us

Karen F Hale, Director

2488 Texas Department of Protective Services

PO Box 149030
Mailcode E-558
Austin, TX 78714-9030   512-438-3412

2489 Texas Health and Human Services Commission

4900 N Lamar Boulevard
Austin, TX 78751   512-424-6500

Utah

2490 Utah Commission on Criminal Justice

101 State Capital
Salt Lake City, UT 84114   801-538-1031
Fax: 801-538-1528

2491 Utah Department of Health

PO Box 142835
Salt Lake Cty, UT 84114-2835   801-538-6151
Fax: 801-538-6694

2492 Utah Department of Health: Health Care Financing
PO Box 242906
Salt Lake City, UT 84114   801-538-6495

2493 Utah Department of Mental Health
2001 S State Street
Suite 2600
Salt Lake City, UT 84190-0001   801-238-7191
                                  Fax: 801-238-7404

Dave Dangerfield, Director

2494 Utah Department of Social Services
120 N 200 W
#4
Salt Lake City, UT 84103-1550
                                  Fax: 801-538-4016

2495 Utah Division of Substance Abuse
120 N 200 W
Suite 201
Salt Lake City, UT 84103-1550   801-538-3939
                                  Fax: 801-538-4696

2496 Utah Health Care Financing Administration
288 S 1460 E
Salt Lake City, UT 84112-8904   801-538-6406
                                  Fax: 801-538-6478

Vermont

2497 Vermont Department of Developmental and Mental Health Services
103 S Main Street
Waterbury, VT 05676   802-241-2604
                                  Fax: 802-241-3052
                                  TTY: 800-253-0191
                                  www.state.vt.us/dmh/

Susan Besio, Commissioner

2498 Vermont Department of Social Welfare: Medicaid Division
103 S Main Street
Waterbury, VT 05676   802-241-2880

2499 Vermont Office of Alchol and Drug Abuse Programs
108 Cherry Street
PO Box 70
Burlington, VT 05402-0070   802-654-1550

Virginia

2500 Virginia Department of Medical Assistance Services
600 E Broad Street
Suite 1300
Richmond, VA 23219-1857   804-786-8099

2501 Virginia Department of Mental Health
PO Box 1797
Richmond, VA 23218-1797   804-786-3915
                                  Fax: 804-786-3824

Ruby-Jean Gould, Director

2502 Virginia Department of Mental Health, Mental Retardation and Substance Abuse Services
1220 Bank Street
Richmond, VA 23219   804-786-3921
                                  Fax: 804-371-6638

2503 Virginia Department of Social Services
730 E Broad Street
Richmond, VA 23219-1849   804-692-1273

2504 Virginina Office of the Secretary of Human Resources
PO Box 1797
Richmond, VA 23218-1797   804-786-3921
                                  Fax: 804-371-6638

Washington

2505 Washington Department of Alcohol and Substance Abuse: Department of Social and Health Service
PO Box 45330
Olympia, WA 98504-5330   360-438-8200
                                  Fax: 360-438-8078

2506 Washington Department of Mental Health
PO Box 592
Olympia, WA 98507-0592   360-438-1900
                                  Fax: 360-902-7691

Dave Novseri, Director

2507 Washington Department of Social & Health Services
14 & Franklin Street
PO Box 45320
Olympia, WA 98504-5320   360-695-3416
                                  Fax: 360-737-1395

2508 Washington Department of Social and Health Services: Mental Health Division
PO Box 45320
Olympia, WA 98504-5320   360-902-8070
                                  Fax: 360-902-7691

West Virginia

2509 West Virginia Department of Health
Building 3, 1900 Capital Complex
Room 206
Charleston, WV 25305   304-558-0684
                                  Fax: 304-558-1130

Taunja Willis-Miller, Secretary

Government Agencies/By State/Wisconsin

2510 West Virginia Department of Health & Human Resources

350 Capitol Street
Room 350
Charleston, WV 25301-3702   304-558-0627
Fax: 304-558-1008

2511 West Virginia Department of Mental Health and Human Services

7012 Maccorkle Avenue SE
Charleston, WV 25304-2943   304-926-1726
Fax: 304-926-1818

2512 West Virginia Department of Welfare

1900 Washington Street E
Charleston, WV 25305-2212   304-926-1700

2513 West Virginia Governor's Commission on Crime

1401 Nottingham Road
Charleston, WV 25314-2433   304-345-5685
Fax: 304-345-5689

2514 West Virginia Office of Behavioral Health Services

Capital Complex, Building 6
Room 717
Charleston, WV 25305   304-558-3717
Fax: 304-558-1008

Wisconsin

2515 Dane County Mental Health Center

625 W Washington
Madison, WI 53703   608-280-2480
Fax: 608-280-2707
www.mhcdc.org

2516 Department of Health and Social Service: Southern Region

3601 Memorial Drive
Madison, WI 53704-1105   608-243-2400

2517 University of Wisconsin Center for Health Policy and Program Evaluation

502 N Walnut
Madison, WI 53705   608-828-9773
800-462-7416
Fax: 608-265-3255

2518 Wisconsin Bureau of Community Mental Health

1 W Wilson Street, Room 433
PO Box 7851
Madison, WI 53707-7851   608-267-7792
Fax: 608-267-7793

2519 Wisconsin Bureau of Health Care Financing

PO Box 309
Madison, WI 53701-0309   608-266-3753
Fax: 608-266-1096

2520 Wisconsin Bureau of Substance Abuse Services

1 W Wilson Street
PO Box 7851
Madison, WI 53707-7851   608-266-2717
Fax: 608-266-1533
www.dhfs.state.wi.us/substance/index.htm

2521 Wisconsin Department of Health and Family Services

PO Box 7851
Madison, WI 53707-7851   608-266-2717
Fax: 608-267-7793

2522 Wisconsin Department of Mental Health

PO Box 7851
1 W Wilson St
Madison, WI 53707-7851   608-266-3249
Fax: 608-267-7793

2523 Wisconsin Division of Community Services

PO Box 7851
Madison, WI 53707-7851   608-266-7576
Fax: 608-266-6836

Wyoming

2524 Wyoming Department of Family Services

2300 Capitol Avenue
Hathaway Bldg Fl 3
Cheyenne, WY 82001-3644   307-777-5994
Fax: 307-777-7747

2525 Wyoming Department of Health: Division of Health Care Finance

6101 Yellowstone Road
Cheyenne, WY 82009-3445   307-777-7531

2526 Wyoming Mental Health Division

Wyoming State Government
6101 Yellowstone Road
Room 259B
Cheyenne, WY 82002-0001   307-777-7094
Fax: 307-777-5580
TDD: 307-777-5581
E-mail: pherna@state.wy.us
www.mentalhealth.state.wy.us

Pablo Hernandez MD, Administrator
Marilyn J Patton MSW, Deputy Administrator

State administrative agency of the Department of Health, for mental health in Wyoming.

Video & Audio

2527 Life Passage in the Face of Death, Volume I: a Brief Psychotherapy

American Psychiatric Publishing
1000 Wilson Boulevard
Suite 1825
Arlington, VA 22209-3901   703-907-7322
                                 800-368-5777
                            Fax: 703-907-1091
                       E-mail: appi@psych.org
                                  www.appi.org

A senior psychoanalyst demonstrates the extraordinary impact of a very brief dynamic psychotherapy on a patient in a time of crisis — the terminal illness and death of a spouse. We not only meet the patient and observe the therapy, but our understanding is guided by the therapist's ongoing explanation of the process. He vividly illustrates concepts such as transference, clarification, interpretation, insight, denial, isolation and above all the relevance of understanding the past for changing the present. This unique opportunity to see a psychotherapy as it is conducted will be of immense value for all mental health clinicians and trainees. *$49.95*

Year Founded: 2002 ISBN 1-585621-01-3

2528 Life Passage in the Face of Death, Volume II : Psychological Engagement of the Physically Ill Patient

American Psychiatric Publishing
1000 Wilson Boulevard
Suite 1825
Arlington, VA 22209-3901   703-907-7322
                                 800-368-5777
                            Fax: 703-907-1091
                       E-mail: appi@psych.org
                                  www.appi.org

Ongoing explanation of therapy from a recogized expert. Valuable to clinicians and students alike. *$49.95*

Year Founded: 2002 ISBN 1-585621-02-1

2529 Rational Emotive Therapy

Research Press
Dept 24 W
PO Box 9177
Champaign, IL 61826   217-352-3273
                                 800-519-2707
                            Fax: 217-352-1221
                  E-mail: rp@researchpress.com
                             www.researchpress.com

Russell Pense, VP Marketing

This video illustrates the basic concepts of Rational Emotive Therapy (RET). It includes demonstrations of RET procedures, informative discussions and unstaged counseling sessions. Viewers will see Albert Ellis and his colleagues help clients overcome such problems as guilt, social anxiety, and jealousy. Also, Dr. Ellis shares his perspectives on the evolution of RET. *$195.00*

Accreditation & Quality Assurance

2530 American Board of Examiners in Clinical Social Work

27 Congress Street #211
Shetland Park
Salem, MA 01970
                                 800-694-5285
                            Fax: 978-740-5395
                       E-mail: abe@abecsw.org
                                  www.abecsw.org

Robert Booth, Executive Director
Michael Brooks, National Marketing Manager

Clinical Social Work certifying and standard setting organization. ABE's no cost online and CD ROM directories (both searchable/sortable) are sources used by the healthcare industry nationwide for network development and referrals. They contain verifyed information about the education, training, experience and practice specialties of over 11,00 Board Certified Diplomates in Clinical Social Work (BCD). Visit our website for the directory, employment resources, contim=nuing education and other services.

2531 American Board of Examiners of Clinical Social Work Regional Office

414 First Street E
Suite 3
Sonoma, CA 95476-2005
                                 888-279-9378
                            Fax: 707-938-3233
                  E-mail: abewest@metro.com

2532 Borgess Behavioral Medicine Services

1521 Gull Road
Kalamazoo, MI 49048   269-226-7000
                            Fax: 269-324-8665
                                  www.borgess.com

2533 CARF: The Rehabilitation Accreditation Commission

4891 E Grant Road
Tucson, AZ 85712-2704   520-325-1044
                            Fax: 520-318-1129
                            TTY: 888-281-6531
                                  www.carf.org

CARF assists organizations to improve the quality of their services, to demonstrate value, and to meet internationally recognized organizational and practice standards.

2534 Cenaps Corporation

6147 Deltona Boulevard
Spring Hill, FL 34606-3700   352-596-8000
                            Fax: 352-596-8002
                       E-mail: info@cenaps.com
                                  www.cenaps.com

Terence T Gorski, President
Tresa Watson, Office Manager

Brief therapy for relapse prevention.

2535 CompHealth Credentialing

PO Box 57910
Salt Lake City, UT 84157-0910   801-264-6466
                                   800-453-3030
                              Fax: 801-284-6811
E-mail: credentialing@comphealth.com
                         www.credentialing.net

Offers reliable temporary coverage, permanent placement, NCQA-certified credentialing, and licensing services.

2536 Consumer Satisfaction Team

1001 Sterigerie Street
Building 6
Norristown, PA 19401   610-270-3685
                         Fax: 610-270-9155
                              www.cstmont.com

2537 Council on Accreditation (COA) of Services for Families and Children

120 Wall Street
New York, NY 10005-3904   212-797-3000
                              866-262-8088
                         Fax: 212-797-1428
E-mail: coanet@aol.com
                              www.coanet.org

David S Liederman, President/CEO

The Council of Accreditation of Services for Families and Children, Inc., is an independent, not-for-profit accreditor of behavioral healthcare and social service organizations in the United States and Canada. COA's mission is to promote standards, champion quality services for children, youth and families, and advocate for the value of accreditation. COA accredits programs in more than 1,000 organizations and publishes standards for the full array of community mental health services.

2538 Council on Social Work Education

1725 Duke Street
Suite 500
Alexandria, VA 22314-3421   703-683-8080
                          Fax: 703-683-8099
E-mail: info@cswe.org
                               www.cswe.org

Donald W Beless, Executive Director
Michael Monti, Director Publications/Media

A national association that preserves and enhances the quality of social work education for the purpose of promoting the goals of individual and community well being and social justice. Pursues this mission through setting and maintaining policy and program standards, accrediting bachelors and masters degree programs in social work, promoting research and faculty development, and advocating for social work education.

2539 HSP Verified

1120 G Street NW
Suite 330
Washington, DC 20005-3801   202-783-1270
                          Fax: 202-783-1269
                              www.hspverified.com

Service which handles credentials verification for health providers.

2540 Healtheast Behavioral Care

69 Exchange Street W
Saint Paul, MN 55102-1004   651-232-3222
                          Fax: 651-232-6414

Assessment and referral for: Psychiatric, Inpatient, Chemical Dependancy.

2541 Joint Commission on Accreditation of Healthcare Organizations

1 Renaissance Boulevard
Oakbrook Terrace, IL 60181-4294   630-792-5000
                                   800-994-6610
                              Fax: 630-792-5005
E-mail: customerservice@jcaho.org
                              www.jcaho.org

The Joint Commission evaluates and accredits nearly 20,000 health care organizations and programs in the United States. An independent, not-for-profit organization, the Joint Commission is the nation's predominant standards-setting and accrediting body in health care. The Joint Commission has developed state-of-the-art, professionally-based standards and evaluated the compliance of health care organizations against these benchmarks.

2542 Lanstat Incorporated

PO Box 1388
Port Townsend, WA 98368   360-379-8628
                               800-672-3166
                          Fax: 360-379-8949
E-mail: info@lanstat.com
                              www.lanstat.com

Landon Kimbrough, President
Sherry Kimbrough, VP

Provides techinical assistance in the areas of CARF accreditation, outcomes and customer satisfaction, program evaluation, policies and procedures, clinical forms and training.

2543 Med Advantage

3452 Lake Lynda Drive
Suite 250
Orlando, FL 32817-1445   407-282-5131
                          Fax: 407-282-9240
                     www.med-advantage.com

John C Barrett, Sr VP

Fully accredited by URAC and certified in all 11 elements by NCQA, Med Advantage is one of the oldest credentials verification organizations in the country. Over the past eight years, they have developed sophisticated computer systems and one of the largest data warehouses of medical providers in the nation, containing information on over 900,000 healthcare providers. Their system is continually updated from primary source data required to meet the standards of the URAC, NCQA and JCAHO.

2544 Mertech

PO Box 787
Norwell, MA 02061   781-659-0701
                          Fax: 781-659-2049
E-mail: admin-info@mertech.org
                              www.mertech.org

2545 National Board for Certified Counselors

3 Terrace Way
Suite D
Greensboro, NC 27403-3660   336-547-0607
                                Fax: 336-547-0017
                          E-mail: nbcc@nbcc.org
                                   www.nbcc.org

Susan E Eubanks NCC, NCSC, LPC Assoc. Executive Director

National voluntary certification board for counselors. Certified counselors have met minimum criteria. Referral lists can to provided to consumers.

2546 National Register of Health Service Providers in Psychology

1120 G Street NW
Suite 330
Washington, DC 20005-3801   202-783-7663
                                Fax: 202-347-0550
                 E-mail: claire@nationalregister.org
                            www.nationalregister.org

Judy Hall PhD, Executive Director
Claire McCardell-Long, Director Administration/Finance

Nonprofit credentialing organization for psychologists; evaluates education, training, and experience of licensed psychologists. Committed to advancing psychology as a profession and improving the delivery of health services to the public.

Year Founded: 1974

2547 SAFY of America: Specialized Alternatives for Families and Youth

10100 Elida Road
Delphos, OH 45833-9056   419-695-8010
                             800-532-7239
                          Fax: 419-695-0004
                      E-mail: safy@safy.org
                               www.safy.org

Christine Pleva, Director Public Relations

2548 SUPRA Management

2424 Eden Born
Metairie, LA 70009-6588   504-837-5557
                              Fax: 504-833-3466

2549 Science Applications International Corporation

10260 Campus Point Drive
San Diego, CA 92121
                               800-430-7629
                          Fax: 858-826-6800
                               www.saic.com

2550 Skypek Group

2528 W Tennessee Avenue
Tampa, FL 33629-6255   813-254-3926
                           Fax: 813-254-3657

2551 Sweetwater Health Enterprises

3939 Belt Line Road
Suite 600
Dallas, TX 75244   972-888-5638
                       Fax: 972-620-7351
           E-mail: mktg@sweetwaterhealth.com
                   www.sweetwaterhealth.com

Cherie Holmes-Henry, VP Sales/Marketing

Associations

2552 AAMR-American Association on Mental Retardation: Religion Division

AAMR
444 N Capitol Street NW
Suite 846
Washington, DC 20001-1508   202-387-1968
                                 800-424-3688
                            Fax: 202-387-2193
                       E-mail: dcroser@aamr.com
                                   www.aamr.org

Doreen Croser, Executive Director

Books, pamphlets, videos of interest to those who support persons with mental and physical disabilities.

2553 APA-Endorsed Psychiatrists Professional Liability Insurance Program

Psychiatrists' Purchasing Group
1515 Wilson Boulevard
Suite 800
Arlington, VA 22209-2402   703-907-3800
                                800-245-3333
                           Fax: 703-276-9637
                   E-mail: theprogram@prms.com
                            www.psychprogram.com

Leslie Davenport, Member Accounts Representative

Specializes in professional liability insurance coverage for psychiatrists and mental health professionals.

2554 Academy of Psychosomatic Medicine

5824 N Magnolia Avenue
Chicago, IL 60660-3416   773-784-2025
                             Fax: 773-784-1304
                   E-mail: apsychmed@aol.com
                                   www.apm.org

Evelyne Hallberg, Executive Director

2555 Advanced Psychotherapy Association

PO Box 7827
Gulfport, MS 39506-7827   228-897-7730
                              Fax: 228-897-2121

2556 Advocate Behavioral Health Partners

485 S Frontage Road
Suite 301
Burr Ridge, IL 60521-7110
                               800-863-0083
                          Fax: 630-655-2836

2557 Agency for Health Care Policy & Research Center for Health Information

2101 E Jefferson Street
Rockville, MD 20852-4908   301-594-6662
                                 Fax: 301-594-2168
                                 www.ahcpr.gov

2558 Alliance for Children and Families

11700 W Lake Park Drive
Milwaukee, WI 53224-3099   414-359-1040
                                 Fax: 414-359-1074
                      E-mail: policy@alliance1.org
                                 www.alliance1.org

Carmen Delgado Votaw, Sr VP
Peter Goldberg, President/CEO
Thomas Harney, VP Membership

International membership association representing more than three hundred fifty private, nonprofit child and family-serving organziations. Their mission is to strengthen members' capacity to serve and advocate for children, families and communities.

2559 American Academy of Child & Adolescent Psychiatry

3615 Wisconsin Avenue NW
Washington, DC 20016-3007   202-966-7300
                                 Fax: 202-966-2891
                                 www.aacap.org

Provides information on childhood psychiatric disorders.

2560 American Academy of Clinical Psychiatrists

PO Box 458
Glastonbury, CT 06033   860-633-5045
                                 Fax: 860-633-6023
                       E-mail: info@aacp.com
                                 www.aacp.com

Alicia A Munoz, Executive Director

Practicing board-eligible or board-certified psychiatrists. Promotes the scientific practice of psychiatric medicine. Conducts educational and teaching research. Publications: Annals of Clinical Psychiatry, quarterly journal. Clinical Psychiatry Quarterly, newsletter. Annual conference and exhibits in fall.

2561 American Academy of Medical Administrators

701 Lee Street
Suite 600
Des Moines, IL 60016-4516   847-759-8601
                                 Fax: 847-759-8602
                      E-mail: info@aameda.org
                                 www.aameda.org

2562 American Academy of Psychiatry and the Law (AAPL)

One Regency Drive
PO Box 30
Bloomfield, CT 06002-0030   860-242-5450
                                 800-331-1389
                                 Fax: 860-286-0787
                       E-mail: office@aapl.org
                                 www.aapl.org

Jacquelyn T Coleman, Executive Director

Seeks to exchange ideas and experience in areas where psychiatry and the law overlap and develop standards of practice in the relationship of psychiatry to the law and encourage the development of training programs for psychiatrists in this area. Publications: Journal of the American Academy of Psychiatry and the Law, quarterly. Scholarly articles on forensic psychiatry. Newsletter of the American Academy of Psychiatry and Law, 3 year. Membership Directory, annual.

2563 American Academy of Psychoanalysis and Dynam ic Psychiatry

One Regency Drive
PO Box 30
Bloomfield, CT 06002   888-691-8281
                                 Fax: 860-286-0787
                       E-mail: info@aapsa.org
                                 www.aapsa.org

Jacquelyn T Coleman CAE, Executive Director

Founded in 1956 to provide an open forum for psychoanalysts to discuss relevant and responsible views of human behavior and to exchange ideas with colleagues and other social behavioral scientists. Aims to develop better communication amoung psychoanalysts and psychodynamic psychiatrists in other disiplines in science and the humanities. Meetings of the Academy provide a forum for inquiry into the phenomena of individual and interpersonal behavior. Advocates an acceptance of all relevant and responsible psychoanalytic views of human behavior, rather than adherence to one particular doctrine.

2564 American Association for Behavioral Healthcare

1101 Pennsylvania Avenue NW
Sixth Floor
Washington, DC 20004   202-756-7308
                                 Fax: 202-756-7308
                                 www.ambha.org

2565 American Association for Marriage and Family Therapy

112 S Alfred Street
Alexandria, VA 22314   703-838-9808
                                 Fax: 703-838-9805
                       E-mail: exec@aamft.org
                                 www.aamft.org

2566 American Association for World Health

1825 K Street NW
Suite 1208
Washington, DC 20006   202-466-5883
                                 Fax: 202-466-5896
                                 www.thebody.com

Private national organization in the US dedicated to funneling a broad spectrum of critical national and international health information to Americans at the grassroots level by developing and distributing practical, easy-to-use health education and promotional materials to those community leaders who can most effectively reach our US citizens at the local level.

2567 American Association of Community Psychiatrists (AACP)

PO Box 570218
Dallas, TX 75357   972-613-0985
Fax: 972-613-5532
www.communitypsychiatry.org

Jacqueline Feldman MD, President
Francis Roton

Psychiatrists and psychiatry residents practicing in community mental health centers or similar programs that provide care to the mentally ill regardless of their ability to pay. Addresses issues faced by psychiatrists who practice within CMHCs. Publications: AACP Membership Directory, annual. Community Psychiatrist, quarterly newsletter. Annual meeting, in conjunction with American Psychiatric Association in May. Annual meeting, in conjunction with Institute on Hospital and Community in fall.

2568 American Association of Chairs of Department s of Psychiatry

UCHC-263 Farmington Avenue LG 066
Farmington, CT 06030-1935   860-679-8113
Fax: 860-679-1246
E-mail: aacdp@psychiatry.uchc.edu
www.aacdp.org

Allan Tasman MD, President

Chairmen of departments of psychiatry in colleges of medicine. Promote medical education, research and patient care; growth and continuing development of psychiatry; forum for discussion and exchange of ideas among the chairmen of departments of psychiatry in medical schools; liaison between chairmen, individuals and organizations whose activities are objectives of the association. Publications: Membership list. Semi-annual meeting.

2569 American Association of Children's Residential Centers

2020 Pennsylvania Avenue NW
Suite 745
Washington, DC 20006   877-332-2272
Fax: 877-362-2272
E-mail: info@aacrc-dc.org
www.aacrc-dc.org

Tammy J Eisenhart, Office Coordinator

Funded by the Mental Health Community Support Program. The purpose of the association is to share information about services, providers and ways to cope with mental illnesses. Available services include referrals, professional seminars, support groups and a variety of publications.

2570 American Association of Community Psychiatrists

492 Wayland Avenue
Providence, RI 02906-4654   401-284-2500

2571 American Association of Community Psychiatri sts

PO Box 570218
Dallas, TX 75228-0218   972-613-0985
Fax: 972-613-5532
E-mail: frdal@airmail.net
www.comm.psych.pitt.edu

Jacqueline M Feldman MD, President

2572 American Association of Directors of Psychiatric Residency Training

263 Farmington Avenue
Farmington, CT 06030-1935   860-679-8112
Fax: 860-679-1246
E-mail: aadprt@psychiatry.uchc.edu
www.aadprt.org

Publications: Academic Psychiatry, quarterly. Newsletter, quarterly. Annual Midwinter Conference in January.

2573 American Association of Geriatric Psychiatry (AAGP)

7910 Woodmont Avenue
Suite 1050
Bethesda, MD 20814-3002   301-654-7850
Fax: 301-654-4137
E-mail: main@aagponline.org
www.aagpgpa.org

Janet L Pailet JD, Executive Director

Members are psychiatrists interested in promoting better mental health care for the elderly. Maintains placement service and speakers' bureau. Publications: AAGP Membership Directory, annual. Geriatric Psychiatry News, bimonthly newsletter. Growing Older and Wiser, covers consumer and general public information. Annual meeting and exhibits in February or March.

2574 American Association of Health Plans

601 Pennsylvania Avenue NW
South Building, Suite 500
Washington, DC 20004   202-778-3206
Fax: 202-778-8486
www.aahp.org

The American Association of Health Plans (AAHP) is the nation's principal association of health plans, representing more than 1,000 plans that provide coverage for approximately 170 million Americans nationwide.

2575 American Association of Healthcare Consultants

5 Revere Drive
Suite 200
Northbrook, IL 60062
888-350-2242
Fax: 847-350-2241
E-mail: info@aahc.net
www.aahc.net

Serve as the preeminent credentialing, professional, and practice development organization for the healthcare consulting profession; to advance the knowledge, quality, and standards of practice for consulting to management in the healthcare industry; and to enhance the understanding and image of the healthcare consulting profession and Member Firms among its various publics.

2576 American Association of Homes and Services for the Aging

2519 Connecticut Avenue NW
Washington, DC 20008-1520
202-783-2242
800-675-9253
Fax: 202-783-2255
E-mail: info@aahsa.org
www.aahsa.org

An association committed to advancing the vision of healty, affordable, ethical long term care for America. The association represents 5,600 million driven, not-for-profit nursing homes, continuing care facilities and community care retirement facilities and community service organizations.

2577 American Association of Mental Health Professionals in Corrections (AAMHPC)

PO Box 160208
Sacramento, CA 95816-0208

John S Zil MD, JD, President

Mental health professionals working in correctional settings. Goals include improving the treatment, rehabilitation and care of the mentally ill, retarded and emotionally disturbed. Promotes research and professional education and conducts scientific meetings to advance the therapeutic community in all institutional settings including hospitals, churches, schools, industry and the family. Publications: Corrective and Social Psychiatry, quarterly. Annual conference and symposium and workshops.

2578 American Association of Pastoral Counselors

9504A Lee Highway
Fairfax, VA 22031-2303
703-385-6967
Fax: 703-352-7725
E-mail: info@aapc.org
www.aapo.org

Douglas M Ronsheim, Director Ministry

Organized in 1963 to promote and support the ministry of pastoral counseling within religious communities and the field of mental health in the United States and Canada.

2579 American Association of Pharmaceutical Scientists

2107 Wilson Boulevard
Suite 700
Arlington, VA 22201-3042
703-243-2800
Fax: 703-243-9650
E-mail: aaps@aaps.org
www.aapspharmaceutica.com

Scott Didawick, Marketing

The American Association of Pharmaceutical Scientists will be the premier organization of all scientists dedicated to the discovery, development and manufacture of pharmaceutical products and therapies through advances in science and technology.

2580 American Association of Retired Persons

601 E Street NW
A-5-146
Washington, DC 20049-0002
202-434-2263

2581 American Association of University Affiliate Programs for Persons With Developmental Disabilities

8630 Fenton Street
Suite 410
Silver Spring, MD 20910-3803
301-588-8252
Fax: 301-588-2842
E-mail: gjesien@aauap.org
www.aauap.org

George Jesien PhD, Executive Director

University based or affiliated clinical service and interdisciplinary training centers for graduate students and others interested in the field of mental retardation and other developmental disabilities. Provides coordination of federal funding for programs, technical assistance to Congress and information exchange among members, educational activites about programs. Publications: Resource Directory, annual.

2582 American Board of Examiners in Clinical Social Work

27 Congress Street #21
Shetland Park
Salem, MA 01970
978-825-9311
800-694-5285
Fax: 978-740-5395
E-mail: abe@abecsw.org
www.abecsw.org

Robert Booth, Executive Director

Clinical social work certification and standards setting organization.

2583 American Board of Professional Psychology (ABPP)

300 Drayton Street
3rd Floor
Savannah, GA 31401
800-255-7792
Fax: 912-644-5655
E-mail: office@abpp.org
www.abpp.org

Russell Bent MD, Executive Director

ABPP serves the public need by providing oversight certifying psychologists competent to deliver high quality services in various specialty areas of psychology.

2584 American Board of Psychiatry and Neurology (ABPN)

500 Lake Cook Road
Suite 335
Deerfield, IL 60015-5249
847-945-7900
Fax: 847-945-1146
www.abpn.com

Stephen C Scheiber MD, Executive Vice President

ABPN is a nonprofit organization that promotes excellence in the practice of psychiatry and neurology through lifelong certification including compentency testing processes.

2585 American College Health Association

PO Box 2837
Baltimore, MD 21240-8937   410-859-1500
Fax: 410-859-1510
E-mail: sfisher@acha.org
www.acha.org

Doyle Randol, Executive Director
Susan L Ainsworth, Member Progams/Services
Sharon Fisher, Communications

Advocate and leadership organization for college and
university health. Provides advocacy, education,
communications, products and services as well as promotes research and culturally competent practices to
enhance its members' ability to advance the health of
all students and the campus community.

2586 American College of Health Care Administrators: ACHCA

300 N Lee Street
Suite 301
Alexandria, VA 22314   703-739-7900
888-882-2422
Fax: 703-739-7901
E-mail: membership@achca.org
www.achca.org

Aileen Holland, Membership
Amber Rashid, Communications

Nonprofit membership organization which provides
educational programming, certification in a variety of
positions and career development. Promotes excellence in leadership among long-term health care administrators.

Year Founded: 1962

2587 American College of Healthcare Executives

One N Franklin Street
Suite 1700
Chicago, IL 60606-4425   312-424-2800
Fax: 312-424-0023
E-mail: ache@ache.org
www.ache.org

Thomas C Dolan PhD, President/CEO
Deborah J Bowen, Executive VP/COO
Peter Weil PhD, Research/Development

International professional society of nearly 30,000
healthcare executives. ACHE is known for its prestigious credentialing and educational programs. ACHE
is also known for its journal, Journal of Healthcare
Management, and magazine, Healthcare Executive, as
well as groundbreaking research and career development programs. Through its efforts, ACHE works toward its goal of improving the health status of society
by advancing healthcare management excellence.

2588 American College of Mental Health Administration: ACMHA

912 Galveston Avenue
Pittsburgh, PA 15233   412-820-0670
Fax: 412-820-0669
E-mail: Executive.Director@acmha.org
www.acmha.org

Carolyn Maue, Executive Director

Advancing the field of mental health and substance
abuse administration and to promote the continuing
education of clinical professionals in the areas of administration and policy. Publication: ACMHA Newsletter, quarterly. Annual Santa Fe Summit,
conference.

Year Founded: 1979

2589 American College of Osteopathic Neurologists & Psychiatrists

28595 Orchard Lake Road
Suite 200
Farmington Hills, MI 48334   810-553-0010
Fax: 810-553-0818
E-mail: acn-aconp@msn.com

Timothy Kowalski DO, President
Louis E Rentz DO, Executive Director

Mission is to promote the art and science of osteopathic medicine in the fields of neurology and psychiatry; to maintain and further elevate the highest
standards of proficiency and training among osteopathic neurologists and psychiatrists; to stimulate
original research and investigation in neurology and
psychiatry; and to collect and disseminate the results
of such work for the benefit of the members of the college, the public, the profession at large, and the ultimate benefit of all humanity.

2590 American College of Psychiatrists

732 Addison Street
Suite C
Berkeley, CA 94710   510-704-8020
Fax: 510-704-0113
E-mail: Barbara@acpsych.org
www.acpsych.org

James H Shore, President
Alice Conde, Executive Director

Nonprofit honorary association of psychiatrists who,
through excellence in their chosen fields, have been
recognized for thier significant contributions to the
profession. The society's goal is to promote and support the highest standards in psychiatry through education, research and clinical practice.

2591 American College of Psychoanalysts: ACPA

434 Fox Run Lane
Hampshire, IL 60140   847-683-7517
Fax: 847-683-7517
www.acopsa.org

Dr. Fred Levin, President
Deborah Quick, Executive Secretary

Honorary, scientific and professional organization
for physician psycholanalysts. Goal is to contribute to
the leadership and support high standards in the practice of psychoanalysis, and understanding the relationship between mind and brain.

2592 American Counseling Association

5999 Stevenson Avenue
Alexandria, VA 22304-3302   703-823-9800
                                 800-347-6647
                            Fax: 703-823-0252
                            TDD: 703-823-6862
               E-mail: aca@counseling.org
                       www.counseling.org

Richard Yep, Executive Director
Janice MacDonald, Professional Services

ACA serves professional counselors in the US and
abroad. Provides a variety of programs and services
that support the personal, professional and program
development goals of its members. ACA works to provide quality services to the variety of clients who use
their services in college, community agencies, in mental health, rehabilitation and related settings. Offers a
large catalog of books, manuals and programs for the
professional counselor.

2593 American Foundation for Psychoanalysis and Psychoanalysis in Groups: AFPPG

4625 Douglas Avenue
c/o Louis E Derosis MD
Bronx, NY 10471   718-796-0308
                            Fax: 718-796-0308

Louis E DeRosis MD, Executive Officer

Raises funds to foster research and education in the
field of psychoanalytic medicine. Holds symposia,
provides lecture service, produces educational motion
pictures on therapy, offers patient placement service
and referral service for psychoanalytic therapy. Quarterly conferences, January, April, October and December.

2594 American Geriatrics Society

350 5th Avenue, Suite 801
Empire State Building
New York, NY 10118   212-308-1414
                            Fax: 212-832-8646
          E-mail: info@americangeriatrics.org
                  www.americangeriatrics.org

Linda Hiddemen Barondess, Executive VP
Kate Eisenburg, Membership
Janis Eisner, Projects

Nationwide, nonprofit association of geriatric health
care professionals, research scientists and other concerned individuals dedicated to improving the health,
independence and quality of life for all older people.
Pivotal force in shaping attitudes, policies and practices regarding health care for older people.

2595 American Group Psychotherapy Association

25 E 21st Street
Floor 6
New York, NY 10010-6207   212-477-2677
                                 877-668-2472
                            Fax: 212-979-6627
               E-mail: info@agpa.org
                       www.agpa.org

Marsha S Block, CEO
Angela Stephens, Professional Development

Interdisciplinary community that has been enhancing
practice, theory and research of group therapy for over
50 years. Provides support to enhance your work as a
mental health care professional, or your life as a member of a therapeutic group.

Year Founded: 1942

2596 American Health Care Association

1201 L Street NW
Washington, DC 20005-4024   202-842-4444
                            Fax: 202-842-3860
               E-mail: astarkey@ahca.org
                       www.ahca.org

Alexis Starkey, Events

Nonprofit federation of affiliated state health organizations, together representing nearly 12,000 nonprofit and for profit assisted living, nursing facility,
developmentally disabled and subacute care providers that care for more than 1.5 million elderly and disabled individuals nationally. AHCA represents the
long term care community at large — to government,
business leaders and the general public. It also serves
as a force for change within the long term care field,
providing information, education, and administrative
tools that enhance quality at every level.

2597 American Health Information Management Association

233 N Michigan Avenue
Suite 2150
Chicago, IL 60601-5088   312-233-1100
                            Fax: 312-233-1090
               E-mail: info@ahima.org
                       www.ahima.org

Marilyn Render, State Association Assistance
Jean Schlichting, Legislative/Public Policy

Dynamic professional association that represents
more than 46,000 specially educated health information management professionals who work throughout
the healthcare industry. Health information management professionals serve the health care industry and
the public by manageing, analyzing and utilizing data
vital for patient care and making it accessible to
healthcare providers when it is needed most.

2598 American Hospital Association: Section for Psychiatric and Substance Abuse

1 N Franklin
Chicago, IL 60606   312-422-3000
                            Fax: 312-422-4796
                       www.aha.org

Barry Johnson, Director

AHA represents and serves all types of hospitals,
health care networks and their patients and communities. Provides education for health care leaders and is
a source of information on health care issues and
trends. The AHA Section for Psychiatric and Substance Abuse Services (SPSAS) provides perspective
on behavioral health issues.

2599 American Humane Association: Children's Services

63 Inverness Drive E
Englewood, CO 80112-5117   303-792-9900
Fax: 303-792-5333
www.americanhumane.org

Charmaine Brittain PhD, Project Director
Myles Edwards PhD, Research Director

Leader in developing programs, policies and services to prevent the abuse and neglect of children, while strengthening families ans communities and enhancing social service systems.

2600 American Managed Behavioral Healthcare Association

1101 Pennsylvania Avenue NW
6th Floor
Washington, DC 20004
Fax: 202-756-7308
www.ambha.org

2601 American Medical Association

515 N State Street
Chicago, IL 60610-4325   312-464-5289
800-621-8335
Fax: 312-464-4184
www.ama-assn.org

Paul Misano MD, President
Janice Shimokubo, Membership

Speaks out in issues important to patients and the nation's health. AMA policy on such issues is decided through its democratic policy making process, in the AMA House of Delegates, which meets twice a year. The House is comprised of physician delegates representing every state; nearly 100 national medical specialty societies, federal service agents, including the Surgeon General of the US; and 6 sections representing hospital and clinic staffs, resident physicians, medical students, young physicians, medical schools and international medical graduates. The AMA's envisioned future is to be a part of the professional life of every physician and an essential force for progress in improving the nation's health.

2602 American Medical Directors Association

1480 Little Patuxent Parkway
Suite 760
Columbia, MD 21044   410-740-9743
800-876-2632
Fax: 410-740-4572
E-mail: info@amda.com
www.amda.com

Lorraine Tarnove, Executive Director
Megan S Brey, Meetings
Cindy N Hock RN, Membership

Professional association of medical directors and physicians practicing in the long-term care continuum, dedicated to excellence in patient care by providing education, advocacy and professional development.

2603 American Medical Group Association

1422 Duke Street
Alexandria, VA 22314-3430   703-838-0033
Fax: 703-548-1890
E-mail: roconnor@amga.org
www.amga.org

Donald W Fisher PhD, President/CEO
Andrea Bartolomeo, Education
Ryan O'Connor, VP Membership

Advocates for the multispecialty group practice model of health care delivery and for the patients served by medical groups, through innovation and information sharing, benchmarking and continuous striving to improve patient care.

2604 American Medical Informatics Association

4915 St. Elmo Avenue
Suite 401
Bethesda, MD 20814   301-657-1291
Fax: 301-657-1296
E-mail: mail@mail.amia.org
www.amia.com

Dennis Reynolds, Executive Director
Ina King, Manager

Nonprofit membership organization of individuals, institutions and corporations dedicated to developing and using information technologies to improve health care. Our members include physicians, nurses, computer and information scientists, biomedical engineers, medical librarians, academic researchers and educators. Holds an annual syposium, 2 congresses, prints a journal and maintains a resource center.

Year Founded: 1990

2605 American Mental Health Counselors Association: AMHCA

801 N Fairfax
Suite 304
Alexandria, VA 22314   703-548-6002
800-326-2642
Fax: 703-548-4775
E-mail: vmoore@amhca.org
www.amhca.org

Gail Adams, President
Virginia Moore, Office Director

Professional counselors employed in mental health services and students. Aims to deliver quality mental health services to children, youth, adults, families and organizations and to improve the availability and quality of services through licensure and certification, training standards and consumer advocacy. Publishes an Advocate Newsletter, Journal of Mental Health Counseling, quarterly, Mental Health Brights, brochures. Annual National Conference.

2606 American Neuropsychiatric Association

4510 W 87th Street
Suite 110
Shawnee Mission, KS 66207-1945   614-447-2077
Fax: 614-263-4366
E-mail: anpa@osu.edu
www.neuropsychiatry.com/ANPA/

Richard Restak MD, President

Our mission is to apply neuroscience for the benefit of people. Three core values have been identified for the association: advancing knowledge of brain-behavior relationships, providing a forum for learning, and promoting excellent, scientific and compassionate health care. Our vision is to be the professional organization of choice for the clinical neurosciences. We publish a journal, hold an annual scientific meeting, and hold joint meetings with international neuropsychiatric associations.

2607 American Nouthetic Psychology Association: A NPA

PO Box 801
Hardwick, GA 31034   478-452-6907
E-mail: biblepsy@alltel.net
www.home.alltel.net/biblepsy/

Dr. David Carnrike, President

Psychologists and other individuals with an interest in nouthetic psychology. Promotes high standards of training, ethics, and practice in the field. Conducts research and educational programs. The Christian psychologist or counselor, by definition, is committed to the Old and New Testaments as the only authoritative rule of faith and practice.

2608 American Nurses Association

600 Maryland Avenue SW
Suite 100W
Washington, DC 20024-2571   202-651-7000
                                    800-274-4262
                              Fax: 202-651-7001
                    E-mail: memberinfo@ana.org
                             www.nursingworld.org

Linda Stierle, CEO
Susan Rimland, Membership Services

Association for psychiatric nurses. Considers nursing's adgenda for the future and workplace advocacy. Offers recertification information, an online journal, state meetings, and an annual convention.

2609 American Pharmacists Association

2215 Constitution Avenue NW
Washington, DC 20037-2985   202-628-4410
                              Fax: 202-783-2351
                  E-mail: membership@aphanet.org
                                www.aphanet.org

James C Appleby, Profesional Education/Relations
Regina C Bethea, Membership Development
Robert Fulcher, Membership/Marketing

National professional society of pharmacists, formerly the American Pharmaceutical Association. Our members include practicing pharmacists, pharmaceutical students, pharmacy scientists, pharmacy technicians, and others interested in advancing the profession. Provides professional information and education for pharmacists and advocates for improved health of the American public through the provision of comprehensive pharmaceutical care.

Year Founded: 1852

2610 American Psychiatric Association: APA

1000 Wilson Boulevard
Suite 1825
Arlington, VA 22209-3901   703-907-7300
                             Fax: 703-907-1095
                    E-mail: apa@psych.org
                             www.psych.org

James Scully MD, President
Susan Cooper, Membership

Members are psychiatrists who seek to further the study of the nature, treatment and prevention of mental disorders. Assists in formulating programs to meet mental health needs. Compiles and disseminates facts and figures about psychiatry and furthers psychiatric eduation and research. Publications: American Journal of Psychiatry, monthly. Psychiatric News, semi-monthly. Psychiatric Services, monthly journal. Membership Directory, biannually. Books and pamphlets. Annual meeting and exhibits in May.

2611 American Psychiatric Nurses Association

1555 Wilson Boulevard
Suite 515
Arlington, VA 22209   703-243-2443
                        Fax: 703-243-3390
               E-mail: hantosiak@apna.org
                        www.apna.org

Jane White, Executive Director
Holly Antosiak, Membership

Provides leadership to promote the psychiatric-mental health nursing profession, improve mental health care for culturally diverse individuals, families, groups and communities and shape health policy for the delivery of mental health services.

2612 American Psychiatric Publishing

1000 Wilson Boulevard
Arlington, VA 22209-3901   703-907-7322
                                   800-368-5777
                             Fax: 703-907-1091
                    E-mail: appi@psych.org
                             www.appi.org

2613 American Psychoanalytic Association (APsaA)

309 E 49th Street
New York, NY 10017-1601   212-752-0450
                            Fax: 212-593-0571
              E-mail: central.office@apsa.com
                           www.apsa.org

Ellen B Fertig, Administrative Director

Professional Membership Organization with approximately 3,500 members nationwide, with 43 Affiliate Societies and 29 Training Institutes. Seeks to establish and maintain standards for the training of psychoanalysts and for the practice of psychoanalysis, fosters the integration of psychoanalysis with other disciplines (psychiatry, psychology, social work), and encourages research. Publications include: Journal of the Psychoanalyst (JAPA), American Psychoanalyst, a quarterly newsletter; Ethics Case Book; and Roster. Twice a year the organization sponsors scientific meetings and exhibits.

2614 American Psychologial Association: Division of Family Psychology

750 1st Street NE
Washington, DC 20002-4241   202-336-6013
                               Fax: 202-218-3599

Roberta Nutt PhD, President

A division of the American Psychological Association. Psychologists intersted in research, teaching, evaluation, and public interest initiatives in family psychology. Seeks to promote human welfare through the development, dissemination, and application of knowledge about the dynamics, structure, and functioning of the family. Conducts research and specialized education programs.

2615 American Psychological Association

750 1st Street NE
Washington, DC 20002-4241   202-336-5500
                               800-374-2721
                               Fax: 202-336-5797
                               www.apa.org

Raymond D Fowler PhD, CEO

Scientific and professional society of psychologists. Students participate as affiliates. Works to advance psychology as a science, as a profession, and as means of promoting human welfare. Annual convention.

2616 American Psychological Association Division of Independent Practice (APADIP)

919 W Marshall Avenue
Phoenix, AZ 85013-1814   602-246-6768
                               Fax: 602-246-6577

Jeannie Beeaff, Administrator

Members of the American Psychological Association engaged in independent practice. Works to ensure that the needs and concerns of independent psychology practitioners are considered by the APA. Gathers and disseminates information on legislation affecting the practice of psychology, managed care, and other developments in the health care industries, office management, malpractice risk and insurance, hospital management. Offers continuing professional and educational programs. Semiannual convention, with board meeting.

2617 American Psychological Association: Applied Experimental and Engineering Psychology

Pacific Science & Engineering
6210 Greenwich Drive
200
San Diego, CA 92122-5913   619-535-1661
                               Fax: 619-535-1665

Wendy A Rogers PhD, President

A division of the American Psychological Association. Individuals whose principal fields of study, research, or work are within the area of applied experimental and engineering psychology. Promotes research on psychological factors in the design and use of environments and systems within which human beings work and live.

2618 American Psychological Society (APS)

1010 Vermont Avenue NW
Suite 110
Washington, DC 20005-4907   202-783-2077
                               Fax: 202-783-2083
                 E-mail: aps@aps.washington.dc.us
                         www.psychologicalscience.org

Alan G Kraut, Contact

Scientists and academics working for the development of the dicipline of psychology and the promotion of human welfare through research and application. Educates policy makers on the role human behavior plays in societal problems. Mailing lists, on-line services, annual convention. Publishes 2 journals, a newsletter, and a book called Lessons Learned: practical advice for teaching psychology.

2619 American Psychology- Law Society (AP-LS)

Medical Colleg of Pennsylvania
Department of Psychology
Broad and Vine Streets
Philadelphia, PA 19102   215-842-6533

Kirk Helibrun

A division of the American Psychological Association. Promotes exchanges between the diciplines of psychology and law in regard to teaching, research, administration of justice, jurisprudence, and other matters at the psychology-law interface; to foster research relevant to legal problems using psychological knowledge and methods; to advance psychological research using the legal setting and related legal research techniques; to promote education of lawyers at all levels regarding psychology, and of psychologists at all levels regarding the law; to encourage legislation and social policies consistent with current states of psychological knowledge; to promote the effective use of psychologists in legal processes.

2620 American Psychosomatic Society

6728 Old McLean Village Drive
McLean, VA 22101-3906   703-556-9222
                               Fax: 703-556-8729
                 E-mail: info@psychosomatic.org
                         www.psychosomatic.org

George Degnon, Executive Director
Laura Degnon, Associate Director

Promotes and advances the scientific understanding of the interrelationships among biological, psychological, social and behavioral factors in human health and disease, and the integration of the fields of science that separately examine each. Publishes a journal, and holds workshops and an annual meeting.

Year Founded: 1942

2621 American Psychosomatic Society Annual Meetin g

6728 Old McLean Village Drive
McLean, VA 22101-3906   703-556-9222
                               Fax: 703-556-8729
                 E-mail: info@psychosomatic.org
                         www.psychosomatic.org

George Degnon, Executive Director
Laura Degnon, Associate Director

Held in a different location each year, workshops, feature presentations and chances to network are key. Promotes and advances the scientific understanding of the interrelationships among biological, psychological, social and behavioral factors in human health and disease, and the integration of the fields of science that separately examine each.

2622 American Society for Adolescent Psychiatry: ASAP

PO Box 570218
Dallas, TX 75357-0218   972-686-6166
                        Fax: 972-613-5532
                  E-mail: info@adolpsych.org
                        www.adolpsych.org

Robert Weinstock MD, President
Stephen Billick MD, VP
Frances Roton, Executive Director

Psychiatrists concerned with the behavior of adolescents. Provides for the exchange of psychiatric knowledge, encourages the development of adequate standards and training facilities and stimulates research in the psychopathology and treatment of adolescents. Publications: Adolescent Psychiatry, annual journal. American Society for Adolescent Psychiatry Newsletter, quarterly. ASAP Membership Directory, biennial. Journal of Youth and Adolescence, bimonthly. Annual conference. Workshops.

Year Founded: 1967

2623 American Society for Clinical Pharmacology & Therapeutics

528 N Washington Street
Alexandria, VA 22314   703-836-6981
                        Fax: 703-836-5223
                    E-mail: info@ascpt.org
                          www.ascpt.org

Sharon J Swan, Executive Director
Kathleen Holmay, Communications

Over 1,900 professionals whose primary interest is to promote and advance the science of human pharmacology and theraputics. Most of the members are physicians or other doctoral scientists. Other members are pharmacists, nurses, research coordinators, fellows in training and other professionals.

Year Founded: 1900

2624 American Society of Consultant Pharmacists

1321 Duke Street
Alexandria, VA 22314   703-739-1300
                               800-355-2727
                        Fax: 703-739-1321
                    E-mail: info@ascp.com
                          www.ascp.com

John Feather, Executive Director
Phylliss M Moret, Associate Executive Director
Robert Appel, Communications

International professional association that provides leadership, education, advocacy and resources to advance the practice of senior care pharmacy. Consultant pharmacists specializing in senior care pharmacy practice are essential participants in the health care system, ensuring that their patients medications are the most appropriate, effective, the safest possible and are used correctly. We identify, resolve and prevent medication related problems that may interfere with the goals of therapy.

2625 American Society of Group Psychotherapy & Psychodrama

301 N Harrison Street
Suite 508
Princeton, NJ 08540   609-452-1339
                        Fax: 609-936-1659
                   E-mail: asgpp@asgpp.org
                          www.asgpp.org

Renee Marineau PhD, President
Eduardo Garcia, Executive Director

Fosters national and international cooperation among all concerned with the theory and practice of psychodrama, sociometry, and group psychotherapy. Promotes research and fruitful application and publication the findings. Maintains a code of professional standards.

Year Founded: 1942

2626 American Society of Health System Pharmacist s

7272 Wisconsin Avenue
Bethesda, MD 20814   301-657-3000
                        Fax: 301-657-1251
                  E-mail: Custserv@ashp.org
                          www.ashp.org

Henri R Manasse Jr. PhD, Executive VP/CEO
Ray Auen, Client Services

Thirty thousand member national professional association that represents pharmacists who practice in hospitals, health maintenance organizations, long-term care facilities, ambulatory care, home care and other components of health care systems. ASHP helps people make the best use of their medications, advances and supports the professional practice of pharmacists in hospitals and health systems and serves as their collective voice on issues related to medication use and public health.

2627 American Society of Psychoanalytic Physicians: ASPP

13528 Wisteria Drive
Germantown, MD 20853   301-540-3197
                        Fax: 301-540-3511
                  E-mail: cfcotter@yahoo.com
                          www.aspp.net

Martin Funk MD, President
Christine Cotter, Executive Secretary

Physicians, psychiatrists and psychoanalysts united to foster a wider understanding and utilization of psychoanalytic concepts, provide an opportunity to study psychoanalytic theory from all schools of thought, encourage clinical and didactic research, promote social and professional fraternalism among members in the field and maintain good relationships with other professional groups. Publications: The Bulletin, semiannual. Annual conference in May.

Year Founded: 1985

2628 American Society of Psychopathology of Expression (ASPE)

74 Lawton Street
Brookline, MA 02446-2501   **617-738-9821**

Dr. Irene Jakab, President

Psychiatrists, psychologists, art therapists, sociologists, art critics, artists, social workers, linguists, educators, criminologists, writers, and histotians. At least two-thirds of the members are physicians. Fosters collaboration among specialists in the United States who are interested in problems of expression and in artistic activities connected with psychiatric, sociological, and pathological research. Disseminates information about research and clinical applications in the field of psychopathology of expression. Sponsors consultations, seminars, and lectures on art therapy.

2629 American Society on Aging

833 Market Street
Suite 511
San Francisco, CA 94103   **415-974-9600**
                                      800-537-9728
                          Fax: 415-974-0300
                   E-mail: info@asaging.org
                          www.asaging.org

Gloria Cavanaugh, President
Jim Emerman, CEO
Susan Markey, VP Membership

Nonprofit organization committed to enhancing the knowledge and skills of those working with older adults and their families. We produce educational programs, publications, conferences and workshops.

2630 Annie E Casey Foundation

701 St. Paul Street
Baltimore, MD 21202   **410-547-6600**
                          Fax: 410-547-6624
                          www.aecf.org

Doug Nelson, President

Working to build better futures for disadvantaged children and their families in the US. The primary mission of the Foundation is to foster policies, human service reforms and community supports that more effectively meet the needs of today's vulnerable children and families. Supports the Making Connections Network, 22 site teams as well as the residents, community leaders, businesses government officials, schools, faith communities, community organizations and others working to revitalize neighborhoods. Together we can connect families to appropriate services, support and opportunity.

Year Founded: 1948

2631 Association for Academic Psychiatry: AAP

725 Concord Avenue
Suite 4200
Cambridge, MA 02138   **617-661-3544**
                          Fax: 617-661-4800
          E-mail: cberney@caregroup.harvard.edu
                   www.academicpsychiatry.org

Carole Berney MA, Administrative Director

Organization for psychiatrists who teach medical students, residents and other physicians.

2632 Association for Advancement of Behavioral Therapy

305 Seventh Avenue
16th Floor
New York, NY 10001-6008   **212-647-1890**
                          Fax: 212-647-1865
                   E-mail: mebrown@aabt.org
                          www.aabt.org

Mary Jane Eimer, Executive Director
Mary Ellen Brown, Administration/Convention
Rosemary Park, Membership Services

Professional, interdisciplinary organization that is concerned with the application of behavioral and cognitive sciences to understanding human behavior, developing interventions to enhance the human condition and promoting the appropriate utilization of these interventions.

2633 Association for Advancement of Psychoanalysi s: Karen Horney Psychoanalytic Institute and Center: AAP

329 E 62nd Street
New York, NY 10021-7755   **212-838-8044**
                          Fax: 212-888-1610

Zoltan Morvay PsyD, President

Certified psychoanalysis disseminating psychoanalytic principles to the medical-psychiatric profession and the general community. Conducts scientific meetings. Maintains a consultation and referral service, placement service and speakers' bureau. Supports research programs, sponsors public educational lectures. Publications: The American Journal of Psychoanalysis, quarterly. Newsletter, semiannual. Annual Karen Horney Lecture in New York City.

2634 Association for Ambulatory Behavioral Healthcare

11240 Waples Mill Road
Suite 200
Fairfax, VA 22030   **703-934-0160**
                          Fax: 703-359-7562
                   E-mail: info@aabh.org
                          www.aabh.org

Karla Gray, President
Jerry Galler, Executive Director

Powerful forum for people engaged in providing mental health services. Promoting the evolution of flexible models of responsive cost-effective ambulatory behavioral healthcare.

2635 Association for Applied Psychophysiology & Biofeedback

10200 W 44th Avenue
Suite 304
Wheat Ridge, CO 80033   303-422-8436
                               Fax: 303-422-8894
                E-mail: aapb@resourcenter.com
                               www.aapb.org

Lynda P Kirk, President
Francine Butler, Executive Director

Formerly the Biofeedback Research Society. Non-profit organization promotes a new understanding of biofeedback and advances the methods used in this practice.

Year Founded: 1969

2636 Association for Behavior Analysis

1219 South Park Street
Kalamazoo, MI 49001   269-492-9310
                             Fax: 269-492-9316
              E-mail: mail@abainternational.org
                             www.abainternational.org

2637 Association for Birth Psychology: ABP

444 E 82nd Street
New York, NY 10028-5903   212-988-6617
                E-mail: bithpsychology@aol.com
                             www.birthpsychology.org

Leslie Feher PhD, Executive Director

Obstetricians, pediatricians, midwives, nurses, psychotherapists, psychologists, counselors, social workers, sociologists, and others interested in birth psychology, a developing discipline concerned with the experience of birth and the correlation between the birth process and personality development. Seeks to promote communication among professionals in the field; encourage commentary, research and theory from different points of view; establish birth psychology as an autonomous science of human behavior; develop guidelines and give direction to the field. Annual conference, regional meetings, workshops.

2638 Association for Child Psychoanalysts: ACP

PO Box 253
Ramsey, NJ 07446-0253   201-825-3138
                               Fax: 201-825-3138
              E-mail: childanalysis@compuserve.com
                             www.childanalysis.org

Nancy Hall, Administrator

Child psychoanalysts united to provide a forum for discussion and dissemination of information in their field. Conducts national and international scientific meetings. Publications: Abstracts, triennial. Association for Child Psychoanalysis-Newsletter, semi-annual. Membership Roster, biennial. Annual Scientific Meeting.

2639 Association for Hospital Medical Education

419 Beulah Road
Pittsburgh, PA 15235   412-244-9302
                              866-617-4780
                         Fax: 412-243-4693
                E-mail: info@ahme.org
                              www.ahme.org

Margie Kleppick, Executive Director
Laurel L Humbert, Meeting Services

National, nonprofit professional association involved in the continuum of medical education — undergraduate, graduate, and continuing medical education. More than 600 members represent hundreds of teaching hospitals, academic medical centers and consortia nationwide. Promotes improvement in medical education to meet health care needs, serves as a forum and resource for medical education information, advocates the value of medical education in health care.

Year Founded: 1956

2640 Association for Humanistic Psychology: AHP

1516 Oak Street
#320A
Alameda, CA 94501-2947   510-769-6495
                                Fax: 510-769-6433
                 E-mail: ahpoffice@aol.com
                                www.ahpweb.org

Bonnie Davenport, Membership Services Director
Luke Lukens, Administrative Coordinator

Psychologists, social workers, clergy, educators, psychiatrists, and others engaged in humanistic practice. Functions as a worldwide network for the development of human sciences in ways that recognize distinctive human qualities and work toward fulfilling the innate capacities of people, both as individuals and in society. Annual midwest conference. Bimonthly magazine/newsletter.

2641 Association for Pre- & Perinatal Psychology and Health

PO Box 1398
Forestville, CA 95436   707-887-2838
                               Fax: 707-887-2838
                E-mail: apppah@aol.com
                               www.birthpsychology.org

Maureen Wolfe, Executive Director

Forum for individuals from diverse backgrounds and disciplines interested in psychological dimensions of prenatal and perinatal experiences. Typically, this includes childbirth educators, birth assistants, doulas, midwives, obstetricians, nurses, social workers, perinatologists, pediatricians, psychologists, counselors researchers and teachers at all levels. All who share these interests are welcome to join. Quarterly journal published.

Year Founded: 1983

2642 Association for Psychoanalytic Medicine (APM)

4560 Delafield Avenue
Bronx, NY 10471-3905   718-548-6088
                              Fax: 718-548-8302
                E-mail: dim1@columbia.edu

Geoc Sagi, President

Organization of physicians who are psychoanalysts. Provides forum on psychoanalytic developments for membership and community. Conducts postgraduate seminars. Sponsors speakers for community or medical groups. Conducts research on psychoanalytic involvement in social issues. Publications: Between Analyst and Patient, book. The Psychology of Men, book. Roster, biennial. Bulletin, every 9 months. Monthly Scientific Meeting, October through June at New York Academy of Medicine.

2643 Association for Psychological Type: APT

4750 W Lake Avenue
Glenview, IL 60025　　　　　**847-375-4717**
　　　　　　　　　　　Fax: 877-734-9374
　　　　　　　　E-mail: info@aptcentral.org
　　　　　　　　　　www.aptcentral.org

Jim Weir, Executive Director
Betsy Bischof, Marketing

Individuals involved in organizational development, religion, management, education and counseling, and who are interested in psychological type, the Myers-Briggs Type Indicator, and the works of Carl G Jung. Purpose is to share ideas related to the uses of MBTI and the application of personality type theory in any area; promotes research, development, and education in the field. Sponsors seminars, conferences, and training sessions on the use of psychological type.

2644 Association for Research in Nervous and Ment al Disease: ARNMD

1300 York Avenue, Box 171
Room F - 1231
New York, NY 10021　　　　　**570-839-0296**
　　　　　　　　　　　Fax: 570-839-0297
　　　E-mail: amgooder@med.cornell.edu
　　　　　　　　　　www.ammd.org

Dr. Anlouise Goodermuth, Executive Director

Keeps practicing physicians in nuerology and psychiatry, and neuroscientists, informed about state of the art research findings of interest to these ever more related disciplines, findings that are beginning to inform the thinking and practice of neurology and psychiatry.

Year Founded: 1920

2645 Association for Women in Psychology: AWP

PO Box 641065
Pullman, WA 99164-1065　　　**310-954-4104**
　　　　　　　　　　E-mail: srose@fiu.edu
　　　　　　　　　　www.awpsych.org

Suzanna Rose PhD, Director
Cassandra Nichols, Treasurer
Karol Dean, Membership

Nonprofit scientific and educational organization committed to encouraging feminist psychological research, theory and activism. We are an organization with a history of affirming and celebrating differences, deepening challenges, and experiencing growth as feminists.

Year Founded: 1969

2646 Association for the Advancement of Psycholog y: AAP

PO Box 38129
Colorado Springs, CO 80937-8129
　　　　　　　　　　　800-869-6595
　　　　　　　　　　Fax: 719-520-0375
　　　　　E-mail: Krivard@AAPNet.org
　　　　　　　　　　www.AAPNet.org

Stephen M Pfeiffer PhD, Executive Officer
Karen Rivard, Administrator

Promotes the interests of all psychologists before public and governmental bodies. AAP's fundamental mission is the support of candidates for the US Congress who are sympathetic to psychology's concerns, through electioneering activities.

Year Founded: 1974

2647 Association of Black Psychologists: ABPsi

PO Box 55999
Washington, DC 20040-5999　　**202-722-0808**
　　　　　　　　　　Fax: 202-722-5941
　　　　　　　E-mail: admin@abpsi.org
　　　　　　　　　　www.abpsi.org

Willie S Williams PhD, President

Members are professional psychologists and others in associated disciplines. Aims to: enhance the psychological well-being of black people in America; define mental health in consonance with newly established psychological concepts and standards, develop policies for local, state, and national decision making that have impact on the mental health of the black community; support established black sister organizations and aid in the development of new, independent black institutions to enhance the psychological educational, cultural, and economic situation. Offers training and information on AIDS. Conducts seminars, workshops and research. Periodic conference, annual convention.

Year Founded: 1968

2648 Association of Community Mental Health Agencies

909 S Fair Oaks Avenue
Pasadena, CA 91105-2625　　**626-584-0204**
　　　　　　　　　　Fax: 626-584-0621

2649 Association of State and Provincial Psychology Boards

PO Box 4389
Montgomery, AL 36103-4389　　**334-832-4580**
　　　　　　　　　　Fax: 334-269-6379
　　　　　　　E-mail: aspbb@asppb.org
　　　　　　　　　　www.asppb.org

Randolph P Reaves, Executive Officer
Amy C Hilson, Associate Executive Officer
Asher R Pacht PhD, Professional Affairs

State boards of psychology from across the US and Canada. Promotes the development and administration of the national Examination for Professional Practice in Psychology examination for certification for the practice of psychology. Provides legal counsel to the member boards as well as keeping them abreast of changes in the field of psychology. Publishes materials for training programs and for students preparing to enter the profession.

Year Founded: 1961

2650 Association of the Advancement of Gestalt Therapy: AAGT

37 Brunswick Road
Montclair, NJ 07042   973-783-0740
                             Fax: 586-314-2490
                   E-mail: bfeder@comcast.net
                             www.aagt.org

Bud Feder, President
Sylvie Falschlunger, Administration

Dynamic, inclusive, energetic nonprofit organization committed to the advancement of theory, philosophy, practice and research in Gestalt Therapy and its various applications. This includes but is not limited to personal growth, mental health, education, organization and systems development, political and social development and change, and the fine and performing arts. Our international member base includes psychiatrists, psychologists, social workers, teachers, academics, artists, writers, organizational consultants, political and social analysts, activists and students.

2651 Bazelon Center for Mental Health Law

1101 15th Street NW
Suite 1212
Washington, DC 20005   202-467-5730
                             Fax: 202-223-0409
                             TDD: 202-467-4232
                     E-mail: info@bazelon.org
                             www.bazelon.org

Robert Bernstein, Executive Director
Lee Carty, Communications Director

Provides technical support to lawyers and advocates on legal issues affecting children and adults with mental disabilities. Website has extensive legal advocacy resources and an online book store with handbooks, manuals and other publications.

2652 Behavioral Health Systems

2 Metroplex Drive
Suite 500
Birmingham, AL 35209   205-879-1150
                             800-245-1150
                             Fax: 205-879-1178
                     E-mail: info@bhs-inc.com
                             www.bhs-inc.com

Deborah L Stephens, Founder/President/CEO
Maureen Gleason, Sr VP/Business Development/COO
Sandy Capps, VP Employee Assistance Programs

Provides managed psychiatric and substance abuse and drug testing services to more than 20,000 employees nationally through a network of 7,600 providers.

2653 Bonny Foundation

PO Box 39355
Baltimore, MD 21212
                             866-345-5465
                E-mail: info@bonnyfoundation.org
                             www.bonnyfoundation.org

Donald Stoner, President
Marilyn Clark, Treasurer/Communications

Nonprofit organization which provides resources and training in the therapeutic use of the arts for professional music therapists, related health professionals, and the general public. The Bonny Foundation Newsletter provides current information on applications of GIM (Guided Imagery and Music), training schedules and publications. Our GIM training program is fully accredited by the Association for Music and Imagery.

2654 CG Jung Foundation for Analytical Psychology

28 E 39th Street
New York, NY 10016-2587   212-697-6430
                             Fax: 212-953-3989
                     E-mail: cgjungny@aol.com
                             www.cgjungny.org

Janet M Careswell, Executive Director
Arnold Devera, Membership

Analysts who follow the precepts of Carl G Jung, a Swiss psychologist, and any other persons interested in analytical psychology. Sponsors public lectures, films, continuing education, courses and professional seminars. Operates book service which provides publications on analytical psychology and related topics, and lectures on audio cassettes. Publishes journal, Quadrant.

Year Founded: 1962

2655 Center for Applications of Psychological Type

2815 NW 13th Street
Suite 401
Gainesville, FL 32609-2868   352-375-0160
                             800-777-2278
                             Fax: 352-378-0503
                   E-mail: development@capt.org
                             www.capt.org

Alecia Perkins, Director Customer Service

Nonprofit organization founded to conduct research and develop applications of the Myers-Briggs Type Indicator for the constructive use of differences. The MBTI is based on CG Jung's theory of psychological types. CAPT provides training for users of the MBTI and the Murphy-Meisgeier Type Indicator for Children, publishes and distributes books and resource materials, and maintains the Isabel Briggs Myers memorial library and the MBTI Bibliography. The MBTI is used in counseling individuals and families, to understand differences in learning styles, and for improving leadership and teamwork in organizations.

Year Founded: 1975

2656 Center for the Study of Psychiatry and Psychology

1036 Park Avenue
Suite 1B
New York, NY 10028   212-585-3758
E-mail: contact@icspp.org
www.icspp.org

Clemmont E Vontress PhD, Chair
Dominick Riccio PhD, Executive Director

Nonprofit research and educational network whose focus is the critical study of the mental health movement. ICSPP is completely independent and at present our funding consists solely of individual memebership dues. Fosters prevention and treatment of mental and emotional disorders. Promotes alternatives to administering psychiatric drugs to children.

2657 Child Welfare League of America: Washington

440 First Street NW
Third Floor
Washington, DC 20001-2085   202-638-2952
Fax: 202-638-4004
E-mail: wtc@cwla.org
www.cwla.org

Floyd Alwon

Provides two national conferences each year: Finding Better Ways and Information Technology: Tools That Work; comprehensive training programs for managers, supervisiors, foster parents, adoptive parents and direct care workers. Also provides a range of published materials and training curricula relating to all facets of child welfare service.

2658 Children's Health Council

650 Clark Way
Palo Alto, CA 94304   650-326-5530
Fax: 650-688-0206
E-mail: intake@chconline.org
www.chconline.org

Christopher Harris, Executive Director
Lucia D' Souza, School Director
Karen Grites, Educational Services

Working to make a measurable difference in the lives of children who face severe or complex behavioral and developmental challenges by providing interdisciplinary educational, assessment and treatment services and professional training.

2659 Christian Association for Psychological Studies

PO Box 310400
New Braunfels, TX 78131-0400   830-629-2277
Fax: 830-629-2342
E-mail: capsintl@compuvision.net
www.caps.net

Randolph Sanders PhD, Executive Director

Psychologists, marriage and family therapists, social workers, educators, physicians, nurses, ministers, researchers, pastoral counselors, and rehabilitation workers and others professionally engaged in the fields of psychology, counseling, psychiatry, pastoring and related areas. Association is based upon a genuine commitment to superior clinical, pastoral and scientific enterprise in the theoretical and applied social sciences and theology, assuming persons in helping professions will be guided to professional and personal growth and a greater contribution to others in this way.

Year Founded: 1956

2660 Clinical Social Work Federation

239 N Highland Street
Arlington, VA 22201   703-522-3866
Fax: 703-522-9441
E-mail: nfscswlo@aol.com
www.cswf.org

Allen DuMont, President
Richard P Yanes, Executive Director
Linda O'Leary, Administration

Thirty one state societies as voluntary associations for the purpose of promoting the highest standards of professional education and clinical practice. Each society is active with legislative advocacy and lobbying efforts for adequate and appropriate mental health services and coverage at their state and national levels of government. The mission of CSWF is to promote excellence in clinical social work practice through development and advancement of the profession.

2661 Commission on Accreditation of Rehabilitation Facilities, Behavioral Health: CARF

4891 E Grant Road
Tucson, AZ 85712   520-325-1044
888-281-6531
Fax: 520-318-1129
TTY: 888-281-6531
www.carf.org

Joanne Finegan, Chair

Promotes the quality, value and optimal outcomes through a consultative accreditation process that centers on enhancing the live of the people served.

2662 Commonwealth Fund

One E 75th Street
New York, NY 10021   212-606-3800
Fax: 212-606-3600
E-mail: info@cmwf.org
www.cmwf.org

Melinda Adams, Program Officer
Anne-Marie Audet, Assistant VP

Private foundation that supports independent research on health and social issues and make grants to improve health care practice and policy.

2663 Community Anti-Drug Coalitions of America: CADCA

625 Slaters Lane
Alexandria, VA 22314   703-706-0560
        800-542-2322
        Fax: 703-706-0565
        E-mail: info@cadca.org
        www.cadca.org

Arthur T Dean, Executive Director
David R Anderson, Communications
Brandi Felser, Meetings

With more than five thousand members across the country, CADCA is working to build and strengthen the capacity of community coalitions to create safe, healthy, and drug free communities. CADCA supports its members with technical assistance and training, public policy, media and marketing, conferences and special events.

2664 Corporate Counseling Associates

475 Park Avenue
Floor 24
New York, NY 10016-6901   212-686-6827

2665 Council of Behavioral Group Practice

1110 Mar West Street E
Tiburon, CA 94920   415-435-9821
        Fax: 415-543-9821

2666 Council on Social Work Education

1725 Duke Street
Suite 500
Alexandria, VA 22314-3421   703-683-8080
        Fax: 703-683-8099
        E-mail: info@cswe.org
        www.cswe.org

Donald W Beless, Executive Director
Michael Monti, Director Publications/Media

A national association that preserves and enhances the quality of social work education for the purpose of promoting the goals of individual and community well being and social justice. Pursues this mission through setting and maintaining policy and program standards, accrediting bachelors and masters degree programs in social work, promoting research and faculty development, and advocating for social work education.

2667 Developmental Disabilities Nurses Association

1733 H Street, Suite 330
PMB 1214
Blaine, WA 98230

        800-888-6733
        Fax: 360-332-2280
        E-mail: ddnahq@aol.com
        www.ddna.org

Mary Kay Moore, President
S Diane Moore-Denton, 1st VP
Ann Smith-Franklin, 2nd VP

National nonprofit professional association for nurses working with individuals with developmental disabilities. Publishes a quarterly newsletter.

Year Founded: 1992

2668 Employee Assistance Professionals Association

2101 Wilson Boulevard
Suite 500
Arlington, VA 22201   703-387-1000
        Fax: 703-522-4585
      E-mail: a.osullivan@eap-association.org
        www.eap-association.org

John Maynard PhD, CEO
Shirley Sringfloat, Credentialing
Allyson O'Sullivan, Membership

International association of approximately 6,200 members who are primarily employee assistance professionals as well as individuals in related fields such as human resources, chemical dependency treatment, mental health treatment, managed behavioral health care, counseling and benefits administration.

Year Founded: 1971

2669 Employee Assistance Society of North America

230 E Ohio Street
Suite 400
Chicago, IL 60611-3265   312-644-0828
        Fax: 312-644-8557
      E-mail: easna@bostrom.com
        www.easna.org

Margaret Altmix, President
Tim Stockert, Credentialing

International group of professional leaders with competencies in such specialties as workplace and family wellness, employee benefits and organizational development. Maintains accreditation program, membership services and professional training opportunities, promotes high standards of employee assistance programs.

2670 Employer Health Care Alliance Cooperative

37 Kessel Court
Suite 201
Madison, WI 53711   608-276-6626
        Fax: 608-210-6677
      www.alliancehealthcoop.com

Christopher Queram, CEO
Mary Borland, Marketing/Member Services

Nonprofit health care purchasing cooperative, owned and directed by employers. We are dedicated to purchasing health care based on high quality at an affordable cost.

2671 Gerontoligical Society of America

1030 15th Street
Suite 250
Washington, DC 20005   202-842-1275
        Fax: 202-842-1150
        E-mail: geron@geron.org
        www.geron.org

Carlo Ann Schutz, Executive Director
Johanna Merryman, Conferences/Education
Robert Harris, Promotion

Nonprofit professional organization with more than 5000 members in the field of aging. GSA provides researchers, educators, practitioners and policy makers with opportunities to understand, advance, integrate and use basic and applied research on aging to improve the quality of life as one ages.

2672 Gorski-Cenaps Corporation Training & Consultation

6147 Deltona Boulevard
Spring Hill, FL 34606   **352-596-8000**
                              Fax: 352-596-8002
                     E-mail: info@cenaps.com
                              www.cenaps.com

Terence T Gorski, President
Tresa J Watson, Office Manager

Cenaps provides advanced clinical skills training for the addiction behavioral health and mental health fields. Our focus is recovery and relapse prevention.

2673 Group Health Association of America

601 Pennsylvania Avenue NW
South Building, Suite 500
Washington, DC 20004   **202-778-3200**
                              Fax: 202-331-7487
                    E-mail: support@aahp.org
                              www.aahp.org

Karen Ignagne, President
Ingrid Reeves, Communications/Membership

National trade association representing the private sector in health care. Nearly 1,300 member companies of AAHP-HIAA provide health, long-term care, dental, disability and supplemental coverage to more than 200 million Americans.

2674 Group for the Advancement of Psychiatry: GAP

PO Box 570218
Dallas, TX 75357-0218   **972-613-3044**
                              Fax: 972-613-5532
                     www.groupadpsych.org

Frances Roton, Communications

Independent psychiatrists organized in working committees interested in applying principles of psychiatry toward the study of human relations. Works closely with specialists in other disciplines. Investigates subjects as school desegregation, use of nuclear energy, religion, psychiatry in the armed forces, mental retardation, cross-cultural communication, medical uses of hypnosis and the college experience. Maintains twenty five committees. Semiannual conference in April and November.

Year Founded: 1946

2675 Health Service Providers Verified

1120 G Street NW
Suite 330
Washington, DC 20005-3801   **202-783-1270**
                              Fax: 202-783-1269
                     www.hspverified.com

2676 Institute for Behavioral Healthcare

4370 Alpine Road
Suite 108
Portola Valley, CA 94028-7927   **415-851-6735**
                              Fax: 415-851-0406

2677 Institute of HeartMath

14700 W Park Avenue
Boulder Creek, CA 95006   **831-338-8500**
                              Fax: 831-338-8504
                     E-mail: info@heartmath.org
                              www.heartmath.org

Sara Paddison, President/CEO
Robert Rees PhD, Director Education

Nonprofit research and education on stress, emotional physiology and heart-brain interactions. Purpose to reduce stress, school violence, improve mental and emotional attitudes, promote harmony within facilities and communities, improve academic performance and improve workplace health and performance. Research facility provides psychometric assessments for both individual and organizational assessment as well as autonomic assessments for physiological assessment and diagnostic purposes. Education initiative currently developing curriculum for rehabilitation of incarcerated teen felons in drug and alcohol recovery program. Seeking funding for development of school-based social-cognitive programs and curricula for grades K-12.

Year Founded: 1991

2678 Institute on Psychiatric Services: American Psychiatric Association

1000 Wilson Boulevard
Suite 1825
Arlington, VA 22209-3901   **703-907-7300**
                              E-mail: apa@psych.org
                              www.psych.org

Jill L Gruber, Coordinator

Open to employees of all psychiatric and related health and educational facilities. Includes lectures by experts in the field and workshops and accredited courses on problems, programs and trends. Offers on-site Job Bank, which lists opportunities for mental health professionals. Organized scientific exhibits. Publications: Psychiatric Services, monthly journal. Annual Institute on Psychiatric Services conference and exhibits in October, Chicago, IL.

2679 Integrated Behavioral Health Consultants

7701 Park Ridge Circle
Fort Collins, CO 80528-8909   **970-223-5633**
                              Fax: 970-223-1697

2680 International Association for the Scientific Study of Intellectual Disabilities

31 Nottingham Way S
Clifton Park, NY 12065-1713
                              Fax: 518-877-3357
                     E-mail: njross@compuserve.com
                              www.isaaid.org

Dr. Neil Ross, President
Stephen Kealy, Secretary

Promotes the scientific study of intellectual disabilities on a multidisciplinary basis throughout the world, meetings held every four years.

2681 International Association of Psychosocial Rehabilitation Services

601 North Hammonds
Suite A
Linthicum, MD 21090   **410-789-7054**
                              Fax: 410-789-7675
                              TDD: 410-789-7682
                              E-mail: iapsrs.org

Ruth Hughes, CEO
David Issing, Conference Coordinator
Paul Seifert, Director Government Affairs

Psychosocial rehabilitation providers offer an integrated, comprehensive array of case management, employment, housing, mental health, and life-skill learning services for adults with serious mental illness.

2682 International Society for Adolescent Psychiatry

730 Soundview Avenue
Bronx, NY 10473-3421   **718-542-0394**
          E-mail: isap.newyork@isap-web.org
                              www.isap-web.org

Rosalie Landy, Administrative Director

Psychiatrists, psychologists, social workers, sociologists, pediatricians, educators and health care professionals involved in the treatment of adolescents. Seeks to advance treatment of psychiatric illnesses of adolescents. Maintains research and educational programs. Publications: International Annals of Adolescent Psychiatry, triennial monograph. Newsletter three times per year. Triennial congress and periodic international conference.

2683 International Society for Comparative Psychology: ISCP

University of California
Department of Psychology
Davis, CA 85618   **530-751-1855**
                        Fax: 530-752-2087
        E-mail: rmurphey@ucdavis.edu
www.pub.naz.edu:900/~mrenner8/iscp/iscp_right
                                    .htm

Robert M Murphey, Secretary/Treasurer

Psychologists, biologists, anthropologists, and neuroscientists who work in or are interested in comparative psychology. Aims: to promote the international development of comparative psychology, establish worldwide communication among comparative psychologists; encourage the study of the development and evolution of behavior. Published quarterly.

Year Founded: 1983

2684 International Society for Developmental Psychology: ISDP

Department Of Psychology: McLean Hospital
115 Mill Street
Belmont, MA 02478   **703-231-5346**
                        Fax: 703-231-3652
                E-mail: licklite@fiu.edu
                              www.isdp.org

Dr. Robert Lickliter, Director
Susan L Anderson, Treasurer/Communications

Members are research scientists in the field of developmental psychobiology and biology and psychology students. Promotes research in the field of developmental psychobiology, the study of the brain and brain behavior throughout the life span and in relation to other biological processes. Stimulates communication and interaction among scientists in the field. Provides the editorship for the journal, Development Psychobiology. Bestows awards. Compiles statistics. Annual conference.

2685 International Society of Political Psychology: ISPP

Pitzer College
1050 N Mills Avenue
Claremont, CA 91711   **909-621-8442**
                        Fax: 909-621-8481
                E-mail: ispp@pitzer.edu
                              www.ispp.org

Dana Ward, Executive Director

Facilitates communication across disciplinary, geographic and political boundaries among scholars, concerned individuals in government and public posts, the communication media and elsewhere who have a scientific interest in the relationship between politics and psychological processes. ISPP seeks to advance the quality of scholarship in political psychology and to increase the usefulness of work in political psychology.

2686 International Society of Sports Psychology: Department of Kinesiology

University of Illinois at Urbana
906 S Goodwin Avenue
Department Of Kinesiology, MC-052
Urbana, IL 61801   **217-265-5425**
                        Fax: 217-333-3124
                E-mail: emcauley@uiuc.edu
www.kines.uiuc.edu/labwebpages/expsych/in-
                                    dex.html

Edward McCauley PhD, Director

Professionally qualified individuals in forty-seven countries interested in sports psychology. Supports and promotes scientific research and professional relations between scholars in the field, participates in information and documentation services in sports psychology, advises and facilitates the establishment of other continental, regional and national societies of sports psychology. Promotes the International Olympic Committee and United States Olympic Committee with information on sport psychology services. Maintains speaker's bureau and bestows awards, operates children's services.

2687 International Transactional Analysis Association (ITAA)
436 14th Street
Suite 1301
Oakland, CA 94612-2710 510-625-7720
Fax: 510-625-7725
E-mail: info@itaa-net.org
www.itaa-net.org

Susan Sevilla, Executive Director

Persons in medical and behavioral sciences, including psychiatrists, psychologists, social workers, nurses, educators, marriage and family counselors, clergy and organizational consultants. Maintains standards of practice and teaching of transactional analysis which involves group therapy, social dynamics and personality theory based on analysis of the interactions between persons. Publications: International Transactional Analysis Association Membership Directory, annual. Annual Conference.

2688 Jean Piaget Society: Society for the Study of Knowledge and Development (JPSSSKD)
Larsen Hall
Harvard GS Education
Cambridge, MA 02138 617-495-3614
Fax: 617-495-3626
www.vanbc.wmsey.com/nchris/JPS/

Michael Chandler, President

Scholars, teachers, and researchers interested in exploring the nature of the developmental construction of human knowledge. Purpose is to further research on knowledge and development, especially in relation to the work of Jean Piaget, a Swiss developmentalist noted for his work in child psychology, the study of human development, and the origin and growth of human knowledge. Conducts small meetings and programs.

2689 Legend Pharmaceutical
510 Broadhollow Road
Suite 306
Melville, NY 11747 516-755-2000
800-755-2000
Fax: 516-755-2007

John A Marmero, COO
Lynn Garitt, Director Membership Services

A network of three hundred independent retail pharmacists. Full, personal service, computerized, delivery, HHC, DME, private label compare to line, and web page.

2690 MCC Behavioral Care
1009 Locust Avenue SE
Huntsville, AL 35801-3109 205-534-0972
Fax: 205-534-0769

2691 MacDermott Foundation
932 W Washginton
Chicago, IL 60607 313-421-3766
Fax: 312-226-0294

2692 Managed Health Care Association
1401 Eye Street NW
Suite 900
Washington, DC 20005-6562 202-218-4121
Fax: 202-478-1734

2693 Med Advantage
3452 Lake Lynda Drive
Suite 250
Orlando, FL 32817-1445 407-282-5131
Fax: 407-282-9240
www.med-advantage.com

John C Barrett, Sr VP

Fully accredited by URAC and certified in all 11 elements by NCQA, Med Advantage is one of the oldest credentials verification organizations in the country. Over the past eight years, they have developed sophisticated computer systems and one of the largest data warehouses of medical providers in the nation, containing information on over 900,000 healthcare providers. Their system is continually updated from primary source data required to meet the standards of the URAC, NCQA and JCAHO.

2694 Medical Group Management Association
104 Inverness Terrace E
Englewood, CO 80112-5306 303-799-1111
877-275-6462
Fax: 303-643-4439
E-mail: service@mgma.com
www.mgma.com

Norma J Plante, Chair

Principal voice for medical group practice.

Year Founded: 1926

2695 Medical Group Management Association: Assemblies & Society
3408 French Park Drive
Suite B
Edmond, OK 73034-7243 405-733-9516
Fax: 405-733-8853

2696 Mental Health Corporations of America
1876-A Eider Court
Tallahassee, FL 32308-3763 850-942-4900
Fax: 850-942-0560
www.mhca.com

2697 Mental Health Materials Center (MHMC)
PO Box 304
Bronxville, NY 10708-0304 914-337-6596
Fax: 914-779-0161

Alex Sareyan, President

Professionals of mental health and health education, seeking to stimulate the development of wider, more effective channels of communication between health educators and the public. Provides consulting services to nonprofit organizations on the implementation of their publishing operations in areas related to mental health and health. Publications: Study on Suicide Training Manual. Survival Manual for Medical Students. Books, booklets and pamphlets. Annual Meeting in New York City.

2698 National Academy of Certified Clinical Mental Health Counselors

5999 Stevenson Avenue
Alexandria, VA 22304-3302   703-823-9800
                                   Fax: 703-823-0252
                                   E-mail: counseling.org
                                   www.counseling.org

Provides standards for the independent practice of mental health counseling. The academy is a corporate affiliate of the American Association for Counseling and Development.

2699 National Academy of Neuropsychology (NAN)

2121 S Oneida Street
Suite 550
Denver, CO 80224-2594   303-691-3694
                               Fax: 303-691-5983
                               E-mail: office@nanonline.org
                               www.nanonlone.org

Josette G Harris PhD, Executive Director

Clinical neuropsychologists and others interested in brain-behavior relationships. Works to preserve and advance knowledge regarding the assessment and remediation of neuropsychological disorders. Promotes the development of neuropsychology as a science and profession; develops standard of practice and training guidelines for the field; fosters communication between members, represents the professional interests of members, serves as an information resource, facilitates the exchange of information among related organizations. Offers continuing education programs, conducts research.

2700 National Association for Children's Behavioral Health

1025 Connecticut Avenue NW
Suite 1012
Washington, DC 20036-5417   202-857-9735
                                   Fax: 202-362-5145
                                   E-mail: nacbc@aol.com

Joy Midman, Executive Director

To promote the availibility and delivery of appropriate and relevant services to children and adolescents with, or at risk of, serious emotional disturbances and their families. Advocate for the full array of mental health and related services necessery, the development and use of assessment and outcome tools based on functional as well as clinical indicators, and the elimination of categorial funding barriers.

2701 National Association for the Advancement of Psychoanalysis: NAAP

80 8th Avenue
Suite 1501
New York, NY 10011-5126   212-741-0515
                                 Fax: 212-366-4347
                                 E-mail: NAAP72@aol.com
                                 www.naap.org

Margery Quackenbush, Administrator
Pearl Appel, President
Sarina Meoves, Editor

Individual psychoanalysts having variety of schools of psychoanalytic thought united for the advancement of psychoanalysis as a profession. Publications: NAAP NEWS, quarterly. National Registry of Psychoanalysts, annual directory. Annual Conference.

2702 National Association in Women's Health

300 Adam Street
Suite 328
Chicago, IL 60606   312-786-1468
                           Fax: 312-786-0376
                           www.nawh.org

Shirley Sachs, Executive Director

2703 National Association of Addiction Treatment Providers

313 W Liberty Street
Suite 129
Lancaster, PA 17603-2748   717-392-8480
                                  Fax: 717-392-8481
                                  E-mail: rhunsicker@naatp.org
                                  www.naatp.org

Ronald J Hunsicker, President/CEO

The mission of the National Association of Addiction Treatment Providers (NAATP) is to promote, assist and enhance the delivery of ethical, effective, research-based treatment for alcoholism and other drug addictions. Provides members and the public with accurate, responsible information and other resources related to the treatment of these diseases, advocates for increased access to and availability of quality treatment for those who suffer from alcoholism and other drug addictions; works in partnership with other organizations and individuals that share NAATP's mission and goals.

2704 National Association of Behavioral Health Directors

1555 Connecticut Avenue NW
Washington, DC 20036-1111   202-234-1360

2705 National Association of Community Action

1100 17th Street NW
Suite 500
Washington, DC 20036-4632   202-265-7546
                                   Fax: 202-265-8850
                                   www.nachc.com

2706 National Association of Community Health Centers

1330 New Hampshire Avenue NW
Suite 122
Washington, DC 20036-6300   202-659-8008
                                   Fax: 202-659-8519

2707 National Association of Psychiatric Health Systems

325 Seventh Street NW
Suite 625
Washington, DC 20004-2802   202-393-6700
Fax: 202-783-6041
E-mail: naphs@naphs.org
www.naphs.org

Mark Covall, Executive Director
Carole Szpak, Director Communications

Merged with Association of Behavioral Group Practices, advocates for behavioral health and represents provider systems that are committed to the delivery of responsive, accountable, and clinically effective prevention, treatment, and care for children, adolescents, and adults with mental and substance use disorders. Working to coordinate a full spectrum of treatment services, including inpatient, residential, partial hospitalization and outpatient programs as well as prevention and management services.

Year Founded: 1933

2708 National Association of School Psychologists (NASP)

4240 EW Highway
Suite 402
Bethesda, MD 20815-5911   310-657-0270
Fax: 301-657-0275
E-mail: ahyman@naspweb.org
www.naspweb.org

Susan Gorin, Executive Director

School psychologists who serve the mental health and educational needs of all children and youth. Encourages and provides opportunites for professional growth of individual members. Informs the public on the services and practice of school psychology, and advances the standards of the profession. Operates national school psychologist certification system. Sponsers children's services.

2709 National Association of Social Workers

750 1st Street NE
Suite 80
Washington, DC 20002-4241   202-336-8244
800-638-8799
Fax: 202-336-8310
E-mail: info@nausuidc.org
www.socialworkers.org

The largest membership organization of professional social workers in the world, with more than one 155,000 members.

2710 National Association of State Mental Health Program Directors (NASMHPD)

66 Canal Center Plaza
Suite 302
Alexandria, VA 22314-1591   703-739-9333
Fax: 703-548-9517
E-mail: roy.praschil@nasmhpd.org
www.nasmhpd.org

Robert W Glover, Executive Director
Roy Praschil, Director Operations
Jackee Williams, Meeting Planner

State commissioners in charge of state mental disability programs for children and youth, aged, legal services, forensic services and adult services. Promotes state government agencies to deliver services to mentally disabled persons and fosters the exchange of scientific and program information in the administration of public mental health programs. Publications: Children and Youth Update, periodic. Federal Agencies, periodic newsletter. State Report, periodic newsletter.

2711 National Association of State Mental Health Program Directors

66 Canal Center Plaza
Suite 302
Alexandria, VA 22317   703-739-9333
Fax: 703-548-9517
E-mail: roy.praschil@nasmhpd.org
www.nasmhpd.org

Robert W Glover PhD, Executive Director
Roy Praschil, Director Operations
Jackee Williams, Meeting Planner

Nonprofit membership organization that adovacates at the national level for the collective interests of state mental health agency commissioners and staff. Operates under a cooperative agreement with the National Governor's Association. NASMHPD is committed to working with other stakeholders to improve public mental health systems and the lives of persons with serious mental illnesses who access these and other systems. Its core services focus on legislative advocacy, technical assistance and information dissemination.

Year Founded: 1959

2712 National Business Coalition Forum on Health

1015 18th Street NW
Suite 450
Washington, DC 20036-5214   202-775-9300
Fax: 202-775-1569
www.nbch.org

2713 National Center on Child Abuse & Neglect

PO Box 1182
Washington, DC 20201-0001   202-205-8306
Fax: 202-401-5917

2714 National Coalition for the Homeless

1012 14th Street NW
Suite 600
Washington, DC 20005-3471   202-737-6444
Fax: 202-737-6445

2715 National Committee of Quality Assurance

2000 L Street NW
Suite 500
Washington, DC 20036-4918   202-955-3517
Fax: 202-955-3599

2716 National Council of Juvenile and Family Court Judges

PO Box 8970
Reno, NV 89507-8970   775-784-6012
                            Fax: 775-784-1084
                            www.ncjfcj.unr.edu

2717 National Council on Aging

409 3rd Street SW
Suite 200
Washington, DC 20024-3204   202-479-1200

2718 National Criminal Justice Association

720 7th Street NW
Third Floor
Washington, DC 20001-3716   202-628-8550
                            Fax: 202-628-0080
                            E-mail: info@ncja.org
                            www.ncja.org

2719 National Eldercare Services Company

2257 Bel Pre Road
Silver Spring, MD 20906-2204 301-340-2851

2720 National Health Enhancement

3200 N Central Avenue
Floor 17
Phoenix, AZ 85012-2425   602-230-7545
                            Fax: 602-274-6158

2721 National Managed Health Care Congress

71 2nd Avenue
Floor 3
Waltham, MA 02451-1107
                            888-446-6422
                            Fax: 781-663-6411

2722 National Mental Health Association

2001 N Beauregard Street
12th Floor
Alexandria, VA 22311   703-684-7722
                            800-969-6642
                            Fax: 703-684-5968
                            TTY: 800-433-5959
                            E-mail: infoctr@nmha.org
                            www.nmha.org

Mike Fienza, Executive Director
Chris Condayn, Communications

Dedicated to improving treatments, understanding and services for adults and children with mental health needs. Working to win political support for funding for school mental health programs. Provides information about a wide range of disorders.

2723 National Mental Illness Screening Project

1 Washington Street
Suite 304
Wellesley, MA 02481-1706   781-239-0071
                            Fax: 781-431-7447
                            www.nmisp.org

Nonprofit organization devoted to assisting people with undiagnosed, untreated mental illness connect with local treatment resources via national screening programs for depression, eating disorders and alcohol problems.

2724 National Nurses Association

1767 Business Center Drive
Suite 330
Reston, VA 20190-5332   703-438-3060
                            Fax: 703-438-3072

2725 National Pharmaceutical Council

1894 Preston White Drive
Reston, VA 20191-5433   703-715-2770
                            Fax: 703-476-0904

2726 National Psychiatric Alliance

3501 Masons Mill Road
Suite 501
Huntingdon Vy, PA 19006-3517 610-627-2640
                            800-486-6721
                            Fax: 215-922-0747

2727 National Psychological Association for Psychoanalysis (NPAP)

150 W 13th Street
New York, NY 10011-7891   212-924-7440
                            E-mail: info@npap.org
                            www.npap.org

Harvey Kaplan, President

Professional society for practicing psychoanalysts. Conducts training program leading to certification in psychoanalysis. Offers information and private referral service for the public. Operates speakers' bureau. Publications: National Psychological Association for Psychoanalysis-Bulletin, biennial. National Psychological Association for Psychoanalysis-News and Reviews, semiannual. Psychoanalytic Review, bimonthly journal.

2728 National Register of Health Service Provider s in Psychology

1120 G Street NW
Suite 330
Washington, DC 20005-3801   202-783-7663
                            Fax: 202-347-0550
                            E-mail: claire@nationalregister.org
                            www.nationalregister.org

Judy Hall PhD, Executive Officer
Claire McCardell-Long, Director Administration/Finance

Psychologists who are licensed or certified by a state/provincial board of examiners of psychology and who have met council criteria as health service providers in psychology.

Year Founded: 1974

2729 National Treatment Alternative for Safe Communities

1500 N Halsted Street
Chicago, IL 60622-2517   312-573-8203
                            Fax: 312-787-9663

2730 National Treatment Consortium

PO Box 1294
Washington, DC 20013-1294   202-434-4780

2731 North American Society of Adlerian Psychology (NASAP)

NASAP
50 NE Drive
Hershey, PA 17033   717-579-8795
                           Fax: 717-533-8616
                  E-mail: nasap@nsn.com
                       www.alfredadler.org

Becky LaFountain, Administrator

NASAP is a professional organization for couselors, educators, physchologists, parent educators, business professionals, researchers and others who are interested in Adler's Individual Psychology. Membership includes journals, newsletters, conferences and training.

2732 Pharmaceutical Care Management Association

2300 9th Street S
Suite 210
Arlington, VA 22204-2320   703-920-8480
                              Fax: 703-920-8491

2733 Physicians for a National Health Program

332 S Michigan Avenue
Suite 500
Chicago, IL 60604-4306   312-554-0382
                           Fax: 312-554-0383
                    E-mail: pnhp@aol.com
                          www.pnhp.org

Physicians for a National Health Program is a nationwide network of doctor-practitioners and academics, residents and students. PNHP gives physicians the power to do collectively what individuals cannot do alone.

2734 PsycINFO

750 1st Street NE
Suite 800
Washington, DC 20002-4241   202-336-8244
                              Fax: 202-336-8310

2735 Psychiatric Society of Informatics

1500 E Medical Center Drive
#Tc3896
Ann Arbor, MI 48109-0005   313-764-5358
                             Fax: 313-936-8907

2736 Psychohistory Forum

627 Dakota Trail
Franklin Lakes, NJ 07417-1043   201-891-7486
                                  Fax: 201-891-6866
                          E-mail: pelovitz@aol.com

Paul H Elovitz PhD, Director

Psychologists, psychiatrists, psychotherapists, social workers, historians, psychohistorians and others having a scholarly interest in the integration of depth psychology and history. Aids individuals in psychohistorical research. Holds lecture series. Publications: Clio's Psyche: Understanding the Why of Current Events and History, quarterly journal. Immigrant Experience: Personal Narrative and Psychological Analysis, monograph. Periodic Meeting.

2737 Psychological Services Index

280 N Central Avenue
Suite 135
Hartsdale, NY 10530-1835   914-271-5435
                             Fax: 914-271-5869

2738 Psychology Society (PS)

100 Beekman Street
New York, NY 10038-1810   212-285-1872

Steven Brown, Executive Director
George E Marcus

Professional membership is limited to psychologists who have a doctorate and are certified/licensed. Associate membership is intended for teachers and researchers as well as persons whose professional status is pending. Seeks to further the use of psychology in therapy, family and social problems, behavior modification, and treatment of drug abusers and prisoners. Encourages the use of psychology in the solution of social and political conflicts.

2739 Psychology of Religion

180 N Oakland Avenue
Fuller Thological Seminary
Pasadena, CA 91101-1714   626-584-5532
                             Fax: 626-584-9630

Siang-Yang Tan, Secretary

A division of the American Psychologial Association. Seeks to encourage and accelerate research, theory, and practice in the psychology of religion and related areas. Facilitates the dissemination of data on religious and allied issues and on the integration of these data with current psychological research, theory and practice.

2740 Psychometric Society

1310 S 6th Street
260C Education Building
Champaign, IL 61820-6925   217-244-3361
                             Fax: 217-244-7620
                    E-mail: tackerma@uiuc.edu

Dr. Terry Ackerman, Secretary

Persons interested in development of quantitative models for psychological phenomena and quantitive methodology in the social and behavioral sciences.

Professional/Associations

2741 Psychonomic Society

University of Texas
Psychology
#195
Arlington, TX 76019-0001

817-272-2775
Fax: 817-272-2364
E-mail: mellsren@uta.edu
www.uta.edu/psychol-
ogy/orgs/skynmx/skyonomx.htm

Dr. Roger L Mellgren, Contact

Persons qualified to conduct and supervise scientific research in psychology or allied sciences; members must hold a PhD degree or its equivalent and must have published significant research other than doctoral dissertation. Promotes the communication of scientific research in psychology and allied sciences.

2742 Radical Caucus in Psychiatry (RCP)

450 Clarkson Avenue #1203
Suny Downstate Medical Center
Brooklyn, NY 11203-2056

718-270-2907
Fax: 718-287-0337

Carl Cohen MD, Coordinator

Members of the American Psychiatric Association and individuals interested in mental health issues who take a politically progressive stand in psychiatry. Objective is to examine the socioeconomic and sociopolitical aspects of mental health issues from a left-oriented perspective. Areas of study have included a critical analysis of biological psychiatry and psychiatric treatment of mental patients in Latin America. Publications: Annual newsletter. Annual conference and symposium. Seminar.

2743 Rapid Psychler Press

3560 Pine Grove Avenue
Suite 374
Port Huron, MI 48060-1994

519-433-7642
888-779-2453
Fax: 888-779-2457
E-mail: rapid@psychler.com
www.psychler.com

David Robinson, Publisher

Produces books and presentation media for educating mental health professionals. Products cover a wide range of learning needs. Where possible, humor is incorporated as an educational aid to enhance learning and retention.

2744 Resource Center for Systems Advocacy

291 Hudson Avenue
Albany, NY 12210-1828

518-427-5056
Fax: 518-427-5059

2745 Risk and Insurance Management Society

655 3rd Avenue
New York, NY 10017-5617

212-286-9292
Fax: 212-986-9716
www.rims.org

2746 Sciacca Comprehensive Services Development

299 Riverside Drive
New York, NY 10025-5278

212-866-5935
Fax: 212-666-1942
E-mail: ksciacca@pobox.com
www.http://pobox.com/~dualdiagnosis

Kathleen Sciacca MA, Executive Director/Consultant

Provides consulting, education and training for treatment and program development for dual diagnosis of mental illness and substance disorders including severe mental illness. Materials available include manuals, videos, articles, book chapters, journals and books. Trains in Motivational Interviewing. Develops programs across the mental health and substance abuse systems.

2747 Sigmund Freud Archives (SFA)

23 The Hemlocks
c/o Harold P Blum, MD
Roslyn, NY 11576-1721

516-621-6850
Fax: 516-621-3014

Harold P Blum MD, Executive Director

Psychoanalysts interested in the preservation and collection of scientific and personal writings of Sigmund Freud. Assists in research on Freud's life and work and the evolution of psychoanalytic thought. Collects and classifies all documents, papers, publications, personal correspondence and historical data written by, to, and on Freud. Transmits all materials collected to the Library of Congress. Annual meeting in New York City.

2748 Society for Behavioral Medicine

7611 Elmwood Avenue
Suite 201
Middleton, WI 53562-3161

301-279-6749
Fax: 301-251-2790

2749 Society for Pediatric Psychology (SPP)

Citadel
Department of Phychiatry
Charleston, SC 29409-0001

843-953-5320
Fax: 843-953-6797

Conway Saylor PhD, Contact

A division of the American Psychological Association. Psychologists working on children's hospitals, developmental clinics, and pediatric and medical group practices. Fosters the development of theory, research, training, and professional practice in pediatric psychology and the application of psychology to medical and psychological problems of children, youths, and their families. Supports legislation benefiting children's health and welfare. Sponsors colloquia and symposia; provides speakers.

2750 Society for Personality Assessment: SPA

6109 Arlington Boulevard
Suite H
Falls Church, VA 22044-2708

703-534-4772
Fax: 703-534-6905
E-mail: manager@spaonline.org
www.personality.org

Paula J Garber, Operations Manager

International professional trade association for psychologists, behavioral scientists, anthropologists, and psychiatrists. Promotes the study, research development and application of personality assessment.

2751 Society for Psychophysiological Research

1010 Vermont Avenue NW
Suite 1100
Washington, DC 20005-4907   202-393-4810
Fax: 202-783-2083
E-mail: spr@aps.washington.dc.us
www.sprweb.org

Louis Shermette, Director Membership

Founded in 1960, the Society for Psychophysiological Research is an international scientific society. The purpose of the society is to foster research on the interrelationship between physiological and phychological aspects of behavior.

2752 Society for Women's Health Research

1828 L Street NW
Suite 625
Washington, DC 20036-5104   202-223-8224
Fax: 202-833-3472
E-mail: information@womens-health.org
www.womens-health.org

The nation's only not-for-profit organization whose sole mission is to improve the health of women through research. Founded in 1990, The Society advocates increased funding for research on women's health, encourages the study of sex differences that may affect the prevention, diagnosis and treatment of disease, and promotes the inclusion of women in medical research studies. Visit the Society's Web site at www.womens-health.org for more information.

2753 Society for the Advancement of Social Psychology (SASP)

Mercer University
Department of Psychology
Macon, GA 31207-0001   912-301-2972
Fax: 912-301-2956
E-mail: dane_fc@mercer.edu

Dr. Frances Dane, Secretary

Social psychologists and students in social psychology. Advances social psychology as a profession by facilitating communication among social psychologists and improving dissemination and utilization of social psychological knowledge.

2754 Society for the Advancement of the Field Theory (SAFT)

903 N 29th Street
Philadelphia, PA 19130-1113   215-232-8088

Martin McGurrin, President

Educators, psychologists, social workers, political scientists, and anthropologists. Promotes the field theory, a concept developed by Kurt Lewin, social psychologist. The field theory explains behavior by describing changes in one's situation, or field. The group focuses on a portion of the field theory referred to as life space, which attempts to schematically represent human motivation.

2755 Society for the Psychological Study of Social Issues (SPPI)

PO Box 1248
Ann Arbor, MI 48106-1248   313-662-9130
Fax: 313-662-5607
E-mail: spssi@umich.edu
www.umich.edu/~sociss

Michelle Agnus, Administrative Assistant

Psychologists, sociologists, anthropologists, psychiatrists, political scientists, and social workers. Works to obtain and disseminate to the public scientific knowledge about social change and other social processes; promotes psychological research on significant theoretical and practical questions of social issues; encourages application of findings to problems of society.

2756 Society of Multivarative Experimental Psychology (SMEP)

University of Virginia
102 Gilmer Hall
Department of Psychology
Charlottesville, VA 22903   804-924-0656
E-mail: jjm@virginia.edu

Jack McArdle, Director

Psychologists interested in the branch of experimental psychology that centers on multivarative designs and associated special forms of analysis. Promotes substantive research and scientific discovery to develop mathematical/statistical models leading to their evaluation and integration into the development of psychological theory.

2757 Society of Teachers of Family Medicine

11400 Tomahawk Creek Parkway
Suite 340
Leawood, KS 66211   913-906-6000
800-274-2234
Fax: 913-906-6096
E-mail: admstaff@stfm.org
www.stfm.org

Mulitdisciplinary, medical organization that offers numerous faculty development opportunities for individuals involved, whether full or part time, in family medicine education. STFM publishes a monthly journal, hosts a web site, distributes books, coordinates CME conferences devoted to family medicine teaching and research and other activities designed to improve teaching skills of family medicine educators.

2758 Taylor Health System

4100 College Avenue
Ellicott City, MD 21043-5506   410-465-3322
800-883-3322
Fax: 410-461-7075
www.taylorhealth.com

Dr. Taylor, President

Independent, private psychiatric hospital with programs for children, adolescents, adults, older adults, crisis intervention and respite for adolescents, adults and older adults, high intensity respite for adolescents, residential treatement for adolescents, intensive outpatient for adolescents, adults and older adults. Treatment includes individual therapy, medication management, recreational therapy, nutritional guidance, physical assessment and care, group therapy, activity therapy, art therapy, behavioral therapy, milieu therapy, family/collateral therapy, somantic therapies, electro-convulsive therapy, cognitive therapy, addiction education and treatment.

2759 Therapeutic Communities of America

1611 Connecticut Avenue NW
Suite 4B
Washington, DC 20009-1033   **202-296-3503**
                                   Fax: 202-518-5475
            E-mail: TCA.office@verizon.net
      www.theraputiccommunitiesofamerica.org

Linda Crawford, Executive Director
Megan Zuckerman, Legislative Associate

National nonprofit membership association representing over 400 abuse treatment programs. The member agencies provide services to substance abuse clients of diverse special needs. Members provide a continum of care including assessment, detoxification, residential care, case management, outpatient treatment, transitional housing, education, vocational and medical care.

2760 Well Mind Association

4649 Sunnyside Avenue N
Suite 344
Seattle, WA 98103   **206-547-6167**
            E-mail: wma@speakeasy.org
                  www.speakeasy.org

Well Mind Association distributes information on current research and promotes alternative therapies for mental illness and related disorders. WMA believes that physical conditions and treatable biochemical imbalances are the causes of many mental, emotional and behavioral problems.

2761 Wellness Councils of America

7101 Newport Avenue
Suite 311
Omaha, NE 68152-2175   **402-572-3590**
                                   Fax: 402-572-3594
                                   www.welcoa.org

2762 WorldatWork

14040 N Northsight Boulevard
Scottsdale, AZ 85260-3627   **877-951-9191**
                                   480-922-2020
                              Fax: 866-816-2962

Books

General

2763 5-HTP: The Natural Way to Overcome Depression, Obesity, and Insomnia

Bantam Doubleday Dell Publishing
1745 Broadway
New York, NY 10019   **212-782-9000**
                              Fax: 212-782-9700

An authorative and comprehensive guide to realizing the health benefits of 5-Htp. Explains how this natural amino acid can safely and effectively regulate low serotonin levels, which have been linked to depression, obesity, insomnia, migraines, and anxiety. 5-HTP is also a powerful antioxidant that can protect the body from free-radical damage, reducing the risk of serious illnesses such as cancer. *$11.95*

304 pages Year Founded: 1999 ISBN 0-553379-46-1

2764 A Family-Centered Approach to People with Mental Retardation

AAMR
444 N Capitol Street NW
Suite 846
Washington, DC 20001-1512   **202-387-1968**
                                   800-424-3688
                              Fax: 202-387-2193
            E-mail: dcroser@aamr.org
                        www.aamr.org

Outlines key principles relevant to a family-centered approach to mental retardation and identifies four components to family-centered practice. *$12.95*

53 pages ISBN 0-940898-59-4

2765 A Guide to Consent

AAMR
444 N Capitol Street NW
Suite 846
Washington, DC 20001-1512   **202-387-1968**
                                   800-424-3688
                              Fax: 202-387-2193
            E-mail: dcroser@aamr.org
                        www.aamr.org

Examines current consent issues and explores legal implications of self-determination topics. Focuses on critical life events for people with mental retardation and practical applications of consent law, such as adult guardianship, consent to sexual activity, program placement and home ownership, capacity for and access to legal representation, capacity and other liberty and autonomy issues. *$27.95*

125 pages ISBN 0-940898-58-6

2766 A History of Nursing in the Field of Mental Retardation

AAMR
444 N Capitol Street NW
Suite 846
Washington, DC 20001-1512
202-387-1968
800-424-3688
Fax: 202-387-2193
E-mail: dcroser@aamr.org
www.aamr.org

For nursing scholars and anyone interested in the history of the treatment of people with mental retardation. *$19.95*

205 pages ISBN 0-940898-68-3

2767 A Primer on Rational Emotive Behavior Therapy

Research Press
Dept 24 W
PO Box 9177
Champaign, IL 61826
217-352-3273
800-519-2707
Fax: 217-352-1221
E-mail: rp@researchpress.com
www.researchpress.com

Russell Pense, VP Marketing

This concise, systematic guide addresses recent developments in the theory and practice of Rational Emotive Behavior Therapy (REBT). The authors discuss rational versus irrational thinking, the ABC framework, the three basic musts that interfere wtih rational thinking and behavior, two basic biological tendencies, two fundamental human disturbances, and the theory of change in REBT. A detailed case example that includes verbatim dialogue between therapist and client illustrates the 18-step REBT treatment sequence. An appendix by Albert Ellis examines the special features of REBT. *$12.95*

114 pages ISBN 0-878224-78-5

2768 A Research Agenda for DSM-V

American Psychiatric Publishing
1000 Wilson Boulevard
Suite 1825
Arlington, VA 22209-3901
703-907-7322
800-368-5777
Fax: 703-907-1091
E-mail: appi@psych.org
www.appi.org

In the ongoing quest to improve our psychiatric diagnostic system, we are now searching for new approaches to understanding the etiological and pathophysiological mechanisms that can improve the validity of our diagnoses and the consequent power of our preventative and treatment interventions-venturing beyond the current DSM paradigm and DSM-IV framework. This volume represents a far-reaching attempt to stimulate research and discussion in the field in preparation for the start of the DSM-V process, still several years away, and to integrate information from a wide variety of sources and technologies. *$38.95*

352 pages Year Founded: 2002 ISBN 0-890422-92-3

2769 Adaptive Behavior and Its Measurement Implications for the Field of Mental Retardation

AAMR
444 N Capitol Street NW
Suite 846
Washington, DC 20001-1512
202-387-1968
800-424-3688
Fax: 202-387-2193
E-mail: dcroser@aamr.org
www.aamr.org

Integrates the concept of adaptive behavior more fully into the AAMR definition of mental retardation.

227 pages ISBN 0-940898-64-0

2770 Addressing the Specific needs of Women with Co-Occuring Disorders in the Criminal Justice System

Policy Research Associates
345 Delaware Avenue
Delmar, NY 12054
518-439-7415
800-444-7415
Fax: 518-439-7612
E-mail: gains@prainc.com
www.prainc.com

Brochure emphasizes the need for gender specific programs to meet the management needs of female offenders. For law enforcement and justice administrators.

2771 Advances in Projective Drawing Interpetation

Charles C Thomas Publisher
2600 S 1st Street
Springfield, IL 62704-4730
217-789-8980
800-258-8980
Fax: 217-789-9130
E-mail: books@ccthomas.com
www.ccthomas.com

Exceptional contributors were chosen for their pertinence, range and inventiveness. This outstanding book assembles the progress in the science and in the clinical art of projective drawings as we enter the twenty-first century. *$95.95*

476 pages Year Founded: 1997 ISBN 0-398067-42-2

2772 Advancing DSM: Dilemmas in Psychiatric Diagnosis

American Psychiatric Publishing
1000 Wilson Boulevard
Suite 1825
Arlington, VA 22209-3901
703-907-7322
800-368-5777
Fax: 703-907-1091
E-mail: appi@psych.org
www.appi.org

Presents case studies from leading clinicians and researchers that illuminate the need for a revamped system. Each chapter presents a diagnostic dilemma from clinical practice that is intriguing, controversial, unresolved and remarkable in its theoretical and scientific complexity. Chapter by chapter, Advancing DSM raises important questions about the nature of diagnosis under the current DSM system and recommends broad changes. *$41.95*

304 pages Year Founded: 2002 ISBN 0-890422-93-1

2773 Adverse Effects of Psychotropic Drugs

Gilford Press
72 Spring Street
New York, NY 10012   212-431-9800

$63.00

2774 Agility in Health Care

Jossey-Bass Publishers
350 Sansome Street
5th Floor
San Francisco, CA 94104   415-394-8677
                                      800-956-7739
                              Fax: 800-605-2665
                              www.josseybass.com

$42.95

250 pages ISBN 0-787942-11-1

2775 American Psychiatric Glossary

American Psychological Press
1400 K Street NW
Washington, DC 20005   202-682-6262
                                   800-368-5777
                           Fax: 202-789-2648
                           E-mail: orders@appi.org
                                   www.appi.org

Hardcover. Paperback also available. *$28.50*

224 pages Year Founded: 1994 ISBN 0-880485-26-4

2776 American Psychiatric Publishing Textbook of Clinical Psychiatry

American Psychiatric Publishing
1000 Wilson Boulevard
Suite 1825
Arlington, VA 22209-3901   703-907-7322
                                       800-368-5777
                               Fax: 703-907-1091
                               E-mail: appi@psych.org
                                       www.appi.org

This densely informative textbook comprises 40 scholarly, authorative chapters by an astonishing 89 experts and combines junior and senior authors alike to enhance the rich diversity and quality of clinical perspectives. *$239.00*

1776 pages Year Founded: 2002 ISBN 1-585620-32-7

2777 Americans with Disabilities Act and the Emerging Workforce

AAMR
444 N Capitol Street NW
Suite 846
Washington, DC 20001-1512   202-387-1968
                                        800-424-3688
                                Fax: 202-387-2193
                                E-mail: dcroser@aamr.org
                                        www.aamr.org

Presents and empirical investigation of ADA issues and their effect on the employment of people with disabilities. Filled with legal cases, court opinions, charts, and tables. *$39.95*

303 pages ISBN 0-940898-52-7

2778 Assesing Problem Behaviors

AAMR
444 N Capitol Street NW
Suite 846
Washington, DC 20001-1512   202-387-1968
                                        800-424-3688
                                Fax: 202-387-2193
                                E-mail: dcroser@aamr.org
                                        www.aamr.org

Shows how to conduct a functional assessment, to link assessment results to interventions, and gives an example of completed fuctional analysis. *$21.95*

44 pages ISBN 0-940898-39-X

2779 Basic Personal Counseling: Training Manual for Counslers

Charles C Thomas Publisher
2600 S 1st Street
Springfield, IL 62704-4730   217-789-8980
                                         800-258-8980
                                 Fax: 217-789-9130
                                 E-mail: books@ccthomas.com
                                         www.ccthomas.com

Contents: Becoming a Counselor; The Counseling Relationship; An Overview of Skills Training; Attending to the Client and the Use of Minimal Responses; Reflection of Feelings; Reflection of Content and Feeling; The Seeing, Hearing, and Feeling Modes; Asking Questions; Summmarizing; Exploring Options; Reframing; Confrontation; Challenging Self-Destructive Beliefs; Termination; Procedure of the Counseling Experience; The Immediacy of the Counseling Experience; The Human Personality as it Emerges in the Counseling Experience; The Angry Client; Loss and Grieg Counseling; The Suicidal Client; Arrangement of the Counseling Room; Keeping Records of Counseling Sessions; Confidentiality; Supervision and Ongoing Training; and The Counselor's Own Well-Being. *$42.95*

214 pages Year Founded: 1989 ISBN 0-398055-40-8

2780 Best of AAMR: Families and Mental Retardation

AAMR
444 N Capitol Street NW
Suite 846
Washington, DC 20001-1512   202-387-1968
                                    800-424-3688
                              Fax: 202-387-2193
                      E-mail: dcroser@aamr.org
                                    www.aamr.org

Provides a comprehensive look at families and mental retardation in the 20th century through the eyes of some of its most respected researchers and service providers. *$59.95*

382 pages ISBN 0-940898-76-4

2781 Boundaries and Boundary Violations in Psychoanalysis

American Psychiatric Publishing
1000 Wilson Boulevard
Suite 1825
Arlington, VA 22209-3901   703-907-7322
                                    800-368-5777
                              Fax: 703-907-1091
                      E-mail: appi@psych.org
                                    www.appi.org

240 pages Year Founded: 2002 ISBN 1-585620-98-X

2782 Brain Calipers: Descriptive Psychopathology and the Mental Status Examination, Second Edition

Rapid Psychler Press
3560 Pine Grove Avenue
Suite 374
Port Huron, MI 48060   519-433-7642
                                888-779-2453
                          Fax: 888-779-2457
                  E-mail: rapid@psychler.com
                                www.psychler.com

David Robinson, Publisher

$34.95

ISBN 1-894328-02-7

2783 Breakthroughs in Antipsychotic Medications: A Guide for Consumers, Families, and Clinicians

WW Norton & Company
500 5th Avenue
New York, NY 10110   212-790-9456
                          Fax: 212-869-0856
              E-mail: admalmud@wwnorton.com
                            www.wwnorton.com

Gives patients and their families needed information about the pros and cons of switching medications, possible side effects. *$ 22.95*

240 pages Year Founded: 1999 ISSN 70303-7

2784 Brief Therapy and Managed Care

Jossey-Bass Publishers
350 Sansome Street
5th Floor
San Francisco, CA 94104   415-394-8677
                                  800-956-7739
                            Fax: 800-605-2665
                            www.josseybass.com

Provides focused, time-sensitive treatment to your patients. Pratical guidelines on psychotherapy that are conscientiously managed, appropriate, and sensitive to a client's needs. *$40.95*

443 pages ISBN 0-787900-77-X

2785 Brief Therapy with Intimidating Cases

Jossey-Bass Publishers
350 Sansome Street
5th Floor
San Francisco, CA 94104   415-394-8677
                                  800-956-7739
                            Fax: 800-605-2665
                            www.josseybass.com

This hands-on guide shows you how to apply the proven principles of brief therapy to a range of complex psychological problems once thought to be treatable only through long-term therapy or with medication. Learn how to focus on your clients' primary complaint and understand how and in what context the undesired behavior is performed. *$34.95*

224 pages ISBN 0-787943-64-9

2786 Challenging Behavior of Persons with Mental Health Disorders and Severe Developmental Disabilities

AAMR
444 N Capitol Street NW
Suite 846
Washington, DC 20001-1512   202-387-1968
                                    800-424-3688
                              Fax: 202-387-2193
                      E-mail: dcroser@aamr.org
                                    www.aamr.org

Provides a valuable compendium of the current knowledge base and empirically tested treatments for individuals with severe developmental disabilities, especially when problematic patterns of behavior are evident. *$39.95*

278 pages ISBN 0-940898-66-7

2787 Changing Health Care Marketplace

Jossey-Bass Publishers
350 Sansome Street
5th Floor
San Francisco, CA 94104   415-394-8677
                                  800-956-7739
                            Fax: 800-605-2665
                            www.josseybass.com

$35.95

366 pages ISBN 0-787902-52-7

2788 Clinical Dimensions of Anticipatory Mourning : Theory and Practice in Working with the Dying, Their Loved Ones, and Their Caregivers

Research Press
Dept 24 W
PO Box 9177
Champaign, IL 61826   217-352-3273
800-519-2707
Fax: 217-352-1221
E-mail: rp@researchpress.com
www.researchpress.com

Russell Pense, VP Marketing

Dr. Therese Rando is joined by 17 contributing authors to present the most comprehensive resource available on the perspectives, issues, interventions, and changing views associated with anticipatory mourning. *$29.95*

616 pages ISBN 0-878223-80-0

2789 Clinical Integration

Jossey-Bass Publishers
350 Sansome Street
5th Floor
San Francisco, CA 94104   415-394-8677
800-956-7739
Fax: 800-605-2665
www.josseybass.com

Learn how to create information systems that can support care coordination and management across delivery sites, develop a case management model program for multi-provider systems, and more. *$41.95*

272 pages ISBN 0-787940-39-9

2790 Cognitive Therapy in Practice

WW Norton & Company
500 5th Avenue
New York, NY 10110   212-790-9456
Fax: 212-869-0856
E-mail: admalmud@wwnorton.com
www.wwnorton.com

Basic text for graduate studies in psychotherapy, psycholgy nursing social work and counseling. *$29.00*

224 pages Year Founded: 1989 ISBN 0-393700-77-1

2791 Collaborative Therapy with Multi-Stressed Families

Guilford Publications
72 Spring Street
New York, NY 10012   212-431-9800
800-365-7006
Fax: 212-966-6708
E-mail: info@guilford.com
www.guilford.com

Written with a clear and fresh style, this is a guide to working in collaboration with clients, therapists and agencies. Experienced and beginning clinicians will appreciate a progressive approach to intricate problems. *$31.50*

358 pages Year Founded: 1999 ISBN 1-572304-90-1

2792 Communicating in Relationships: A Guide for Couples and Professionals

Research Press
Dept 24 W
PO Box 9177
Champaign, IL 61826   217-352-3273
800-519-2707
Fax: 217-352-1221
E-mail: rp@researchpress.com
www.researchpress.com

Russell Pense, VP Marketing

Addresses the behavioral, affective and cognitive aspects of communicating in relationships. The book can be used by couples as a self-help guide, by professionals as an adjunct to therapy, or as a supplementary text for related college courses. Numerous readings are interspersed with 44 exercises that provide a hands-on approach to learning. The authors outline 18 steps for developing communication skills and describe procedures for integrating the skills into relationships. *$29.95*

280 pages ISBN 0-878223-42-8

2793 Community-Based Instructional Support

AAMR
444 N Capitol Street NW
Suite 846
Washington, DC 20001-1512   202-387-1968
800-424-3688
Fax: 202-387-2193
E-mail: dcroser@aamr.org
www.aamr.org

Offers practical guidelines for applying instructional strategies for adults who are learning community-based tasks. *$12.95*

34 pages ISBN 0-940898-43-8

2794 Computerization of Behavioral Healthcare: How to Enhance Clinical Practice, Management, and Communications

Jossey-Bass Publishers
350 Sansome Street
5th Floor
San Francisco, CA 94104   415-433-1767
800-956-7739
Fax: 800-605-2665
www.josseybass.com

How computers and networked interactive information systems can help to contain costs, improve clinical outcomes, make your organizations more competitive using practical guidelines. *$27.95*

304 pages Year Founded: 1996 ISBN 0-787902-21-7

2795 Concise Guide to Marriage and Family Therapy

American Psychiatric Publishing
1000 Wilson Boulevard
Suite 1825
Arlington, VA 22209-3901   **703-907-7322**
                                       800-368-5777
                               Fax: 703-907-1091
                       E-mail: appi@psych.org
                               www.appi.org

Developed for use in the clinical setting, presents the core knowledge in the field in a single quick-reference volume. With brief, to-the-point guidance and step-by-step protocols, it's an invaluable resource for the busy clinician. *$29.95*

240 pages Year Founded: 2002 ISBN
1-585620-77-7

2796 Concise Guide to Mood Disorders

American Psychiatric Publishing
1000 Wilson Boulevard
Suite 1825
Arlington, VA 22209-3901   **703-907-7322**
                                       800-368-5777
                               Fax: 703-907-1091
                       E-mail: appi@psych.org
                               www.appi.org

Designed for daily use in the clinical setting, the Concise Guide to Mood Disorders is a fingertip library of the latest information, easy to understand and quick to access. This practical reference summarizes everything a clinician needs to know to diagnose and treat unipolar and bipolar mood disorders. *$29.95*

320 pages Year Founded: 2002 ISBN
1-585620-56-4

2797 Concise Guide to Psychiatry and Law for Clinicians

American Psychiatric Publishing
1000 Wilson Boulevard
Suite 1825
Arlington, VA 22209-3901   **703-907-7322**
                                       800-368-5777
                               Fax: 703-907-1091
                       E-mail: appi@psych.org
                               www.appi.org

Katie Duffy, Marketing Assistant

Practical information for psychiatrists in understanding legal regulations, legal decisions and present managed care applications. *$29.95*

296 pages Year Founded: 1998 ISBN
0-880483-29-6

2798 Concise Guide to Psychopharmacology

American Psychiatric Publishing
1000 Wilson Boulevard
Suite 1825
Arlington, VA 22209-3901   **703-907-7322**
                                       800-368-5777
                               Fax: 703-907-1091
                       E-mail: appi@psych.org
                               www.appi.org

Packed with practical information that is easy to access via detailed tables and charts, this pocket-sized volume (it literally fits into a lab coat or jacket pocket) is designed to be immediately useful for students, residents and clinicians working in a variety of treatment settings, such as inpatient psychiatry units, outpatient clinics, consultation-liaison services and private offices. *$29.95*

224 pages Year Founded: 2002 ISBN
1-585620-75-0

2799 Consent Handbook for Self-Advocates and Support Staff

AAMR
444 N Capitol Street NW
Suite 846
Washington, DC 20001-1512   **202-387-1968**
                                        800-424-3688
                               Fax: 202-387-2193
                       E-mail: dcroser@aamr.org
                               www.aamr.org

Offers options for self-advocates and those for people who cannot consent on their own. *$14.95*

36 pages ISBN 0-904898-69-1

2800 Countertransference Issues in Psychiatric Treatment

American Psychiatric Publishing
1000 Wilson Boulevard
Suite 1825
Arlington, VA 22209-3901   **703-907-7322**
                                       800-368-5777
                       Fax: 703-907-1091
                       E-mail: appi@psych.org
                               www.appi.org

Katie Duffy, Marketing Assistant

Overview of countertransference: theory and technique. *$37.50*

160 pages Year Founded: 1999 ISBN
0-880489-59-6

2801 Crisis: Prevention and Response in the Community

AAMR
444 N Capitol Street NW
Suite 846
Washington, DC 20001-1512   **202-387-1968**
                                        800-424-3688
                               Fax: 202-387-2193
                       E-mail: dcroser@aamr.org
                               www.aamr.org

Provides a look at crisis services for people with developmental disabilities and how they impact the surrounding community. *$49.95*

240 pages ISBN 0-940898-74-8

2802 Cross -Cultural Perspectives on Quality of Life

AAMR
444 N Capitol Street NW
Suite 846
Washington, DC 20001-1512   **202-387-1968**
                                       800-424-3688
                            Fax: 202-387-2193
                E-mail: dcroser@aamr.org
                            www.aamr.org

Provides a ground-breaking global outlook on quality-of-life issues for people with mental retardation. *$47.95*

380 pages ISBN 0-940898-70-5

2803 Cruel Compassion: Psychiatric Control of Society's Unwanted

John Wiley & Sons
605 3rd Avenue
New York, NY 10058-0180   **212-850-6000**
                            Fax: 212-850-6008
                E-mail: info@wiley.com
                            www.wiley.com

Demonstrates that the main problem that faces mental health policy makers today is adult dependency. A sobering look at some of our most cherished notions about our humane treatment of society's unwanted, and perhaps more importantly, about ourselves as a compassionate and democratic people. *$19.95*

264 pages Year Founded: 1994 ISBN 0-471010-12-X

2804 Culture & Psychotherapy: A Guide to Clinical Practice

American Psychiatric Publishing
1000 Wilson Boulevard
Suite 1825
Arlington, VA 22209-3901   **703-907-7322**
                                       800-368-5777
                            Fax: 703-907-1091
                E-mail: appi@psych.org
                            www.appi.org

Katie Duffy, Marketing Assistant

Case presentations, analysis, special issues and populations are covered. *$51.50*

320 pages Year Founded: 2001 ISBN 0-880489-55-3

2805 Cybermedicine

Jossey-Bass Publishers
350 Sansome Street
5th Floor
San Francisco, CA 94104   **415-394-8677**
                                       800-956-7739
                            Fax: 800-605-2665
                            www.josseybass.com

A passionate plea for the use of computers for initial diagnosis and assessment, treatment decisions, and for self-care, research, prevention, and above all, patient empowerment. *$25.00*

235 pages ISBN 0-787903-43-4

2806 DRG Handbook

Dorland Healthcare Information
1500 Walnut Street
Suite 1000
Philadelphia, PA 19102   **215-875-1212**
                                       800-784-2332
                            Fax: 215-735-3966
                E-mail: info@dorlandhealth.com
                            www.dorlandhealth.com

Diagnosis-related groups are the building blocks of hospital reimbursement under the Medicare Prospective Payment System. Also provides the ability to forecast and manage information at DRG-specific levels using comparison groups of like hospitals, a critical tool for both providers and payers. *$399.00*

1 per year Year Founded: 1998 ISBN 1-573721-39-5

2807 DSM: IV Diagnostic & Statistical Manual of Mental Disorders

American Psychiatric Publishing
1000 Wilson Boulevard
Suite 1825
Arlington, VA 22209-3901   **703-907-7322**
                                       800-368-5777
                            Fax: 703-907-1091
                E-mail: appi@psych.org
                            www.appi.com

Katie Duffy, Marketing Assistant

Focuses on clinical, research and educational findings. Practical and useful for clinicians and researchers of many orientations. Leatherbound. Hardcover and paperback also available. *$75.00*

886 pages Year Founded: 1994 ISBN 0-890420-64-5

2808 DSM: IV Personality Disorders

Rapid Psychler Press
3560 Pine Grove Avenue
Suite 374
Port Huron, MI 48060   **519-433-7642**
                                       888-779-2453
                            Fax: 888-779-2457
                E-mail: rapid@psychler.com
                            www.psychler.com

David Robinson, Publisher

$9.95

ISBN 1-894328-23-x

2809 Designing Positive Behavior Support Plans

AAMR
444 N Capitol Street NW
Suite 846
Washington, DC 20001-1512   **202-387-1968**
                                       800-424-3688
                            Fax: 202-387-2193
                E-mail: dcroser@aamr.org
                            www.aamr.org

Provides a conceptual framework for understanding, designing, and evaluating positive behavior support plans. *$21.95*

43 pages ISBN 0-940898-55-1

2810 Developing Mind: Toward a Neurobiology of Interpersonal Experience

Guilford Publications
72 Spring Street
New York, NY 10012   212-431-9800
800-365-7006
Fax: 212-966-6708
E-mail: info@guilford.com
www.guilford.com

Concise research results as to the origins of our behavior based on cognitive neuroscience.

2811 Disaility at the Dawn of the 21st Century and the State of the States

AAMR
444 N Capitol Street NW
Suite 846
Washington, DC 20001-1512   202-387-1968
800-424-3688
Fax: 202-387-2193
E-mail: dcroser@aamr.org
www.aamr.org

Consumate source book on the analysis of financing services and supports for people with developmental disabilities in the United States. A detailed state-by-state analysis of public financial support for persons with MR/DD, mental illness, and physical disabilities.

512 pages ISBN 0-940898-85-3

2812 Diversity in Psychotherapy: The Politics of Race, Ethnicity, and Gender

Praeger
2727 Palisade Avenue
Suite 4H
Bronx, NY 10463-1020   718-796-0971
Fax: 718-796-0971
www.vd6@columbia.edu

Dr. Victor De La Cancela, President/CEO Salud Management

This challenging and insightful work wrestles with difficult treatment problems confronting both culturally and socially oppressed clients and psychotherapists. Case studies offer highly valuable resource material and insights into challenging perpsectives on behavioral health services. *$49.95*

224 pages Year Founded: 1993 ISBN 0-275941-80-9

2813 Doing What Comes Naturally: Dispelling Myths and Fallacies About Sexuality and People with Developmental Disabilities

High Tide Press
3650 W 183rd Street
Homewood, IL 60430   708-206-2054
888-487-7377
Fax: 708-206-2044
E-mail: managing.editor@hightidepress.com
www.hightidepress.com

Diane J Bell, Managing Editor

Uncovers misconceptions about adults whose sexual needs vary greatly, and yet are often treated as children or non-sexual people. Includes heartwarming success stories from adults Mrs. Anderson has supported, as well as suggestions for teaching and a guide to sexual incident reporting. *$19.95*

119 pages ISBN 1-892696-13-4

2814 Dynamic Psychotherapy: An Introductory Approach

American Psychiatric Publishing
1000 Wilson Boulevard
Suite 1825
Arlington, VA 22209-3901   703-907-7322
800-368-5777
Fax: 703-907-1091
E-mail: appi@psych.org
www.appi.org

Katie Duffy, Marketing Assistant

Principles and techniques. *$33.50*

229 pages Year Founded: 1990

2815 Efficacy of Special Education and Related Services

AAMR
444 N Capitol Street NW
Suite 846
Washington, DC 20001-1512   202-387-1968
800-424-3688
Fax: 202-387-2193
E-mail: dcroser@aamr.org
www.aamr.org

Provides an objective, explicit, and clear evaluation of the existing literature of special education. Also evaluates general education practices adapted and modified for special education. *$31.95*

123 pages ISBN 0-940898-51-9

2816 Electroconvulsive Therapy: A Guide

Madison Institute of Medicine
7617 Mineral Point Road
Suite 300
Madison, WI 53717-1623   608-827-2470
Fax: 608-827-2479
E-mail: mim@miminc.org
www.miminc.org

ECT is an extremely effective method of treatment for severe depression that does not respond to medication. This guidebook explains what ECT is and how it is used today to help patients overcome depression and other serious, treatment resistant psychiatric disorders. *$5.95*

19 pages

2817 Embarking on a New Century: Mental Retardation at the end of the Twentieth Century

AAMR
444 N Capitol Street NW
Suite 846
Washington, DC 20001-1512   202-387-1968
                                     800-424-3688
                          Fax: 202-387-2193
               E-mail: dcroser@aamr.org
                          www.aamr.org

This volume of 18 essays summarizes major public policy and servuce delivery advancements from 1975 to 2000. These changes can be summarized as a siginificant shift in many areas — from services to supports; from passive to active consumer roles; from normalization to quality. *$29.97*

265 pages

2818 Emergencies in Mental Health Practice

Guilford Publications
72 Spring Street
New York, NY 10012   212-431-9800
                              800-365-7006
                    Fax: 212-966-6708
          E-mail: info@guilford.com
                    www.guilford.com

Focusing on acute clinical situations in which there is an imminent risk of serious harm or death to self or others, this practical resource helps clinicians evaluate and manage a wide range of mental health emergencies. The volume provides guidelines for interviewing with suicidal patients, potentially violent patients, vulnerable victims of violence, as well as patients facing life-and-death medical decisions, with careful attention to risk management and forensic issues. *$24.95*

450 pages ISBN 1-572305-51-7

2819 Essential Guide to Psychiatric Drugs

St. Martin's Press
175 5th Avenue
New York, NY 10010   212-674-5151
          E-mail: webmaster@stmartins.com
                    www.stmartins.com

Information not found in other drug references. Lists many common drugs and not so common side effects, including drug interaction and the individual's reaction, including sexual side effects. Expert but nontechnical narrative. *$6.99*

416 pages Year Founded: 98 ISBN 0-312954-58-1

2820 Ethical Way

Jossey-Bass Publishers
350 Sansome Street
5th Floor
San Francisco, CA 94104   415-394-8677
                                   800-956-7739
                         Fax: 800-605-2665
                         www.josseybass.com

Leads you through a maze of ethical principles and crucial issues confronting mental health professionals. *$38.95*

254 pages ISBN 0-787907-41-X

2821 Executive Guide to Case Management Strategies

Jossey-Bass Publishers
350 Sansome Street
5th Floor
San Francisco, CA 94104   415-394-8677
                                   800-956-7739
                         Fax: 800-605-2665
                         www.josseybass.com

A guide to plan, organize, develop, improve and help case management programs reach their full potential in the clinical and financial management of care. *$58.00*

160 pages ISBN 1-556481-28-4

2822 Exemplar Employee: Rewarding & Recognizing Direct Contact Employees

High Tide Press
3650 W 183rd Street
Homewood, IL 60430   708-206-2054
                              888-487-7377
                    Fax: 708-206-2044
     E-mail: managing.editor@hightidepress.com
                    www.hightidepress.com

Diane J Bell, Managing Editor

With staff turnover as high as 90 percent in some agencies, you need to provide direct contact employees with as many incentives to excel as you can. This successful recognition program for non-management, direct contact employees is broken down and explained, with specific advice on how to implement it in your own organization from the people who developed the program. *$10.95*

48 pages ISBN 1-892696-03-7

2823 Family Approach to Psychiatric Disorders

American Psychiatric Publishing
1000 Wilson Boulevard
Suite 1825
Arlington, VA 22209-3901   703-907-7322
                                    800-368-5777
                          Fax: 703-907-1091
               E-mail: appi@psych.org
                          www.appi.org

Katie Duffy, Marketing Assistant

Examines how treatment can and should involve the family of the patient. *$67.50*

404 pages Year Founded: 1996

2824 Family Stress, Coping, and Social Support

Charles C Thomas Publisher
2600 S 1st Street
Springfield, IL 62704-4730
217-789-8980
800-258-8980
Fax: 217-789-9130
E-mail: books@ccthomas.com
www.ccthomas.com

$48.95

294 pages Year Founded: 1982 ISSN 0-398-06275-7ISBN 0-398046-92-1

2825 Family Therapy Progress Notes Planner

John Wiley & Sons
10475 Crosspoint Boulevard
Indianapolis, IN 46256
877-762-2974
Fax: 800-597-3299
E-mail: consumers@wiley.com
www.wiley.com

Extends the line into the growing field of family therapy. Included is critical information about HIPAA guidelines, which greatly impact the privacy status of patient progress notes. Helps mental health practitioners reduce the amount of time spent on paperwork by providing a full menu of pre-written progress notes that can be easily and quickly adapted to fit a particular patient need or treatment situation. *$ 49.95*

352 pages ISBN 0-471484-43-1

2826 Fifty Ways to Avoid Malpractice: a Guidebook for Mental Health Professionals

Professional Resource Press
PO Box 15560
Sarasota, FL 34277-1560
941-343-9601
800-443-3364
Fax: 941-343-9201
E-mail: orders@prpress.com
www.prpress.com

Debra Fink, Managing Editor

Offers straightforward guidance on providing legally safe and ethically appropriate services to your clients. *$18.95*

158 pages Year Founded: 1988 ISBN 0-943158-54-0

2827 First Therapy Session

Jossey-Bass Publishers
350 Sansome Street
5th Floor
San Francisco, CA 94104
415-394-8677
800-956-7739
Fax: 800-605-2665
www.josseybass.com

Presents an effective, straightforward approach for conducting first therapy sessions, showing step-by-step, how to identify client problems and help solve them within families. *$27.95*

ISBN 1-555421-94-6

2828 Flawless Consulting

Jossey-Bass Publishers
350 Sansome Street
5th Floor
San Francisco, CA 94104
415-394-8677
800-956-7739
Fax: 800-605-2665
www.josseybass.com

This book offers advice on what to say and what to do in specific situations to see your recommendations through. *$39.95*

214 pages ISBN 0-893840-52-1

2829 Forgiveness: Theory, Research and Practice

Guilford Publications
72 Spring Street
New York, NY 10012
212-431-9800
800-365-7006
Fax: 212-966-6708
E-mail: info@guilford.com
www.guilford.com

Scholarly, up-to-date examination of forgiveness ranges many disiplines for mental health professionals. *$35.00*

334 pages Year Founded: 2000 ISBN 1-572305-10-X

2830 Foundations of Mental Health Counseling

Charles C Thomas Publisher
2600 S 1st Street
Springfield, IL 62704-4730
217-789-8980
800-258-8980
Fax: 217-789-9130
E-mail: books@ccthomas.com
www.ccthomas.com

The latest writings regarding the explosive growth of mental health counseling over the past twenty years. Leading experts discuss the past, present, and future of the field from their unique positions as practitioners, theoreticians, and educators. Major issues such as professional identity, ethics, assessment, research, and theory are joined with the contemporary problems of managed health care, insurance reimbursement, and private practice. An up-to-date resource in the field of mental health counseling. *$89.95*

446 pages Year Founded: 1996 ISBN 0-398066-69-8

2831 Fundamentals of Psychiatric Treatment Planning

American Psychiatric Publishing
1000 Wilson Boulevard
Suite 1825
Arlington, VA 22209-3901
703-907-7322
800-368-5777
Fax: 703-907-1091
E-mail: appi@psych.org
www.appi.org

Professional discussion of important basics. *$49.00*

368 pages Year Founded: 2002 ISBN 1-585620-61-0

2832 Group Involvement Training

New Harbinger Publications
5674 Shattuck Avenue
Oakland, CA 94609-1662   510-652-2002
                                800-748-6273
                            Fax: 510-652-5472
E-mail: customerservice@newharbinger.com
                    www.newharbinger.com

This book shows how training chronically ill mental patients in a series of structured group tasks can be used to treat the symptoms of apathy, withdrawl, poor interpersonal skills, helplessness, and the inability to structure leisure time constructively. *$24.95*

160 pages Year Founded: 1988 ISBN 0-934986-65-7

2833 Guide to Possibility Land: Fifty One Methods for Doing Brief, Respectful Therapy

WW Norton & Company
500 5th Avenue
New York, NY 10110   212-790-9456
                        Fax: 212-869-0856
E-mail: admalmud@wwnorton.com
                    www.wwnorton.com

The creator of Possibility therapy, William O'Hanlon, outlines acknowledging patient's experience and opinions about their lives while seeing that possibilites for change are explored and underlined. *$13.00*

94 pages Year Founded: 1999 ISBN 0-393702-97-9

2834 Guide to Treatments That Work

Oxford University Press/Oxford Reference
198 Madison Avenue
New York, NY 10016   212-726-6000
                            800-451-7556
                        Fax: 919-677-1303
                    www.oup-usa.org/orbs/

A systematic review of various treatments currently in use for virtually all of the recognized mental disorders. *$75.00*

624 pages Year Founded: 1997 ISBN 0-195102-27-4

2835 Handbook on Quality of Life for Human Service Practitioners

AAMR
444 N Capitol Street NW
Suite 846
Washington, DC 20001-1512   202-387-1968
                                    800-424-3688
                                Fax: 202-387-2193
E-mail: dcroser@aamr.org
                    www.aamr.org

Revolutionary generic model for quality of life that integrates core domains and indicators with a cross-cultural systems prespective that can be used in all human services. *$59.95*

429 pages ISBN 0-940898-77-2

2836 Helper's Journey: Working with People Facing Grief, Loss, and Life-Threatening Illness

Research Press
Dept 24 W
PO Box 9177
Champaign, IL 61826   217-352-3273
                            800-519-2707
                        Fax: 217-352-1221
E-mail: rp@researchpress.com
                    www.researchpress.com

Russell Pense, VP Marketing

Written for both professional and volunteer caregivers, this unique manual provides exercises, activities and specific strategies for more successful caregiving, increased personal growth and effective stress management. The author explores the theory and practice of helping. He includes numerous case examples and verbatim disclosures of fellow caregivers that powerfully convey the joys and sorrows of the helper's journey. Cited as a "Book of the Year" by the American Journal of Nursing. *$21.95*

292 pages ISBN 0-878223-44-4

2837 High Impact Consulting

Jossey-Bass Publishers
350 Sansome Street
5th Floor
San Francisco, CA 94104   415-394-8677
                                800-956-7739
                            Fax: 800-605-2665
                        www.josseybass.com

Offers a new model for consulting services that shows how to produce short-term successes and use them as a springboard to larger accomplishments and, ultimately, to organization-wide continuous improvement. Also includes specific guidance to assist clients in analyzing their situation, identifying their real needs, and choosing an appropriate consultant. *$26.00*

256 pages ISBN 0-787903-41-8

2838 Home Maintenance for Residential Service Providers

High Tide Press
3650 W 183rd Street
Homewood, IL 60430   708-206-2054
                            888-487-7377
                        Fax: 708-206-2044
E-mail: managing.editor@hightidepress.com
                    www.hightidepress.com

Diane J Bell, Managing Editor

What happens when a human service organization becomes a large, commercial landlord, not unlike a real estate firm or condominium management company? Property management for homes supporting persons with disabilities requires a unique blend of human services and physical plant expertise. Provides detailed checklists for all house systems, fixtures and furnishings. Includes a discussion of maintaining an attractive residence that blends with the neighborhood. *$10.95*

42 pages ISBN 0-965374-46-7

2839 How to Partner with Managed Care: a Do It Yourself Kit for Building Working Relationships & Getting Steady Referrals

John Wiley & Sons
605 3rd Avenue
New York, NY 10058-0180   212-850-6000
Fax: 212-850-6008
E-mail: info@wiley.com
www.wiley.com

366 pages Year Founded: 1996

2840 Improving Clinical Practice

Jossey-Bass Publishers
350 Sansome Street
5th Floor
San Francisco, CA 94104   415-394-8677
800-956-7739
Fax: 800-605-2665
www.josseybass.com

Enhance your organization's clinical decision making, and ultimately improve the quality of patient care. *$41.95*

342 pages ISBN 0-787900-93-1

2841 Improving Therapeutic Communication

Jossey-Bass Publishers
350 Sansome Street
5th Floor
San Francisco, CA 94104   415-394-8677
800-956-7739
Fax: 800-605-2665
www.josseybass.com

Improve your communication technique with this definitive guide for counselors, therapists, and caseworkers. Focuses on the four basic skills that facilitate communication in therapy: empathy, respect, authenticity, and confrontation. *$62.95*

394 pages ISBN 0-875893-08-2

2842 Increasing Variety in Adult Life

AAMR
444 N Capitol Street NW
Suite 846
Washington, DC 20001-1512   202-387-1968
800-424-3688
Fax: 202-387-2193
E-mail: dcroser@aamr.org
www.aamr.org

Step-by-step guidelines for implementing the general-case instructional process and shows how the process can be used across a variety of activities. *$12.95*

38 pages ISBN 0-940898-43-2

2843 Independent Practice for the Mental Health Professional

Brunner/Mazel
325 Chestnut Street
Philadelphia, PA 19106
800-821-8312
Fax: 215-269-0363

Ralph H Earle PhD
Dorothy J Barnes MC

An excellent resource for beginning therapists considering private practice or for experienced therapists moving from agency or institutional settings into private practice. Offers practical, down-to-earth suggestions for practice settings, marketing and working with clients. The authors provide worksheets and examples of successful planning for the growth of a practice. *$24.95*

141 pages ISBN 0-876308-38-8

2844 Infanticide: Psychosocial and Legal Perspectives on Mothers Who Kill

American Psychiatric Publishing
1000 Wilson Boulevard
Suite 1825
Arlington, VA 22209-3901   703-907-7322
800-368-5777
Fax: 703-907-1091
E-mail: appi@psych.org
www.appi.org

Written to help remedy today's dearth of up-to-date, research-based literature, this unique volume brings together a multidisciplinary group of 17 experts who focus on the psychiatric perspective of this tragic cause of infant death. Balanced perspective on a highly emotional issue will find a wide audience among psychiatric and medical professionals, legal professionals, public health professionals and interested laypersons. *$53.50*

304 pages Year Founded: 2002 ISBN 1-585620-97-1

2845 Innovative Approaches for Difficult to Treat Populations

American Psychiatric Publishing
1000 Wilson Boulevard
Suite 1825
Arlington, VA 22209-3901   703-907-7322
800-368-5777
Fax: 703-907-1091
E-mail: appi@psych.org
www.appi.org

Katie Duffy, Marketing Assistant

Alternate methods when the usual approaches are not helpful. *$86.95*

512 pages Year Founded: 1997

2846 Insider's Guide to Mental Health Resources Online

Guilford Publications
72 Spring Street
New York, NY 10012   212-431-9800
800-365-7006
Fax: 212-966-6708
E-mail: info@guilford.com
www.guilford.com

This guide helps readers take full advantage of Internet and world-wide-web resources in psychology, psychiatric, self-help and patient education. The book explains and evaluates the full range of search tools, newsgroups, databases and describes hundreds of specific disorders, find job listings and network with other professionals, obtain needed articles and books, conduct grant searches and much more. *$21.95*

338 pages ISBN 1-572305-49-5

2847 Instant Psychoparmacology

WW Norton & Company
500 5th Avenue
New York, NY 10110   **212-790-9456**
                    Fax: 212-869-0856
          E-mail: admalmud@wwnorton.com
                    www.wwnorton.com

Revision of the best selling guide to all the new medications. Straightforward book teaches non medical therapists, clients and their families how the five different clases of drugs work, advice on side effects, drug interaction warnings and much more practical information. *$18.95*

168 pages Year Founded: 2002 ISBN 0-393703-91-6

2848 Integrated Treatment of Psychiatric Disorders

American Psychiatric Publishing
1000 Wilson Boulevard
Suite 1825
Arlington, VA 22209-3901   **703-907-7322**
                    800-368-5777
          Fax: 703-907-1091
          E-mail: appi@psych.org
                    www.appi.org

Katie Duffy, Marketing Assistant

Psychodynamic therapy and medication. *$34.95*

208 pages Year Founded: 2001 ISBN 1-585620-27-0

2849 Integrative Brief Therapy: Cognitive, Psychodynamic, Humanistic & Neurobehavioral Approaches

Impact Publishers
PO Box 6016
Atascadero, CA 93423-6016   **805-466-5917**
                    800-246-7228
                    Fax: 805-466-5919
          E-mail: info@impactpublishers.com
                    www.impactpublishers.com

Thorough discussion of the factors that contribute to effectiveness in therapy carefully integrates key elements from diverse theoretical viewpoints. *$17.95*

272 pages Year Founded: 1998 ISBN 1-886230-09-9

2850 International Handbook on Mental Health Policy

Greenwood Publishing Group
88 Post Road W
PO Box 5007
Westport, CT 06880-4208   **203-226-3571**
                    Fax: 203-222-1502

Major reference book for academics and practitioners that provides a systematic survey and analysis of mental health policies in twenty representative countries. *$125.00*

512 pages Year Founded: 1993 ISBN 0-313275-67-X

2851 Interpersonal Psychotherapy

American Psychiatric Publishing
1000 Wilson Boulevard
Suite 1825
Arlington, VA 22209-3901   **703-907-7322**
                    800-368-5777
          Fax: 703-907-1091
          E-mail: appi@psych.org
                    www.appi.org

Katie Duffy, Marketing Assistant

An overview of interpersonal psychotherapy for depression, preventative treatment for depression, bulimia nervosa and HIV positive men and women. *$37.50*

156 pages Year Founded: 1998 ISBN 0-880488-36-0

2852 Introduction to Time: Limited Group Psychotherapy

American Psychiatric Publishing
1000 Wilson Boulevard
Suite 1825
Arlington, VA 22209-3901   **703-907-7322**
                    800-368-5777
          Fax: 703-907-1091
          E-mail: appi@psych.org
                    www.appi.org

Katie Duffy, Marketing Assistant

Do more with limited time and sessions. *$57.95*

317 pages Year Founded: 1997

2853 Introduction to the Technique of Psychotherapy: Practice Guidelines for Psychotherapists

Charles C Thomas Publisher
2600 S 1st Street
Springfield, IL 62704-4730   **217-789-8980**
                    800-258-8980
                    Fax: 217-789-9130
          E-mail: books@ccthomas.com
                    www.ccthomas.com

A basic, simply written book, with a minimum of theory, helpful to the beginning therapist. Discuss how to conduct psychotherapy: by having a format in mind, taking a comprehensive history, and a careful, observing examination of the patient. *$34.95*

122 pages Year Founded: 1998 ISSN 0-398-06905-0ISBN 0-398069-04-2

2854 Languages of Psychoanalysis

Analytic Press
101 W Street
Hillsdale, NJ 07642-1421　　**201-358-9477**
　　　　　　　　　　　　　　800-926-6579
　　　　　　　　　Fax: 201-358-4700
　　　　　E-mail: TAP@analyticpress.com
　　　　　　　www.analyticpress.com

Paul E Stepansky PhD, Managing Director
John Kerr PhD, Sr Editor

A guide to understanding the full range of human discourse, especially how behavioral conflicts and communicational deficits as they impinge upon the transactions of the analytic dyad. Available in hardcover. *$39.95*

224 pages Year Founded: 1996 ISBN 0-881631-86-8

2855 Leadership and Organizational Excellence

AAMR
444 N Capitol Street NW
Suite 846
Washington, DC 20001-1512　　**202-387-1968**
　　　　　　　　　　　　　　800-424-3688
　　　　　　　　　Fax: 202-387-2193
　　　　　E-mail: dcroser@aamr.org
　　　　　　　　www.aamr.org

Examines key managerial and organizational strategies that can be used to help ensure high-quality work environments for both staff and service delivery for people with developmental disabilities. *$ 14.95*

65 pages ISBN 0-940898-78-0

2856 Life Course Perspective on Adulthood and Old Age

AAMR
444 N Capitol Street NW
Suite 846
Washington, DC 20001-1512　　**202-387-1968**
　　　　　　　　　　　　　　800-424-3688
　　　　　　　　　Fax: 202-387-2193
　　　　　E-mail: dcroser@aamr.org
　　　　　　　　www.aamr.org

Experts in gerontology, sociology, and cognitive disability share the latest research, trends, and thoughtful insights into old age. *$19.95*

229 pages ISBN 0-940898-31-4

2857 Making Money While Making a Difference: Achieving Outcomes for People with Disabilities

High Tide Press
3650 W 183rd Street
Homewood, IL 60430　　　　**708-206-2054**
　　　　　　　　　　　　　　888-487-7377
　　　　　　　　　Fax: 708-206-2044
　　E-mail: managing.editor@hightidepress.com
　　　　　　　www.hightidepress.com

Diane J Bell, Managing Editor

Unique handbook for corporations and nonprofits alike. The authors guide readers through a step-by-step process for implementing strategic alliances between nonprofit organizations and corporate partners. Learn the tenets of cause related marketing and much more. *$14.95*

231 pages ISBN 0-965374-49-1

2858 Managed Mental Health Care in the Public Sector: a Survival Manual

Harwood Academic Publishers

Manual for administrators, planners, clinicians and consumers with concepts and strategies to maneuver in public sector managed mental healthcare system. *$35.00*

410 pages Year Founded: 1996 ISBN 9-057025-37-X

2859 Managing Client Anger: What to Do When a Client is Angry with You

New Harbinger Publications
5674 Shattuck Avenue
Oakland, CA 94609-1662　　**510-652-2002**
　　　　　　　　　　　　　　800-748-6273
　　　　　　　　　Fax: 510-652-5472
　　E-mail: customerservice@newharbinger.com
　　　　　　　www.newharbinger.com

Guide to help therapists understand their reactions and make interventions when clients express anger toward them. *$49.95*

261 pages Year Founded: 1998 ISBN 1-572241-23-3

2860 Manual of Clinical Psychopharmacology

American Psychiatric Publishing
1000 Wilson Boulevard
Suite 1825
Arlington, VA 22209-3901　　**703-907-7322**
　　　　　　　　　　　　　　800-368-5777
　　　　　　　　　Fax: 703-907-1091
　　　　　E-mail: appi@psych.org
　　　　　　　　www.appi.org

Examines the recent changes and standard treatments in psychopharmacology. *$63.00*

736 pages Year Founded: 2002 ISBN 0-880488-65-4

2861 Mastering the Kennedy Axis V: New Psychiatric Assessment of Patient Functioning

American Psychiatric Publishing
1000 Wilson Boulevard
Suite 1825
Arlington, VA 22209-3901   703-907-7322
                                 800-368-5777
                        Fax: 703-907-1091
                    E-mail: appi@psych.org
                            www.appi.org

Professional evaluation methods. *$44.00*

*320 pages Year Founded: 2002 ISBN
1-585620-62-9*

2862 Meditative Therapy Facilitating Inner-Directed Healing

Impact Publishers
PO Box 6016
Atascadero, CA 93423-6016   805-466-5917
                                   800-246-7228
                          Fax: 805-466-5919
        E-mail: info@impactpublishers.com
                www.impactpublishers.com

Offers to the professional therapist a full description of the therapeutic procedures that facilitate inner-directed healing and explains the therapist's role in guiding clients' growth psychologically, physiologically and spiritually. *$27.95*

*230 pages Year Founded: 1999 ISBN
1-886230-11-0*

2863 Mental Disability Law: Primer, a Comprehensive Introduction

Commission on the Mentally Disabled
1800 M Street NW
Washington, DC 20036-5802   202-331-2240

An updated and expanded version of the 1984 edition provides a comprehensive overview of mental disability law. Part I of the Primer examines the scope of mental disability law, defines the key terms and offers tips on how to provide effective representation for clients. Part II reviews major federal legislative initiatives including the Americans with Disabilities Act. *$15.00*

2864 Mental Health Rehabilitation: Disputing Irrational Beliefs

Charles C Thomas Publisher
2600 S 1st Street
Springfield, IL 62704-4730   217-789-8980
                                    800-258-8980
                          Fax: 217-789-9130
          E-mail: books@ccthomas.com
                www.ccthomas.com

Applicable to a wide variety of disciplines involved with therapeutic counseling of people with mental and/or physical disabilities such as rehabilitation counseling, mental health counseling, pastoral counseling, school counseling, clinical social work, clinical and counseling psychology, and behavioral science oriented medical specialities and related health and therapeutic professionals. *$36.95*

*106 pages Year Founded: 1995 ISBN
0-398065-31-4*

2865 Mental Health Resources Catalog

Paul H Brookes Company
PO Box 10624
Baltimore, MD 21285-0624   410-337-9580
                                  800-638-3775
                        Fax: 410-337-8539
   E-mail: custserv@brookespublishing.com
           www.brookespublishing.com

This catalog offers practical resources for mental health professionals serving young children and their families, including school psychologists, teachers and early intervention professionals, FREE.

2 per year

2866 Mental Retardation: Definition, Classification, and Systems of Supports

AAMR
444 N Capitol Street NW
Suite 846
Washington, DC 20001-1512   202-387-1968
                                   800-424-3688
                          Fax: 202-387-2193
             E-mail: dcroser@aamr.org
                     www.aamr.org

Presents a complete system to define and diagnose mental retardation, classify and describe strenghts and limitations, and plan a supports needs profile. *$79.95*

250 pages ISBN 0-940898-81-0

2867 Metaphor in Psychotherapy: Clinical Applications of Stories and Allegories

Impact Publishers
PO Box 6016
Atascadero, CA 93423-6016   805-466-5917
                                   800-246-7228
                          Fax: 805-466-5919
        E-mail: info@impactpublishers.com
                www.impactpublishers.com

Comprehensive resource aids therapists in helping clients change distorted views of the human experience. Dozens of practical therapeutic activities involving metaphor, drama, fantasy, and meditation. *$29.95*

*320 pages Year Founded: 1998 ISBN
1-886230-10-2*

2868 Microcounseling: Innovations in Interviewing, Counseling, Psychotherapy, and Psychoeducation

Charles C Thomas Publisher
2600 S 1st Street
Springfield, IL 62704-4730   217-789-8980
800-258-8980
Fax: 217-789-9130
E-mail: books@ccthomas.com
www.ccthomas.com

$91.95

624 pages Year Founded: 1978 ISSN 0-398-06175-0ISBN 0-398037-12-4

2869 Natural Supports: A Foundation for Employment

AAMR
444 N Capitol Street NW
Suite 846
Washington, DC 20001-1512   202-387-1968
800-424-3688
Fax: 202-387-2193
E-mail: dcroser@aamr.org
www.aamr.org

Step-by-step strategy for developing a network of natural supports aimed at promoting the goals and interests of all individuals in the work setting. *$12.95*

34 pages ISBN 0-940898-65-9

2870 Negotiating Managed Care: Manual for Clinicians

American Psychiatric Publishing
1000 Wilson Boulevard
Suite 1825
Arlington, VA 22209-3901   703-907-7322
800-368-5777
Fax: 703-907-1091
E-mail: appi@psych.org
www.appi.org

Katie Duffy, Marketing Assistant

Help for professionals to successfully present a case during clinical review. *$26.95*

120 pages Year Founded: 2002 ISBN 1-585620-42-4

2871 Neurobiology of Violence

American Psychiatric Publishing
1000 Wilson Boulevard
Suite 1825
Arlington, VA 22209-3901   703-907-7322
800-368-5777
Fax: 703-907-1091
E-mail: appi@psych.org
www.appi.org

Important information on the basic science of violence, including genetics, with topics of great practical value to today's clinician, including major mental disorders and violence; alcohol and substance abuse and violence; and psychopharmacological approaches to managing violent behavior. *$69.00*

368 pages Year Founded: 2002 ISBN 1-585620-81-5

2872 Neurodevelopment & Adult Psychopathology

Cambridge University Press
40 W 20th Street
New York, NY 10011-4221   212-924-3900
Fax: 212-691-3239
E-mail: marketing@cup.org
www.cup.org

2873 Neuropsychiatry and Mental Health Services

American Psychiatric Publishing
1000 Wilson Boulevard
Arlington, VA 22209-3901   703-907-7322
800-368-5777
Fax: 703-907-1091
E-mail: appi@psych.org
www.appi.org

Katie Duffy, Marketing Assistant

Cognitive therapy practices in conjunction with mental health treatment. *$79.95*

448 pages Year Founded: 1999 ISBN 0-880487-30-5

2874 Neuropsychology of Mental Disorders: Practical Guide

Charles C Thomas Publisher
2600 S 1st Street
Springfield, IL 62704-4730   217-789-8980
800-258-8980
Fax: 217-789-9130
E-mail: books@ccthomas.com
www.ccthomas.com

Discusses the advances in diverse areas such as biology, electrophysiology, genetics, neuroanatomy, pharmacology, psychology, and radiology which are increasingly important for a practical understanding of behavior and its pathology. *$70.95*

338 pages Year Founded: 1994 ISBN 0-398059-05-5

2875 New Roles for Psychiatrists in Organized Systems of Care

American Psychiatric Publishing
1000 Wilson Boulevard
Suite 1825
Arlington, VA 22209-3901   703-907-7322
800-368-5777
Fax: 703-907-1091
E-mail: appi@psych.org
www.appi.org

Katie Duffy, Marketing Assistant

Comprehensive view of opportunities, challenges and roles for psychiatrists who are working for or with new organized systems of care. Discusses the ethical dilemmas for psychiatrists in managed care settings and training and identity of the field as well as historical overviews of health care policy. *$50.00*

312 pages Year Founded: 1998 ISBN 0-880487-58-5

2876 Of One Mind: The Logis of Hypnosis, the Practice of Therapy

WW Norton & Company
500 5th Avenue
New York, NY 10110   212-790-9456
                           Fax: 212-869-0856
          E-mail: admalmud@wwnorton.com
                           www.wwnorton.com

A new approch to an old treatment, the author explains his ideas on connecting with patients in hypno and brief therapies. *$30.00*

240 pages Year Founded: 2001 ISSN 70382-7

2877 On Being a Therapist

Jossey-Bass Publishers
350 Sansome Street
5th Floor
San Francisco, CA 94104   415-394-8677
                                 800-956-7739
                           Fax: 800-605-2665
                           www.josseybass.com

This thoroughly revised and updated edition shows you how to use the insights gained from your clients' experiences to solve your own problems, realize positive change in yourself, and become a better therapist. *$22.00*

320 pages ISBN 1-555425-55-0

2878 On the Counselor's Path: a Guide to Teaching Brief Solution Focused Therapy

New Harbinger Publications
5674 Shattuck Avenue
Oakland, CA 94609-1662   510-652-2002
                                 800-748-6273
                           Fax: 510-652-5472
     E-mail: customerservice@newharbinger.com
                           www.newharbinger.com

A teacher's guide for conducting training sessions on solution focused techniques. *$24.95*

92 pages Year Founded: 1996 ISBN 1-572240-48-2

2879 Opportunities for Daily Choice Making

AAMR
444 N Capitol Street NW
Suite 846
Washington, DC 20001-1512   202-387-1968
                                   800-424-3688
                           Fax: 202-387-2193
          E-mail: dcroser@aamr.org
                           www.aamr.org

Provides strategies for increasing choice-making opportunities for people with developmental disabilities. It describes basic principles of choice-making, shows how to teach choice-making skills to the passive learner, describes how to build in multiple choice-making opportunities within daily routines, introduces self-scheduling, and addresses common questions. *$12.95*

48 pages ISBN 0-904898-44-6

2880 Out of Darkness and Into the Light: Nebraska's Experience In Mental Retardation

AAMR
444 N Capitol Street NW
Suite 846
Washington, DC 20001-1512   202-387-1968
                                   800-424-3688
                           Fax: 202-387-2193
          E-mail: dcroser@aamr.org
                           www.aamr.org

The Nebraska model for dealing with the condition of mental retardation has been so successful that it has been emulated throughout the United States and other countries. The inspiring story of how this change occured, written by those who made it happen. It is an account of both the changing approach to those once considered less the human. and their successful movement from despondency to hope, and from patient to people. *$29.97*

267 pages

2881 Participatory Evaluation for Special Education and Rehabilitation

AAMR
444 N Capitol Street NW
Suite 846
Washington, DC 20001-1512   202-387-1968
                                   800-424-3688
                           Fax: 202-387-2193
          E-mail: dcroser@aamr.org
                           www.aamr.org

Nine-step method for identifying and weighting the importance of disparate goals and outcomes. *$31.95*

90 pages ISBN 0-940898-73-X

2882 Person-Centered Foundation for Counseling and Psychotherapy

Charles C Thomas Publisher
2600 S 1st Street
Springfield, IL 62704-4730   217-789-8980
                                    800-258-8980
                           Fax: 217-789-9130
          E-mail: books@ccthomas.com
                           www.ccthomas.com

Focusing on counseling and psychotherapy, its goals are to renew interest in the person-centered approach in the US, make a signigicant contribution to extending person-centered theory and practice, and promote fruitful dialogue and futher development of person-centered theory. Presents: the rationale for an eclectic application of person-centered counseling; the rationale and process for reflecting clients' feelings; the importance of the theory as the foundation for the counseling process; the importance of values and their influence on the counseling relationship; the modern person-centered counselor's role; and the essential characteristics of a person-centered counseling relationship.

260 pages Year Founded: 1999 ISSN 0-398-06966-2ISBN 0-398069-64-6

2883 PharmaCoKinetics and Therapeutic Monitering of Psychiatric Drugs

Charles C Thomas Publisher
2600 S 1st Street
Springfield, IL 62704-4730   217-789-8980
                                    800-258-8980
                              Fax: 217-789-9130
                    E-mail: books@ccthomas.com
                              www.ccthomas.com

$52.95

226 pages Year Founded: 1993 ISBN 0-398058-41-5

2884 Positive Bahavior Support for People with Developmental Disabilities: A Research Synthesis

AAMR
444 N Capitol Street NW
Suite 846
Washington, DC 20001-1512   202-387-1968
                                    800-424-3688
                              Fax: 202-387-2193
                    E-mail: dcroser@aamr.org
                              www.aamr.org

Offers a careful analysis documenting that positive behavioral procedures can produce important change in the behavior and lives of people with disabilities. *$31.95*

108 pages ISBN 0-940898-60-8

2885 Positive Behavior Support Training Curriculum

AAMR
444 N Capitol Street NW
Suite 846
Washington, DC 20001-1512   202-387-1968
                                    800-424-3688
                              Fax: 202-387-2193
                    E-mail: dcroser@aamr.org
                              www.aamr.org

Designed for training supervisors of direct support staff, as well as direct support professionals themselves in the values and practices of positive behavior support.

2886 Practical Guide to Cognitive Therapy

WW Norton & Company
500 5th Avenue
New York, NY 10110   212-790-9456
                      Fax: 212-869-0856
            E-mail: admalmud@wwnorton.com
                      www.wwnorton.com

Based on highly successful workshops by the author, this book provides a framework to apply cognitive therapy model to office practices. *$22.95*

200 pages Year Founded: 1991 ISBN 0-393701-05-0

2887 Practical Psychiatric Practice Forms and Protocols for Clinical Use

American Psychological Publishing
1400 K Street NW
Washington, DC 20005   202-682-6262
                               800-368-5777
                         Fax: 202-789-2648
                E-mail: appi@psych.org
                         www.appi.org

Katie Duffy, Marketing Assistant

Designed to aid psychiatrists in organizing their work. Provides rating scales, model letters, medication tracking forms, clinical pathology requests and sample invoices. Handouts on disorders and medication are provided for patients and their families. Spiralbound. *$47.50*

312 pages Year Founded: 1998 ISBN 0-880489-43-X

2888 Practice Guidelines for Extended Psychiatric Residential Care: From Chaos to Collaboration

Charles C Thomas Publisher
2600 S 1st Street
Springfield, IL 62704-4730   217-789-8980
                                    800-258-8980
                              Fax: 217-789-9130
                    E-mail: books@ccthomas.com
                              www.ccthomas.com

Patrick W Corrigan, Author/Editor
Stanley McCracken, Author/Editor
Joseph Mehr, Author/Editor

Presents a set of practice guidelines that represent state-of-the-art treatments for consumers of extended residential care. Written for line-level staff charged with the day-to-day services: psychiatrists, psychologists, social workers, activity therapists, nurses, and psychiatric technicians who work closely with consumers in residential programs and program administrators who have immediate responsibility for supervising treatment teams. *$47.95*

176 pages Year Founded: 1995 ISSN 0-398-06536-5 ISBN 0-398065-35-7

2889 Primer of Brief Psychotherapy

WW Norton & Company
500 5th Avenue
New York, NY 10110   212-790-9456
                      Fax: 212-869-0856
            E-mail: admalmud@wwnorton.com
                      www.wwnorton.com

Positive guide to brief therapy is a task oriented aid with emphasis on the first session and details of procedures afterward. *$19.55*

160 pages Year Founded: 1995 ISBN 0-393701-89-1

Professional/Books/General

2890 Primer of Supportive Psychotherapy

Analytic Press
101 W Street
Hillsdale, NJ 07642-1421   201-358-9477
                                    800-926-6579
                          Fax: 201-358-4700
          E-mail: TAP@analyticpress.com
                www.analyticpress.com

Paul E Stepansky PhD, Managing Director
John Kerr PhD, Sr Editor

Focuses on the rationale for and techniques of supportive psychotherapy as a form of dyadic intervention distinct from expressive psychotherapies. The realities, ironies, conundrums and opportunities of the therapeutic encounter are vividly portrayed in scores of illustrative dialogues drawn from actual treatments. Among the topics covered are how to provide reassurance in the realistic way, how to handle requests for advice, the role of praise and reinforcement, the appropriate use of reframing techniques and of modeling, negotiating patients' concerns about medication and other collateral forms of treatment. *$45.00*

296 pages Year Founded: 1997 ISBN
0-881632-74-0

2891 Psychiatry in the New Millennium

American Psychiatric Publishing
1000 Wilson Boulevard
Suite 1825
                                    703-907-7322
                                    800-368-5777
                          Fax: 703-907-1091
          E-mail: appi@psych.org
                www.appi.org

Katie Duffy, Marketing Assistant

Keeping the standards and utilizing advances in diagnosis and treatment. *$66.50*

352 pages Year Founded: 1999 ISBN
0-880489-38-3

2892 Psychoanalysis, Behavior Therapy & the Relational World

American Psychological Association
750 1st St NE
Washington, DC 20002-4241   202-336-5647
                          Fax: 202-216-7610
                www.apa.org

Carolyn Valliere, Marketing Specialist

2893 Psychoanalytic Therapy as Health Care Effectiveness and Economics in the 21st Century

Analytic Press
101 W Street
Hillsdale, NJ 07642-1421   201-358-9477
                                    800-926-6579
                          Fax: 201-358-4700
          E-mail: TAP@analyticpress.com
                www.analyticpress.com

Paul E Stepansky PhD, Managing Director
John Kerr PhD, Sr Editor

Drawing on a wide range of clinical and empirical evidence, authors argue that contemporary psychoanalytic approaches are applicable to seriously distressed persons in a variety of treatment contexts. Failure to include such long term therapies within health care delivery systems, they conclude, will deprive many patients of help they need, and help from which they can benefit in enduring ways that far transcend the limited treatment goals of managed care. Available in hardcover. *$49.95*

312 pages Year Founded: 1999 ISBN
0-881632-02-3

2894 Psychologists' Desk Reference

Oxford University Press/Oxford Reference Book Society
198 Madison Avenue
New York, NY 10016   212-726-6000
                             800-451-7556
                   Fax: 919-677-1303
                www.oup-usa.org/orbs/

For the practicing psychologist; easily accessible, current information on almost any topic by some of the leading thinkers and innovators in the field. *$65.00*

672 pages Year Founded: 1998 ISBN
0-195111-86-9

2895 Psychoneuroendocrinology: The Scientific Basis of Clinical Practice

American Psychiatric Publishing
1000 Wilson Boulevard
Suite 1825
Arlington, VA 22209-3901   703-907-7322
                                    800-368-5777
                          Fax: 703-907-1091
          E-mail: appi@psych.org
                www.appi.org

Applications of scientific research.

752 pages Year Founded: 2003 ISBN
0-880488-57-3

2896 Psychopharmacology Desktop Reference

Manisses Communications Group
208 Governor Street
Providence, RI 02906   401-831-6020
                               800-333-7771
                     Fax: 401-861-6370
          E-mail: manissescs@manisses.com
                www.manisses.com

Karienne Stovell, Editor

Covers medications for all types of mental disorders. Provides detailed information on all the latest drugs as well as colored photographs of the different kinds of drugs. Helps you spot side effects and avoid drug interactions. Includes revealing case studies and outcomes data. *$159.00*

ISBN 1-864937-69-1

2897 Psychopharmacology Update

Manisses Communications Group
208 Governor Street
Providence, RI 02906   401-831-6020
                             800-333-7771
                        Fax: 401-861-6370
          E-mail: manissescs@manisses.com
                        www.manisses.com

Karienne Stovell, Editor

Offers psychopharmacology advice for general practitioners and nonprescribing professionals in the mental health field. Covers child psychopharmacology and street drugs. Contains case reports. Recurring features include news of research and book reviews. *$147.00*

12 per year   ISSN 1068-5308

2898 Psychotherapist's Duty to Warn or Protect

Charles C Thomas Publisher
2600 S 1st Street
Springfield, IL 62704-4730   217-789-8980
                               800-258-8980
                          Fax: 217-789-9130
          E-mail: books@ccthomas.com
                        www.ccthomas.com

Alan R Felthous, Author

$47.95

194 pages Year Founded: 1989 ISBN 0-398055-46-7

2899 Psychotherapist's Guide to Cost Containment: How to Survive and Thrive in an Age of Managed Care

Sage Publications
2455 Teller Road
Thousand Oaks, CA 91320   805-499-9774
                               800-818-7243
                          Fax: 800-583-2665
          E-mail: info@sagepub.com
                        www.sagepub.com

$23.50

Year Founded: 1998 ISBN 0-803973-81-0

2900 Psychotherapy Indications and Outcomes

American Psychiatric Publishing
1000 Wilson Boulevard
Suite 1825
Arlington, VA 22209-3901   703-907-7322
                               800-368-5777
                          Fax: 703-907-1091
          E-mail: appi@psych.org
                        www.appi.org

Katie Duffy, Marketing Assistant

Clinical approaches to different symptoms. *$66.50*

416 pages Year Founded: 1999 ISBN 0-880487-61-5

2901 Quality of Life: Volume II

AAMR
444 N Capitol Street NW
Suite 846
Washington, DC 20001-1512   202-387-1968
                               800-424-3688
                          Fax: 202-387-2193
          E-mail: dcroser@aamr.org
                        www.aamr.org

Focuses on how the concepts and research on quality of life can be applied to people with mental retardation. *$19.95*

267 pages ISBN 0-940898-41-1

2902 Questions of Competence

Cambridge University Press
40 W 20th Street
New York, NY 10011-4221   212-924-3900
                          Fax: 212-691-3239
          E-mail: marketing@cup.org
                        www.cup.org

2903 Reaching Out in Family Therapy: Home Based, School, and Community Interventions

Guilford Publications
72 Spring Street
New York, NY 10012   212-431-9800
                               800-365-7006
                          Fax: 212-966-6708
          E-mail: info@guilford.com
                        www.guilford.com

Practical framework for clinicians using multisystems intervention. *$27.00*

244 pages Year Founded: 2000 ISBN 1-572305-19-3

2904 Recognition and Treatment of Psychiatric Disorders: Psychopharmacology Handbook for Primary Care

American Medical Association
515 N State Street
Chicago, IL 60610-4325   312-464-5000
                               800-621-8335
                          Fax: 312-464-5600
          E-mail: apsychmed@aol.com
                        www.ama-assn.org

Provides the primary care physician with practical and timely strategies for screening and treating patients who have psychiatric disorders. Includes an overview of the epidemiology, pathophysiology, presentation, diagnostic criteria and screening tests for common psychiatric disorders including anxiety, mood, substance abuse, somatization and eating disorders, as well as insomnia, dementia and schizophrenia. *$35.00*

324 pages

2905 Recognition of Early Psychosis

Cambridge University Press
40 W 20th Street
New York, NY 10011-4221   212-924-3900
                                 Fax: 212-691-3239
                     E-mail: marketing@cup.org
                                 www.cup.org

2906 Review of Psychiatry

American Psychiatric Publishing
1000 Wilson Boulevard
Suite 1825
Arlington, VA 22209-3901   703-907-7322
                                 800-368-5777
                     Fax: 703-907-1091
                     E-mail: appi@psych.org
                                 www.appi.org

Katie Duffy, Marketing Assistant

Cognitive therapy, repressed memories and obsessive-compulsive disorder across the life cycle. *$59.95*

928 pages Year Founded: 1997 ISBN 0-880484-43-8

2907 Sandplay Therapy: Step By Step Manual for Physchotherapists of Diverse Orientations

WW Norton & Company
500 5th Avenue
New York, NY 10110   212-790-9456
                                 Fax: 212-869-0856
                E-mail: admalmud@wwnorton.com
                                 www.wwnorton.com

Change often occurs on a non-verbal level. This book is for psychotherapists with alternative methods. *$35.00*

256 pages Year Founded: 2000 ISSN 70319-3

2908 Selecting Effective Treatments: a Comprehensive, Systematic, Guide for Treating Mental Disorders

Jossey-Bass Publishers
350 Sansome Street
5th Floor
San Francisco, CA 94104
                                 800-956-7739
                     Fax: 800-605-2665
                     www.josseybass.com

$39.95

416 pages Year Founded: 1998 ISBN 0-787943-07-X

2909 Social Work Dictionary

National Association of Social Workers
750 1st Street NE
Suite 700
Washington, DC 20002-4241   202-408-8600
                                 800-638-8799
                     Fax: 202-336-8312
                     E-mail: press@naswdc.org
                                 www.naswpress.org

Paula Delo, Executive Editor, NASW Press

More than 8,000 terms are defined in this essential tool for understanding the language of social work and related disciplines. The resulting reference is a must for every human services professional. *$34.95*

620 pages Year Founded: 1999 ISBN 0-871012-98-7

2910 Strategic Marketing: How to Achieve Independence and Prosperity in Your Mental Health Practice

Professional Resource Press
PO Box 15560
Sarasota, FL 34277-1560   941-343-9601
                                 800-443-3364
                     Fax: 941-343-9201
                E-mail: orders@prpress.com
                                 www.prpress.com

Debra Fink, Managing Editor

Presents ways to reshape your practice to capitalize on new opportunities for success in today's healthcare marketplace. *$21.95*

152 pages Year Founded: 1997 ISBN 1-568870-31-0

2911 Supports Intensity Scale

AAMR
444 N Capitol Street NW
Suite 846
Washington, DC 20001-1512   202-387-1968
                                 800-424-3688
                     Fax: 202-387-2193
                E-mail: dcroser@aamr.org
                                 www.aamr.org

Designed to help you plan meaningful supports for adults with mental retardation. Consists of a comprehensive scoring system that measures the needs of persons with mental retardation in 57 key life activities based on 7 areas of competence. *$125.00*

128 pages

2912 Surviving & Prospering in the Managed Mental Health Care Marketplace

Professional Resource Press
PO Box 15560
Sarasota, FL 34277-1560   941-343-9601
                                 800-443-3364
                     Fax: 941-343-9201
                E-mail: orders@prpress.com
                                 www.prpress.com

Debra Fink, Managing Editor

Includes examples of different managed care models, extensive references, and checklists. Offers examples of the typical steps in providing outpatient treatment in a managed care milieu, and other extremely useful resources. *$14.95*

106 pages Year Founded: 1994 ISBN 1-568870-04-3

2913 Suzie Brown Intervention Maze: Training Tool for Staff Working with People with Developmental Disabilities who Have Challenging Needs

High Tide Press
3650 W 183rd Street
Homewood, IL 60430　　　　708-206-2054
　　　　　　　　　　　　　888-487-7377
　　　　　　　　Fax: 708-206-2044
E-mail: managing.editor@hightidepress.com
　　　　　　www.hightidepress.com

Diane J Bell, Managing Editor

Suzie Brown, age 25, has severe developmental disabilities. She lives in a staffed house for six adults, where you work as a team. She has major communication difficulties, is prone to self-injurious behavior, and no longer responds to all the usual calming methods. What can you do? This workbook offers a practical blueprint for group decision making. Each option page presents a new scenario and ideas for moving forward. Decision logs keep track of decisions as they are made. The binder format allows for easy photocopying. *$69.99*

ISBN 1-892696-09-6

2914 Teaching Buddy Skills to Preschoolers

AAMR
444 N Capitol Street NW
Suite 846
Washington, DC 20001-1512　　　202-387-1968
　　　　　　　　　　　　　　　800-424-3688
　　　　　　　　　Fax: 202-387-2193
　　　　　　E-mail: dcroser@aamr.org
　　　　　　　　　www.aamr.org

Shows how the rewards of social interactions must outweigh the costs to encouraging friendships between pre-schoolers with and without disabilities. *$12.95*

40 pages　ISBN 0-940898-45-4

2915 Teaching Goal Setting and Decision-Making to Students with Developmental Disabilities

AAMR
444 N Capitol Street NW
Suite 846
Washington, DC 20001-1512　　　202-387-1968
　　　　　　　　　　　　　　　800-424-3688
　　　　　　　　　Fax: 202-387-2193
　　　　　　E-mail: dcroser@aamr.org
　　　　　　　　　www.aamr.org

Link four basic steps of goal setting and decision making to twelve instructional principles that engage students in activities. *$12.95*

34 pages　ISBN 0-940898-97-7

2916 Teaching Practical Communication Skills

AAMR
444 N Capitol Street NW
Suite 846
Washington, DC 20001-1512　　　202-387-1968
　　　　　　　　　　　　　　　800-424-3688
　　　　　　　　Fax: 202-387-2193
　　　　　　E-mail: dcroser@aamr.org
　　　　　　　　　www.aamr.org

Discusses strategies for teaching students to request their preferences, protest non-preferred activities, and clarify misunderstandings. *$12.95*

30 pages　ISBN 0-940898-42-X

2917 Teaching Problem Solving to Students with Mental Retardation

AAMR
444 N Capitol Street NW
Suite 846
Washington, DC 20001-1512　　　202-387-1968
　　　　　　　　　　　　　　　800-424-3688
　　　　　　　　Fax: 202-387-2193
　　　　　　E-mail: dcroser@aamr.org
　　　　　　　　　www.aamr.org

Gives clear teaching strategies for social problem-solving, including role-playing, modeling, and training sequences. *$12.95*

30 pages　ISBN 0-940898-62-4

2918 Teaching Self-Management to Elementary Students with Developmental Disabilities

AAMR
444 N Capitol Street NW
Suite 846
Washington, DC 20001-1512　　　202-387-1968
　　　　　　　　　　　　　　　800-424-3688
　　　　　　　　Fax: 202-387-2193
　　　　　　E-mail: dcroser@aamr.org
　　　　　　　　　www.aamr.org

This book will help you design and implement self-management systems for elementary students with disabilities including self-monitoring and self-evaluation. *$12.95*

51 pages　ISBN 0-940898-48-9

2919 Teaching Students with Severe Disabilities in Inclusive Settings

AAMR
444 N Capitol Street NW
Suite 846
Washington, DC 20001-1512　　　202-387-1968
　　　　　　　　　　　　　　　800-424-3688
　　　　　　　　Fax: 202-387-2193
　　　　　　E-mail: dcroser@aamr.org
　　　　　　　　　www.aamr.org

Presents student-specific strategies for teaching students with severe disabilities in inclusive settings. Strategies include how to write IEPs in inclusive settings; effective scheduling; planning for adaptations of objectives; materials, responses, and settings; and anticipating the need for support. *$12.95*

50 pages　ISBN 0-940898-49-7

2920 Textbook of Family and Couples Therapy: Clinical Applications

American Psychiatric Publishing
1000 Wilson Boulevard
Suite 1825
Arlington, VA 22209-3901   703-907-7322
                                  800-368-5777
                          Fax: 703-907-1091
                    E-mail: appi@psych.org
                                 www.appi.org

Blending theoretical training and up-to-date clinical strategies. It's a must for clinicians who are currently treating couples and families, a major resource for training future clinicians in these highly effective therapeutic techniques. *$63.00*

448 pages Year Founded: 2002 ISBN 0-880485-18-3

2921 Theory and Technique of Family Therapy

Charles C Thomas Publisher
2600 S 1st Street
Springfield, IL 62704-4730   217-789-8980
                                    800-258-8980
                            Fax: 217-789-9130
                    E-mail: books@ccthomas.com
                                www.ccthomas.com

Charles P Barnard, Author
Ramon Garrido Corrales, Author

Contents: The Family as an Interactional System; The Family as an Intergenerational System; A Model for the Therapeutic Relationship in Family Theory, The Therapeutic Process and Related Concerns; Therapeutic Intervention Techniques and Adjuncts; Marital Group and Multiple Family Therapy; Counseling at Two Critical Stages of Family Development, Formation and Termination of Marriage. Useful information for students and practitioners of family therapy, social workers, the clergy, psychiatrists, psychologists, counselors, and related professionals. *$55.95*

352 pages Year Founded: 1981 ISBN 0-398038-59-7

2922 Thesaurus of Psychological Index Terms

American Psychological Association Database Department/PsycINFO
750 1st Street NE
Washington, DC 20002-4241   202-336-5650
                                   800-374-2722
                           Fax: 202-336-5633
                           TDD: 202-336-6123
                    E-mail: psycinfo@apa.org
                          www.apa.org/psycinfo

Reference to the PsycINFO database vocabulary of over 5,400 descriptors. Provides standardized working to represent each concept for complete, efficient and precise retrieval of psychological information and is updated regularly. 9th edition published 2001. *$60.00*

379 pages ISBN 1-557987-75-0

2923 Three Spheres: Psychiatric Interviewing Primer

Rapid Psychler Press
3560 Pine Grove Avenue
Suite 374
Port Huron, MI 48060   519-433-7642
                              888-779-2453
                      Fax: 888-779-2457
                E-mail: rapid@psychler.com
                          www.psychler.com

David Robinson, Publisher

$16.95

ISBN 0-968032-49-4

2924 Through the Patient's Eyes

Jossey-Bass Publishers
350 Sansome Street
5th Floor
San Francisco, CA 94104   415-394-8677
                                 800-956-7739
                         Fax: 800-605-2665
                            www.josseybass.com

Jennifer Daley, Editor
Thomas Delbanco, Editor

Learn how providers can improve their ability to meet patient's needs and enhance the quality of care by bringing the patient's perspective to the design and delivery of health services. *$36.95*

347 pages ISBN 7-555425-44-5

2925 Total Quality Management in Mental Health and Mental Retardation

AAMR
444 N Capitol Street NW
Suite 846
Washington, DC 20001-1512   202-387-1968
                                   800-424-3688
                           Fax: 202-387-2193
                    E-mail: dcroser@aamr.org
                                 www.aamr.org

Describes how this leadership philosophy helps an organization identify and achive quality outcomes for all its cistomers. *$14.95*

64 pages ISBN 0-940898-67-5

2926 Training Families to do a Successful Intervention: a Professional's Guide

Hazelden
15251 Pleasant Valley Road
PO Box 176
Center City, MN 55012-0176   651-213-2121
                                    800-328-9000
                            Fax: 651-213-4590
                              www.hazelden.org

Helps professionals explain basic intervention concepts and give clients step-by-step instructions. *$15.95*

152 pages ISBN 1-562461-16-8

2927 Transition Matters-From School to Independence

Resources for Children with Special Needs
116 E 16th Street
5th Floor
New York, NY 10003   212-677-4650
                           Fax: 212-254-4070
                    E-mail: info@resourcenyc.org
                           www.resourcenyc.org

This new guide and directory to the transition from school to adult life for youth with disabilities takes you through the systems involved and covers rights, entitlements, options, and programs. More than 1000 organization descriptions cover college, specialized education, job training, supported work, indpendent living and much more. In collaboration with New York Lawyers for the Public Interest. *$35.00*

ISBN 0-967836-56-5

2928 Treating Complex Cases: Cognitive Behavioral Therapy Approach

John Wiley & Sons
605 3rd Avenue
New York, NY 10058-0180   212-850-6000
                           Fax: 212-850-6008
                    E-mail: info@wiley.com
                           www.wiley.com

Amy Bazarnik, Conventions Coordinator

2929 Treatment of Complicated Mourning

Research Press
Dept 24 W
PO Box 9177
Champaign, IL 61826   217-352-3273
                           800-519-2707
                    Fax: 217-352-1221
                E-mail: rp@researchpress.com
                       www.researchpress.com

Russell Pense, VP Marketing

This is the first book to focus specifically on complicated mourning, often referred to as pathological, unresolved or abnormal grief. It provides caregivers with practical therapeutic strategies and specific interventions that are necessary when traditional grief counseling is insufficient. The author provides critically important information on the prediction, identification, assessment, classification and treatment of complicated mourning. *$39.95*

768 pages ISBN 0-878223-29-0

2930 Treatments of Psychiatric Disorders

American Psychiatric Publishing
1000 Wilson Boulevard
Suite 1825
Arlington, VA 22209-3901   703-907-7322
                           800-368-5777
                    Fax: 703-907-1091
                E-mail: appi@psych.org
                       www.appi.org

Katie Duffy, Marketing Assistant

Examines customary approaches to the major psychiatric disorders. Diagnostic, etiologic and therapeutic issues are clearly addressed by experts on each topic. *$307.00*

2800 pages Year Founded: 1995 ISBN 0-880487-00-3

2931 Values Clarification for Counselors: How Counselors, Social Workers, Psychologists, and Other Human Service Workers Can Use Available Techniques

Charles C Thomas Publisher
2600 S 1st Street
Springfield, IL 62704-4730   217-789-8980
                           800-258-8980
                    Fax: 217-789-9130
                E-mail: books@ccthomas.com
                       www.ccthomas.com

Gordon M Hart, Author

$24.95

104 pages Year Founded: 1978 ISBN 0-398038-47-3

2932 What Psychotherapists Should Know About Disability

Guilford Publications
72 Spring Street
New York, NY 10012   212-431-9800
                           800-365-7006
                    Fax: 212-966-6708
                E-mail: info@guilford.com
                       www.guilford.com

Available in alternate formats for people with disabilities, this guide confronts biases and relates the human dimesions of disability. Stereotypes and discomfort can get in the way of even a well intentioned therapist, this helps achieve a clearer professional relationship with clients of special need. *$35.00*

368 pages Year Founded: 1999 ISBN 1-572302-27-5

2933 Where to Start and What to Ask: Assessment Handbook

WW Norton & Company
500 5th Avenue
New York, NY 10110   212-790-9456
                           Fax: 212-869-0856
                E-mail: admalmud@wwnorton.com
                       www.wwnorton.com

Framework for gathering information from the client and using that information to formulate an accurate assessment. *$15.95*

Year Founded: 1993 ISSN 70152-2

2934 Women's Mental Health Services: Public Health Perspecitive

Sage Publications
2455 Teller Road
Thousand Oaks, CA 91320   805-499-9774
                                 800-818-7243
                            Fax: 800-583-2665
              E-mail: info@sagepub.com
                      www.sagepub.com

Paperback, hardcover also available. *$29.95*

Year Founded: 1998 ISBN 0-761905-09-X

2935 Workbook: Mental Retardation

AAMR
444 N Capitol Street NW
Suite 846
Washington, DC 20001-1512   202-387-1968
                                   800-424-3688
                              Fax: 202-387-2193
                E-mail: dcroser@aamr.org
                        www.aamr.org

Presents key components from a practical point of view. *$29.95*

64 pages ISBN 0-940898-82-9

2936 Working with the Core Relationship Problem in Psychotherapy

Jossey-Bass Publishers
350 Sansome Street
5th Floor
San Francisco, CA 94104   415-394-8677
                                 800-956-7739
                            Fax: 800-605-2665
                      www.josseybass.com

Learn to reveal, understand, and use the core relationship problem, which is formed from earliest childhood and creates an image of the self in relation to others so it can aid in understanding the underlying conflict that repeatedly plays out in a client's behavior. *$39.95*

256 pages ISBN 0-787943-01-0

2937 Writing Behavioral Contracts: A Case Simulation Practice Manual

Research Press
Dept 24 W
PO Box 9177
Champaign, IL 61826   217-352-3273
                             800-519-2707
                        Fax: 217-352-1221
          E-mail: rp@researchpress.com
                  www.researchpress.com

Russell Pense, VP Marketing

The most difficult aspect of using contingency contracting is designing a contract acceptable to and appropriate for all involved parties. This unusually versatile book improves contract-writing skills through practice with typical cases. Valuable for social workers, mental health professionals and educators. *$10.95*

94 pages ISBN 0-878221-23-9

2938 Writing Psychological Reports: a Guide for Clinicians

Professional Resource Press
PO Box 15560
Sarasota, FL 34277-1560   941-343-9601
                                 800-443-3364
                            Fax: 941-343-9201
              E-mail: orders@prpress.com
                      www.prpress.com

Debra Fink, Managing Editor

Presents widely accepted structured format for writing psychological reports. Numerous useful suggestions for experienced clinicians, and qualifies as essential reading for all clinical psychology students. *$15.95*

128 pages Year Founded: 1993 ISBN 0-943158-93-1

Adjustment Disorders

2939 Ambiguous Loss: Learning to Live with Unresolved Grief

Harvard University Press
79 Garden Street
Cambridge, MA 02138   800-405-1619
                        Fax: 800-406-9145
          E-mail: CONTACT_HUP@harvard.edu
                  www.hup.harvard.edu

$22.00

192 pages Year Founded: 1999 ISBN 0-674017-38-2

2940 Attachment and Interaction

Jessica Kingsley
47 Runway Drive
Suite G
Levittown, PA 19057-4738   215-269-0400
                             Fax: 215-269-0363
                  www.taylorandfrancis.com

Available in paperback. *$29.95*

238 pages Year Founded: 1998 ISBN 1-853025-86-0

2941 Body Image: Understanding Body Dissatisfaction in Men, Women and Children

Routledge
2727 Palisade Avenue
Suite 4H
Bronx, NY 10463-1020   718-796-0971
                         Fax: 718-796-0971
               www.vdg@columbia.edu

$75.00

208 pages Year Founded: 1998 ISBN 0-415147-84-0

Alcohol Abuse & Dependence

2942 An Elephant in the Living Room: Leader's Guide for Helping Children of Alcoholics

Hazelden
15251 Pleasant Valley Road
PO Box 176
Center City, MN 55012-0176   651-213-2121
800-328-9000
Fax: 651-213-4590
www.hazelden.org

Marion H Typpo PhD, Co-Author
Jill M Hastings PhD, Co-Author

Practical guidance for education and health professionals who help young people cope with a family member's chemical dependency. *$9.95*

129 pages ISBN 1-568380-34-8

2943 Narrative Means to Sober Ends: Treating Addiction and Its Aftermath

Guilford Publications
72 Spring Street
New York, NY 10012   212-431-9800
800-365-7006
Fax: 212-966-6708
E-mail: info@guilford.com
www.guilford.com

This eloquently written volume illuminates the devastating power of addiction and describes an array of innovative approaches to facilitating clients' recovery. Demonstrated are creative ways to help clients explore their relationship to drugs and alcohol, take the first steps toward sobriety and develop meaningful ways of living without addiction. *$37.95*

386 pages ISBN 1-572305-66-5

2944 Psychological Theories of Drinking and Alcoholism

Guilford Publications
72 Spring Street
New York, NY 10012   212-431-9800
800-365-7006
Fax: 212-966-6708
E-mail: info@guilford.com
www.guilford.com

Multidisciplinary approach discusses biological, pharmacological and social factors that influence drinking and alcoholism. Contributors review established and emerging approaches that guide research into the psychological processes influencing drinking and alcoholism. *$47.95*

460 pages Year Founded: 1999 ISBN 1-572304-10-3

2945 Relapse Prevention Maintenance: Strategies in the Treatment of Addictive Behaviors

Guilford Publications
72 Spring Street
New York, NY 10012   212-431-9800
800-365-7006
Fax: 212-966-6708
E-mail: info@guilford.com
www.guilford.com

Research on relapse prevention to problem drinking, smoking, substance abuse, eating disorders and compulsive gambling. Analyzes factors that may lead to relapse and offers practical techniques for maintaining treatment gains. *$55.00*

558 pages Year Founded: 1985 ISBN 0-898620-09-0

2946 Treating the Alcoholic: Developmental Model of Recovery

John Wiley & Sons
605 3rd Avenue
New York, NY 10058-0180   212-850-6000
Fax: 212-850-6008
E-mail: info@wiley.com
www.wiley.com

376 pages Year Founded: 1985

Anxiety Disorders

2947 Anxiety Disorders: a Scientific Approach for Selecting the Most Effective Treatment

Professional Resource Press
PO Box 15560
Sarasota, FL 34277-1560   941-343-9601
800-443-3364
Fax: 941-343-9201
E-mail: orders@prpress.com
www.prpress.com

Debra Fink, Managing Editor

Presents descriptive and empirical information on the differential diagnosis of DSM-IV and DSM-III-R categories of anxiety disorders. Explicit decision rules are provided for developing treatment plans based on both scientific research and clinical judgement. *$13.95*

114 pages Year Founded: 1994 ISBN 1-568870-00-0

2948 Applied Relaxation Training in the Treatment of PTSD and Other Anxiety Disorders

New Harbinger Publications
5674 Shattuck Avenue
Oakland, CA 94609-1662   510-652-2002
800-748-6273
Fax: 510-652-5472
E-mail: customerservice@newharbinger.com
www.newharbinger.com

Comes with a one hundred five minute video tape and a 52 page paperback manual. *$100.00*

Year Founded: 1998 ISBN 1-889287-08-3

2949 Assimilation, Rational Thinking, and Suppression in the Treatment of PTSD and Other Anxiety Disorders

New Harbinger Publications
5674 Shattuck Avenue
Oakland, CA 94609-1662   510-652-2002
                                   800-748-6273
                    Fax: 510-652-5472
    E-mail: customerservice@newharbinger.com
                    www.newharbinger.com

Comes with two videotapes and a ninety four page paperback manual. *$150.00*

Year Founded: 1998 ISBN 1-889287-06-7

2950 Client's Manual for the Cognitive Behavioral Treatment of Anxiety Disorders

New Harbinger Publications
5674 Shattuck Avenue
Oakland, CA 94609-1662   510-652-2002
                                   800-748-6273
                    Fax: 510-652-5472
    E-mail: customerservice@newharbinger.com
                    www.newharbinger.com

$10.00

106 pages Year Founded: 1994 ISBN 1-889287-99-7

2951 Cognitive Therapy

American Psychiatric Publishing
1000 Wilson Boulevard
Suite 1825
Arlington, VA 22209-3901   703-907-7322
                                     800-368-5777
                      Fax: 703-907-1091
          E-mail: appi@psych.org
                          www.appi.org

Katie Duffy, Marketing Assistant

Cognitive therapy for anxiety, substance abuse, personality, eating and mental disorders. *$37.50*

176 pages Year Founded: 1997 ISBN 0-880484-45-4

2952 Gender Differences in Mood and Anxiety Disorders: From Bench to Bedside

American Psychiatric Publishing
1000 Wilson Boulevard
Suite 1825
Arlington, VA 22209-3901   703-907-7322
                                     800-368-5777
                      Fax: 703-907-1091
          E-mail: appi@psych.org
                          www.appi.org

Katie Duffy, Marketing Assistant

Gender differences in neuroimaging. Discusses women, stress and depression, sex differences in hypothalamic-pituitary-adrenal axis regulation, modulation of anxiety by reproductive hormones. Questions if hormone replacement and oral contraceptive therapy induce or treat mood symptoms. *$37.50*

224 pages Year Founded: 1999 ISBN 0-880489-58-8

2953 Generalized Anxiety Disorder: Diagnosis, Treatment and Its Relationship to Other Anxiety Disorders

American Psychiatric Publishing
1000 Wilson Boulevard
Suite 1825
Arlington, VA 22209-3901   703-907-7322
                                     800-368-5777
                      Fax: 703-907-1091
          E-mail: appi@psych.org
                          www.appi.org

Katie Duffy, Marketing Assistant

Historical introduction, diagnosis, classification and differential diagnosis. Relationship with depression, panic and OCD. Treatments. *$74.95*

96 pages Year Founded: 1998 ISBN 1-853176-59-1

2954 Integrative Treatment of Anxiety Disorders

American Psychiatric Publishing
1000 Wilson Boulevard
Suite 1825
Arlington, VA 22209-3901   703-907-7322
                                     800-368-5777
                      Fax: 703-907-1091
          E-mail: appi@psych.org
                          www.appi.org

Katie Duffy, Marketing Assistant

Up-to-date look at combined pharmacotherapy and cognitive behavioral therapy in the treatment of anxiety disorders. *$41.50*

320 pages Year Founded: 1995 ISBN 0-880487-15-1

2955 Long-Term Treatments of Anxiety Disorders

American Psychiatric Publishing
1000 Wilson Boulevard
Suite 1825
Arlington, VA 22209-3901   703-907-7322
                                     800-368-5777
                      Fax: 703-907-1091
          E-mail: appi@psych.org
                          www.appi.org

Katie Duffy, Marketing Assistant

Treatment of anxiety disorders encapsulating important advances made over the past two decades. *$56.00*

464 pages Year Founded: 1996 ISBN 0-880486-56-2

2956 Overcoming Agoraphobia and Panic Disorder

New Harbinger Publications
5674 Shattuck Avenue
Oakland, CA 94609-1662
510-652-2002
800-748-6273
Fax: 510-652-5472
E-mail: customerservice@newharbinger.com
www.newharbinger.com

A twelve to sixteen session treatment. *$11.95*

88 pages Year Founded: 1998 ISBN 1-572241-46-2

2957 Panic Disorder: Clinical Diagnosis, Management and Mechanisms

American Psychiatric Publishing
1000 Wilson Boulevard
Suite 1825
Arlington, VA 22209-3901
703-907-7322
800-368-5777
Fax: 703-907-1091
E-mail: appi@psych.org
www.appi.org

Katie Duffy, Marketing Assistant

Novel and important new discoveries for biological research together with up to date information for the diagnosis and treatment for the practicing clinician. *$75.00*

264 pages Year Founded: 1998 ISBN 1-853175-18-8

2958 Panic Disorder: Theory, Research and Therapy

John Wiley & Sons
605 3rd Avenue
New York, NY 10058-0180
212-850-6000
Fax: 212-850-6008
E-mail: info@wiley.com
www.wiley.com

364 pages Year Founded: 1989

2959 Phobias: Handbook of Theory, Reseach and Treatment

John Wiley & Sons
605 3rd Avenue
New York, NY 10058-0180
212-850-6000
Fax: 212-850-6008
E-mail: info@wiley.com
www.wiley.com

Provides an up-to-date summary of current knowledge of phobias. Psychological treatments availible for specific phobias have been refined considerabley in recent years. This extensive handbook acknowledges these treatments and includes the description and nature of prevalent phobias, details of symptoms, prevalence rates, individual case histories, and a brief review of of our knowledge of the etiology of phobias.

470 pages Year Founded: 1995

2960 Practice Guideline for the Treatment of Patients with Panic Disorder

American Psychiatric Publishing
1000 Wilson Boulevard
Suite 1825
Arlington, VA 22209-3901
703-907-7322
800-368-5777
Fax: 703-907-1091
E-mail: appi@psych.org
www.appi.org

Katie Duffy, Marketing Assistant

Summarizes data, evaluation of the patient for coexisting mental disorders and issues specific to the treatment of panic disorders in children and adolescents. *$22.50*

160 pages Year Founded: 1998 ISBN 0-890423-11-3

2961 Shy Children, Phobic Adults: Nature and Trea tment of Social Phobia

American Psychiatric Publishing
1000 Wilson Boulevard
Suite 1825
Arlington, VA 22209-3901
703-907-7322
800-368-5777
Fax: 703-907-1091
E-mail: appi@psych.org
www.appi.org

Katie Duffy, Marketing Assistant

Describes the similiarities and differences in the syndrome across all ages. Draws from the clinical, social and developmental literatures, as well as from extensive clinical experience. Illustrates the impact of developmental stage on phenomenology, diagnoses and assessment and treatment of social phobia. *$39.95*

321 pages Year Founded: 1998 ISBN 1-557984-61-1

2962 Social Phobia: Clinical and Research Perspectives

American Psychiatric Publishing
1000 Wilson Boulevard
Suite 1825
Arlington, VA 22209-3901
703-907-7322
800-368-5777
Fax: 703-907-1091
E-mail: appi@psych.org
www.appi.org

Katie Duffy, Marketing Assistant

Comprehensive and practice guide for mental health professionals who encounter individuals with social phobia. *$48.00*

384 pages Year Founded: 1995 ISBN 0-880486-53-8

2963 Treating Anxiety Disorders

Jossey-Bass Publishers
350 Sansome Street
5th Floor
San Francisco, CA 94104
415-394-8677
800-956-7739
Fax: 800-605-2665
www.josseybass.com

$30.95

288 pages ISBN 0-787903-16-7

2964 Treating Anxiety Disorders with a Cognitive: Behavioral Exposure Based Approach and the Eye Movement Technique

New Harbinger Publications
5674 Shattuck Avenue
Oakland, CA 94609-1662   510-652-2002
                                 800-748-6273
                           Fax: 510-652-5472
E-mail: customerservice@newharbinger.com
                  www.newharbinger.com

Comes with a fifty eight minute videotape and a fifty one page paperback manual. *$100.00*

Year Founded: 1998 ISBN 1-889287-02-4

2965 Treating Panic Disorder and Agoraphobia: a Step by Step Clinical Guide

New Harbinger Publications
5674 Shattuck Avenue
Oakland, CA 94609-1662   510-652-2002
                                 800-748-6273
                           Fax: 510-652-5472
E-mail: customerservice@newharbinger.com
                  www.newharbinger.com

Treatment program covering breath control training, changing automatic thoughts and underlying beliefs. *$49.95*

296 pages Year Founded: 1997 ISBN 1-572240-84-9

ADHD

2966 ADHD in Adolesents: Diagnosis and Treatment

Guilford Publications
72 Spring Street
New York, NY 10012   212-431-9800
                                 800-365-7006
                           Fax: 212-966-6708
          E-mail: info@guilford.com
                  www.guilford.com

Practical reference with a down to earth approach to diagnosing and treatment of ADHD in adolesents. A structured intervention program with guidelines to using educational, psycholgical and medical components to help patients. Many reproducible handouts, checklists and rating scales. *$24.95*

461 pages Year Founded: 1999 ISBN 1-572305-45-2

2967 ADHD in Adulthood: Guide to Current Theory, Diagnosis and Treatment

Health Source
1404 K Street NW
Washington, DC 20005-2401   202-789-7303
                                     800-713-7122
                               Fax: 202-789-7899
          E-mail: healthsource@appi.org
                  www.healthsourcebooks.org

Discusses how ADHD manifests itself in adult life and answers popular questions posed by physicians and by adults with ADHD. Provides health professionals with a practical approach for treatment and diagnosis in adult ADHD patients. *$49.95*

392 pages Year Founded: 1999 ISBN 0-801861-41-1

2968 All About ADHD: Complete Practical Guide for Classroom Teachers

ADD WareHouse
300 NW 70th Avenue
Suite 102
Plantation, FL 33317   954-792-8100
                                   800-233-9273
                             Fax: 954-792-8545
          E-mail: sales@addwarehouse.com
                  www.addwarehouse.com

Brings together both the art and science of effective teaching for students with ADHD using the Parallel Teaching Model as the base for blending behavior management and teaching, particularly in regular classroom settings. Real-life examples are used throughout the book and are intended to help you design strategies for you own classrooms to help your students be the best they can be. *$17.00*

175 pages

2969 Attention Deficit Disorder ADHD and ADD Syndromes

Pro-Ed Publications
8700 Shoal Creek Boulevard
Austin, TX 78757-6816   512-451-3246
                                    800-897-3202
                              Fax: 800-397-7633
          E-mail: info@proedinc.com
                  www.proedinc.com

This book enters its third edition with even more complete explanations of how ADHD and ADD interfere with: classroom learning, behavior at home, job performance, and social skills development. *$19.00*

216 pages Year Founded: 1998 ISBN 0-890797-42-0

2970 Attention Deficit Disorder and Learning Disabilities: Realities, Myths and Controversial Treatments

ADD WareHouse
300 NW 70th Avenue
Suite 102
Plantation, FL 33317   954-792-8100
                                   800-233-9273
                             Fax: 954-792-8545
          E-mail: sales@addwarehouse.com
                  www.addwarehouse.com

Designed to help parents and professionals recognize symptoms of learning disabilities and attentional disorders. Covers in detail conventional treatments that have been scientifically validated plus more controversial methods of treatment such as orthomolecular therapies, amino acid supplementation, dietary interventions, EEG biofeedback, cognitive therapy and visual training. *$13.00*

240 pages

2971 Attention Deficit/Hyperactivity Disorder: Cl inical Guide to Diagnosis and Treatment for Health and Mental Health Professionals

American Psychiatric Publishing
1000 Wilson Boulevard
Suite 1825
Arlington, VA 22209-3901   **703-907-7322**
                              800-368-5777
                         Fax: 703-907-1091
                    E-mail: appi@psych.org
                              www.appi.org

Making the proper diagnosis, and treatment strategies. *$29.95*

298 pages Year Founded: 1999 ISBN 0-880489-40-5

2972 Attention-Deficit Hyperactivity Disorder: a Handbook for Diagnosis and Treatment

Guilford Publications
72 Spring Street
New York, NY 10012   **212-431-9800**
                              800-365-7006
                         Fax: 212-966-6708
                    E-mail: info@guilford.com
                              www.guilford.com

This second edition incorporated the latest finding on the nature, diagnosis, assessment and treatment of ADHD. Includes select chapters by seasoned colleagues covering their respective areas of expertise and providing clear guidelines for practice in clinical, school and community settings. *$56.95*

602 pages Year Founded: 1998 ISBN 1-572302-75-5

2973 Attention-Deficit/Hyperactivity Disorder in the Classroom

Pro-Ed Publications
8700 Shoal Creek Boulevard
Austin, TX 78757-6816   **512-451-3246**
                              800-897-3202
                         Fax: 800-397-7633
                    E-mail: info@proedinc.com
                              www.proedinc.com

Provides educators with a complete guide on how to deal effectively with students with attention deficits in their classroom. Emphasizes practical applications for teachers to use that will facilitate the success of students, both academically and socially, in a school setting. *$29.00*

291 pages Year Founded: 1998 ISBN 0-890796-65-3

2974 Complete Learning Disabilities Handbook

ADD WareHouse
300 NW 70th Avenue
Suite 102
Plantation, FL 33317   **954-792-8100**
                              800-233-9273
                         Fax: 954-792-8545
                    E-mail: sales@addwarehouse.com
                              www.addwarehouse.com

Provides a wealth of useful, practical suggestions and ready-to-use materials for meeting the special needs of students with learning disabilities and attention deficit disorders. Outlines an effective referral and identification process utilizing the concept of student study teams to provide data and formulate effective intervention strategies to assist the student in class. *$30.00*

206 pages

2975 Family Therapy for ADHD: Treating Children, Adolesents and Adults

Guilford Publications
72 Spring Street
New York, NY 10012   **212-431-9800**
                              800-365-7006
                         Fax: 212-966-6708
                    E-mail: info@guilford.com
                              www.guilford.com

ADHD affects the entire family. This book helps the clinician evaluate its impact on marital dynamics, parent/sibling/child relationships and the complex treatment of ADHD in a larger context. Includes session by session plans and clinical material. *$32.95*

270 pages Year Founded: 1999 ISBN 1-572304-38-3

2976 How to Operate an ADHD Clinic or Subspecialty Practice

ADD WareHouse
300 NW 70th Avenue
Suite 102
Plantation, FL 33317   **954-792-8100**
                              800-233-9273
                         Fax: 954-792-8545
                    E-mail: sales@addwarehouse.com
                              www.addwarehouse.com

This book goes beyond academic discussions of ADHD and gets down to how to establish and manage an ADHD practice. In addition to practice guidelines and suggestions, this guide presents a compendium of clinic forms and letters, interview formats, sample reports, tricks of the trade and resource listings, all of which will help you develop or refine your clinic/counseling operation. *$65.00*

325 pages

2977 Medications for Attention Disorders and Related Medical Problems: A Comprehensive Handbook

ADD WareHouse
300 NW 70th Avenue
Suite 102
Plantation, FL 33317
954-792-8100
800-233-9273
Fax: 954-792-8545
E-mail: sales@addwarehouse.com
www.addwarehouse.com

ADHD and ADD are medical conditions and often medical intervention is regarded by most experts as an essential component of the multimodal program for the treatment of these disorders. This text presents a comprehensive look at medications and their use in attention disorders. *$37.00*

420 pages

2978 Parenting a Child With Attention Deficit/Hyperactivity Disorder

Pro-Ed Publications
8700 Shoal Creek Boulevard
Austin, TX 78757-6816
512-451-3246
800-897-3202
Fax: 800-397-7633
E-mail: info@proedinc.com
www.proedinc.com

Offers proven parenting approaches for helping children between the ages of 5-11 years improve their behavior. *$29.00*

150 pages Year Founded: 1999 ISBN 0-890797-91-9

2979 Pretenders: Gifted People Who Have Difficulty Learning

High Tide Press
3650 W 183rd Street
Homewood, IL 60430
708-206-2054
888-487-7377
Fax: 708-206-2044
E-mail: managing.editor@hightidepress.com
www.hightidepress.com

Diane J Bell, Managing Editor

Profiles of 8 adults with dyslexia and/or ADD with whom the author has worked. Informative, facinating, at times heartbreaking, but ultimately inspiring. *$24.50*

177 pages ISBN 0-965374-41-6

Autistic Disorder

2980 Asperger Syndrome: a Practical Guide for Teachers

ADD WareHouse
300 NW 70th Avenue
Suite 102
Plantation, FL 33317
954-792-8100
800-233-9273
Fax: 954-792-8545
E-mail: sales@addwarehouse.com
www.addwarehouse.com

A clear and concise guide to effective classroom practice for teachers and support assistants working with children with Asperger Syndrome in school. The authors explain characteristics of children with Asperger Syndrome, discusse methods of assessment and offer practical strategies for effective classroom interventions. *$24.95*

90 pages

2981 Biological Treatments for Autism & PDD: What's Going On? What Can You Do About It?

Sunflower Publications

An authoritative, comprehensive, and easy-to-read resource guide to a wide range of therapies that have been useful in the treatment of autism including antifungal and antibacterial therapies, gluten and casein restriction, homeopathy, vitamin therapy, gamma globulin treatment, transfer factor therapies, treatment of food allergies, and alternatives to antibiotic therapy. Useful not only in the field of autism but also in virtually any disorder in which some of the symptons of autism are sometimes or frequently present. *$19.95*

303 pages Year Founded: 1998 ISBN 0-966123-80-8

Cognitive Disorders

2982 Cognitive-Behavioral Strategies in Crisis Intervention

Guilford Publications
72 Spring Street
New York, NY 10012
212-431-9800
800-365-7006
Fax: 212-966-6708
E-mail: info@guilford.com
www.guilford.com

This text brings together leading cognitive-behavioral practitioners to describe effective intervention for a broad crisis situations. Covers panic disorder, Cluster B personality disorders, suicidal depression, substance abuse, rape, sexual abuse, family crises, natural disasters, medical problems, problems of the elderly and much more. This book presents proven short-term approaches to helping patients weather the immediate crisis and build needed coping and problem-solving skills. *$46.95*

470 pages ISBN 1-572305-79-7

2983 Geriatric Mental Health Care: a Treatment Guide for Health Professionals

Guilford Publications
72 Spring Street
New York, NY 10012
212-431-9800
800-365-7006
Fax: 212-966-6708
E-mail: info@guilford.com
www.guilford.com

Designed for mental health practitioners and primary care providers without advanced training in geriatric psychiatry. Covers depression, anxiety, the dementias, psychosis, mania, sleep disturbances, personality and pain disorders, adapting principles, sexuality, elder issues, alcohol and substance abuse, suicide risk, consultation, legal and ethic issues, exercise and much more. *$39.00*

347 pages ISBN 1-572305-92-4

2984 Guidelines for the Treatment of Patients with Alzheimer's Disease and Other Dementias of Late Life

American Psychiatric Publishing
1000 Wilson Boulevard
Suite 1825
Arlington, VA 22209-3901   703-907-7322
                                  800-368-5777
                             Fax: 703-907-1091
                    E-mail: appi@psych.org
                                  www.appi.org

Katie Duffy, Marketing Assistant

Diagnosis and treatment strategies. *$22.50*

40 pages Year Founded: 1995 ISBN 0-890423-04-0

2985 Loss of Self: Family Resource for the Care of Alzheimer's Disease and Related Disorders

WW Norton & Company
500 5th Avenue
New York, NY 10110   212-790-9456
                      Fax: 212-869-0856
        E-mail: admalmud@wwnorton.com
                       www.wwnorton.com

How to help a relative and also meet a family's own needs during the long and tragic period of care involved with Alzheimer's Disease. Challenges are more than medical and can be emotional, involve family conflict, sexuality, abuse, and eventually, dealing with death. As well as the emotional challenges, the latest treatments, drugs and diagnosis information, plus causes and preventative measures are included. *$27.95*

432 pages Year Founded: 2001 ISBN 0-393050-16-5

2986 Neurobiology of Primary Dementia

American Psychiatric Publishing
1000 Wilson Boulevard
Suite 1825
Arlington, VA 22209-3901   703-907-7322
                                  800-368-5777
                             Fax: 703-907-1091
                    E-mail: appi@psych.org
                                  www.appi.org

Katie Duffy, Marketing Assistant

Study of aging and Alzheimer's. Contains investigations of the basic neurobiologic aspects of the etiology of dementia, clear discussions of the diagnostic process with regard to imaging and other laboratory tests, psychopharmacologic treatment and genetic counseling. *$61.50*

440 pages Year Founded: 1998 ISBN 0-880489-15-4

2987 Strange Behavior Tales of Evolutionary Nuerolgy

WW Norton & Company
500 5th Avenue
New York, NY 10110   212-790-9456
                      Fax: 212-869-0856
        E-mail: admalmud@wwnorton.com
                       www.wwnorton.com

Both educational and entertaining, the author presents an array of people with unusual problems who have one thing in common, brain disorder. Carefully constructed, this book outlines the functioning of the brain and evolution of language skills. *$13.95*

256 pages Year Founded: 2001 ISBN 0-393321-84-3

Conduct Disorder

2988 Behavioral Risk Management

Jossey-Bass Publishers
350 Sansome Street
5th Floor
San Francisco, CA 94104   415-394-8677
                                 800-956-7739
                            Fax: 800-605-2665
                             www.josseybass.com

Learn to identify potential mental health and behavioral problems on the job and apply effective intervention strategies for behavioral risk. *$41.95*

432 pages ISBN 0-787902-20-9

2989 Beyond Behavior Modification: Cognitive-Behavioral Approach to Behavior Management in the School

Pro-Ed Publications
8700 Shoal Creek Boulevard
Austin, TX 78757-6816   512-451-3246
                               800-897-3202
                          Fax: 800-397-7633
                 E-mail: info@proedinc.com
                               www.proedinc.com

Focuses on traditional behavior modification, and presents a social learning theory approach. *$39.00*

643 pages Year Founded: 1995 ISBN 0-890796-63-7

2990 Effective Discipline

Pro-Ed Publications
8700 Shoal Creek Boulevard
Austin, TX 78757-6816　　　　　512-451-3246
　　　　　　　　　　　　　　　800-897-3202
　　　　　　　　　　　　　Fax: 800-397-7633
　　　　　　　E-mail: info@proedinc.com
　　　　　　　　　　　　www.proedinc.com

Designed to provide principals, counselors, teachers, and college students preparing to become educators with information about research-based techniques that reduce or eliminate school behavior problems. Provides the knowledge to prevent discipline problems, identify specific behaviors that disrupt the environment, match interventions with behavioral infractions, implement a variety of intervention tactics, and evaluate the effectiveness of the intervention program. *$28.00*

220 pages Year Founded: 1993 ISBN 0-890795-79-7

2991 Helping Parents, Youth, and Teachers Understand Medications for Behavioral and Emotional Problems

American Psychiatric Press
1000 Wilson Boulevard
Suite 1825
Arlington, VA 22209-3901　　　　703-907-7322
　　　　　　　　　　　　　　　800-368-5777
　　　　　　　　　　　　　Fax: 703-907-1091
　　　　　　　E-mail: appi@psych.org
　　　　　　　　　　　　　www.appi.org

Katie Duffy, Marketing Assistant

Valuable resource for anyone involved in evaluating psychiatric disturbances in children and adolescents. Provides a compilation of information sheets to help promote the dialogue between the patient's family, caregivers and the treating physician. *$39.95*

196 pages Year Founded: 1999 ISBN 0-880487-94-1

2992 Inclusion Strategies for Students with Learning and Behavior Problems

Pro-Ed Publications
8700 Shoal Creek Boulevard
Austin, TX 78757-6816　　　　　512-451-3246
　　　　　　　　　　　　　　　800-897-3202
　　　　　　　　　　　　　Fax: 800-397-7633
　　　　　　　E-mail: info@proedinc.com
　　　　　　　　　　　　www.proedinc.com

Provides the components necessary to implement successful inclusion by presenting the experience of those directly impacted by inclusion: an individual with a disability; parents of a student with a disbility; teachers who implement inclusion; and researchers of best practices. Integrates theory and practice in an easy, how-to manner. *$36.00*

416 pages Year Founded: 1997 ISBN 0-890796-98-X

2993 Outrageous Behavior Mood: Handbook of Strategic Interventions for Managing Impossible Students

Pro-Ed Publications
8700 Shoal Creek Boulevard
Austin, TX 78757-6816　　　　　512-451-3246
　　　　　　　　　　　　　　　800-897-3202
　　　　　　　　　　　　　Fax: 800-397-7633
　　　　　　　E-mail: info@proedinc.com
　　　　　　　　　　　　www.proedinc.com

This handbook is for educators who have had success in managing difficult students. Introduces such methods as planned confusion, disruptive word pictures, unconscious suggestion, double-bind predictions, off the wall interpretations, and even some straight faced paradoxical assignments. *$26.00*

154 pages Year Founded: 1999 ISBN 0-890798-17-6

Depression

2994 A Woman Doctor's Guide to Depression: Essential Facts and Up-to-the-Minute Information on Diagnosis, Treatment, and Recovery

Hyperion

Includes information on what depression feels like and how it affects daily life, women's unique risks of developing depression throughout the life cycle from puberty to menopause and current treatment strategies and their risks and benefits, preventive measures and warning signs. *$9.95*

176 pages Year Founded: 1997 ISBN 0-786881-46-1

2995 Active Treatment of Depression

WW Norton & Company
500 5th Avenue
New York, NY 10110　　　　　212-790-9456
　　　　　　　　　　　　　Fax: 212-869-0856
　　　　　E-mail: admalmud@wwnorton.com
　　　　　　　　　　　　www.wwnorton.com

A candid discussion on depression and effective, hopeful therapy strategies. *$35.00*

272 pages Year Founded: 2001 ISSN 70322-3

2996 Anitdepressant Fact Book: What Your Doctor Won't Tell You About Prozac, Zoloft, Paxil, Celexa and Luvox

Perseus Books Group
550 Central Avenue
Boulder, CO 80301
　　　　　　　　　　　　　800-386-5656
　　　　　　　　　　　　Fax: 720-406-7336
　　E-mail: westview.orders@perseusbooks.com
　　　　　　　　www.perseusbooksgroup.com

What antidepressants will and won't treat, documented side and withdrawl effects, plus what parents need to know about teenagers and antidepressants. The author has been a medical expert in many cout cases involving the use and misuse of psychoactive drugs. *$13.00*

240 pages Year Founded: 2001 ISBN 0-738204-51-X

2997 Antipsychotic Medications: A Guide

Madison Institute of Medicine
7617 Mineral Point Road
Suite 300
Madison, WI 53717-1623   **608-827-2470**
Fax: 608-827-2479
E-mail: mim@miminc.org
www.miminc.org

A number of medications are available today to treat schizophrenia and other illnesses that may lead to psychotic behaviors. This concise guide covers antipsychotic medications available today and provides information about correct dosing and possible side effects. *$5.95*

39 pages

2998 Brief Therapy for Adolescent Depression

Professional Resource Press
PO Box 15560
Sarasota, FL 34277-1560   **941-343-9601**
800-443-3364
Fax: 941-343-9201
E-mail: orders@prpress.com
www.prpress.com

Debra Fink, Managing Editor

Useful book for practicing clinicians and advanced students interested in building new skills for working with depressed young people. Written from the perspective that adaptations of cognitive therapy are necessary when working with adolescents both because of the difference in thinking (relative verses absolute) between adults and adolescents, and because adolescents are deeply embedded in their families of origin and effective treatment rarely can be conducted without intervening with the family. Includes detailed clinical vignettes to illustrate key principles and techniques of this treatment model. *$13.95*

112 pages Year Founded: 1997 ISBN 1-568870-28-0

2999 Changing Lanes

Accent
PO Box 700
Bloomington, IL 61702-0700   **309-378-2961**
800-787-8444
Fax: 309-378-4420

A guide to help when aging, illness or disability forces us into the slow lane. Addressing such topics as grieving our losses, how to recognize depression, how to control our moods, overcome loneliness, appreciate life in the slow lane and more. *$6.50*

3000 Cognitive Therapy of Depression

Guilford Publications
72 Spring Street
New York, NY 10012   **212-431-9800**
800-365-7006
Fax: 212-966-6708
E-mail: info@guilford.com
www.guilford.com

Shows how psychotherapists can effectively treat depressive disorders. Case examples illustrate a wide range of strategies and techniques. Chapter topics include the role of emotions in cognitive therapy, application of behavioral techniques and cognitive therapy and antidepressant medications. Hardcover. Paperback also available. *$ 46.95*

425 pages Year Founded: 1979 ISBN 0-898620-00-7

3001 Concise Guide to Women's Mental Health

American Psychiatric Publishing
1000 Wilson Boulevard
Suite 1825
Arlington, VA 22209-3901   **703-907-7322**
800-368-5777
Fax: 703-907-1091
E-mail: appi@psych.org
www.appi.org

Katie Duffy, Marketing Assistant

Examines the biological, psychological, and sociocultural factors that influence a woman's mental health and often contribute to psychiatric disorders. Supplies clinicians with important information on gender related differences on differential diagnosis, case formulation and treatment planning. Topics include premenstrual dysphoric disorder, hormonal contraception and effects on mood, psychiatric disorders in pregnancy, postpartum psychiatric disorders and perimenopause and menopause. *$21.95*

187 pages Year Founded: 1997 ISBN 0-880483-43-1

3002 Depression & Antidepressants

Madison Institute of Medicine
7617 Mineral Point Road
Suite 300
Madison, WI 53717-1623   **608-827-2470**
Fax: 608-827-2479
E-mail: mim@miminc.org
www.miminc.org

A concise, up-to-date guide to the wide range of medications available today for the treatment of depression. *$5.95*

48 pages ISBN 1-890802-19-0

3003 Depression in Context: Strategies for Guided Action

WW Norton & Company
500 5th Avenue
New York, NY 10110   **212-790-9456**
Fax: 212-869-0856
E-mail: admalmud@wwnorton.com
www.wwnorton.com

Description of Behavioral Activation, a new treatment for Depression. *$32.00*

224 pages Year Founded: 2001 ISSN 70350-9

3004 Evaluation and Treatment of Postpartum Emotional Disorders

Professional Resource Press
PO Box 15560
Sarasota, FL 34277-1560　　　**941-343-9601**
　　　　　　　　　　　　　　　　　800-443-3364
　　　　　　　　　　　　　Fax: 941-343-9201
　　　　　　　E-mail: orders@prpress.com
　　　　　　　　　　　　www.prpress.com

Debra Fink, Managing Editor

Teaches how to recognize and treat postpartum emotional disorders. Procedures for clinical assessment, psychotherapeutic interventions, and medical - psychiatric treatments are described. *$ 13.95*

110 pages Year Founded: 1997 ISBN 1-568870-24-8

3005 Handbook of Depression

Guilford Publications
72 Spring Street
New York, NY 10012　　　　**212-431-9800**
　　　　　　　　　　　　　　　800-365-7006
　　　　　　　　　　　　Fax: 212-966-6708
　　　　　　　E-mail: info@guilford.com
　　　　　　　　　　www.guilford.com

Brings together well-known authorities who address the need for a comprehensive review of the most current information available on depression. Surveys current theories and treatment models, covering both what the MD and non-MD needs to know. *$65.00*

628 pages Year Founded: 1995 ISBN 0-898628-41-5

3006 Interpersonal Psychotherapy

American Psychiatric Publishing
1000 Wilson Boulevard
Suite 1825
Arlington, VA 22209-3901　　　**703-907-7322**
　　　　　　　　　　　　　　　800-368-5777
　　　　　　　　　　　　Fax: 703-907-1091
　　　　　　　E-mail: appi@psych.org
　　　　　　　　　　www.appi.org

Katie Duffy, Marketing Assistant

An overview of interpersonal psychotherapy for depression, preventative treatment for depression, bulimia nervosa and HIV positive men and women. *$26.00*

156 pages Year Founded: 1998 ISBN 0-880488-36-0

3007 Mother's Tears: Understanding the Mood Swings That Follow Childbirth

Seven Stories Press

A clinical psychologist specializing in mood disorders provides a primer on the causes and cures of postpartum depression, a common but long-overlooked illness. *$16.77*

256 pages Year Founded: 1998 ISBN 1-888363-70-3

3008 Postpartum Mood Disorders

American Psychiatric Publishing
1000 Wilson Boulevard
Suite 1825
Arlington, VA 22209-3901　　　**703-907-7322**
　　　　　　　　　　　　　　　800-368-5777
　　　　　　　　　　　　Fax: 703-907-1091
　　　　　　　E-mail: appi@psych.org
　　　　　　　　　　www.appi.org

Katie Duffy, Marketing Assistant

$38.50

280 pages Year Founded: 1999 ISBN 0-880489-29-4

3009 Premenstrual Dysphoric Disorder: A Guide

Madison Institute of Medicine
7617 Mineral Point Road
Suite 300
Madison, WI 53717-1623　　　**608-827-2470**
　　　　　　　　　　　　Fax: 608-827-2479
　　　　　　　E-mail: mim@miminc.org
　　　　　　　　　　www.miminc.org

This new 41 page booklet explains what Premenstrual Dysphoric Disorder (PMDD) is, how it is diagnosed, how it differs from PMS, and how it is treated. Anyone seeking information about PMDD and its treatments will find this concise guide of great benefit in their search for accurate, up-to-date information. *$5.95*

41 pages

3010 Scientific Foundations of Cognitive Theory and Therapy of Depression

John Wiley & Sons
605 3rd Avenue
New York, NY 10058-0180　　　**212-850-6000**
　　　　　　　　　　　　Fax: 212-850-6008
　　　　　　　E-mail: info@wiley.com
　　　　　　　　　　www.wiley.com

A synthesis of decades of research and practice, this semminal book presents and critically evaluates this scientific and emprical status of co author Aaron Beck's revised cognitive theory and therapy of depression. The authors explore the evolution of cognitive theory and therapy of depression and discuss the future directions for the treatment of depression.

400 pages Year Founded: 1999

3011 Symptoms of Depression

John Wiley & Sons
605 3rd Avenue
New York, NY 10058-0180　　　**212-850-6000**
　　　　　　　　　　　　Fax: 212-850-6008
　　　　　　　E-mail: info@wiley.com
　　　　　　　　　　www.wiley.com

336 pages Year Founded: 1993

3012 Treating Depressed Children: a Theraputic Manual of Proven Cognitive Behavioral Techniques

New Harbinger Publications
5674 Shattuck Avenue
Oakland, CA 94609-1662   **510-652-2002**
                                  800-748-6273
                        Fax: 510-652-5472
E-mail: customerservice@newharbinger.com
                        www.newharbinger.com

A full twelve session treatment program incorporates cartoons and role playing games to help children recognize emotions, change negative thoughts, gain confidence and learn crucial interpersonal skills. *$49.95*

160 pages Year Founded: 1996 ISBN 1-572240-61-X

3013 Treating Depression

Jossey-Bass Publishers
350 Sansome Street
5th Floor
San Francisco, CA 94104   **415-394-8677**
                                  800-956-7739
                        Fax: 800-605-2665
                        www.josseybass.com

$27.95

244 pages ISBN 0-787915-85-8

3014 Treatment of Recurrent Depression

American Psychiatric Publishing
1000 Wilson Boulevard
Suite 1825
Arlington, VA 22209-3901   **703-907-7322**
                                  800-368-5777
                        Fax: 703-907-1091
                        E-mail: appi@psych.org
                                  www.appi.org

Katie Duffy, Marketing Assistant

Five topics covered are, Lifetime Impact of Gender on Recurrent Major Depressive Disorder in Women, Treatment Stategies, Prevention of Recurrences in Bipolar Patients, Potential Applications and Updated Recommendations. *$29.95*

208 pages Year Founded: 2001 ISBN 1-585620-25-4

Dissociative Disorders

3015 Dissociative Identity Disorder: Diagnosis, Clinical Features, and Treatment of Multiple Personality

John Wiley & Sons
605 3rd Avenue
New York, NY 10058-0180   **212-850-6000**
                        Fax: 212-850-6008
                        E-mail: info@wiley.com
                                  www.wiley.com

Comprehensive and interesting, this account of the history of MPD dispells many myths and presents new insight into the treatment of MPD. Perfect for sexual abuse clinics, child abuse agencies, correctional facilities and clinicians of all fields. *$64.50*

Year Founded: 1996 ISBN 0-471132-65-9

3016 Handbook of Dissociation: Theoretical, Empirical, and Clinical Perspectives

Kluwer Academic/Plenum Publishers
233 Spring Street
New York, NY 10013   **212-620-8000**
                        Fax: 212-463-0742
                        www.kluweronline.com

Covers both current and emerging theories, research and treatment of dissociative phenomena. Discusses historic, epidemiologic, phenomenologic, etiologic, normative and cross-cultural dimensions of dissociation, providing an empirical foundation for the last chapters. Eight case studies apply dissociation theory and research to specific treatment modalities. *$132.00*

615 pages Year Founded: 1996 ISBN 0-306451-50-6

Eating Disorders

3017 American Psychiatric Association Practice Guideline for Eating Disorders

American Psychiatric Publishing
1000 Wilson Boulevard
Suite 1825
Arlington, VA 22209-3901   **703-907-7322**
                                  800-368-5777
                        Fax: 703-907-1091
                        E-mail: appi@psych.org
                                  www.appi.org

James Scully MD, President
Katie Duffy, Marketing

With up to 3 hours of Category 1 CME Credit. *$22.50*

38 pages Year Founded: 1993 ISBN 0-890423-00-8

3018 Drug Therpay and Eating Disorders

Mason Crest Publishers
370 Reed Road
Suite 302
Broomall, PA 19008   **866-627-2665**
                        Fax: 610-543-3878

Provides a clear, concise account of the history, symptoms, and current treatment of anorexia nervosa and bulimia nervosa. It is estimated the eating disorders affect five million Americans each year, and many more millions among other nations.

ISBN 1-590845-65-X

3019 Handbook of Treatment for Eating Disorders

Guilford Publications
72 Spring Street
New York, NY 10012

212-431-9800
800-365-7006
Fax: 212-966-6708
E-mail: info@guilford.com
www.guilford.com

Includes coverage of binge eating and examines pharmacological as well as therapeutic approaches to eating disorders. Presents cognitive behavioral, psychoeducational, interpersonal, family, feminist, group and psychodynamic approaches, as well as the basics of pharmacological management. Features strategies for handling sexual abuse, substance abuse, concurrent medical conditions, personality disorder, prepubertal eating disorders and patients who refuse therapy. $56.95

540 pages Year Founded: 1997 ISBN 1-572301-86-4

3020 Interpersonal Psychotherapy

American Psychiatric Publishing
1000 Wilson Boulevard
Suite 1825
Arlington, VA 22209-3901

703-907-7322
800-368-5777
Fax: 703-907-1091
E-mail: appi@psych.org
www.appi.org

Katie Duffy, Marketing Assistant

An overview of interpersonal psychotherapy for depression, preventative treatment for depression, bulimia nervosa and HIV positive men and women. $26.00

156 pages Year Founded: 1998 ISBN 0-880488-36-0

3021 Sexual Abuse and Eating Disorders

200 E Joppa Road
Suite 207
Baltimore, MD 21286

410-825-8888
888-825-8249
Fax: 410-337-0747
E-mail: sidran@sidran.org
www.sidran.org

This is the first book to explore the complex relationship between sexual abuse and eating disorders. Sexual abuse is both an extreme boundary violation and a disruption of attachment and bonding; victims of such abuse are likely to exhibit symptoms of self injury, including eating disorders. This volume is a discussion of the many ways that sexual abuse and eating disorders are related, also has accounts by a survivor of both. Investigates the prevalence of sexual abuse amoung individuals with eating disorders. Also examines how a history of sexual violence can serve as a predictor of subsequent problems with food. Looks at related social factors, reviews trauma based theories, more controversial territory and discusses delayed memory versus false memory. $34.95

228 pages

Gender Identification Disorder

3022 Gender Loving Care

WW Norton & Company
500 5th Avenue
New York, NY 10110

212-790-9456
Fax: 212-869-0856
E-mail: admalmud@wwnorton.com
www.wwnorton.com

Understanding and treating gender identity disorder, especially transexuals, who may feel stuck in the wrong-sexed body. $25.00

196 pages Year Founded: 1999 ISBN 0-393703-40-5

3023 Homosexuality and American Psychiatry: The Politics of Diagnosis

Princeton University Press
Princeton University
Princeton, NJ 08544

800-777-4726
Fax: 800-999-1958
www.pup.princeton.edu

$18.00

249 pages Year Founded: 1987 ISBN 0-691028-37-0

3024 Identity Without Selfhood

Cambridge University Press
40 W 20th Street
New York, NY 10011-4221

212-924-3900
Fax: 212-691-3239
E-mail: marketing@cup.org
www.cup.org

Mariam Fraser

Situated at the crossroads of feminism, queer theory and poststructuralist debates around identity, this is a book that shows how key Western concepts such as individuality constrain attempts to deconstruct the self and prevent bisexuality being understood as an identity. $64.95

226 pages Year Founded: 1999

3025 Principles and Practice of Sex Therapy

Guilford Publications
72 Spring Street
New York, NY 10012

212-431-9800
800-365-7006
Fax: 212-966-6708
E-mail: info@guilford.com
www.guilford.com

Many new developments in theory, diagnosis and treatment of sexual disorders have occured in the past decade. The authors set clear guidlines for assessment and treatment with fresh clinical material. A text for professionals and students in a wide range of mental health fields; sexual disorders, male and female, paraphilias, gender identity disorders, vasoactive drugs and more are covered. $50.00

518 pages Year Founded: 2000 ISBN 1-572305-74-6

3026 Psychoanalytic Therapy & the Gay Man

Analytic Press
101 W Street
Hillsdale, NJ 07642-1421   201-358-9477
                                 800-926-6579
                              Fax: 201-358-4700
                     E-mail: TAP@analyticpress.com
                            www.analyticpress.com

Paul E Stepansky PhD, Managing Director
John Kerr PhD, Sr Editor

Explores of the subjectivities of gay men in psychoanalytic psychotherapy. It is a vitally human testament to the richly varied inner experiences of gay men. Offers that sexual identity, which encompass a spectrum of possibilities for any gay man, must be addressed in an atmosphere of honest encounter that allows not only for exploration of conflict and dissasociation but also for restitutive conformation of the patient's right to be himself. Available in hardcover. *$55.00*

384 pages Year Founded: 1998 ISBN 0-881632-08-2

3027 Transvestites and Transsexuals: Toward a Theory of Cross-Gender Behavior

Kluwer Academic/Plenum Publishers
233 Spring Street
New York, NY 10013   212-620-8000
                        Fax: 212-463-0742
                     www.kluweronline.com

This book proposes a theory of transvestism and transexualism presented with a large amount of important raw data collected from interviews with one hundred ten transvestites and thirty five of their wives. *$54.00*

266 pages Year Founded: 1988 ISBN 0-306428-78-4

Impulse Control Disorders

3028 Abusive Personality: Violence and Control in Intimate Relationships

Guilford Publications
72 Spring Street
New York, NY 10012   212-431-9800
                           800-365-7006
                        Fax: 212-966-6708
                  E-mail: info@guilford.com
                        www.guilford.com

A study of domestic violence, especially male perpetrators. *$26.95*

214 pages Year Founded: 1998 ISBN 1-572303-70-0

3029 Coping With Self-Mutilation: a Helping Book for Teens Who Hurt Themselves

Rosen Publishing Group
29 E 21st Street
New York, NY 10010-6209
                              800-237-9932
                         Fax: 888-436-4643
                  E-mail: info@rosenpub.com
                     www.rosenpublishing.com

Examines the reasons for this phenomenon, and ways one might seek help. *$17.95*

Year Founded: 1999 ISBN 0-823925-59-5

3030 Dealing with Anger Problems: Rational-Emotive Therapeutic Interventions

Professional Resource Press
PO Box 15560
Sarasota, FL 34277-1560   941-343-9601
                                 800-443-3364
                              Fax: 941-343-9201
                     E-mail: orders@prpress.com
                            www.prpress.com

Debra Fink, Managing Editor

Demonstrates ways to apply rational-emotive therapy techniques to help your clients control their anger. Offers step-by-step anger control treatment program that includes a variety of cognitive, emotive, and behavioral homework assignments, and procedures for modifying behaviors and facilitating change. *$11.95*

68 pages Year Founded: 1990 ISBN 0-943158-59-1

3031 Domestic Violence 2000: Integrated Skills Program for Men

WW Norton & Company
500 5th Avenue
New York, NY 10110   212-790-9456
                        Fax: 212-869-0856
                  E-mail: admalmud@wwnorton.com
                        www.wwnorton.com

Various theories are examined to deal with this difficult social problem. For group classes. *$23.20*

224 pages Year Founded: 1999 ISSN 70314-2

3032 Sex Murder and Sex Aggression: Phenomenology Psychopathology, Psychodynamics and Prognosis

Charles C Thomas Publisher
2600 S 1st Street
Springfield, IL 62704-4730   217-789-8980
                                    800-258-8980
                                 Fax: 217-789-9130
                     E-mail: books@ccthomas.com
                            www.ccthomas.com

By Eugene Revitch, Robert Wood Johnson School of Medicine, Piscataway, New Jersey, and Louis B Schlesinger, New Jersey Medical School, Newark. With a foreword by Robert R Hazelwood. Contents: The Place of Gynocide and Sexual Aggression in the Classification of Crime; Catathymic Gynocide; Compulsive Gynocide; Psychodynamics, Psychopathology and Differential Diagnosis; Prognostic Considerations. *$43.95*

152 pages Year Founded: 1989 ISSN 0-398-06346-XISBN 0-398055-56-4

3033 Teaching Behavioral Self Control to Students

Pro-Ed Publications
8700 Shoal Creek Boulevard
Austin, TX 78757-6816
512-451-3246
800-897-3202
Fax: 800-397-7633
E-mail: info@proedinc.com
www.proedinc.com

Demonstrates how teachers, counselors and parents can help children of all ages and ability levels to modify their own behavior. Clear step-by-step methods describe how common childhood problems can be solved by helping children become more responsible and independent. $ 21.00

*122 pages Year Founded: 1995 ISBN
0-890796-17-3*

Movement Disorders

3034 Movement Disorders:Neuropsychiatric Approach

Gilford Press
72 Spring Street
New York, NY 10012
212-431-9800

$63.00

3035 Tardive Dyskinesia: Task Force Report of the American Psychiatric Association

American Psychiatric Publishing
1000 Wilson Boulevard
Suite 1825
Arlington, VA 22209-3901
703-907-7322
800-368-5777
Fax: 703-907-1091
E-mail: appi@psych.org
www.appi.org

Katie Duffy, Marketing Assistant

Obsessive Compulsive Disorder

3036 Current Treatments of Obsessive-Compulsive Disorder

American Psychiatric Publishing
1000 Wilson Boulevard
Suite 1825
Arlington, VA 22209-3901
703-907-7322
800-368-5777
Fax: 703-907-1091
E-mail: appi@psych.org
www.appi.org

Helps clinicians better match treatment approaches with each patients unique needs.

Year Founded: 01 ISBN 0-880487-79-8

3037 Handbook of Pathological Gambling

Charles C Thomas Publisher
2600 S 1st Street
Springfield, IL 62704-4730
217-789-8980
800-258-8980
Fax: 217-789-9130
E-mail: books@ccthomas.com
www.ccthomas.com

Contents: The Diagnosis and Scope of Pathological Gambling; The Pathological Gambler: Salient Personality Variables; The Psychodynamics of Pathological Gambling: A Review of the Literature; Family Dynamics of Pathological Gamblers; Gambling, Pathological Gambling and Crime; Physiological Determinants of Pathological Gambling; Psychological Testing of Pathological Gamblers: Research, Uses and New Directions; The Pathological Gambler in Treatment; A General Theory of Addictions: Application to Treatment and Rehabilitation Planning for Pathological Gamblers; Forensic Issues in Pathological Gambling. $ 47.95

*228 pages Year Founded: 1987 ISSN
0-398-06142-4ISBN 0-398052-68-9*

3038 Motivational Interviewing: Prepare People to Change Addictive Behavior

Hazelden
15251 Pleasant Valley Road
PO Box 176
Center City, MN 55012-0176
651-213-2121
800-328-9000
Fax: 651-213-4590
www.hazelden.org

William K Miller, Co-Author
Stephen Rollnick, Co-Author

A key resource for clinical psychologists, social workers and chemical dependency counselors for mastering interviewing skills and working with resistant clients. *$21.95*

348 pages ISBN 0-898624-69-X

3039 Obsessive-Compulsive Disorder: Contemporary Issues in Treatment

Lawrence Erlbaum Associates
10 Industrial Avenue
Mahwah, NJ 07430-2262
201-825-3200
800-926-6577
Fax: 201-236-0072
E-mail: orders@erlbaum.com
www.erlbaum.com

Hardcover.

Year Founded: 00 ISBN 0-805828-37-0

3040 Obsessive-Compulsive and Related Disorders in Adults: a Comprehensive Clinical Guide

Cambridge University Press
40 W 20th Street
New York, NY 10011-4221
212-924-3900
Fax: 212-691-3239
E-mail: marketing@cup.org
www.cup.org

The author challenges the current implicit models used in alcohol problem prevention and demonstrates an ecological perspective of the community as a complex adaptive systems composed of interacting subsystems. This volume represents a new and sensible approach to the prevention of alcohol dependence and alcohol-related problems. *$65.00*

380 pages Year Founded: 1999 ISBN 0-521559-75-8

3041 Overcoming Obsessive-Compulsive Disorder

New Harbinger Publications
5674 Shattuck Avenue
Oakland, CA 94609-1662   510-652-2002
                                    800-748-6273
                        Fax: 510-652-5472
E-mail: customerservice@newharbinger.com
                        www.newharbinger.com

A fourteen session treatment. *$11.95*

72 pages Year Founded: 1998 ISBN 1-572241-29-2

3042 Psychotherapy and Couples Communicaton

1745 Saratoga Avenue
Suite 201
San Jose, CA 95129-5207   408-562-4878
                        Fax: 408-358-8535
                E-mail: MGodfreyTx@aol.com

Obsessive compulsive and related anxiety disorders, using exposure and response prevention integrated with cognitive and wholistic modalities. Collaborate with MD-prescribed medication, when appropriate. Couples counseling, coach communication skills to enhance relationships at home and in the workplace. Executive stress and its management. Brief therapy as needed. Publications: Biannual newsletter.

3043 Treatment of Obsessive Compulsive Disorder

Guilford Publications
72 Spring Street
New York, NY 10012   212-431-9800
                                800-365-7006
                        Fax: 212-966-6708
                E-mail: info@guilford.com
                        www.guilford.com

Provides everything the mental health professional needs for working with clients who suffer from obsessions and compulsions. Supplies background by describing in detail up-to-date clinically relevant information and a step-by-step guide for conducting behavioral treatment. *$39.95*

224 pages Year Founded: 1993 ISBN 0-898621-84-4

Personality Disorders

3044 Bad Boys, Bad Men: Confronting Antisocial Personality Disorder

Oxford University Press
198 Madison Avenue
New York, NY 10016   212-726-6000
                                800-451-7556
                        Fax: 919-677-1303
                        www.oup-usa.org

This book examines the mental condition characterized by a serial pattern of bad behavior. Draws on case studies, scientific data, and current events. *$25.00*

256 pages Year Founded: 1999 ISBN 0-195121-13-9

3045 Biological Basis of Personality

Charles C Thomas Publisher
2600 S 1st Street
Springfield, IL 62704-4730   217-789-8980
                                        800-258-8980
                        Fax: 217-789-9130
                E-mail: books@ccthomas.com
                        www.ccthomas.com

H J Eysenck, Author

$70.95

420 pages Year Founded: 1977 ISBN 0-398005-38-9

3046 Biology of Personality Disorders

American Psychiatric Publishing
1000 Wilson Boulevard
Suite 1825
Arlington, VA 22209-3901   703-907-7322
                                        800-368-5777
                        Fax: 703-907-1091
                E-mail: appi@psych.org
                        www.appi.org

Katie Duffy, Marketing Assistant

Content topics include neurotransmitter function in personality disorders, new biological researcher strategies for personality disorders, the genetics psychobiology of the seven - factor model of personality disorders, and significance of biological research for a biopsychosocial model of personality disorders. *$25.00*

166 pages Year Founded: 1998 ISBN 0-880488-35-2

3047 Borderline Personality Disorder: Tailoring the Psychotherapy to the Patient

American Psychiatric Publishing
1000 Wilson Boulevard
Suite 1825
Arlington, VA 22209-3901   703-907-7322
                                        800-368-5777
                        Fax: 703-907-1091
                E-mail: appi@psych.org
                        www.appi.org

Katie Duffy, Marketing Assistant

$34.00

256 pages Year Founded: 1996 ISBN 0-880486-89-9

3048 Borderline Personality Disorder: Therapists Guide to Taking Control

WW Norton & Company
500 5th Avenue
New York, NY 10110   **212-790-9456**
          Fax: 212-869-0856
          E-mail: admalmud@wwnorton.com
          www.wwnorton.com

From identifacation to relapse prevention, this guide helps therapists manage a patient's treatment for the rather complex problem of Borderline Personality Disorder, an often difficult and sometimes life threatening condition. *$27.50*

224 pages Year Founded: 2002 ISBN 0-393703-52-5

3049 Cognitive Therapy for Personality Disorders: a Schema-Focused Approach

Professional Resource Press
PO Box 15560
Sarasota, FL 34277-1560   **941-343-9601**
          800-443-3364
          Fax: 941-343-9201
          E-mail: orders@prpress.com
          www.prpress.com

Debra Fink, Managing Editor

A guide to treating the most difficult cases in your practice: personality disorders and other chronic, self - defeating problems. Contains rationale, theory, practical applications, and active cognitive behavioral techniques. *$13.95*

96 pages Year Founded: 1999 ISBN 1-568870-47-7

3050 Cognitive Therapy of Personality Disorders

Guilford Publications
72 Spring Street
New York, NY 10012   **212-431-9800**
          800-365-7006
          Fax: 212-966-6708
          E-mail: info@guilford.com
          www.guilford.com

Focuses on the use of cognitive therapy to treat people with personality disorders who do not usually engage in therapy. Emanates the research and practical experience of Beck and his associates and is the first to focus specifically on this diverse and clinically demanding population. Case vignettes are used throughout. *$43.00*

396 pages Year Founded: 1990 ISBN 0-989624-34-7

3051 Dealing With the Problem of Low Self-Esteem: Common Characteristics and Treatment

Charles C Thomas Publisher
2600 S 1st Street
Springfield, IL 62704-4730   **217-789-8980**
          800-258-8980
          Fax: 217-789-9130
          E-mail: books@ccthomas.com
          www.ccthomas.com

Robert P Rugel, Author

Considers the practice of psychotherapy from the self-esteem perspective. Describes the common characteristics of low self-esteem that are manifested in clients with diverse problems; focuses on the functions the therapist performs in addressing these characteristics. The third is to consider the modalities of treatment through which the therapist delivers these therapeutic functions. *$ 48.95*

228 pages Year Founded: 1995 ISSN 0-398-05951-9ISBN 0-398059-36-5

3052 Disorders of Personality: DSM-IV and Beyond

John Wiley & Sons
605 3rd Avenue
New York, NY 10058-0180   **212-850-6000**
          Fax: 212-850-6008
          E-mail: info@wiley.com
          www.wiley.com

Clarifies the distictions between the vast array of personality disorders and helps clinicians make accurate diagnoses; thoroughly updated to incorporate the recent change in the DSM - IV. Guides the clinicians throught the intricate maze of personality disorders, with special attention on changes in their conceptualization over the last decade. *$85.00*

Year Founded: 1995 ISBN 0-471011-86-X

3053 Expressive and Functional Therapies in the Treatment of Multiple Personality Disorder

Charles C Thomas Publisher
2600 S 1st Street
Springfield, IL 62704-4730   **217-789-8980**
          800-258-8980
          Fax: 217-789-9130
          E-mail: books@ccthomas.com
          www.ccthomas.com

Estelle S Kluft, Author

Addresses the use of creative arts, play and other modalities in the psychotherapy of victims of multiple personality disorder. Contains the collected insights and observations of a group of pioneers who have made seminal presentations and have written groundbreaking articles in their areas of expertise. Recognized by their peers as innovators and significant contributors to this emerging field. *$71.95*

332 pages Year Founded: 1993 ISSN 0-398-06207-2ISBN 0-398058-26-1

3054 Group Exercises for Enhancing Social Skills & Self-Esteem

Professional Resource Press
PO Box 15560
Sarasota, FL 34277-1560   941-343-9601
                                 800-443-3364
                              Fax: 941-343-9201
                     E-mail: orders@prpress.com
                                 www.prpress.com

Debra Fink, Managing Editor

Includes exercises for enhancing self-esteem utilizing proven social, emotional, and cognitive skill-building techniques. These exercises are useful in therapeutic, psychoeducational, and recreational settings. *$24.95*

150 pages Year Founded: 1996 ISBN
1-568870-20-5

3055 Personality Characteristics of the Personality Disordered

John Wiley & Sons
605 3rd Avenue
New York, NY 10058-0180   212-850-6000
                              Fax: 212-850-6008
                     E-mail: info@wiley.com
                                 www.wiley.com

340 pages Year Founded: 1995

3056 Personality Disorders and Culture: Clinical and Conceptual Interactions

John Wiley & Sons
605 3rd Avenue
New York, NY 10058-0180   212-850-6000
                              Fax: 212-850-6008
                     E-mail: info@wiley.com
                                 www.wiley.com

Discusses two of the most timely and complex areas in mental health, personality disorders and the impact of cultural variables. Treading on the timeless nature - nurture debate, it suggests that social variables have a dramatic impact on the definition, development, and manifestation of personality disorders.

310 pages Year Founded: 1998

3057 Personality and Stress: Individual Differences in the Stress Process

John Wiley & Sons
605 3rd Avenue
New York, NY 10058-0180   212-850-6000
                              Fax: 212-850-6008
                     E-mail: info@wiley.com
                                 www.wiley.com

302 pages Year Founded: 1991

3058 Psychotherapy for Borderline Personality

John Wiley & Sons
605 3rd Avenue
New York, NY 10058-0180   212-850-6000
                              Fax: 212-850-6008
                     E-mail: info@wiley.com
                                 www.wiley.com

Based on the work of a research team, this manual offers techniques and strategies for treating patients with Borderline Personality Disorder using Transference Focused Psychology. Provides therapists with an overall strategy for treating BPD patients and helpful tactics for working with individual patients on a session by session basis.

400 pages Year Founded: 1999

3059 Role of Sexual Abuse in the Etiology of Borderline Personality Disorder

200 E Joppa Road
Suite 207
Baltimore, MD 21286   410-825-8888
                                 888-825-8249
                              Fax: 410-337-0747
                     E-mail: sidran@sidran.org
                                 www.sidran.org

Presenting the latest generation of research findings about the impact of traumatic abuse on the development of BPD. This book focuses on the theoretical basis of BPD, including topics such as childhood factors associated with the development, the relationship of child sexual abuse to dissociation and self mutilation, severity of childhood abuse, borderline symptoms and family environment. Twenty six contributors cover every aspect of BPD as it relates to childhood sexual abuse. *$42.00*

248 pages

3060 Shorter Term Treatments for Borderline Personality Disorders

New Harbinger Publications
5674 Shattuck Avenue
Oakland, CA 94609-1662   510-652-2002
                                 800-748-6273
                              Fax: 510-652-5472
          E-mail: customerservice@newharbinger.com
                                 www.newharbinger.com

This guide offers approaches designed to help clients stabilize emotions, decrease vulnerability and work toward a more adaptive day to day functioning. *$49.95*

184 pages Year Founded: 1997 ISBN
1-572240-92-X

3061 Treating Difficult Personality Disorders

Jossey-Bass Publishers
350 Sansome Street
5th Floor
San Francisco, CA 94104   415-394-8677
                                 800-956-7739
                              Fax: 800-605-2665
                                 www.josseybass.com

In this essential resource, experts in the field provide the most current information for the successful assessment and clinical treatment of this challenging client population. This book presents flexible treatment options for clients suffering from borderline, narcissistic, and antisocial personality disorders. *$28.95*

288 pages ISBN 0-787903-15-9

Post Traumatic Stress Disorder

3062 Body Remembers: Psychophysiology of Trauma and Trauma Treatment

WW Norton & Company
500 5th Avenue
New York, NY 10110
212-790-9456
Fax: 212-869-0856
E-mail: admalmud@wwnorton.com
www.wwnorton.com

Unites traditional verbal therapy and body oriented therapies for Post Traumatic Stress Disorder patients, as memories sometimes present in a physical disorder. $30.00

224 pages Year Founded: 2000 ISSN 70327-4

3063 Brief Therapy for Post Traumatic Stress Disorder

John Wiley & Sons
605 3rd Avenue
New York, NY 10058-0180
212-850-6000
Fax: 212-850-6008
E-mail: info@wiley.com
www.wiley.com

Discusses a new and exciting treatment technique that has proven to be more effective than the widely used direct theraputic exposure technique. Fills the growing need for a step by step practical treatment manual for PTSD using Tramatic Incident Reduction. It is an ideal companion to training workshops.

192 pages Year Founded: 1998

3064 Cognitive Processing Therapy for Rape Victims

Sage Publications
2455 Teller Road
Thousand Oaks, CA 91320
805-499-9774
800-818-7243
Fax: 800-583-2665
E-mail: info@sagepub.com
www.sagepub.com

Information regarding the assessment and treatment of rape victims. Discusses disorders that result from rape and add to a victim's suffering such as post traumatic stress, depression, poor self-esteem, interpersonal difficulties and sexual dysfunction. $46.00

192 pages Year Founded: 1993 ISBN 0-803949-01-4

3065 Concise Guide to Brief Dynamic Psychotherapy

American Psychiatric Publishing
1000 Wilson Boulevard
Suite 1825
Arlington, VA 22209-3901
703-907-7322
800-368-5777
Fax: 703-907-1091
E-mail: appi@psych.org
www.appi.org

Katie Duffy, Marketing Assistant

Seven brief psychodynamic therapy models including supportive, time - limited, interpersonal, time - limited dynamic, short term dynamic for post traumatic stress disorder and brief dynamic for substance abuse. $21.00

224 pages Year Founded: 1997 ISBN 0-880483-46-6

3066 EMDR: Breakthrough Therapy for Overcoming Anxiety, Stress and Trauma

200 E Joppa Road
Suite 207
Baltimore, MD 21286
410-825-8888
888-825-8249
Fax: 410-337-0747
E-mail: sidran@sidran.org
www.sidran.org

EMDR - Eye Movement Desensitization and Reprocessing, has successfully relieved symptoms like depression, phobias and nightmares of PTSD survivors, with a rapidity that almost defies belief. Dr. Shapiro, the originator of EMDR, explains how she created the groundbreaking therapy, how it works and how it can help people who feel stuck in negative reactions and behaviors. Included with the text are a variety of compelling case studies. $16.00

284 pages

3067 Effective Treatments for PTSD: Practice Guidelines from the International Society for Traumatic Stress Studies

Guilford Publications
72 Spring Street
New York, NY 10012
212-431-9800
800-365-7006
Fax: 212-966-6708
E-mail: info@guilford.com
www.guilford.com

Developed under the auspices of the PTSD Treatment Guidelines Task Force of the International Society for Traumatic Stress Studies, this comprehensive volume brings together leading authorities on psychological trauma to offer best practice guidelines for the treatment of PTSD. Approaches covered include acute interventions, cognitive-behavior therapy, pharmacotherapy, EMDR, group therapy, psychodynamic therapy, impatient treatment, psychosocial rehabilitation, hypnosis, creative therapies, marital and family treatment. $42.00

388 pages ISBN 1-572305-84-3

3068 Even from a Broken Web: Brief, Respectful Solution Oriented Therapy for Sexual Abuse and Trauma

WW Norton & Company
500 5th Avenue
New York, NY 10110
212-790-9456
Fax: 212-869-0856
E-mail: admalmud@wwnorton.com
www.wwnorton.com

Recent years have shown more people than ever coming to therapy with the afer affects of sexual abuse. The authors provide therapists solution oriented treatment that considers a person's inner healing abilities. This method is less traumatic and disruptive to the patient's life than traditional therapies. *$16.95*

208 pages Year Founded: 2002 ISBN 0-393703-94-0

3069 Eye Movement Desensitization and Reprocessing: Basic Principles, Protocols, and Procedures

Guilford Publications
72 Spring Street
New York, NY 10012   212-431-9800
                                    800-365-7006
                              Fax: 212-966-6708
              E-mail: info@guilford.com
                      www.guilford.com

Reviews research and development, discusses theoretical constructs and possible underlying mechanisms, and presents protocols and procedures for treatment of adults and children with a range of presenting complaints. Material is applicable for victims of sexual abuse, crime, combat and phobias. *$45.00*

398 pages Year Founded: 1995 ISBN 0-898629-60-8

3070 Group Treatments for Post-Traumatic Stress Disorder

Brunner/Mazel
325 Chestnut Street
Philadelphia, PA 19106
                                    800-821-8312
                              Fax: 215-269-0363

Contains contributions from renowned PTSD experts who provide group treatment to trauma survivors. It reviews the state-of-the-art applications of group therapy for such survivors of trama as rape victims, combat veterans, adult survivors of childhood abuse, motor vehicle accident survivors, survivors of disaster, homicide witnesses and disaster relief workers. *$34.95*

216 pages ISBN 0-876309-83-X

3071 Life After Trauma: Workbook for Healing

Guilford Publications
72 Spring Street
New York, NY 10012   212-431-9800
                                    800-365-7006
                              Fax: 212-966-6708
              E-mail: info@guilford.com
                      www.guilford.com

Useful exercises for clinicians and trauma survivors, very empowering. *$17.95*

352 pages Year Founded: 1999 ISBN 1-572302-39-9

3072 Memory, Trauma and the Law

WW Norton & Company
500 5th Avenue
New York, NY 10110   212-790-9456
                              Fax: 212-869-0856
        E-mail: admalmud@wwnorton.com
                      www.wwnorton.com

Professionals need to be informed of memory in the legal context to avoid malpractice liability suits. Recovered memory research, trauma treatment and the controversy of false memory in some cases are covered. *$100.00*

960 pages Year Founded: 1998 ISSN 70254-5

3073 Overcoming Post-Traumatic Stress Disorder

New Harbinger Publications
5674 Shattuck Avenue
Oakland, CA 94609-1662   510-652-2002
                                    800-748-6273
                              Fax: 510-652-5472
    E-mail: customerservice@newharbinger.com
                      www.newharbinger.com

An eleven to twenty four session treatment. *$11.95*

95 pages Year Founded: 1998 ISBN 1-572241-47-0

3074 PTSD in Children and Adolesents

American Psychiatric Publishing
1000 Wilson Boulevard
Suite 1825
Arlington, VA 22209-3901   703-907-7322
                                    800-368-5777
                              Fax: 703-907-1091
              E-mail: appi@psych.org
                      www.appi.org

Katie Duffy, Marketing Manager

Mental health and other professionals who work with Post Traumatic Stress Disorder and the young people who suffer from it will find discussions of evaluation, biological treatment strategies, the need for an integrated approach to juvenille offenders who suffer from PTSD and more. *$29.95*

208 pages Year Founded: 2001

3075 Perturbing the Organism: the Biology of Stressful Experience

University of Chicago Press
5801 S Ellis
Chicago, IL 60637   773-702-7700
                              Fax: 773-702-9756
        E-mail: marketing@press.uchicago.edu
                      www.press.uchicago.edu

Critical analysis of the entire range of research and theory on stress in animals and humans, from the earliest studies in the 30's to present day. Includes empirical and conceptual advances of recent years, but also supplies a new working definition of stressful experience. Hardcover. *$40.50*

358 pages Year Founded: 1992 ISBN 0-226890-41-4

3076 Post Traumatic Stress Disorder

New Harbinger Publications
5674 Shattuck Avenue
Oakland, CA 94609-1662
510-652-2002
800-748-6273
Fax: 510-652-5472
E-mail: customerservice@newharbinger.com
www.newharbinger.com

Includes techniques for managing flashbacks, anxiety attacks, nightmares, insomnia, and dissociation; working through layers of pain; and handling survivor guilt, secondary wounding, low self esteem, victim thinking, anger, and depression. *$49.95*

384 pages Year Founded: 1994 ISBN
1-879237-68-7

3077 Post Traumatic Stress Disorder: Complete Treatment Guide

200 E Joppa Road
Suite 207
Baltimore, MD 21286
410-825-8888
888-825-8249
Fax: 410-337-0747
E-mail: sidran@sidran.org
www.sidran.org

For clinicians who want to work more effectively with trauma survivors, this textbook provides a step by step description of PTSD treatment strategies. Includes chapters on definitions, diagnostic criteria and the biochemistry of PTSD. Reflects a generalized 'ideal' structure of the healing process. Includes cognitive and behavioral techniques for managing flashbacks, anxiety attacks, sleep disturbances and dissociation; a comprehensive program for working through deeper layers of pain; plus PTSD related problems such as survivor guilt, secondary wounding, low self esteem, victim thinking, anger and depression. Presents trauma issues clearly for both general audiences and trauma professionals. *$49.95*

345 pages

3078 Rebuilding Shattered Lives: Responsible Treatment of Complex Post-Traumatic and Dissociative Disorders

John Wiley & Sons
605 3rd Avenue
New York, NY 10058-0180
212-850-6000
Fax: 212-850-6008
E-mail: info@wiley.com
www.wiley.com

The most up-to-date, integrative and emperically sound account of trauma theory and practice availible. Based on more than a decade of clinical research and treatment experience at the Harvard Medical School, this comprehensive and nontechnical text offers a stage oriented approach to understanding and treating complex and difficult traumatized patients, integrating modern trauma theory with traditional theraputic interventions. *$47.50*

256 pages Year Founded: 1998 ISBN
0-471247-32-4

3079 Remembering Trauma: Psychotherapist's Guide to Memory & Illusion

John Wiley & Sons
605 3rd Avenue
New York, NY 10058-0180
212-850-6000
Fax: 212-850-6008
E-mail: info@wiley.com
www.wiley.com

Amy Abzarnik, Conventions Coordinator

3080 Standing in the Spaces: Essays on Clinical Process, Trauma, and Dissociation

Analytic Press
101 W Street
Hillsdale, NJ 07642-1421
201-358-9477
800-926-6579
Fax: 201-358-4700
E-mail: TAP@analyticpress.com
www.analyticpress.com

Paul E Stepansky PhD, Managing Director
John Kerr PhD, Sr Editor

Bromberg's essays are delightfully unpredictable, as they strive to keep the reader continually abreast of how words can and cannot capture the subtle shifts in relatedness that characterize the clinical process. Radiating clinical wisdom infused with compassion and wit, Standing in the Spaces, is a classic destined to be read and reread by anlysts and therapists for decades to come. *$55.00*

376 pages Year Founded: 1998 ISBN
0-881632-46-5

3081 Transforming Trauma: EMDR

WW Norton & Company
500 5th Avenue
New York, NY 10110
212-790-9456
Fax: 212-869-0856
E-mail: admalmud@wwnorton.com
www.wwnorton.com

Has helped thousands of people dealing with abuse histories or recent traumatic events. The author has a unique perspective, as she is both a client of EMDR and a therapist. *$14.95*

288 pages Year Founded: 1996 ISSN 31757-9

3082 Trauma Response

WW Norton & Company
500 5th Avenue
New York, NY 10110
212-790-9456
Fax: 212-869-0856
E-mail: admalmud@wwnorton.com
www.wwnorton.com

Different causes of psychological trauma and modes of recovery. *$22.36*

240 pages Year Founded: 1993

3083 Traumatic Events & Mental Health

Cambridge University Press
40 W 20th Street
New York, NY 10011-4221
212-924-3900
Fax: 212-691-3239
E-mail: marketing@cup.org
www.cup.org

Psychosomatic Disorders

3084 Anatomy of a Psychiatric Ilness: Healing the Mind and the Brain

American Psychiatric Publishing
1000 Wilson Boulevard
Suite 1825
Arlington, VA 22209-3901
703-907-7322
800-368-5777
Fax: 703-907-1091
E-mail: appi@psych.org
www.appi.org

Katie Duffy, Marketing Assistant

$22.95

232 pages Year Founded: 1993

3085 Concise Guide to Neuropsychiatry and Behavioral Neurology

American Psychiatric Publishing
1000 Wilson Boulevard
Suite 1825
Arlington, VA 22209-3901
703-907-7322
800-368-5777
Fax: 703-907-1091
E-mail: appi@psych.org
www.appi.org

Katie Duffy, Marketing Assistant

Provides brief synopsis of the major neuropsychiatric and neurobehavioral syndromes, discusses their clinical assessment, and provides guidelines for management. *$21.00*

368 pages Year Founded: 1995 ISBN 0-880483-43-1

3086 Concise Guide to Psychodynamic Psychotherapy: Principles and Techniques in the Era of Managed Care

American Psychiatric Publishing
1000 Wilson Boulevard
Suite 1825
Arlington, VA 22209-3901
703-907-7322
800-368-5777
Fax: 703-907-1091
E-mail: appi@psych.org
www.appi.org

Katie Duffy, Marketing Assistant

Thoroughly updated coverage of all the major principles and important issues in psychodynamic psychotherapy and issues not commonly addressed in the standard training curriculum, including the office setting, suicidal and dangerous patients, and what to do when the therapist makes an error. *$21.00*

272 pages Year Founded: 1998 ISBN 0-880483-47-4

3087 Functional Somatic Syndromes

Cambridge University Press
40 W 20th Street
New York, NY 10011-4221
212-924-3900
Fax: 212-691-3239
E-mail: marketing@cup.org
www.cup.org

3088 Manual of Panic: Focused Psychodynamic Psychotherapy

American Psychiatric Publishing
1000 Wilson Boulevard
Suite 1825
Arlington, VA 22209-3901
703-907-7322
800-368-5777
Fax: 703-907-1091
E-mail: appi@psych.org
www.appi.org

Katie Duffy, Marketing Assistant

A psychodynamic formulation applicable to many or most patients with Axis 1 panic disorders. *$28.00*

112 pages Year Founded: 1997 ISBN 0-880488-71-9

3089 Overcoming Specific Phobia

New Harbinger Publications
5674 Shattuck Avenue
Oakland, CA 94609-1662
510-652-2002
800-748-6273
Fax: 510-652-5472
E-mail: customerservice@newharbinger.com
www.newharbinger.com

$9.95

72 pages Year Founded: 1998 ISBN 1-572241-15-2

3090 Somatization, Physical Symptoms and Psychological Illness

American Psychiatric Publishing
1000 Wilson Boulevard
Suite 1825
Arlington, VA 22209-3901
703-907-7322
800-368-5777
Fax: 703-907-1091
E-mail: appi@psych.org
www.appi.org

Katie Duffy, Marketing Assistant

$99.95

351 pages Year Founded: 1990 ISBN 0-632028-39-4

3091 Somatoform and Factitious Disorders

American Psychiatric Publishing
1000 Wilson Boulevard
Suite 1825
Arlington, VA 22209-3901
703-907-7322
800-368-5777
Fax: 703-907-1091
E-mail: appi@psych.org
www.appi.org

Katie Duffy, Marketing Assistant

Consise yet thorough, this book covers Factitious disorders, Somatization disorder, Conversion disorder, Hypochondriasis and Body dysmorphic disorder. Explores the latest on these conditions and emphasises the need for further research to improve patient treament and understanding. *$29.95*

208 pages Year Founded: 2001 ISBN 1-585620-29-7

Schizophrenia

3092 Behavioral High-Risk Paradigm in Psychopathology

Springer-Verlag New York
175 5th Avenue
New York, NY 10010-2485   212-460-1500
                                 800-777-4643
                                 Fax: 212-533-3503
                   E-mail: custserv@springer-ny.com
                                 www.springer-ny.com

Examines both traditional clinical research on psychopathology and psychophysiological research on psychopathology, with an emphasis on risk for schizophrenia and for mood disorders. Complementing treatments of risk for psychopathology in other sources which emphasize either genetic factors or large-scale psychosocial factors, chapters focus on research in specific areas of each disorder. Hardcover. $98.00

304 pages Year Founded: 1995 ISBN 0-387945-04-0

3093 Cognitive Therapy for Delusions, Voices, and Parinoia

John Wiley & Sons
605 3rd Avenue
New York, NY 10058-0180   212-850-6000
                                 Fax: 212-850-6008
                        E-mail: info@wiley.com
                                 www.wiley.com

A cognitive view of delusions and voices. The practice of therapy and the problem of engagement.

230 pages Year Founded: 1995

3094 Delusional Beliefs

John Wiley & Sons
605 3rd Avenue
New York, NY 10058-0180   212-850-6000
                                 Fax: 212-850-6008
                        E-mail: info@wiley.com
                                 www.wiley.com

Unique collection of ideas and empirical data provided by leading experts in a variety of disciplines. Each offers perspectives on questions such as: What criteria should be used to identify, describe and classify delusions? How can delusional individuals be identified? What distinguishes delusions from normal beliefs? $95.00

352 pages Year Founded: 1988 ISBN 0-471836-35-4

3095 Families Coping with Schizophrenia: Practitioner's Guide to Family Groups

John Wiley & Sons
605 3rd Avenue
New York, NY 10058-0180   212-850-6000
                                 Fax: 212-850-6008
                        E-mail: info@wiley.com
                                 www.wiley.com

294 pages Year Founded: 1995

3096 Practice Guideline for the Treatment of Patients with Schizophrenia

American Psychiatric Publishing
1000 Wilson Boulevard
Suite 1825
Arlington, VA 22209-3901   703-907-7322
                                  800-368-5777
                             Fax: 703-907-1091
                        E-mail: appi@psych.org
                                  www.appi.org

Katie Duffy, Marketing Assistant

$22.00

146 pages Year Founded: 1997

3097 Schizophrenia Revealed: From Nuerons to Social Interactions

WW Norton & Company
500 5th Avenue
New York, NY 10110   212-790-9456
                             Fax: 212-869-0856
                   E-mail: admalmud@wwnorton.com
                                 www.wwnorton.com

Helps explain some of the former mysteries of Schizophrenia that are now possible to study through advances in neuroscience. $ 10.80

Year Founded: 1979 ISBN 0-393090-17-5

Sexual Disorders

3098 Erectile Dysfunction: Integrating Couple Therapy, Sex Therapy and Medical Treatment

WW Norton & Company
500 5th Avenue
New York, NY 10110   212-790-9456
                             Fax: 212-869-0856
                   E-mail: admalmud@wwnorton.com
                                 www.wwnorton.com

Helpful to marriage and couple therapists, very up to date and encompassing, with simple and professional writing. $30.00

208 pages Year Founded: 2000 ISSN 70330-4

3099 Hypoactive Sexual Desire: Integrating Sex and Couple Therapy

WW Norton & Company
500 5th Avenue
New York, NY 10110   212-790-9456
                             Fax: 212-869-0856
                   E-mail: admalmud@wwnorton.com
                                 www.wwnorton.com

Discussion of treating the couple, not the individual with lack of desire, the authors include distinguishing between organic and psychogenic problems plus how to combine relational and sex therapy. Although lack of desire is one of the most common problems couples face, it is one of the most challenging to treat. $30.00

288 pages Year Founded: 2002 ISSN 70344-4

Substance Abuse & Dependence

3100 Addictive Behaviors Across the Life Span

Sage Publications
2455 Teller Road
Thousand Oaks, CA 91320   805-499-9774
                                 800-818-7243
                            Fax: 800-583-2665
                      E-mail: info@sagepub.com
                                 www.sagepub.com

Leading scholars, researchers and clinicians in the field of addictive behavior provide and examination of drug dependency from a life span perspective in this authoritative volume. Four general topic areas include: etiology; early intervention; integrated treatment; and policy issues across the life span. Other topics include biopsychosocial perspectives on the intergenerational transmission of alcoholism to children and reducing the risks of addictive behaviors. *$59.95*

358 pages Year Founded: 1993 ISBN 0-803950-78-0

3101 Addictive Thinking: Understanding Self-Deception

Health Communications
292 Fernwood Avenue
Edison, NJ 08837   732-346-0027
                         Fax: 732-346-0442
                              www.hcomm.com

Exposes the irrational and contradictory patterns of addictive thinking, and shows how to overcome them and barries they create; low self-esteem and relapse.

140 pages ISBN 1-568381-38-7

3102 Addition Treatment Homework Planner

John Wiley & Sons
10475 Crosspoint Boulevard
Indianapolis, IN 46256   877-762-2974
                           Fax: 800-597-3299
                  E-mail: consumers@wiley.com
                                www.wiley.com

Helps clients suffering from chemical and nonchemical additions develops the skills they need to work through problems. *$ 49.95*

370 pages ISBN 0-471274-59-3

3103 Addition Treatment Planner

John Wiley & Sons
10475 Crosspoint Boulevard
Indianapolis, IN 46256   877-762-2974
                           Fax: 800-597-3299
                  E-mail: consumers@wiley.com
                                www.wiley.com

Provides all the elements necessary to quickly and easily develop formal treatment plans that satisfy the demands of HMOs, managed care companies, third-party payers, and state and federal review agencies. *$49.95*

384 pages ISBN 0-471418-14-5

3104 Adolescents, Alcohol and Drugs: a Practical Guide for Those Who Work With Young People

Charles C Thomas Publisher
2600 S 1st Street
Springfield, IL 62704-4730   217-789-8980
                                800-258-8980
                           Fax: 217-789-9130
                  E-mail: books@ccthomas.com
                                www.ccthomas.com

$41.95

210 pages Year Founded: 1988 ISBN 0-398053-93-6

3105 Adolescents, Alcohol and Substance Abuse: Reaching Teens through Brief Interventions

Guilford Press
72 Spring Street
New York, NY 10012   212-431-9800
                                800-365-7006
                           Fax: 212-966-6708
                   E-mail: info@guilford.com
                                www.guilford.com

Reviews a range of empirically supported approachs to dealing with the growing problems of substance use and abuse among young people. While admission to specialized treatment programs is relatively rare in today's health care climate, there are many opportunities for brief interventions. Brief interventions also allow the clinician to work with the teen on his or her home turf, emphasize autonomy and personal responsibility, and can be used across the full range of teens who are engainging in health risk-behavior.

350 pages ISBN 1-572306-58-0

3106 American Psychiatric Press Textbook of Substance Abuse Treatment

American Psychiatric Publishing
1000 Wilson Boulevard
Suite 1825
Arlington, VA 22209-3901   703-907-7322
                                800-368-5777
                           Fax: 703-907-1091
                    E-mail: appi@psych.org
                                www.appi.org

Katie Duffy, Marketing Assistant

Comprehensive view of basic science and psychology underlying addiction and coverage of all treatment modalities. New topics include the neurobiology of alcoholism, stimulants, marijuana, opiates and hallucinogens, club drugs, and addiction in women. *$95.00*

608 pages Year Founded: 1999 ISBN 0-880488-20-4

3107 Before It's Too Late: Working with Substance Abuse in the Family

WW Norton & Company
500 5th Avenue
New York, NY 10110   212-790-9456
                           Fax: 212-869-0856
                 E-mail: admalmud@wwnorton.com
                                www.wwnorton.com

Sometimes, the problem a patient or the family of the patient's root cause to the problem they seek help for, is actually substance abuse. How to present the problem, and step-by-step models for working with families dealing with substance abuse are examined. *$ 23.95*

224 pages Year Founded: 1989 ISBN 0-393700-68-2

3108 Behind Bars: Substance Abuse and America's Prison Population

National Center on Addiction and Substance Abuse at Columbia Univ
633 3rd Avenue
19th Floor
New York, NY 10017-6706   **212-841-5200**
          Fax: 212-956-8020
          www.casacolumbia.org

Steven Belenko

Results of a three year study of American prisons and the reason drugs are responible for the booming prison population and escalating costs. *$25.00*

Year Founded: 1998

3109 Blaming the Brain: The Truth About Drugs and Mental Health

Free Press
866 3rd Avenue
New York, NY 10022-6221   **212-832-2101**
          800-323-7445
          Fax: 800-943-9831
          www.simonsays.com

Exposes weaknesses inherent in the scientific arguments supporting the theory that biochemical imbalances are the main cause of mental illness. It discusses how the accidental discover of mood-altering drugs stimulated an interest in psychopharmacology. *$25.00*

320 pages Year Founded: 1998 ISBN 0-684849-64-X

3110 Building Bridges: States Respond to Substance Abuse and Welfare Reform

National Center on Addiction and Substance Abuse at Columbia Univ
633 3rd Avenue
19th Floor
New York, NY 10017-6706   **212-841-5200**
          Fax: 212-956-8020
          www.casacolumbia.org

Prepared in partnership with the American Public Human Services Association, this two year study among the front line workers in the nation's welfare offices, job training programs and substance abuse agencies reveals what they find works and does not work in helping clients. *$15.00*

Year Founded: 1999

3111 CASAWORKS for Families: Promising Approach to Welfare Reform and Substance-Abusing Women

National Center on Addiction and Substance Abuse at Columbia Univ
633 3rd Avenue
19th Floor
New York, NY 10017-6706   **212-841-5200**
          Fax: 212-956-8020
          www.casacolumbia.org

Designed for TANF recipients, this promising approach to welfare reform is used in 11 cities and nine states. *$5.00*

3112 Clinician's Guide to the Personality Profiles of Alcohol and Drug Abusers: Typological Descriptions Using the MMPI

Charles C Thomas Publisher
2600 S 1st Street
Springfield, IL 62704-4730   **217-789-8980**
          800-258-8980
          Fax: 217-789-9130
          E-mail: books@ccthomas.com
          www.ccthomas.com

Donald J Tosi, Author
Dennis M Eshbaugh, Author
Michael A Murphy, Author

$39.95

156 pages Year Founded: 1993 ISSN 0-399-06463-6ISBN 0-398058-85-7

3113 Critical Incidents: Ethical Issues in Substance Abuse Prevention and Treatment

Hazelden
15251 Pleasant Valley Road
PO Box 176
Center City, MN 55012-0176   **651-213-2121**
          800-328-9000
          Fax: 651-213-4590
          www.hazelden.org

Two hundred critical situations for health care professionals to sharpen their decision-making skills about everyday ethical dilemmas that arise in their field. *$17.95*

276 pages ISBN 0-938475-03-7

3114 Dangerous Liaisons: Substance Abuse and Sex

National Center on Addiction and Substance Abuse at Columbia Univ
633 3rd Avenue
19th Floor
New York, NY 10017-6706   **212-841-5200**
          Fax: 212-956-8020
          www.casacolumbia.org

An intensive report on the dangerous and sometimes life-threatening connection between alcohol, drug abuse and sexual activity. Parents, guidance professionals and others will find this useful. *$22.00*

170 pages Year Founded: 1999

3115 Determinants of Substance Abuse: Biological, Psychological, and Environmental Factors

Kluwer Academic/Plenum Publishers
233 Spring Street
New York, NY 10013
212-620-8000
Fax: 212-463-0742
www.kluweronline.com

Hardcover. *$90.00*

454 pages Year Founded: 1985 ISBN 0-306418-73-8

3116 Drug Information for Teens: Health Tips about the Physical and Mental Effects of Substance Abuse

Omnigraphics
615 Giswold
Detroit, MI 48226
313-961-1340
Fax: 313-961-1383
E-mail: info@omnigraphics.com
www.omnigraphics.com

Provides students with facts about drug use, abuse, and addiction. It describes the physical and mental effects of alcohol, tobacco, marijuana, ecstasy, inhalants and many other drugs and chemicals that are often abused. It includes information about the process that leads from casual use to addiction and offers suggestions for resisting peer pressure and helping friends stay drug free.

452 pages ISBN 0-780804-44-9

3117 Empowering Adolesent Girls

WW Norton & Company
500 5th Avenue
New York, NY 10110
212-790-9456
Fax: 212-869-0856
E-mail: admalmud@wwnorton.com
www.wwnorton.com

Strategies and activities for professionals who work with adolesent girls (teachers, counselors, therapists) to offer support and encouagement through the Go Girls program. *$32.00*

256 pages Year Founded: 2001 ISSN 70347-9

3118 Ethics for Addiction Professionals

Hazelden
15251 Pleasant Valley Road
PO Box 176
Center City, MN 55012-0176
651-213-2121
800-328-9000
Fax: 651-213-4590
www.hazelden.org

The first on ethics written by and for addiction professionals that addresses complex issues such as patient confidentiality versus mandatory reporting, clinician relapse, personal and social relationships with clients and other important related issues. *$14.95*

60 pages ISBN 0-894864-54-8

3119 Hispanic Substance Abuse

Charles C Thomas Publisher
2600 S 1st Street
Springfield, IL 62704-4730
217-789-8980
800-258-8980
Fax: 217-789-9130
E-mail: books@ccthomas.com
www.ccthomas.com

Addresses the concerns of students and professionals who work with Hispanics. Brings together current research on this problem by well-known experts in the fields of alcohol and drug abuse. Useful for scholars and researchers, practitioners in the human services, and the general public. There is shown the extent of substance abuse problems in Hispanic communities, the differences amount the Hispanic subgroups and casual factors that are involved. There are detailed strategies for prevention and the necessary approaches to treatment. *$57.95*

258 pages Year Founded: 1993 ISSN 0-398-06274-9ISBN 0-398058-49-0

3120 Jail Detainees with Co-Occurring Mental Health and Substance Use Disorders

Policy Research Associates
345 Delaware Avenue
Delmar, NY 12054
518-439-7415
800-444-7415
Fax: 518-439-7612
E-mail: gains@prainc.com
www.prainc.com

Brief report that discusses the issue of keeping federal benefits for jail detainees.

3121 Love First: A New Approach to Intervention for Alcoholism and Drug Addiction

Hazelden
15245 Pleasant Valley Road
PO Box 11-CO 3
Center City, MN 55012-0011
651-213-4000
800-257-7810
Fax: 651-213-4411
www.hazelden.org

A straightforward, simple and practical resource written specifically for families seeking to help a love one struggling with substance addiction.

280 pages ISBN 1-568385-21-8

3122 Malignant Neglect: Substance Abuse and America's Schools

National Center on Addiction and Substance Abuse at Columbia Univ
633 3rd Avenue
19th Floor
New York, NY 10017-6706
212-841-5200
Fax: 212-956-8020
www.casacolumbia.org

Six years of exhaustive research of focus groups, schools, parent and professionals. Findings of the costs of drug abuse in dollars, student behavior, truancy and more. *$22.00*

117 pages Year Founded: 2001

3123 Missed Opportunity: National Survey of Primary Care Physicians and Patients on Substance Abuse

National Center on Addiction and Substance Abuse at Columbia Univ
633 3rd Avenue
19th Floor
New York, NY 10017-6706   212-841-5200
                                   Fax: 212-956-8020
                                   www.casacolumbia.org

Findings and recomendations based on a CASA report that revealed 94% of primary care physicians fail to diagnose symptoms of alcohol abuse in adult patients, and 41% of pediatricians missed a diagnosis of drug abuse when presented with a classic description of a teenage patient with these symptoms. The report also sheds light on the fact that many physicians feel unprepared to diagnose substance abuse and have little confidence in the effectiveness of treatments available. *$22.00*

Year Founded: 2000

3124 Narrative Means to Sober Ends: Treating Addiction and Its Aftermath

Guilford Publications
72 Spring Street
New York, NY 10012   212-431-9800
                              800-365-7006
                              Fax: 212-966-6708
                              E-mail: info@guilford.com
                              www.guilford.com

This eloquently written volume illuminates the devastating power of addiction and describes an array of innovative approaches to facilitating clients' recovery. Demonstrated are creative ways to help clients explore their relationship to drugs and alcohol, take the first steps toward sobriety and develop meaningful ways of living without addiction. *$37.95*

386 pages ISBN 1-572305-66-5

3125 No Place to Hide: Substance Abuse in Mid-Size Cities and Rural America

National Center on Addiction and Substance Abuse at Columbia Univ
633 3rd Avenue
19th Floor
New York, NY 10017-6706   212-841-5200
                                   Fax: 212-956-8020
                                   www.casacolumbia.org

Surprisingly to some, young people in smaller cities and rural areas are more likely to use many forms of illegal substances. Tobacco use is also higher away from the major cities. The findings on other statistics of drugs and rural adolescent and teenager use are included. *$10.00*

Year Founded: 2000

3126 No Safe Haven: Children of Substance-Abusing Parents

National Center on Addiction and Substance Abuse at Columbia Univ
633 3rd Avenue
19th Floor
New York, NY 10017-6706   212-841-5200
                                   Fax: 212-956-8020
                                   www.casacolumbia.org

Jeanne Reid, Author
Peggy Macchetto, Author
Susan Foster, Author

Comprehensive report with shattering facts and figures reveals the impact of substance abuse on parenting skills and child neglect. The number of children affected by their parent's substance abuse driven behavior has more than doubled in the last ten years, greater than the rise in children's overall population. This report calls for a reworking of the child welfare system, and provides guidelines to when the child should be permanently remove from the home. *$22.00*

Year Founded: 1999

3127 Non Medical Marijuana: Rite of Passage or Russian Roulette?

National Center on Addiction and Substance Abuse at Columbia Univ
633 3rd Avenue
19th Floor
New York, NY 10017-6706   212-841-5200
                                   Fax: 212-956-8020
                                   www.casacolumbia.org

The most recent numbers available find that more teens from 19 years old and younger enter treatment for marijuana abuse than for any other drug, including alcohol. Many teens also have a problem with secondary drugs. This report released by CASA at Columbia University, concludes that non medical marijuana is indeed a dangerous substance. *$20.00*

Year Founded: 1999

3128 Perfect Daughters

Health Communications
292 Fernwood Avenue
Edison, NJ 08837   732-346-0027
                            Fax: 732-346-0442
                            www.hcomm.com

Identifies what differentiates the adult daughters of alcoholics from other women. Adult daughters of alcoholics operate from a base of harsh and limiting views of themselves and the world. Having learned that they must function perfectly in order to avoid unpleasant situations, these women often assume responsibility for the failures of others. They are drawn to chemically dependent men and are more likely to become addicted themselves. These book collects the thoughts, feelings and experience of twelve hundred perfect daughters, offering readers an opportunity to explore their own life's dynamics and thereby heal and grow.

350 pages ISBN 1-558749-52-7

3129 Prescription Drug Abuse and Dependence

Charles C Thomas Publisher
2600 S 1st Street
Springfield, IL 62704-4730   217-789-8980
                                    800-258-8980
                              Fax: 217-789-9130
                       E-mail: books@ccthomas.com
                                www.ccthomas.com

Discusses prescription drug abuse dependence from a variety of perspectives, in three broad sections. Presents material in a practical biopsychosocial, and broad perspective and addresses an important aspect of health care; one which is more often an impediment to good health care than providers might realize or acknowledge. *$33.95*

184 pages Year Founded: 1995 ISBN 0-398059-54-3

3130 Proven Youth Development Model that Prevents Substance Abuse and Builds Communities

National Center on Addiction and Substance Abuse
at Columbia Univ
633 3rd Avenue
19th Floor
New York, NY 10017-6706   212-841-5200
                            Fax: 212-956-8020
                            www.casacolumbia.org

How-to manual developed with nine years of research. The program is a collaboration of local school, law enforcement, social service and health teams to help high risk youth between the ages of 8 - 13 years old and their families prevent substance abuse and violent behavior. Used in 23 urban and rural communities in 11 states and the District of Columbia. *$50.00*

79 pages Year Founded: 2001

3131 Relapse Prevention Maintenance: Strategies in the Treatment of Addictive Behaviors

Guilford Publications
72 Spring Street
New York, NY 10012   212-431-9800
                            800-365-7006
                      Fax: 212-966-6708
                 E-mail: info@guilford.com
                       www.guilford.com

Research on relapse prevention to problem drinking, smoking, substance abuse, eating disorders and compulsive gambling. Analyzes factors that may lead to relapse and offers practical techniques for maintaining treatment gains. *$55.00*

558 pages Year Founded: 1985 ISBN 0-898620-09-0

3132 So Help Me God: Substance Abuse, Religion and Spirituality

National Center on Addiction and Substance Abuse
at Columbia Univ
633 3rd Avenue
19th Floor
New York, NY 10017-6706   212-841-5200
                            Fax: 212-956-8020
                            www.casacolumbia.org

Results of a 2 year study, finding that spirituality has enormous power to potentially lower the risks of substance abuse. When this is combined with professional treatment, an individual's religion helps greatly with recovery. *$10.00*

Year Founded: 2001

3133 Solutions Step by Step: Substance Abuse Treatment Manual

WW Norton & Company
500 5th Avenue
New York, NY 10110   212-790-9456
                      Fax: 212-869-0856
             E-mail: admalmud@wwnorton.com
                       www.wwnorton.com

Quick tips, questions and examples focusing on successes that can be experienced helping substance abusers help themselves. *$25.00*

192 pages Year Founded: 1997 ISSN 70251-0

3134 Substance Abuse and Learning Disabilities: Peas in a Pod or Apples and Oranges?

National Center on Addiction and Substance Abuse
at Columbia Univ
633 3rd Avenue
19th Floor
New York, NY 10017-6706   212-841-5200
                            Fax: 212-956-8020
                            www.casacolumbia.org

Report originating from a conference in 1999 sponsored by CASA, the relationship between learning disabilities that are not addressed, and possible substance abuse by these same children is examined. Attention Deficit/Hyperactivity Disorder and Conduct Disorder and the link to substance abuse is also considered. *$10.00*

00 pages

3135 Substance Abuse: A Comprehensive Textbook

Lippincott Williams & Wilkins
PO Box 1600
Hagerstown, MD 21741-1600   301-714-2300
                                    800-638-3030
                              Fax: 301-824-7390

$162.00

956 pages Year Founded: 1997 ISBN 0-683181-79-3

3136 Teens and Alcohol: Gallup Youth Survey Major Issues and Trends

Mason Crest Publishers
370 Reed Road
Suite 302
Broomall, PA 19008   **866-627-2665**
                              Fax: 610-543-3878
                              www.masoncrest.com

Eighty-seven percent of high school seniors have tried alcohol and, according to a Gallup Youth Survey, 27 percent of teenagers say it is very easy for them to get alcoholic beverages. Alcohol is a contributor to the three leading causes of death for teens and young adults: automobile crashes, homicide and suicides.

112 pages ISBN 1-590847-23-7

3137 Therapeutic Communities for Addictions: Reading in Theory, Research, and Practice

Charles C Thomas Publisher
2600 S 1st Street
Springfield, IL 62704-4730   **217-789-8980**
                                        800-258-8980
                              Fax: 217-789-9130
                              E-mail: books@ccthomas.com
                              www.ccthomas.com

George De Leon, Author
James T Ziegenfuss Jr, Author

Contents: The Therapeutic Community (TC) for Substance Abuse; Democratic TCs or Programmatic TCs or Both?; Motivational Aspects of Heroin Addicts in TCs; A Sociological View of the TC; Psychodynamics of TCs for Treatment of Heroin Addicts; Britain and the Psychoanalytic Tradition in TCs; TC Research; Outcomes of Drug Abuse Treatment; 12-Year Follow-up Outcomes, College Training in a TC; Client Evaluations of TCs and Retention; Side Bets and Secondary Adjustments; Measuring Program Implementation; The TC Looking Ahead; TCs within Prisons; Uses and Abuses of Power and Authority. *$51.95*

282 pages Year Founded: 1986 ISBN
0-398052-06-9

3138 Under the Rug: Substance Abuse and the Mature Woman

National Center on Addiction and Substance Abuse
at Columbia Univ
633 3rd Avenue
19th Floor
New York, NY 10017-6706   **212-841-5200**
                              Fax: 212-956-8020
                              www.casacolumbia.org

Discusses the fact that millions of mature women are robbed of a healthy and longer lifespan due to a substance abuse problem that they discreetly hide. Their reluctance to get help costs them and the health systems billions. *$25.00*

Year Founded: 1998

3139 Understanding Psychiatric Medications in the Treatment of Chemical Dependency and Dual Diagnoses

Charles C Thomas Publisher
2600 S 1st Street
Springfield, IL 62704-4730   **217-789-8980**
                                        800-258-8980
                              Fax: 217-789-9130
                              E-mail: books@ccthomas.com
                              www.ccthomas.com

Designed to address coexisting chemical dependency and psychiatric disorder (dual diagnoses) and specifically to focus on the appropriate role of psychotropic medications in the treatment of dual diagnonsis patients. The text presents a comprehensive overview of psychiatric medication treatment for dual diagnoses that speaks to a broad professional audience while being sensitive to the values and beliefs of the chemical dependents. *$39.95*

134 pages Year Founded: 1995 ISSN
0-398-05964-0ISBN 0-398059-63-2

3140 Your Drug May Be Your Problem: How and Why to Stop Taking Pyschiatric Medications

Perseus Books Group
550 Central Avenue
Boulder, CO 80301
                              800-386-5656
                              Fax: 720-406-7336
                   E-mail: westview.orders@perseusbooks.com
                              www.perseusbooksgroup.com

In a very short time, a doctor may prescribe a drug which an individual may take for months, years, even the rest of their lives. This book provides up-to-date, descriptions of the pros and cons of taking psychiatric medication, dangers involved, and explains a safe method of withdrawl if needed. *$17.00*

288 pages Year Founded: 2000 ISBN
0-738203-48-3

Suicide

3141 Comprehensive Textbook of Suicidology

Guilford Publications
72 Spring Street
New York, NY 10012   **212-431-9800**
                                800-365-7006
                              Fax: 212-966-6708
                              E-mail: info@guilford.com
                              www.guilford.com

This volume presents an authoritative overview of current scientific knowledge about suicide and suicide prevention. Multidisciplinary and comprehesive in scope, the book provides a solid foundation in theory, research and clinical applications. Topics covered include the classification and prevalence of suicidal behaviors, psychiatric and medical factors, ethical and legal issues in intervention as well as the social, cultural and gender context of suicide. *$70.00*

650 pages ISBN 1-572305-41-X

3142 Practical Art of Suicide Assessment: A Guide for Mental Health Professionals and Substance Abuse Counselors

John Wiley & Sons
10475 Crosspoint Boulevard
Indianapolis, IN 46256   877-862-2974
                                800-597-3299
          E-mail: consumers@wiley.com
                                www.wiley.com

Covers the critical elements of suicide assessment, from risk factor analysis to evaluating clients with borderline personality disorders or psychotic process.

316 pages ISBN 0-471237-61-2

3143 Suicide From a Psychological Prespective

Charles C Thomas Publisher
2600 S 1st Street
Springfield, IL 62704-4730   217-789-8980
                                    800-258-8980
                          Fax: 217-789-9130
          E-mail: books@ccthomas.com
                                www.ccthomas.com

$39.95

142 pages Year Founded: 1988 ISBN 0-398057-09-5

3144 Teens and Suicide

Mason Crest Publishers
370 Reed Road
Suite 302
Broomall, PA 19008   866-627-2665
                          Fax: 610-543-3878
                          www.masoncrest.com

Suicide is the third-leading cause of death among adolescents in the United States; in a recent study by The Gallup Organization, 47 percent of teenagers between the ages of 13 and 17 said they know someone who has tried to take their own lives. This volume examines the cause of teen-age suicide and explores such issues as teens and guns as well as suicide rates among minorities.

3145 Treatment of Suicidal Patients in Managed Care

American Psychiatric Publishing
1000 Wilson Boulevard
Suite 1825
Arlington, VA 22209-3901   703-907-7322
                                800-368-5777
                          Fax: 703-907-1091
          E-mail: appi@psych.org
                                www.appi.org

Katie Duffy, Marketing Assistant

Suicide is an all too common cause of death and preventable, but the managed care concerns of cost control with rapid diagnosis and treatment of depression puts the clinician in a dilemma. This book guides the professional with advice on knowing who to contact, and getting more of what is needed from the patient's managed care provider. *$39.00*

240 pages Year Founded: 2001 ISBN 0-880488-28-x

Pediatric & Adolescent Issues

3146 Acquired Brain Injury in Childhood and Adolescence

Charles C Thomas Publisher
2600 S 1st Street
Springfield, IL 62704-4730   217-789-8980
                                    800-258-8980
                          Fax: 217-789-9130
          E-mail: books@ccthomas.com
                                www.ccthomas.com

Designed to increase professionals' understanding of the educational dimensions of acquired brain injury; its goal is not simply to help readers understand the often tricky realities of acquired brain injury in children, but more importantly to help them work effectively with these children and their families. Topics include a summary of basic information related to brain injury and its varied effects on behavior, a review of the history of special education law, procedural regulations, options for educational service delivery, and practical discussions. For rehabilitation professionals, educators, vocational specialists, attorneys, and parents. *$60.95*

262 pages Year Founded: 1996 ISSN 0-398-06590-XISBN 0-398065-89-6

3147 Adolescents in Psychiatric Hospitals: a Psychodynamic Approach to Evaluation and Treatment

Charles C Thomas Publisher
2600 S 1st Street
Springfield, IL 62704-4730   217-789-8980
                                    800-258-8980
                          Fax: 217-789-9130
          E-mail: books@ccthomas.com
                                www.ccthomas.com

A short history of adolescent inpatient psychiatry and its clinical methods, and a month-long, running account of the morning meetings of a typical inpatient ward. For trainees in child and adolescent psychiatry, nurses, social workers, administrators, and psychologists working in the field of adolescent inpatient psychiatry. *$32.95*

208 pages Year Founded: 1998 ISBN 0-398068-60-7

3148 Adolesent in Family Therapy: Breaking the Cycle of Conflict and Control

Guilford Publications
72 Spring Street
New York, NY 10012   212-431-9800
                            800-365-7006
                          Fax: 212-966-6708
          E-mail: info@guilford.com
                                www.guilford.com

Family relationships that are troubled can be catalysts for change. A guide to treating a wide range of parent/adolescent problems with straightforward advice. *$19.95*

336 pages Year Founded: 1998 ISBN 1-572305-88-6

3149 At-Risk Youth in Crises

Pro-Ed Publications
8700 Shoal Creek Boulevard
Austin, TX 78757-6816   512-451-3246
                                          800-897-3202
                                   Fax: 800-397-7633
                          E-mail: info@proedinc.com
                                    www.proedinc.com

This edition has updated material in the chapters covering divorce, loss, abuse, severe depression and suicide. *$31.00*

268 pages Year Founded: 1994 ISBN 0-890795-74-6

3150 Attachment, Trauma and Healing: Understanding and Treating Attachment Disorder in Children and Families

200 E Joppa Road
Suite 207
Baltimore, MD 21286   410-825-8888
                                          888-825-8249
                                   Fax: 410-337-0747
                          E-mail: sidran@sidran.org
                                     www.sidran.org

An in depth look at the causes of attachment disorder, explains the normal development of attachment, examines the research in this area and present treatment plans. Numerous appendices include a sample intake packet, two brief day in the life accounts of children with attachment disorder, assessment guides, treatment plans and references. *$34.95*

313 pages

3151 Basic Child Psychiatry

American Psychiatric Publishing
1000 Wilson Boulevard
Suite 1825
Arlington, VA 22209-3901   703-907-7322
                                          800-368-5777
                                   Fax: 703-907-1091
                          E-mail: appi@psych.org
                                       www.appi.org

Katie Duffy, Marketing Assistant

$46.95

416 pages Year Founded: 1995 ISBN 0-632037-72-5

3152 Behavior Modification for Exceptional Children and Youth

Pro-Ed Publications
8700 Shoal Creek Boulevard
Austin, TX 78757-6816   512-451-3246
                                          800-897-3202
                                   Fax: 800-397-7633
                          E-mail: info@proedinc.com
                                    www.proedinc.com

An authoritative textbook for courses in behavior modification. Serves as a practical, comprehensive reference work for clinicians working with people with disabilities and behavior problems. *$37.00*

296 pages Year Founded: 1993 ISBN 1-563720-42-6

3153 Behavior Rating Profile

Pro-Ed Publications
8700 Shoal Creek Boulevard
Austin, TX 78757-6816   512-451-3246
                                          800-897-3202
                                   Fax: 800-397-7633
                          E-mail: info@proedinc.com
                                    www.proedinc.com

Provides different evaluations of a student's behavior at home, at school, and in interpersonal relationships from the varied perpsectives of parents, teachers, peers, and the target students themselves. Identifies students whose behavior is perceived to be deviant, the settings in which behavior problems are prominent, and the persons whose perceptions of student's behavior are different from those of other respondents. *$194.00*

Year Founded: 1990

3154 Behavioral Approach to Assessment of Youth with Emotional/Behavioral Disorders

Pro-Ed Publications
8700 Shoal Creek Boulevard
Austin, TX 78757-6816   512-451-3246
                                          800-897-3202
                                   Fax: 800-397-7633
                          E-mail: info@proedinc.com
                                    www.proedinc.com

This new book addresses one of the most challenging aspects of special education: evaluating students referred for suspected emotional/behavioral disorders. Geared to the practical needs and concerns of school-based practitioners, including special education teachers, school psychologists and social workers. *$44.00*

729 pages Year Founded: 1996 ISBN 0-890796-25-4

3155 Behavioral Approaches: Problem Child

Cambridge University Press
40 W 20th Street
New York, NY 10011-4221   212-924-3900
                                   Fax: 212-691-3239
                          E-mail: marketing@cup.org
                                       www.cup.org

3156 Candor, Connection and Enterprise in Adolesent Therapy

WW Norton & Company
500 5th Avenue
New York, NY 10110   212-790-9456
                                   Fax: 212-869-0856
                          E-mail: admalmud@wwnorton.com
                                    www.wwnorton.com

Suggestions and troubleshooting for therapists dealing with uncooperative adolescent patients. Avoiding the appearance of trying too hard, dialouges that seem to go nowhere, and gaining the faith of a child who may not appreciate efforts on their behalf. *$35.00*

208 pages Year Founded: 2001 ISSN 70356-8

3157 Child Friendly Therapy: Biophysical Innovations for Children and Families

WW Norton & Company
500 5th Avenue
New York, NY 10110   212-790-9456
                                  Fax: 212-869-0856
              E-mail: admalmud@wwnorton.com
                              www.wwnorton.com

Family centered treatment for children. Suggestions and case studies, therapy room set up and session structure, multi sensory skill building leading to a fresh understanding of often misunderstood children. Family members can be incorporated to work as a team to help with therapy. *$32.00*

256 pages Year Founded: 2002 ISSN 70355-X

3158 Child Psychiatry

American Psychiatric Publishing
1000 Wilson Boulevard
Suite 1825
Arlington, VA 22209-3901   703-907-7322
                                        800-368-5777
                                  Fax: 703-907-1091
                         E-mail: appi@psych.org
                                      www.appi.org

Katie Duffy, Marketing Assistant

Provides the essential facts and concepts for everyone involved in child psychiatry, the book includes 200 questions and answers for trainees approaching professional examinations. *$46.95*

336 pages Year Founded: 1987 ISBN 0-632038-85-3

3159 Child Psychopharmacology

American Psychiatric Publishing
1000 Wilson Boulevard
Suite 1825
Arlington, VA 22209-3901   703-907-7322
                                        800-368-5777
                                  Fax: 703-907-1091
                         E-mail: appi@psych.org
                                      www.appi.org

Katie Duffy, Marketing Assistant

Includes: Tic disorders and obsessive-compulsive disorder; Attention-deficit/hyperactivity disorder; Children and adolescents with psychotic disorders; Affective disorders in children and adolescents; Anxiety disorders; Eating disorders. *$26.00*

200 pages ISBN 0-880488-33-6

3160 Child and Adolescent Mental Health Consultation in Hospitals, Schools and Courts

American Psychiatric Publishing
1000 Wilson Boulevard
Suite 1825
Arlington, VA 22209-3901   703-907-7322
                                        800-368-5777
                                  Fax: 703-907-1091
                         E-mail: appi@psych.org
                                      www.appi.org

Katie Duffy, Marketing Assistant

Leading experts present a practical guide for mental health professionals. *$38.50*

316 pages Year Founded: 1993 ISBN 0-880484-18-7

3161 Child and Adolescent Psychiatry: Modern Approaches

American Psychiatric Publishing
1000 Wilson Boulevard
Suite 1825
Arlington, VA 22209-3901   703-907-7322
                                        800-368-5777
                                  Fax: 703-907-1091
                         E-mail: appi@psych.org
                                      www.appi.org

Katie Duffy, Marketing Assistant

ISBN 0-632028-21-1

3162 Child-Centered Counseling and Psychoterapy

Charles C Thomas Publisher
2600 S 1st Street
Springfield, IL 62704-4730   217-789-8980
                                        800-258-8980
                                  Fax: 217-789-9130
              E-mail: books@ccthomas.com
                              www.ccthomas.com

Topics include an introduction to child-centered counseling, counseling as a three-phase process, applying the reflective process, phase three alternatives, counseling through play, consultation, and professional issues. It represents the status of child-centered counseling which also indentifies ideas which can influence its future. *$62.95*

262 pages Year Founded: 1995 ISSN 0-398-06522-5ISBN 0-398065-21-7

3163 Childhood Behavior Disorders: Applied Research and Educational Practice

Pro-Ed Publications
8700 Shoal Creek Boulevard
Austin, TX 78757-6816   512-451-3246
                                        800-897-3202
                                  Fax: 800-397-7633
              E-mail: info@proedinc.com
                              www.proedinc.com

Provides the balance of theory, research and practical relevance needed by students in graduate and undergraduate introductory courses, as well as practicing teachers and other professionals. *$ 39.00*

550 pages Year Founded: 1998 ISBN 0-890797-19-6

3164 Childhood Disorders

Brunner/Mazel
325 Chestnut Street
Philadelphia, PA 19106
                                        800-821-8312
                                  Fax: 215-269-0363

Provides an up-to-date summary of the current information about thepsychological disorders of childhood as well as their causes, nature and course. Together with discussion and evaluation of the major models that guide psychological thinking about the disorders. Gives detailed consideration of the criteria used to make the diagnoses, a presentation of the latest research findings on the nature of the disorder and an overview of the methods used and evaluations conducted for the treatment of the disorders. *$26.95*

240 pages ISBN 0-863776-09-4

3165 Childs Work/Childs Play

135 Dupont Street
PO Box 760
Plainview, NY 11803-0760

800-962-1141
Fax: 800-262-1886
E-mail: info@Childswork.com
www.Childswork.com

Catalog of books, games, toys and workbooks relating to child development issues such as recognizing emotions, handling uncertainty, bullies, ADD, shyness, conflicts and other things that children may need some help navigating.

3166 Clinical & Forensic Interviewing of Children & Families

Jerome M Sattler
PO Box 3557
La Mesa, CA 91944-3557

619-460-3667
Fax: 619-460-2489

3167 Clinical Application of Projective Drawings

Charles C Thomas Publisher
2600 S 1st Street
Springfield, IL 62704-4730

217-789-8980
800-258-8980
Fax: 217-789-9130
E-mail: books@ccthomas.com
www.ccthomas.com

On its way to becoming the classic in the field of projective drawings, this book provides a grounding in fundamentals and goes on to consider differential diagnosis, appraisal of psychological resources as treatment potentials and projective drawing usage in therapy. *$65.95*

688 pages Year Founded: 1980 ISBN 0-398007-68-3

3168 Clinical Child Documentation Sourcebook: Comprehensive Collection of Forms and Guidelines for Efficient Record Keeping in Child Mental Health

John Wiley & Sons
605 3rd Avenue
New York, NY 10058-0180

212-850-6000
Fax: 212-850-6008
E-mail: info@wiley.com
www.wiley.com

This easy to use resource offers child psychologists and therapists a full array of forms, inventories, checklists, client handouts, and clinical records essential to a successful practice in either and organizational or clinical setting. *$49.95*

256 pages Year Founded: 1999 ISBN 0-471291-11-0

3169 Cognitive Behavior Therapy Child

Cambridge University Press
40 W 20th Street
New York, NY 10011-4221

212-924-3900
Fax: 212-691-3239
E-mail: marketing@cup.org
www.cup.org

3170 Concise Guide to Child and Adolescent Psychiatry

American Psychiatric Publishing
1000 Wilson Boulevard
Suite 1825
Arlington, VA 22209-3901

703-907-7322
800-368-5777
Fax: 703-907-1091
E-mail: appi@psych.org
www.appi.org

Katie Duffy, Marketing Assistant

Topics include evaluation and treatment planning, axis I disorders usually first diagnosed in infancy, childhood or adolescence, attention deficit and disruptive behavior disorders, developmental disorders, special clinical circumstances, psychopharmacology, and psychosocial treatments. *$21.95*

400 pages Year Founded: 1998 ISBN 0-880489-05-7

3171 Controlling Stress in Children

Charles C Thomas Publisher
2600 S 1st Street
Springfield, IL 62704-4730

217-789-8980
800-258-8980
Fax: 217-789-9130
E-mail: books@ccthomas.com
www.ccthomas.com

$39.95

210 pages Year Founded: 1985 ISBN 0-398050-50-3

3172 Counseling Children with Special Needs

American Psychiatric Publishing
1000 Wilson Boulevard
Suite 1825
Arlington, VA 22209-3901

703-907-7322
800-368-5777
Fax: 703-907-1091
E-mail: appi@psych.org
www.appi.org

Katie Duffy, Marketing Assistant

$29.95

224 pages Year Founded: 1997 ISBN 0-632041-51-

3173 Creative Therapy with Children and Adolescents

Impact Publishers
PO Box 6016
Atascadero, CA 93423-6016

805-466-5917
800-246-7228
Fax: 805-466-5919
E-mail: info@impactpublishers.com
www.impactpublishers.com

Encourages creativity in therapy, assists therapists in talking with children to facilitate change. From simple ideas to fresh innovations, the activities are to be used as tools to supplement a variety of therapeutic approaches, and can be tailored to each child's needs. $21.95

*192 pages Year Founded: 1999 ISBN
1-886230-19-6*

3174 Defiant Teens

Guilford Publications
72 Spring Street
New York, NY 10012

212-431-9800
800-365-7006
Fax: 212-966-6708
E-mail: info@guilford.com
www.guilford.com

Guidelines for best practices in working with families and their teenaged children.

*250 pages Year Founded: 1999 ISBN
1-572304-40-5*

3175 Developmental Therapy/Developmental Teaching

Pro-Ed Publications
8700 Shoal Creek Boulevard
Austin, TX 78757-6816

512-451-3246
800-897-3202
Fax: 800-397-7633
E-mail: info@proedinc.com
www.proedinc.com

Constance Quirk, Editor

Provides extensive applications for teachers, counselors, parents and other adults concerned about the behavior and emotional stability of children and teens. The focus is on helping children and youth to cope effectively with the stresses of comtemporary life, with an emphasis on the positive effects adults can have on students when they adjust strategies to the social emotional needs of children. $41.00

*398 pages Year Founded: 1996 ISBN
0-890796-64-5*

3176 Enhancing Social Competence in Young Students

Pro-Ed Publications
8700 Shoal Creek Boulevard
Austin, TX 78757-6816

512-451-3246
800-897-3202
Fax: 800-397-7633
E-mail: info@proedinc.com
www.proedinc.com

Addresses conceptual and practical issues of providing social competence-enhancing interventions for young students in schools, based on research findings. Summarizes recent advances in social skills programming for at-risk students and prevention interventions for all students. Discussions of developmental issues of childhood maladjustment, intervention strategies, implementation issues and assessment/evaluation issues are provided. $28.00

*281 pages Year Founded: 1995 ISBN
0-890796-20-3*

3177 Group Therapy With Children and Adolescents

American Psychiatric Publishing
1000 Wilson Boulevard
Suite 1825
Arlington, VA 22209-3901

703-907-7322
800-368-5777
Fax: 703-907-1091
E-mail: appi@psych.org
www.appi.org

Explores a major treatment modality often used with adult populations and rarely considered for child and adolescent treatments. With contributions from international experts, this book looks at the effectiveness of treatment and cost of group therapy as it applies to this particular age group. $52.00

400 pages ISBN 0-880484-06-3

3178 Handbook of Child Behavior in Therapy and in the Psychiatric Setting

John Wiley & Sons
605 3rd Avenue
New York, NY 10058-0180

212-850-6000
Fax: 212-850-6008
E-mail: info@wiley.com
www.wiley.com

512 pages Year Founded: 1994

3179 Handbook of Infant Mental Health

Guilford Publications
72 Spring Street
New York, NY 10012

212-431-9800
800-365-7006
Fax: 212-966-6708
E-mail: info@guilford.com
www.guilford.com

Included are chapters on neurobiology, diagnostic issues, parental mental health issues and family dynamics. $60.00

*588 pages Year Founded: 2000 ISBN
1-572305-15-0*

3180 Handbook of Parent Training: Parents as Co-Therapists for Children's Behavior Problems

John Wiley & Sons
605 3rd Avenue
New York, NY 10058-0180

212-850-6000
Fax: 212-850-6008
E-mail: info@wiley.com
www.wiley.com

This completely revised handbook shows professionals who work with troubled children how to teach parents to become co-therapists. It presents various techniques and behavior modification skills that will help parents to better relate, communicate, and respond to their child. Updates are provided on such problems as noncompliance, ADHD, and conduct disorder, and a new section on special needs parents which includes adolescent mothers, aggressive parents, substance abusing parents, and more.

594 pages Year Founded: 1994

3181 Handbook of Psychiatric Practice in the Juvenile Court

American Psychiatric Press
1000 Wilson Boulevard
Suite 1825
Arlington, VA 22209-3901   703-907-7322
                                  800-368-5777
                             Fax: 703-907-1091
                    E-mail: appi@psych.org
                             www.appi.org

Katie Duffy, Marketing Assistant

Examines the role that psychiatrists and other mental health professionals are asked to play when children, adolescents, and their families end up in court. *$12.95*

198 pages ISBN 0-890422-33-8

3182 Helping Parents, Youth, and Teachers Understand Medications for Behavioral and Emotional Problems

American Psychiatric Publishing
1000 Wilson Boulevard
Suite 1825
Arlington, VA 22209-3901   703-907-7322
                                  800-368-5777
                             Fax: 703-907-1091
                    E-mail: appi@psych.org
                             www.appi.org

Katie Duffy, Marketing Assistant

Valuable resource for anyone involved in evaluating psychiatric disturbances in children and adolescents. Provides a compilation of information sheets to help promote the dialogue between the patient's family, caregivers, and the treating physician. *$39.95*

196 pages Year Founded: 1999 ISBN 0-880487-94-1

3183 How to Teach Social Skills

Pro-Ed Publications
8700 Shoal Creek Boulevard
Austin, TX 78757-6816   512-451-3246
                               800-897-3202
                          Fax: 800-397-7633
                 E-mail: info@proedinc.com
                          www.proedinc.com

$8.00

ISBN 0-890797-61-7

3184 In the Long Run... Longitudinal Studies of Psychopathology in Children

American Psychiatric Publishing
1000 Wilson Boulevard
Suite 1825
Arlington, VA 22209-3901   703-907-7322
                                  800-368-5777
                             Fax: 703-907-1091
                    E-mail: appi@psych.org
                             www.appi.org

$29.95

224 pages Year Founded: 1999 ISBN 0-873182-11-1

3185 Infants, Toddlers and Families: Framework for Support and Intervention

Guilford Publications
72 Spring Street
Department 4E
New York, NY 10012-9902
                    E-mail: exam@guilford.com
                             www.guilford.com

Examines the complex development in a child's first 3 years of life. Instead of preaching or judging, this book acknowledges the challenges facing all families, especially vulnerable ones, and offers straightforward advice. *$28.95*

204 pages Year Founded: 1999 ISBN 1-572304-87-1

3186 Interventions for Students with Emotional Disorders

Pro-Ed Publications
8700 Shoal Creek Boulevard
Austin, TX 78757-6816   512-451-3246
                               800-897-3202
                          Fax: 800-397-7633
                 E-mail: info@proedinc.com
                          www.proedinc.com

This graduate textbook for special education students advocates an eclectic approach toward teaching children with social adjustment problems. Provides how-to information for implementing various techniques to successfully enhance positive sociobehavioral development in children with emotional disorders. *$36.00*

212 pages Year Founded: 1991 ISBN 0-890792-96-8

3187 Interviewing Children and Adolesents: Skills and Strategies for Effective DSM-IV Diagnosis

Guilford Publications
72 Spring Street
New York, NY 10012   212-431-9800
                             800-365-7006
                        Fax: 212-966-6708
               E-mail: info@guilford.com
                        www.guilford.com

Guide to developmentally appropriate interviewing. *$ 45.00*

482 pages Year Founded: 99 ISBN 1-572305-01-0

3188 Interviewing the Sexually Abused Child

American Psychiatric Publishing
1000 Wilson Boulevard
Suite 1825
Arlington, VA 22209-3901　　　**703-907-7322**
800-368-5777
Fax: 703-907-1091
E-mail: appi@psych.org
www.appi.org

Katie Duffy, Marketing Assistant

A guide for mental health professionals who need to know if a child has been sexually abused. Presents guidelines on the structure of the interview and covers the use of free play, toys, and play materials by focusing on the investigate interview of the suspected victim. *$15.00*

80 pages Year Founded: 1993 ISBN 0-880486-12-0

3189 Learning Disorders and Disorders of the Self in Children and Adolesents

WW Norton & Company
500 5th Avenue
New York, NY 10110　　　**212-790-9456**
Fax: 212-869-0856
E-mail: admalmud@wwnorton.com
www.wwnorton.com

Clinicians who work with learning disabled children need to understand the complex, integrated framework of learning and self image problems. Specific problems and treatments are discussed. *$32.00*

332 pages Year Founded: 2001 ISSN 70377-0

3190 Living on the Razor's Edge: Solution-Oriented Brief Family Therapy with Self-Harming Adolesents

WW Norton & Company
500 5th Avenue
New York, NY 10110　　　**212-790-9456**
Fax: 212-869-0856
E-mail: admalmud@wwnorton.com
www.wwnorton.com

Research supported stagies and a therapy model for self harming adolesents and their families to devlop closer and more meaningful relationships. *$25.60*

320 pages Year Founded: 2002 ISSN 70335-5

3191 Making the Grade: Guide to School Drug Prevention Programs

Drug Strategies
1150 Connecticut Avenue NW
Suite 800
Washington, DC 20036　　　**202-289-9070**
Fax: 202-414-6199
E-mail: dspoilcy@aol.com

Updated and expanded from the 1996 original, this guide to drug prevention programs in America helps parents and educators make informed decisions with often limited budgets. *$14.95*

3192 Manual of Clinical Child and Adolescent Psychiatry

American Psychiatric Publishing
1000 Wilson Boulevard
Suite 1825
Arlington, VA 22209-3901　　　**703-907-7322**
800-368-5777
Fax: 703-907-1091
E-mail: appi@psych.org
www.appi.org

Katie Duffy, Marketing Assistant

Addresses current issues such as cost containment, insurance complications, and legal and ethical issues, as well as neuropsychology, alcohol, and substance abuse, and mental retardation and genetics. *$42.50*

528 pages ISBN 0-880485-28-0

3193 Mental Affections Childhood

Cambridge University Press
40 W 20th Street
New York, NY 10011-4221　　　**212-924-3900**
Fax: 212-691-3239
E-mail: marketing@cup.org
www.cup.org

$30.00

185 pages Year Founded: 1991

3194 Myth of Maturity: What Teenagers Need from Parents to Become Adults

WW Norton & Company
500 5th Avenue
New York, NY 10110　　　**212-790-9456**
Fax: 212-869-0856
E-mail: admalmud@wwnorton.com
www.wwnorton.com

Debunking outdated and misguided ideas about maturity, the author discusses the amount of support teens need from their parents, what is too much for independence, or not enough. *$24.95*

256 pages Year Founded: 2001 ISBN 0-393049-42-6

3195 Narrative Therapies with Children and Adolescents

Guilford Publications
72 Spring Street
New York, NY 10012　　　**212-431-9800**
800-365-7006
Fax: 212-966-6708
E-mail: info@guilford.com
www.guilford.com

Many renowned, creative contributors collaborate to bring this professional resource to the shelf. Transcripts of case examples, using many different methods and mediums are shown to engage children of different perspectives and ages. This book can serve as a text for child/adolesent psychotherapy, or is a useful guide for mental health professionals. *$39.95*

469 pages Year Founded: 1997 ISBN 1-572302-53-4

3196 National Survey of American Attitudes on Substance Abuse VI: Teens

National Center on Addiction and Substance Abuse at Columbia Univ
633 3rd Avenue
19th Floor
New York, NY 10017-6706
212-841-5200
Fax: 212-956-8020
www.casacolumbia.org

Results of the sixth annual CASA National Survey of teens 12 - 17 years old reveals that parents that are more involved with their children's activities and have house rules and expectations can greatly influence teen behavior choices. Other statistics about availability of illegal substances and who may use them. *$22.00*

3197 No-Talk Therapy for Children and Adolescents

WW Norton & Company
500 5th Avenue
New York, NY 10110
212-790-9456
Fax: 212-869-0856
E-mail: admalmud@wwnorton.com
www.wwnorton.com

Creative approach to treatment of young people who cannot respond to conversation based therapy. Seemingly sullen patients can be helped to find a voice of their own. *$.27*

288 pages Year Founded: 1999 ISSN 70286-3

3198 Ordinary Families, Special Children: Systems Approach to Childhood Disability

Guilford Publications
72 Spring Street
New York, NY 10012
212-431-9800
800-365-7006
Fax: 212-966-6708
E-mail: info@guilford.com
www.guilford.com

Families, including siblings and grandparents are impacted by the special needs of a child's disability. The authors explore personal accounts that shape a family's response to childhood disability and how they come to adapt these unique needs to a satisfactory lifestyle. Available in hardcover and paperback. *$35.00*

324 pages Year Founded: 1999 ISBN 1-572301-55-4

3199 Outcomes for Children and Youth with Emotional and Behavioral Disorders and their Families

Pro-Ed Publications
8700 Shoal Creek Boulevard
Austin, TX 78757-6816
512-451-3246
800-897-3202
Fax: 800-397-7633
E-mail: info@proedinc.com
www.proedinc.com

This new book addresses one of the most challenging aspects of serving children and youth with emotional and behavioral disorders-evaluating the outcomes of the services you've provided. Also includes information on such topics as: child and family outcomes, system level anaylsis, case study analysis, cost analysis, cultural diversity, managed care, and consumer satisfaction. *$44.00*

730 pages Year Founded: 1998 ISBN 0-890797-50-1

3200 Play Therapy with Children in Crisis: Individual, Group and Family Treatment

Guilford Publications
72 Spring Street
New York, NY 10012
212-431-9800
800-365-7006
Fax: 212-966-6708
E-mail: info@guilford.com
www.guilford.com

$45.00

506 pages Year Founded: 1999 ISBN 1-572304-85-5

3201 Power and Compassion: Working with Difficult Adolesents and Abused Parents

Guilford Publications
72 Spring Street
New York, NY 10012
212-431-9800
800-365-7006
Fax: 212-966-6708
E-mail: info@guilford.com
www.guilford.com

Useful as a supplemental text, or for mental health professionals dealing with aggressive teenagers and their parents. Pragmatic guide to help demoralized parents be more understanding, but more decisive. *$16.95*

196 pages Year Founded: 1999 ISBN 1-572304-70-7

3202 Practical Charts for Managing Behavior

Pro-Ed Publications
8700 Shoal Creek Boulevard
Austin, TX 78757-6816
512-451-3246
800-897-3202
Fax: 800-397-7633
E-mail: info@proedinc.com
www.proedinc.com

$29.00

160 pages Year Founded: 1998 ISBN 0-890797-36-6

3203 Psychological Examination of the Child

John Wiley & Sons
605 3rd Avenue
New York, NY 10058-0180
212-850-6000
Fax: 212-850-6008
E-mail: info@wiley.com
www.wiley.com

279 pages Year Founded: 1991

3204 Psychotherapies with Children and Adolescents

American Psychiatric Publishing
1000 Wilson Boulevard
Suite 1825
Arlington, VA 22209-3901
703-907-7322
800-368-5777
Fax: 703-907-1091
E-mail: appi@psych.org
www.appi.org

Katie Duffy, Marketing Assistant

Illustrated with case histories and demonstrates how psychoanalytic techniques can be modified to meet the therapeutic needs of children and adolescents in specific clinical situations. *$47.50*

346 pages ISBN 0-880484-06-3

3205 Safe Schools/Safe Students: Guide to Violence Prevention Stategies

Drug Strategies
1150 Connecticut Avenue NW
Suite 800
Washington, DC 20036
202-289-9070
Fax: 202-414-6199
E-mail: dspoilcy@aol.com

Practical assistance in rating over 84 violence prevention programs for classroom use, helps examine school policies and possible changes for student protection. *$14.95*

3206 Severe Stress and Mental Disturbance in Children

American Psychiatric Publishing
1000 Wilson Boulevard
Suite 1825
Arlington, VA 22209-3901
703-907-7322
800-368-5777
Fax: 703-907-1091
E-mail: appi@psych.org
www.appi.org

Katie Duffy, Marketing Assistant

Uniquely blends current research and clinical data on the effects of severe stress on children. Each chapter is written by international experts in their field. *$69.95*

708 pages ISBN 0-880486-57-0

3207 Structured Adolescent Pscyhotherapy Groups

Professional Resource Press
PO Box 15560
Sarasota, FL 34277-1560
941-343-9601
800-443-3364
Fax: 941-343-9201
E-mail: orders@prpress.com
www.prpress.com

Debra Fink, Managing Editor

Provides specific techniques for use in the beginning, middle, and end phase of time-limited structured psychotherapy groups. Offers concrete suggestions for working with hard to reach and difficult adolescents, providing feedback to parents, and dealing with administrative, legal, and ethical issues. Examples of pre/post evaluation forms, therapy contracts, evaluation feedback letters, parent response forms, therapist rating scales, co-therapist rating forms, problem identification forms, supervision and session records, client and patient handouts, and specific group exercises. Solidly anchored to research on the curative factors in group therapy, this book includes empirical data, references, theoretical formulations and examples of group sessions. *$19.95*

164 pages Year Founded: 1994 ISBN 0-943158-74-5

3208 Textbook of Child and Adolescent Psychiatry

American Psychiatric Publishing
1000 Wilson Boulevard
Suite 1825
Arlington, VA 22209-3901
703-907-7322
800-368-5777
Fax: 703-907-1091
E-mail: appi@psych.org
www.appi.org

Katie Duffy, Marketing Assistant

Includes chapter on changes in DSM-IV classification and discusses the latest research and treatment advances in the areas of epidemiology, fenetics, developmental neurobiology, and combined treatments. A special section covers essential issues such as HIV and AIDS, gender identity disorders, physical and sexual abuse, and substance abuse, for the child and adolescent psychiatrist. *$140.00*

960 pages ISBN 1-882103-03-3

3209 Textbook of Pediatric Neuropsychiatry

American Psychiatric Publishing
1000 Wilson Boulevard
Suite 1825
Arlington, VA 22209-3901
703-907-7322
800-368-5777
Fax: 703-907-1091
E-mail: appi@psych.org
www.appi.org

Katie Duffy, Marketing Assistant

Comprehensive textbook on pediatric medicine. *$175.00*

1632 pages Year Founded: 1998 ISBN 0-880487-66-6

3210 Through the Eyes of a Child

WW Norton & Company
500 5th Avenue
New York, NY 10110 212-790-9456
Fax: 212-869-0856
E-mail: admalmud@wwnorton.com
www.wwnorton.com

Comprehensive and helpful, this book helps therapists work with children and parents in the application of EMDR with children. $ 37.00

288 pages Year Founded: 1999 ISSN 70287-1

3211 Treating Depressed Children: a Therapeutic Manual of Proven Cognitive Behavior Techniques

New Harbinger Publications
5674 Shattuck Avenue
Oakland, CA 94609-1662 510-652-2002
800-748-6273
Fax: 510-652-5472
E-mail: customerservice@newharbinger.com
www.newharbinger.com

Program invorporating cartoons and role playing games to help children recognize emotions, change negative thoughts, gain confidence, and learn interpersonal skills. $49.94

160 pages Year Founded: 1996 ISBN 1-572240-61-

3212 Treating the Aftermath of Sexual Abuse: a Handbook for Working with Children in Care

Child Welfare League of America

A handbook for working with children in care who have been sexually abused. The authors review the impact of sexual abuse on a child's physical and emotional development and describe the effect of abuse on basic life experiences. Paperback. $18.95

176 pages Year Founded: 1998 ISBN 0-878686-93-2

3213 Treating the Tough Adolesent: Family Based Step by Step Guide

Guilford Publications
72 Spring Street
New York, NY 10012 212-431-9800
800-365-7006
Fax: 212-966-6708
E-mail: info@guilford.com
www.guilford.com

Model for effective family therapy, with reproducible handouts. $35.00

320 pages Year Founded: 1998 ISBN 1-572304-22-7

3214 Troubled Teens: Multidimensional Family Therapy

WW Norton & Company
500 5th Avenue
New York, NY 10110 212-790-9456
Fax: 212-869-0856
E-mail: admalmud@wwnorton.com
www.wwnorton.com

Based on 17 years of research, this treatment manual is for therapists who work with youth referred for substance abuse and behavior counseling. Treatment ivolves drug counseling, family and individual sessions and interventions. People or systems of influence outside the family are also considered. $35.00

320 pages Year Founded: 2002 ISBN 0-393703-40-1

3215 Understanding and Teaching Emotionally Disturbed Children and Adolescents

Pro-Ed Publications
8700 Shoal Creek Boulevard
Austin, TX 78757-6816 512-451-3246
800-897-3202
Fax: 800-397-7633
E-mail: info@proedinc.com
www.proedinc.com

Shows how diverse theoretical perspectives translate into practice by exploring forms of therapy and types of interventions currently employed with children and adolescents. $41.00

620 pages Year Founded: 1993 ISBN 0-890795-75-4

3216 Ups & Downs: How to Beat the Blues and Teen Depression

Price Stern Sloan Publishing

Andy Cooke, Illustrator

This book discusses how to recognize depression in teens and what to do about it. Informal, yet informative, using quotes and case studies representing typical young people who are dealing with mood swings, eating disorders and problems at school or at home. The book also demystifies therapy and advises readers on how to seek help, particularly if they, or their friends, have suicidal thoughts. Reading level ages nine to twelve. $4.99

90 pages Year Founded: 1999 ISBN 0-843174-50-1

3217 Youth Violence: Prevention, Intervention, and Social Policy

American Psychiatric Publishing
1000 Wilson Boulevard
Suite 1825
Arlington, VA 22209-3901 703-907-7322
800-368-5777
Fax: 703-907-1091
E-mail: appi@psych.org
www.appi.org

Katie Duffy, Marketing Assistant

Based on more than a decade of clinical research and treatment experience, this comprehensive and non-technical book offers a stage-oriented approach to understanding and treating complex and difficult traumatized patients, integrating modern trauma theory with traditional therapeutic interventions. *$48.50*

336 pages Year Founded: 1998 ISBN 0-880488-09-3

Conferences & Meetings

3218 AAMR-American Association on Mental Retardation Conference: Annual Meeting at the Crossroads

AAMR
444 N Capitol Street NW
Suite 846
Washington, DC 20001-1512   202-387-1968
                                800-424-3688
                          Fax: 202-387-2193
                    E-mail: dcroser@aamr.com
                               www.aamr.org

Paula A Hirt, Meetings Director Programs
Malene S Ward, Meeting Coordinator

The annual meeting offers a full compliment of workshops, symposia, and multidisciplinary sessions that fill five days including social events. Ethics, Genetics, Leadership, and Self-Determination. *$245.00*

3219 American Academy of Child and Adolescent Psychiatry (AACAP): Annual Meeting

3615 Wisconsin Avenue NW
Washington, DC 20016-3007   202-966-7300
                                800-333-7636
                          Fax: 202-966-2891
                               www.aacap.org

Virginia Q Anthony, Executive Director

Professional society of physicians who have completed an additional five years of stimulate and advance medical contributions to the knowledge and treatment of psychiatric illnesses of children and adolescents. Annual meeting.

3220 American Academy of Addiction Psychiatry: Annual Meeting

7301 Mission Road
Suite 252
Prairie Village, KS 66208-3075   913-262-6161
                                Fax: 913-262-4311
                          E-mail: info@aaap.org
                               www.aaap.org

Jeanne G Trumble, Executive Director
Becky Stien, Deputy Executive Director

3221 American Academy of Child & Adolescent Psychiatry Annual Conference

American Academy of Child & Adolescent Psychiatry
3615 Wisconsin Avenue NW
Washington, DC 20016-3007   202-966-7300
                                800-333-7636
                          Fax: 202-966-2891

October, Sheraton Inn, Chicago, IL.

3222 American Academy of Psychiatry & Law Annual Conference

American Academy of Psychiatry & Law
1 Regency Drive
PO Box 30
Bloomfield, CT 06002-0030   860-447-9408
                                800-331-1389
                          Fax: 860-286-0787
                               www.aapl.org

October, Renaissance Harbour Place, Baltimore, MD; May, Semi-Annual Conference.

3223 American Academy of Psychoanalysis Preliminary Meeting

American Academy of Psychoanalysis and Dynamic Psychiatry
One Regency Drive
PO Box 30
Bloomfield, CT 06002   888-691-8281
                    Fax: 860-286-0787
               E-mail: info@aapsa.org
                    www.aapsa.org

Jacquelyn T Coleman CAE, Executive Director

January, Plaza Hotel, New York, NY 'Paradigm Shifts.' The meeting will present advances and challenges within psychoanalysis, psychiatry, and other related fields. Explores changes in methods of practice and in organizations. This meeting will maintain a strong clinical orientation.

3224 American Association of Children's Residential Center Annual Conference

American Association of Children's Residential Centers
51 Monroe Place
Suite 1603
Rockville, MD 20850   301-738-6460
                    Fax: 301-738-6431
               E-mail: info@aacrc-dc.org
                    www.aacrc-dc.org

Elissa Schwartz, Association Director

Funded by the Mental Health Community Support Program. The purpose of the association is to share information about services, providers and ways to cope with mental illnesses. Available services include referrals, professional seminars, support groups and a variety of publications.

3225 American Association of Geriatric Psychiatry Annual Meetings

7910 Woodmont Avenue
Suite 1050
Bethesda, MD 20814-3004   301-654-7850
        Fax: 301-654-4137
        E-mail: main@aagponline.org
        www.aagpgpa.org

Annual Meetings: March, Fontaine Blue, Miami Beach, FL; February, San Diego, CA.

3226 American Association of Health Care Consultants Annual Fall Conference

American Association of Health Care Consultants
11208 Waples Mill Road
Suite 109
Fairfax, VA 22030-6077   703-691-2242
        Fax: 703-691-2247

Association host an Annual Fall Conference: October, LaQuinta Resort and Club, LaQuinta, CA.

3227 American Association of Homes & Services for the Aging Annual Convention

American Association of Homes & Services for the Aging
901 E Street NW
Washington, DC 20004-2037   202-508-9473
        Fax: 202-783-2255
        www.aahsa.org

October, Navy Pier.

3228 American College of Health Care Administrators: ACHCA Annual Meeting

300 N Lee Street
Suite 301
Alexandria, VA 22314   703-739-7900
        888-882-2422
        Fax: 703-739-7901
        E-mail: meetings@achca.org
        www.achca.org

Aileen Holland, Membership
Marguerite Leishman, Meetings
Amber Rashid, Communications

Professional society for nearly 6,300 administrators in long-term care, assisted living and subacute care. Our mission is to be the premier organization serving as a catalyst to empower administrators who will define professionalism throughout the continuum of care.

3229 American College of Healthcare Executives Educational Events

American College of Healthcare Executives
One N Franklin Street
Suite 1700
Chicago, IL 60606-0023   312-424-9388
        Fax: 312-424-0023
        E-mail: ache@ache.org
        www.ache.org

Benjamin A Reed, Education Program Registration
Charles J Macfarlane, Education
Amber Rashid, Communications

October, Advanced Negotiating, San Diego, CA; October, Lessons Learned Innovative Strategies for Managed Care and Physician Integration, Pittsburgh, PA; October, Public Policy Institute; November, Leadership Development Institute, Lisle, IL; November, Fall Fellows Conference New Directions in Physician Integration, Palm Springs, CA; November, CEO Circle Forum, Phoenix, AZ; November, New Directions in Physician Integration, San Antonio, TX; and December, Aligning Competing Interests: The Key to Successful Integrations.

3230 American College of Psychiatrists Annual Meeting

732 Addison Street
Suite C
Berkeley, CA 94710   510-704-8020
        Fax: 510-704-0113
        E-mail: Barbara@acpsych.org
        www.acpsych.org

James H Shore, President
Alice Conde, Executive Director

Nonprofit honorary association of psychiatrists who, through excellence in their chosen fields, have been recognized for their significant contributions to the profession. The society's goal is to promote and support the highest standards in psychiatry through education, research and clinical practice.

3231 American Group Psychotherapy Association Annual Conference

American Group Psychotherapy Association
25 E 21st Street
6th Floor
New York, NY 10010   212-477-2677
        877-668-2472
        Fax: 212-979-6627
        E-mail: info@agpa.org
        www.agpa.org

Marsha S Block, CEO
Angela Stephens, Professional Development

Educational conference with a changing annual focus.

Year Founded: 1942

3232 American Health Care Association Annual Meeting

1201 L Street NW
Washington, DC 20005-4024   202-842-4444
        Fax: 202-842-3860
        E-mail: astarkey@ahca.org
        www.ahca.org

Alexis Starkey, Events

Exhibits and educational workshops from the non-profit federation of affiliated state health organizations, together representing nearly 12,000 nonprofit and for profit assisted living, nursing facility, developmentally disabled and subacute care providers that care for more than 1.5 million elderly and disabled individuals nationally. AHCA represents the long term care community at large — to government, business leaders and the general public. It also serves as a force for change within the long term care field, providing information, education, and administrative tools that enhance quality at every level.

3233 American Health Information Management Association Annual Exhibition and Conference

233 N Michigan Avenue
Suite 2150
Chicago, IL 60601-5088   312-233-1100
                               Fax: 312-233-1090
                    E-mail: info@ahima.org
                               www.ahima.org

Marilyn Render, State Association Assistance
Jean Schlichting, Legislative/Public Policy

Exhibits, business and educational conferences of the dynamic professional association that represents more than 46,000 specially educated health information management professionals who work throughout the healthcare industry. Health information management professionals serve the health care industry and the public by manageing, analyzing and utilizing data vital for patient care and making it accessible to healthcare providers when it is needed most.

3234 American Medical Association Annual and Interim Conferences

American Medical Association
515 N State Street
Chicago, IL 60610-4325   312-464-5000
                               800-621-8335
                               Fax: 312-464-5600
                    E-mail: apsychmed@aol.com
                               www.ama-assn.org

Paul Misano MD, President
Janice Shimokubo, Membership

AMA Meetings: Interim San Diego, CA, December; Annual Chicago, IL, June; Interim Orlando, FL, December; Annual Chicago, Il, June; Interim San Francisco, CA, December; Academy of Psychosomatic Medicine New Orleans, LA, November, Information: Phone (773)784-2025; Fax (773)784-1304; State of the Art in Addiction Medicine, Washington, DC; November, Information: Phone (301) 656-3920.

3235 American Society for Adolescent Psychiatry: Annual Meeting

PO Box 570218
Dallas, TX 75357-0218   972-686-6166
                               Fax: 972-613-5532
                    E-mail: info@adolpsych.org
                               www.adolpsych.org

Robert Weinstock MD, President
Stephen Billick MD, VP
Frances Roton, Executive Director

Feature presentations by prominent members of the professional community, exhibits, workshops, receptions, award ceremony and installation of officers.

3236 Annual AAMA Conference & Convocation

American Academy of Medical Administrators
30555 Southfield Road
Suite 105
Southfield, MI 48076-1221   248-540-4310
                               Fax: 248-645-0590
                    E-mail: info@aameda.org
                               www.aameda.org

Annual AAMA Conference and Convocation including ACCA National Management Conference, ACOA Annual National Symposium: Atlanta, GA November.

3237 Annual Summit on International Managed Care Trends

Academy for International Health Studies
621 Georgetown Place
Davis, CA 95616-1821   530-758-8600
                               Fax: 530-758-8686
                               www.aihs.com

December, Sheraton Bal Harbour Hotel, Bal Harbour, FL. Global healthcare meeting; 500 people, 47 nations attended previous summits.

3238 Association for Ambulatory Behavioral Healthcare: Training Conference

11240 Waples Mill Road
Suite 200
Fairfax, VA 22030   703-934-0160
                               Fax: 703-359-7562
                    E-mail: info@aabh.org
                               www.aabh.org

Karla Gray, President
Jerry Galler, Executive Director

Powerful forum for people engaged in providing mental health services. Promoting the evolution of flexible models of responsive cost-effective ambulatory behavioral healthcare.

3239 Association of Black Psychologists Annual Convention

PO Box 55999
Washington, DC 20040-5999   202-722-0808
                               Fax: 202-722-5941
                    E-mail: admin@abpsi.org
                               www.abpsi.org

Willie S Williams PhD, President

Feature presentations, exhibits and workshops held over a four day period focusing on the unique concerns of Black professionals.

3240 Behavioral Healthcare Tomorrow: Spring Calender of Events

Institute for Advancement of Human Behavior/Centralink
4370 Alpine Road
Suite 209
Portola Valley, CA 94028-7927   650-851-8411
                                       800-258-8411
                                  Fax: 650-851-0406
                                       www.ibh.com

Host 10-15 meetings a year.

3241 Institute for Behavioral Healthcare & Expert Knowledge Systems

4370 Alpine Road
Suite 108
Portola Valley, CA 94028-7927   415-482-5005
                                  Fax: 415-851-0406

3242 NAMI Convention

National Alliance for the Mentally Ill
200 N Glebe Road
Suite 1015
Arlington, VA 22203-3728   703-524-7600
                                       800-950-6264
                                  Fax: 703-524-9094
                                  TDD: 703-516-7227
                               E-mail: ann@nami.org
                                       www.nami.org

Ann Nagle

Annual meeting that draws more than 2,000 people from across the country. Presentations by top researchers, physicians, policymakers. Different location each year.

3243 National Dialogue Conference on Mental Health and Addiction Treatment-Sustaining Entrepreneurship and Value

Partnership for Behavioral Healthcare/Centralink
1110 Mar W Street
Suite E
Tiburon, CA 94920-1879   415-435-9821
                                       415-435-9092
                         E-mail: info@centralink.com
                                  www.centralink.com

Industry Leadership Banquet and Panel; September, San Francisco, CA.

3244 National Summit of Mental Health Consumers and Survivors

National Mental Health Consumer's Self-Help Clearinghouse
1211 Chestnut Street
Suite 1207
Philadelphia, PA 19107   215-751-1810
                                       800-553-4539
                                  Fax: 215-636-6312
                          E-mail: info@mhselfhelp.org
                                  www.mhselfhelp.org

3245 Public/Private Behavioral Healthcare Summit

Institute of Behavioral Healthcare & CentraLink
1110 Mar W Street
Suite E
Belvedere Tiburon, CA 94920   415-435-9821

National Leadership Conference on integerating public and private behavioral healthcare funding streams and delivery systems.

3246 Spring ABDA Conference

American Board of Medical Psychotherapists and Psychodiagnosticians
345 24th Avenue N, Suite 201
Park Plaza Medical Building
Nashville, TN 37203-1595   615-327-2984
                                  Fax: 615-327-9235

Hosting three conferences in 2004, Febuary, Juneo, October.

3247 Winter ABDA Conference

American Board of Medical Psychotherapists and Psychodiagnosticians
345 24th Avenue N, Suite 201
Park Plaza Medical Bldg
Nashville, TN 37203-1595   615-327-2984
                                  Fax: 615-327-9235
                      E-mail: americanbd@aol.com

ABMPP holds interdisciplinary continuing education meetings in the US and abroad each year. A calendar of events is available by contacting the central office.

3248 YAI/National Institute for People with Disabilities

YAI
460 W 34th Street
New York, NY 10001-2382   212-273-6100
                                       www.yai.org

Joel M Levy, CEO
Philip H Levy, President/COO
Aimee Matza, Conference Manager

Consulting Services

3249 American Society of Addiction Medicine

4601 N Park Avenue
Apartment 101
Chevy Chase, MD 20815-4520   301-656-3920
                                  Fax: 301-656-3815

Increase access to and improve the quality of addictions treatment. Educate physicians, medical and osteopathic, and the public.

3250 Healthcare Forum

180 Montgomery Street
Suite 1520
San Francisco, CA 94104   415-248-8400
                                  Fax: 415-248-0400
                          www.hospitalconnect.com

John King, Chair
George Bennett, Director
Catherine Mecker, Director

Provides communications, information, education and research products and services that advance leadership for health. These services empower health care providers, suppliers, payers and consumers with new knowledge toward the advancement of organizational, market, clinical, medical and community leadership.

3251 Info Management Associates

1595 Lincoln Highway
Edison, NJ 08817   732-572-2253
                          800-572-2256
                    Fax: 732-572-3039
            E-mail: info@imasys.com
                       www.imasys.com

Mike Samel, President

Custom software applications for a variety of industries, with a special focus on systems and services for human services organizations.

3252 MHM Services

1593 Spring Hill Road
Suite 610
Vienna, VA 22182   703-749-4600
                          800-416-3649
                    Fax: 703-749-4604
              www.mhm-services.com

National specialist in providing on-site mental health services to correctional systems, including state and local prison, jails and juvenile detention centers. Also is a leader in the management of behavioral health programs in the community

3253 McManis Associates

1300 Parkwood Circle
Atlanta, GA 30339   770-737-6950
                     Fax: 770-980-1680

Craig Savage, Principal
Rob Gershon, Managing Associate

Management consulting firm specializing in strategic planning and organizational development for healthcare providers and systems. Particular expertise in facilitating mergers, acquisitions, and affiliations of behavioral health providers.

3254 Mental Health Consultants

1878 Sugar Bottom Road
Furlong, PA 18925-1525   215-345-6838
                         Fax: 215-345-8488
                www.mhconsultants.com

Edward Haaz, President

Workplace behavioral specialty network in southeastern Pennsylvania and New Jersey. 850+ licensed professionals/trainers, 45 inpatient and alternative care facilities under contract. Provides Employee Assistance Services on a case rate or capitated basis. In addition, MHC offers the following workplace services: employee education workshops/seminars, executive coaching, team building, communication enhancement, trauma intervention, critical incident stress debriefing, workplace behavioral assessments, risk management assessments.

3255 River Valley Behavioral Health

1100 Walnut Street
Owensboro, KY 42301   270-683-4039
                       Fax: 270-689-6664

Professional management company for behavioral health and mental retardation/developmental disability service providers; offering training, evaluation, substance abuse, supported employment, community support, case management, professional placement, and organizational management. Training topics include consumer advocacy, juvenile justice, elder abuse, and estate planning for people with disabilities.

Periodicals & Pamphlets

3256 AACAP News

AACAP
3615 Wisconsin Avenue NW
Washington, DC 20016-3007   202-966-7300
                              Fax: 202-966-2891
                                  www.aacap.org

Michelle Morse, Production Editor

The American Academy of Child and Adolescent Psychiatry, (AACAP) publishes a newsletter which focuses events within the Academy, child and adolescent psychiatrists, and AACAP members.

36-64 pages 6 per year

3257 AAMI Newsletter

Arizona Alliance for the Mentally Ill (NAMI Arizona)
2210 N 7th Street
Phoenix, AZ 85006   602-244-8166
                          800-626-5022
                    Fax: 602-244-9264
           E-mail: azami@aol.com
                     www.az.nami.org

Sue Davis, Executive Director
Mary Robson, Education Director
Joanne Abbott, Education Coordinator

Provides support, education, research, and advocacy for individuals and families affected by mental illness. Reports on legislative updates, conventions, psychiatry/psychological practices, and activities of the alliance. Newsletter with membership. *$10.00*

8 pages 4 per year

3258 AAPL Newsletter

American Academy of Psychiatry and the Law
One Regency Drive
PO Box 30
Bloomfield, CT 06002-0030   860-242-5450
                              800-331-1389
                        Fax: 860-286-0787
             E-mail: office@aapl.org
                         www.aapl.org

Newsletter that discusses psychiatry as it relates to the law. Recurring features include recent legal cases, legislative updates, letters to the editor, notices of publications available, news of educational opportunities, job listings, a calendar of events, and editorial columns. *$25.00*

20 pages 3 per year

3259 ACP Newsletter

Association for Child Psychoanalysis (ACP)
320 Glendale Drive
Chapel Hill, NC 27514-5914   **919-967-5819**
Fax: 919-929-0988
E-mail: brinich@unc.edu

Discusses child analysis methods, child psychoanalysis training, and the treatment and education of children throughout the world. Recurring features include news of members, announcements of research training programs, meetings, lectures, and committees concerned with child psychoanalysis.

24-36 pages 2 per year ISSN 1077-0305

3260 AJMR-American Journal on Mental Retardation

AAMR
444 N Capitol Street NW
Suite 846
Washington, DC 20001-1512   **202-387-1968**
800-424-3688
Fax: 202-387-2193
E-mail: dcroser@aamr.org
www.aamr.org

Provides updates on the latest program advances, current research, and information on products and services in the developmental disabilities field. *$10.50*

24 per year ISSN 0047-6765

3261 AMIA News

American Medical Informatics Association
4915 St. Elmo Avenue
Suite 401
Bethesda, MD 20814-6052   **301-657-1291**
Fax: 301-657-1296
www.amia.org

3262 AMOS Realm

Ancient Mystic Order of Samaritans
17 Heil Street
Bushnell, IL   **309-772-2403**

Promotes centers for the mentally retarded. Reports on organization's activities and fundraising projects. Recurring features include inspirational items, profiles of members and their efforts, and a calendar of events. *$3.00*

4-6 pages 4 per year

3263 APA Monitor

American Psychological Association
750 1st Street NE
Washington, DC 20002-4242   **202-336-5500**
800-374-2721
Fax: 202-336-6103
E-mail: letters.monitor@apa.org
www.apa.org/monitor

Magazine of the American Psychological Association.

12 per year ISSN 1529-4978

3264 ARC News

Association for Retarded Citizens-Pennsylvania
329 1/2 Stanton Street
S Williamsport, PA 17702-7034   **570-326-6997**

Publicizes work of the Association, which is committed to securing for all people with mental retardation the opportunity to choose and realize their goals; promotes reducing the incidence and limiting the consequence of mental retardation through education, research, advocacy, and the support of family, friends, and the community; provides leadership in the field and strives for development of necessary human and financial resources to succeed.

4 pages 12 per year

3265 ASAP Newsletter

American Psychological Association
PO Box 28218
Dallas, TX 75228-0218   **972-686-6166**
Fax: 972-613-5532

Contains articles about adolescent psychiatry and society news. Recurring features include news of research, a calendar of events, and book reviews. *$10.00*

16-20 pages 4 per year

3266 Advocate: Autism Society of America

Autism Society of America
7910 Woodmont Avenue
Suite 300
Bethesda, MD 20814-3067   **301-657-0881**
800-328-8476
Fax: 301-657-0869
www.autism-society.org

Reports news and information of national significance for individuals, families, and professionals dealing with autism. Recurring features include personal features and profiles, research summaries, government updates, book reviews, statistics, news of research, and a calendar of events.

32-36 pages 6 per year ISSN 0047-9101

3267 Alcohol & Drug Abuse Weekly

Manisses Communications Group
PO Box 9758
Providence, RI 02906   **401-831-6020**
800-333-7771
Fax: 401-861-6370
E-mail: mhweekly@bdol.com
www.manisses.com

William Kanapaux, Managing Editor

Economic and policy issues for mental health professionals. *$549.00*

8 pages 48 per year Year Founded: 1992 ISSN 10581103

3268 American Academy of Child and Adolescent Psychiatry (AACAP)

3615 Wisconsin Avenue NW
Washington, DC 20016-3007   **202-966-7300**
800-333-7636
Fax: 202-966-2891
www.aacap.org

Virginia Q Anthony, Executive Director

Professional society of physicians who have completed an additional five years of stimulate and advance medical contributions to the knowledge and treatment of psychiatric illnesses of children and adolescents. Publications: AACAP News, bimonthly. Journal of the AACAP, monthly. Bulletin, periodic. Membership Directory, periodic. Catalog and Manuals. Annual meeting.

36-34 pages 6 per year

3269 American Academy of Child and Adolescent Psychiatry News

AACAP
3615 Wisconsin Avenue NW
Washington, DC 20016-3007   **202-966-7300**
Fax: 202-966-2891
www.aacap.org

Publishes news of the Academy, child and adolescent psychiatrists, and AACAP members. Focuses on the practice of child and adolescent psychiatry. Recurring features include letters to the editor, legislative updates, news of research, statistics, announcements of open positions, and columns.

3270 American Association of Community Psychiatrists (AACP)

PO Box 570218
Dallas, TX 75357   **972-613-0985**
Fax: 972-613-5532
www.communitypsychiatry.org

Jacqueline Feldman MD, President
Francis Roton

Psychiatrists and psychiatry residents practicing in community mental health centers or similar programs that provide care to the mentally ill regardless of their ability to pay. Addresses issues faced by psychiatrists who practice within CMHCs. Publications: AACP Membership Directory, annual. Community Psychiatrist, quarterly newsletter. Annual meeting, in conjunction with American Psychiatric Association in May. Annual meeting, in conjunction with Institute on Hospital and Community in fall.

4 per year

3271 American Institute for Preventive Medicine

American Institute for Preventive Medicine Press
30445 Northwestern Highway
Suite 350
Farmington Hills, MI 48334-3107   **248-539-1800**
Fax: 248-539-1808
E-mail: aipm@healthy.net
www.HealthyLife.com

Don R Powell, President
Sue Jackson, VP

AIPM is an internationally renowned developer and provider of wellness programs and publications that address both mental and physical health issues. It works with over 11,500 corporations, hospitals, MCOs, universities, and goverment agencies to reduce health care costs, lower absenteeism, and improve productivity. The Institute has a number of publications that address mental health issues, including stress management, depression, self - esteem, and EAP issues.

96 pages Year Founded: 1999

3272 American Journal of Hypertension

PO Box 945
New York, NY 10159-0945   **212-633-3730**
888-437-4336
Fax: 212-633-3680
www.usinfo-f@alsevier.com

16 per year   ISSN 0895-7061

3273 American Psychiatric Association: Psychiatri c News

1000 Wilson Boulevard
Suite 1825
Arlington, VA 22209-3901   **703-907-7300**
Fax: 703-907-1095
E-mail: apa@psych.org
www.psych.org

James Scully MD, President
Katie Duffy, Marketing

Official newspaper of the American Psychiatric Association, features informative articles on the latest treatment approaches for practicing psychiatrists.

3274 American Psychoanalyst Newsletter

American Psychological Association
750 1st Street NE
Washington, DC 20002-4241   **202-336-5500**
800-374-2721
Fax: 202-336-5568
E-mail: webmaster@apa.org

Covers developments in psychoanalysis for those in the profession. Presents news of the Association, announces winners of grants and awards, and reports on the conferences and other institutes.

32-36 pages 4 per year ISSN 1052-7958

3275 American Psychological Association

750 1st Street NE
Washington, DC 20002-4241   202-336-5500
                                    800-374-2721
                              Fax: 202-336-5723
                    E-mail: webmaster@apa.org
                                    www.apa.org

Covers developments in psychoanalysis for those in the profession. Presents news of the Association, announces winners of grants and awards, and reports on conferences and other institutes. *$27.50*

32-36 pages 4 per year ISSN 1052-7958

3276 American Society for Adolescent Psychiatry (ASAP)

ASAP Newsletter
PO Box 28218
Dallas, TX 75228-0218   972-686-6166
                          Fax: 972-613-5532

Leonard Henschel, Editor

Contains articles about adolescent psychiatry and Society news. Recurring features include news of research, a calendar of events, and book reviews. *$10.00*

16-20 pages 4X per year

3277 Analytic Press

101 W Street
Hillsdale, NJ 07642-1421   201-358-9477
                          Fax: 201-358-4700

3278 Arts in Psychotherapy

Customer Support Department
PO Box 945
New York, NY 10159-0945   212-633-3730
                                    888-437-4636
                          Fax: 212-633-3680
              www.elsevier.nl/locate/artspsycho

ISSN 0197-4556

3279 Assessment and Prediction of Suicide

Guilford Publications
72 Spring Street
New York, NY 10012   212-431-9800
                                    800-365-7006
                          Fax: 212-966-6708
                    E-mail: info@guilford.com
                                    www.guilford.com

Comprehensive reference volume that includes contributions from top suicide experts of the current knowledge in the field of suicide. Covers concepts and theories, methods and quantification, in-depth case histories, specific single predictors applied to the case histories and comorbidity. *$69.95*

697 pages Year Founded: 1992 ISBN 0-898627-91-5

3280 Association for Child Psychoanalysis Newsletter

Association for Child Psychoanalysis
320 Glendale Drive
Chapel Hill, NC 27514-5914   919-967-5819
                              Fax: 919-929-0988
                    E-mail: brinich@unc.edu

Paul Brinich, Editor

Discusses child analysis methods, child psycholanalysis training, and the treatment and education of children throughout the world. Recurring features include news of members and the Association and announcements of research training programs, meetings, lectures, and committees concerned with child psychoanalysis.

24-36 pages 2 per year ISSN 1077-0305

3281 Because Kids Grow Up

National Alliance for the Mentally Ill
200 N Glebe Road
Suite 1015
Arlington, VA 22203-3728   703-524-7600
                                    800-950-6264
                          Fax: 703-524-9094
                          TDD: 703-516-7227
                    E-mail: brenda@nami.org
                                    www.nami.org

A quarterly newsletter focusing on children and adolescents, also availible online.

4 per year

3282 Behavior Research and Therapy

Customer Service Department
PO Box 945
New York, NY 10159-0945   212-633-3730
                                    888-437-4636
                          Fax: 212-633-3680
                    www.elsevier.nl/locate/bbr

ISSN 0005-7967

3283 Behavioral & Cognitive Psychotherapy

Cambridge University Press
40 W 20th Street
New York, NY 10011-4221   212-924-3900
                          Fax: 212-691-3239
                    E-mail: marketing@cup.org
                                    www.cup.org

3284 Behavioral Brain Research

Customer Service Department
PO Box 945
New York, NY 10159-0945   212-633-3730
                                    888-437-4636
                          Fax: 212-633-3680
                    www.elsiver.nl/locate/bbr

3285 Behavioral Health Accreditation & Accountability Alert

Manisses Communications Group
208 Governor Street
PO Box 9758
Providence, RI 02906   401-831-6020
                             800-333-7771
                        Fax: 401-861-6370
        E-mail: manissescs@manisses.com
                      www.manisses.com

Outcomes, best practices, performance measures, re-imbursement coding. *$549.00*

8 pages 12 per year Year Founded: 1992 ISSN 1529-7055

3286 Behavioral Health Management

Open Minds and Behavioral Health Practice Advisor
PO Box 20179
Cleveland, OH 44120   216-391-9100
                        Fax: 216-391-9200
                        www.behavioral.net

3287 Behavioral Healthcare Management

Medquest Communications LLC
3800 Lakeside Avenue
Suite 201
Cleveland, OH 44114   216-391-9100
                        Fax: 216-391-9200

ISSN 1075-6701

3288 Behavioral Healthcare Tomorrow

Manisses Communications Group
208 Governor Street
PO Box 9758
Providence, RI 02906-3246   401-831-6020
                             800-333-7771
                        Fax: 401-861-6370
        E-mail: manissescs@manisses.com
                      www.manisses.com

Peter Sanderson, Director Operations

National dialogue journal on mental health and addiction treatment benefits and services in the era of managed care. Readers include mental health professionals, managed care executives, public and private sector integrated delivery system managers, medical directors, EAP and benefits administrators and others involved in the provision, purchasing or management of behavioral healthcare benefits and services. Institutional price $104.00. Individual price $74.00.

48 pages 6 per year

3289 Behavioral Processes

Customer Support Department
PO Box 945
New York, NY 10159-0945   212-633-3730
                             888-437-4636
                        Fax: 212-633-3680
        www.elsiver.nl/locate/behavproc

ISSN 0376-6357

3290 Brain Research Bulletin

Customer Support Department
PO Box 945
New York, NY 10159-0945   212-633-3730
                             888-437-4636
                        Fax: 212-633-3680
        www.elsevier.nl/locate/brainresbull

ISSN 0361-9230

3291 Briefings on Behavioral Accreditation

Opus Communications
100 Hoods Lane
Marblehead, MA 01945-2578   781-639-1872
                        Fax: 781-639-2982

3292 Brown University: Child & Adolescent Behavior Letter

Manisses Communications Group
208 Governor Street
PO Box 9758
Providence, RI 02906   401-831-6020
                             800-333-7771
                        Fax: 401-861-6370
        E-mail: manissescs@manisses.com
                      www.manisses.com

Karienne Stovell, Managing Editor

Practical counseling techniques and authoritative summaries of research on development and behavior of children and adolescents. *$117.00*

12 per year ISSN 10581103

3293 Brown University: Digest of Addiction Theory and Application (DATA)

Manisses Communications Group
PO Box 9758
Providence, RI 02940-9758   401-831-6020
                             800-333-7771
                        Fax: 401-861-6370
        E-mail: manissescs@manisses.com
                      www.manisses.com

Lindaam Watts Jakim, Sr Managing Editor

Highlights of articles in leading medical and addiction journals written in news style. *$129.00*

8 pages 48 per year Year Founded: 1992 ISSN 10581103

3294 Brown University: Geriatric Psychopharmacology Update

Manisses Communications Group
PO Box 9758
Providence, RI 02940-9758   401-831-6020
                             800-333-7771
                        Fax: 401-861-6370
        E-mail: manissescs@manisses.com
                      www.manisses.com

Kariene Stovell, Managing Editor

Updates on research, use of psychotropic medications and specific interventions with the aging. *$197.00*

12 per year ISSN 1529-2584

3295 Brown University: Long-Term Care Quality Advisor

Manisses Communications Group
PO Box 9758
Providence, RI 02940-9758   401-831-6020
                                   800-333-7771
                            Fax: 401-861-6370
           E-mail: manissescs@manisses.com
                            www.manisses.com

William Kanapaux, Managing Editor

Public policy, treatment and management issues for health professionals in long-term care settings. *$199.00*

12 per year   ISSN 10581103

3296 Bull Publishing Company

110 Gilbert Avenue
Menlo Park, CA 94025-2865
                                   800-676-2855
                            Fax: 650-327-3300

3297 Bulletin of Menninger Clinic

Menninger Clinic Department of Research
PO Box 829
Topeka, KS 66601-0829   785-380-5000
                                   800-288-3950
                            Fax: 785-273-8625
                            www.menninger.edu

Valuable, practical information for clincans. Recent topical issues have focused on rekindling the psychodynamic vision, treatment of different clinical populations with panic disorder, and treatment of complicated personality disorders in an era of managed care. All in an integrated, psychodynamic approach. *$82.00*

3298 Bulletin of Psychological Type

Association for Psychological Type
4700 W Lake Avenue
Glenview, IL 60025   847-375-4717
                            Fax: 877-734-9374
           E-mail: info@aptcentral.com
                            www.aptcentral.com

Jim Weir, Executive Directoe

Provides information on regional, national, and international events to keep professionals up-to-date in the study and application of psychological type theory and the Myers-Briggs Type Indicator. Contains announcements of training workshops; international, national, and regional conferences; and awards, along with articles on issues directly related to type theory.

40 pages   4 per year

3299 Business & Health

Medical Economics
5 Paragon Drive
Montvale, NJ 07645-1725   201-358-7276
                                   800-526-4870
                            Fax: 201-722-2686
           E-mail: B&H@medec.com
                            www.businessandhealth.com

Jeanne Sabatiec, Production Editor

Magazine serving an audience of nearly 50,000 Business & Health aims to influence the restructuring of the U.S.health care system by showing employers of all sizes how to provide high-quality, cost efficient health benefits. B&H reports and interprets provider and corporate innovations as well as developments in federal and state regulation and legislation through analytical articles, case histories, opinion pieces, surveys and news briefs. B&H is published monthly by Medical Economics Co.

3300 Buyers Guide for Health Care Market

American Hospital Publishing
737 N Michigan Avenue
Suite 700
Chicago, IL 60611-6661   312-226-5880
                                   800-621-6902
                            Fax: 312-787-9663

3301 CNS Spectrums

MBL Communications
665 Broadway
New York, NY 10012-2302   212-328-0800
                            Fax: 212-328-0600
                            www.medicalbroadcast.com

The journal addresses issues that are of interest to both psychiatrists and neurologists.

80+ pages   12 per year   ISSN 1092-8529

3302 California Healthcare Association (CHA)

Center for Behavioral Health
1215 K Street
Suite 800
Sacramento, CA 95814-3906   916-552-7576
                            Fax: 916-552-7585
           E-mail: pryan@calhealth.org

Patricia Ryan, VP Behavioral Health

3303 Cambridge Handbook of Psychology, Health and Medicine

Cambridge University Press
40 W 20th Street
New York, NY 10011-4221   212-924-3900
                            Fax: 212-691-3239
           E-mail: marketing@cup.org
                            www.cup.org

$80.00

678 pages   Year Founded: 1997 ISBN 0-521436-86-9

3304 Capitation Report

National Health Information
PO Box 15429
Atlanta, GA 30333-0429   404-607-9500
                                   800-597-6300
                            Fax: 404-607-0095
                            www.nhionline.net

3305 Child and Adolescent Psychiatry

American Academy of Child and Adolescent Psychiatry
3615 Wisconsin Avenue NW
Washington, DC 20016-3007   202-966-7300
                                   Fax: 202-966-2891
                                   www.aacap.org

A journal with good research notes.

3306 Children's Services Report

Manisses Communications Group
208 Governor Street
PO Box 9758
Providence, RI 02940-9758   401-831-6020
                                   800-333-7771
                      Fax: 401-861-6370
          E-mail: manissescs@manisses.com
                            www.manisses.com

Coverage and analysis of developments affecting child and adolescent programs. *$247.00*

12 per year

3307 Chronicle

Association for the Help of Retarded Children (AHRC)
200 Park Avenue S
New York, NY 10003-1503   212-780-2500
                                   Fax: 212-777-5893
             E-mail: ahrcnyc@ahrcnyc.org
                            www.ahrcnyc.org

Covers developmental disabilities, includes legislation and entitlements updates, field news, accessing information and services, advocacy issues, and current research. Recurring features include interviews, news of research, a calendar of events, reports of meetings, book reviews, and notices of publications available.

16-28 pages 4 per year

3308 Claiming Children

Federation of Families for Children's Mental Health
1101 King Street
Suite 420
Alexandria, VA 22314   703-684-7710
                                   Fax: 703-836-1040
                 E-mail: ffcmh@ffcmh.org
                            www.ffcmh.org

Barbara Huff, Executive Director
Cynthia Warger, Editor

Dedicated to children and adolescents with mental health needs and their families.

4 per year

3309 Clinical Psychiatry News

International Medical News Group
12230 Wilkins Avenue
Rockville, MD 20852-1834   301-816-8700
                                   Fax: 301-816-8712

3310 Clinical Psychiatry Quarterly

AACP
PO Box 458
Glastonbury, CT 06033   860-633-5045
                                   Fax: 860-633-6023
                         E-mail: info@aacp.com
                                   www.aacp.com

Informs members of of news and events. Recurring features include letters to the editor, news of research, a calendar of events, reports of meetings, and book reviews.

4 per year

3311 Clinical Psychology Review

Customer Support Department
PO Box 945
New York, NY 10159-0945   212-633-3730
                                   888-437-4636
                      Fax: 212-633-3680
          www.elsevier.nl/locate/clinpsychrev

ISSN 0272-7358

3312 Cognitive Brain Research

Customer Support Department
PO Box 945
New York, NY 10159-0945   212-633-3730
                                   888-437-4636
                      Fax: 212-633-3680
             www.elsevier.nl/locate/cogbri

ISSN 0926-6410

3313 Couples Therapy in Managed Care

Haworth Press
10 Alice Street
Binghamton, NY 13904-1580   607-722-5857
                                   800-429-6784
                      Fax: 607-722-1424
        E-mail: getinfo@haworthpressinc.com
                       www.Haworthpress.com

Provides social workers, psychologists and counselors with an overview of the negative effects of the managed care industry on the quality of marital health care.

ISBN 7-890078-86-6

3314 Creative Training Techniques

Bill Communications
50 S 9th Street
Minneapolis, MN 55402-3118   612-340-4903
                                   800-707-7749
                      Fax: 612-340-4819
              www.trainingsupersite.com/ctt

Newsletter of tips, tactis and how-to's for delivering effective training. *$109.00*

12 per year

3315 Decade of the Brain

National Alliance for the Mentally Ill
200 N Glebe Road
Suite 1015
Arlington, VA 22203-3728   703-524-7600
                                 800-950-6264
                            Fax: 703-524-9094
                            TDD: 703-516-7227
                                 www.nami.org

A quarterly newsletter about research.

3316 Development & Psychopathology

Cambridge University Press
40 W 20th Street
New York, NY 10011-4221   212-924-3900
                            Fax: 212-691-3239
                    E-mail: marketing@cup.org
                                 www.cup.org

This multidisciplinary journal is devoted to the publication of original, empirical, theoretical and review papers which address the interrelationship of normal and pathological development in adults and children. It is intended to serve and intergrate the emerging field of developmental psychopathology which strives to understand patterns of adaptation and maladaptation throughout the lifespan. This journal is of vital interest to psychologists, psychiatrists, social scientists, neuroscientists, pediatricians and researchers. $66.00

4 per year   ISSN 0954-5794

3317 Developmental Brain Research

Customer Support Department
PO Box 945
New York, NY 10159-0945   212-633-3730
                                 888-437-4636
                            Fax: 212-633-3680
                    www.elsevier.nl/locate/devbri

ISSN 0165-3806

3318 Disability Funding News

CD Publications
8204 Fenton Street
Silver Spring, MD 20910-4509   301-588-6380
                                 800-666-6380
                            Fax: 301-588-6385
                    E-mail: cdpubs@clark.net
                         www.cdpublications.com

Wayne Welch, Editor

Up to date news for mental health professionals. $259.00

*14-18 pages 24 per year Year Founded: 1992
ISSN 1069-1359*

3319 Disease Management News

Business Information Services
12811 N Point Lane
Laurel, MD 20708-2341   301-604-4001
                                 800-559-8550
                            Fax: 301-604-5126
                    E-mail: businfosvc@aol.com

James H Gutman, Publisher

Devoted exclusively to disease management, business news and analysis including: start-ups, shutdowns, acquisitions, partnerships, rollouts, contracting, financing and investing, clinical and cost outcomes, new disease and geographic markets, technology, names and phone numbers of contacts, demand management, provider compliance and more. *$387.00*

8 pages 26 per year   ISSN 1084-7146

3320 Drug and Crime Prevention Funding News

Government Information Services
4301 Fairfax Drive
Suite 875
Arlington, VA 22203-1635   703-920-7600
                                 800-876-0226
                            Fax: 800-426-2012
                    www.grantsandfunding.com

Provides federal and private drug and crime funding information, including congressional legislation and appropriations. Also features grant alert a weekly compilation of federal grants and contracts. Recurring features include a collection, reports of meetings, and notices of publications available. *$289.00*

10-12 pages 56 per year   ISSN 1076-1519

3321 Drugs in the Workplace

Warren, Gorham, & Lamont
31 St. James Avenue
Boston, MA 02116-4101   914-225-2935
                            Fax: 914-225-5395

3322 EAPA Exchange

Employee Assistance Professionals Association
2101 Wilson Boulevard
Arlington, VA 22201-3062   703-522-6272
                            Fax: 703-522-4585

3323 EBSCO Publishing

10 Estes Street
Ipswich, MA 01938   978-356-6500
                                 800-653-2726
                            Fax: 978-356-6565
                                 www.epnet.com

*Robert Preston, Medical Inside Sales Manager
Daniel Boutchie, Inside Sales Representative
Jeffery Greaves, Inside Sales Representative*

EBSCO Publishing offers electronic access to a variety of health data: full text databases containing aggregate journals, access to publishers' electronic journals, and the citational databases produced by the American Psychiatric Association to name just a few. Contact us for a free, nonobligation, on-line trial today.

3324 ETR Associates

Health Education, Research, Training Curriculum
4 Carbonero Way
Scotts Valley, CA 95066   831-438-4060
                                 800-321-4407
                            Fax: 831-438-4284
                                 www.etr.org

John Henry Ledwith, National Sales Director

Publishes a complete line of innovative materials covering the full spectrum of health education topics, including maternal/child health, HIV/STD prevention, risk and injury prevention, self esteem, fitness and nutrition, college health, and wellness education, engaging in both extensive training and research endeavors and a comprehensive K-12 health curriculum.

3325 Edgewood Children's Center

330 N Gore Avenue
Saint Louis, MO 63119-1699   314-968-2060
                                  Fax: 314-968-8308

3326 Elsevier Science BV

655 Avenue of the Americas
New York, NY 10010-5107   212-633-3980
                                Fax: 212-633-3975

3327 Employee Benefit News

Securities Data Publishing
1483 Chain Bridge Road
Suite 202
McLean, VA 22101-5703   703-448-0336
                              Fax: 703-448-0270

3328 Employee Benefit Plan Review

Charles D Spencer & Associates
250 S Wacker Drive
Suite 600
Chicago, IL 60606-5800   312-993-7900
                               Fax: 312-993-7910

3329 Employee Benefits Journal

International Foundation of Employee Benefit Plans
PO Box 69
Brookfield, WI 53008-0069   414-786-6700
                                  Fax: 414-786-8670
                          E-mail: marybr@ifebp.org
                                    www.ifebp.org

Contains articles on all aspects of employee benefits and related topics. *$70.00*

32-48 pages   4 per year   ISSN 0361-4050

3330 Employer's Guide to HIPAA

Thompson Publishing Group
1725 K Street NW
Suite 7
Washington, DC 20006-1401   202-739-9698
                                  Fax: 202-739-9686

3331 Exceptional Parent

PO Box 5446
Pittsfield, MA 01203-5446   201-634-6550
                                   800-372-7368
                             Fax: 740-389-6845
                             www.eparent.com

Magazine for parents and professionals involved in the care and development of children and young adults with special needs, including physical disabilities, developmental disabilities, mental retardation, autism, epilepsy, learning disabilities, hearing/vision impairments, emotional problems, and chronic illnesses. *$36.00*

12 per year

3332 Family Experiences Productions

PO Box 5879
Austin, TX 78763   512-494-0338
                        Fax: 512-494-0340
                 E-mail: FEPIrag@aol.com
                          www.fepi.com

R Geyer, Executive Producer

Consumers Health videos; available individually, or in large volume (private branded) for health providers to give to patients, professionals, staff. Postpartum Emotions, Parenting Preschoolers, Facing Death (4-tape series) English and Spanish.

ISSN 1-930772-00-9

3333 Family Services Report

CD Publications
8204 Fenton Street
Silver Spring, MD 20910-4509   301-588-6380
                                      800-666-6380
                                 Fax: 301-588-6385
                      E-mail: fsr@cdpublications.com
                              www.cdpublications.com

Mark Sherman, Editor

Designed to help organizations working with families to identify and win financial support for the families. Concerned with funding for families experiencing abandonment, sexual abuse, child abuse, elder abuse, adoption, child care, runaways and divorce. *$269.00*

18 pages   24 per year   ISSN 1524-9484

3334 Focal Point

Regional Research Institue-Portland State University
PO Box 751
Portland, OR 97207-0751   503-725-4040
                                  800-628-1696
                             Fax: 503-725-4180
                       E-mail: janetw@pdx.edu
                               www.rtc.pdx.edu

Janet Walker, Editor

Features information on support groups, organizations, strategies, and conferences to aid families that have children with emotional, mental, and/or behavioral disorders. Recurring features include news of research, reports of meetings, and notices of publications available.

24 pages

3335 Forty Two Lives in Treatment: a Study of Psychoanalysis and Psychotherapy

Guilford Publications
72 Spring Street
New York, NY 10012   212-431-9800
                               800-365-7006
                               Fax: 212-966-6708
                               E-mail: info@guilford.com
                               www.guilford.com

Comprehensive results of the study of 42 patients undergoing psychoanalysis and analytic psychotherapy. *$79.95*

784 pages Year Founded: 1986 ISBN 0-898623-25-1

3336 Franklin Electronic Publishers

1 Franklin Plaza
Burlington, NJ 08016   609-239-4333
                                 800-266-5626
                                 Fax: 609-387-1787
                                 www.franklin.com

3337 From the Couch

Behavioral Health Record Section-AMRA
919 N Michigan Avenue
Suite 1400
Chicago, IL 60611-1692   312-787-2672
                                   Fax: 312-787-5926

From the couch, the newsletter for the Behavioral Health Record section of the American Medical Record Association, covers aspects of the medical records industry that pertain to mental health records.

4 per year

3338 Frontiers of Health Services Management

American College of Healthcare Executives
1 N Franklin Street
Chicago, IL 60606-3421   312-424-2800
                                   Fax: 312-424-0023

Enhanced by special access to today's healthcare leaders. Frontiers provides you with the cutting edge insight you want. Each quarterly issue engages you in a vigorous debate on a hot healthcare topic. One stimulating article leads the debate, followed by commentaries and perspectives from recognized experts. Unique combination of opinion, practice and research stimulate you to develop new management strategies. *$70.00*

4 per year ISSN 0748-8157

3339 General Hospital Psychiatry: Psychiatry, Medicine and Primary Care

Elsevier Science
725 Concord Avenue
Suite 4200
Cambridge, MA   617-661-3544
                          Fax: 617-661-4800
                          E-mail: don_lipsitt@hms.harvard.edu

Journal that explores the linkages and interfaces between psychiatry, medicine and primary care. As a peer-reviewed journal, it provides a forum for communication among professionals with clinical, academic and research interests in psychiatry's essential function in the mainstream of medicine. *$195.00*

84 pages 6 per year ISSN 01638343

3340 Geriatrics

Advanstar Communications
7500 Old Oak Boulevard
Cleveland, OH 44130-3343   440-243-8100
                                     Fax: 440-891-2733
                     E-mail: arossetti@advanstar.com
                                     www.geri.com

David Briemer, Sales Manager
Rich Ehrlich, Associate Publisher

Peer-reviewed clinical journal for primary care physicians who care for patients age 50 and older.

100 pages 12 per year

3341 Groden Center

86 Mount Hope Avenue
Providence, RI 02906   401-274-6310
                                 Fax: 401-421-3280
                 E-mail: grodencenter@grodencenter.org
                                 www.grodencenter.org

Andrea Pingitore, Administrative Assistant

Groden Center has been providing day and residential treatment and educational services to children and youth who have developmental and behavioral difficulties and their families. By providing a broad range of individualized services in the most normal and least restrictive settings possible, children and youth learn skills that will help them engage in typical experiences and interact more successfully with others. Education and treatment take place in Groden Center classrooms, in the student's homes, and in the community with every effort made to maintain typical family and peer relationships. Call or visit our web site for more information about the Center and the publications and materials we have available. *$195.00*

Year Founded: 1976

3342 Group Practice Journal

Amerian Medical Group Association
1422 Duke Street
Alexandria, VA 22314-3403   703-838-0033
                                      Fax: 703-548-1890
                          E-mail: tflatt@amga.org
                                      www.amga.org

Fred Haig, VP Communications
Donald Fisher, Publisher

Adresses the vital business information needs of the medical group industry with practical, timely articles about everything from implementing best practices to negotiating managed care delivery systems. Written by physician leaders and industry professionals, the Group Practice Journal provides solutions to health care leaders at every medical group in the country, with a circulation of aproximately 60,000.

10 per year

3343 HR Magazine

Society for Human Resource Management
1800 Duke Street
Alexandria, VA 22314   703-548-3440
                             Fax: 703-836-0367
                             www.shrm.org

3344 Habilitative Mental Healthcare Newsletter

Psych-Media
PO Box 57
Bear Creek, NC 27207-0057   910-581-3700
                             Fax: 910-581-3766

Publishes articles concerning the diagnosis and treatment of psychological disturbances in individuals with developmental disabilities. Recurring features include news of research and a collection. *$57.00*

24 per year

3345 Harvard Mental Health Letter

Harvard Health Publications
10 Shattuck Street
Suite 612
Boston, MA 02115-6011   617-432-1485
                             Fax: 617-432-1506
                   E-mail: hhp@hms.harvard.edu
                             www.health.harvard.edu

Research and treatment regarding mental health. *$48.00*

8 pages 12 per year Year Founded: 1983 ISSN 08843783

3346 Harvard Review of Psychiatry

Mosby
11830 Westline Industrial Drive
Saint Louis, MO 63146   314-872-8370
                             800-325-4177
                             Fax: 314-432-1380

3347 Hazelden Publishing & Education

15251 Pleasant Valley Road
Center City, MN 55012-9640
                             800-328-9000
                             Fax: 612-257-1331

3348 Health & Social Work

National Association of Social Works
750 1st Street NE
Suite 700
Washington, DC 20002-4241   202-336-8236
                             Fax: 202-336-8312

3349 Health Data Management

Faulkner & Gray
11 Penn Plaza
New York, NY 10001-2006   212-967-7000
                             Fax: 212-239-4993

3350 Health Facilities Management

American Hospital Publishing
737 N Michigan Avenue
Suite 700
Chicago, IL 60611-6661   312-226-5880
                             800-621-6902
                             Fax: 312-951-8491

3351 Health Grants & Contracts Weekly

Capitol Publications
1101 K Street
Suite 444
Alexandria, VA 22314   703-583-4100
                             Fax: 703-739-6517

3352 Health Management Technology

Intertec Publishing
6151 Powers Ferry Road NW
Atlanta, GA 30339-2959   770-955-2500
                             Fax: 770-618-0343

3353 Health Network Letter

Capitol Publications
1101 K Street
Suite 444
Alexandria, VA 22314   703-583-4100
                             Fax: 703-739-6517

3354 Health Plan Business Advisor

Capitol Publications
1101 K Street
Suite 444
Alexandria, VA 22314   703-583-4100
                             Fax: 703-739-6517

3355 Health Plan Magazine

American Assciation of Health Plans
1129 20th Street NW
Suite 600
Washington, DC 20036-3455   202-778-8496
                             Fax: 202-778-8508

3356 Health Services Research

American College of Healthcare Executives
1 N Franklin Street
Chicago, IL 60606-3421   312-424-2800
                             Fax: 312-424-0023

This leading journal provides researchers, policymakers, and healthcare executives with cutting edge research findings on the important issues associated with accesss, cost, quality, and outcomes of healthcare delivery. The jouurnal features original empirical articles, a public policy and managerial impact section, and occasional debates.

6 per year

3357 Health System Leader

Capitol Publications
1101 K Street
Suite 444
Alexandria, VA 22314   703-583-4100
                             Fax: 703-739-6517

3358 HealthCare Leadership Review

COR Healthcare Resources
PO Box 40959
Santa Barbara, CA 93140-0959   805-564-2177
                                  Fax: 805-564-2146

3359 Healthcare Executive Magazine

American College of Healthcare Executives
1 N Franklin Street
Chicago, IL 60606-3421   312-424-2800
                             Fax: 312-424-0023

3360 Healthcare Forum

180 Montgomery Street
Suite 1520
San Francisco, CA 94104   415-248-8400
                             Fax: 415-248-0400
                             www.hospitalconnect.com

John King, Chair
George Bennett, Director
Catherine Mecker, Director

Provides communications, information, education and research products and services that advance leadership for health.

3361 Healthcare Marketing Abstracts

COR Healthcare Resources
PO Box 40959
Santa Barbara, CA 93140-0959   805-564-2177
                                  Fax: 805-564-2146

3362 Healthcare Pratice Management News

Business Information Services
9811 Mallard Drive
Suite 220
Laurel, MD 20708-3199   301-604-4001
                             Fax: 301-604-5126

3363 HealthyLife Mental Fitness Guide

American Institute for Preventive Medicine
30445 Northwestern Highway
Suite 350
Farmington Hills, MI 48334   248-539-1800
                                 Fax: 248-539-1808
                                 E-mail: aipm@healthy.net
                                 www.HealthyLife.com

Don R Powell, President
Sue Jackson, VP

Providers of EAP health promotion programs and self-care publications. Materials are designed to lower mental health care costs, decrease absenteeism, improve morale and increase visiblity for hospitals, HMOs, corporations and government agencies. The HealthyLife Mental Fitness Guide teaches employees when to seek professional help and when self care is appropriate. *$5.25*

96 pages 1 per year Year Founded: 1999

3364 Home Health Focus

Mosby
11830 Westline Industrial Drive
Saint Louis, MO 63146   314-872-8370
                             800-325-4177
                             Fax: 314-432-1380

3365 Homosexuality: Research Implications for Public Policy

Sage Publications
2455 Teller Road
Thousand Oaks, CA 91320   805-499-9774
                             800-818-7243
                             Fax: 800-583-2665
                             E-mail: info@sagepub.com
                             www.sagepub.com

Up-to-date discussions of the crucial issues of gay and lesbian populations: myths, prejudices and issues of policy and the scientific research. Summarizes what science knows about homosexuality and its relevance for public policy. *$62.00*

312 pages Year Founded: 1991 ISBN 0-803942-44-3

3366 Hospitals & Health Networks

American Hospital Publishing
737 N Michigan Avenue
Suite 700
Chicago, IL 60611-6661   312-226-5880
                             800-621-6902
                             Fax: 312-951-8491

3367 IABMCP Newsletter

IABMCP
3208 N Academy Boulevard, Suite 160
Colorado Springs, CO 80917   719-597-5959
                                 Fax: 719-597-0166
                                 E-mail: iabmcp@att.net

The International Academy of Behavioral Medicine, Counseling, and Psychotherapy, (IABMCP) publishes research articles in the field of behavioral medicine, 'the systematic application of various principles of behavioral science to health care problems.' Contains news of the Academy and its members. Recurring features include book reviews, letters to the editor, and a calendar of events. *$60.00*

4-8 pages 4 per year

3368 Insider

Alliance for Children and Families
1701 K Street NW
Suite 200
Washington, DC 20006-1523   202-223-3447
                                 Fax: 202-331-7476
                                 E-mail: policy@alliance1.org
                                 www.alliance1.org

Carmen Delgado Votaw, Sr VP
Peter Goldberg, President/CEO
Thomas Harney, VP Membership

Alliance for Children and Families' tool for providing members with accurate and up-to-date information on current legislation, issues the Alliance is advocating on Capitol Hill, summaries of how proposed bills will affect member organizations and the people they serve, and suggestions for local advocacy efforts.

3369 Internal Medicine News

International Medical News Group
12230 Wilkins Avenue
Rockville, MD 20852-1834   301-816-8778
                                 Fax: 301-816-8738

3370 International Benefits Information System

Charles D Spencer & Associates
250 S Wacker Drive
Suite 600
Chicago, IL 60606-5800   312-993-7900
                                Fax: 312-993-7910

3371 International Drug Therapy Newsletter

Lippincott Williams & Wilkins
351 W Camden Street
Baltimore, MD 21201-7912   410-528-8517
                                  800-882-0483
                             Fax: 410-528-4312
                   E-mail: korourke@lww.com
                                  www.lww.com

Newsletter that focuses on psychotropic drugs, discussing individual drugs, their effectiveness, and history. Examines illnesses and the drugs used to treat them, studies done on various drugs, their chemical make-up, and new developments and changes in drugs. *$149.00*

8 pages ISSN 0020-6571

3372 International Journal of Neuropsychopharmacology

Cambridge University Press
40 W 20th Street
New York, NY 10011-4221   212-924-3900
                            Fax: 212-691-3239
                 E-mail: marketing@cup.org
                                 www.cup.org

3373 International Journal of Aging and Human Developments

Baywood Publishing Company
26 Austin Avenue
Box 337
Amityville, NY 11701   631-691-1270
                              800-638-7819
                         Fax: 631-691-1770
              E-mail: info@baywood.com
                          www.baywood.com

$218.00

8 per year Year Founded: 1973 ISSN 0091-4150

3374 International Journal of Health Services

Baywood Publishing Company
26 Austin Avenue
Box 337
Amityville, NY 11701   631-691-1270
                              800-638-7819
                         Fax: 631-691-1770
              E-mail: info@baywood.com
                          www.baywood.com

$160.00

4 per year Year Founded: 1970

3375 International Journal of Psychiatry in Medicine

Baywood Publishing Company
26 Austin Avenue
Box 337
Amityville, NY 11701   631-691-1270
                              800-638-7819
                         Fax: 631-691-1770
              E-mail: info@baywood.com
                          www.baywood.com

$160.00

4 per year Year Founded: 1970 ISSN 0091274

3376 Journal of AHIMA

American Health Information Management Association
233 N Michigan Avenue
Suite 2150
Chicago, IL 60601-5800   312-233-1100
                           Fax: 312-233-1090
                 E-mail: info@ahima.org
                                www.ahima.org

Jessica Squazzo, Editor
Jean Schlichting, Legislative/Public Policy

Monthly magazine with articles, news and event annoucements from the nonprofit federation of affiliated state health organizations, together representing nearly 12,000 nonprofit and for profit assisted living, nursing facility, developmentally disabled and sub-acute care providers that care for more than 1.5 million elderly and disabled individuals nationally.

3377 Journal of American Health Information Management Association

American Health Information Management Association
233 N Michigan Avenue
Suite 2150
Chicago, IL 60601-5800   312-233-1100
                           Fax: 312-233-1090
                 E-mail: info@ahima.org
                                www.ahima.org

3378 Journal of American Medical Information Association

Hanley & Befus
210 S 13th Street
Philadelphia, PA 19107-5467   215-546-4656

3379 Journal of Behavior Therapy and Experimental Psychiatry

Customer Support Department
PO Box 945
New York, NY 10159-0945   212-633-3730
                                 888-347-4636
                            Fax: 212-633-3680
                      www.elsevier.nl/locate/jbtep

ISSN 0005-7916

3380 Journal of Drug Education

Baywood Publishing Company
26 Austin Avenue
Box 337
Amityville, NY 11701   631-691-1270
                                 800-638-7819
                            Fax: 631-691-1770
                      E-mail: info@baywood.com
                            www.baywood.com

$160.00

4 per year Year Founded: 1970

3381 Journal of Education Psychology

American Psychological Association
750 1st Street NE
Washington, DC 20002-4241   202-336-5510
                                 800-374-2721
                            Fax: 202-336-5502
                            TDD: 202-336-6123
                            TTY: 202-336-6123
                      E-mail: order@apa.org
                            www.apa.org/books

Carole Beal, Associate Editor

$102.00

4 per year   ISSN 0022-0663

3382 Journal of Emotional and Behavioral Disorders

Pro-Ed Publications
8700 Shoal Creek Boulevard
Austin, TX 78757-6816   512-451-3246
                                 800-897-3202
                            Fax: 800-397-7633
                      E-mail: info@proedinc.com
                            www.proedinc.com

Lisa Tippett, Managing Production Editor

An international, multidisciplinary journal featuring articles on research, practice and theory related to individuals with emotional and behavioral disorders and to the professionals who serve them. Presents topics of interest to individuals representing a wide range of disciplines including corrections, psychiatry, mental health, counseling, rehabilitation, education, and psychology. *$39.00*

64 pages 4 per year ISSN 1063-4266

3383 Journal of Healthcare Management

American College of Healthcare Executives
1 N Franklin Street
Chicago, IL 60606-3421   312-424-2800
                            Fax: 312-424-0023

Presents cutting edge health care management research in a concise, reader friendly format that practitioners, educators, and researchers will find useful. JHM also contains regular columns written by leaders in the field that discuss timely topics such as leadership and managed care. Issues also contain interviews, case studies, and book reviews.

6 per year

3384 Journal of Intellectual & Development Disability

Taylor & Francis Publishing
875 Massachusetts Avenue
Suite 81
Cambridge, MA 02139-3067   215-625-8900
                            Fax: 215-269-0363
                      www.taylorandfrancis.com

3385 Journal of Neuropsychiatry and Clinical Neurosciences

American Neuropsychiatric Association
4510 W 87th Street
Suite 110
Shawnee Mission, KS 66207-1945   614-447-2077
                            Fax: 614-263-4366
                      E-mail: anpa@osu.edu
                      www.neuropsychiatry.com/ANPA/

Richard Restak MD, President

Official publication of the organization and a benefit of membership. Our mission is to apply neuroscience for the benefit of people. Three core values have been identified for the association: advancing knowledge of brain-behavior relationships, providing a forum for learning, and promoting excellent, scientific and compassionate health care.

3386 Journal of Positive Behavior Interventions

Pro-Ed Publications
8700 Shoal Creek Boulevard
Austin, TX 78757-6816   512-451-3246
                                 800-897-3202
                            Fax: 800-397-7633
                      E-mail: info@proedinc.com
                            www.proedinc.com

Lisa Tippett, Managing Production Editor

Deals with principles of positive behavioral support in school, home, and community settings for people with challenges in behavioral adaptation. *$39.00*

64 pages 4 per year ISSN 1098-3007

3387 Journal of Practical Psychiatry

Williams & Wilkins
351 W Camden Street
Baltimore, MD 21201-7912   410-528-4000
                            Fax: 410-528-4312

3388 Journal of Psychiatric Research

Customer Support Department
PO Box 945
New York, NY 10159-0945   212-633-3730
                                 888-437-4636
                            Fax: 212-633-3680
                      www.elsevier.nl/locate/jpsychores

ISSN 0022-3956

3389 Journal of the American Psychiatric Nurses Association

Mosby
11830 Westline Industrial Drive
Saint Louis, MO 63146   314-872-8370
800-325-4177
Fax: 314-432-1380

3390 Journal of the American Psychoanalytic Association

Analytic Press
101 W Street
Hillsdale, NJ 07642-1421   201-358-9477
800-926-6579
Fax: 201-358-4700
E-mail: TAP@analyticpress.com
www.analyticpress.com

Paul E Stepansky PhD, Managing Director
John Kerr PhD, Sr Editor

JAPA is one of the preeminent psychoanalytic journals. Recognized for the quality of its clinical and theoretical contributions, JAPA is now a major publication source for scientists and humanists whose work elaborates, applies, critiques or impinges on psychoanalysis. Topics include child psychoanalysis and the effectiveness of the intensive treatment of children, boundary violations, problems of memory and false memory syndrome, the concept of working through, the scientific status of psychoanalysis and the relevance or irrevance of infant observation for adult analysis. *$115.00*

300 pages 4 per year Year Founded: 1952
ISSN 0003-0651

3391 Journal of the International Neuropsychological Society

Cambridge University Press
40 W 20th Street
New York, NY 10011-4221   212-924-3900
Fax: 212-691-3239
E-mail: marketing@cup.org
www.cup.org

3392 Just the Facts

Children and Adolescent Psychopharmacology Information
6001 Research Park Boulevard, Suite 1568
Wisconsin Psychiatric Institute
Madison, WI 53719-1176   608-263-6171

A newsletter for physicians, and various guides.

3393 Key

National Mental Health Consumers Self-Help
1211 Chestnut Street
Lobby 100
Philadelphia, PA 19107-4114   215-751-1810
800-553-4539
Fax: 215-636-6310
TTY: 215-751-9655
E-mail: info@mhselfhelp.org
www.mhselfhelp.org

Violet Phillips, Editor

Provides information for consumers of mental health services/psychiatric survivors on mental health issues, including advocacy and alternative mental health services. *$15.00*

12 pages 4 per year

3394 Managed Care Interface

Medicom International
66 Palmer Avenue
Suite 49
Bronxville, NY 10708-3420   914-337-7878
Fax: 914-337-5023
E-mail: stan.mehr@medicomint.com
www.medicomint.com

Irene Rosen, Managing Editor

Medicom International publishes two monthly journals, Managed Care Interface and Product Management Today. The former is a peer-reviewed jounral sent to nearly 40,000 professionals working within the managed care industry. The latter provides approximately 11,000 members of product management teams nationwide the practical solutions to today's marketing challenges. Manage Care Interface, $80 individual one year, $100 institutional one year. Product Management Today, $65 individual one year, $80 institutional one year.

12 per year ISSN 1096-5645

3395 Managed Care Outlook

Capitol Publications
1101 K Street
Suite 444
Alexandria, VA 22314   703-583-4100
Fax: 703-739-6517

3396 Managed Care Register

Dorland Healthcare Information
1500 Walnut Street
Suite 1000
Philadelphia, PA 19102   215-875-1212
800-784-2332
Fax: 215-735-3966
E-mail: info@dorlandhealth.com

Directory of organziations that provide products and services to health and managed care executives. *$45.00*

1 per year Year Founded: 1999

3397 Managed Care Reporter

BNA's
1231 25th Street NW
Washington, DC 20037-1157   202-452-4200
Fax: 202-452-4610

3398 Managed Care Strategies

Managed Care Strategies & Psychotherapy Finances
13901 US Highway 1
Suite 5
Juno Beach, FL 33408-1612   561-624-1155
Fax: 561-624-6006

3399 Managed Healthcare

Advanstar Communications
545 Boylston Street
Boston, MA 02116   617-267-6500
                     Fax: 617-267-6900
          E-mail: info@advanstar.com
               www.advanstar.com

3400 Managed Pharmaceutical Report

Capitol Publications
1101 K Street
Suite 444
Alexandria, VA 22314   703-583-4100
                     Fax: 703-739-6517

3401 Marketing Homecare Services & Products to Managed Care

Dorland Healthcare Information
1500 Walnut Street
Suite 1000
Philadelphia, PA 19102   215-875-1212
                          800-784-2332
                     Fax: 215-735-3966
     E-mail: info@dorlandhealth.com
              www.dorlandhealth.com

Managed care primer with detailed marketing and sales training manual. Presents the landscape and terminology of managed care from a homecare marketing perspective. Each step of managed care is explained, with hundreds of specific, practical recommendations useful for both managed care veterans and novices. Over 40 guidelines, check lists and case histories are included. Hardcover. *$295.00*

Year Founded: 1995

3402 Materials Management in Health Care

American Hospital Publishing
737 N Michigan Avenue
Suite 700
Chicago, IL 60611-6661   312-226-5880
                          800-621-6902
                     Fax: 312-951-8491

3403 Mayo Clinic Health Letter

Mayo Clinic
200 1st Street SW
Rochester, MN 55905-0002   507-284-2511
                     Fax: 507-266-0230
       E-mail: healthletter@mayo.edu
               www.mayoclinic.com

Helping our subscribers achieve healthier live by providing useful, easy to understand health information that is timely and of broad interest.

ISSN 0741-6245

3404 Mayo Clinic Women's Health Source

Mayo Clinic
200 1st Street SW
Rochester, MN 55905-0001   507-284-2511
                     Fax: 507-284-5410

3405 Medical Group Management Journal

Medical Group Management Association
104 Inverness Terrace E
Englewood, CO 80112-5313   303-799-1111
                          877-275-6462
                     Fax: 303-643-4439
        E-mail: service@mgma.com
               www.mgma.com

Norma J Plante, Chair

Principal voice for medical group practice.

3406 Medical Psychotherapist

Americal Board of Medical Psychotherapists & Psychodiagnosticians
345 24th Avenue N
Suite 201
Nashville, TN 32703-1520   615-327-2984
                     Fax: 615-327-9235

Official newsletter of the American Board of Medical Psychotherapists and Psychodiagnosticians.

3407 Medications

National Institute of Mental Health
6001 Executive Boulevard
Room 8184
Bethesda, MD 20892-9663
                          866-615-6464
                     Fax: 301-443-4279
                     TTY: 301-443-8431
         E-mail: nimhinfo@nih.gov
               www.nimh.nih.gov

This booklet is designed to help mental health patients and their families understand how and why medications can be used as part of the treatment of mental health problems.

36 pages

3408 Mental & Physical Disability Law Reporter

American Bar Association
740 15th Street NW
9th Floor
Washington, DC 20005-1022 202-662-1570
                     Fax: 202-662-1032
                     TTY: 202-662-1012
    E-mail: CMPDL@staff.abanet.org
               www.abanet.org/disability

Amy Allbright, Managing Editor
Renee Dexter, Production/Marketing Manager

Contains bylined articles and summaries of federal and state court opinions and legislative developments addressing persons with mental and physical disabilities.

6 per year Year Founded: 1976 ISSN 0883-7902

3409 Mental Health Aspects of Developmental Disabilities

Psych-Media
PO Box 57
Bear Creek, NC 27207-0057   336-581-3700
Fax: 336-581-3766
E-mail: mhdd@amji.net
www.mhaspectsofdd.com

Margaret Zwilling, Managing Editor
Linda Vollmoeller, Assistant Managing Editor

A practical clinical reference for the hands on clinician. This is a peer-reviewed journal covering the diagnosis, treatment and rehabilitation needs of persons with developmental disabilities. *$ 58.00*

40 pages 4 per year ISSN 1057-3291

3410 Mental Health Law News

Interwood Publications
3 Interwood Place
Suite 20241
Cincinnati, OH 45220-1821   513-221-3715

Mental health case law summaries - malpractice, patient rights, discrimination, alcoholism, guardianship, negligence, professional liability, commitment, drug dependency and conservatorship. *$89.00*

6 pages ISBN 0-88901 -0 -

3411 Mental Health Law Reporter

Business Publishers
8737 Colesville Road
Suite 1100
Silver Spring, MD 20910-3956   301-587-6300
800-274-6737
Fax: 301-587-1081
E-mail: jbond@bpinews.com
www.bpinews.com

Nancy Biglin, Director Marketing

Summary of court cases pertaining to mental health professionals. *$273.00*

12 per year ISSN 0741-5141

3412 Mental Health Report

Business Publishers
8737 Colesville Road
Suite 1100
Silver Spring, MD 20910-3928   301-587-6300
800-274-6737
Fax: 301-587-4530
E-mail: jbond@bpinews.com
www.bpinews.com

Nancy Biglin, Director Marketing

Independent, inside Washington coverage of mental health administration, legislation and regulation, state policy plus research and trends. *$396.00*

26 per year ISSN 0191-6750

3413 Mental Health Special Interest: Section Quarterly

American Occupational Therapy Association (AOTA)
PO Box 31220
Bethesda, MD 20824-1220   301-652-2682
800-877-1383
Fax: 301-652-7711
TDD: 800-377-8555
E-mail: ajotsis@aota.org
www.aota.org

Occupational therapy and other approaches. *$20.00*

4 pages 4 per year Year Founded: 1978 ISSN 1093-7226

3414 Mental Health Views

CD Publications
8204 Fenton Street
Silver Spring, MD 20910-4509   301-588-6380
Fax: 301-588-6385

3415 Mental Health Weekly

Manisses Communications Group
PO Box 9758
Providence, RI 02940-9758   401-831-6020
800-333-7771
Fax: 401-861-6370
E-mail: manissescs@manisses.com
www.manisses.com

William Kanapaux, Managing Editor

Economic and policy issues for mental health professionals. *$499.00*

48 per year ISSN 10581103

3416 Mental Retardation

AAMR
444 N Capitol Street NW
Suite 846
Washington, DC 20001-1512   202-387-1968
800-424-3688
Fax: 202-387-2193
E-mail: dcroser@aamr.org
www.aamr.org

Newsletter that provides information on the latest program advances, current research, and information on products and services in the developmental disabilities field. Free with membership.

24 per year ISSN 0895-8033

3417 Mentally Disabled and the Law

William S Hein & Company
1285 Main Street
Buffalo, NY 14209-1911   716-882-2600
800-828-7571
Fax: 716-883-8100

Offers information on treatment rights, the provider-patient relationship, and the rights of mentally disabled persons in the community. *$80.00*

3418 Modern Healthcare

Crain Communications
740 N Rush Street
Chicago, IL 60611-2546　　312-649-5200
　　　　　　　　　　　　　　Fax: 312-280-3183

3419 NAMI Advocate

National Alliance for the Mentally Ill
200 N Glebe Road
Suite 1015
Arlington, VA 22203-3728　　703-524-7600
　　　　　　　　　　　　　　800-950-6264
　　　　　　　　　　　　Fax: 703-524-9094
　　　　　　　　　　　　TDD: 703-516-7227
　　　　　　　　　E-mail: frieda@nami.org
　　　　　　　　　　　　　　www.nami.org

Newsletter that provides information on latest research, treatment, and medications for brain disorders. Reviews status major policy and legislation at federal, state, and local levels. Recurring features include interviews, news of research, news of educational opportunities, book reviews, politics, legal issues, and columns titled President's Column, Ask the Doctor, and News You Can Use. Included as NAMI membership benefit.

24-28 pages 24 per year

3420 NASW News

National Association of Social Works
750 1st Street NE
Suite 700
Washington, DC 20002-4241　　202-336-8236
　　　　　　　　　　　　　　Fax: 202-336-8312

3421 National Psychologist

Ohio Psychology Publications Incorporated
6100 Channingway Boulevard
Suite 303
Columbus, OH 43232　　614-861-1999
　　　　　　　　　　　　Fax: 614-861-1996
　　　　　　　E-mail: natlpsych@aol.com
　　　　　　　www.nationalpsychologists.com

Martin Saeman, Marketing/Advertising Sales

Practitioner oriented newspaper which focuses on nonclinical issues such as legal and legislative issues, confidentiality, ethics, cyberspace, reimbursement, marketing, etc. *$30.00*

28-40 pages 6 per year ISSN 1058-6776

3422 National Resource Center on Homelessness & Mental Illness

345 Delaware Avenue
Delmar, NY 12054　　518-439-7415
　　　　　　　　　　　　800-444-7415
　　　　　　　　　　Fax: 518-439-7612
　　　　　　　E-mail: nrc@prainc.com
　　　　　　　www.nrchmi.samsa.gov

Francine Williams, Director
Deborah Dennis, VP/Project Director

Provides technical assistance and comprehensive information concerning the treatment, services and housing needs of persons who are homeless and who have serious mental illnesses. The Resource Center provides technical assistance to CHS grantees, provides or arranges technical assistance on the development of housing and services for special needs populations; maintains an extensive bibliographic database of published and unpublished materials, develops workshops and training institutes on the coordination of services and housing for homeless persons with mental illnesses, and responds to requests for information.

3423 Neuropsychology Abstracts

American Psychological Association Database Department/PsycINFO
750 1st Street NE
Washington, DC 20002-4241　　202-336-5650
　　　　　　　　　　　　　　800-374-2722
　　　　　　　　　　　　Fax: 202-336-5633
　　　　　　　E-mail: psycinfo@apa.org
　　　　　　　　www.apa.org/psycinfo

Bibliographic with current research on the relationship between the brain and behavior. Citations and abstracts are taken from the PsycINFO database.

4 per year ISSN 1083-4915

3424 New Ideas in Psychology

Customer Support Department
PO Box 945
New York, NY 10159-0945　　212-633-3730
　　　　　　　　　　　　　　888-437-4636
　　　　　　　　　　　　Fax: 212-633-3680
　　　　　　www.elsevier.nl/locate/newideapsych

ISSN 0732-118X

3425 News & Notes

AAMR
444 N Capitol Street NW
Suite 846
Washington, DC 20001-1512　　202-387-1968
　　　　　　　　　　　　　　800-424-3688
　　　　　　　　　　　　Fax: 202-387-2193
　　　　　　　E-mail: dcroser@aamr.org
　　　　　　　　　　　　www.aamr.org

Doreen Croser, Executive Director

Covers legislative, program, and research developments of interest to the field, as well as international news, Association activities, job ads and other classifieds and upcoming events.

3426 Newsletter of the American Psychoanalytic Association

Analytic Press
101 W Street
Hillsdale, NJ 07642-1421　　201-358-9477
　　　　　　　　　　　　　　800-926-6579
　　　　　　　　　　　　Fax: 201-358-4700
　　　　　　　E-mail: TAP@analyticpress.com
　　　　　　　　www.analyticpress.com

Paul E Stepansky PhD, Managing Director
John Kerr PhD, Sr Editor

A scholarly and clinical resource for all analytic practitioners and students of the field. Articles and essays focused on contemporary social, political and cultural forces as they relate to the practice of psychoanalysis, regular interviews with leading proponents of analysis, essays and reminiscences that chart the evolution of anlaysis in America. The newsletter publishes articles that are rarely if ever found in the journal literature. Sample copies available. *$29.50*

4 per year

3427 North American Society of Adlerian Psychology Newsletter

NASAP
50 NE Drive
Hershey, PA 17033   717-579-8795
Fax: 717-533-8616
E-mail: nasap@msn.com
www.alfredadler.org

Becky LaFountain, Administrator

Relates news and events of the North American Society of Alderian Psychology and regional news of affiliated associations. Recurring features include lists of courses and workshops offered by affiliated associations, reviews of new publications in the field, professional employment opportunities, a calendar of events, and a column titled President's Message. *$20.00*

8 pages 24 per year ISSN 0889-9428

3428 ORTHO Update

American Orthopsychiatric Association
2001 Beauregard Street
12th Floor
Alexandria, VA 22311   703-797-2584
Fax: 703-684-5968
E-mail: amerortho@aol.com
www.amerortho.org

Intended for members of the Association, who are concerned with the early signs of mental and behavioral disorder and preventive psychiatry. Provides news notes and feature articles on the trends, issues and events that concern mental health, as well as Association news.

6-16 pages 3 per year

3429 Open Minds

Behavioral Health Industry News
10 York Street
Suite 200
Gettysburg, PA 17325-2301   717-334-1329
Fax: 717-334-0538
E-mail: openminds@openminds.com
www.openminds.com

Provides information on marketing, financial, and legal trends in the delivery of mental health and chemical dependency benefits and services. Recurring features include interviews, news of research, a calendar of events, job listings, book reviews, notices of publications available, and industry statistics. *$185.00*

12 pages 12 per year ISSN 1043-3880

3430 Policy Research Associates

345 Delaware Avenue
Delmar, NY 12054-1123   518-439-7415
800-444-4715
Fax: 518-439-7612
E-mail: pra@prainc.com
www.prainc.com

Joseph J Cocozza, VP Research/Development
Pamela Clark Robbins, VP Technical Assistance

Offers comprehensive services for the application of rigorous social science research methods to crucial policy issues at the federal, state and local levels. Conducts short and long term research and evaluations on a wide range of topics that inform policy decisions in the area of human services. Special expertise in planning and evaluating programs and policies in such specific areas as the relationship between the mental health and criminal justice systems, the housing and service need of homeless mentally ill persons, the issues confronting at-risk children, youth and their families and the cause and impacts of violence.

3431 Professional Counselor

3201 SW 15th Street
Deerfield Beach, FL 33442   954-360-0909
800-851-9100
Fax: 954-360-0034
www.professionalcounselor.com

The number one publication serving the addictions and mental health fields.

3432 Professional Resource Press

Professional Resource Press
PO Box 15560
Sarasota, FL 34277-1560   941-343-9601
800-443-3364
Fax: 941-343-9201
E-mail: orders@prpress.com
www.prpress.com

Debra Fink, Managing Editor

Publisher of books, continuing education programs and other applied resources for mental health professionals, including psychologists, psychiatrists, clinical social workers, counselors, OTs, and recreational therapists.

3433 Provider Magazine

American Health Care Association
1201 L Street NW
Washington, DC 20005-4024   202-842-4444
Fax: 202-842-3860
E-mail: astarkey@ahca.org
www.ahca.org

Alexis Starkey, Events

Of interest to the professionals who work for the nearly 12,000 nonprofit and for profit assisted living, nursing facility, developmentally disabled and subacute care providers that care for more than 1.5 million elderly and disabled individuals nationally. Provides information, education, and administrative tools that enhance quality at every level.

3434 PsycINFO News

American Psychological Association Database Department/PsycINFO
750 1st Street NE
Washington, DC 20002-4241   202-336-5650
                                   800-374-2722
                              Fax: 202-336-5633
                              TDD: 202-336-6123
                              TTY: 202-336-6123
                        E-mail: psycinfo@apa.org
                              www.apa.org/psycinfo

Free newsletter that keeps you up to date on enhancements to PsycINFO products.

4 per year

3435 PsycSCAN Series

PsycINFO/American Psychological Association
750 1st Street NE
Washington, DC 20002-4242   202-336-5650
                                   800-374-2722
                              Fax: 202-336-5633
                              TDD: 202-336-6123
                        E-mail: psycinfo@apa.org
                              www.apa.org/psycinfo

Quarterly current awareness print publications in the fields of clinical, developmental, and applied psychology, as well as learning disorders/mental retardation and behavior analysis and therapy. Contains relevant citations and abstracts from the PsycINFO database. PyscScan: Psychopharmacology is an electronic only publication.

4 per year

3436 Psych Discourse

Association of Black Psychologists
PO Box 55999
Washington, DC 20040-5999   202-722-0808
                              Fax: 202-722-5941
                        E-mail: admin@abpsi.org
                              www.abpsi.org

Halford Fairchild, Editor

Publishes news of the Association. Recurring features include editorials, news of research, letters to the editor, a calendar of events, and columns titled Social Actions, Chapter News, Publications, and Members in the News. *$110.00*

32-64 pages 12 per year Year Founded: 1969
ISSN 1091-4781

3437 Psychiatric Home Health

Aspen Publishers
1185 Avenue of the Americas
New York, NY 10036   212-597-0200
                              Fax: 212-597-0338

3438 Psychiatric News

American Psychiatric Publishing
1000 Wilson Boulevard
Suite 1825
Arlington, VA 22209-3901   703-907-7322
                                   800-368-5777
                              Fax: 703-907-1091
                        E-mail: appi@psych.org
                              www.appi.org

Katie Duffy, Marketing Assistant

Psychiatric News is the official newspaper for the American Psychiatric Association. It is published twice a month and mailed to all APA members as a member benefit as well as to about 2,000 subscribers.

3439 Psychiatric Nursing Administration

Aspen Publishers
1185 Avenue of the Americas
New York, NY 10036   212-597-0200
                              Fax: 212-597-0338

3440 Psychiatric Rehabilitation Journal

International Association of Psychosociology
10025 Gover
Columbia, MD 21044   410-730-5965

3441 Psychiatric Times

Continuing Medical Education
2801 McGaw Avenue
Irvine, CA 92614-5835   949-250-1008
                                   800-993-2632
                              Fax: 949-250-0445
                        E-mail: pt@mhsource.com
                              www.mhsource.com

John Schwartz MD, Editor-in-Chief

Allows you to earn CME credit every month with a clinical article, as well as keeping you up to date on the current news in the field. *$54.95*

12 per year

3442 Psychiatry Drug Alerts

MJ Powers & Company
65 Madison Avenue
Ssite 220
Morristown, NJ 07960-7307   973-898-1200
                                   800-875-0058
                              Fax: 973-898-1201
                        E-mail: psych@alertpubs.com
                              www.alertpubs.com

Jenny Marie DeJesus, Circulation Manager

Discusses drugs used in the psychiatric field, including side effects and risks. *$63.00*

8 pages 12 per year   ISSN 0894-4873

3443 Psychiatry Research

Customer Support Department
PO Box 945
New York, NY 10159-0945   212-633-3730
                                   888-437-4636
                              Fax: 212-633-3680
                              www.elsevier.nl/locate/psychres

ISSN 0165-1781

3444 Psychohistory News

International Psychohistorical Assocation (IPA)
34 Plaza Street E
Suite 1109
Brooklyn, NY 11238-5061   **718-638-1414**

Includes news of Association events, conference announcements, events in the psychohistorical field, and interviews and reviews. *$15.00*

8-10 pages 4 per year

3445 Psychological Abstracts

PsycINFO/American Psychological Association
750 1st Street NE
Washington, DC 20002-4242   **202-336-5650**
                                      800-374-2722
                                 Fax: 202-336-5633
                                 TDD: 202-336-6123
                   E-mail: psycinfo@apa.org
                          www.apa.org/psycinfo

Print index containing citations and abstracts for journal articles, books, and book chapters in psychology and related disciplines. Annual indexes.

12 per year

3446 Psychological Assessment Resources

PO Box 998
Odessa, FL 33556-0998   **813-968-3003**
                              Fax: 813-968-2598

3447 Psychological Science Agenda

Science Directorate-American Psychological Association
750 1st Street NE
Washington, DC 20002-4241   **202-336-6000**
                                      800-374-2721
                                 Fax: 202-336-5953
                    E-mail: science@apa.org
            www.apa.org/science/psa/psacover.html

This newsletter disseminates information on scientific psychology, including news on activities of the Association and congressional and federal advocacy efforts of the Directorate. Recurring features include reports of meetings, news of research, notices of publications available, interviews, and the columns titled Science Directorate News, On Behalf of Science, Science Briefs, Announcements, and Funding Opportunities.

16-20 pages   6 per year   ISSN 1040-404X

3448 Psychology Teacher Network Education Directorate

750 1st Street NE
Washington, DC 20002-4241   **202-336-6021**
                                 Fax: 202-336-5962
                 E-mail: jrg.apa@email.apa.org

Provides descriptions of experiments and demonstrations aimed at introducing topics as a basis for classroom lectures or discussion. Recurring features include news and announcements of courses, workshops, funding sources, and meetings; reviews of teaching aids; and reports of innovative programs or curricula occurring in schools, interviews and brief reports from prominent psychologists. *$15.00*

16 pages 5 per year

3449 Psychophysiology

Cambridge University Press
40 W 20th Street
New York, NY 10011-4221   **212-924-3900**
                             Fax: 212-691-3239
                 E-mail: marketing@cup.org
                          www.cup.org

3450 Psychosomatic Medicine

American Psychosomatic Society
6728 Old McLean Village Drive
McLean, VA 22101-3906   **703-556-9222**
                             Fax: 703-556-8729
              E-mail: info@psychosomatic.org
                       www.psychosomatic.org

George Degnon, Executive Director
Laura Degnon, Associate Director

News and event annoucements, examines the scientific understanding of the interrelationships among biological, psychological, social and behavioral factors in human health and disease, and the integration of the fields of science that separately examine each.

3451 Psychotherapy Bulletin

American Psychological Association
750 First Street NE
Washington, DC 20002-4242   **202-336-5500**
                                      800-374-2721
                                 Fax: 202-336-5708
                                      www.apa.org

Recurring features include letters to the editor, news of research, reports of meetings, news of educational opportunities, committee reports, legislative issues, and columns titled Washington Scene, Finance, Marketing, Professional Liability, Medical Psychology Update, and Substance Abuse. *$8.00*

50 pages 4 per year

3452 Psychotherapy Finances

Managed Care Strategies & Psychotherapy Finances
13901 US Highway 1
Suite 58979
Juno Beach, FL 33408-1612   **561-624-1155**
                                      800-869-8450
                                 Fax: 561-624-6006

3453 Quality Letter for Healthcare Leaders

Capitol Publications
1101 K Street
Suite 444
Alexandria, VA 22314   **703-583-4100**
                            Fax: 703-739-6517

3454 Report on Healthcare Information Management

Capitol Publications
1101 K Street
Suite 444
Alexandria, VA 22314   703-583-4100
                              Fax: 703-739-6517

3455 Report on Medical Guidelines & Outcomes Research

Capitol Publications
1101 K Street
Suite 444
Alexandria, VA 22314   703-583-4100
                              Fax: 703-739-6517

3456 Research Reports

Charles D Spencer & Associates
250 S Wacker Drive
Suite 600
Chicago, IL 60606-5800   312-993-7900
                              Fax: 312-993-7910

3457 Research and Training for Children's Mental Health-Update

University of South Florida
13301 Bruce B Downs Boulevard
Florida Mental Health Institute
Tampa, FL 33612-3807   813-974-4661
                              Fax: 813-974-6257
                              www.rtckids.fmhi.usf.edu

Services and research on children with emotional disorders.

2 per year

3458 Research in Developmental Disabilities

Customer Support Department
PO Box 945
New York, NY 10159-0945   212-633-3730
                              888-437-4636
                              Fax: 212-633-3680
                              www.elsevier.nl/locate/redevdis

ISSN 0891-4222

3459 Smooth Sailing

Depression and Related Affective Disorders Association
600 N Wolfe Street
John Hopkins Hospital Meyer 3-181
Baltimore, MD 21287-7381
                              Fax: 410-614-3241
                              www.med.jhu.edu/drada/

Outreach to students and parents through schools.

4 per year

3460 Social Work

National Association of Social Works
750 1st Street NE
Suite 700
Washington, DC 20002-4241   202-336-8236
                              Fax: 202-336-8312

3461 Social Work Abstracts

National Association of Social Works
750 1st Street NE
Suite 700
Washington, DC 20002-4241   202-336-8236
                              Fax: 202-336-8312

3462 Social Work Research

National Association of Social Works
750 1st Street NE
Suite 700
Washington, DC 20002-4241   202-336-8236
                              Fax: 202-336-8312

3463 Social Work in Education

National Association of Social Works
750 1st Street NE
Suite 700
Washington, DC 20002-4241   202-336-8236
                              Fax: 202-336-8312

3464 Society for Adolescent Psychiatry Newsletter

PO Box 570218
Dallas, TX 75357-0218   972-686-6166
                              Fax: 972-613-5532
                              E-mail: info@adolpsych.org
                              www.adolpsych.org

Frances Roton, Executive Director
Leonard Henschel MD, Editor

Puts psychiatrists in touch with an informed cross-section of the profession from all over North America. Dedicated to education development and advocacy of adolescents and the adolescent psychiatric field.

3465 Strategic Medicine

Medical Economics
5 Paragon Drive
Montvale, NJ 07645-1725   201-358-7200
                              Fax: 201-722-2490

3466 Stress Management Research

10609 Grant Road
Suite B
Houston, TX 77070-4462   281-890-8575
                              E-mail: relax@stresscontrol.com
                              www.stresscontrol.com

Stress management books and tapes, seminars and training in relaxation and stress management.

3467 Training Magazine

Bill Communications
50 S 9th Street
Minneapolis, MN 55402   612-333-0471
                              800-328-4329
                              Fax: 612-333-6526
                              E-mail: edit@trainingmag.com
                              www.trainingsupersite.com

Focuses on human performance and productivity in the workplace; employer-sponsored training and education; it's about workplace issues and the relationships between organizations and the people who make them work; it's about managing people, the environments in which they do their jobs, and the systems that affect the way those jobs are done. *$78.00*

12 per year

3468 Trustee

American Hospital Publishing
737 N Michigan Avenue
Suite 700
Chicago, IL 60611-6661   312-226-5880
                               800-621-6902
                          Fax: 312-951-8491

3469 World Federation for Mental Health Newslette r

World Federation for Mental Health
PO Box 16810
Alexandria, VA 22302-0810   703-838-7525
                               Fax: 703-519-7648
                          E-mail: info@wfmh.com
                               www.wfmh.com

Gwen Dixon, Office Administrator

World-wide mental health reports. Education and advocacy on mental health issues. Working to protect the human rights of those defined as mentally ill.

8 pages 1 per year Year Founded: 1984

Testing & Evaluation

3470 Adolescent Substance Abuse: Assessment, Prevention, and Treatment

John Wiley & Sons
605 3rd Avenue
New York, NY 10058-0180   212-850-6000
                               Fax: 212-850-6008
                          E-mail: info@wiley.com
                               www.wiley.com

Extensive, up-to-date coverage includes theoretical models of drug abuse and abusers, contributing biological and genetic factors, social pressures, family and environmental variable, classification, diagnosis and more. *$69.95*

260 pages Year Founded: 1995 ISBN 0-471550-80-9

3471 Aging and Neuropsychological Assessment

Kluwer Academic/Plenum Publishers
233 Spring Street
New York, NY 10013   212-620-8000
                          Fax: 212-463-0742
                          www.kluweronline.com

Clincal introduction to the neural effects of aging provides new insights into the effects of aging on the brain and behavior and serves as a guide to the psychological assessment of older patients. Focuses on common neuropsychiatric disorders and uses numerous case studies to demonstrate the applications of different treatment techniques. *$64.00*

361 pages Year Founded: 1992 ISBN 0-306440-62-8

3472 Assessment and Treatment of Anxiety Disorders in Persons with Mental Retardation

NADD
132 Fair Street
Kingston, NY 12401   845-331-4336
                          Fax: 845-331-4569
                     E-mail: thenadd@aol.com
                          www.thenadd.org

$19.95

104 pages Year Founded: 1996 ISBN 1-572560-01-0

3473 Assessment of Neuropsychiatry and Mental Health Services

American Psychiatric Publishing
1000 Wilson Boulevard
Suite 1825
Arlington, VA 22209-3901   703-907-7322
                               800-368-5777
                          Fax: 703-907-1091
                     E-mail: orders@appi.org
                          www.appi.org

Katie Duffy, Marketing Assistant

Examines the importance of an integrated approach to neuropsychiatric conditions and looks at ways to overcome the difficulties in assessing medical disorders in psychiatric populations. Addresses neuropsychiatric disorders and their costs and implications on policy. *$59.95*

448 pages Year Founded: 1999 ISBN 0-880487-30-5

3474 Attention-Deficit/Hyperactivity Disorder Test: a Method for Identifying Individuals with ADHD

Pro-Ed Publications
8700 Shoal Creek Boulevard
Austin, TX 78757-6816   512-451-3246
                               800-897-3202
                          Fax: 800-397-7633
                     E-mail: info@proedinc.com
                          www.proedinc.com

An effective instrument for identifying and evaluating attention - deficit disorders in persons ages three to twenty-three. Designed for use in schools and clinics, the test is easily completed by teachers, parents and others who are knowledgeable about the referred individual. *$79.00*

Year Founded: 1995

3475 Behavioral and Emotional Rating Scale

Pro-Ed Publications
8700 Shoal Creek Boulevard
Austin, TX 78757-6816   512-451-3246
                              800-897-3202
                         Fax: 800-397-7633
              E-mail: info@proedinc.com
                       www.proedinc.com

Helps to measure the personal strengths of children ages five through eighteen. Contains 52 items that measure five aspects of a child's strength: interpersonal strength, involvement with family, intrapersonal strength, school functioning, and affective strength. Provides overall strength score and five subtest scores. Identifies individual behavioral and emotional strengths of children, the areas in which individual strengths need to be developed, and the goals for individual treatment plans. *$79.00*

Year Founded: 1998

3476 Childhood History Form for Attention Disorders

ADD WareHouse
300 NW 70th Avenue
Suite 102
Plantation, FL 33317   954-792-8100
                              800-233-9273
                         Fax: 954-792-8545
        E-mail: sales@addwarehouse.com
                 www.addwarehouse.com

This form is completed by parents prior to a history taking session. It is designed to be used in conjunction with standardized assessment questionaires utilized in the evaluation of attention disorders. 25 per package. *$35.00*

10 pages

3477 Children's Depression Inventory

ADD WareHouse
300 NW 70th Avenue
Suite 102
Plantation, FL 33317   954-792-8100
                              800-233-9273
                         Fax: 954-792-8545
        E-mail: sales@addwarehouse.com
                 www.addwarehouse.com

Maria Kovac PhD

A self-report, symptom-oriented scale which requires at least a first grade reading level and was designed for school-aged children and adolescents. The CDI has 27 items, each of which consists of three choices. Quickscore form scoring make the inventories easy and economical to administer. The profile contains the following five factors plus a total score normed according to age and sex: negative mood, interpersonal problems, ineffectiveness, anhedonia and negative self-esteem. Contains ten items and provides a general indication of depressive symptoms. *$105.00*

3478 Clinical Evaluations of School Aged Children

Professional Resource Press
PO Box 15560
Sarasota, FL 34277-1560   941-343-9601
                                 800-443-3364
                            Fax: 941-343-9201
                 E-mail: orders@prpress.com
                          www.prpress.com

Debra Fink, Managing Editor

This book delineates the specific symptoms and behaviors associated with each DSM - IV diagnostic syndrome and provides an exceptionally well designed system for communicating diagnostic findings with great clarity when working with parents and professionals from different disciplines. *$39.95*

376 pages Year Founded: 1998 ISBN 1-568870-27-2

3479 Clinical Interview of the Adolescent: From Assessment and Formulation to Treatment Planning

Charles C Thomas Publisher
2600 S 1st Street
Springfield, IL 62704-4730   217-789-8980
                                    800-258-8980
                               Fax: 217-789-9130
                 E-mail: books@ccthomas.com
                          www.ccthomas.com

This book addresses the process of interviewing troubled and psychologically disturbed adolescents who are seen in hospital settings, schools, courts, clinics, and residential facilities. Interviews with adolescents, younger children or adults should follow a logical, sequential and integrated procedure, accomplishing diagnostic closure and the development of a treatment formulation. The nine chapters cover the theoretical and developmental concerns of adolescence; the initial referral; meeting with parents; the therapist; getting acquainted; getting to the heart of the matter; making order out of disorder; the reasons and rationale for the behavior problems. *$59.95*

234 pages Year Founded: 1997 ISBN 0-398067-79-1

3480 Concise Guide to Assessment and Management of Violent Patients

American Psychiatric Publishing
1000 Wilson Boulevard
Suite 1825
Arlington, VA 22209-3901   703-907-7322
                                  800-368-5777
                             Fax: 703-907-1091
                   E-mail: appi@psych.org
                            www.appi.org

Katie Duffy, Marketing Assistant

Written by an expert on violence, this edition provides current information on psychopharmacology, safety of clinicians and how to deal with threats of violence to the clinician. *$21.00*

180 pages Year Founded: 1996 ISBN 0-880483-44-X

3481 Conducting Insanity Evaluations

Guilford Publications
72 Spring Street
New York, NY 10012   212-431-9800
                            800-365-7006
                    Fax: 212-966-6708
            E-mail: info@guilford.com
                    www.guilford.com

Great resource for both psychologists and lawyers. Covers legal standards and their applications to clinical work. Mental health professionals who evaluate defendants or consult to courts on criminal matters will find this a useful resource. *$40.00*

371 pages ISBN 1-572305-21-5

3482 Conners' Rating Scales

Pro-Ed Publications
8700 Shoal Creek Boulevard
Austin, TX 78757-6816   512-451-3246
                               800-897-3202
                       Fax: 800-397-7633
             E-mail: info@proedinc.com
                     www.proedinc.com

Conner's Rating Scales are a result of 30 years of research on childhood and adolescent psychopathology and problem behavior. This revision adds a number of enhancements to a set of measures that has long been the standard instruments for the measurement of attention-deficit/hyperactivity disorder in children and adolescents. *$114.00*

Year Founded: 1997

3483 Depression and Anxiety in Youth Scale

Pro-Ed Publications
8700 Shoal Creek Boulevard
Austin, TX 78757-6816   512-451-3246
                               800-897-3202
                       Fax: 800-397-7633
             E-mail: info@proedinc.com
                     www.proedinc.com

A unique battery of three norm-referenced scales useful in identifying major depressive disorder and overanxious disorders in children and adolescents. *$129.00*

Year Founded: 1994

3484 Diagnosis and Treatment of Alcoholism

Charles C Thomas Publisher
2600 S 1st Street
Springfield, IL 62704-4730   217-789-8980
                                    800-258-8980
                            Fax: 217-789-9130
              E-mail: books@ccthomas.com
                      www.ccthomas.com

Recent advances are presented along with new perspectives on the individual and social problems associated with alcoholism; information is included on personality characteristics, developmental stages, sociological and physiological considerations, and diagnosis. Contents also include current treatment strategies. All mental health professionals concerned with alcoholism will find this book readable, informative and provocative, providing understanding and the tools required to succeed in alcoholism rehabilitation. *$46.95*

362 pages Year Founded: 1978 ISBN 0-398037-80-9

3485 Diagnosis and Treatment of Multiple Personality Disorder

Guilford Publications
72 Spring Street
New York, NY 10012   212-431-9800
                            800-365-7006
                    Fax: 212-966-6708
            E-mail: info@guilford.com
                    www.guilford.com

Comprehensive and integrated approach to a complex psychotherapeutic process. From first interview to crisis management to final post-integrative treatment each step is systematically reviewed, with detailed instructions on specific diagnostic and therapeutic techniques and examples of clinical applications. Specially geared to the needs of therapists, novice or expert alike, struggling with their first MPD case. *$42.00*

351 pages Year Founded: 1989 ISBN 0-898621-77-1

3486 Diagnosis and Treatment of Sociopaths and Clients with Sociopathic Traits

New Harbinger Publications
5674 Shattuck Avenue
Oakland, CA 94609-1662   510-652-2002
                                800-748-6273
                        Fax: 510-652-5472
        E-mail: customerservice@newharbinger.com
                        www.newharbinger.com

This text presents a full course of treatment, with special attention to safety issues and other concerns for different client populations in a range of treatment settings. *$49.95*

208 pages Year Founded: 1996 ISBN 1-572240-47-4

3487 Diagnostic Interview Schedule for Children: DISC

Columbia DISC Development Group
Columbia University
1051 Riverside Drive, Unit 78
New York, NY 10032   212-543-2285
                            888-814-3472
                    Fax: 212-795-2488
        E-mail: DISC@childpsych.columbia.edu

David Shaffer MD, Executive Director
Christopher Lucas MD, Reseach Director
Prudence Fisher PhD, Editorial Director

Automated diagnostic interview assessing 34 common child and adolescent mental health disorders, using DSM-IV criteria. A valuable aid to research, as well as clinical and school assessments.

3488 Draw a Person: Screening Procedure for Emotional Disturbance

Pro-Ed Publications
8700 Shoal Creek Boulevard
Austin, TX 78757-6816   **512-451-3246**
                                   800-897-3202
                          Fax: 800-397-7633
                E-mail: info@proedinc.com
                          www.proedinc.com

Helps identify children and adolescents ages six through seventeen who have emotional problems and require further evaluation. *$96.00*

Year Founded: 1991

3489 Educational Testing Service

Tests In Microfiche
The Test Collection
Princeton, NJ 08541-0001   **609-734-5689**
                            Fax: 609-683-7186
                E-mail: pstanley@ets.org
                      www.ets.org/testcoll/

Pauline Stanley, Communications Assistant

Provides 1,100 plus tests available in microfiche for use in research.

3490 Erectile Disorders: Assesment and Treatment

Guilford Publications
72 Spring Street
New York, NY 10012   **212-431-9800**
                                800-365-7006
                       Fax: 212-966-6708
             E-mail: info@guilford.com
                       www.guilford.com

In-depth analysis of the many developments in the assessment and treatment of erectile dysfunction. Represents a definitive critique of theory and practice in the field. Diagnostic procedures are described in detail, as well as various medical, surgical and psychological treatments. Provides a carefully balanced integration of biomedical, behavioral and systemic factors in erectile dysfunction. *$45.00*

*378 pages Year Founded: 1992 ISBN
0-898627-92-3*

3491 Functional Assessment and Intervention: Guide to Understanding Problem Behavior

High Tide Press
3650 W 183rd Street
Homewood, IL 60430   **708-206-2054**
                                888-487-7377
                       Fax: 708-206-2044
E-mail: managing.editor@hightidepress.com
                       www.hightidepress.com

Diane J Bell, Managing Editor

These experienced practitioners in behavior analyses provide a hands-on, practical approach to recognizing, analyzing, understanding and modifying problem behaviors. Learn the fundamentals of functional assessment and behavior management. *$10.95*

50 pages ISBN 0-965374-45-9

3492 Handbook of Psychological Assessment

John Wiley & Sons
605 3rd Avenue
New York, NY 10058-0180   **212-850-6000**
                            Fax: 212-850-6008
                E-mail: info@wiley.com
                          www.wiley.com

Classic, revised and new psychological tests are all considered for validity and overall reliability in the light of current clinical thought and scientific development. The new edition has expanded coverage of neuropsychological assessment and reports on assessment and treatment planning in the age of managed care. *$59.95*

*816 pages Year Founded: 1997 ISBN
0-471052-20-5*

3493 Harvard Medical School Guide to Suicide Assessment and Intervention

Jossey-Bass Publishers
350 Sansome Street
Floor 5
San Francisco, CA 94104   **415-394-8677**
                                      800-956-7739
                             Fax: 800-605-2665
                          www.josseybass.com

The definitive guide for helping mental health professionals determine the risk for suicide and appropriate treatment strategies for suicidal or at-risk patients. *$59.95*

656 pages ISBN 0-787943-03-7

3494 Health Watch

28 Maple Avenue
Medford, MA 02155   **781-395-5515**
                                800-643-2757
                       Fax: 781-395-6547
                       www.healthwatch.cc

William Gauvastus, Executive Director

On site performer of preventative health screening services and disease risk management programming. Specializing in point of care testing, we perform fast and accurate health screening tests and services to assist in indentifying participant's risk for developing future disease.

Year Founded: 1987

3495 Neuropsychological Assessment and Intervention

Charles C Thomas Publisher
2600 S 1st Street
Springfield, IL 62704-4730

217-789-8980
800-258-8980
Fax: 217-789-9130
E-mail: books@ccthomas.com
www.ccthomas.com

This book is an introduction for the graduate students, advanced undergraduate, and interested professionals to the state of neuropsychlogy today. While it reflects the diversity of approaches within the field, it emphasizes those which are common. Topics include theories of brain function; functional neuroanatomy; Luria's functional systems; issues in neuropsychological assessment, test batteries: Wechler Audlt Intelligence Scale-Revised, Standardized Version of Luria's Neuropsychological Test Battery; individual tests of neuropsychological function; neurological disorders; rehabilitation; planning the rehabilitation program; and rehabilitation technique. *$56.95*

319 pages Year Founded: 1992 ISBN 0-398057-54-0

3496 Psychological and Biological Assessment

American Psychiatric Publishing
1000 Wilson Boulevard
Suite 1825
Arlington, VA 22209-3901

703-907-7322
800-368-5777
Fax: 703-907-1091
E-mail: appi@psych.org
www.appi.org

Katie Duffy, Marketing Assistant

Guidelines for selecting psychological instruments for treatment outcome assessment, performance measurement in healthcare delivery systems. *$25.00*

144 pages Year Founded: 1997 ISBN 0-880484-49-7

3497 Psychotherapy, Counseling, and Primary Mental Health Care: Assessment for Brief or Longer-Term Care

John Wiley & Sons
605 3rd Avenue
New York, NY 10058-0180

212-850-6000
Fax: 212-850-6008
E-mail: info@wiley.com
www.wiley.com

270 pages Year Founded: 1998

3498 Scale for Assessing Emotional Disturbance

Pro-Ed Publications
8700 Shoal Creek Boulevard
Austin, TX 78757-6816

512-451-3246
800-897-3202
Fax: 800-397-7633
E-mail: info@proedinc.com
www.proedinc.com

Helps you identify children and adolescents who qualify for the federal special education category Emotional Disturbance. *$79.00*

Year Founded: 1998

3499 School Social Behavior Scales

Pro-Ed Publications
8700 Shoal Creek Boulevard
Austin, TX 78757-6816

512-451-3246
800-897-3202
Fax: 800-397-7633
E-mail: info@proedinc.com
www.proedinc.com

A behavior rating scale designed specifically for use by professionals in school settings. It provides an integrated rating of both social skills and antisocial problem behaviors through ratings of students. Designed to be used as a screening instrument for early detection of developing social behavioral problems and as part of a multimethod assessment battery for conducting comprehensive assessments, determining program eligibility and developing intervention plans. *$42.00*

Year Founded: 1993

3500 Screening for Brain Dysfunction in Psychiatric Patients

Charles C Thomas Publisher
2600 S 1st Street
Springfield, IL 62704-4730

217-789-8980
800-258-8980
Fax: 217-789-9130
E-mail: books@ccthomas.com
www.ccthomas.com

This book presents how medical diseases can be misdiagnosed as psychiatric disorders and how clinicians without extensive training in the neurosciences can do a competent job of screening psychiatric clients for possible brain disorders. The research cited in this book, dating back to the 1890's, establishes beyond a doubt that such misdiagnoses are more common than most clinicians would guess. This book focuses on one type of medical condition that is likely to be misdiagnosed: brain injuries and illnesses. *$36.95*

148 pages Year Founded: 1998 ISBN 0-398069-21-2

3501 Sexual Dysfunction: Guide for Assessment and Treatment

Guilford Publications
72 Spring Street
New York, NY 10012

212-431-9800
800-365-7006
Fax: 212-966-6708
E-mail: info@guilford.com
www.guilford.com

Designed as a succinct guide to contemporary sex therapy, this book provides an empirically based overview of the most common sexual dysfunctions and a step-by-step manual for their assessment and treatment. Provides a biopsychosocial model of sexual function and dysfunction and describes the authors' general approach to management of sexual difficulties. *$49.95*

212 pages Year Founded: 1991 ISBN 0-898622-07-7

3502 Social-Emotional Dimension Scale

Pro-Ed Publications
8700 Shoal Creek Boulevard
Austin, TX 78757-6816 512-451-3246
800-897-3202
Fax: 800-397-7633
E-mail: info@proedinc.com
www.proedinc.com

A rating scale for teachers, counselors, and psychologists to screen age 5 1/2 through 18 1/2 who are at risk for conduct disorders, behavior problems, or emotional disturbance. It assesses physical/fear reaction, depressive reaction, avoidance of peer interaction, avoidance of teacher interaction, aggressive interaction, and inappropriate behaviors. *$76.00*

Year Founded: 1986

3503 Weinberg Depression Scale for Children and Adolescents

Pro-Ed Publications
8700 Shoal Creek Boulevard
Austin, TX 78757-6816 512-451-3246
800-897-3202
Fax: 800-397-7633
E-mail: info@proedinc.com
www.proedinc.com

Use this quick, effective tool to assess depression in children and adolescents. The only self-report instrument for depression designed for children and adolescents that is based on established criteria for depression. *$94.00*

Year Founded: 1998

Training & Recruitment

3504 Ackerman Institute for the Family

149 E 78th Street
New York, NY 10021-0486 212-879-4900
Fax: 212-744-0206
E-mail: ackerman@ackerman.org
www.ackerman.org
Marcia Sheinberg CSW, Director Clinic/Training
Miranda Aaron CSW, Director Intake

Provides family counseling and therapy.

3505 Active Intervention

735 Whitney Avenue
Gretna, LA 70056 504-367-5766
Fax: 504-367-5755

3506 Advocate Ravenswood Hospital Medical Center

2025 Windsor Avenue
Oakbrook, IL 60523 603-572-9393
Fax: 630-990-4752
www.http://www.advocatehealth.com
Anil Godbole MD, Chairman Department Psychiatric
Carroll Cradock PhD, Director Mental Health Center
Sandie Cleckner RN, MS, Director, Impatient Psy. and PHP

Provides a comprehensive array of services for impatient (Adult, Adolescent, Substance Abuse), Partial Hospital, Intensive Outpatient, Psychological Rehabilitation, Emergency-Crisis, Assertive Community Outreach, Case Management, Program for Deaf and Hard of Hearing at multiple sites on the Northside of Chicago.

3507 Affiliated Counseling Clinic

925 12th Street E
Glencoe, MN 55336 320-864-6139
Fax: 320-864-6130

3508 Affiliates for Evaluation and Therapy

290 NW 165th Street
Suite P300
Miami, FL 33169-6477 305-274-4437
Fax: 305-274-4347

General mental services for children, adults and couples including testing for school placement and general clinical services.

3509 Alfred Adler Institute (AAI)

594 Broadway
Suite 1213
New York, NY 10012 212-254-1048
Fax: 212-254-8271
E-mail: alfredadler@ny.com
www.alfredadler-ny.org
Robert Ellenbogen PhD, Executive Director

Offers training in psychotherapy and analysis to psychiatrists, psychologists, social workers, teachers, clergymen and other related professional persons. Conducts three-year program to provide an understanding of the dynamics of personality and interpersonal relationships and to teach therapeutic methods and techniques. Presents the theory of Individual Psychology as formulated by Alfred Adler. Publications: Journal of Individual Psychology, quarterly. Annual meeting. Semi-annual seminar.

3510 Allegheny Behavioral Health Services

3200 Henry Avenue
Philadelphia, PA 19129-1137 215-842-4559
Fax: 215-843-0371

3511 Alliance Behavioral Care: University of Cincinnati Psychiatric Services

222 Piedmont Avenue
Suite 3300
Cincinnati, OH 45219-4218 513-475-7611
Fax: 513-475-8023

3512 Alternative Associates Therapies

417 N Main Street
Suite 108
Mitchell, SD 57301-2600   605-995-0243
  Fax: 605-995-0243

3513 Alton Ochsner Medical Foundation, Psychiatry Residency

1516 Jefferson Highway
New Orleans, LA 70121-2484   504-842-4178
  Fax: 504-842-3236

3514 American Academy of Child and Adolescent Psychiatry

3615 Wisconsin Avenue NW
Washington, DC 20016-3007   202-966-7300
  Fax: 202-966-2891
  www.aacap.org

3515 American Association of General Hospital Psychiatrists

725 Concord Avenue
Suite 200
Cambridge, MA 02138   617-661-3544
  Fax: 617-661-4800
E-mail: don_lipsitt@hms.harvard.edu
  www.aaghp.org

Don R Lipsitt MD, Communications Secretary

Founded to disseminate clinical and organizational knowledge important to general hospital psychiatrists in fields of consultation-liaison, emergency, inpatient, outpatient, substance abuse and primary care psychiatry. Communication through annual meetings, newsletter, and journal. Dues of $125 ($70 for residents/fellows) includes subscription to General Hospital Psychiatry.

Year Founded: 1978

3516 American College of Healthcare Executives

One N Franklin Street
Suite 1700
Chicago, IL 60606-4425   312-424-2800
  Fax: 312-424-0023
  E-mail: ache@ache.org
  www.ache.org

Thomas C Dolan PhD, President/CEO
Deborah J Bowen, Executive VP/COO
Peter Weil PhD, VP Research & Development

International professional society of nearly 30,000 healthcare executives. ACHE is known for its prestigious credentialing and educational programs. ACHE is also known for its journal, Journal of Healthcare Management, and magazine, Healthcare Executive, as well as groundbreaking research and career development programs. Through its efforts, ACHE works toward its goal of improving the health status of society by advancing healthcare management excellence.

3517 American College of Women's Health Physicians

1111 N Plaza Drive
Suite 550
Schaumburg, IL 60173-4946   847-517-7402
  Fax: 847-517-7229

3518 American Foundation of Counseling

130 E Walnut Street
Suite 706
Green Bay, WI 54301-4236   920-437-8256
  Fax: 920-437-1188
  E-mail: afes@itol.com
  www.americanfoundation.net

Robert Johnson, Executive Director
Keith Hammond, Directions Operations

3519 Anxiety & Mood Disorders Clinic: Department of Psychiatry & Behavioral Medicine

University of Illinois College of Medicine at Peoria
5407 N University
Suite C
Peoria, IL 61614-2025   309-671-8222
  Fax: 309-691-9316
  E-mail: sasaeed@uic.edu
  www.uicomp.uic.edu/psychiatry

Specializes in the evaluation and treatment of anxiety and mood disorders, including panic disorder, social anxiety disorder, obsessive-compulsive disorder, generalized anxiety disorder, post traumatic stress disorder, various phobias, and both unipolar and bipolar mood disorders. We also evaluate and treat other psychiatric difficulties including eating disorders, hypochondriasis, and other obsessive-compulsive spectrum disorders such as body dysmorphic disorder and tricotillomania. Our providers have particular expertise in empirically-supported pharmocotherapy and psychotherapies. We see children, adolesents, and adults and offer individual or group formats.

3520 Asian Pacific Development Center

1825 York Street
Denver, CO 80206-1213   303-393-0304
  Fax: 303-388-1172

3521 BMC Division of Psychiatry, Boston University

One BMC Place
Boston, MA 02118   617-414-4230
  Fax: 617-414-4517

3522 Baystate Medical Center

140 High Street
Springfield, MA 01199-1000   413-794-4286
  Fax: 413-794-4333

3523 Behavioral Healthcare Center

725 Concord Avenue
Cambridge, MA 02138   617-661-3544
  Fax: 617-661-4800

Don R Lipsitt MD, President

A behavorial health facility providing consultation in psychiatry, psychopharmacology and psychotherapy to primary care physicians and their patients.

3524 Behavioral Medicine and Biofeedback

150 SW 12th Avenue
Suite 480
Pompano Beach, FL 33069   954-783-5100
  Fax: 954-783-5176
  E-mail: behmed@aol.com

3525 Berkshire Farm Center and Services for Youth

13640 State Route 22
Canaan, NY 12029-3504   518-781-4567
                              Fax: 518-781-4577
                              www.berkshirefarm.org

3526 Blue Springs Psychological Service

1200 NW S Outer Road
Blue Springs, MO 64015-3072   816-224-6500
                              Fax: 816-224-6500
E-mail: bsshrink@discoverynet.com
          www.jeff@1200corpicon

Jeffery L Miller PhD, Psychologist/Owner

Offers a full range of outpatient mental health services including individuals, couples and family therapy. Offers psychological testing and evaluation. Adults, adolescents and children served.

3527 Brandeis University/Heller School

415 South Street
Waltham, MA 02453-2700   781-736-3800
                              Fax: 781-736-3905

3528 Breining Institute College for the Advanced Study of Addictive Disorders

8880 Greenback Lane
Suite A
Orangevale, CA 95662-4019   916-987-2007
                              Fax: 916-987-8823
        E-mail: college@breining.edu
                www.breining.edu

Kathy Breining, Dean of Students

3529 Brown Schools Behavioral Health System

PO Box 150459
Austin, TX 78715-0459   512-464-0200
                                800-848-9090
                              Fax: 512-464-0220

3530 California Institute of Behavioral Sciences

701 Welch Road
Suite 203
Palo Alto, CA 94304-1705   650-325-1501
                              Fax: 650-462-6755
        www.psychiatryexpert.com

Sanjay Jasuja MD, Medical Director
Ann Bala, Adminsitrative Assistant

Provides the following services for children, adolescents, adults and families on national and international level: Objective testing and comprehensive treatment for ADHD/ADD, depression, manic depressive disorder or Bipolar disorder, anxiety disorders, including obsessive compulsive disorder, panic attacks, phobias, post-traumatic stress disorder, Tourette's syndrome, stuttering, psychopharmacology, stress and anger control, violence and workplace issues, learning and behavior problems, and parenting support groups.

3531 Cambridge Hospital: Department of Psychiatry

1493 Cambridge Street
Cambridge, MA 02139-1099   617-498-1013
                              Fax: 617-498-1390

3532 Cartesian Solutions: Department of Internal Medicine

200 Hawkins Drive
C429-1 GH
Iowa City, IA 52242-1009   319-356-3131
                              Fax: 319-356-2587

3533 Cedars-Sinai Medical Center: Psychiatry and Mental Health

8730 Alden Drive
Suite E339
Los Angeles, CA 90048   310-855-3406
                              Fax: 310-968-0114

3534 Center for Family Counseling

215 W 20th Street
Anniston, AL 36201-3103   205-236-2661
                              Fax: 205-236-9565

3535 Center for Health Policy Studies

10440 Little Patuxent Parkway
10th Floor
Columbia, MD 21044-3561   410-715-9400
                              Fax: 410-715-9718

3536 Changing Your Mind

Hazelden
15251 Pleasant Valley Road
PO Box 176
Center City, MN 55012-0176   651-213-2121
                                800-328-9000
                              Fax: 651-213-4590
                              www.hazelden.org

Clients learn the physical, behavioral and cognitive effects of alcohol and other drug use. Fifty leaflet handouts and a facilitator's guide provide clients with the maximum product benefit. Video is 17 minutes.
$100.00

3537 Children and Adolescents with Emotional and Behavioral Disorders

Virginia Commonwealth University, Medical College
PO Box 980489
Richmond, VA 23298-0489   804-828-4393
                              Fax: 804-828-2645

Cynthia R Eillis MD, Program Chair

3538 College of Health and Human Services: SE Missouri State

1 University Plaza
Mail Stop 8000
Cape Girardeau, MO 63701-4710   573-651-2178
                              Fax: 573-651-5113

3539 College of Southern Idaho

PO Box 1238
Twin Falls, ID 83303-1238   208-733-9554
Fax: 208-736-4743
www.csi.edu

3540 Colonial Services Board

1657 Merrimac Trail
Williamsburg, VA 23185-5624   757-220-3200
Fax: 757-229-7173

3541 Columbia Counseling Center

900 St. Andrews Road
Columbia, SC 29210-5816   803-731-4708
Fax: 803-798-7607

3542 Copper Hills Youth Center

5899 Rivendell Drive
W Jordan, UT 84088-5700   801-561-3377
Fax: 801-569-2959

3543 Corphealth

1300 Summit Avenue
6th Floor
Fort Worth, TX 76102-4414   817-332-2519
800-240-8388
Fax: 817-335-9100
E-mail: businessdevelopment@corphealth.com
www.corphealth.com

Paul J Floyd, Sr VP
Jack Moore, National Director

Privately owned and managed behavioral health care company which serves its customers by facilitating the resolution of behavioral health problems in a manner which balances the needs of purchasers, patients and providers. Provides services that bring added value to insurers and health plans while delivering quality care for their members and customers.

3544 Counseling Program of Pennsylvania Hospital

210 W Washington Square
Floor 11
Philadelphia, PA 19106-3510   215-829-7639
Fax: 215-829-7672

3545 Counseling Services

18 W Colony Plaza
Suite 250
Durham, NC 27705-5582   919-493-2674
Fax: 919-493-1923

3546 Daniel Memorial Institute

3725 Belfort Road
Jacksonville, FL 32216-5899   904-296-1055
Fax: 904-296-1953

3547 Daniel and Yeager Healthcare Staffing Solutions

200 Clinton Avenue W
Suite 400
Huntsville, AL 35801-4919   256-551-1070
800-955-1919
Fax: 256-551-1075
E-mail: info@daniel-yeager.com
www.daniel-yeager.com

Torrie Gentry, Psychiatry Team Leader

3548 Department of Psychiatry: Dartmouth University

Dartmouth Medical School
Lebanon, NH 03756   603-650-5834
Fax: 603-650-5842
E-mail: ben.lewis@dartmouth.edu

Benjamin Lewis EdD, Director Administration

3549 Distance Learning Network

111 W Main Street
Boalsburg, PA 16827   814-466-7808
800-326-9166
Fax: 814-466-7509
E-mail: dlnstaff@dlnetwork.com
www.dlnetwork.com

Eric Porterfield, President/CEO
Sandy Weaver, VP Program Development
Sheri Mills, Marketing

Broadcast and multimedia company dedicated solely to meeting the medical education and communications needs of physicians through the use of both traditional and innovative media formats. More than 150,000 physicians, nurses and pharmacists turn to DLN each year for their medical education.

Year Founded: 1996

3550 Downstate Mental Hygiene Association

370 Lenox Road
Brooklyn, NY 11226-2206   718-287-4806
Fax: 718-287-0337

3551 East Carolina University Department of Psychiatric Medicine

600 Moye Boulevard, Brody Building
Room 4E-100
Greenville, NC 27858   252-816-2660
Fax: 252-816-3815

3552 Education Research Laboratories

226 Bailey Avenue
Suite 102
Fort Worth, TX 76107-1260   817-336-5751

3553 Emory University School of Medicine, Psychology and Behavior

1639 Pierce Drive
Suite 4000
Atlanta, GA 30322-0001   404-778-5526
Fax: 404-727-3233

3554 Emory University: Psychological Center

1462 Clifton Road NE
Atlanta, GA 30322-1013   404-727-7451
                                 Fax: 404-727-1284

Cynthia Messing PhD, Associate Director

Nonprofit community clinic providing low cost counseling and psychological testing services for children and adults.

3555 Enterprise Health Solutions

2 Alba Avenue
Salem, MA 01970

                                     800-484-5113
                              Fax: 978-744-9860
                        E-mail: EHealthS@aol.com

David R Selden, President

Operational consulting services for behavioral health organizations.

3556 Essentials of Clinical Psychiatry: Based on the American Psychiatric Press Textbook of Psychiatry

American Psychiatric Publishing
1000 Wilson Boulevard
Suite 1825
Arlington, VA 22209-3901   703-907-7322
                                     800-368-5777
                              Fax: 703-907-1091
                        E-mail: appi@psych.org
                                   www.appi.org

Katie Duffy, Marketing Assistant

Key points professionals need to know. *$84.95*

1092 pages Year Founded: 1999 ISBN 0-880488-48-4

3557 Essentials of Consultation-Liaison Psychiatry: Based on the American Psychiatric Press Textbook of Consultation-Liaison Psychiatry

American Psychiatric Publishing
1000 Wilson Boulevard
Suite 1825
Arlington, VA 22209-3901   703-907-7322
                                     800-368-5777
                              Fax: 703-907-1091
                        E-mail: appi@psych.org
                                   www.appi.org

Katie Duffy, Marketing Assistant

Important key points and ideas for your practice. *$79.00*

704 pages Year Founded: 1999 ISBN 0-880488-01-8

3558 Family Resources

1214 King Street
PO Box 787
Beaufort, SC 29901-0787   843-521-8409
                                 Fax: 843-521-8410

3559 Family and Children Center Counseling and Development Services

612 John Glenn Court
Mishawaka, IN 46544   219-256-0010
                                 Fax: 219-256-0043

3560 Finch University of Health Sciences

3333 Green Bay Road
N Chicago, IL 60064-3037   847-578-3330
                                 Fax: 847-578-3328

3561 Fletcher Allen Health Care

111 Colchester Avenue
Burlington, VT 05401-1416   802-847-0000
                                 Fax: 802-847-5312
                                       www.fahc.org

3562 Focus Center EEG Neurofeedback

747 S Brea Boulevard
Suite 33
Brea, CA 92821-5379   949-990-3240

3563 Genesis Learning Center

430 Allied Drive
Nashville, TN 37211-3304   615-832-4222
                                 Fax: 615-832-4577

3564 George Washington University

1011 22nd Street NW
Suite 700
Washington, DC 20037-1807   202-994-1000

3565 Gerard Treatment Programs

6009 Wayzata Boulevard
Suite 114
Saint Louis Park, MN 55416-1223   612-546-6996
                                 Fax: 614-546-4749

3566 Harper House: Change Alternative Living

2940 E Eight Mile Road
Detroit, MI 48234-1017   313-891-4976
                                 Fax: 313-891-4204

3567 Haymarket Center, Professional Development

120 N Sangamon Street
Chicago, IL 60607-2202   312-226-7984
                                 Fax: 312-226-8048

3568 Heartshare Human Services

191 Joralemon Street
Brooklyn, NY 11201-4306   718-330-0600
                                 Fax: 718-237-2040

3569 Indiana University Psychiatric Management

5610 Crawfordsville Road
Suite 1200
Indianapolis, IN 46224-3784   317-274-2760
                                     800-230-4876
                                 Fax: 317-484-1250

3570 Inner Health Incorporated

Christopher Alsten, PhD
1260 Lincoln Avenue
San Diego, CA 92103-2322   619-299-7273
                                 800-283-4679
                            Fax: 619-291-7753
          E-mail: sleepenhancement@aol.com

Provides a series of prerecorded therpeutic audio programs for anxiety, insomnia and chemical dependency, both for adults and children. Developed over a 15 year period by a practicing psychiatrist and recording engineer they employ state-of-the-art 3-D sound technologies and the latest relaxation and psychological techniques (but no suliminals). Clients include: US Air Force, US Navy, National Institute of Health, National Institute of Aging and various psychiatric and chemical dependency facilities and companies with shiftworkers.

3571 Institute for Behavioral Healthcare

4370 Alpine Road
Suite 209
Portola Valley, CA 94028
                                 800-258-8411
                            Fax: 415-851-0406
                                 www.ibh.com

Innovative clinical training for behavioral health care professionals.

3572 Institute for Health Policy

415 S Street
Suite MS35
Waltham, MA 02453-2728   781-736-3900
                            Fax: 781-736-3905

3573 Jacobs Institute of Women's Health

409 12th Street SW
Washington, DC 20024-2125   202-863-2468
                            Fax: 202-484-7480

3574 Jefferson Drug/Alcohol

1201 Chestnut Street
Floor 14
Philadelphia, PA 19107-4123   215-955-8856
                            Fax: 215-568-3596

3575 John A Burns School of Medicine Department of Psychiatry

1356 Lusitana Street
Floor 4
Honolulu, HI 96813-2421   808-586-2900
                                 800-872-8760
                            Fax: 808-586-2940
          E-mail: dop@dop.hawaii.edu
                       www.dop.hawaii.edu

Rodante Baysa, Administrative Officer

Medical School Programs and Residency Programs, general, geriatric, addictive and, child and adolescent.

3576 Julia Dyckman Andrus Memorial

1156 N Broadway
Yonkers, NY 10701-1108   914-965-3700
                            Fax: 914-965-3883

3577 Langley Porter Psych Institute - University of California

401 Parnassus Avenue
San Francisco, CA 94143-0984   415-476-7500
                            Fax: 415-502-6361
          E-mail: info@lppi.ucsf.edu

3578 Laurelwood Hospital and Counseling Centers

35900 Euclid Avenue
Willoughby, OH 44094   440-953-3000
                                 800-438-4673
                            Fax: 440-953-3344

3579 Life Science Associates

1 Fenimore Road
Bayport, NY 11705-2115   631-472-2111
                            Fax: 631-472-8146
          E-mail: lifesciassoc@pipeline.com
              www.lifesciassoc.home.pipeline.com

Publishes over fifty computer programs for individuals impaired by head trauma and stroke. Also produces EDS, a software/hardware system for assessing driving.

3580 Living Center

PO Box 65124
Shoreline, WA 98155-9124   206-362-6222
                            Fax: 206-440-9017

3581 Locumtenens.com

500 Northridge Road
Suite 500
Atlanta, GA 30350-3322   770-643-5638
                                 800-562-8663
                            Fax: 770-643-5797
                                 www.locumtenens.com

Davis, VP

Specializing in temporary and permanant placement of psychiatrists. Physicians tell us where and when they want to work and locumtenens.com will find a jop that fits those needs.

3582 MCG Telemedicine Center

1120 15th Street
EA - 100
Augusta, GA 30912-0004   706-721-6616
                            Fax: 706-721-8892
          E-mail: lweisser@mail.mcg.edu
              www.mcg.edu/telemedicine/index.html

Lydia Weisser DO, Telepsychiatrist
Dora Norton, Web Editor

Involved in the delivery of mental health services via telemedicine. In addition, the Telemedicine Center maintains the Georgia Mental Health Network website, a comprehensive listing of mental health resources in the State.

3583 MCW Department of Psychiatry and Behavioral Medicine

8701 Watertown Plank
Milwaukee, WI 53226   414-456-8990
                            Fax: 414-456-6299
          E-mail: aodya@mcw.edu

3584 MDA, Staffing Consultants

145 Technology Parkway
Norcross, GA 30092
770-246-9191
800-780-3500
Fax: 770-246-0882

3585 MS Hershey Medical Center

500 University Drive
PO Box 850
Hershey, PA 17033-0850
717-531-8136
Fax: 717-531-6491

3586 Management Recruiters of Washington, DC

12520 Prosperity Drive
Suite 220
Silver Spring, MD 20904
301-625-5100
Fax: 301-625-3001
E-mail: info@mr-twg.com

3587 Marsh Foundation

1229 Lincoln Highway
PO Box 150
Van Wert, OH 45891-0150
419-238-1695
Fax: 419-238-3986
www.themashfoundation.com

Jan H Giesen MSW, LSW, Assistant Director

Nonprofit center serving children and families with special emphasis in juvenile sex offender population. Services include individual therapy, group therapy, case management and diagnostic assessment.

3588 Masters of Behavioral Healthcare Management

California School of Professional Psychology
Los Angeles Campus
San Francisco, CA 94109
415-346-4500
800-457-1273
E-mail: pmullen@mail.cspp.edu
www.cspp.edu

Offers industry-specific training to mid-management and supervisory personnel employed in behavioral healthcare organizations.

3589 Medical College of Georgia

1140 Parkside Trail
Evans, GA 30809-5234
706-721-6616
Fax: 706-721-7270

3590 Medical College of Ohio, Psychiatry

3000 Arlington Avenue
PO Box 10008
Toledo, OH 43699-0008
419-381-5695
Fax: 419-383-3031

3591 Medical College of Pennsylvania

3200 Henry Avenue
Philadelphia, PA 19129-1137
215-842-4340
Fax: 215-843-9028

3592 Medical College of Virginia

Division of Substance Abuse Medic
PO Box 980109
Richmond, VA 23298-0109
804-828-3584
Fax: 804-828-4800

3593 Medical College of Wisconsin

8701 Watertown Plank
Milwaukee, WI 53226
414-456-8990
Fax: 414-456-6299

3594 Medical University of South Carolina Institute of Psychiatry, Psychiatry Access Center

171 Ashley Avenue
Charleston, SC 29425-0100
843-792-9888
Fax: 843-792-5818

3595 Meharry Medical College

1005-David B Todd Boulevard
Nashville, TN 37208
615-327-6111
Fax: 615-327-6568

3596 Menninger Division of Continuing Education

Menninger Clinic Department of Research
PO Box 829
Topeka, KS 66601-0829
785-380-5000
800-288-3950
Fax: 785-273-8625
www.menninger.edu

Offers continuing medical education programs for a multidisciplinary audience including psychiatrists, psychologists, social workers, marriage and family therapists, pastoral counselors, nurses, and others who practice in the mental health arena.

3597 Mental Health Center

Sheridan County Courthouse
Plentywood, MT 59254
406-765-2550
Fax: 406-228-4553

3598 Mental Health Services Training Collaborative

University of Maryland
685 W Redwood Street
Room 300
Baltimore, MD 21201-1542
410-706-6669
Fax: 410-706-0022

Catherine Z Bailey JD, Program Director

Provides technical assistance to local mental health authorities on the development, operation, and financing supports for mentally ill persons.

3599 NE Ohio Universities College of Medicine

4209 State Route 44
PO Box 95
Rootstown, OH 44272-0095
330-325-2511
Fax: 330-996-2943

3600 Nathan S Kline Institute for Psychiatric Research

140 Old Orangeburg Road
Orangeburg, NY 10962
845-398-5500
Fax: 845-398-5510
E-mail: webmaster@nki.rfmh.org
www.rfmh.org/nki

Robert Cancro MD, Director
Jerome Levine MD, Deputy Director

Research programs in Alzheimers disease, analytical psychopharmacology, basic and clinical neuroimaging, cellular and molecular neurobiology, clinical trail data management, co-occuring disorders and many other mental health studies.

3601 National Association of Alcholism and Drug Abuse Counselors

901 N Washington Street
Suite 600
Alexandria, VA 22314-1535
703-741-7686
800-548-0497
Fax: 703-741-7698
E-mail: rdavis@naadac.org
www.naadac.org

Pat Ford-Roegner, Executive Director
Bill Malone, COO
Rhonda A Davis, Public Affairs

NAADAC is the only professional membership organization that serves counselors who specialize in addiction treatment. With 14,000 members and 47 state affiliates representing more than 80,000 addiction counselors, it is the nation's largest network of alcoholism and drug abuse treatment professionals. Among the organization's national certifacation programs are the National Certified Addiction Counselor and the Masters Addiction Counselor designations.

3602 National Association of School Psychologists

4340 E West Highway
Suite 402
Bethesda, MD 20814
301-657-0270
Fax: 301-657-0275
www.nasponline.org

3603 New York University Behavioral Health Programs

530 1st Avenue
Suite 7D
New York, NY 10016-6481
212-263-7419
Fax: 212-263-7460
www.med.nyu.edu/nyubhp

David Ginsburg MD, Director

Outpatient psychiatry group for Tisch Hospital at NYU Medical Center. Our multidisciplinary team of licensed psychiatrists and social workers offers you the most up-to-date and scientifically validated treatments.

3604 Nickerson Center

7025 N Lombard Street
Portland, OR 97203-3203
503-289-9071
Fax: 503-289-9281

3605 Northwestern University Medical School

303 E Chicago Avenue
Chicago, IL 60611-3072
312-908-8972
Fax: 312-503-0466
E-mail: jsl329@nwu.edu

The Mental Health Services and Policy Program is a multidisciplinary research/educational program on the development and implementation of outcomes management technology.

3606 Northwestern University, Feinberg School of Medicine

303 E Chicago Avenue
Chicago, IL 60611-3008
312-503-8649

3607 Onslow County Behavioral Health

301 Johnson Boulevard
Jacksonville, NC 28540
910-938-3546
Fax: 910-938-4618

3608 PRIMA A D D

4004 Belt Line Road
Suite 250
Dallas, TX 75244
972-386-8599
Fax: 972-386-8597

3609 Parent Child Center

2500 Metrocentre Boulevard
Suite 3
W Palm Beach, FL 33407-3190
561-688-9113
Fax: 561-689-4188

3610 Penelope Price

Cindy Hide
4281 MacDuff Plaza
Dublin, OH 43016
614-793-0165
Fax: 614-793-0443
www.penelope.com

3611 Pepperdine University, Graduate School of Education and Psychology

6100 Center Drive
Los Angeles, CA 90045
310-568-5600
800-347-4849
Fax: 310-568-5755

Crystal Guy, Public/Media Relations Coord.

Offers graduate degree programs designed to prepare psychologists, marriage and family therapists, and mental health practitioners. Many programs accommodate a full-time work schedule with evening and weekend classes available in a trimester schedule. The average class size is 15. There are five educational centers in southern California and three community counseling clinics available to the surrounding community.

3612 Pittsburgh Health Research Institute

600 Forbes Avenue
Pittsburgh, PA 15282-0001
412-766-0300
Fax: 412-396-4519

Professional/Training & Recruitment

3613 Postgraduate Center for Mental Health
124 E 28th Street
New York, NY 10016-8402
212-689-7700
Fax: 212-696-1679

Leona Mackler, Director

Information on mental health.

3614 Pressley Ridge Schools
530 Marshall Avenue
Pittsburgh, PA 15214-3098
412-442-2892
Fax: 412-321-5313

3615 Professional Horizons, Mental Health Service
PO Box 20078
Fountain Hills, AZ 85269
602-246-3311
Fax: 602-482-0156

3616 Psych-Med Association, St. Francis Medical
2616 Wilmington Road
Suite A
New Castle, PA 16105-1530
724-652-2323
Fax: 724-654-3461

3617 PsychTemps
2404 Auburn Avenue
Cincinnati, OH 45219-2735
513-651-9500
Fax: 513-651-9558
E-mail: marilyn@psychtemps.com
www.psychtemps.com

Marilyn Tribbe, Associate Director

Specialized recruiting and staffing company that fills temporary, permanent, and temp-to-hire job placement for the behavioral healthcare field.

3618 Psychiatric Associates
PO Box 6504
Kokomo, IN 46904-6504
765-453-9338
Fax: 765-455-2710

3619 Psychological Associates-Texas
10609 Grant Road
Houston, TX 77070
281-469-6395

3620 Psychological Center
180 N Oakland Avenue
Pasadena, CA 91101-1714
626-395-7100
Fax: 626-395-7270

3621 Psychological Diagnostic Services
10850 E Traverse Highway
Suite 2204
Traverse City, MI 49684-1363
616-947-6634
Fax: 616-947-3340

3622 Psychology Department
Bowling Green, OH 43403-0001
419-372-2540

3623 QuadraMed Corporation
12110 Sunset Hills Road
Reston, VA 20190
703-709-2300
800-393-0278
Fax: 703-709-2490
www.quadramed.com

3624 Regional Research Institute for Human Services of Portland University
1912 SW Sixth Avenue
Suite 120
Portland, OR 97207-0751
503-725-4040
Fax: 503-725-4186
www.rri.pdx.edu

3625 Research Center for Children's Mental Health, Department of Children and Family
University of South Florida
13301 Bruce B Downs Boulevard
Tampa, FL 33612-3807
813-974-4661
Fax: 813-974-4406

3626 River City Mental Health Clinic
2265 Como Avenue
Suite 201
Saint Paul, MN 55108-1700
651-646-8985
Fax: 651-646-3959

Mark Hansen PhD, LP, CEO
Doug Jensen MSW, LISW, Executive Director

Psychotherapy and assessment for all ages.

3627 Riveredge Hospital
8311 Roosevelt Road
Forest Park, IL 60130-2500
708-771-7000
800-252-2540
Fax: 708-209-2280

Mark R Russell, Chairman/CEO
Robin S Scott, Administrative Director

210 bed behavioral health facility.

3628 Riverside Center
PO Box 2033
Winston, OR 97496-2033
541-679-6129
Fax: 541-679-5285

3629 Rockland Children's Psychiatric Center
599 Convent Road
Orangeburg, NY 10962
845-359-7400
800-597-8481
Fax: 845-359-7461
E-mail: RocklandCPC@Omh.State.Ny.Us
www.omh.state.ny.us/omhweb/facilities/rcph/facility

David J Woodlock, CEO
Sadhana Sardana MD, Clinical Director
Agatha Caton, Admissions Coordinator

RCPC is a JCAHO accredited children's psychiatric center. We provide inpatient care to youngsters 10 - 18 years of age from the lower Hudson Valley. An array of local, school-based outpatient services are available in each of the seven counties in the area.

3630 Rosemont Center

2440 Dawnlight Avenue
Columbus, OH 43211-1999   614-471-2626
                              Fax: 614-478-3234

3631 SAFY of America

10100 Elida Road
Delphos, OH 45833-9056   419-695-8010
                               800-532-7239
                          Fax: 419-695-0004
                      E-mail: safy@safy.org
                              www.safy.org

3632 SUNY

1001 Humboldt Parkway
Buffalo, NY 14208-2221   716-887-8230
                          Fax: 716-887-8124

3633 School of Nursing, UCLA

PO Box 951702
Los Angeles, CA 90095-1702   310-825-7181
                          Fax: 310-267-0330
             E-mail: sonsaff@sonnet.ucla.edu
                       www.nursing.ucla.edu

3634 Sonia Shankman Orthogenic School

1365 E 60th Street
Chicago, IL 60637-2890   773-702-1203
                          Fax: 773-702-1304

3635 Southern Illinois University School of Medicine: Department of Psychiatry

PO Box 19642
Springfield, IL 62702   217-545-8229
                          Fax: 217-545-2275
          www.siumed.edu/psych/main/SIUpsych.htm

3636 Southern Illinois University School of Medicine

PO Box 19230
Springfield, IL 62794-9230   217-785-3847
                          Fax: 217-524-2275

3637 St. Francis Medical Center

400 45th Street
Pittsburgh, PA 15233   412-622-4343
                          Fax: 412-622-6756

3638 St. Joseph Behavioral Medicine Network

861 Corporate Drive
Suite 103
Lexington, KY 40503-5433   859-224-2022
                          Fax: 859-224-2024

3639 St. Louis Behavioral Medicine Institute

1129 Macklind Avenue
Saint Louis, MO 63110-1440   314-534-0200
                          Fax: 314-534-7996
                              www.slbmi.com

3640 Stonington Institute

75 Swantown Hill Road
N Stonington, CT 06359   860-535-1010
                               800-832-1022
                          Fax: 860-535-8538
        E-mail: info@stoningtoninstitute.com
                  www.stoningtoninstitute.com

3641 Success Day Training Program

Skills Unlimited
2060 Ocean Avenue
Suite 3
Ronkonkoma, NY 11779-6533   631-580-5319
                          Fax: 631-580-5327
             E-mail: success@systec.com

SUCCESS is a socialization, recreation and prevocational day program for persons with chronic mental illness. Transportation is provided for attenees from Islip, Babylon, and Brookhaven townships. There is no cost to consumers. An evening and weekend program is also available to Islip residents.

3642 Texas Tech Health Sciences Center-Department of Corrections, Education Resources

3601 4th Street
Lubbock, TX 79430-0001   806-743-2820
                          Fax: 806-743-2784

3643 Three Springs LEAPS

Three Springs
PO Box 297
Centerville, TN 37033   931-729-5040
                          Fax: 931-729-9525

Robert Moore, Director Admissions
Susan Hardy, Program Administrator
Glenn Drew, Program Director

The 90-day outdoor therapeutic program near Centerville, Tennessee is accredited by JCAHO. Boys ages 13-17 just beginning to have difficulty with behavioral issues, substance abuse, and school difficulties will be considered for admission. The program offers intensive adventure based bimonthly trips such as canoeing, hiking, and mountain biking. Family therapy modules are offered to family members. Specialty groups for such issues as grief or substance abuse are offered. The boys attend the private SACS accredited school on campus. Price: $180 per diem; $16,200 for 90 days. Work with some third-party payors.

3644 Topeka Institute for Psychoanalysis

PO Box 829
Topeka, KS 66601-0829   785-380-5000
                               800-288-3950
                          Fax: 785-273-8625
                              www.menninger.edu

A training facility for health care professionals, the Topeka Institute for Psychoanalysis has the tripartite mission of promoting research to expand the knowledge base in its field of expertise; providing didactic education and clinical supervision to trainees; and caring for patients in need of its services through a low-fee clinic.

3645 Training Behavioral Healthcare Professionals: Higher Learning in an Era of Managed Care

Wiley Europe and Jossey-Bass Publications
1110 Mar Street
Suite E
Tiburon, CA 94920　　　　415-435-9821
　　　　　　　　　　　　Fax: 415-435-9092
　　　　　　　　　　　　www.wileyeurope.com

Identifies best practices and a model curriculum for training the next generation of behavioral healthcare providers. *$ 32.95*

208 pages Year Founded: 1997 ISBN 0-787907-95-2

3646 Training Behavioral Healthcare Professionals

Jossey-Bass Publishers
350 Sansome Street
5th Floor
San Francisco, CA 94104　　　415-394-8677
　　　　　　　　　　　　　800-956-7739
　　　　　　　　　　Fax: 800-605-2665
　　　　　　　　　　www.josseybass.com

$36.95

200 pages ISBN 0-787907-95-2

3647 UC Berkeley

School of Business
Berkeley, CA 94720-0001　　510-642-6000

3648 UCLA Neuropsychiatric Institute and Hospital

300 UCLA Medical Plaza
Suite 2414
Los Angeles, CA 90095-8346　　310-825-0051

3649 UCSF-Department of Psychiatry, Cultural Competence

1001 Potrero Avenue
Suite 7M
San Francisco, CA 94110-3518　　415-206-8984
　　　　　　　　　　　　Fax: 415-206-8942

3650 USC Psychiatry and Psychology Associates

1640 Marengo Street
Suite 510
Los Angeles, CA 90033-4586
　　　　　　　　E-mail: ericknun@usc.edu

3651 USC School of Medicine

Health Sciences Campuses
Name/Department USC
Los Angeles, CA 90033　　　323-442-1100
　　　　　　　　　　　　Fax: 323-442-2722
　　www.usc.edu/schools/medicine/ksom.html

3652 Ulster County Mental Health Department

239 Golden Hill Lane
Kingston, NY 12401-6441　　845-340-4174
　　　　　　　　　　　Fax: 845-340-4094

3653 Union County Psychiatric Clinic

117 Roosevelt Avenue
Suite 119
Plainfield, NJ 07060-1331　　973-263-8070
　　　　　　　　　　　Fax: 973-263-8666

3654 Universal Behavioral Service

820 Fort Wayne Avenue
Indianapolis, IN 46204-1309　　317-684-0442
　　　　　　　　　　　Fax: 317-684-0679

3655 University Behavioral Healthcare

671 Hoes Lane
PO Box 1392
Piscataway, NJ 08855-1392
　　　　　　　　　　　800-969-5300
　　　　　　　　　　Fax: 732-235-5867

3656 University of California at Davis

2230 Stockton Boulevard
Sacramento, CA 95817-1445　　916-734-3574
　　　　　　　　　　　Fax: 916-734-0849

3657 University of Cincinnati College of Medical Department of Psychiatry

PO Box 670559
Cincinnati, OH 45267-0001　　513-558-4247
　　　　　　　　　　　Fax: 513-558-0187

3658 University of Colorado Health Sciences Center

4455 E 9th Avenue
Denver, CO 80262　　　　303-372-0000
　　　　　　　　　　　www.uchsc.edu

3659 University of Connecticut Health Center

263 Farmington Avenue
Farmington, CT 06030-0002　　860-679-7692
　　　　　　　　　　　800-535-6232
　　　　　　　　　　Fax: 860-679-2374
　　　　E-mail: hmark@nsoz.uchc.edu
　　　　　　　　　　　www.uchc.edu

Hal Mark, Director

3660 University of Illinois at Chicago

912 S Wood Street
M/C 913
Chicago, IL 60612-7325　　312-996-7383
　　　　　　　　　　　Fax: 312-996-7658

3661 University of Iowa Hospital

200 Hawkins Drive
C429-1 GH
Iowa City, IA 52242-1009　　319-356-3131
　　　　　　　　　　　Fax: 319-356-2587

3662 University of Kansas Medical Center
3901 Rainbow Boulevard
Kansas City, KS 66160-0003   913-588-6418
                                    Fax: 913-588-6414

3663 University of Kansas School of Medicine
1010 N. Kansas
Wichita, KS 67214-3199   316-293-2635
                                    Fax: 316-293-2628
                                    www.wichita.kumc.edu

3664 University of Louisville School of Medicine
PO Box 35070
Louisville, KY 40232-5070   502-893-9271
                                    Fax: 502-629-7788

3665 University of Maryland Medical Systems
701 W Pratt Street
Suite 388
Baltimore, MD 21201-1023   410-328-6771
                                    Fax: 410-328-3693

3666 University of Maryland School of Medicine
645 W Redwood Street
Baltimore, MD 21201-1542   410-328-6735
                                    Fax: 410-328-3693

3667 University of Massachusetts Medical Center
55 Lake Avenue N
Worcester, MA 01655-0002   508-856-1477
                                    Fax: 508-856-1710

3668 University of Miami - Department of Psychology
5202 University Drive
Miami, FL 33146   305-284-2814
                                    Fax: 305-284-3402

3669 University of Michigan
400 E Eisenhower Parkway
Suite A
Ann Arbor, MI 48108-3318   734-764-1817
                                    Fax: 734-763-9506
                                    E-mail: info@umich.edu
                                    www.umich.edu

3670 University of Minnesota Health Systems
PO Box 393
Minneapolis, MN 55480-0393   612-626-5078

3671 University of Minnesota Press Test Division
111 3rd Avenue S
Suite 290
Minneapolis, MN 55401-2552   612-627-1970
                                    Fax: 612-627-1980

3672 University of Minnesota, Family Social Science
290 McNeal Street
Saint Paul, MN 55108   612-625-1900
                                    Fax: 612-625-4227

3673 University of Minnesota-Media Distribution
420 Delaware Street SE
Mayo Memorial Building
Minneapolis, MN 55455-0374   612-624-7906

3674 University of Nebraska
PO Box 880227
Lincoln, NE 68588-0227   402-472-9084

3675 University of New Mexico, School of Medicine
Albuquerque, NM 87131-0001   505-272-5416
                                    Fax: 505-272-4639

3676 University of North Carolina School of Social Work, Behavioral Healthcare
301 Pittsboro Street
Suite 3550
Chapel Hill, NC 27516-2911   919-962-4372
                                    Fax: 919-962-6562

3677 University of North Carolina, School of Medicine
CB 7160
Chaple Hill, NC 27399   909-966-4738
                                    Fax: 919-966-7659

3678 University of Pennsylvania Health System
2002 Penn Tower
399 S. 34th Street
Philadelphia, PA 19104-4385   215-662-4000
                                    800-789-7366
                                    Fax: 215-349-8120
                                    www.uphs.upenn.edu

3679 University of Pennsylvania, Department of Psychiatry
7 William Charles Drive
Glen Mills, PA 19342-8829   215-662-2899
                                    Fax: 215-662-6911

3680 University of Pittsburgh
3500 Victoria Street
415 Victoria Building
Pittsburgh, PA 15261-0001   412-624-2215
                                    Fax: 412-624-9176

3681 University of Psychiatric Center
2751 E Jefferson Avenue
Suite 200
Detroit, MI 48207-4100   313-993-3434
                                    Fax: 313-993-3421

3682 University of Tennessee Medical Group: Department of Medicine and Psychiatry

135 N Pauline Street
Floor 6
Memphis, TN 38105-4619　　901-448-2400
Fax: 901-448-2481
www.utmedicalgroup.com/pages/depts/Psych_ho
me.html

3683 University of Texas Medical Branch Managed Care

301 University Boulevard
Galveston, TX 77555-5302　　409-772-1011
Fax: 409-772-8698
www.utmb.edu

3684 University of Texas, Southwestern Medical Center

5323 Harry Hines Boulevard
Dallas, TX 75390　　214-648-3111
Fax: 214-648-8955
www.utsouthwestern.edu/index.html

3685 University of Texas-Houston Health Science Center

2800 S Macgregor Way
Suite 3A18
Houston, TX 77021-1032　　713-741-7803
Fax: 713-741-7832

3686 University of Utah Neuropsychiatric

501 Chipeta Way
Salt Lake City, UT 84108-1222　　801-583-2500

3687 Utica Psychiatric Service

1145 S Utica Avenue
Suite 1000
Tulsa, OK 74104-4002　　918-587-2104
Fax: 918-579-2991

3688 VA Medical Center

10 N Greene Street
Baltimore, MD 21201-1524　　410-605-7410
Fax: 410-605-7942

3689 Wake Forest University

1834 Wake Forest Road
Winston Salem, NC 27106　　336-758-5255
Fax: 336-716-6841

3690 Wayne State University School of Medicine

2751 E Jefferson Avenue
Suite 200
Detroit, MI 48207-4100　　313-577-0147
Fax: 313-993-3421

3691 West Jefferson Medical Center: Behavioral Medical Center

229 Bellemeade Boulevard
Gretna, LA 70056-7153　　504-391-2440
Fax: 504-398-4339

3692 Western Psychiatric Institute and Clinic

3811 Ohara Street
Room E-607
Pittsburgh, PA 15213-2593　　412-624-2215
Fax: 412-624-9176

3693 Wordsworth

Pennsylvania Avenue & Camphill Road
Fort Washington, PA 19034-2913　　215-643-5400
800-769-0088
Fax: 215-643-0595

The mission of Wordsworth, a not-for-profit institution, is to provide quality education, treatment and care to children and families with special needs.

Year Founded: 1952

3694 Yale University School of Medicine: Child Study Center

230 S Frontage Road
PO Box 207900
New Haven, CT 06520-7900　　203-785-6252
Fax: 203-737-5455
E-mail: paula.armbruster@yale.edu

Paula Armbruster MSW, Director

Provides a comprehensive range of in-depth diagnostic and treatment services for children with psychiatric and developmental disorders. These services include specialized developmental evaluations for children ages zero-four, and psychological and psychiatric evaluations for children 5-18. Individualized treatment plans following evaluation make use for a range of theraputic interventions, including psychotherapy, group therapy, family therapy, psycho-pharmacological treatment, parent couseling, consultation and service planning. Immediate access for children needing to be seen within 24 hours and walk-in serrvice is also available.

Video & Audio

3695 Changing Your Mind

Hazelden
15251 Pleasant Valley Road
PO Box 176
Center City, MN 55012-0176　　651-213-2121
800-328-9000
Fax: 651-213-4590
www.hazelden.org

Clients learn the physical, behavioral and cognitive effects of alcohol and other drug use. Fifty leaflet handouts and a facilitator's guide provide clients with the maximum product benefit. *$100.00*

3696 Cognitive Behavioral Assessment

New Harbinger Publications
5674 Shattuck Avenue
Oakland, CA 94609-1662　　510-652-2002
800-748-6273
Fax: 510-652-5472
E-mail: customerservice@newharbinger.com
www.newharbinger.com

A videotape that guides three clients through PAC (Problem, Antecedents, Consequences) method of cognitive behavioral assessment. *$49.95*

3697 Couples and Infertility - Moving Beyond Loss

Guilford Publications
72 Spring Street
New York, NY 10012
212-431-9800
800-365-7006
Fax: 212-966-6708
E-mail: info@guilford.com
www.guilford.com

A VHS video explores the biological and resulting psychological and social issues of infertility. *$95.00*

Year Founded: 1995 ISBN 1-572302-86-0

3698 Educating Clients about the Cognitive Model

New Harbinger Publications
5674 Shattuck Avenue
Oakland, CA 94609-1662
510-652-2002
800-748-6273
Fax: 510-652-5472
E-mail: customerservice@newharbinger.com
www.newharbinger.com

Videotape that helps three clients understand their symptoms as they work toward developing a working contract to begin cognitive restructing. *$49.95*

3699 Gender Differences in Depression: Marital Therapy Approach

Guilford Publications
72 Spring Street
New York, NY 10012
212-431-9800
800-365-7006
Fax: 212-966-6708
E-mail: info@guilford.com
www.guilford.com

Male-female treatment team is shown working with a markedly depressed couple to improve communication and sense of well being in their marriage. *$85.50*

Year Founded: 1996 ISBN 1-572302-87-9

3700 Group Work for Eating Disorders and Food Issues

American Counseling Association
5999 Stevenson Avenue
Alexandria, VA 22304-3300
800-422-2648
Fax: 703-823-0252
www.counseling.org

A plan for working with high school and college age females who are at risk for eating disorders. This video provides a method for identifying at-risk clients, a session-by-session desciption of the group, exercises and information on additional resources. *$89.95*

Year Founded: 1995 ISSN 79801

3701 Help This Kid's Driving Me Crazy - the Young Child with Attention Deficit Disorder

Pro-Ed Publications
8700 Shoal Creek Boulevard
Austin, TX 78757-6816
512-451-3246
800-897-3202
Fax: 800-397-7633
E-mail: info@proedinc.com
www.proedinc.com

This videotape provides information about the behavior and special needs of young children with ADD and offers suggestions on fostering appropriate behaviors. *$89.00*

3702 I Love You Like Crazy: Being a Parent with Mental Illness

Mental Illness Education Project
PO Box 470813
Brookline Village, MA 02247-0244
617-562-1111
800-343-5540
Fax: 617-779-0061
E-mail: miep@tiac.net
www.miepvideos.org

Christine Ledoux, Executive Director

In this videotape, eight mothers and fathers who have mental illness discuss the challenges they face as parents. Most of these parents have faced enormous obstacles from homelessness, addictions, legal difficulties and hospitalizations, yet have maintained a positive and loving relationship with their children. The tape introduces issues of work, fear, stigma, relationships with children and the rest of the family, with professionals, and with the community at large. Discounted price for families/consumers. *$79.95*

Year Founded: 1999

3703 Know Your Rights: Mental Health Private Practice & the Law

American Counseling Association
5999 Stevenson Avenue
Alexandria, VA 22304-3300
800-347-6647
Fax: 703-823-0252
E-mail: webmaster@counseling.org
www.counseling.org

Whether you are in private practice or are thinking about opening your own practice, this forum lead by national experts, offers answers to important questions and provides invaluable information for every practitioner. Helps to orientate practitioners on the legally permissible boundaries, legal liabilities that are seldom known and how to respond in the face of legal action. *$145.00*

ISSN 79062

3704 Life Is Hard: Audio Guide to Healing Emotional Pain

Impact Publishers
PO Box 6016
Atascadero, CA 93423-6016
805-466-5917
800-246-7228
Fax: 805-466-5919
E-mail: info@impactpublishers.com
www.impactpublishers.com

Professional/Web Sites

In a very warm and highly personal style, psychologist Preston offers listeners powerful advice — realistic, practical, effective, on dealing with the emotional pain life often inflicts upon us. *$11.95*

Year Founded: 1996 ISBN 0-915166-99-2

3705 Medical Aspects of Chemical Dependency
Active Parenting Publishers

Hazelden
15251 Pleasant Valley Road
PO Box 176
Center City, MN 55012-0176   651-213-2121
                                 800-328-9000
                                 Fax: 651-213-4590
                                 www.hazelden.org

This interactive curriculum helps professionals educate clients in treatment and other settings about medical effects of chemical use and abuse. The program includes a video that explains body and brain changes that can occur when using alcohol or other drugs, a workbook that helps clients apply the information from the video to their own situations, a handbook that provides in-depth information on addiction, brain chemistry and the physiological effects of chemical dependency and a pamphlet that answers critical questions clients have about the medical effects of chemical dependency. Total price of $244.70, available to purchase separately. Program value packages available for $395.00, with 25 workbooks, two handbooks, two video and 25 pamphlets.

3706 Mental Illness Education Project

PO Box 470813
Brookline Village, MA 02447-0813   617-562-1111
                                    800-343-5540
                                    Fax: 617-779-0061
                                    E-mail: info@miepvideos.org
                                    www.miepvideos.org

Christine Ledoux, Executive Director

Engaged in the production of video-based educational and support materials for the following specific populations: people with psychiatric disabilities; families, mental health professionals, special audiences, and the general public. The Project's videos are designed to be used in hospital, clinical and educational settings, and at home by individuals and families.

3707 Personality and Stress Center for
Applications of Psychological Type

2815 NW 13th Street
Suite 401
Gainesville, FL 32609-2868   352-375-0160
                                  800-777-2278
                                  Fax: 352-378-0503
                                  E-mail: development@CAPT.org
                                  www.catp.org

Alecia Perkins, Director Customer Service

Humorous and energetic presentation of the use of type and rational-emotive therapy concepts in stress management. The authors share years of experience using this model in a hospital setting. Useful to the counselor, educator, or anyone working with stress management. *$11.00*

audio pages Year Founded: 1989

3708 Physicians Living with Depression

American Psychiatric Publishing
1000 Wilson Boulevard
Suite 1825
Arlington, VA 22209-3901   703-907-7322
                                  800-368-5777
                                  Fax: 703-907-1091
                                  E-mail: appi@psych.org
                                  www.appi.org

Michael F Myers MD, Producer
Katie Duffy, Marketing Assistant

Designed to help doctors see the signs of depression in their fellow physicians and to alert psychiatrists to the severity of the illness in their physician patients, the tape contains two fifteen-minute interviews, one with an emergency physician and one with a pediatrician. *$25.00*

ISBN 0-890422-78-8

3709 Solutions Step by Step - Substance Abuse
Treatment Videotape

WW Norton & Company
500 5th Avenue
New York, NY 10110   212-790-9456
                                  Fax: 212-869-0856
                                  E-mail: admalmud@wwnorton.com
                                  www.wwnorton.com

Quick tips, questions and examples focusing on successes that can be experienced helping substance abusers help themselves. *$ 100.00*

Year Founded: 1997 ISSN 70260-X

3710 Testing Automatic Thoughts with
Thought Records

New Harbinger Publications
5674 Shattuck Avenue
Oakland, CA 94609-1662   510-652-2002
                                  800-748-6273
                                  Fax: 510-652-5472
                                  E-mail: customerservice@newharbinger.com
                                  www.newharbinger.com

Videotape that helps a client explore the hot thoughts that contribute to depression. *$49.95*

3711 Treating Trauma Disorders Effectively

200 E Joppa Road
Suite 207
Baltimore, MD 21286   410-825-8888
                                  888-825-8249
                                  Fax: 410-337-0747
                                  E-mail: sidran@sidran.org
                                  www.sidran.org

This video illustrates two fundamental treatment principles: attachment to the perpetrator and locus of control shift. For clinicians, the program provides immediatley usable techniques for their practices; for the layperson it provides a clear explanation for two consequences of childhood trauma. *$85.00*

Web Sites

Includes information about the Association's history and objectives, contact and member information, upcoming events, and publications of interest.

3712 www.TheAtlantic.com/politics/family/divorce

Divorce and the Family in America

Historical perspective on the family and divorce.

3713 www.aacap.org

American Academy of Child and Adolescent Psychiatry

Represents over 6,000 child and adolescent psychiatrists, brochures availible online which provide concise and up-to-date material on issues ranging from children who suffer from depression and teen suicide to stepfamily problems and child sexual abuse.

3714 www.aan.com

American Academy of Neurology

Provides information for both professionals and the public on neurology subjects, covering Alzheimer's and Parkinson's diseases to stroke and migraine, includes comprehensive fact sheets.

3715 www.aapb.org

Association for Applied Psychophysiology and Biofeedback

Represents clinicians interested in psychopsysiology or biofeedback, offers links to their mission statement, membership information, research, FAQ about biofeedback, conference listings, and links.

3716 www.abecsw.org/

American Board of Examiners in Clinical Social Work

Information about the American Board of Examiners, credentialing, and ethics.

3717 www.about.com

About.Com

Network of comprehensive Web sites for over 600 mental health topics.

3718 www.abpsi.org/

American Association of Black Psychologists

3719 www.ama-assn.org

American Medical Association

Offers a wide range of medical information and links, full-text abstracts of each journal's current and past articles.

3720 www.americasdoctor.com

AmericasDoctor.com

3721 www.apa.org/

American Psychological Association

Information about journals, press releases, professional and consumer information related to the psychological profession; resources include ethical principles and guidelines, science advocacy, awards and funding programs, testing and assessment information, other on-line and real world resources.

3722 www.apa.org/ethics/ethics.html

American Psychological Association-Ethics Division

APA Ethics Committee Rules and Procedures, ethical principles converted into Web-based format.

3723 www.apa.org/journels/anton.html

Psychotherapy versus Medication for Depression

Article reviews range of studies comparing psychological with pharmacological treatments.

3724 www.apna.org

American Psychiatric Nurses Association

Includes membership information, contact information, organizational information, announcements and related links.

3725 www.appi.org

American Psychiatric Association

Informational site about mental disorders, 'Lets Talk Facts' brochure series.

3726 www.apsa.org/

American Psychoanalytic Asssociation

Includes searchable bibliographic database containing books, reviews and articles of a psychoanalytical orientation, links and member information.

3727 www.assc.caltech.edu/

Association for the Scientific Study of Consciousness

Electronic journal dedicated to interdisciplinary exploration on the nature of consciousness and its relationship to the brain, congnitive science, philosophy, psychology, physics, neuroscience, and artificial intelligence.

3728 www.bewell.com

HealthGate MEDLINE Data Corporation

Offers patient and consumer information, both advanced and simple searches in MEDLINE database. Webpage includes Health Resources, Search Tools, Active Press, In the Know Health Tips, What's New, Information for Health Living, All of Today's Headlines, Healthy Webzines, Wellness Center, Drugs and Vitamins, Symptoms and Medical Tests, Health News, and About Healthcare.

3729 www.blarg.net/~charlatn/voices/voices.html

Compilation of Writings by People Suffering from Depression

3730 www.bpso.org

BPSO-Bipolar Significant Others

3731 www.bpso.org.ourfavs.htm

Construction of Your Own Life Chart: The NIMH Life Chart Method

How to collect data and improve diagnostic accuracy.

3732 www.bpso.org/nomania.htm

How to Avoid a Manic Episode

3733 www.cape.org/

Cape Cod Institute

Offers symposia every summer for keeping mental health professionals up-to-date on the latest developments in psychology, treatment, psychiatry, and mental health, outlines available workshops, links and other relevant information.

3734 www.chadd.org

CHADD

Peg Nichols, Director Communications

National non-profit organization representing children and adults with attention deficit/hyperactivity disorder (AD/HD).

3735 www.chandra.astro.indiana.edu/bipolar/physical.html

Primer on Depression and Bipolar Disorder

Useful for those struggling with committing to treatment.

3736 www.closetoyou.org/eatingdisorders/disthink. htm

15 Styles of Distorted Thinking

Reference useful for cognitive therapy.

3737 www.cnn.com/Health

CNN Health Section

Updated with health and mental health-related stories three to four times weekly.

3738 www.compuserve.com

IQuest/Knowledge Index

On-line research and database information provider.

3739 www.couns.uiuc.edu/depression.htm

Understanding and Treating Depression

Complete overview.

3740 www.counseling.com

American Counseling Association

Hosts information about the American Counseling Association, membership, legislative and news updates, a conference and workshop calendar, and links to related resources and publications.

3741 www.counselingforloss.com

Counseling for Loss and Life Changes

Look under articles for reprints of writings and links.

3742 www.cyberpsych.org

CyberPsych

Hosts the American Psychoanalyists Foundation, American Association of Suicideology, Society for the Exploration of Psychotherapy Intergration, and Anxiety Disorders Association of America. Also subcategories of the anxiety disorders, as well as general information, including panic disorder, phobias, obsessive compulsive disorder (OCD), social phobia, generalized anxiety disorder, post traumatic stress disorder, and phobias of childhood. Book reviews and links to web pages sharing the topics.

3743 www.depression.com/health_library/treatments /cognitive.html

Cognitive Therapy

A complete introduction.

3744 www.disabilitynews.net

Psych-Media

A collaboration of an internationally renowned group of physicians and human service professionals in the field of mental retardation and mental health; custom taylored for multiple target audiences, including human services professionals and providers, families of people with disabilities, educators and students and people with disabilities.

3745 www.ericae.net

ERIC Clearinghouse on Assessment and Evaluation

National information system designed to provide users an extensive body of education-related literature, supported by the US Department of Education, Office of Educational Research and Improvement, and the National Library of Education. Provides direct on-line, free access to the ERIC database, allows users to locate citations and reviews of educational and psychological tests and measurements.

3746 www.factsforhealth.org

Madison Institute of Medicine

Resource to help identify, understand and treat a number of medical conditions, including social anxiety disorder and posttraumatic stress disorder.

747 www.fathermag.com

Fathering Magazine

Hundreds of articles online.

748 www.gamma.rug.nl/sibhome.html

Software Information Bank

Software information bank contains information on computer applications for the social and behavioral sciences; submitting a program description and retrieving information are free of charge. Entries include functional descriptions, technical and data requirements, prices, availablility of manual and interface, literature references, and purchase addresses.

3749 www.gasou.edu/psychweb

Psych Web

Hosts a wide variety of professional and lay resources, and includes specific categories for psychology students, psychology-related information for students and teachers of psychology. Includes: methods of research, notable people, graduate study programs, publication resources, links to related sites, and the full text of William James' Varieties of Religious Experience.

3750 www.geocities.com/EnchantedForest/1068

Bipolar Kids Homepage

Set of links.

3751 www.geocities.com/HotSprings/3628/index.html

Have a Heart's Depression Home

Several fine essays and seven triggers for suicide.

3752 www.goaskalice.columbia.edu

GoAskAlice/Healthwise Columbia University

Oriented toward students, information on sexuality, sexual health, general health, alcohol and other drugs, fitness and nutrition, emotional wellbeing and relationships.

3753 www.grieftalk.com/help1.html

Grief Journey

Short readings for clients.

3754 www.habitsmart.com/cogtitle.html

Cognitive Therapy Pages

Offers accessible explanations.

3755 www.health-center.com/mentalhealth/schizophrenia/default.htm

Schizophrenia

Basic information for beginners.

3756 www.healthgate.com/

HealthGate

On-line reference and database information service, $.75/record.

3757 www.healthguide.com/english/brain.bipolar

Bipolar Disorder

Covers symptoms, diagnoses, and medications.

3758 www.healthtouch.com

Healthtouch Online

Healthtouch Online is a resource that brings together valuable information from trusted health organizations.

3759 www.healthy.net/

HealthWorld Online

Consumer-oriented articles on a wide range of health and mental health topics, including: Welcome Center, QuickN'Dex, Site Search, Free Medline, Health Conditions, Alternative Medicine, Referral Network, Health Columns, Global Calendar, Discussion, Cybrarian, Professional Center, Free Newsletter, Opportunities, Healthy Travel, Homepage, Library, University, Marketplace, Health Clinic, Wellness Center, Fitness Center, News Room, Association Network, Public Health, Self Care Central, and Nutrition Center.

3760 www.helix.com

Helix MEDLINE: Glaxo SmithKline

Helix is an Education, Learning and Information exchange. Developed especially for healthcare practitioners by Glaxo SmithKline, HELIX is a premire source of on-line education and professional resources on a range of therapeutic and practice-management issues.

3761 www.human-nature.com/odmh/index.html

On-line Dictonary of Mental Health

Global information resource and research tool. It is compiled by Internet mental health resource users for Internet mental health resource users, and covers all the disciplines contributing to our understanding of mental health.

3762 www.ianr.unl.edu/pubs/NebFacts/nf223.htm

Supporting Stepfamilies: What Do the Children Feel

Deals with emotions of children in blended families.

3763 www.infotrieve.com

Infotrieve Medline Services Provider

Infotrieve is a library services company offering full-service document delivery, databases on the web and a variety of tools to simplify the process of identifying, retrieving and paying for published literature.

3764 www.intelihealth.com

InteliHealth

3765 www.interport.net/nypsan

FreudNet Abraham A Brill Library, Psychoanalyitic Institute

Information about Sigmund Freud and psychoanalysis.

3766 www.irisphone.com

Iris Systems

Mental health related software.

3767 www.jumbo.com

Jumbo

100,000 shareware and freeware programs available from one location.

3768 www.klis.com/chandler/pamphlet/bipolar/bipolarpamphlet.html

Bipolar Affective Disorder in Children and Adolescents

An introduction for families.

3769 www.klis.com/chandler/pamphlet/dep/depressionpamphlet.htm

Depression in Children and Adolescents

3770 www.krinfo.com

DataStar/Dialog

Information provider: reference and databases.

3771 www.lemoyne.edu/academic_affairs/depa rtments /psychology/psychindex.html

LeMoyne College Psychology Department

Oriented toward professionals within the mental health field; teaching topics in psychology, clinical and abnormal psychology, behavioral science and neuropsychology.

3772 www.lollie.com/suicide.html

Comprehensive Approach to Suicide Prevention

Readings for anyone contemplating suicide.

3773 www.mayohealth.org/mayo

Mayo Clinic Health Oasis Library

Healthcare library and resources.

3774 www.med.jhu.edu.drada/ref/goldstein.ht ml

Pharmacological Treatment of Mood Disorders

A review of medications.

3775 www.med.jhu.edu/drada/creativity.html

Creativity and Depression and Manic-Depression

3776 www.med.nyu.edu/Psych/index.html

NYU Department of Psychiatry

General mental health information, screening tests, reference desk, continuing educations in psychiatry program, interactive testing in psychiatry, augmentation of antidepressants, NYU Psychoanalytic Institute, Psychology Internship Program, Internet Mental Health Resources links.

3777 www.medinfosource.com

CME, Medical Information Source

Medical information and education, fully accredited for all medical specialties.

3778 www.medscape.com

Medscape

Oriented toward physicians and medical topics, but also carries information relevant to the field of psychology and mental health.

3779 www.medweb.emory.edu/MedWeb/

MedWeb Emory University Health Sciences Center Library

Hundreds of links for mental health, psychology, and pscyhiatry. Recognized nationally for clinical, educational and research programs, and its hospitals and professional schools are ranked among the top in the nation. Webpage includes General Information Links, Emory Healthcare, Schools and Research Centers, Libraries and Research Tools, Health Sciences Communications Office, Employment Opportunities, Frequently Requested Contact Information, and much more.

3780 www.members.aol.com/dswgriff/suicide.h tml

Now Is Not Forever: A Survival Guide

Print out a no-suicide contract, do problem solving, and other exercises.

3781 www.members.tripod.com/~suicidepreven tion/ index

Suicide Prevention Help

Coping with suicidal thoughts and friends.

3782 www.mentalhealth.com/book/p40-sc01.ht ml

Schizophrenia: A Handbook for Families

Mostly unique information.

3783 www.mentalhealth.com/book/p40-sc02.ht ml

Schizophrenia: Youth's Greatest Disabler

Comprehensive and realistic coverage of schizophrenia.

3784 www.mentalhealth.com/p20-grp.html

Manic-Depressive Illness

Click on Bipolar and then arrow down to Booklets.

3785 www.mentalhealth.com/story/p52-dps2.ht ml

How to Help a Person with Depression

Valuable family education.

3786 www.metanoia.org/suicide/

If You Are Thinking about Suicide...Read This First

Excellent suggestions, information and links for the suicidal.

3787 www.mhnet.org/perspectives/

Perspectives: A Mental Health Magazine

Online journal for professionals and laypeople, features articles related to mental health.

3788 www.mhnet.org/pni/

PsychNews International

Newsletter dedicated to keeping readers up-to-date about psychology, psychiatry, and the social sciences online.

3789 www.mhsource.com

CME Mental Health InfoSource

Mental health information and education, fully accredited for all medical specialties.

3790 www.mhsource.com/

CME Psychiatric Time

Select articles published online from the Psychiatric Times, topics relevant to all mental health professionals.

3791 www.mhsource.com/narsad.schiz.html

Understanding Schizophrenia

Available in Spanish.

3792 www.mhsource.com/wb/thow9903.html

Steven Thos Mental Health Resources-Depression and Bipolar Disorder

About 40 questions asked by patients.

3793 www.mindfreedom.org

Support Coalition Human Rights & Psychiatry Home Page

Support Coalition is an independent alliance of several dozen grassroots groups in the USA, Canada, Europe, New Zealand; has used protests, publications, letter-writing, e-mail, workshops, Dendron News, the arts and performances. Led by psychiatric survivors, and open to the public, membership is open to anyone who supports its mission and goals.

3794 www.mindstreet.com/synopsis.html

Cognitive Therapy: A Multimedia Learning Program

The basics of cognitive therapy are presented.

3795 www.mindstreetcom/mindstreet/cbt.html

Basics of Cognitive Therapy

3796 www.mirror-mirror.org/eatdis.htm

Mirror, Mirror

Relapse prevention for eating disorders.

3797 www.moodswing.org/bdfaq.html

Bipolar Disorder Frequently Asked Questions

Excellent for those newly diagnosed.

3798 www.naphs.org

National Association of Psychiatric Health Systems

The NAPHS advocates for behavioral health and represents provider systems that are committed to the delivery of responsive, accountable and clinically effective prevention, treatment and care for children, adolescents and adults with mental and substance use disorders.

3799 www.naswdc.org/

National Associaton of Social Workers

Central resource for clinical social workers, includes information about the federation, a conference and workshop calender, information on how to subscribe to social worker mailing lists, legislative and news updates, links to state agencies and social work societies, and publications.

3800 www.ndmda.org/justmood.htm

Just a Mood...or Something Else

A brochure for teens.

3801 **www.nimh.nih.gov/about/about.htm**
National Institute of Mental Health (NIMH)

The mission of NIMH is to diminish the burden of mental illness through research of the biological, behavioral, clinical, epidemiological, economic, and social science aspects of mental illnesses.

3802 **www.nimh.nih.gov/publicat/depressionmenu.cfm**

Depression

National Institute of Mental Health offers brochures organized by topic.

3803 **www.nimh.nih.gov/publicat/schizoph.htm**

Schizophrenia

National Institute of Mental Health.

3804 **www.nlightn.com**

NlightN

Online reference and database information provider, $.50/record.

3805 **www.nmha.org**
National Mental Health Association

Dedicated to promoting mental health, preventing mental disorders and achieving victory over mental illness through advocacy, education, research and service. NMHA's collaboration with the National GAINS Center for People with Co-Occuring Disorders in the Justice System has produced the Justice for Juveniles Initiative. This program battles to reform the juvenile justice system so that the inmates mental needs are addressed. Envisions a just, humane and healthy society in which all people are accorded respect, dignity and the opportunity to achieve their full potential free from stigma and prejudice.

3806 **www.oclc.org/**

EPIC

On-line reference and database information provider, $40/hour (plus connection fees) and $.75/record.

3807 **www.odp.od.nih.gov/consensus/cons/110/**

110 Diagnosis/Treatment of Attention Deficit Hyperactivity Disorder

Scientific data on diagnosis, effective treatments, effects, risks of treatments.

3808 **www.onhealth.com**
On Health Network Company

3809 **www.oznet.ksu.edu/library/famlf2/**
Family Life Library

3810 **www.pace-custody.org**
Professional Academy of Custody Evaluators

Nonprofit corporation and membership organization to acknowledge and strengthen the professionally prepared comprehensive custody evaluation; psychologicals legal knowledge base, assessment procedures, courtroom testimony, provides continuing education courses, conferences, conventions and seminars.

3811 **www.paperchase.com**
PaperChase

Searches may be conducted through a browsable list of topics, search engine recognizes queries made in natural language.

3812 **www.parenthoodweb.com/parent_cfmfiles/pros. cfm/155**
Blended Families

Resolving conflicts.

3813 **www.pendulum.org/alternatives/lisa_alternatives.htm**
Alternative Approaches to the Treatment of Manic-Depression

Introduction to uses of nutrients.

3814 **www.pendulum.org/articles/Worst_to_say.html**
99 Worst Things to Say to Someone Who is Depressed

3815 **www.pendulum.org/articles/best_to_say.html**
23 Best Things to Say to Someone Who is Depressed

3816 **www.planetpsych.com**
Planetpsych.com

Learn about disorders, their treatments and other topics in psychology. Articles are listed under the related topic areas. Ask a therapist a question for free, or view the directory of professionals in your area. If you are a therapist sign up for the directory. Current features, self-help, interactive, and newsletter archives.

3817 www.positive-way.com/step.htm

Stepfamily Information

Introduction and tips for stepfathers, stepmothers and remarried parents.

3818 www.princeton.edu/~harnad/psych.html

American Psychological Association

Unique psychology journal online.

3819 www.priory.com/sex.htm

Sexual Disorders

Diagnoses and treatments.

3820 www.psych.org

American Psychiatric Association

A medical specialty society recognized world-wide. Its 40,500 US and international physicians specializing in the diagnosis and treatment of mental and emotional illness and substance use disorders.

3821 www.psych.org/apa_members/ethics.html

American Psychiatric Association-Membership Ethics

Relavent information for professionals within the psychiatric field, includes the 'Principles of Medical Ethics.'

3822 www.psychcentral.com

Psych Central

Personalized one-stop index for psychology, support, and mental health issues, resources, and people on the Internet.

3823 www.psychcrawler.com

American Psychological Association

Indexing the web for the links in psychology.

3824 www.psychguides.com/bphe.html

Expert Consensus Treatment Guidelines for Bipolar Disorder

3825 www.psychology.com/therapy.htm

Therapist Directory

Therapists listed geographically plus answers to frequently asked questions.

3826 www.psycom.net/depression.central.html

Dr. Ivan's Depression Central

Medication-oriented site.

3827 www.psycom.net/depression.central.suicide. html

Suicide and Suicide Prevention

List of links to material on suicide.

3828 www.pwc.org

Physicians Who Care

Devoted to protecting the traditional doctor-patient relationship while ensuring quality health care, offers newsletters and complete information about Physicians Who Care and Patients Who Care.

3829 www.rebt.org

Information on rational emotive behavior therapy (REBT), includes a directory of REBT-trained therapists throughout the world, an FAQ file, a schedule of upcoming seminars and additional resources

3830 www.recovery-inc.com

Recovery

Describes the organizations approach.

3831 www.reutershealth.com

Reuters Health

Relevant and useful clinical information on mental disorders, news briefs updated daily.

3832 www.save.org

SA/VE - Suicide Awareness/Voices of Education

3833 www.schizophrenia.com

Schizophrenia.com

Offers basic and in-depth information, discussion and chat.

3834 www.schizophrenia.com/ami

Alliance for the Mentally Ill

Information on mental disorders, reducing the stigmatization of them in our society today, and how you can be more active in your local community. Includes articles, press information, media kits, mental disorder diagnostic and treatment information, coping issues, advocacy guides and announcements.

3835 www.schizophrenia.com/newsletter

Schizophrenia.com

Comprehensive psychoeducational site on schizophrenia.

3836 www.schizophrenia.com/newsletter/buckets/ success.html

Schizophrenia.com

Success stories including biographical accounts, links to stories of famous people who have schizophrenia, and personal web pages.

3837 www.shpm.com

Self-Help and Psychology Magazine

General psychology and self-help magazine online, offers informative articles on general well being and psychology topics. Features Author of the Month, Breaking News Stories of the Month, Most Popular Pages, What's Hot, Departments, and Soundoff (articles and opinion page). This online compendium of hundreds of readers and professionals.

3838 www.shpm.com/articles/depress/antidprs. html

Placebo Effect Accounts for Fifty Percent of Improvement

3839 www.shpm.com/articles/depress/negfeed.html

People with Depression Tend to Seek Negative Feedback

A brief handout.

3840 www.siop.org

Society for Industrial and Organizational Psychology

Home to the Industrial-Organizational Pyschologist newsletter, links and resources, member information, contact information for doctoral and master's level program in I/O psychology, and announcements of various events and conferences.

3841 www.snowcrest.net/skiing/stepmom.htm

Wicked Stepmothers, Fact or Fiction

Details the harm done by stereotyping stepmothers.

3842 www.something-fishy.com/cry.htm

Poetry from People Living with Depression

3843 www.spsp.clarion.edu/tposs/topss.html

American Psychological Association

For secondary school teachers interested in helping to promote the introduction of students in high school to psychology through curriculum suggestions, essay contests, and teacher workshops.

3844 www.stange.simplenet.com/psycsite

Department of Psychology, Nipissing University

Information about psychology related software available on the internet, links to shareware and commercial software.

3845 www.stepfamily.org/tensteps.htm

Ten Steps for Steps

Guidelines for stepfamilies.

3846 www.stepfamilyinfo.org/sitemap.htm

Stepfamily in Formation

3847 www.thriveonline.com

ThriveOnline

3848 www.twhj.com

Wounded Healer Journal

Online journal, published daily for therapists, healers and victims of abuse.

3849 www.uhs.bsd.uchicago.edu/~bhsiung/men tal

Dr. Bob's Mental Health Links

Includes hypertext links for professionals, but open to the public.

3850 www.usatoday.com/

USA Today

'Mental Health' category includes news and in-depth reports.

3851 www.users.interport.net/~mpullier/

Pulier's Personal Psychiatric and Behavioral Healthcare Resources

A link to a resource of over 2900 mental health organizations all over the world indexed by name and location. Professional organization to provide education and networking opportunities for administrators of psychiatric programs in academic settings, site offers organizational information and select articles from quarterly newsletter.

3852 www.uta.edu/cussn.html

Computer Use in Social Services Network (CUSSN)

Informal association of professionals interested in exchanging information and experiences on using computers in the human services. Provides users with descriptions of human service freeware, shareware, and demonstration programs; topics include clinical and theraputic, welfare and child protection, aging, deveopmental disabilities, education and training, management, accounting, billing and fund raising and data analysis.

3853 www.utexas.edu/student/cmhc/meds.html

Are You Considering Medication for Depression

3854 www.vcc.mit.edu/comm/samaritans/broch ure. html

How to Help Someone You Care About

Guidelines for family.

3855 www.vvc.mit.edu/comm/samaritans/warni ng. html

Signs of Suicide Risk

3856 www.webmd.com

WebMD

3857 www.wingofmadness.com

Wing of Madness: A Depression Guide

Accurate information, advice, support, and personal experiences.

3858 www.wynja.com/personality/theorists.ht ml

Personality and Consciousness

Site devoted to discussing the major theorists in personality psychology, including Alfred Adler, Sigmund Freud, Carl Jung, George Kelly, Abraham Maslow, Carl Rogers, BF Skinner and Charles T Tart, offers their respective theories and philosophies on psychotherapy.

3859 www.york.ac.uk/inst/ctipsych/dir/treat.ht ml

CTI Dirctory of Psychology Software

Works to support the use of communication and information technologies in UK higher education with academic sites of interest to students and teachers of psychology. Information about psychological software programs, divided into general psychology, practicals and methodology, mainstream courses, specialized courses, assessment and treatment, studying and teaching tools, and administration.

3860 www1.tpgi.com.au/users/revolve/ncprepo rt/ furstenberg

Parenting Apart: Patterns of Childrearing after Marital Disruption

National survey of family relations.

Workbooks & Manuals

3861 Activities for Adolescents in Therapy: Handbook of Facilitating Guidelines and Planning Ideas for Group Therapy With Troubled Adolescents

Charles C Thomas Publisher
2600 S 1st Street
Springfield, IL 62704-4730   217-789-8980
                                   800-258-8980
                              Fax: 217-789-9130
                    E-mail: books@ccthomas.com
                              www.ccthomas.com

In this practical resource manual, professionals will find more than 100 therapeutic group activities for use in counseling troubled adolescents. This new edition provides specifics on establishing an effective group program while, at the same time, outlining therapeutic activities that can be used in each phase of a therapy group. Has step-by-step instructions have been provided for setting up, planning and facilitating adolescent groups with social and emotional problems. The interventions provided have been designed specifically for initial, middle and termination phases of group. $39.95

264 pages Year Founded: 1998 ISBN 0-395068-07-0

3862 Activities for Children in Therapy: Guide for Planning and Facilitating Therapy with Troubled Children

Charles C Thomas Publisher
2600 S 1st Street
Springfield, IL 62704-4730   217-789-8980
                                        800-258-8980
                              Fax: 217-789-9130
              E-mail: books@ccthomas.com
                          www.ccthomas.com

Provides the mental health professional with a wide variety of age-appropriate activities which are simultaneously fun and therapeutic for the five-to-twelve-year-old troubled child. Activities have been designed as enjoyable games in the context of therapy. Provides a comprehensive listing of books with other therapeutic intervention ideas, bibliotherapy materials, assessment scales for evaluating youngsters, and a sample child assessment for individual therapy. For professionals who provide counseling to children, such as social workers, psychologists, guidance counselors, speech/language pathologists, and art therapists. *$45.95*

302 pages Year Founded: 1999 ISBN 0-398067-91-9

3863 Chemical Dependency Treatment Planning Handbook

Charles C Thomas Publisher
2600 S 1st Street
Springfield, IL 62704-4730   217-789-8980
                                        800-258-8980
                              Fax: 217-789-9130
              E-mail: books@ccthomas.com
                          www.ccthomas.com

Provides the entry-level clinician with a broad data base of treatment planning illustrations from which unpretentious treatment plans for the chemically dependent client can be generated. They are simple, largely measurable, and purposefully, with language that is cognizant of comprehension and learning needs of clients. It will be of interest to drug and alcohol counselors. *$29.95*

174 pages Year Founded: 1997 ISBN 0-398067-76-7

3864 Clinical Manual of Supportive Psychotherapy

American Psychiatric Publishing
1000 Wilson Boulevard
Suite 1825
Arlington, VA 22209-3901   703-907-7322
                                        800-368-5777
                              Fax: 703-907-1091
                 E-mail: appi@psych.org
                             www.appi.org

Katie Duffy, Marketing Assistant

New approaches and ideas for your practice. *$64.00*

362 pages Year Founded: 1993

3865 Clinician's Manual for the Cognitive - Behavioral Treatment of Post Traumatic Stress Disorder

New Harbinger Publications
5674 Shattuck Avenue
Oakland, CA 94609-1662   510-652-2002
                                        800-748-6273
                              Fax: 510-652-5472
    E-mail: customerservice@newharbinger.com
                        www.newharbinger.com

$20.00

150 pages Year Founded: 1994 ISBN 1-889287-00-8

3866 Comprehensive Directory: Programs and Services for Children with Disabilities and Their Families in The Metro New York Area

Resources for Children with Special Needs
116 E 16th Street
Fifth Floor
New York, NY 10003   212-677-4550
                              Fax: 212-254-4070
           E-mail: info@resourcesnyc.org
                        www.resourcesnyc.org

This directory includes up-to-date information about agencies, schools, after-school social, recreational and cultural programs, camps and summer pgrams, family support and respite services, plus legal, advocacy, medical, evaluation, diagnostic, therapeutic services- and much more. This directory lists services taht cover your child's needs at every age, from early intervention through vocational and job-training programs. Everything you need to know to provide support and assistance to children. *$55.00*

ISBN 0-967836-51-4

3867 Concise Guide to Laboratory and Diagnostic Testing in Psychiatry

American Psychiatric Publishing
1000 Wilson Boulevard
Suite 1825
Arlington, VA 22209-3901   703-907-7322
                                        800-368-5777
                              Fax: 703-907-1091
                 E-mail: appi@psych.org
                             www.appi.org

Katie Duffy, Marketing Assistant

Basic strategies for applying laboratory testing and evaluation. *$19.50*

176 pages Year Founded: 1989 ISBN 0-880483-33-4

3868 Conducting Training Workshops

Jossey-Bass Publishers
350 Sansome Street
5th Floor
San Francisco, CA 94104　　　**415-394-8677**
　　　800-956-7739
Fax: 800-605-2665
www.josseybass.com

This easy-to-follow guide makes for effortless planning and delivery.

3869 Creating and Implementing Your Strategic Plan: Workbook for Public and Nonprofit Organizations

Jossey-Bass and CentraLink Publications
1110 Mar Street
Suite E
Tiburon, CA 94920　　　**415-435-9821**
Fax: 415-435-9092
www.centralink.com

Step-by-step workbook to conducting strategic planning in public and nonprofit organizations. *$24.95*

139 pages Year Founded: 1995 ISBN 0-787901-42-3

3870 Handbook for the Study of Mental Health

Cambridge University Press
40 W 20th Street
New York, NY 10011-4221　　　**212-924-3900**
Fax: 212-691-3239
E-mail: marketing@cup.org
www.cup.org

Offers the first comprehensive presentation of the sociology of mental health illness, including original, contemporary contributions by experts in the relevant aspects of the field. Divided into three sections, the chapters cover the general perspectives in the field, the social determinants of mental health and current policy areas affecting mental health services. Designed for classroom use in sociology, social work, human relations, human services and psychology. With its useful definitions, overview of the histroical, social and institutional frameworks for understanding mental health and illness, and nontechnical style, the text is suitable for advanced undergraduate or lower level graduate students. *$90.00*

694 pages Year Founded: 1999 ISBN 0-521561-33-7

3871 Handbook of Clinical Psychopharmacology for Therapists

New Harbinger Publications
5674 Shattuck Avenue
Oakland, CA 94609-1662　　　**510-652-2002**
　　　800-748-6273
Fax: 510-652-5472
E-mail: customerservice@newharbinger.com
www.newharbinger.com

This newly revised classic includes updates on new medications, and expanded quick reference section, and new material on bipolar illness, the treatment of psychosis, and the effect of severe trauma. *$49.95*

264 pages Year Founded: 1999 ISBN 1-572240-94-6

3872 Handbook of Constructive Therapies

Jossey-Bass Publishers
350 Sansome Street
5th Floor
San Francisco, CA 94104　　　**415-394-8677**
　　　800-956-7739
Fax: 800-605-2665
www.josseybass.com

Learn techniques that focus on the strengths and resources of your clients and look to where they want to go rather than where they have been. *$49.95*

500 pages ISBN 0-787940-44-5

3873 Handbook of Counseling Psychology

John Wiley & Sons
605 3rd Avenue
New York, NY 10058-0180　　　**212-850-6000**
Fax: 212-850-6008
E-mail: info@wiley.com
www.wiley.com

880 pages Year Founded: 1992

3874 Handbook of Managed Behavioral Healthcare

Jossey-Bass Publishers
350 Sansome Street
5th Floor
San Francisco, CA 94104　　　**415-394-8677**
　　　800-956-7739
Fax: 800-605-2665
www.josseybass.com

A comprehensive curriculum to understanding managed care. *$32.95*

240 pages ISBN 0-787941-53-0

3875 Handbook of Medical Psychiatry

Mosby
11830 Westline Industrial Drive
Saint Louis, MO 63146　　　**314-872-8370**
　　　800-325-4177
Fax: 314-432-1380

This large-format handbook covers almost every psychiatric, neurologic and general medical condition capable of causing disturbances in thought, feeling, or behavior and includes almost every psychopharmacologic agent available in America today. *$49.95*

545 pages Year Founded: 1996 ISBN 0-815164-84-X

3876 Handbook of Mental Retardation and Development

Cambridge University Press
40 W 20th Street
New York, NY 10011-4221   **212-924-3900**
                              Fax: 212-691-3239
                    E-mail: marketing@cup.org
                              www.cup.org

This book reviews theoretical and empirical work in the developmental approach to mental retardation. Armed with methods derived from the study of typically developing children, developmentalists have recently learned about the mentally retarded child's own development in a variety of areas. These now encompass many aspects of cognition, language, social and adaptive functioning, as well as of maladaptive behavior and psychopathology. In addition to a focus on individuals with mental retardation themselves, other ecological factors have influenced developmental approaches to mental retardation. Comprised of twenty seven chapters on various aspects of development, this handbook provides a comprehensive guide to understanding mental retardation. *$80.00*

764 pages Year Founded: 1998

3877 Handbook of Psychiatric Education and Faculty Development

American Psychiatric Publishing
1000 Wilson Boulevard
Suite 1825
Arlington, VA 22209-3901   **703-907-7322**
                              800-368-5777
                    Fax: 703-907-1091
                    E-mail: appi@psych.org
                              www.appi.org

Katie Duffy, Marketing Assistant

Putting education to work in the real world. *$68.50*

496 pages Year Founded: 1999 ISBN 0-880487-80-1

3878 Handbook of Psychiatric Practice in the Juvenile Court

American Psychiatric Publishing
1000 Wilson Boulevard
Suite 1825
Arlington, VA 22209-3901   **703-907-7322**
                              800-368-5777
                    Fax: 703-907-1091
                    E-mail: appi@psych.org
                              www.appi.org

Katie Duffy, Marketing Assistant

How your practice can work with the court system, so your patients can get the help they need. *$27.95*

198 pages Year Founded: 1992 ISBN 0-890422-33-8

3879 Handbook of Solution Focused Brief Therapy

Jossey-Bass Publishers
350 Sansome Street
5th Floor
San Francisco, CA 94104   **415-394-8677**
                              800-956-7739
                    Fax: 800-605-2665
                    www.josseybass.com

Develop the skills necessary to deliver effective solution focused therapy across a variety of treatment settings. *$42.95*

384 pages ISBN 0-787902-17-9

3880 Healthy People 2010 Toolkit: Field Guide to Healthy Planning

Public Health Foundation
PO Box 753
Waldorf, MD 20604   **301-645-7773**
                              877-252-1200
                    Fax: 301-843-0159
                    E-mail: info@phf.org
                    www.bookstore.phf.org

Stacy Baker, Senior Project Manager
Dianna Conrad, Analyst

Contains practical guidance, technical tools, and resources for states, territories, tribes, and others involved in health planning. State examples and ideas in the toolkit can help professionals effectively integrate mental health objectives into state and local Healthy People initiatives. The guide includes checklists and tips to get started, engage partners, identify resources, set objectives, market plans, manage and sustain efforts, and measure progress. *$39.00*

Year Founded: 1999

3881 Living Skills Recovery Workbook

Elsevier Science
11830 Westline Industrial Drive
St. Louis, MO 63146   **314-453-7010**
                              800-545-2522
                    Fax: 314-453-7095
                    E-mail: orders@bhusa.com or
                    custserv@bhusa.com
                    www.bh.com

Katie Hennessy, Medical Promotions Coordinator

Provides clinicians with the tools necessary to help patients with dual diagnoses acquire basic living skills. Focusing on stress management, time management, activities of daily living, and social skills training, each living skill is taught in relation to how it aids in recovery and relapse prevention for each patient's individual lifestyle and pattern of addiction.

224 pages ISBN 0-750671-18-1

3882 Managing Diversity in Health Care Manual

Jossey-Bass Publishers
350 Sansome Street
5th Floor
San Francisco, CA 94104　　　　415-394-8677
800-956-7739
Fax: 800-605-2665
www.josseybass.com

Provides the hands-on resources to turn strategy into immediate action. Focused specifically to meet the needs of trainers, managers, and in-service or consulting educators, these ready-to-use tools are ideal for creating customized training agendas. *$99.95*

160 pages ISBN 0-787943-93-2

3883 Managing Outcomes

Manisses Communications Group
208 Governor Street
PO Box 9758
Providence, RI 02940-9758　　　　401-831-6020
800-333-7771
Fax: 401-861-6370
E-mail: Manissescs@manisses.com
www.manisses.com

$149.00

ISBN 8-84937-66-7

3884 Medical Aspects of Chemical Dependency Active Parenting Publishers

Hazelden
15251 Pleasant Valley Road
PO Box 176
Center City, MN 55012-0176　　　　651-213-2121
800-328-9000
Fax: 651-213-4590
www.hazelden.org

This interactive curriculum helps professionals educate clients in treatment and other settings about medical effects of chemical use and abuse. The program includes a video that explains body and brain changes that can occur when using alcohol or other drugs, a workbook that helps clients apply the information from the video to their own situations, a handbook that provides in-depth information on addiction, brain chemistry and the physiological effects of chemical dependency and a pamphlet that answers critical questions clients have about the medical effects of chemical dependency. Total price of $244.70, available to purchase separately. Program value packages available for $395.00, with 25 workbooks, two handbooks, two video and 25 pamphlets.

3885 On the Client's Path: a Manual for the Practice of Brief Solution - Focused Therapy

New Harbinger Publications
5674 Shattuck Avenue
Oakland, CA 94609-1662　　　　510-652-2002
800-748-6273
Fax: 510-652-5472
E-mail: customerservice@newharbinger.com
www.newharbinger.com

Provides everything you need to master the solution - focused model. *$49.95*

157 pages Year Founded: 1995 ISBN 1-572240-21-0

3886 PACT Manual

National Alliance for the Mentally Ill
200 N Glebe Road
Suite 1015
Arlington, VA 22203-3728　　　　703-524-7600
800-950-6264
Fax: 703-524-9094
TDD: 703-516-7227
www.nami.org

A comprehensive, how to manual that spells out in detail how to effectively start up and operate a successful PACT team. *$10.00*

Year Founded: 1998

3887 Relaxation & Stress Reduction Workbook

New Harbinger Publications
5674 Shattuck Avenue
Oakland, CA 94609-1662　　　　510-652-2002
800-748-6273
Fax: 510-652-5472
E-mail: customerservice@newharbinger.com
www.newharbinger.com

Matthew McKay, Editor

Details effective stress reduction methods such as breathing exercises, meditation, visualization, and time management. Widely recomended by therapists, nurses, and physicians throughout the US, this fourth edition has been substantially revised and updated to reflect current research. Line drawings and charts. *$14.36*

276 pages Year Founded: 1998 ISBN 1-879237-82-2

3888 Skills Training Manual for Treating Borderline Personality Disorder, Companion Workbook

Guilford Publications
72 Spring Street
New York, NY 10012　　　　212-431-9800
800-365-7006
Fax: 212-966-6708
E-mail: info@guilford.com
www.guilford.com

A vital component in Dr. Linehan's comprehensive treatment program, this step-by-step manual details precisely how to implement the skills training procedures and includes practical pointers on when to use the other treatment strategies described. It includes useful, clear-cut handouts that may be readily photocopied. *$27.95*

180 pages Year Founded: 1993 ISBN 0-898620-34-1

3889 Step Workbook for Adolescent Chemical Dependency Recovery

American Psychiatric Publishing
1000 Wilson Boulevard
Suite 1825
Arlington, VA 22209-3901   703-907-7322
                                          800-368-5777
                              Fax: 703-907-1091
                        E-mail: appi@psych.org
                                     www.appi.org

Katie Duffy, Marketing Assistant

Strategies for younger patients in your practice. $ 62.00

72 pages Year Founded: 1990 ISBN 0-882103-00-9

3890 Stress Management Training: Group Leader's Guide

Professional Resource Press
PO Box 15560
Sarasota, FL 34277-1560   941-343-9601
                                          800-443-3364
                              Fax: 941-343-9201
                      E-mail: orders@prpress.com
                                     www.prpress.com

Debra Fink, Managing Editor

This practical guide will help you define the concept of stress for group members and teach them various intervention techniques ranging from relaxation training to communication skills. Includes specific exercises, visual aids, stress response index, stress analysis form and surveys for evaluating program effectiveness. *$13.95*

96 pages Year Founded: 1990 ISBN 0-943158-33-8

3891 Stress Owner's Manual: Meaning, Balance and Health in Your Life

Impact Publishers
PO Box 6016
Atascadero, CA 93423-6016   805-466-5917
                                          800-246-7228
                              Fax: 805-466-5919
                E-mail: info@impactpublishers.com
                              www.impactpublishers.com

Offers specific solutions: maps, checklists and rating scales to help you assess your life; dozens of stress buffer activities to help you deal with stress on the spot; life-changing strategies to prepare you for a lifetime of effective stress management. *$15.95*

208 pages Year Founded: 1996 ISBN 0-915166-84-4

3892 Therapist's Workbook

Jossey-Bass Publishers
350 Sansome Street
5th Floor
San Francisco, CA 94104   415-394-8677
                                          800-956-7739
                              Fax: 800-605-2665
                              www.josseybass.com

This workbook nourishes and challenges counselors, guiding them on a journey of self-reflection and renewal. *$19.95*

192 pages ISBN 0-787945-23-4

3893 Treating Alcohol Dependence: a Coping Skills Training Guide

Guilford Publications
72 Spring Street
New York, NY 10012   212-431-9800
                                          800-365-7006
                              Fax: 212-966-6708
                        E-mail: info@guilford.com
                                     www.guilford.com

Treatment program based on a cognitive-social learning theory of alcohol abuse. Presents a straight-forward treatment strategy that copes with how to stop drinking and provides the training skills to make it possible. *$21.95*

240 pages Year Founded: 1989 ISBN 0-898622-15-8

Directories & Databases

3894 AAHP/Dorland Directory of Health Plans

Dorland Healthcare Information
1500 Walnut Street
Suite 1000
Philadelphia, PA 19102   215-875-1212
                                          800-784-2332
                              Fax: 215-735-3966
                E-mail: info@dorlandhealth.com
                              www.dorlandhealth.com

Paperback, published yearly. *$215.00*

3895 Alcoholism Information & Treatment Directory

American Business Directories
5711 S 86th Circle
PO Box 27347
Omaha, NE 68127-0347   402-593-4600
                                          800-555-6124
                              Fax: 402-331-5481
                        E-mail: directory@abii.com
                                     www.abii.com

1 per year

3896 American Academy of Child and Adolescent Psychiatry - Membership Directory

3615 Wisconsin Avenue NW
Washington, DC 20016-3007   202-966-7300
                                          800-333-7636
                              Fax: 202-966-2891
                E-mail: membership@aacap.org
                                     www.aacap.org

Laurie Thomas, Membership Coordinator

$30.00

179 pages 2 per year

3897 American Academy of Psychoanalysis-Membership Roster

American Academy of Psychoanalysis and Dynamic
Psychiatry
One Regency Drive
PO Box 30
Bloomfield, CT 06002

888-691-8281
Fax: 860-286-0787
E-mail: info@aapsa.org
www.aapsa.org

Jacquelyn T Coleman CAE, Executive Director

The journal of the American Academy of Psychoanalysis. Publishes articles by members and other authors who have a significant contribution to make to the community of scholars or practitioners interested in a psychodynamic understanding of human behavior. *$50.00*

70 pages

3898 American Drug Index

Facts and Comparisons
111 Westport Plaza
Suite 300
Saint Louis, MO 63146-3014

314-878-2515
800-223-0554
Fax: 314-878-1574
www.drugfacts.com

Laura Hartel, Marketing Manager

Most exhaustive list of 22,000 drugs and drug products; includes trade and generic drug names, phonetic pronunciations, indications, manufacturers and schedule information.

ISBN 1-574391-08-9

3899 American Network of Community Options and Resources-Directory of Members

ANCOR
1101 King Street
Suite 380
Alexandria, VA 22314

703-535-7850
Fax: 703-535-7860
E-mail: ancor@ancor.org
www.ancor.org

Covers 650 agencies serving people with mental retardation and other developmental disabilities. *$25.00*

179 pages 1 per year

3900 American Psychiatric Association-Membership Directory

Harris Publishing
2500 Westchester Avenue
Suite 400
Purchase, NY 10577

800-326-6600
Fax: 914-641-3501
www.bcharrispub.com

$59.95

816 pages

3901 American Psychoanalytic Association - Roster

American Psychological Association
750 1st Street NE
Washington, DC 20002-4241

202-336-5500
800-374-2721
Fax: 202-336-5568
E-mail: webmaster@apa.org
www.apa.org

$40.00

194 pages

3902 American Society of Psychoanalytic Physicians: Membership Directory

13528 Wisteria Drive
Germantown, MD 20853

301-540-3197
Fax: 301-540-3511
E-mail: cfcotter@yahoo.com
www.aspp.net

Martin Funk MD, President
Christine Cotter, Executive Secretary

Directory of member psychoanalysts and psychoanalytically oriented phychiatrists and physicians and others interested in the field.

15 pages 1 per year

3903 Association for Advancement of Behavior Therapy: Membership Directory

305 Seventh Avenue
16th Floor
New York, NY 10001-6008

212-647-1890
Fax: 212-647-1890
E-mail: mebrown@aabt.org
www.aabt.org

Mary Jane Eimer, Executive Director
Mary Ellen Brown, Administration/Convention
Rosemary Park, Membership Services

Covers over 4,500 psychologists, psychiatrists, social workers and other interested in behavior therapy. *$50.00*

240 pages 2 per year

3904 At Health Incorporated

1370 116th Avenue NE, Suite 206
Eastview Professional Building
Bellevue, WA 98004-3825

425-451-4399
888-284-3258
Fax: 425-451-7399
E-mail: support@athealth.com
www.athealth.com

John E Cebhart III, CEO
John L Miller MD, CMIO

Mental health information, directory of mental health practitioners and treatment facilities, and online continuing education for mental health professionals and other healthcare providers.

3905 Behavioral Measurement Database Services

PO Box 110287
Pittsburgh, PA 15232-0787   412-687-6850
Fax: 412-687-5213
E-mail: bmds@aol.com

Service health and psychosocial instruments, a database of over 75,000 records on measurement instruments enriching the health and psychosocial sciences. Records include questionnaires, interview schedules, vignettes/scenarios, coding schemes, rathing and other scales, checklists, indexes, and tests in medicine, nursing, public health, psychology, social work, sociology, and communicaiton. Also provides copies of selected instruments cited in the HAPI database through its instrument delivery service. Contact Ovid Technologies 1-800-950-2035

3906 Behavioral Outcomes & Guidelines Sourcebook

Faulkner & Gray
11 Penn Plaza
New York, NY 10001   212-967-7000
800-535-8403
Fax: 212-967-7180
E-mail: order@faulknergray.com
www.faulknergray.com

Sourcebook profiles engineering outcomes measurement and guideline development initiatives and provides in-depth articles on how to implement an outcomes or guidelines project. Includes a detailed guide to one hundred thirty leading outcomes measurement instruments and a comprehensive directory of behavioral practice guidelines. Special focus on client-centered outcomes. A must for any agency embarking on an outcomes or guidelines project. $325.00

769 pages Year Founded: 1999

3907 CARF Directory of Organizations with Accredited Programs

Rehabilitation Accreditation Commission
4891 E Grant Road
Tucson, AZ 85712   520-325-1044
Fax: 520-318-1129
TTY: 888-281-6531
www.carf.org

Joanne Finegan, Chair
Kari Kjersti, Document Production

Covers about three thousand organizations in seven thousand locations offering more than eighteen hundred medical rehabilitation, behavioral health, and employment and community support services that have been accredited by CARF. *$100.00*

200 pages 1 per year Year Founded: 1999

3908 Case Management Resource Guide

Dorland Healthcare Information
1500 Walnut Street
Suite 1000
Philadelphia, PA 19102   215-875-1212
800-784-2332
Fax: 215-735-3966
E-mail: info@dorlandhealth.com
www.dorlandhealth.com

Extensive directory of healthcare services used by case managers, discharge planners, managed care contracting staff, sales and marketing professionsal, search firms and information and referral agencies. $175 for four-volume set or $49 for each regional edition.

1 per year

3909 Case Management Resource Guide (Health Care)

Dorland Healthcare Information
1500 Walnut Street
Suite 1000
Philadelphia, PA 19102   215-875-1212
800-784-2332
Fax: 215-735-3966
E-mail: info@dorlandhealth.com
www.dorlandhealth.com

In four volumes, over 110,000 health care facilities and support services are listed, including homecare, rehabilitation, psychiatric and addiction treatment programs, hospices, adult day care and burn and cancer centers.

5,200 pages 1 per year ISBN 1-880874-84-9

3910 Case Manager Database

Dorland Healthcare Information
1500 Walnut Street
Suite 1000
Philadelphia, PA 19102   215-875-1212
800-784-2332
Fax: 215-735-3966
E-mail: info@dorlandhealth.com
www.dorlandhealth.com

Largest database of information on case managers in US, especially of case managers who work for health plans and health insurers. Covers over 15,000 case managers and includes detailed data such as work setting and clinical specialty, which can be used to carefully target marketing communications. $2500 for full database, other prices available.

3911 ClinPSYC

American Psychological Association Database Department/PsycINFO
750 1st Street NE
Washington, DC 20002-4242   202-336-5650
800-374-2722
Fax: 202-336-5633
TDD: 202-336-6123
E-mail: psycinfo@apa.org
www.apa.org/psycinfo

ClinPSYC is a database that contains citations and summaries of the international journal literature in clinical pschology and behavioral medicine, including neuropsychology, psychopharmacology, psychological disorders, psychological aspects of physical disorders, treatment, prevention, assessment, diagnosis and professional issues for mental health and health personnel. Coverage spans the most recent ten years and includes material selected from 1,800 periodicals written in over 30 languages. Approximately 30,000 references are added annually through quarterly updates.

4 per year

Professional/Directories & Databases

3912 Community Mental Health Directory

Department of Community Health
320 S Walnut
Suite 6
Lansing, MI 48913-0001   517-373-3740
                                Fax: 517-335-3090
                                www.mdch.state.mi.us

Covers about 51 public community mental health services and programs in Michigan.

20 pages 2 per year

3913 Complete Directory for People with Disabilities

Grey House Publishing
185 Millerton Road
PO Box 860
Millerton, NY 12546   518-789-8700
                             800-562-2139
                        Fax: 518-789-0545
                 E-mail: books@greyhouse.com
                        www.www.greyhouse.com

Leslie Mackenzie, Publisher
Laura Mars-Proietti, Editor

This one-stop resource provides immediate access to the latest products and services available for people with disabilities, such as Periodicals & Books, Assistive Devices, Employment & Education Programs, Camps and Travel Groups. *$165.00*

1200 pages ISBN 1-592370-07-1

3914 Complete Learning Disabilities Directory

Grey House Publishing
185 Millerton Road
PO Box 860
Millerton, NY 12546   518-789-8700
                             800-562-2139
                        Fax: 518-789-0545
                 E-mail: books@greyhouse.com
                        www.www.greyhouse.com

Leslie Mackenzie, Publisher
Laura Mars-Proietti, Editor

Includes information about Associations & Organizations, Schools, Colleges & Testing Materials, Government Agencies, Legal Resources and much more. *$195.00*

745 pages ISBN 1-930956-79-7

3915 Complete Mental Health Directory

Grey House Publishing
185 Millerton Road
PO Box 860
Millerton, NY 12546   518-789-8700
                             800-562-2139
                        Fax: 518-789-0545
                 E-mail: books@greyhouse.com
                        www.www.greyhouse.com

Leslie Mackenzie, Publisher
Laura Mars-Proietti, Editor

This directory offers understandable descriptions of 25 Mental Health Disorders as well as detailed information on Associations, Media, Support Groups and Mental Health Facilities. *$165.00*

800 pages ISBN 1-592370-46-2

3916 DSM-IV Psychotic Disorders: New Diagnostic Issue

American Psychiatric Publishing
1000 Wilson Boulevard
Suite 1825
Arlington, VA 22209-3901   703-907-7322
                                  800-368-5777
                             Fax: 703-907-1091
                      E-mail: appi@psych.org
                                  www.appi.org

Nancy Andreasen, Moderator
Katie Duffy, Marketing Assistant

Updates on clinical findings. *$39.95*

Year Founded: 1995

3917 Detwiler's Directory of Health and Medical Resources

Dorland Healthcare Information
1500 Walnut Street
Suite 1000
Philadelphia, PA 19102   215-875-1212
                                800-784-2332
                           Fax: 215-735-3966
                E-mail: info@dorlandhealth.com
                        www.dorlandhealth.com

An invaluable guide to healthcare information sources. This directory lists information on over 2,000 sources of information on the medical and healthcare industry. *$195.00*

1 per year Year Founded: 1999 ISBN 1-880874-57-1

3918 Directory of Developmental Disabilities Services

Nebraska Health and Human Services System
PO Box 94728
Department of Services
Lincoln, NE 68509-4728   402-471-2851
                                800-833-7352
                           Fax: 402-479-5094

Covers agencies and organizations that provide developmental disability services and programs in Nebraska.

28 pages

3919 Directory of Health Care Professionals

Dorland Healthcare Information
1500 Walnut Street
Suite 1000
Philadelphia, PA 19102   215-875-1212
                                800-784-2332
                           Fax: 215-735-3966
                E-mail: info@dorlandhealth.com
                        www.dorlandhealth.com

Helps you easily locate the key personnel and facilities you want by hospital name, system head-quarters, or job title. Valuable for locating industry professionals, recruiting, networking, and prospecting for industry business. *$299.00*

1 per year Year Founded: 1998 ISBN 1-573721-40-9

3920 Directory of Hospital Personnel

Grey House Publishing
85 Millerton Road
PO Box 860
Millerton, NY 12546   **518-789-8700**
                                  800-562-2139
                       Fax: 518-789-0545
          E-mail: books@greyhouse.com
                  www.greyhouse.com

Leslie MacKenzie, Publisher
Laura Mars, Editor

Best resource for researching or marketing a product or service to the hospital industry. *$275.00*

2400 pages ISBN 1-592370-26-8

3921 Directory of Physician Groups & Networks

Dorland Healthcare Information
1500 Walnut Street
Suite 1000
Philadelphia, PA 19102   **215-875-1212**
                                     800-784-2332
                        Fax: 215-735-3966
          E-mail: info@dorlandhealth.com
                  www.dorlandhealth.com

This directory offers the most comprehensive and current data on these fast-changing organizations. Includes valuable lists and rankings such as the top 200 group practices, plus, five industry experts provide exclusive reviews of current dynamics and trends in the physician marketplace. *$349.00*

3922 Directory of Physician Groups and Networks

Dorland Healthcare Information
1500 Walnut Street
Suite 1000
Philadelphia, PA 19102   **215-875-1212**
                                     800-784-2332
                        Fax: 215-735-3966
          E-mail: info@dorlandhealth.com
                  www.dorlandhealth.com

Reference tool with over 4,000 entries covering IPAs, PHOs, large medical group practices with 20 or more physicians, MSOs and PPMCs. Paperback, published yearly. *$345.00*

Year Founded: 1998 ISBN 1-880874-50-4

3923 Directory of the American Psychological Association

750 1st Street NE
Washington, DC 20002-4241   **202-336-5500**
                                        800-374-2721
                           Fax: 202-336-5568
             E-mail: webmaster@apa.org
                     www.apa.org

$70.00

1,968 pages 4 per year

3924 Dorland's Medical Directory

Dorland Healthcare Information
1500 Walnut Street
Suite 1000
Philadelphia, PA 19102   **215-875-1212**
                                     800-784-2332
                        Fax: 215-735-3966
          E-mail: info@dorlandhealth.com
                  www.dorlandhealth.com

Contains expanded coverage of healthcare facilities with profiles of 616 group practices, 661 hospitals and 750 rehabilitation, subacute, hospice and long term care facilities. *$699.00*

1 per year ISBN 1-880874-82-2

3925 Drug Information Handbook for Psychiatry

Lexi-Comp
1100 Terex Road
Hudson, OH 44236-3771   **330-650-6506**
                                    800-837-5394
                       Fax: 330-656-4307
                           www.lexi.com

Katie Seabeck, Marketing

Written specifically for mental health professionals. Addresses the fact that mental health patients may be taking additional medication for the treatment of another medical condition in combination with their psychtropic agents. With that in mind, this book contains information on all drugs, not just the psychotropic agents. Specific fields of information contained within the drug monograph include Effects on Mental Status and Effects on Psychiatric Treatment. *$38.75*

1 per year ISBN 1-591950-64-3

3926 HMO & PPO Database & Directory

Dorland Healthcare Information
1500 Walnut Street
Suite 1000
Philadelphia, PA 19102   **215-875-1212**
                                     800-784-2332
                        Fax: 215-735-3966
          E-mail: info@dorlandhealth.com
                  www.dorlandhealth.com

Delivers comprehensive and current information on senior-level individuals at virtually all US HMOs and PPOs at an affordable price. *$400.00*

3927 HMO/PPO Directory

Grey House Publishing
85 Millerton Road
PO Box 860
Millerton, NY 12546   **518-789-8700**
                                  800-562-2139
                       Fax: 518-789-0545
          E-mail: books@greyhouse.com
                  www.greyhouse.com

Leslie MacKenzie, Publisher
Laura Mars, Editor

Provides detailed information about health maintenance organizations and preferred provider organizations nationwide. *$275.00*

500 pages ISBN 1-592370-22-5

3928 Innovations in Clinical Practice: Source Book - Volume 17

Professional Resource Press
PO Box 15560
Sarasota, FL 34277-1560   **941-343-9601**
800-443-3364
Fax: 941-343-9201
E-mail: orders@prpress.com
www.prpress.com

Debra Fink, Managing Editor

Provides a comprehensive source of practical information and applied techniques that can be put to immediate use in your practice. *$59.95*

524 pages Year Founded: 1999 ISSN 0737125xISBN 1-568870-49-3

3929 Managing Chronic Behavioral Disorders: Desktop Reference for Mental Health and Addiction Professionals

Manisses Communications Group
PO Box 9758
Providence, RI 02906   **401-831-6020**
800-333-7771
Fax: 401-861-6370
E-mail: manissescs@manisses.com

Covers the full range of chronic disorders from substance abuse and schizophrenia to depression, obsessive-compulsive disorders, ADHD, dementia, post-traumatic stress syndrome and more. *$159.00*

3930 Medi-Pages (Health and Medical Care) On-line Directory-Medipages.Com

Medi-Pages
719 Main Street
Niagara Falls, NY 14301-1703   **716-284-4277**
800-554-6661
Fax: 716-284-4401
E-mail: marilyn@medipages.com
www.medipages.com

Marilyn Gould, Executive Assistant

On-line service covers more than 1.5 million listings of hospitals, nursing homes, clinics, home healthcare providers, HMOs, PPOs, CPOs, health associations, professional associations, federal government agencies, international health organizations, medical libraries, hospital management companies, case managers, HFCA offices, AT&T numbers as well as an online medical product locater.

3931 Medicaid Managed Behavioral Care Sourcebook

Faulkner & Gray
11 Penn Plaza
Basement 17
New York, NY 10001-2006   **212-967-7000**
800-535-8403
Fax: 212-967-7180
E-mail: order@faulknergray.com
www.faulknergray.com/

Covers medicaid, managed behavioral care, state agencies, providers, MCOs and others. *$60.00*

1 per year

3932 Medical & Healthcare Marketplace Guide Directory

Dorland Healthcare Information
1500 Walnut Street
Suite 1000
Philadelphia, PA 19102   **215-875-1212**
800-784-2332
Fax: 215-735-3966
E-mail: info@dorlandhealth.com
www.dorlandhealth.com

Contains valuable data on pharmaceutical, medical advice, and clinical and non-clinical healthcare service companies worldwide. *$499.00*

3933 Mental Health Directory

Office of Consumer, Family & Public Information
5600 Fishers Lane, Room 15-99
Center For Mental Health Services
Rockville, MD 20857-0002   **301-443-2792**
Fax: 301-443-5163

Covers hospitals, treatment centers, outpatient clinics, day/night facilities, residential treatment centers for emotionally disturbed children, residential supportive programs such as halfway houses, and mental health centers offering mental health assistance. *$23.00*

468 pages

3934 Mental Health and Social Work Career Directory

Gale Research
27500 Drake Road
Farmington Hills, MI 48331-3535   **248-699-4253**
800-877-4253
Fax: 248-699-8069
E-mail: galeord@gale.com
www.gale.com

Covers over three hundred agencies, organizations, and companies offering entry-level positions in mental health, social work, counseling, psychology, etc.; sources of help-wanted ads, professional associations, producers of videos, databases, career guides, and professional guides and handbooks. *$17.95*

360 pages

3935 National Association of Psychiatric Health Systems: Membership Directory

325 Seventh Street NW
Suite 625
Washington, DC 20004-2802   202-393-6700
                                  Fax: 202-783-6041
                                  E-mail: naphs@naphs.org
                                  www.naphs.org

Mark Covall, Executive Director
Carole Szpak, Director Communications

Contact information of professional groups working to coordinate a full spectrum of treatment services, including inpatient, residential, partial hospitalization and outpatient programs as well as prevention and management services. *$32.10*

48 pages 1 per year Year Founded: 1933

3936 National Directory of Medical Psychotherapists and Psychodiagnosticians

345 24th Avenue N
Park Plaza Medical Building Suite 201
Nashville, TN 37203-1595   615-327-2984
                                  Fax: 615-327-9235
                                  E-mail: americanbd@aol.com

Includes the following: Disability Analysis in Practice: Fundamental Framework for an Interdiciplinary Science, and The Disability Handbook: Tools for Independent Practice. *$45.00*

240 pages 1 per year

3937 National Register of Health Service Providers in Psychology

1120 G Street NW
Suite 330
Washington, DC 20005-3873   202-783-7663
                                  Fax: 202-347-0550
                                  E-mail: claire@nationalregister.org
                                  www.nationalregister.org

Judy Hall PhD, Executive Officer
Claire McCardell-Long, Director Administration/Finance

Psychologists who are licensed or certified by a state/provincial board of examiners of psychology and who have met council criteria as health service providers in psychology.

Year Founded: 1974

3938 National Registry of Psychoanalysts

National Association for the Advancement of Psychoanalysis
80 8th Avenue
Suite 1501
New York, NY 10011-5126   212-741-0515
                                 Fax: 212-366-4347
                                 E-mail: naap72@aol.com
                                 www.naap.org

Margery Quackenburh, Administrator
Pearl Appel, President

Psychoanalysis provides information to the public on psychoanalysis. Publishes quarterly NAAP News, annual Registry of Psychoanalysis. *$15.00*

175 pages

3939 Patient Guide to Mental Health Issues: Desk Chart

Lexi-Comp
1100 Terex Road
Hudson, OH 44236-3771   330-650-6506
                               800-837-5394
                               Fax: 330-656-4307
                               www.lexi.com

Katie Seabeck, Marketing

Designed specifically for healthcare professionals dealing with mental health patients. Combines eight of our popular Patient Chart titles into one, convienient desktop presentation. This will assist in explaining the most common mental health issue to your patients on a level that they will understand. *$38.75*

1 per year ISBN 1-591950-54-6

3940 PsycINFO Database

PsycINFO, American Psychological Association
750 1st Street NE
Washington, DC 20002-4242   202-336-5650
                                   800-374-2722
                                   Fax: 202-336-5633
                                   TDD: 202-336-6123
                                   E-mail: psycinfo@apa.org
                                   www.apa.org/psychinfo

PsycINFO is a database that contains citations and summaries of journal articles, book chapters, books, dissertations and technical reports in the field of psychology and the psychological aspects of related disciplines, such as medicine, psychiatry, nursing, sociology, education, pharmacology, physiology, linguistics, anthropology, business and law. Journal coverage, spanning 1887 to present, includes international material from 1,800 periodicals written in over 30 languages. Current chapter and book coverage includes worldwide English language material published from 1987 to present. Over 75,000 references are added annually through weekly updates.

52 per year

3941 Psychotherapists Directory

American Business Directories
5711 S 86th Circle
PO Box 27347
Omaha, NE 68127-0347   402-593-4600
                              800-555-6124
                              Fax: 402-331-5481
                              E-mail: directory@abii.com
                              www.abii.com

1 per year

485

3942 Psychotropic Drug Information Handbook

Lexi-Comp
1100 Terex Road
Hudson, OH 44236-3771 330-650-6506
800-837-5394
Fax: 330-656-4307
www.lexi.com

Katie Seabeck, Marketing

Concise handbook, designed to fit into your lab coat, is a current and portable psychotropic drug reference with 150 drugs and 35 herbal monographs. Perfect companion to Drug Information Handbook for Psychiatry. *$38.75*

1 per year ISBN 1-591950-65-1

3943 Rating Scales in Mental Health

Lexi-Comp
1100 Terex Road
Hudson, OH 44236-3771 330-650-6506
800-837-5394
Fax: 330-656-4307
www.lexi.com

Katie Seabeck, Marketing

Ideal for clinicians as well as administrators, this title provides an overview of over 100 recommended rating scales for mental health assessment. This book is also a great tool to assist mental healthcare professionals determine the appropriate psychiatric rating scale when assessing their clients. *$38.75*

1 per year ISBN 1-591950-52-X

3944 Roster: Centers for the Developmentally Disabled

Nebraska Health and Human Services
301 Centennial Mall S
Lincoln, NE 68509-5007 402-471-4363
Fax: 402-471-0555
TDD: 070-119-99
www.2.hhs.state.ne.us/

Joann Erickson RN, Program Manager

Covers approximately 160 licensed facilities in Nebraska for the developmentally disabled.

40 pages 1 per year

3945 Roster: Health Clinics

Nebraska Health and Human Services
301 Centennial Mall S
Lincoln, NE 68509 402-471-0309
Fax: 402-471-0555
www.2.hhs.state.ne.us/

Nancy L Brown RN, Program Manager

Covers approximately 46 licensed health clinic facilities in Nebraska.

11 pages 1 per year

3946 Roster: Substance Abuse Treatment Centers

Nebraska Health and Human Services
301 Centennial Mall S
Lincoln, NE 68509-5007 402-471-4363
Fax: 402-471-0555
www.2.hhs.state.ne.us/

Joann Erickson RN, Program Manager

Covers approximately 56 licensed substance abuse treatment centers in Nebraska.

12 pages 1 per year

3947 Yellow Pages of Oklahoma Department of Mental Health and Substance Abuse Services

Oklahoma State Dept. of Mental Health & Substance Abuse Services
PO Box 53277
Oklahoma City, OK 73152-3277 405-522-3908
800-522-9054
Fax: 405-522-3650
www.odmhsas.org

Service directory listing publicly funded. Mental Health, Substance Abuse, and Domestic Violence Services.

36 pages 1 per year

By State

Alabama

3948 Bryce Hospital
200 University Boulevard
Tuscaloosa, AL 35401-1294   205-759-0750
                                   Fax: 205-759-0845

James F Redroch Jr, Contact

3949 Greil Memorial Psychiatric Hospital
2140 Upper Wetumpka Road
Montgomery, AL 36107-1398   334-262-0363
                                   Fax: 334-262-5192

Susan P Chambers MPA, Contact

3950 Lincoln Regional Center
2705 S Folsom
Montgomery, AL 36107-1398   334-262-0363
                                   Fax: 334-262-5192

Barb Ramsey, Contact

3951 Mary Starke Harper Geriatric Psychiatry Center
201 University Boulevard
Tuscaloosa, AL 35402   205-759-0900
                                   Fax: 205-759-0931

Kathy R Grissom, Contact

3952 North Alabama Regional Hospital
Highway 31 S
Decatur, AL 35609   256-560-2200
                                   Fax: 256-560-2338

Kay V Greenwood, Contact

3953 Searcy Hospital
Coy Smith Highway
PO Box 1001
Mount Vernon, AL 35660   251-662-6700

John T Bartlett, Contact

3954 Taylor Hardin Secure Medical Facility
1301 Jack Warner Parkway NE
Tuscaloosa, AL 35405-1098   205-556-7060
                                   Fax: 205-556-1198

James F Reddach Jr, JD, Facility Director

Alaska

3955 Alaska Psychiatric Hospital
2900 Providence Drive
Anchorage, AK 99508-4677   907-269-7100
                                   Fax: 907-269-7128

Randall Burns, Contact

Arizona

3956 Arizona State Hospital
2500 E Van Buren
Phoenix, AZ 85008-6079   602-220-6271
                                   Fax: 602-220-6292

Jack Silver MPA, Contact

Arkansas

3957 Arkansas State Hospital
4313 W Markham Street
Little Rock, AR 72205-4096   501-686-9410
                                   Fax: 501-686-9483

Glen Sago, Contact

California

3958 Atascadero State Hospital
10333 El Camino Real
PO Box 7001
Atascadero, CA 93423-5808   805-468-2035
                                   Fax: 805-468-3000

Jon Demorales, Contact

3959 Augustus F Hawkins Community Mental Health Center
Los Angeles County Department of Mental Health
1720 E 120th Street
Los Angeles, CA 90059-3097   310-668-4186
                                   Fax: 310-223-0712

Provides community and client crisis intervention, case management, community promotion and outpatient services. Clinical facilities for professional field training.

3960 Department of Mental Health Psychiatric Program: Vacaville
PO Box 2297
Vacaville, CA 95696-2297   707-449-6554
                                   Fax: 707-453-7047

Sylvia Blount, Contact

3961 Fremont Hospital
39001 Sundale Drive
Fremont, CA 94538   510-796-1100
                                   Fax: 510-574-4801
                                   www.fremonthospital.com

3962 Lincoln Child Center
4368 Lincoln Avenue
Oakland, CA 94602   510-531-3111
                                   Fax: 510-530-8083
                                   E-mail: info@lincolncc.org
                                   www.lincolncc.org

Jack Soares, Development

Nonprofit organization that provides mental health services for children and families living in Oakland and the Bay Area through our residential, education and community based programs.

3963 Merit Behavioral Care of California

400 Oyster Point Boulevard
Suite 306
S San Francisco, CA 94080-1919   650-615-5119
Fax: 650-742-0988

3964 Metropolitan State Hospital

11401 Bloomfield Avenue
Norwalk, CA 90650   562-863-7011
Fax: 562-929-3131
TDD: 562-863-1743

William G Silva, Contact

3965 Mills-Peninsula Hospital: Behavioral Health

1783 El Camino Real
Burlingame, CA 94010-3205   650-696-5909
Fax: 650-696-5472
www.mills-peninsula.org/behavioralhealth

Community hospital mental health and chemical dependency care. Our team is uniquely qualified to evaluate, diagnose and treat a wide range of behavioral conditions.

3966 Napa State Hospital

2100 Napa-Vallejo Highway
Napa, CA 94558-6293   707-253-5000
Fax: 707-253-5411

Frank Turley PhD, Contact

3967 Orange County Mental Health

822 Town & Country Road
Orange, CA 92868-4712   714-547-7559
Fax: 717-543-4431
E-mail: info@mhaoc.org
www.mhaoc.org

The Mental Health Association of Orange County is a nonprofit organization dedicated to improving the quality of life of Orange County residents impacted by mental illness through direct service, advocacy, education and information dissemination.

3968 PacifiCare Behavioral Health

PO Box 31053
Laguna Hills, CA 92654-1053

800-999-9585
www.pbhi.com

Richard J Kelliher PsyD, Clinical Director

Provides behavioral health services to children, adolescents, adults, and seniors.

3969 Patton State Hospital

3102 E Highland Avenue
Patton, CA 92369   909-425-7321
Fax: 909-425-6169

William L Summers, Contact

3970 Pine Grove Hospital

7011 Shoup Avenue
Conoga Park, CA 91307

800-843-4768
www.pinegrovehospital.com

3971 Presbyterian Intercommunity Hospital Mental Health Center

12401 Washington Boulevard
Whittier, CA 90602-1099   562-698-0811
www.whittierpres.com

Offers an inpatient program for those with a variety of menatl disorders.

Colorado

3972 Colorado Mental Health Institute at Fort Logan

3520 W Oxford Avenue
Denver, CO 80236-3197   303-866-7066
Fax: 303-866-7048

Garry Toerber PhD, Contact

3973 Colorado Mental Health Institute at Pueblo

1600 W 24th Street
Pueblo, CO 81003-1499   719-546-4000
Fax: 719-546-4484

Robert Hawkins, Contact

3974 Emily Griffith Center

PO Box 95
Larkspur, CO 80118-0095   303-681-2400
Fax: 303-681-2400

Howard Shiffman, CEO
Beth Miller, Program Director
John Smrcka, Clinical Director

A non-profit organization committed to meeting the needs of children. EGC operates a sixty seven RTC facility in rural Larkspur, CO and a twenty one bed RTC in Colorado springs, CO. Our RTC facilities provide treatment for boys between the ages of ten and twenty one. Emily Griffith Center provides treatment for a diverse population, but also provides specialized treatment for sex offenders.

Connecticut

3975 Cedarcrest Hospital

525 Russell Road
Newington, CT 06111-1595   860-666-7603
Fax: 860-666-7642

John Simsarian MSW, Contact

3976 Greater Bridgeport Community Mental Health Center

1635 Central Avenue
PO Box 5117
Bridgeport, CT 06610-2700   203-551-7400
Fax: 203-551-7446

James M LeHene MPH, Contact

3977 Health Center Community Mental Health Center

PO Box 351
Middletown, CT 06457-7023   860-262-5887
Fax: 860-262-5895

Garrel S Mulany CEO, Contact

3978 Klingberg Family Centers

370 Linwood Street
New Britain, CT 06052-1998   860-224-9113
Fax: 860-832-8221
E-mail: lynner@klingberg.org
www.klingberg.org

To uphold, preserve and restore families in a therapeutic environment, valuing the absolute worth of every child, while adhering to the highest ethical principles in accordance with our Judaeo-Christian heritage. Offers an array of programs designed to help children and families whose lives have been affected by abuse in its various forms, emotional/behavioral difficulties and more.

3979 Silver Hill Hospital

208 Valley Road
New Canaan, CT 06840

800-899-4455
www.silverhospital.com

Delaware

3980 Delaware State Hospital

1901 N Dupont Highway
New Castle, DE 19720   302-577-4000
Fax: 302-255-4459

Jiro Shimono, Contact

District of Columbia

3981 St. Elizabeth's Hospital

2700 Martin Luther King Jr Avenue SE
Washington, DC 20032-2698   202-562-4000
Fax: 202-673-4386

Elizabeth Jones, Contact

Florida

3982 Florida State Hospital

100 N Main Street
Chattahoochee, FL 32324   850-663-7536
Fax: 850-663-7326

Robert B Williams, Contact

3983 G Pierce Wood Memorial Hospital

5847 SE Highway 31
Arcadia, FL 33821-9627   863-494-3323

Myers R Kurtz, Contact

3984 Manatee Glens

391 6th Avenue W
Bradenton, FL 34206-9478   941-741-3111
Fax: 941-741-3112
E-mail: mccartyn@manateeglens.com
www.manateeglens.com

Mary Ruiz, CEO/President
Deborah Kostroun, COO
John Denaro, CFO

Charitable organization that is the area's oldest and largest provider of mental health and addiction treatment services.

3985 Manatee Palms Youth Services

4480 51st Street W
Bradenton, FL 34210-2855   941-792-2222
Fax: 941-795-4359

Committed to providing the highest quality comprehensive mental health care and education services for at-risk children, adolescents, families and our community.

3986 North Florida Evaluation and Treatment Center

1200 NE 55th Boulevard
Gainesville, FL 32641-2783   352-375-8484
Fax: 352-955-2094

Dennis Gies, Contact

3987 North Star Centre

9033 Galdes Road
Boca Raton, FL 33434   561-361-0500
877-779-2448
E-mail: info@northstar-centre.com
www.northstar-centre.com

Ira Kaufman, Executive Director
Mark Alper, Associate Executive Director

Uniquely comprehensive facility dedicated to restoring your sense of emotional and physical well being. Because our staff consists of South Florida's well known and respected professionals, one can be assured that each patient will be matched to a professional that best suits their needs and personality.

3988 Northeast Florida State Hospital

S State Road 121
MacClenny, FL 32063-9777   904-259-6211
Fax: 904-259-7101

CV Stotler, Administrator

543 bed licensed mental health facility. Provides individuals with a variety of person centered services within a residential setting. Core services include health care, psychiatric treatment, psychiatric rehabilitation, vocational programming, behavior analysis, community reintegration, and care coordination. Assessment, diagnostic, and treatment services are provided in concert with community mental health systems to transition individuals through the system of care in the smoothest, most theraputic, and least traumatic manner possible.

3989 Renaissance Manor

1401 16th Street
Sarasota, FL 34236-2519   941-365-8645
Fax: 941-955-0520

Heather Eller, Administrator

Community based assisted living facility with a limited mental health license, specializes in serving adults with neuro-biological disorders and mood disorders along with other special mental health needs. Our not-for-profit organization is a program designed to encourage positive mental health while meeting the various interest of our residents.

3990 South Florida Evaluation and Treatment Center

2200 NW 7th Avenue
Miami, FL 33127-2491   305-637-2500

Cheryl Brantley, Contact

3991 South Florida State Hospital

1000 SW 84th Avenue
Pembroke Pines, FL 33025-1499   954-967-7589
                                  Fax: 954-985-4709

Andrew Reid, Contact

3992 University Pavilion Psychiatric Services

7425 N University Drive
Tamarac, FL 33321-2901   954-722-9933
                                Fax: 954-722-8416
                                www.uhmchealth.com

Offers psychiatric services on an inpatient and outpatient basis for all individuals.

3993 Willough Healthcare System

9001 Tamiami Trail E
Naples, FL 34113   800-722-0100
                     E-mail: willough1@aol.com
                              www.thewillough.com

Georgia

3994 Candler General Hospital: Rehabilitation Unit

5353 Reynolds Street
Savannah, GA 31405-6013   912-354-9211
                               Fax: 912-697-6566

Virginia Donaldson, Admissions Director

3995 Central State Hospital

620 Broad Street
Milledgeville, GA 31062-9989   478-445-4128
                                Fax: 478-445-6034
          E-mail: info@centralstatehospital.org
                  www.centralstatehospital.org

Joe T Hodge, Contact

3996 Georgia Regional Hospital at Atlanta

3073 Panthersville Road
Decatur, GA 30034-3800   404-243-2110
                                Fax: 404-212-4228

Ron Hogan, Contact

3997 Georgia Regional Hospital at Augusta

3405 Old Savannah Road
Augusta, GA 30906-3897   706-792-7019
                                Fax: 706-792-7041

Ben Waker EdD, Contact

3998 Georgia Regional Hospital at Savannah

1915 Eisenhower Drive
PO Box 13607
Savannah, GA 31416-0607   912-356-2045
                                Fax: 912-356-2691

Douglas Osborne, Contact

3999 Northwest Georgia Regional Hospital

1305 Redmond Circle
Rome, GA 30165-1307   706-295-6246
                                Fax: 706-802-5454

Thomas Muller, Contact

4000 Southwestern State Hospital

400 Pinetree Boulevard
Thomasville, GA 31799-6859   912-227-3032
                                Fax: 912-227-2883

David Sofferin, Contact

4001 West Central Georgia Regional Hospital

3000 Schatulga Road
PO Box 12435
Columbus, GA 31907-1035   706-568-5203
                                Fax: 706-568-5339

Marvin Bailey, Contact

Hawaii

4002 Hawaii State Hospital

45-710 Keaahala Road
Kaneohe, HI 96744-3597   808-247-2191
                                Fax: 808-247-7335

Marvin O Saint Clair, Contact

Idaho

4003 Children of Hope Family Hospital

PO Box 2353
Boise, ID 83701   208-658-8013
                     E-mail: chfhosp@juno.net
                              www.chfhosp.dmi.net

4004 State Hospital North

300 Hospital Drive
Orofino, ID 83544-9034   208-476-4511
                                Fax: 208-476-7898

Jay Kessinger, Contact

4005 State Hospital South

700 E Alice Street
PO Box 400
Blackfoot, ID 83221-0400   208-785-8401
                                Fax: 208-785-8448

Raymond Laible, Contact

Illinois

4006 Alton Mental Health Center

4500 College Avenue
Alton, IL 62002-5099   618-474-3209
                                Fax: 618-474-4800

Thomas H Johnson, Contact

4007 Andrew McFarland Mental Health Center

901 Southwind Road
Springfield, IL 62703-5195   217-786-6994
                                Fax: 217-786-7167

G. Scott Viniard, Hospital Administrator

4008 Chester Mental Health Center

PO Box 31
Chester, IL 62233-0031 618-826-4571
Fax: 618-826-3229

Stephen Hardy PhD, Contact

4009 Choate Mental Health and Development Center

1000 N Main Street
Anna, IL 62906-1699 618-833-5161
Fax: 618-833-4191

Tom Richards, Contact

4010 Elgin Mental Health Center

750 S State Street
Elgin, IL 60123-7692 847-742-1040
Fax: 847-429-4911

Nancy Staples, Contact

4011 H Douglas Singer Mental Health Center

4402 N Main Street
Rockford, IL 61103-1200 815-987-7302
Fax: 815-987-7559

Angelo Campagna, Contact

4012 Jane Addams Community Mental Health Center

1133 W Stephenson Street
Suite 401
Freeport, IL 61032-4866 815-232-4183
Fax: 815-232-4193

4013 John J Madden Mental Health Center

1200 S 1st Avenue
Hines, IL 60141 708-338-7249
Fax: 708-338-7057

Patricia Madden, Contact

4014 John R Day and Associates

3716 W Brighton Avenue
Peoria, IL 61615-2938 309-692-7755
Fax: 306-692-7755

4015 MacNeal Hospital

3231 South Euclid Avenue
Berwyn, IL 60402 708-783-3094
888-622-6325
Fax: 708-783-3656
TTY: 708-783-3058
E-mail: inf@macnealfp.com
www.macnealfp.com/hospital.htm

Donna Lawlor MD, Program Director
Davis Yang, Center Director
John Gong, Clinical Faculty
Edward C Foley MD, Director Of Research

The MacNeal Family Practice Residency Program was one of the first family practice programs in rhe country and the first in Illinois. We have continue a progressive tradition in all aspects of our curriculum. Our program is at the forefront of contemporary family medicine offering diverse academic and clinical opportunites and building on the innovative ideas of our residents.

4016 McHenry County Mental Health Board

101 N Virginia Street
Suite 150
Crystal Lake, IL 60014-3439 815-455-2828
Fax: 815-455-2925

4017 Read Mental Health Center: Chicago

4200 N Oak Park Avenue
Chicago, IL 60634-1457 773-794-4010
Fax: 773-794-4046

James Brunner MD, Hospital Administrator
Randy Thompson, Medical Director
Thomas Simpatico MD, Facility Director

An important psychiatric hospital which is part of the Department of Human Services of the State of Illinois. Provides comprehensive psychiatric inpatient services for adults in cooperation with a broad spectrum of community mental health service providers.

4018 Salem Children's Home

15161 N 400 E Road
Flanagan, IL 61740 815-796-4561
Fax: 815-796-4565
E-mail: salem@salemhome.org
www.salemhome.org

Salem Children's Home is a Christian organization which provides a variety of individualized services od superior quality to meet the spiritual, social, educational, emotional and psysical needs of children, adolescents and their familes. We gladly accept the responsibility to provide this care in a personal, nurtuing manner to reconcile familes, develop positive self-images and build health relationships among those we serve.

4019 Tinley Park Mental Health Center

7400 W 183rd Street
Tinely Park, IL 60477-3695 708-614-4008
Fax: 708-614-4495

Janice Thomas, Contact

4020 Transitions Mental Health Rehabilitation

805 19th Street
Rock Island, IL 61204-4238 309-793-4993
Fax: 309-793-9053
E-mail: transitions@revealed.net
www.transrehab.org

Betsy McLeland, Associate Director Marketing

Transitions is dedicated to promoting, enhancing and improving the health and well-being of individuals, families and the community impacted by mental health issues.

Indiana

4021 Community Hospital: Anderson and Madison County

1515 N Madison Avenue
Anderson, IN 46011-3457 765-298-4242
Fax: 765-298-5848
www.communityanderson.com

William C VanNess II MD, President and CEO

The mission of Community Hospital is to serve the medical, health and human service needs to the people in Anderson-Madison County and contiguous counties with compassion dignity, repect and excellence. Service, although focused on injury, illness and disease will also embrace prevention, education and alternative systems of health care delivery.

4022 Crossroad: Fort Wayne's Children's Home

2525 Lake Avenue
Fort Wayne, IN 46805-5457   **260-484-4153**
                              Fax: 260-484-2337
                              www.crossroad-fwch.org

Imogene Nusbaum Snyder, President/CEO
John Link, VP Clinical Services/COO
Randy Rider, VP Professional Services

Crossroad provides a variety of programs and continues to expand its services. Over the past 30 years, Crossroad has created a residentiail Diagnostic Program, opened the Intensive Treatment Center and estbalished specialized treatment programs including both individual and group therapy for youth with serious, emotional needs. Services now include day-treatment, day-treatment education and home-bassed programming.

4023 Evansville Psychiatric Children's Center

3300 E Morgan Avenue
Evansville, IN 47715   **812-477-6436**
                          Fax: 812-474-4247
              E-mail: trich@fssa.state.in.us
                          www.epcckids.com

Tom Rich, Contact

4024 Evansville State Hospital

3400 Lincoln Avenue
Evansville, IN 47715-0146   **812-473-2100**
                               Fax: 812-473-2109

Ralph Nichols, Contact

4025 Fort Wayne State Development Center

4900 St. Joe Road
Fort Wayne, IN 46835-3299   **219-485-7554**
                               Fax: 219-485-2863

Ajit Mukherjee, Contact

4026 Hamilton Center

620 Eighth Avenue
PO Box 4323
Terre Haute, IN 47804   **812-231-8323**
                          www.hamiltoncenter.org

Louise Anderson, President
Dianna Lancaster, Vice president
Thomas Harris, Treasurer
Doug Samuleson, Secretary

Services are provided to children, adolescents and adults with specialized progams for pregnant women, infants, and people with drug and alcohol problems. Counseling services are provided for people that may be stuggling with stress, life, changes, relationship issues as well as more serious problems such as depression, anxiety disorders, or other serious mental illnesses.

4027 Indiana Family Support Network, MHA Indiana

55 Monument Circle
Suite 455
Indianapolis, IN 46204-2918   **317-638-3501**
                                 800-555-6424
                            Fax: 317-638-3401
E-mail: mha@mentalhealthassociation.com
                            www.nmha.org

Elizabeth Jewell

The National Mental Associatio is dedicated to promoting mental health, preventing mental diorders and achieving victory over mental illnesses through advocacy, education, research and service.

4028 LaRue D Carter Memorial Hospital

2601 Cold Spring Road
Indianapolis, IN 46222-2273   **314-941-4000**
                                 Fax: 317-941-4085

Diana Haugh RN, Contact

4029 Logansport State Hospital

1098 S State Road 25
Logansport, IN 46947-6723   **219-722-4141**
                               Fax: 219-735-2414

Jeffery Smith, Contact

4030 Madison State Hospital

711 Green Road
Madison, IN 47250-2199   **812-265-2611**
                            Fax: 812-265-7227

Steven Covington, Contact

4031 Muscatatuk State Developmental Center

PO Box 77
Butlerville, IN 47223-0077   **812-346-4401**
                                Fax: 812-346-6308

Michael Coppol, Contact

4032 New Castle State Developmental Center

100 Van Nuys Road
New Castle, IN 47362-9277   **765-529-0900**
                               Fax: 765-521-3168

Claudia Ciotroski, Contact

4033 Northern Indiana State Developmental Center

1234 N Notre Dame Avenue
S Bend, IN 46617-1399   **219-234-2101**
                           Fax: 219-288-7869

Dan Mohnke, Contact

4034 Parkview Hospital Rehabilitation Center

2200 Randilla Drive
Ft. Wayne, IN 46805   **260-373-6450**
                         888-480-5151
                    Fax: 260-373-4548
E-mail: vicki.maisonneuve@parkview.com
                    www.parkview.com

Paulette Fisher RN, CRRN, Admissions Specialist
Barbara Gregorey RN, Operational Lead

31 bed inpatient rehabilitation unit serving a wide variety of diagnoses. CARF accredited for both comprehensive and B1 programs. Outpatient services are offered at several sites throughout the community.

4035 Richmond State Hospital

498 NW 18th Street
Richmond, IN 47374-2898   765-966-0511
                          Fax: 765-966-4593
              www.richmondstatehospital.org
Jeff Butler, CEO/Superintendent

4036 William C Weber and Associates

Constitution Hill Office Park
6201 Constitution Drive
Fort Wayne, IN 46804   260-432-0696
                                 800-729-3971
                            Fax: 260-436-5795
              E-mail: info@webereap.com
                      www.webereap.com

William C Weber, Director
Linda Young, Probation Officer
John P Crowley, Psychotheraputic Services

We are Employee Assistance and Managed Behavioral Health Care Specialists. Unlike other EAP Providers affiliated with treatment programs, we are an independent firm specializing in the delivery of EAP and manages care services to employers. Our independence and single-minded focus assures your employees recieve the highest quality care in the most cost effecive way.

Iowa

4037 Cherokee Mental Health Institute

1251 W Chedar Loop
Cherokee, IA 51012-1599   712-225-2594
                            Fax: 712-225-6925

Tom Deiker PhD, Contact

4038 Clarinda Mental Health Treatment Complex

1800 N 16th Street
PO Box 338
Clarinda, IA 51632-1165   712-542-2161
                            Fax: 712-542-2012

Mark Lund, Contact

4039 Four Seasons Counseling Clinic

116 E 2nd Street
Muscatine, IA 52761-4003   563-263-3869
                            Fax: 563-263-3869

4040 Independence Mental Health Institute

2277 Iowa Avenue
PO Box 111
Independence, IA 50644-0111   319-334-2583
                            Fax: 319-334-5252

Dave Bhasker MD, Contact

4041 Mount Pleasant Mental Health Institute

1200 E Washington Street
Mount Pleasant, IA 52641-1898   319-385-7231
                            Fax: 319-385-8465

Ken Burger, Contact

Kansas

4042 Beacon Behavioral Health Group

6740 Antioch Road
Suite 260
Shawnee Mission, KS 66204-1261   913-384-7655
                            Fax: 913-362-3901

Kim Hegemen, Practice Administrator

Offers comprehensive mental health services by licensed clinical social workers, PhD psychologists and psychiatrists. Services include psychiatric evaulations, medication management, neuropsychological testing, ADHD evaluations and individual psychotherapy.

4043 Larned State Hospital

Route 3
PO Box 89
Larned, KS 67550-9365   316-285-2131
                            Fax: 316-285-4357

Mani Lee PhD, Contact

4044 Osawatomie State Hospital

PO Box 500
Osawatomie, KS 66064-0500   913-755-7000
                            Fax: 913-755-2637

Don Jordan, Superintendent

JCAHO accredited state psychiatric hospital.

4045 Rainbow Mental Health Facility

2205 W 36th Avenue
Kansas City, KS 66103-2198   913-384-1880
                            Fax: 913-384-1948
              www.kumc.edu/rainbow

Roz Underdahl, Contact

Kentucky

4046 ARH Psychiatric Center

100 Medical Center Drive
Hazard, KY 41701-9429   606-439-1331
                            Fax: 606-439-6701

Geoffry Duckworth, Contact

4047 ARH Psychiatric Hospital

100 Medical Center Drive
Hazard, KY 41701-9429   606-439-1331
                            Fax: 606-439-6701

Goeffry Duckworth, Contact

4048 Central State Hospital

10510 La Grange Road
Louisville, KY 40223-1228   502-245-4121
                            Fax: 502-253-7049

Paula Tamee-Cook, Contact

4049 Cumberland River Regional Board

American Greeting Road
Corbin, KY 40701   606-528-7010
Fax: 606-528-5401

For children with emotional, behavioral and/or mental challenges.

4050 Eastern State Hospital

627 W Fourth Street
Lexington, KY 40508-9990   859-246-7000
Fax: 859-246-7025
E-mail: kjsusman@bluegrass.org
www.bluegrass.org/easternst.html

Daniel J Luchtefeld, Contact

4051 Kentucky Correctional Psychiatric Center

1612 Dawkins Road
PO Box 67
La Grange, KY 40031-0067   502-222-7161
Fax: 502-222-7798

Gregory Taylor, Contact

4052 Our Lady of Bellefonte Hospital

St. Christopher Drive
Ashland, KY 41101   606-833-3333
www.olbh.com

4053 Western State Hospital

2400 Russeville Road
PO Box 2200
Hopkinsville, KY 42240-2200   502-886-4431
Fax: 502-886-4487

Steven Wiggins, Contact

Louisiana

4054 Central Louisiana State Hospital

PO Box 5031
Pineville, LA 71361-5031   318-484-6200
Fax: 318-484-6501

Gary S Grand, Contact

4055 East Louisiana State Hospital

PO Box 498
Highway 10
Jackson, LA 70748   225-634-0100
Fax: 225-634-5827

Warren Taylor-Price, Contact

4056 Feliciana Forensic Facility

PO Box 888
Jackson, LA 70748   225-634-0100
Fax: 225-634-5827

Warren Taylor-Price, Contact

4057 Greenwell Springs Hospital

PO Box 549
Greenwell Springs Road
Greenwell Springs, LA 70739   225-261-2730
Fax: 225-261-9080

Warren Taylor-Price, Contact

4058 Medical Center of LA: Mental Health Services

1532 Tulane Avenue
New Orleans, LA 70140   504-568-2869

William Malone, Contact

4059 New Orleans Adolescent Hospital

210 State Street
New Orleans, LA 70118   504-897-3400
Fax: 504-896-4959

Walter W Shervington MD, Contact

4060 River Oaks Hospital

1525 River Oaks Road W
New Orleans, LA 70123   504-734-1740
Fax: 504-733-7020
E-mail: mjroh@cmq.com
www.riveroakhospital.com

4061 Southeast Louisiana Hospital

PO Box 3850
Mandeville, LA 70470-3850   985-626-6300
Fax: 985-626-6658

Joseph Vinturella, Contact

Maine

4062 Augusta Mental Health Institute

Arsenal Street
PO Box 724
Augusta, ME 04330-0742   207-287-7200
Fax: 207-287-6123

Lisa Kavanaugh, Superintendent

Acute care psychiatric hospital owned and operated by the state of Maine.

4063 Bangor Mental Health Institute

PO Box 926
Bangor, ME 04401-0926   207-941-4000
Fax: 207-941-4062

N Lawrence Ventura, Contact

4064 Good Will-Hinckley Homes for Boys and Girls

PO Box 159
Hinckley, ME 04944   207-238-4000
Fax: 207-453-2515
E-mail: info@gwh.org
www.gwh.org

John Willey, Secretary
David Kimball, Chairman

Provides a home for the reception and support of needy boys and girls who are in needs maintaing and operates a school for them; attends to the physical, industrial, moral and spiritual development of those who shall be placed in its care.

4065 Spring Harbor Hospital

175 Running Hill Road
S Portland, ME 04106-3272   207-761-2000
Fax: 207-761-2108
TTY: 207-761-2224
E-mail: wilkersong@springharbor.org
www.springharbor.org

Gail Wilkeman, Dir. Communications/Marketing

Spring Harbor is southern Maine's premier provider
of inpatient services for individuals who experience
acute mental illness or dual disorders issues.

Maryland

4066 Clifton T Perkins Hospital Center

8450 Dorsey Run Road
PO Box 1000
Jessup, MD 20794-1000   410-724-3001
Fax: 410-724-3249

Richard Fragala, Contact

4067 Crownsville Hospital Center

1520 Crownsville Road
Crownsville, MD 21032   410-729-6000
800-937-0938
Fax: 410-729-6800
TDD: 410-987-0416

Ron Hendler, Contact

4068 Eastern Shore Hospital

PO Box 800
Cambridge, MD 21613-0800   410-221-2310
Fax: 410-221-2534

Mary K Noren, Contact

4069 John L. Gildner Regional Institute for Children and Adolescents

15000 Broschart Road
Rockville, MD 20850-3392   301-251-6800
Fax: 301-309-9004
www.dhmh.state.md.us/jlgrica/

Thomas E. Pukalski, CEO
Claudette Bernstein, Medical Director
Debrak K. VanHorn, Director of Comm. Res. & Dev.

John L. Gildner Regional Institute for Children and
Adolescents (JLG-RICA) is a community-based, public residential, clinical, and educational facility serving children and adolescents with severe emotional
disabilities. The program is designed to provide residential and day treatment for students in grades 5-12.
JLG-RICA's goal is to successfully return its students
to an appropriate family, community, and academic or
vocational setting that will lead to happy and successful lives.

4070 Laurel Regional Hospital

7300 Van Dusen Road
Laurel, MD 20707-9266   301-725-4300
Fax: 410-792-2270
www.dimensionshealth.org

Laurel Regional Hospital is a full-service community
hospital serving northern Prince George's County and
Montgomery, Howard, and Anne Arundel Counties
with 185 beds and 747 employees.

4071 Northville Regional Psychiatric Hospital

41001 Seven Mile Road
Northville, MD 48167-2698   248-349-1800
Fax: 248-349-9022

Shobhana Joshi MD, Contact

4072 RICA- Baltimore

605 S Chapel Gate Lane
Baltimore, MD 21229-3999   410-368-7800
877-203-5179
Fax: 410-368-7886
E-mail: pmakris@dhmh.state.md.us

Penny Makris, Contact

4073 RICA: Southern Maryland

9400 Surratts Road
Cheltenham, MD 20623-1324   301-372-1800
Fax: 301-372-1906

Audry Chase, Contact

4074 Spring Grove Hospital Center

Wade Avenue
Catonsville, MD 21228   410-402-6000
Fax: 410-402-7094

Mark Pecevich MD, Contact

4075 Springfield Hospital Center

Route 32
Sykesville, MD 21784   410-795-2100
Fax: 410-795-6048

Paula Langmead, Contact

4076 Thomas B Finan Cetner

Country Club Road
PO Box 1722
Cumberland, MD 21502-1722   301-777-2260
Fax: 301-777-2364

Archie Wallace, Contact

4077 Upper Shore Community Mental Health Center

Scheeler Road
PO Box 229
Chestertown, MD 21620-0229   410-778-6800
888-784-0137
Fax: 410-778-1648
TTY: 410-810-0285

Mary K Noren, CEO

4078 Walter P Carter Center

630 W Fayette Street
Baltimore, MD 21201-1585   410-209-6000
Fax: 410-209-6020

Patricia Kendall PhD, Contact

Massachusetts

4079 Baldpate Hospital
83 Baldpate Road
Georgetown, MA 01833

978-352-2131
www.baldpate.com

4080 Berkshire Center
PO Box 160
Lee, MA 01238-0160

413-243-2576
E-mail: bcenter@bcn.net

Gary Shaw, Admissions Director

A postsecondary program for young adults with learning disabilities ages eighteen - twenty six. Half the students attend Berkshire Community College part-time while others go directly into the working world. Services include: vocational and academic preparation, tutoring, college liaison, life skills instruction, drivers education, money management, psychotherapy and more. The program is year-round with a two year average stay.

4081 New England Home for Little Wanderers: Planning and Programs
271 Huntington Avenue
Boston, MA 02115

617-267-3700
888-466-3321
Fax: 617-267-8142
www.thehome.org

Joan Wallace-Benjamin, President/CEO
Alan Berns, VP for Programs

The home is a nationally renowned, private non-profit child and family service agency providing services to more than 10,000 children and families each year through over 30 programs that are measurably changing lives.

4082 Taunton State Hospital
PO Box 4007
Taunton, MA 02780-0997

508-977-3000
Fax: 508-977-3341

Katherine Chmiel, Contact

4083 Westboro State Hospital
Lyman Street
PO Box 288
Westboro, MA 01581-0288

508-616-2100
Fax: 508-616-2857

Steve Scheibel, Contact

Michigan

4084 Caro Center
2000 Chambers Road
Caro, MI 48723-9296

989-672-9261
Fax: 989-673-6749

Rose Laskowski, Hospital Director

4085 E Lansing Center for Family
425 W Grand River Avenue
E Lansing, MI 48823-4201

517-332-8900
Fax: 517-332-8149

Provides mental health treatment.

4086 Hawthorn Center
18741 Haggerty Road
Northville, MI 48167

248-349-3000
Fax: 248-349-6893

Hubert A Carbone MD, Interim Director

4087 Kalamazoo Psychiatric Hospital
1312 Oakland Drive
PO Box A
Kalamazoo, MI 49008

269-337-3000
Fax: 269-337-3007

James J Coleman EdD, Contact

4088 Mount Pleasant Center
1400 W Pickard
Mount Pleasant, MI 48858

989-773-7921
Fax: 989-773-6527

George Garland, Contact

4089 Samaritan Counseling Center
29887 W Eleventh Mile Road
Farmington Hills, MI 48336-1309

248-474-4701
Fax: 248-474-1518
E-mail: samaritaneesemi@juno.com
www.samaritancounselingmichigan.com

Dr. Wesley L Brun, Executive Director

The Samaritan Counseling Center is a pastoral counseling center. We provide counseling and psychotherapy that integrates the best in psychological and psychiatric theory and practice with the resources of the client's religous/faith tradition.

4090 Walter P Ruther Psychiatric Hospital
30901 Palmer Road
Westland, MI 48186-5389

734-722-4500
Fax: 734-722-5562

Norma Joses MD, Contact

4091 Westlund Child Guidance Clinic
3253 Congress Avenue
Saginaw, MI 48602-3199

989-793-4790
Fax: 989-793-1641

Provides mental health services.

Minnesota

4092 Brainerd Regional Human Services Center
1777 Highway 18 E
Brainerd, MN 56401-7389

218-828-2698
Fax: 218-828-2207

Harcey G Cakdwell, Contact

4093 Fergus Falls Regional Treatment Center
1400 N Union Avenue
Fergus Falls, MN 56537-1200

218-739-7200
Fax: 218-739-7243

Michael Ackley, Contact

4094 Metro Regional Treatment Center: Anoka

3300 4th Avenue N
Anoka, MN 55303-1119 763-576-5500
Fax: 763-712-4013

Judith Krohn, Contact

4095 St. Peter Regional Treatment Center

100 Freeman Drive
Saint Peter, MN 56082-1599 507-931-7128
Fax: 507-931-7711
TDD: 507-931-7825

Larry Te Brake, Forensic Site Director
Jim Behrends, Regional Administrator

4096 Willmar Regional Treatment Center

1550 Highway 71 NE
Willmar, MN 56201 320-231-5100
Fax: 320-231-5329

Sandra J Butturff, Site Director

Mississippi

4097 East Mississippi State Hospital

PO Box 4128, W Station
Meridian, MS 39304-4128 601-482-6186
Fax: 601-483-5543

Ramiro Martinez, Contact

4098 Mississippi State Hospital1

PO Box 157-A
Whitfield, MS 39193-0157 601-351-8000
Fax: 601-939-0647
E-mail: chastain@state.ms.us
www.msh.state.ms.us

James Chastain, Contact

4099 North Mississippi State Hospital

PO Box 86
Whitfield, MS 39193 662-690-4200
Fax: 662-690-4227

Wynona Winfield, Contact

4100 South Mississippi State Hospital

PO Box 86
Whitfield, MS 39193 601-351-8400
Fax: 601-351-8300

Wynona Winfield, Contact

Missouri

4101 Cottonwood Residential Treatment Center

1025 N Sprigg Street
Cape Girardeau, MO 63701-4831 573-290-5888
Fax: 573-290-5895

Martha Cassel, Contact

4102 Fulton State Hospital

600 E 5th Street
Fulton, MO 65251-1798 573-592-4100
Fax: 573-592-3000

Stephen Reeves, Contact

4103 Hawthorn Children's Psychiatric Hospital

1901 Pennsylvania Avenue
Saint Louis, MO 63133-1325 314-513-7800
Fax: 314-512-7812

Cary Drennen, Contact

4104 Hyland Behavioral Health System

10020 Kennerly Road
Sappington, MO 63128-2106 314-525-7200
800-525-2032
Fax: 314-525-4420

Adult and pediatric psychiatric inpatient/partial services located at St. Anthony's Medical Center.

4105 Metropolitan Saint Louis Psychiatric Center

5351 Delmar Boulevard
Saint Louis, MO 63112-3416 314-877-0524
Fax: 314-877-0553

Greg Dale, Contact

4106 Mid-Missouri Mental Health Center

3 Hospital Drive
Columbia, MO 65201-5296 573-884-1300
573-874-1209

Dennis Canote, Contact

4107 Northwest Missouri Psychiatric Rehabilitation Center

3505 Frederick Avenue
Saint Joseph, MO 64506-2914 816-387-2300
Fax: 816-387-2329

Donna Buchanan, PhD, COO

Inpatient care for long-term psychiatric/adult.

4108 Southeast Missouri Mental Health Center

1010 W Columbia Street
Farmington, MO 63640 573-218-6792
Fax: 573-218-6807

Donald Barton, Contact

4109 Southwest Missouri Mental Health Center

1301 Industrial Parkway E
El Dorado Springs, MO 64744 417-876-1002
Fax: 417-876-1004

Richard Scotten, Contact

4110 St. Louis Psychiatric Rehabilitation Center

5300 Arsenal Street
Saint Louis, MO 63139-1463 314-644-8000
Fax: 314-644-8115

Roberta Gardine, Contact

4111 Western Missouri Mental Health Center
1000 E 24th Street
Kansas City, MO 64108 816-512-7000
Fax: 816-512-7509

Gloria Joseph, Contact

Montana

4112 Montana State Hospital
Warmsprings Campus
Warmsprings, MT 59756 406-693-7000
Fax: 406-693-7023

Debra Dirkson, Contact

Nebraska

4113 Hastings Regional Center
4200 W 2nd Street
PO Box 579
Hastings, NE 68902-0579 402-463-2471
Fax: 402-460-3134

Michael Sheehan, Contact

4114 Norfolk Regional Center
1700 N Victory Road
PO Box 1209
Norfolk, NE 68701-6859 402-370-3400
Fax: 402-370-3194

Dan Sturgis, Contact

Nevada

4115 Nevada Mental Health Institute
480 Galletti Way
Sparks, NV 89431-5573 775-688-2001
Fax: 775-688-2052

David Rosin MD, Contact

4116 Southern Nevada Adult Mental Health Services
6161 W Charleston Boulevard
Las Vegas, NV 89102-1126 702-486-6000
Fax: 702-486-6248

Jim Northrop PhD, Contact

New Hampshire

4117 New Hampshire State Hospital
36 Clinton Street
Concord, NH 03301-2359 603-271-5200
Fax: 603-271-5395

Chester Batchelder, CHE

New Jersey

4118 Ancora Psychiatric Hospital
202 Spring Garden Road
Ancora, NJ 08037-9699 609-561-1700
Fax: 609-561-2509

Greg Roberts, Contact

4119 Arthur Brisbane Child Treatment Center
Allaire Road
PO Box 625
Farmingdale, NJ 07727-0625 732-938-5061
Fax: 732-938-3102

Raymond Grimaldi, Contact

4120 Forensic Psychiatric Hospital
PO Box 7717
W Trenton, NJ 08628-0717 609-633-0900
Fax: 609-633-0971

John Main, Contact

4121 Greystone Park Psychiatric Hospital
Greystone Park, NJ 07950 973-538-1800
Fax: 973-993-8782

Michael Greenstein, Contact

4122 Jersey City Medical Center Behavioral Health Center
50 Baldwin Avenue
Jersey City, NJ 07304 201-915-2000
Fax: 201-915-2038

4123 Senator Garrett Hagedorm Center for Geriatrics
200 Sanitarium Road
Glen Gardner, NJ 08826-3291 908-537-2141
Fax: 908-537-3149

Edna Volpeway, Contact

New Mexico

4124 Hampstead Hospital
218 E Road
Hamptead, NM 03841 603-229-5311
Fax: 603-329-4746
www.hampsteadhospital.com

4125 Life Transition Therapy
110 Delgado Street
Santa Fe, NM 87501-2781 505-982-4183
800-547-2574
Fax: 505-982-9219
E-mail: info@lifetransition.com
www.lifetransition.com

Sabina Schultze, Therapist
Ralph Steele, Therapist

Promotes individual and social healing through meditation practice, education and research.

4126 New Mexico State Hospital
Las Vegas Medical Center
PO Box 1388
Las Vegas, NM 87701-1388 505-454-2100
Fax: 505-454-2346

Felix Alderete, Contact

4127 Northern New Mexico Rehabilitation Center

Las Vegas Medical Center
PO Box 1388
Las Vegas, NM 87701-1388   505-454-5100

Felix Alderete, Contact

4128 Sequoyah Adolescent Treatment Center

3405 W Pan American Freeway NE
Albuquerque, NM 87107-4786   505-344-4673
Fax: 505-344-4676
E-mail: hgardner@health.state.nm.us

WH Gardner PhD, Contact

A facility of the Department of Health, State of New Mexico, Sequoyah is a thirty six bed residential treatment center. The purpose of Sequoyah is to provide care, treatment and reintegration in to society for adolesents whao are violent or who have a mental disorder and who are amenable to treatment. Services are provided based upon the client's needs and integrated within the continuum of services offered throughout the state.

New York

4129 Binghamton Psychiatric Center

425 Robinson Street
Binghamton, NY 13901-4198   607-724-1391
Fax: 607-773-4387
E-mail: binghamton@Omh.State.Ny.Us
www.omh.state.ny.us/omhweb/facilities/bipc/

Margaret R Dugan, Executive Director

Comprehensive outpatient and inpatient services for individuals who are seriously mentally ill. BPC is a teaching and learning institution which provides many opportunities for clinical internships to a variety of students training for professional careers in social work, psychology, nursing, theraputic recreation, dietary and health information management.

130 Bronx Children's Psychiatric Center

1000 Waters Place
Bronx, NY 10461-2799   718-239-3600
Fax: 718-239-3669

Mark Bienstock, Contact

131 Bronx Psychiatric Center

1500 Waters Place
Bronx, NY 10461-2796   718-931-0600
Fax: 718-597-8015

Leroy Carmichael, Contact

132 Brooklyn Children's Psychiatric Center

1819 Bergen Street
Brooklyn, NY 11233-4513   718-221-4500
Fax: 718-221-4581

Mark Bienstock, Contact

4133 BryLin Hospitals

1263 Delaware Avenue
Buffalo, NY 14209   716-886-8200
800-727-9546
Fax: 716-889-1986
E-mail: mis@brylin.com
www.brylin.com

4134 Buffalo Psychiatric Center

400 Forest Avenue
Buffalo, NY 14213-1298   716-885-2261
Fax: 716-885-4852

George Molnar MD, Contact

4135 Capital District Psychiatric Center

75 New Scotland Avenue
Albany, NY 12208-3474   518-447-9611
Fax: 518-434-0041

Jesse Nixon PhD, Contact

4136 Central New York Forensic Psychiatric Center

PO Box 300
Marcy, NY 13404-0300   315-736-8271
Fax: 315-768-7210

Harold E Smith, Contact

4137 Creedmoor Psychiatric Center

80-45 Winchester Boulevard
Queens Village, NY 11427-2199   718-464-7500
Fax: 718-264-3636

Charlotte Seltzer CSW, Contact

4138 Elmira Psychiatric Center

100 Washington Street
Elmira, NY 14901-2898   607-737-4739
Fax: 607-737-9080

William L Benedict, Executive Director

4139 Graham-Windham Services for Children and Families: Manhattan Mental Health Center

151 W 136th Street
Lenox & 7th Avenue
New York, NY   212-368-4100
Fax: 212-614-9811
E-mail: info@graham-windham.org

Offers mental health services to children from birth through 18 years and their families: individual, family and group therapy, psychiatric evaluation and medication management, psychological assessment. Family support services program offering advocacy, support and referrals to families with seriously emotionally disturbed children.

4140 Hudson River Psychiatric Center

10 Ross Circle
Poughkeepsie, NY 12601-1197   845-452-8000
Fax: 845-452-8040

James Regan PhD, Contact

4141 Hutchings Psychiatric Center
620 Madison Street
Syracuse, NY 13210-2319   315-473-4980
                                 Fax: 315-473-4984

Bryan Rudes, Contact

4142 Kingsboro Psychiatric Center
681 Clarkson Avenue
Brooklyn, NY 11203-2199   718-221-7700
                                 Fax: 718-221-7206

John Palmer PhD, Contact

4143 Kirby Forensic Psychiatric Center
600 E 125th Street
New York, NY 10035   646-672-5800
                                 Fax: 646-672-6893

Renate Wack PhD, Contact

4144 Manhattan Psychiatric Center
600 E 125th Street
New York, NY 10035-6098   646-672-6000
                                 Fax: 646-672-6446

Horace Belton, Contact

4145 Mid-Hudson Forensic Psychiatric Center
Box 158, Route 17-M
New Hampton, NY 10958   845-374-3171
                                 Fax: 845-374-3961

Rich Bennett, Contact

4146 Middletown Psychiatric Center
122 Dorothea Dix Drive
Middletown, NY 10940-6198   845-342-5511
                                 Fax: 845-342-4975

James Bopp, Contact

4147 Mohawk Valley Psychiatric Center
1400 Noyes at York
Utica, NY 13502-3802   315-797-6800
                                 Fax: 315-738-4412

Sarah Rudes, Contact

4148 Nathan S Kline Institute
140 Old Orangeburg Road
Orangeburg, NY 10962-1197   845-398-5500
                                 Fax: 845-398-5510
                    E-mail: webmaster@nki.rfmh.org
                                 www.rfmh.org/nki

Robert Cancro MD, Director
Jerome Levine MD, Deputy Director

Research programs in Alzheimer's disease, analytical psychopharmacology, basic and clinical neuroimaging, cellular and molecular neurobiology, clinical trail data management, co-occuring disorders and many other mental health studies.

4149 New York Psychiatric Institute
1051 Riverside Drive
New York, NY 10032-2695   212-543-5000
                                 Fax: 212-543-6012

John Oldham MD, Contact

4150 Pilgrim Psychiatric Center
998 Crooked Hill Road
West Brentwood, NY 11717-1087   631-761-3500
                                 Fax: 631-761-2600

Kathleen Kelly, Contact

4151 Queens Children's Psychiatric Center
74-03 Commonwealth Boulevard
Bellerose, NY 11426-1890   718-264-4500
                                 Fax: 718-740-0968

Gloria Faretra, Contact

4152 Rochester Psychiatric Center
1111 Elmwood Avenue
Rochester, NY 14620-3972   585-241-1200
                                 Fax: 585-241-1424

Bryan Rudes, Contact

4153 Rockland Children's Psychiatric Center
599 Convent Road
Orangeburg, NY 10962-1199   845-359-7400
                                 800-597-8481
                                 Fax: 845-359-7461
              E-mail: RocklandCPC@Omh.State.Ny.Us
              www.omh.state.ny.us/omhweb/facility/rcph/facility

David Woodlock, Contact

RCPC is a JCAHO accredited children's psychiatric center. We provide inpatient care to youngsters 10 - 18 years of age from the lower Hudson Valley. An array of local, school - based outpatient services are available in each of the seven counties in the area.

4154 Rockland Psychiatric Center
140 Old Orangeburg Road
Orangeburg, NY 10962-1196   845-359-1000
                                 Fax: 845-359-1744

James Bopp, Contact

4155 Sagamore Children's Psychiatric Center
197 Half Hollow Road
Dix Hills, NY 11746   631-673-7700
                                 Fax: 631-673-7816

Robert Schwitzer EdD, Contact

4156 South Beach Psychiatric Center
777 Seaview Avenue
Staten Island, NY 10305-3499   718-667-2300
                                 Fax: 718-667-2344
                                 E-mail: y.htm
              www.omh.state.ny.us/omhweb/facilities/sbpc/facilit

William F. Henry, Executive Director
Marion S. Schaal, Director Of Customer Services

South Beach Psychiatric Center is a New York State Ofice of Mental Health comprehensive psychiatric facility providing inpatient service on the Staten Island campus and outpatient service in local community sites in Brooklyn and Staten Island boroughs of New York City.

4157 St. Lawrence Psychiatric Center

1 Chimney Point Drive
Ogdensburg, NY 13669   315-541-2001
     Fax: 315-541-2013

John Scott, Contact

4158 Western New York Children's Psychiatric Center

1010 E & W Road
W Seneca, NY 14224-3698   716-674-6300
     Fax: 716-675-6455

Jed Cohen, Contact

North Carolina

4159 Broughton Hospital

1000 S Sterling Street
Morganton, NC 28655   828-433-2111
     Fax: 828-438-6396
E-mail: BH.Information@NCMail.net
www.broughtonhospital.org

Seth P Hunt, Contact

4160 Cherry Hospital

201 Stevens Mill Road
Goldsboro, NC 27530-1057   919-731-3204
     Fax: 919-731-3785

Jerry Edwards, Contact

4161 Dorthea Dix Hospital

S Boylan Avenue
Raleigh, NC 27603-2176   919-733-5324
     Fax: 919-715-0707

Mike Pedneau, Contact

4162 John Umstead Hospital

1003 12th Street
Butner, NC 27509-1626   919-575-7229
     Fax: 919-575-7643

Patricia Christian, Contact

North Dakota

4163 North Dakota State Hospital

PO Box 476
Jamestown, ND 58402-0476   701-328-2060
     Fax: 701-253-3999

Alex Schweitzer EdD, Contact

Ohio

4164 Appalachian Behavioral Healthcare System

Athens Campus
100 Hospital Drive
Athens, OH 45701-2301   740-594-5000
     800-372-8862
     Fax: 740-594-3006

Don W Mobley, CEO
Mark McGee MD, CCO
Kelly Douglas-Markins, Hospital Manager

40 Bed inpatient psychiatric facility.

4165 Appalachian Psychiatric Healthcare System

Cambridge Campus
66737 Old Twenty One Road
Cambridge, OH 43725-9298   740-439-1381
     Fax: 740-432-7567

Steven Pierson PhD, Contact

4166 Hannah Neil Center for Children

301 Obetz Road
Columbus, OH 43207-4092   614-491-5784
     E-mail: suzan@worldofchildren.org

Randy Copas, Director

The Hannah Neil Center for Children serves children who suffer from severe behavioral and emotional difficulties.

4167 Massillon Psychiatric Center

3000 Erie Street S
Massillon, OH 44648-0540   330-833-3135
     Fax: 330-929-6656

Cathy Cincinat, Contact

4168 Millcreek Children's Services

6600 Paddock Road
PO Box 16006
Cincinnati, OH 45237-3983   513-948-3983
     Fax: 513-948-0443

Peter Steele, Contact

4169 Northcoast Behavioral Healthcare System

Cleveland Campus
1708 Southpoint Drive
Cleveland, OH 44109-1999   216-787-0500
     Fax: 216-787-0633

George P Gintoli, Contact

4170 Northcoast Behavioral Healthcare System

Northfield Campus
PO Box 305
Northfield, OH 44067-0305   330-467-7131
     Fax: 330-467-2420

George P Gintoli, Contact

4171 Northwest Psychiatric Hospital

930 S Detroit Avenue
Caller Number 10002
Toledo, OH 43614-2701   419-381-1881
     Fax: 419-389-1361

Terrance Smith, Contact

4172 Paulene Warfield Lewis Center

1101 Summit Road
Cincinnati, OH 45237-2652   513-948-3600
     Fax: 513-821-5034

Liz Banks, Contact

4173 Sagamore Children's Services: Woodside CSN

Sagamore Children's CSN
3076 Remsen Road
Medina, OH 44256   330-722-0750
                      Fax: 330-723-0068

Charles Johnson, Contact

4174 Sagamore Children's Services: Woodside CSN

Woodside CSN
419 Main Avenue SW
Warren, OH 44481   330-742-2593
                      Fax: 330-742-2598

Charles Johnston, Contact

4175 Twin Valley Behavioral Healthcare

Dayton Campus, 2611 Wayne Avenue
Dayton, OH 45420-1800   937-258-0440
                      Fax: 937-258-6218
                      TDD: 937-258-6257

James Ignelzi, CEO

4176 Twin Valley Psychiatric System

Columbus Campus, 1960 W Broad Street
Columbus, OH 43223   614-752-0333
                      Fax: 614-752-0385

James Ignelzi, Contact

Oklahoma

4177 Eastern State Hospital

PO Box 69
Vinita, OK 74301-0069   918-256-7841
                      Fax: 918-256-4491

William Burkett, Contact

4178 Griffin Memorial Hospital

900 E Main Street
PO Box 151
Norman, OK 73070-0151   405-321-4880
                      Fax: 405-522-8320

Don Bowen, Contact

4179 Oklahoma Youth Center

1120 E Main Street
PO Box 1008
Norman, OK 73070-1008   405-364-9004
                      Fax: 405-573-3804

Paul Bouffard, Contact

4180 Western State Psychiatric Center

1222 10th Street
Woodward, OK 73801   580-571-3233
                      Fax: 580-256-8609
                      www.odmhsas.org

Steve Norwood, Contact

Comprehensive regional behavioral health center.

4181 Willow Crest Hospital

Miami, OK   918-542-1836
                      www.willowcresthospital.com

Oregon

4182 Eastern Oregon Psychiatric Hospital

2575 Westgate
Pendleton, OR 97801-9613   541-246-0810
                      Fax: 541-276-1147

Steve Shambaugh, Contact

4183 Oregon State Hospital: Portland

1225 NE 2nd Avenue
Portland, OR 97232   503-731-8620
                      www.omhs.mhd.hr.state.or.us

4184 Oregon State Hospital: Salem

2600 Center Street NE
Salem, OR 97301-2682   503-945-2800
                      Fax: 503-945-2807

David Freed   PhD, Interim Superintendent

4185 St. Mary's Home for Boys

16535 SW Tualatin Valley Highway
Beaverton, OR 97006-5199   503-649-5651
                      Fax: 503-649-7405
E-mail: reception@stmaryshomeforboys.org
                      www.stmaryshomeforboys.org

Founded in 1889 as an orphanage for abandoned and wayward children, today St. Mary's offers residential treatment and services to at-risk boys between the ages of 10 and 17 who are emotionally disturbed and behaviorally delinquent.

Pennsylvania

4186 Allentown State Hospital

1600 Hanover Avenue
Allentown, PA 18103-2498   610-740-3400
                      Fax: 610-740-3413

Gregory Smith, Contact

4187 Clarks Summit State Hospital

1451 Hillside Drive
Clarks Summit, PA 18411-9505   570-587-7250
                      Fax: 570-587-7415

Thomas P Comerford Jr, Contact

4188 Mayview State Hospital

1601 Mayview Road
Bridgeville, PA 15017-1599   412-257-6200
                      Fax: 412-257-6800

Shirley Dumpman MPH, Contact

4189 Norristown State Hospital

Stanbridge & Sterigere Streets
Norristown, PA 19401-5397   610-313-1000
                      Fax: 610-313-1013

Aidan Altenor PhD, Contact

4190 Renfrew Center Foundation

475 Spring Lane
Philadelphia, PA 19128   877-367-3383
Fax: 215-482-2695
E-mail: foundation@renfrew.org
www.renfrew.org

This facility is a tax exempt, nonprofit organization advancing the education , prevention, research and treatment of the mental illness eater disorders.

4191 State Correctional Institution at Waymart

Forensic Treatment Center
PO Box 256
Waymart, PA 18472-0256   570-488-5811
Fax: 570-488-2550

Martin Andrews, Contact

4192 Torrance State Hospital

PO Box 111
Torrance, PA 15779-0111   724-459-4511
Fax: 724-459-4498

Richard Stillwagon, Contact

4193 Warren State Hospital

33 Main Drive
N Warren, PA 16365-5099   814-723-5500
Fax: 814-726-4119

Carmen Ferranto, Contact

4194 Wernersville State Hospital

PO Box 300
Wernersville, PA 19565-0300   610-678-3411
Fax: 610-670-4101

Kenneth Ehrhart, Contact

Rhode Island

4195 Butler Hospital

345 Blackstone Boulevard
Providence, RI 02906   401-455-6200
www.butler.org

South Carolina

4196 CM Tucker Jr Nursing Care Center

2200 Harden Street
Columbia, SC 29203-7199   803-737-5300
Fax: 803-737-5364

Laura W Hughes, RN, BSN, MPH, Director
Robert Miller, NHA
Frances F Corley, NHA

Five hundred sixty bed nursing care center providing skilled and intermediate level of care. Operated by the South Carolina Department of Mental Health.

4197 Coastal Carolina Hospital

152 Waccamaw Medical Park Drive
Conway, SC 29526-8922   843-347-7156
Fax: 843-347-7176

4198 Earle E Morris Jr Alcohol & Drug Treatment Center

610 Faison Drive
Columbia, SC 29203   803-935-7100
Fax: 803-935-7781

Louis Haynes, Contact

4199 G Werber Bryan Psychiatric Hospital

220 Faison Drive
Columbia, SC 29203-3295   803-935-7140
Fax: 803-935-7110

Beverly Wood MD, Contact

4200 James F Byrnes Medical Center

2100 Bull Street
Box 119
Columbia, SC 29202-0119   803-254-9325
Fax: 803-734-0779

Jaime E Condom MD, Contact

4201 Patrick B Harris Psychiatric Hospital

PO Box 2907
Anderson, SC 29622-2907   864-231-2600
Fax: 864-225-3297

Arthur Robarge PhD, Contact

4202 South Carolina State Hospital

2100 Bull Street
Columbia, SC 29202   803-898-2038
Fax: 803-898-2048

Jaime E Condon MD, Contact

Psychiatric hospital

4203 William S Hall Psychiatric Institute

1800 Colonial Drive
PO Box 202
Columbia, SC 29292-0202   803-898-1693
Fax: 803-898-2048

Dalmer Sercy, Contact

South Dakota

4204 South Dakota Human Services Center

3515 Broadway Avenue
PO Box 76
Yankton, SD 57078-0076   605-668-3100
Fax: 605-668-3460

Cory Nelson, Interim Administrator

Tennessee

4205 Camelot Care Center: Bridge Therapeutic Foster Care

659 Emory Valley Road
Suite B
Oak Ridge, TN 37830   423-481-3972

Treatment option for severely troubled children who have been referred for out-of-home placement or who are in need of a step-down from a more intensive level of care. The goal is to tech troubled children how to be successfull in a family and community to facilitate the child's return to a more permanent placement.

4206 Lakeshore Mental Health Institute

5908 Lyons View Drive
Knoxville, TN 37919-7598   865-584-1561
                                  Fax: 423-450-5222

Lee Thomas, Contact

4207 Memphis Mental Health Institute

865 Poplar Avenue
Memphis, TN 38105-4626   901-524-1200
                                Fax: 901-524-1332

Russell Davidson, Contact

4208 Middle Tennessee Mental Health Institute

221 Stewarts Ferry Pike
Nashville, TN 37214-3325   615-902-7400
                                  Fax: 615-902-7541

Joseph Carobene, Contact

4209 Moccasin Bend Mental Health Institute

100 Moccasin Bend Road
Chattanooga, TN 37405-4496   423-265-2271
                                    Fax: 423-785-3347

Russell Vatter, Contact

4210 Western Mental Health Institute

Highway 64 W
Bolivar, TN 38074-9999   731-228-2000
                                Fax: 731-658-2044

Elizabeth Littlefield MD, Contact

4211 Woodridge Hospital

403 State of Franklin Road
Johnson City, TN 37604   423-928-7111
                                800-346-8899
                                Fax: 423-979-7492
       E-mail: kcudebec@frontierhealth.org
                          www.frontierhealth.org

Dr. Donald W Larkin, Administrator
Kim Cudebec, Clinical Director

Texas

4212 Austin State Hospital

4110 Guadalupe Street
Austin, TX 78751-4296   512-452-0381
                               Fax: 512-323-6150

Carl Schock, Superintendent

4213 Big Spring State Hospital

Highway 87 N
PO Box 231
Big Spring, TX 79721-0231   432-268-8216
                                   Fax: 432-268-7259

Edward Moghon, Contact

4214 Dallas Mental Health Connection

5909 Harry Hines Boulevard
Dallas, TX 75235   214-879-2826
                          Fax: 214-879-2834

Mary Nguyen, Contact

4215 Dallas Metrocare Services

1380 Riverbend Drive
Dallas, TX 75247   214-743-1200
                          Fax: 214-630-3642

Serves the mentally ill community

4216 El Paso Psychiatric Center

4615 Alameda
El Paso, TX 79905   915-532-2202
                           Fax: 915-534-5587

Josie Herrera, Contact

Hospital serving El Paso and the surrounding community. Dedicated to treatment conducted in an environment of compassion, respect, and on addressing individual and family needs. For adults and children, both high and low functioning.

4217 Harris County Psychiatric Center

2800 S MacGregor
Houston, TX 77021   713-741-5000
                           Fax: 713-741-7832

David R Small, Contact

4218 Kerrville State Hospital

721 Thompson Drive
Kerrville, TX 78028-5199   830-896-2211
                                  Fax: 830-825-6269

Gloria P Olson PhD, Contact

4219 New Horizons Ranch and Center

PO Box 549
Goldthwaite, TX 76844   915-938-5518
                               Fax: 915-938-5665
                               www.newhorizonsinc.com

To provide an environment where children, families and staff are able to heal and grow through caring relationships and unconditional love and acceptance.

4220 Rio Grande State Center for Mental Health & Mental Retardation

PO Box 2668
Harlingen, TX 78551-2668   956-425-8900
                                  Fax: 956-430-2496

Sonia Hernandez-Keeble, Contact

4221 Rusk State Hospital

Highway 69 N
PO Box 318
Rusk, TX 75785-0318   903-683-3421
                             Fax: 903-683-4303

Harrold R Parrish Jr, Contact

4222 San Antonio State Hospital
PO Box 23991
San Antonio, TX 78223-0991   210-531-8128
                                      Fax: 210-534-0067
E-mail: robert.arizpe@mhmrstatetx.us
www.mhmr.state.tx.us/hospitals/sanantonioSH
Robert Arizpe, Contact

4223 Terrell State Hospital
PO Box 70
Terrell, TX 75160-9000   972-563-6452
                                 Fax: 972-551-1094

Beatrice Butler, Contact

4224 Vernon State Hospital
PO Box 2231
Vernon, TX 76385-2231   940-552-9901
                                Fax: 940-553-2500

Jim Smith, Contact

4225 Waco Center for Youth
3501 N 19th Street
Waco, TX 76708   254-754-5174
                         Fax: 254-745-5369

Dana Renschler, Contact

4226 Wichita Falls State Hospital
PO Box 300
Wichita Falls, TX 76307-0300   940-692-1220
                                        Fax: 940-689-5538

Jim Smith, Contact

Utah

4227 Utah State Hospital
1300 E Center Street
Provo, UT 84603-3554   801-344-4400
                               Fax: 801-344-4291

Mark Payne, Contact

Vermont

4228 Brattleboro Retreat
Anna Marsh Lane
PO Box 803
Brattleboro, VT 05302   802-257-7785
                                Fax: 802-258-3791
www.bratretreat.org

4229 Spring Lake Ranch
PO Box 310
Cuttingville, VT 05738   802-492-3322
                                 Fax: 802-492-3331
E-mail: springlakeranch@mindspring.com
www.springlakeranch.org

Seventy-five-year-old residential treatment facility for men and women over the age of 17. Also offers aftercare and supported apartment program.

4230 Vermont State Hosptial
103 S Main Street
Waterbury, VT 05671-2501   802-241-1000
                                   Fax: 802-241-3001

Bertold Francke MD, Contact

Virginia

4231 Catawba Hospital
PO Box 200
Catawba, VA 24070-2006   540-375-4200
                                 Fax: 540-375-4394

James S Reinhard MD, Contact

4232 Central State Hospital
PO Box 4030
Petersburg, VA 23803-0030   804-524-7373
                                    Fax: 504-524-4571

Daniel O'Donnel MD, Contact

4233 De Jarnette Center
PO Box 2309
Staunton, VA 24402-2309   540-332-2100
                                  Fax: 540-332-2201

Andrea C Newsome, Contact

4234 Dominion Hospital
2960 Sleepy Hollow Road
Falls Church, VA 22044   703-536-2000
                                 Fax: 703-536-6601
E-mail: catherine.morse@hcahealthcare.com
www.dominionhospital.com
Catherine Morse, Admissions

Psychiatric hospital serving children, adolesents, adults and senior adults with age specific inpatient and partial hospitalization programs. Teams of psychiatrists, nurses and therapists offer patients short term crisis intervention, stabilization, evaluation and discharge planning. Dominion participates in most major insurance and managed care health plans.

4235 Eastern State Hospital
PO Box 8791
Williamsburg, VA 23187-8791   757-253-5241
                                       Fax: 757-253-5065

John M Favret, Contact

4236 Hiram W Davis Medical Center
PO Box 4030
Petersburg, VA 23803-0030   804-524-7344
                                    Fax: 804-524-7148

David A Rosenquist, Contact

4237 Nothern Virginia Mental Health Institute
3302 Gallows Road
Falls Church, VA 22042-3398   703-207-7100
                                       Fax: 703-207-7146

John C Russotto, Contact

4238 Piedmont Geriatric Hospital
PO Box 427
Burkeville, VA 23922-0427   434-767-4404
                                   Fax: 434-767-4951
                                   www.pgh.state.va.us

Willard R Pierce Jr, Contact

4239 Southern Virginia Mental Health Institute
382 Taylor Drive
Danville, VA 24541-4023   434-799-6220
                                 Fax: 434-773-4274
              E-mail: ngibson@svmhi.state.va.us
                        www.svmhi.state.va.us

Constance N Fletcher PhD, Contact

4240 Southwestern Virginia Mental Health Institute
340 Bagley Circle
Marion, VA 24354-3390   267-783-1200
                               Fax: 540-783-9712
              E-mail: sveselik@swvmhi.state.va.us
                        www.swvmhi.state.va.us

Gerald E Deans, Contact

4241 Western State Hospital
PO Box 2500
Staunton, VA 24401-9124   540-332-8200
                                 Fax: 540-332-8197

Jack Barber, Contact

Washington

4242 Child Study & Treatment Center
8805 Steilacoom Boulevard SW
Tacoma, WA 98498-4771   253-756-2504
                               Fax: 253-756-3911

Mary Lafond, Contact

4243 Eastern State Hospital
PO Box A
Medical Lake, WA 99022-0045   509-299-3121
                                     Fax: 509-299-4596

Jan Gregg, Contact

4244 Ryther Child Center
2400 NE 95th Street
Seattle, WA 98115-2499   206-525-5050
                                Fax: 206-525-9795
                                www.ryther.org

Ryther Child Center provides family support and education, early childhood and family services, intensive residential treatment, chemical dependency treatment, mental health counseling, training and consultation to nearly 5,000 children, families and community members each year.

4245 Western State Hospital
9601 Steilacoom Boulevard SW
Tacoma, WA 98498-7213   253-582-8900
                               Fax: 253-756-2963

Jerry Dennis MD, Contact

West Virginia

4246 Highland Hospital
300 56th Street SE
Charleston, WV 25304   800-250-3806
                              www.highlandhosp.com

4247 Mildred Mitchell-Bateman Hospital
1530 Norway Avenue
PO Box 448
Huntington, WV 25709-0448   304-525-7801
                                   800-644-9318
                                   Fax: 304-525-7249
              E-mail: carolwellman@wvdar.org
Carol Wellman, Administrator

4248 Weirton Medical Center
601 Colliers Way
Weirton, WV 26062-5091   304-797-6000

Provider of inpatient and outpatient mental health services.

4249 Weston State Hospital
PO Box 1127
Weston, WV 26452-1127   304-269-1210
                               Fax: 304-269-6235

Jack Clohan Jr, Contact

Wisconsin

4250 Bellin Psychiatric Center
301 E St. Joseph Street
PO Box 23725
Green Bay, WI 54305   920-433-3630
              E-mail: lsroet@bellin.org
                        www.bellin.org/psych

4251 Elmbrook Memorial Hospital
19333 W North Avenue
Brookfield, WI 53045-4198   262-785-2000
                                   Fax: 262-785-2485
              www.http://207.198.127.147/affiliat/elmbr.shtml

4252 Mendota Mental Health Institute
301 Troy Drive
Madison, WI 53704-1599   608-301-1000
                                Fax: 608-301-1358
              www.dhfs.state.wi.us/MH_Mendota/
Steve Walters, Contact

4253 Winnebago Mental Health Institute
PO Box 9
Winnebago, WI 54985-0009   920-235-4910
                                  Fax: 920-237-2043

Joan O'Connor, Contact

Wyoming

4254 Wyoming State Hospital
PO Box 177
Evanston, WY 82931-0177   307-789-3464
                              Fax: 307-789-5277

Pablo Hernandez MD, Contact

Management Companies

4256 100 Top Series

Dorland Healthcare Information
1500 Walnut Street
Suite 1000
Philadelphia, PA 19102   215-875-1212
                                800-784-2332
                           Fax: 215-735-3966
          E-mail: info@dorlandhealth.com
                 www.dorlandhealth.com

A leader in health and managed care business information. *$495.00*

Year Founded: 1999

4257 ABE

21 Merchants Row
Boston, MA 02109-2005   617-742-9406
                               800-694-5285
                          Fax: 800-694-7882

4258 ACORN Behavioral Care Management Corporation

134 N Narberth Avenue
Narberth, PA 19072-2299   610-664-8350
                                 800-223-7050

4259 ADA/EAP Consulting

PO Box 60348
Sacramento, CA 95860-0348   916-974-1436

4260 ADAPS

1154 Fort Street Mall
Suite 209
Honolulu, HI 96813-2712   808-528-1184
                            Fax: 808-566-1885

4261 APOGEE

900 West Valley Forge Road
Box 61846
King of Prussia, PA 19406-1336   610-337-3200
                                        877-337-3200
                                   Fax: 610-337-2337
          E-mail: info@apogeeinsgroup.com
                 www.apogeeinsgroup.com

4262 Academy of Managed Care Providers

1945 Palo Verde Avenue
Suite 202
Long Beach, CA 90815-3445   562-596-8660
                                   800-297-2627
                              Fax: 562-799-3355
          E-mail: staff@academymcp.org
                 www.academymcp.org

Dr. John Russell, President
Mary McConnell, Director Member Services

National organization of clinicans and MCO professionals. Provides many services to members including continuing education, diplomate certification, notification of panel openings and practice opportunities, newsletter, group health insurance and many other benefits.

4263 Access Behavioral Care

117 S 17th Street
Suite 900
Philadelphia, PA 19103-5009   215-567-3638
                                Fax: 215-567-5572

4264 Accountable Oncology Associates

1430 Spring Hill Road
Suite 106
Mc Lean, VA 22102-3013   703-506-8244
                                800-482-2280
                           Fax: 703-506-0623

4265 Acorn Behavioral Healthcare Management Corporation

134 N Narberth Avenue
Narberth, PA 19072-2299   215-664-8350

4266 Action Healthcare

301 E Bethany Home Road
Phoenix, AZ 85012-1263   602-277-4748
                                800-433-0681

4267 Adanta Group-Behavioral Health Services

259 Parkers Mill Road
Somerset, KY 42501   606-678-2768
                       Fax: 606-678-5296

4268 Adult Learning Systems

1954 S Industrial Highway
Suite A
Ann Arbor, MI 48104-4625   734-668-7447
                             Fax: 734-668-2772
          E-mail: a.roelofs@internetmci.com

4269 Advanced Clinical Systems

49 Music Square W
Suite 502
Nashville, TN 37203-3272   615-231-5577
                             Fax: 615-321-5566

Provide managed behavioral healthcare services to employers and payors nationally. Services include capitated carveouts, employee assistance programs, provider networks, and utilization management programs.

4270 Advanced Healthcare Services Group

105 Bristol Lane
Alpharetta, GA 30022-6382   404-813-1859

4271 Aetna-US HealthCare

151 Farmington Avenue
Stop 21 F
Hartford, CT 06156
860-273-0123
800-323-9930
www.aetna.com

4272 Aldrich and Cox

3075 Southwestern Boulevard
Suite 202
Orchard Park, NY 14127-1287
716-675-6300
Fax: 716-675-2098

4273 Alexander Consulting Group

225 N Michigan Avenue
Chicago, IL 60601-7601
312-346-8822

4274 Alliance Behavioral Care

222 Piedmont Avenue, Suite 3300
Med Arts Building ML 665
Cincinnati, OH 45219-4231
513-375-8710
Fax: 513-475-7614

4275 Allied Center for Therapy

2495 Caring Way
Suite A
Port Charlotte, FL 33952-5380
941-764-0444
Fax: 941-764-0774
E-mail: ccmhs@sunline.net

4276 Allina Hospitals & Clinics Behavioral Health Services

Abbot Northwestern Hospital
710 E 24th Street
Minneapolis, MN 55407-3723
612-863-8873
Fax: 612-775-9733
www.allina.com

Provides clinically and geographically integrated care delivery. Innovative programs and services across comprehensive continuum of care. Practicing guideline development, outcomes data and quality managment programs to enhance care delivery.

4277 Ameen Consulting and Associates

7025 Noffke Drive
Caledonia, MI 49316-8806
616-891-9339
Fax: 616-891-9339

4278 AmeriChoice

8045 Leesburg Pike, Ste.650
Wanamaker Building
Vienna, VA 22182
703-506-3555
Fax: 212-898-7967
E-mail: webmaster@americhoice.com
www.americhoice.com

4279 American Behavioral Systems

70 W Red Oak Lane
White Plains, NY 10604-3602
914-697-7535
Fax: 914-697-7529
E-mail: MRABS@worldnet.att.net

ABS develops and manages behavioral health care Integrated Delivery Systems. The company works with provider groups and with payers seeking to retool their existing networks.

4280 American Guidance Service (AGS)

4201 Woodland Road
Circle Pines, MN 55014-1796
651-287-7220
800-328-2560
Fax: 800-471-8457
E-mail: agsmail@agsnet.com
www.agsnet.com

AGS is a publisher of assessment tools and instructional materials in the special needs behavior management, speech, language, and mental health markets. Among their numerous products are the Behavior Assessment System for Children (BASC), BASC Monitor for ADHD, Vineland Adaptive Behavior Scales, and the Peabody Picture Vocabulary Test (PPVT-3).

4281 American Healthware Systems

4522 Fort Hamilton Parkway
Brooklyn, NY 11219-2410
718-435-6300

4282 American Managed Behavioral Healthcare Association

1101 Pennsylvania Avenue NW
6th Floor
Washington, DC 20004
Fax: 202-756-7308
www.ambha.org

A non-profit trade association representing the nation's leading managed behavioral healthcare organizations. These organizations collectively manage mental health and substance abuse services for its over 100 million individuals.

Year Founded: 1994

4283 Analysis Group Economics

1 Brattle Square
Suite 5
Cambridge, MA 02138-3723
617-349-2100
Fax: 617-864-3742

4284 Aon Consulting Group

125 Chubb Avenue
Lyndhurst, NJ 07071-3504
201-460-6600
Fax: 201-460-6999

4285 Arizona Center For Mental Health PC

3352 E Camelback Road
Suite I
Phoenix, AZ 85018-2310
602-954-6700

4286 Arthur S Shorr and Associates

4710 Desert Drive
Suite 100
Woodland Hills, CA 91364-3720
818-225-7055
Fax: 818-225-7059

4287 Associated Claims Management

390 N Wiget Lane
Walnut Creek, CA 94598-2406
510-930-9883

4288 Associated Counseling Services
8 Roberta Drive
South Dartmouth, MA 02748-2020 508-992-9376

4289 B&W Associates Health and Human Services Consultants
8 Captain Parker Arms
Lexington, MA 02421-7039 781-862-1588

4290 BB Consulting Group
PO Box 7570
Berkeley, CA 94707-0570 510-528-2263
Fax: 510-524-2533
E-mail: bbconsults@aol.com

Betty Bleicher LCSW, Principal

Works with behavioral healthcare organizations to develop and promote programs, negotiate contracts and create a service delivery system that is sensitive to the managed care environment. Specializes in assisting organizations to obtain their necessary accreditation.

4291 BROOKS and Associates
680 Boston Post Road
Weston, MA 02493-1522 781-891-1306

4292 Babylon Consultation Center
534 Deer Park Avenue
Babylon, NY 11702-1929 516-587-1924

4293 Barbanell Associates
3629 Sacramento Street
San Francisco, CA 94118-1709 415-929-1155

4294 Barry Associates
PO Box 586
Kokomo, IN 46903-0586 765-459-5761
Fax: 765-459-5779
E-mail: barryaso@netusa1.net
www.barry-online.com

John S Barry MSW, MBA, President

Provides technical assistance services to behavioral health and social service organizations in the areas of performance measurement, survey research, program evaluation, compensation system design and other selected human resource management areas.

4295 Behavioral Health Care
6801 S Yosemite Street
Englewood, CO 80112-1406 303-793-9657
Fax: 303-779-6038

4296 Behavioral Health Management Group
Hawley Building
Suite 708
Wheeling, WV 26003 304-232-7232
Fax: 304-232-7245

4297 Behavioral Health Network
1 Pillsbury Street
Suite 300
Concord, NH 03301-3556 603-225-6633
888-386-4343
Fax: 603-228-2246

4298 Behavioral Health Partners
2200 Century Parkway NE
Suite 675
Atlanta, GA 30345-3156 404-315-9325
800-845-6505
Fax: 404-315-0786
www.bhpi.com

Gary Larig, President
Tracey Roxby, VP Business Development

Management consultants to integrated delivery systems, professional practices and public mental health agencies as well as the developers of Connex-a behavioral health software package enabling health care systems, MCOs and EAPs to manage financial, clinical and contract information. Specialize in tailoring partnerships with health care organizations that positively impact the delivery of behavioral health services in their communities.

4299 Behavioral Health Services
800 E 28th Street
Minneapolis, MN 55407-3723 612-863-8633
Fax: 612-863-8876
www.allina.com

Provides clinically and geographically integrated delivery system, innovative programs and services across comprehensive continuum of care, practice guidelines development, outcomes data and quality management programs to enhance care delivery systems.

4300 Behavioral Health Services - Allina Health
800 E 28th Street
Minneapolis, MN 55407-3723 763-717-8727

4301 Behavioral Health Systems
2 Metroplex Drive
Suite 500
Birmingham, AL 35209 205-879-1150
800-245-1150
Fax: 205-879-1178
E-mail: info@bhs-inc.com
www.bhs-inc.com

Deborah L Stephens, Founder/President/CEO
Maureen Gleason, Sr VP/Business Development/COO
Sandy Capps, VP Employee Assistance Programs

Provides managed psychiatric and substance abuse and drug testing services to more than 20,000 employees nationally through a network of 7,600 providers.

4302 Behavioral Healthcare Consultants
12 Windham Lane
Beverly, MA 01915-1568 978-921-5968
Fax: 978-921-5968

4303 BehavioralCare

18881 Von Karman Avenue
Suite 250
Irvine, CA 92612-1572   714-752-1510

4304 Birch and Davis Associates

12 Seven Oaks Lane
Ewing, NJ 08628-1616   609-882-6023

4305 Boylston Group

377 Elliot Street
Newton, MA 02464-1126   617-327-7735

4306 Bright Consulting

2201 Santiago Drive
Newport Beach, CA 92660-3618   949-548-6166
                              Fax: 949-548-6639
                          E-mail: brithcon@aol.com

Kent Dunlop, President

Public sector contracting and business development consultation. System of care design and inter-agency linkage development. Operations management services and consultation.

4307 Broward County Healthcare Management

101 NE 3rd Avenue
Suite 4
Fort Lauderdale, FL 33301-1162   954-765-4610

4308 Brown and Associates

121 N Erie Street
Toledo, OH 43624   419-241-8547
                          800-495-6786
                     Fax: 419-241-8689
     E-mail: info@danbrownconsulting.com
              www.danbrownconsulting.com

4309 CAFCA

1766 S Franklin Street
Denver, CO 80210-3340   303-698-1876

4310 CARE

53 Otter Cove Drive
Old Saybrook, CT 06475-1339   203-433-1092

4311 CBI Group

310 Basse Highway
Park Ridge, IL 60068-3251   847-292-6676
                              Fax: 847-823-0740
                          www.cbipartners.com

4312 CHPS Consulting

40 Beaver Street
Albany, NY 12207-1511   518-426-4315
                          Fax: 518-426-4316

4313 CIGNA Behavioral Care

11095 Viking Drive
Suite 350
Eden Prairie, MN 55344-7234
                              800-433-5768
                  www.apps.cignabehavioral.com

4314 CIGNA Corporation

1601 Chestnut Street
M/B TL378
Philadelphia, PA 19192-0004   215-761-8362
                              Fax: 215-761-5602

4315 CLF Consulting

47 Plaza Street W
Suite 15B
Brooklyn, NY 11217-3905   718-783-5334

4316 CNR Health

2514 S 102nd Street
Suite 100
Milwaukee, WI 53227-2154   262-787-2200
                              800-654-5160
                          Fax: 262-787-2503

Specializes in quality, cost-effective case management services. Services include an EAP; behavioral health, medical, disability and prenatal case management.

4317 CORE Management

200 Wheeler Road
Suite 5
Burlington, MA 01803-5501   781-229-9400

4318 CORE/Peer Review Analysis

2 Copley Place
Boston, MA 02116-6502   617-375-7767
                              Fax: 617-375-7683

4319 CPP Incorporated

3803 E Bayshore Road
PO Box 10096
Palo Alto, CA 94303-4300   650-969-8901
                              800-624-1765
                          Fax: 650-969-8608
                              www.cpp.com

4320 Calland and Company

2296 Henderson Mill Road
Suite 222
Atlanta, GA 30345-2739   770-270-9100
                              Fax: 770-270-9300

4321 Cameron and Associates

6100 Lake Forrest Drive NW
Suite 550
Atlanta, GA 30328-3889   404-843-3399
                              Fax: 404-843-3572

4322 Capital Behavioral Health Company
125 Wolf Road
Suite 205
Albany, NY 12205-1221   518-452-6701
Fax: 518-452-6753

4323 Caregivers Consultation Services
368 Veterans Memorial Highway
Commack, NY 11725-4322   516-269-5392

4324 Carewise
701 5th Avenue
Suite 2600
Seattle, WA 98104-7015   206-749-1100
Fax: 206-749-1125

4325 Casey Family Services
127 Church Street
New Haven, CT 06510   203-929-3837
Fax: 203-401-6901
www.caseyfamilyservices.org

4326 Centennial Mental Health Center
211 W Main Street
Sterling, CO 80751-3142   970-522-4549
Fax: 970-522-9544

Linda Dettmer, Resource Specialist

4327 Center For Prevention And Rehabilitation
26 Conneaut Lake Road
Greenville, PA 16125-2167   724-588-3001
Fax: 724-588-9620

4328 Center for Outcomes Research and Effectiveness
5800 W 10th Street
Suite 605
Little Rock, AR 72204-1773   501-660-7550
Fax: 501-660-7543

4329 Center for Psychology and Behavioral Medicine
9033 Glades Road
Suite B
Boca Raton, FL 33434-3939   561-241-7741

4330 Center for State Policy Research
1911 Fort Myer Drive
Suite 702
Arlington, VA 22209-1605   703-525-7100
Fax: 703-525-5335

4331 Center for the Advancement of Health
2000 Florida Avenue NW
Suite 210
Washington, DC 20009-1231   202-387-2829
Fax: 202-387-2857

4332 Centers for Mental Healthcare Research
5800 W 10th Street
Suite 605
Little Rock, AR 72204-1773   501-660-7559

4333 Central Behavioral Healthcare
6620 W Central Avenue
Suite 101
Toledo, OH 43617-1017   419-841-5934
Fax: 419-841-9447

4334 Century Financial Services
185 NW Spanish River Boulevard
Boca Raton, FL 33431-4227   407-362-0111

4335 Chaisson and Berkowitz
8635 W 3rd Street
Suite 685W
Los Angeles, CA 90048-6109   310-659-3823

4336 Cherokee Health Systems
6350 W Andrew Johnson Highway
Talbott, TN 37877-8605   423-586-5031
Fax: 423-586-0614
www.cherokeehealth.com

Uses an integrated model to provide behavioral health and primary care services in a community-based setting.

4337 Chi Systems
1035 Virginia Drive
Suite 300
Fort Washington, PA 19034   215-542-1400
Fax: 215-542-1400
E-mail: info.pa@chisystems.com
www.chiinc.com

4338 Children's Home of the Wyoming Conference, Quality Improvement
1182 Chenango Street
Binghamton, NY 13901-1653   607-772-6904
Fax: 607-723-2617

Child care agency referred to various departments of social services, court systems, school systems for children who at risk, have trouble in the home, or have been abused or abandoned.

4339 Choate Health Management
500W Cummings Park
Suite 3900
Woburn, MA 01801-6505   781-933-6700
Fax: 781-469-5013

4340 Choice Behavioral Health Partnership
PO Box 551188
Jacksonville, FL 32255-1188   904-996-2000
800-700-8646
Fax: 904-996-2056

4341 ChoiceCare

655 Eden Park Drive, Suite 400
Grand Baldwin Building
Cincinnati, OH 45202-6000   513-241-1400
                                   800-543-7158
                              Fax: 513-684-7461

4342 College Health IPA

7711 Center Avenue
Suite 300
Huntington Beach, CA 92647-3067   562-467-5555
                                   800-779-3825
                              Fax: 562-402-2666
                     E-mail: info@chipa.com
                                   www.chipa.org

Ruth Bikes, Communications

Culturally sensitive mental health referral service.

4343 College of Dupage

22nd and Lambert Road
Glen Ellyn, IL 60137   630-942-2800
                              Fax: 630-858-9399

4344 College of Southern Idaho

PO Box 1238
Twin Falls, ID 83303-1238   208-733-9554
                              Fax: 208-736-4743
                                   www.csi.edu

4345 Columbia Hospital M/H Services

2201 45th Street
W Palm Beach, FL 33407-2095   561-881-2670
                              Fax: 561-881-2668

4346 Columbia/HCA Behavioral Health

1 Park Plaza
Nashville, TN 37203-6527   615-344-5715
                              Fax: 615-344-1561
         E-mail: deborah.cagle@columbia.net
         www.medtropolis.com/behavioralhealth

4347 ComPsych

455 N City Front Plaza Drive
NBC Tower Floor 24
Chicago, IL 60611-5503   312-595-4000
                                   800-755-3050
                              Fax: 312-595-4029
         E-mail: mpaskell@compsych.com
                                   www.compsych.com

Mary Paskell, Directo Marketing

Worlwide leader in guidance resources, including employee assistance programs, managed behavioral health, work-life, legal, financial, and personal convenience services. ComPsych provides services worldwide covering millions of individuals. Clients range from Fortune 100 to smaller public and private concerns, government entities, health plans and Taft-Hartley groups. Guidance Resources transforms traditionally separate services into a seamless integration of information, resources and creative solutions that address personal life challenges and improve workplace productivity and performance.

4348 Community Companions

2001 The Alameda
San Jose, CA 95126-1136   408-261-7777
                              Fax: 408-248-6520

4349 Compass Health Systems

1065 NE 125th Street
Suite 409
N Miami, FL 33161-5834   305-891-0050
                                   888-852-6672
                              Fax: 305-891-6275
                     www.compasshealthsystems.com

4350 Compass Information Services

10625 Jacobs Drive
Mount Vernon, OH 43050   740-397-3997
         E-mail: training@compassinformation.com
                     www.compassinformation.com

A research-based, scientifically-valid management system that provides real-time clinical and management information for behavioral health organizations.

4351 Comprehensive Behavioral Care

200 South Hoover Boulevard
Building 219
Tampa, FL 33609-1512   813-288-4808
                              Fax: 813-288-4844
                                   www.compcare.com

4352 Comprehensive Care Corporation

200 South Hoover Boulevard
Building 219, Suite 200
Tampa, FL 33609   813-288-4808
                              Fax: 813-288-4844
                     www.comprehensivecare.com

Pauline A Macdonald MEd, Business Development

Offers a flexible system of services to provide comprehensive, compassionate and cost-effective mental health and substance abuse services to managed care organizations both public and private. CompCare is committed to providing state-of-the-art comprehensive care management services for all levels and phases of behavioral health care.

4353 Comprehensives Services

1555 Bethel Road
Columbus, OH 43220-2091   614-442-0664
                                   800-551-0664
                              Fax: 614-442-0620

Richard C Davis PhD, President
MaryAnne Booer, Practice Administrator

A multi-disciplinary private behavioral health practice with 30+ clinicians and five locations in central Ohio.

4354 Comsort

2300 N Charles Street
Baltimore, MD 21218-5137   410-785-1900
                              Fax: 410-785-7760
                     E-mail: info@comsort.com
                                   www.comsort.com

4355 Consultation Service of the American Pscyhological Association
1400 K Street NW
Washington, DC 20005-2403   202-682-6203
Fax: 202-682-6348

4356 Consumer Credit Counseling
111 Founders Plaza
Suite 1400
E Hartford, CT 06108-3241   860-282-2000
Fax: 860-291-2765

4357 Consumer Credit Counseling Services of Sacramento Valley
8795 Folsom Boulevard Suite 250
Suite E
Rancho Cordova, CA 95826   916-379-3600
Fax: 916-379-0626

2 per year

4358 Contact
1400 E Southern Avenue
Suite 800
Tempe, AZ 85282-8007   480-807-8168
Fax: 480-807-8268

4359 Corporate Benefit Consultants
300 Cahaba Park S
Suite 207
Birmingham, AL 35242-5043   205-969-1155
Fax: 205-969-1199

4360 Corporate Health Systems
33 Tenth Avenue South
Suite 260
Hopkins, MN 55343   952-939-0911
Fax: 952-939-0990

4361 Counseling Associates
109 High Street
Salisbury, MD 21801-4276   410-546-1692

4362 Counseling and Consultation Services
182 Highland Avenue
S Portland, ME 04106-4506   207-767-3031

4363 Covenant Home Healthcare
4709 66th Street
Lubbock, TX 79414   806-797-8125
Fax: 806-797-1023

4364 Coventry Health Care of Iowa
4600 Westtown Parkway
Suite 200
W Des Moines, IA 50266   515-225-1234
Fax: 515-223-0097
www.chia.cvty.com

4365 Craig Academy
751 N Negley Avenue
Pittsburg, PA 15206   412-361-2801
Fax: 412-536-5675
www.craigacademy.org

4366 Creative Management Strategies
305 Madison Avenue
Suite 2033
New York, NY 10165-0006   212-697-7207

4367 Creekside Consultants
5190 Bayou Boulevard
Suite 6
Pensacola, FL 32503-2162   850-476-0977

4368 Crystal Clinic
3975 Embassy Parkway
Akron, OH 44333-8319   330-668-4070
Fax: 216-621-4015

4369 DD Fischer Consulting
8105 White Oak Road
Quincy, IL 62301-8148   217-656-3000

4370 DML Training and Consulting
4228 Boxelder Place
Davis, CA 95616-5071   530-753-4300
Fax: 530-753-7500
www.dmlmd.com

4371 Dannenbaum Associates
110 Paseo de La Playa
Redondo Beach, CA 90277-5346
    800-424-1565

4372 David Group
14416 Myer Terrace
Rockville, MD 20853-2301   301-460-0088
Fax: 301-460-0088

4373 DeLair Systems
2639 N 33rd Avenue
Phoenix, AZ 85009-1427   602-269-8373
800-443-3811
Fax: 602-269-6462

4374 Decker Professional Group
1412 17th Street
Suite 220
Bakersfield, CA 93301-5219   661-324-1982
Fax: 661-324-1220

4375 Deloitte and Touche LLP Management Consulting
1700 Market Street
Floor 24
Philadelphia, PA 19103-3922   215-246-2300
Fax: 215-569-2441
www.deloitte.com

4376 DeltaMetrics

225 Market Street
Suite 1120
Philadelphia, PA 19106-4502   215-665-2880
                                     800-238-2433
                                Fax: 215-665-2894

4377 Devon Hill Associates

1535 El Paso Real
La Jolla, CA 92037-6303   858-456-7800
                                Fax: 818-790-9815
                        www.devonhillassociates.com

4378 Dougherty Management Associates

9 Meriam Street
Suite 4
Lexington, MA 02420-5312   781-863-8003
                                Fax: 781-863-1519
        E-mail: public@doughertymanagement.com
                     www.doughertymanagement.com

Richard H Dougherty, President
Wendy Holt, Sr Associate
Sara L Nochasek, Sr Associate

Providing the public and private sectors with superior management conusulting services to improve healthcare delivery systems and manage complex organizational change.

4379 Dupage County Health Department

111 N County Farm Road
Wheaton, IL 60187   630-682-7400
                                Fax: 630-462-9249

4380 Echo Management Group

Kaile Mansir
15 Washington Street
PO Box 2150
Conway, NH 03813-4117   603-447-8600
                                     800-635-8209
                                Fax: 603-447-8680
                    E-mail: sales@echoman.com
                              www.echoman.com

Michael Lachapelle, Director Sales/Marketing

Provides financial, clinical, and administrative software applications for behavioral health and social service agencies; comprehensive, fully-intergrated Human Service Information System is a powerful management tool that enables agencies to successfully operate their organizations within the stringent guidelines of managed care mandates. Provides implementation planning, training, support and systems consulting services.

4381 Elon Homes for Children

103 Antioch Street
PO Box 157
Elon College, NC 27244-0157   336-584-0091
                                Fax: 336-584-4026
                    E-mail: FGosse@aol.com
                              www.elon.homes.com

4382 Employee Assistance Professionals

1234 Summer Street
Stamford, CT 06905-5510   203-977-2446

4383 Employee Benefit Specialists

9351 Grant Street
Suite 300
Denver, CO 80229-4364   303-280-1215
                                Fax: 303-280-1821
                              www.clickebs.com

4384 Employee Network

1040 Vestal Parkway E
Vestal, NY 13850-1748   607-754-1043
                                Fax: 607-754-1629

4385 Entropy Limited

345 South Great Road
Lincoln, MA 01773   781-259-8901
                                Fax: 781-259-1255
                        www.entropylimited.com

Uses pattern recognition, statistics, and computer simulation to track past behavior, see current behavior and predict future behavior. Used by insuranch companies and the healthcare industry.

4386 Essi Binder Systems

70 Otis Street
Floor 2
San Francisco, CA 94103-1236   415-252-8224
                                     800-252-3774
                                Fax: 415-252-5732

4387 Ethos Consulting

50 California Street
Suite 1500
San Francisco, CA 94111   415-277-5450
                                Fax: 415-277-5451
                        www.ethosconsulting.com

4388 Evaluation Center at HSRI

2336 Massachusetts Avenue
Cambridge, MA 02140-1813   617-876-0426
                                Fax: 617-492-7401

4389 Executive Consulting Group

401 Edgewater Plaza
Suite 640
Wakefield, MA 01880-6200   781-246-2900

4390 FCS

1711 Ashley Circle
Suite 6
Bowling Green, KY 42104-5801   502-782-9152
                                     800-783-9152
                                Fax: 502-782-1055

4391 FPM Behavioral Health: Corporate Marketing

1276 Minnesota Avenue
Winter Park, FL 32789-4833   407-647-6153
                                Fax: 407-647-0668

4392 Family Managed Care

5745 Esson Lane
Suite 100
Baton Rouge, LA 70810

800-572-6983
Fax: 225-765-6572
www.calaishealth.com

Kristy Carriere, Business Development
John Chioce, VP Managed Care/Behavioral Hlth.

Provider of managed behavioral healthcare and employee assistance programs.

4393 Findley, Davies and Company

300 Madison Avenue
Suite 1000
Toledo, OH 43604-1596

419-255-1360
Fax: 419-259-5685

4394 First Consulting Group

111 W Ocean Boulevard
Suite 4
Long Beach, CA 90802-4632

562-624-5200
800-345-0957
Fax: 562-432-5774
www.fcg.com

4395 First Corp-Health Consulting

38 W Fulton Street
Suite 300
Grand Rapids, MI 49503-2644

616-676-3258
Fax: 616-676-0846

4396 First Things First

2125 Heights Drive
Suite 2D
Eau Claire, WI 54701-6146

715-832-8432
Fax: 715-832-5007

4397 Foundation for Behavioral Health

University of California, Berkeley
Berkeley, CA 94720-0001

510-642-1715
Fax: 510-643-6981

4398 Fowler Healthcare Affiliates

2800 Riveredge Parkway
Suite 920
Atlanta, GA 30328

770-261-6363
800-784-9829
Fax: 770-261-6361
www.fowler-consulting.com

4399 Freedom To Fly

27871 Medical Center Road
Suite 285
Mission Viejo, CA 92691-6440

949-364-1833

4400 Full Circle Programs

70 Skyview Terrace
San Rafael, CA 94903-1845

415-499-3320
Fax: 415-499-1542

4401 G Murphy and Associates

1151 E Warrenville Road
Suite 106
Naperville, IL 60563-9339

630-682-0030
Fax: 630-577-0169

4402 GMR Group

1301 Virginia Drive
Suite 301
Fort Washington, PA 19034-3231

215-653-7401
Fax: 215-653-7982

4403 Gadrian Corporation

5680 Greenwood Plaza Boulevard
Englewood, CO 80111-2414

303-930-2600

4404 Garner Consulting

799 E Colorado Boulevard
Suite 720
Pasadena, CA 91101-2104

626-440-0399
Fax: 626-440-0496

4405 Gaynor and Associates

396 Orange Street
New Haven, CT 06511-6405

203-865-0865
Fax: 203-865-0093
E-mail: MLg110@columbia.edu

Mack Gaynor LCSW, Principle

Clinical social work provider, EAP services, and clinical practice.

4406 Geauga Board of Mental Health, Alcohol and Drug Addiction Services

13244 Ravenna Road
Chardon, OH 44024-9012

440-285-2282
Fax: 440-285-9617

4407 Glazer Medical Solutions

100 Beach Plum Lane
Menemsha, MA 02552

508-645-9635
Fax: 308-645-3212
www.antispsychotic.com

4408 Goucher College

1021 Dulaney Valley Road
Baltimore, MD 21204-2780

410-337-6389
Fax: 410-337-6576

4409 Green Spring Health Services

5565 Sterrett Plaza
Suite 500
Columbia, MD 21044-2679

301-621-4245
800-346-5491

Expert management for managed behavioral health care.

4410 Green Spring Health Services' AdvoCare Program

5565 Sterrett Plaza
Suite 500
Columbia, MD 21044-2679

410-992-0720
800-346-5491

Clinical Management/Management Companies

This team of professionals applies the latest systems and technology to bring together the best of the public and private health care systems.

4411 HBO and Company
303 Perimeter Center N
Atlanta, GA 30346-2402
404-338-6000
Fax: 404-338-6101

4412 HPN Worldwide
180 W Park Avenue
Suite 300
Elmhurst, IL 60126-3368
630-941-9030
Fax: 630-941-9064

4413 HSP Verified
1120 G Street NW
Suite 330
Washington, DC 20005-3801
202-783-1270
Fax: 202-783-1269
www.hspverified.com

Offers comprehensive, innovative credential verification services designed to help you find that precious time. It relieves health care providers and management of tedious administrative activities-leaving time and resources to focus on quality health care. Provides valuable information and cultivates alliances between cutting edge health care organizations/plans and qualified health care providers.

4414 Hay Group:Washington, DC
4301 N Fairfax Drive
Suite 500
Arlington, VA 22203
703-841-3100
Fax: 703-908-3000

4415 Hay/Huggins Company: Philadelphia
220 S 18th Street
Philadelphia, PA 19103
215-861-2000
Fax: 215-861-2000

4416 Health Alliance Plan
2850 W Grand Boulevard
Detroit, MI 48202-2692
313-664-8314

4417 Health Assist
490 Whittingham Plaza
Lake Mary, FL 32746-3781
407-324-7249

4418 Health Capital Consultants
33 Dunwoody Park
Suite 103
Atlanta, GA 30338-6716
404-396-6334
Fax: 404-393-0522

4419 Health Capital Consultants
10420 Old Olive Street Road
Suite 200
Saint Louis, MO 63141-5938
314-994-7641
800-394-8258
Fax: 314-991-3435

4420 Health Connection Network
360 Brittany Court
Apartment B
Geneva, IL 60134-3615
708-208-1778

4421 Health Decisions
409 Plymouth Road
Suite 220
Plymouth, MI 48170-1834
734-451-2230
Fax: 734-451-2835
www.healthdecisions.com

4422 Health Management Associates
5811 Pelican Bay Boulevard
Suite 500
Naples, FL 34108-2710
239-403-3857
Fax: 941-594-2705
www.hma-corp.com

4423 Health Marketing and Management
1738 Windjammer Court
Lodi, CA 95242-4287
209-339-4943

4424 Health Marketing and Management
PO Box 2392
Mill Valley, CA 94942-2392
415-381-2953
Fax: 415-380-8241

4425 Health Net Services
404 Baltimore Street
PO Box 1060
Gettysburg, PA 17325-1060
717-334-9247
800-497-4421
Fax: 717-334-5509

4426 Health Review Services
1205 W Sherwin Avenue
Apatment 708
Chicago, IL 60626-2291
312-761-9869

4427 Health Risk Management (HRM)
10900 Hampshire Avenue S
Bloomington, MN 55438-2306
612-829-3500
800-824-3882
Fax: 612-946-7694
www.prnewswire.com

Provides total health plan management including 24 hours a day, seven days a week patient access and demand management, care management, behavioral health care management, disease management and disability workers' compensation management, all supported by QualityFIRST clinical decision guidelines. These services are electronically integrated with HRM's national provider networks and electronic claims management. HRM's clients include HMOs, hospital systems, insurance and self-insured plans, workers' compensation and disability plans and Medicare/Medicaid plans throughout the US, Canada and New Zealand.

4428 Health Systems Research

2021 L Street NW
Suite 400
Washington, DC 20036-4929   202-828-5100
                                   Fax: 202-728-9469

4429 HealthPartners

2701 University Avenue SE
Minneapolis, MN 55414-3233   612-627-3500
                                   Fax: 612-627-3535

4430 Healthcare America

1201 Claridge Road
Glenside, PA 19038-7537   610-940-1658

4431 Healthcare Management Solutions

1824 Atlantic Boulevard
Jacksonville, FL 32207-3404   904-399-2766
                                   Fax: 904-399-2712
                        E-mail: caphelp@msn.com
                        www.contactcapsolutions.com

Clifford R Frank, President

Consulting and training firm, with experience working with physicians, hospitals and payers to successfully develop global capitation programs, single specialty capitation and mental health capitation products.

4432 Healthcare Network Systems

1691 NW 93rd Terrace
Fort Lauderdale, FL 33322-4331   305-987-4100

4433 Healthcare Providers Strategies

7700 Irvine Center Drive
Suite 800
Irvine, CA 92618-3047   949-753-2853

4434 Healthcare Southwest

2016 S 4th Avenue
Tucson, AZ 85713-3509   520-795-0755
                                    520-458-8767
                               TDD: 520-458-8767

4435 Healthcare Value Management Group

100 River Ridge Drive
Norwood, MA 02062-5217   781-762-5511
                                    800-922-4286
                               Fax: 781-762-5518
                        E-mail: jwhoule@neaccess.net
                                www.hcvm.com

John W Houle, President

Consulting practice providing information technology, operations and provider contracting consultitative services.

4436 Healthcare in Partnership, LLC

3230 73rd Avenue SE
Mercer Island, WA 98040-3415   206-232-6300
                               Fax: 206-236-8110
                        E-mail: mhrnllc@ccmcajt.net

Health care consulting including managed care contract negotiation, IPA development, provider support. Specializes in behavioral health.

4437 Healthsource Provident Administrators Administration

2 Fountain Square
Suite 1-W
Chattanooga, TN 37402-0300   423-755-8335
                                   Fax: 423-642-4023

4438 Healthwise

PO Box 8525
Bend, OR 97708-8525   541-389-2711
                                   Fax: 541-388-3832

4439 Healthy Companies

1420 16th Street NW
Washington, DC 20036-2218   202-234-9288
                                   Fax: 202-234-9289

4440 HeartMath

14700 W Park Avenue
Boulder Creek, CA 95006-9318   831-338-8700
                                    800-450-9111
                               Fax: 831-338-9861
                       E-mail: info@heartmath.com
                               www.heartmath.com

Specializing in individual and organizational transformation. Programs, and resources are based on the research of the nonprofit Institute of HeartMath, which has spent over a decade researching the physiological and psychological mechanisms by which the heart communicates with the brain, thereby influencing information processing, perceptions, emotions and health. Provides research ased programs, products, coaching, and consulting. Human performance tools and technology for mental and emotional health, stability and well being.

4441 Hellman Health Strategies

134 Mount Auburn Street
Cambridge, MA 02138-5736   617-864-5247
                                   Fax: 617-864-4354

4442 Horizon Behavioral Services

1500 Waters Ridge Drive
Lewisville, TX 75057-6011   972-420-8200
                                    800-931-4646
                               Fax: 972-420-8282

Robert A Lefton, President

Provider of national managed care, utilization management and employee assistance programs. Horizon will work in collaboration with HMOs, insurance companies, employers and hospitals to develop seamless, cost-effective managed care services including practitioner panel formation, information system development, utilization management services, EAPs, outcomes measurement systems and sales and marketing functions.

4443 Horizon Management Services

PO Box 1623
Ventura, CA 93002-1623   805-644-1560
                                   Fax: 805-644-0484

Neal Andrews, President

Consultants, business planning, corporate strategies, marketing and public relations.

4444 Horizon Mental Health Management

1500 Waters Ridge Drive
Lewisville, TX 75057-6011   972-420-8350
800-727-2407
Fax: 972-420-8383

Gary A Kagan, Executive VP Development

Inpatient, outpatient, partial hospitalization and home health psychiatric programs.

4445 How to Operate an ADHD Clinic or Subspecialty Practice

ADD WareHouse
300 NW 70th Avenue
Suite 102
Plantation, FL 33317   954-792-8100
800-233-9273
Fax: 954-792-8545
E-mail: sales@addwarehouse.com
www.addwarehouse.com

This book goes beyond academic discussions of ADHD and gets down to how to establish and manage an ADHD practice. In addition to practice guidelines and suggestions, this guide presents a compendium of clinic forms and letters, interview formats, sample reports, tricks of the trade and resource listings, all of which will help you develop or refine your clinic/counseling operation. *$65.00*

325 pages

4446 Human Affairs International

10150 Centennial Parkway
PO Box 57896
Sandy, UT 84070-4170   801-256-7000
Fax: 801-256-7669

4447 Human Affairs International

332 5th Avenue
Suite 300
Pittsburgh, PA 15222-2411   412-281-7724
800-424-1533

4448 Human Affairs International: Illinois

100 N Riverside Plaza
Chicago, IL 60606-1501   312-441-5648

4449 Human Affairs International: Ohio

7476 E US Route 40
New Carlisle, OH 45344   937-845-2121
Fax: 937-846-0628

4450 Human Affairs International: Pennsylvania

1100 1st Avenue
Suite 300
King of Prussia, PA 19406-1312   610-251-6479

4451 Human Affairs International: Utah

488 E 4600 S
Suite 300
Murray, UT 84107-3948   810-578-7336

4452 Human Behavior Associates

191 Military E
Suite A
Benicia, CA 94510-2744   707-747-0117
800-937-7770
Fax: 707-747-6646
E-mail: humanbeh@ix.netcom.com

James B Wallace PhD, President
Yolanda Calderon MAT, Operations Manager

National provider of employee assistance programs, managed behavioral healthcare services, critical incident debriefing services, conflict mediation and organizational consultation. Maintains a network of 6500 licensed mental health care providers and 650 hospitals, treatment centers.

4453 Human Resources Projects/Consulting

212 Devonshire Road
Savannah, GA 31410-4208   912-897-1788

4454 Human Service Collaborative

2262 Hall Place NW
Suite 204
Washington, DC 20007-1841   202-333-1892
Fax: 202-333-8217

4455 Human Services Research Institute

2336 Massachusetts Avenue
Cambridge, MA 02140-1813   617-876-0426
Fax: 617-492-7401

4456 Hyde Park Associates

1515 E 52nd Place
3rd Floor
Chicago, IL 60615-4111   773-493-8212
Fax: 773-955-2166

4457 ID Entity

PO Box 1686
Brea, CA 92822-1686   800-355-9817
Fax: 800-355-9814

4458 IHC Behavioral Health Network

36 S State Street
Suite 21
Salt Lake City, UT 84111-1401   801-442-3125
Fax: 801-442-3821

4459 IMC Studios

1222 E 14th Street
Russellville, AR 72802   479-968-1731
Fax: 479-968-2034
E-mail: info@imcstudios.com
www.imcstudios.com

John Montgomery, General Partner

IMC Studios provides affordable, effective video, audio, graphics design and web services for mental health facilities. We can also provide support services for presentations to audiences from five to 5,000 members. Member of the National Leadership Council.

4460 INTEGRA

Stonebridge Plaza I
9606 N MoPac Expressway, Suite 600
Austin, TX 78759
512-347-7900
888-638-7491
Fax: 610-992-7033
E-mail: ningram@integraease.com
www.integra-ease.com

Greg Santore, President Corporate Services
Nicole Ingram, Director Communications

Health care management and solutions company providing employee assistance programs (EAP), work life programs, managed behavioral health care and consulting services.

4461 In Behavorial Health

5132 Bird Lane
Winter Haven, FL 33884-2601
941-324-3993

4462 Inclusion

1436 Independence Avenue SE
Washington, DC 20003-1536
202-543-4464
Fax: 202-546-4465

4463 Inroads Behavioral Health Services

PO Box 660696
Dallas, TX 75266-0696
800-565-9013

Fully integrated behavorial health care company.

4464 Insurance Management Institute

6007 Deer Run
Fort Myers, FL 33908-4314
813-433-4390

4465 Intech

3776 Via Picante
La Mesa, CA 91941-7326
619-452-2100

4466 Integrated Behavioral Health

1347 Rue Bayonne
Mandeville, LA 70471-1229
504-626-4893

4467 Integrated Behavioral Healthcare

140 S Arthur Street
Suite 690
Spokane, WA 99202-2260
509-534-1731
Fax: 509-535-7073

4468 Integrated Behavioral Systems

165 S Wellwood Avenue
Lindenhurst, NY 11757-4902
516-951-1121

4469 Interface EAP

7670 Woodway Drive
Suite 350
Houston, TX 77063-6500
713-781-3364
Fax: 713-781-4954

4470 Interim Personnel

15145 W 22nd Street, Suite 750
Regency Towers
Oak Brook, IL 60521
630-571-3900
Fax: 630-571-1629

4471 Interim Physicians

1601 Sawgrass Corporate Parkway
Sunrise, FL 33323
954-858-6000
800-338-7786
Fax: 954-858-2820
www.interimphysicians.com

4472 Interlink Health Services

4950 NE Belknap Court, Suite 205
Hillsboro, OR 97124
503-640-2000
800-599-9119
Fax: 503-640-2028
www.interlinkhealth.com

4473 International Technology Corporation

2790 Mosside Boulevard
Monroeville, PA 15146-2743
412-372-7701

4474 JDA

1340 Treat Boulevard
Suite 600
Walnut Creek, CA 94596-7581
415-434-1014

4475 JGK Associates

14464 Kerner Drive
Sterling Heights, MI 48313-2372
313-247-9055

4476 JM Oher and Associates

10 Tanglewild Plaza
Suite 100
Chappaqua, NY 10514-2528
914-238-0607
Fax: 914-238-3161

4477 JS Medical Group

Two Penn Center Plaza
Suite 200
Philadelphia, PA 19102-1706
215-854-6446
Fax: 215-893-8909
E-mail: information@jsmg.com
www.jsmg.com/main

4478 Jennings Ryan and Kolb

80 Capital Drive
W Springfield, MA 01089-1331
413-586-7606
Fax: 413-732-7711

4479 Jeri Davis Marketing Consultants

11622 Yeatman Terrace
Silver Spring, MD 20902-3057
301-593-9663
Fax: 301-539-4359

4480 John Maynard and Associates

58 Spruce Street
Boulder, CO 80302-4906   303-444-6300

4481 Johnson, Bassin and Shaw

8630 Fenton Street
Silver Spring, MD 20910-3806   301-495-1080
                              Fax: 301-587-4352

4482 Juniper Healthcare Containment Systems

110 Great Neck Road
Suite 604
Great Neck, NY 11021-3304   516-829-3090
                              Fax: 516-829-4691

4483 KAI Associates

6001 Montrose Road
Suite 920
Rockville, MD 20852-4874   301-770-2730
                              Fax: 301-770-4183

4484 KAMFT/Managed Care Coordinators

2840 Jefferson Street
Paducah, KY 42001-4170   502-442-5738

4485 KPMG Peat Marwick

99 High Street
Boston, MA 02110-2320   617-988-1170
                              Fax: 617-988-0802

4486 Kelly, Waldron and Company

330 Milltown Road
Suite W-5
E Brunswick, NJ 08816-2267   732-257-1777
                              Fax: 908-257-7368
                              E-mail: sfox@kwsp.com

4487 Krepack and Associates

260 California Street
Suite 801
San Francisco, CA 94111-4382   415-381-4751
                              Fax: 415-381-5738

4488 Kushner and Company

1050 17th Street NW
Suite 810
Washington, DC 20036   202-887-0958
                              Fax: 269-342-1606
                              www.kushnerco.com

4489 Kwasha Lipton

2100 N Central Road
Fort Lee, NJ 07024-7558   201-592-1300

4490 LAB Research and Development

755 Avery Street
San Bernardino, CA 92404-1801   909-882-7007

4491 LMS Consultation Network

5800 Arlington Avenue
Suite 11 V
Bronx, NY 10471-1414
                              800-597-3070

4492 Lake Mental Health Consultants

PO Box 115
Osage Beach, MO 65065-0115   573-348-3010
                              Fax: 573-348-1858

4493 Lakshmi Enterprises

3309 Juanita Street
San Diego, CA 92105-3809   619-286-6614

4494 Lanstat Resources

PO Box 259
Southworth, WA 98386-0259
                              800-672-3166
                              Fax: 360-769-7308

4495 Legacy Enterprises

7400 Shoreline Drive
Suite 3
Stockton, CA 95219-5498   209-957-3185
                              Fax: 209-957-7843

4496 Lewin Group

3130 Fairview Park Drive
Suite 800
Falls Church, VA 22042-4504   703-269-5721
                              Fax: 703-269-5501
                              E-mail: dwoodruff@lewin.com
                              www.lewin.com

4497 Liberty Healthcare Management Corporation

1841 Broadway
New York, NY 10023-7603
                              800-989-9118
                              Fax: 212-399-7068

4498 Lifelink Corporation

331 S York Road
Suite 206
Bensenville, IL 60106-2600   630-521-8061
                              Fax: 630-521-8844
                              E-mail: kmocasio@lifelink.org
                              www.lifelink.org

Kenny Martin-Ocasio, Dir. Latino Family Health Svcs.

Provides therapy services in Spanish for children, families and couples. Offers substance abuse treatment and educational groups for men who batter in English and Spanish. Provides comprehensive services to Latina victims of domestic violence and their children in Spanish.

4499 Lifespan Care Management Agency

600 Frederick Street
Santa Cruz, CA 95062-2203   831-469-4900
                              Fax: 831-469-4950
                              E-mail: info@lifespancare.com
                              www.lifespancare.com

Comprehensive care management for adults who need care.

4500 MACRO International

3 Corporate Square NE
Suite 370
Atlanta, GA 30329-2010   404-321-3211
                                Fax: 404-321-3688

4501 MCF Consulting

25 Bragg Drive
E Berlin, PA 17316-9342   717-259-6631
                                Fax: 717-259-6537
                                E-mail: mcfcom@cvm.net

Mark C Fox, President

MCF Consulting has demonstrated accomplishments in: developing managed care and management service organization (MSO) capabilities; managed Medicaid strategic planning efforts; Information System analysis and design contracts; product development projects; pricing and product positioning; business plan and marketing plan development; proposal development; organizational change; and creating joint ventures and partnerships. Clients have included managed care firms, provider groups, hospital systems, state and county governments and diverse contract agencies.

4502 MCG Telemedicine Center

1120 15th Street
EA - 100
Augusta, GA 30912-0004   706-721-6616
                                Fax: 706-721-8892
                                E-mail: lweisser@mail.mcg.edu
                                www.mcg.edu/telemedicine/Index.html

Lydia Weisser DO, Telephychiatrist
Dora Norton, Web Editor

Involved with the delivery of mental health services via telemedicine. In addition, the Telemedicine Center maintains the Georgia Mental Health Network website, a comprehensive listing of mental health resources in the State.

4503 MCW Department of Psychiatry and Behavioral Medicine

8701 Watertown Plank
Milwaukee, WI 53226   414-456-8990
                                Fax: 414-456-6299
                                E-mail: aodya@mcw.edu

4504 MMHR

2550 University Avenue W
Suite 335N
Saint Paul, MN 55114-2005   651-647-1900
                                Fax: 651-647-1861
                                www.mentalhealthinc.com

Tim Quesnell, Administrator

4505 MP Associates

16641 Calle Brittany
Pacific Palisades, CA 90272-1967   818-242-6290
                                   Fax: 818-242-0767

4506 MSI International

245 Peachtree Center Avenue NE
Suite 2500
Atlanta, GA 30303-1224   404-659-5236
                                800-438-6086

4507 MTS

307 Chase Lane
Marietta, GA 30068-3516   404-565-3736

4508 Magellan Behavioral Health

3850 Priority Way S Drive
Suite 200
Indianapolis, IN 46240-3813
                                800-727-6227
                                Fax: 317-573-3789

4509 Magellan Health Service

6950 Columbia Gateway Drive
Columbia, MD 21046-3308   410-964-3222
                                800-458-2740
                                Fax: 410-953-1251
                                www.magellanhealth.com

John J Wider Jr, President/COO
Danna Mauch PhD, CEO
Alan M Elkins MD, Sr VP
Linda Deloach Weaver PhD, Executive VP

Provides members with high quality, clinically appropriate, affordable health care which is tailored to each individual's needs.

4510 Magellan Health Services

3414 Peachtree Road NE
Suite 1400
Atlanta, GA 30326-1114   404-869-5646

4511 Magellan Public Solutions

222 Berkeley Street
Suite 1350
Boston, MA 02116-3733   617-661-2851
                                800-947-0071
                                Fax: 617-790-4848

4512 Maki and Associates

PO Box 1469
Ridgecrest, CA 93556-1469   760-939-2480

4513 Managed Care Concepts

PO Box 812032
Boca Raton, FL 33481-2032   561-750-2240
                                800-899-3926
                                Fax: 561-750-4621
                                www.theemployeesassistanceprogram.com

Beth Harrell, Corporate Contacts Director
Ginger Minnelonica, Administrative Assistant

Provides comprehensive EAP services to large and small companies in the United States and parts of Canada. Also provides child/elder care referrals, drug free workplace program services, consultation and training services.

4514 Managed Care Consultants

8260 E Raintree Drive
Scottsdale, AZ 85260-2516   602-998-1103

4515 Managed Health Network

1600 Los Gamos Drive
Suite 300
San Rafael, CA 94903-1807   415-491-7225
                              800-327-7526
                         Fax: 415-472-8187

Provides high-quality, cost-effective behavioral
health care services to the public sector.

4516 Managed Healthcare Consultants

1907 London Lane
Wilmington, NC 28405-4210   910-256-6196
                         Fax: 910-256-6196

4517 Managed Networks of America

1206 Laskin Road
Suite 207
Virginia Beach, VA 23451-5263   757-428-7200
                             Fax: 757-428-8185
                    E-mail: mnamerica@aol.com
                         www.mnamerica.com

Matthew Weinstein, President
Richard Edley PhD, COO

Management services that include strategic and business plan development, new corporate formations and
contractual affiliations, product and infrastructure development, implementation, and management. Organizes cost effective provider networks which include a
full continuum of care and services while supplying
the necessary clinical, administrative, and financial
systems to enable effective management of populations across varied geographic areas.

4518 Managed Psychiatric Benefits Company

2001 L Street NW
Suite 200
Washington, DC 20036-4948   202-466-8981
                         Fax: 202-955-3996

4519 Maniaci Insurance Services

916 Silver Spur Road
Suite 206
Rolling Hills Estates, CA 90274-3844 310-541-4824
                             Fax: 310-377-2016

4520 Marin Institute

24 Belvedere Street
San Rafael, CA 94901-4817   415-456-5692

4521 Market Pulse Research Services

PO Box 1686
Brea, CA 92822-1686
                              800-203-7076
                         Fax: 800-355-9814

4522 Marketing Directions

15702 Rosehaven Lane
Santa Clarita, CA 91351-1880   805-252-4493

4523 May Mental Health Service

780 American Legion Highway
Roslindale, MA 02131-3908   617-325-6700
                         Fax: 617-325-6581

4524 Mayes Group

Daisy Point
PO Box 399
Saint Peters, PA 19470-0399   610-469-6900
                              800-469-5274
                         Fax: 610-469-6088
                         www.mayesgroup.com

Abby Mayes, President

Retained executive search firm that specializes exclusively in managed care/behavioral healthcare since
1986. Offices in Pennsylvania and Florida.

4525 McGladery and Pullen CPAs

800 Marquette Avenue
Suite 1300
Minneapolis, MN 55402-2877   612-376-9544
                         Fax: 612-376-9876

4526 McGraw Hill Healthcare Management

1221 Avenue of the Americas
Floor 41
New York, NY 10020-1001   212-512-2000
                            800-544-8168

4527 Menninger Care Systems

6404 International Parkway
Suite 2000
Plano, TX 75093-8223   972-588-2500
                         800-492-4357
                    Fax: 972-588-2775
                    www.menningercare.com

4528 Mercer, Meidinger and Hansen

200 Clarendon Street
Floor 35
Boston, MA 02116-5021   617-421-5300

4529 Meridian Resource Corporation

1401 Enclave Parkway
Suite 300
Houston, TX 77077   281-597-7000
                 Fax: 281-558-5744
                      www.tmrc.com

4530 Merit Behavioral Care Tricare

15451 N 28th Avenue
Phoenix, AZ 85053-4067   602-564-2330
                      Fax: 602-564-2336

4531 Merit Behavorial Care Corporation

1 Maynard Drive
Park Ridge, NJ 07656-1878   201-391-8700

Provides high-quality, cost-effective managed behavioral health care and employee assistance programs.

4532 Mesa Mental Health

6723 Academy Road NE
Albuquerque, NM 87109-3345   505-858-1585
                                    Fax: 505-858-1779

4533 Mihalik Group

1048 W Oakdale Avenue
Chicago, IL 60657-4318   773-929-4276
                                    Fax: 773-929-4466

4534 Milliman and Robertson

1099 18th Street
Suite 3100
Denver, CO 80202-2431   303-672-9093
                                  Fax: 303-299-9018
          E-mail: stevemelek@milliman.com

Stephen P Melek, Principal and Consulting Actuary

4535 Mind Body Connection

19742 MacArthur Boulevard
Suite 101
Irvine, CA 92612-2447   949-442-1660

4536 Minimize & Manage Risk

1515 Wilson Boulevard
Suite 800
Arlington, VA 22209

                                  800-245-3333
          E-mail: walter@prms.com
                  www.prms.com

4537 Missouri Institute of M/H

5247 Fyler Avenue
Saint Louis, MO 63139-1361   314-644-8629
                                  Fax: 614-644-8834

4538 Multnomah Co. Behavioral Health

421 SW 6th Avenue
Suite 500
Portland, OR 97204-1620   503-248-3999
                                  Fax: 503-248-3328

4539 Murphy-Harpst-Vashti

740 Fletcher Street
Cedartown, GA 30125-3249   770-748-2214
                                  Fax: 770-749-1094

4540 NASW JobLink

9200 E Panorama Circle
Suite 120
Englewood, CO 80112-3482

                                  888-261-2265
                                  Fax: 800-595-2929

4541 National Behavioral Health Consulting Practice

Cristi Cohn, William M Mercer
2390 E Camelback Road
Suite 435
Phoenix, AZ 85016-3452   602-955-9682
                                  Fax: 602-957-9573

Assists you with all aspects of delivery system integration.

4542 National Empowerment Center

599 Canal Street
Lawrence, MA 01840-1233   617-491-6775
                                  800-769-3728
                                  Fax: 978-681-6426
                                  www.power2u.org

Daniel B Fisher, Executive Director
Laurie Ahern, Educator

Consumer/survivor/ex-patient run organization that carries a message of recovery, empowerment, hope and healing to people who have been diagnosed with mental illness.

4543 National Healthcare Solutions

6946 Rosewood Street
Pittsburgh, PA 15208-2639   412-362-6950
                                  Fax: 412-362-6954

4544 Network Behavioral Health

275 North Street
Harrison, NY 10528-1524   914-967-6500
                                  888-224-2273
                                  Fax: 914-925-5175

4545 New Day

49 Music Square W
Suite 502
Nashville, TN 37203-3230   615-321-5577
                                  800-786-6211
                                  Fax: 615-321-5566
                                  E-mail: retter@acs4.com
                                  www.acs4.com

James Harper, VP

Develops and manages successful mental health units by utilizing clinical operations and information systems to set quality, low cost standards in diagnosing treating psychiatric conditions.

4546 New England Psych Group

10 Langley Road
Suite 202
Newton Center, MA 02459-1972   617-527-4055
                                  Fax: 617-527-2571

4547 New Standards

4663 Chatsworth Street N
Suite 101
Shoreview, MN 55126-5813

                                  800-755-6299
                                  Fax: 401-231-2055

4548 Newbride Consultation

585 Stewart Avenue
Suite L70
Garden City, NY 11530-4701   516-222-1221
                                  Fax: 516-222-2915

4549 North American Computer Services

14828 W 6th Avenue
Suite 16B
Golden, CO 80401-5000   303-278-1501
                                  Fax: 303-278-1173

4550 Northland Health Group

7 Ocean Street
S Portland, ME 04106-2800
207-767-7500
Fax: 207-767-7504

4551 Northpointe Behavioral Healthcare Systems

715 Pyle Drive
Kingsford, MI 49802-4456
906-774-9522
Fax: 906-774-1570
E-mail: info@nbhs.org
www.nbhs.org

Michigan Community Mental Health agency serving Dickinson, Menominee and Iron counties. Provides a full spectrum of managed behavioral healthcare services to the chronically mentally ill and developmentally disabled. A corporate services division provides employee assistance programs both in Michigan and outside the state.

4552 Northridge Hospital Medical Center

18300 Roscoe Boulevard
Northridge, CA 91325-4167
818-885-5348

4553 OPTIONS Health Care-California

525 Oregon Street
Vallejo, CA 94590-3201
707-648-2200

4554 OPTIONS Health Care-Texas

100 Congress Avenue
Suite 2100
Austin, TX 78701-4042
512-469-3540
Fax: 512-469-3711

555 Oklahoma Mental Health Consumer Council

5131 N Classen Boulevard
Suite 200
Oklahoma City, OK 73118-4433
405-634-5644
Fax: 405-634-2075

556 Open Minds

Behavioral Health Industry News
10 York Street
Suite 200
Gettysburg, PA 17325-2301
717-334-1329
Fax: 717-334-0538
E-mail: openminds@openminds.com
www.openminds.com

Provides information on marketing, financial, and legal trends in the delivery of mental health and chemical dependency benefits and services. Recurring features include interviews, news of research, a calendar of events, job listings, book reviews, notices of publications available, and industry statistics. $185.00

12 pages 12 per year ISSN 1043-3880

4557 Optimum Care Corporation

3011 Ivy Glenn Drive
Suite 219
Laguna Niguel, CA 92677
800-995-4410
Fax: 949-495-4316

4558 Options Health Care

240 Corporate Boulevard
Norfolk, VA 23502-4948
757-459-5200
Fax: 757-892-5729
www.optionshealthcare.com

Specializes in creating innovative services for a full range of at-risk and administrative services only benefits, including behavioral health programs, customized provider and facility networks, utilization and case management, EAPs and youth services.

4559 PMCC

250 W 57th Street
Suite 901
New York, NY 10107-0999
212-564-2295

4560 PRO Behavioral Health

950 S Cherry Street
Suite 200
Denver, CO 80246
303-315-9330
800-962-1037

A managed behavioral health care company dedicated to containing psychiatric and substance abuse costs while providing high-quality health care. Owned and operated by mental health care professionals, PRO has exclusive, multi-year contracts with HMOs and insurers on both coasts and in the Rocky Mountain region.

4561 PSC

1147 Starmount Court
Suite B
Bel Air, MD 21015-5650
410-569-6106
Fax: 410-569-6364

4562 PSIMED Corporation

1221 E Dyer Road
Suite 260
Santa Ana, CA 92705-5654
714-979-7670
E-mail: sales@psimed-ambs.com
www.psimed-ambs.com

4563 Paris International Corporation

2 Linden Place
Great Neck, NY 11021-2646
516-487-2630
Fax: 516-466-6255

4564 Persoma Management

400 Penn Center Boulevard
Suite 777
Pittsburgh, PA 15235-5607
800-500-6622
Fax: 412-823-8262

Clinical Management/Management Companies

4565 Perspectives

111 N Wabash Avenue
Suite 1620
Chicago, IL 60602-2002   630-932-7788
800-456-6327
Fax: 312-558-1570

4566 Philadelphia Health Management

260 S Broad Street
Philadelphia, PA 19102-5021   215-985-2500
Fax: 215-985-2550

4567 Philadelphia Mental Health Care Corporation

123 S Broad Street
Floor 23
Philadelphia, PA 19109-1029   215-546-0300
Fax: 215-732-1606

4568 PhyCor

30 Burton Hills Boulevard
Suite 400
Nashville, TN 37215-6140   615-665-7425
Fax: 615-665-7840

4569 Pinal Gila Behavioral Health Association

2066 W Apache Trail
Suite 116
Apache Junction, AZ 85220-3733   602-982-1317

4570 Porras and Associates, Healthcare Consulting

351 Pleasant Street
Suite 143
Northampton, MA 01060-3900   716-842-4571
Fax: 413-585-1522
E-mail: mrkcon@javanet.com
www.javanet.com/mrkcon

4571 Porter Novelli

1120 Connecticut Avenue NW
Washington, DC 20036-3902   202-973-5800
Fax: 202-973-5858

4572 Posen Consulting Group

5274 Langlewood Drive
W Bloomfield, MI 48322-2018   248-661-0663
Fax: 248-661-6279

4573 Practice Integration Team

107 Fairview Drive
Lansdale, PA 19446-6363   215-855-3572

4574 Practice Management Institute

19762 MacArthur Boulevard
Suite 300
Irvine, CA 92612-2410   949-253-3435

4575 Practice Management Resource Group

700 Larkspur Landing Circle
Suite 199
Larkspur, CA 94939-1754   415-925-4334
Fax: 415-331-7479

4576 Pragmatix

5650 Greenwood Plaza Boulevard
Suite 250A
Greenwood Village, CO 80111-2309   303-779-0812
Fax: 303-779-1335

4577 Preferred Mental Health Management

8535 East 21 Street N
Wichita, KS 67206-3413   316-609-2345
Fax: 316-609-2481
E-mail: pmhm@southwind.net
www.pmhm.com

Offers managed care services and EAP services.

4578 Prime Care Consultants

297 Knollwood Road
White Plains, NY 10607   914-686-6891
800-933-8629
Fax: 914-682-7518

4579 ProAmerica Managed Care

PO Box 202008
Arlington, TX 76006-8008

800-523-3669

4580 ProMetrics CAREeval

480 American Avenue
King of Prussia, PA 19406-1405   610-265-6344
Fax: 610-265-8377
E-mail: admin@prometrics.com
www.careeval.com

Ron Thompson PhD, Director Research, Boys Town
David Doty PhD, President, Susqueha. Pathfinders
Marc Duey, President, ProMetrics Consulting

A joint venture formed by Father Flanagan's Home (Boys Town), Susquehanna Pathfinders and ProMetrics Consulting. These organizations combine years of experience as service providers and technical resource developers. Provides innovative ways to collect, store and analyze service outcome data to improve the effectiveness of your services.

4581 ProMetrics Consulting & Susquehanna PathFinders

480 American Avenue
King of Prussia, PA 19406-1405   610-265-6344
Fax: 610-265-8377
E-mail: admins@prometrics.com

4582 Process Strategies Institute

PO Box 3146
Charleston, WV 25331-3146   304-345-0880
Fax: 304-345-3312

4583 Professional Services Consultants

1147 Starmount Center
Suite B
Bel Air, MD 21015-5650   410-569-6106
Fax: 410-569-6364
E-mail: psc@netgsi.com
www.netgsi.com/~psc.

Professional Services Consultants (PSC), a unique nationally-recognized management consulting company, assists behavioral health care programs with policies, procedures, accreditation, licensure, reimbursement, documentation, infection control, credentialing, performance improvement, legal, risk management and employment issues. The PSC Healthcare Consultant is a subscription newsletter bringing you the latest on accreditation, licensure and management issues affecting health care. PSC's benchmarking system (NBN) provides an easy, low-cost approach to state-of-the-art outcome measurement. Call for more information. *$ 99.00*

4584 Providence Behavioral Health Connections

10300 SW Eastridge Street
Portland, OR 97225-5004   503-216-4984
                            Fax: 503-216-4987

4585 Psy Care

4550 Kearny Villa Road
Suite 116
San Diego, CA 92123   858-279-1223
                        Fax: 858-279-8150

4586 PsycHealth

PO Box 5312
Evanston, IL 60204-5312   847-864-4961
                            Fax: 847-864-9930

Specialists providing mental health services, managed care and referrals.

4587 Psychiatric Associates

PO Box 6504
Kokomo, IN 46904-6504   765-453-9338
                          Fax: 765-455-2710

4588 Psycho Medical Chirologists

11612 Lockwood Drive
Suite 103
Silver Spring, MD 20904-2314   301-681-6614
                                 Fax: 301-681-0738

Robert F Spiegel, Director

What part of your body...in all seriousness!...is most revealing about yourself? (Health, character, personality, intelligence, creativity, latent strengths and hidden potential.) Is it your face, eyes, smile, voice, or body language. Absolutely not. Without any doubt, it is your hands. Hands speak a language with a vocabulary three times richer than basic English! Just listen to what they have to say. 18,000 references of medical and psychological literature (researched at NIH), have proven hands to be the most extraordinary repository of over 2,500 'bits' of diagnostic information. Do you know what your hands are silently trying to tell you? Free information (taught in Departments of Medicine, Psychiatry, Psychology and Law).

4589 Psychology Consultants

1001 Cherry Street
Suite 304
Columbia, MO 65201-7931   314-874-6777
                            Fax: 614-874-9867

4590 Public Consulting Group

294 Washington Street
Suite 1006
Boston, MA 02108-4608   617-426-2026

4591 Pyrce Healthcare Group

7627 Lake Street
Suite 205
River Forest, IL 60305-1878   708-383-7700
                                Fax: 708-383-7746
          E-mail: phg-inc@ix.netcom.com
                 www.netcom.com/~phg-inc

Janice M Pyrce, President
Linda R Coen, VP
Christine C Duffy, Market Analyst

A national consulting firm, founded in 1990, with a focus on behavioral health. The firm specializes in strategic planning, market research, integrated delivery systems, business development, retreat facilitation and management/organizational development. PHG offers significant depth of resources, with direct involvement of experienced senior staff. Clients include hospitals, healthcare systems, academic medical centers, human service agencies, physician/allied practices, professional/trade associations and investor groups. The firm has over 200 organizations with locations in over 40 states.

4592 QK Consulting Resources

3159 N Mount Curve Avenue
Altadena, CA 91001-1766   626-797-1699
                            Fax: 626-797-1496

4593 QualChoice Health Plan

6000 Parkland Boulevard
Cleveland, OH 44124-6119   440-460-4121
                             Fax: 261-460-4006

4594 Quality Management Audits

4553 N Shallowford Road
Suite 80C
Atlanta, GA 30338-6415   404-451-4214
                           Fax: 404-457-8590

4595 Quinco Behavioral Health Systems

720 N Marr Road
Columbus, IN 47201   812-379-2341
                        800-266-2341
                  Fax: 812-376-4875
                  TTY: 812-379-2341
           E-mail: qbhs@quinco.com
                  www.quincobhs.org

Robert S Williams, CEO
Amy Matheny, Marketing/Communications Manager

Nonprofit mental health care provider serving south central Indiana. 24 hour crisis line and full continum of mental health services.

4596 REC Management

1640 Powers Ferry Road SE
Suite 350
Marietta, GA 30067-5491   770-955-7715
                            Fax: 770-956-9325

4597 Ramsay Health Care
592 W 1350 S
Woods Cross, UT 84010-8180   801-299-9966
Fax: 801-299-9965

4598 Resource Management Consultants
59 Stiles Road
Salem, NH 03079-2885   603-372-5940
800-332-7998

4599 Resource Opportunities
3070 Bristol Street
Suite 610
Costa Mesa, CA 92626-3071   805-985-6633
Fax: 805-984-9303

4600 Risk Management Group
PO Box 36
Newtown Square, PA 19073-0036   215-359-1776
Fax: 215-359-9676

4601 Roger Rose Consulting
PO Box 811
Bloomfield, CT 06002-0811   413-786-8457

4602 SIGMA Assessment Systems
511 Fort Street
Suite 435
Port Huron, MI 48060-3939   810-982-3713
800-265-1285
Fax: 800-361-9411

4603 SJ Hughes Consulting
2047 W Gila Lane
Chandler, AZ 85224-8390   602-963-0659
Fax: 602-963-3098

4604 SLA Consulting
1008 Balmoral Drive
Silver Spring, MD 20903-1303   301-445-6548
Fax: 301-445-6548

4605 SM Hart and Associates
3975 Madison Road
La Canada, CA 91011-3951   818-790-1707
Fax: 818-790-9815

4606 SUMMIT Behavioral Partners
1300 Summit Avenue
6th Floor
Fort Worth, TX 76102-4414   817-332-2519
Fax: 817-335-9100
E-mail: businessdevelopment@corphealth.com
www.corphealth.com

Paul J Floyd, Sr VP
Jack Moore, National Director

4607 Sachs Group
1800 Sherman Avenue
Evanston, IL 60201-3777   847-475-7526
Fax: 847-475-7830

4608 Salud Mangement Associates
2727 Palisade Avenue
Suite 4H
Riverdale, NY 10463-1020   718-796-0971
800-765-1209
Fax: 718-796-0971
www.vd6@columbia.edu

Dr. Victor De La Cancela, President/CEO

Clinical Psichology and Community Health Services. Bilingual Spanish-English culturally competent providers, trainers and organizational consultants.

4609 Sandra Fields-Neal and Associates
535 S Burdick Street
Suite 165
Kalamazoo, MI 49007-5261   616-381-5213
Fax: 616-381-4375

4610 Sarmul Consultants
1 Strawberry Hill Court
Stamford, CT 06902-2548   203-327-1596
Fax: 203-325-1639

4611 Savant Health
PO Box 419257
Kansas City, MO 64141-6257
800-444-8898
Fax: 816-756-2247

4612 Schafer Consulting
602 Hemlock Road
Coraopolis, PA 15108-9140   412-695-0652
Fax: 412-695-0180

4613 Scheur Mangement Group
255 Washington Street
Suite 100
Newton, MA 02458-1611   617-969-7500
Fax: 617-969-7508

4614 Schwab, Bennett and Associates
9000 W Sunset Boulevard
Suite 700
Los Angeles, CA 90069-5807   310-274-8787

4615 Sciacca Comprehensive Service Development for MIDAA
299 Riverside Drive
New York, NY 10025-5278   212-866-5935
Fax: 212-666-1942
E-mail: ksciacca@pobox.com
www.pobox.com/~dualdiagnosis

Kathleen Sciacca MA, Executive Director/Consultant

Provides consulting, education, and training for treatment and program development for dual diagnosis of mental illness and substance disorders including severe mental illness. Materials available include manuals, videos, articles, book chapters, journals, and books. Trains in Motivational Interviewing.

4616 Seelig and Company: Child Welfare and Behavioral Healthcare

1300 Patrio Drive
Suite 201
Campbell, CA 95008   408-377-0123
                            Fax: 408-377-0123

4617 Sentinent Systems

10410 Kensington Parkway
Kensington, MD 20895-2943   301-929-7600
                            Fax: 301-929-7680

4618 Sheldon I Dorenfest and Associates

515 N State Street
Floor 18
Chicago, IL 60610-4325   312-464-3000
                            Fax: 312-464-3030

4619 Sheppard Pratt Health Plan

PO Box 6815
Baltimore, MD 21285-6815   410-938-3200
                            Fax: 410-938-4099
            E-mail: shahn@sheppardpratt.org
                    www.sheppardpratt.org

4620 Shueman and Associates

PO Box 90024
Pasadena, CA 91109-5024   626-585-8248

4621 Skypek Group

2528 W Tennessee Avenue
Tampa, FL 33629-6255   813-254-3926
                            Fax: 813-254-3926

4622 Smith Kazazian

790 E Colorado Boulevard
Suite 720
Pasadena, CA 91101-2189   818-409-0821

4623 South Coast Medical Center

31872 S Coast Highway
Laguna Beach, CA 92651-6775   949-499-7146
                            Fax: 949-499-7582

4624 Southeast Nurse Consultants

5424 Saffron Drive
Atlanta, GA 30338-3115   404-395-6731
                            Fax: 770-668-0706

4625 Specialized Alternatives for Families & Youth of America (SAFY)

10100 Elida Road
Delphos, OH 45833-9058   419-695-8010
                                 800-532-7239
                            Fax: 419-695-0004
                   E-mail: safy@safy.org
                           www.safy.org

Not-for-profit managerial service organization providing a full continuum of quality care to families and youth across the nation.

4626 Specialized Therapy Associates

83 Summit Avenue
Hackensack, NJ 07601-1262   201-488-6678
                            Fax: 201-488-6224

4627 Specialty Healthcare Management

1500 Waters Ridge Drive
Lewisville, TX 75057-6011   972-420-8350
                                 800-456-6785
                            Fax: 303-793-0771

4628 Spring Harbor Hospital

175 Running Hill Road
S Portland, ME 04106-3272   207-761-2200
                            Fax: 207-761-2108
                            TTY: 207-761-2224
            E-mail: wilkerson@springharbor.org
                        www.springharbor.org

Gail Wilkeman, Dir. Communications/Marketing

Mental health hospital.

4629 St. Anthony Behavioral Medicine Center, Behavioral Medicine

1000 N Lee Avenue
Oklahoma City, OK 73102-1036   405-272-6000
                            Fax: 405-272-6208

4630 St. John Health System

2210 Jackson Street
Anderson, IN 46016-4363   765-646-8464
                            Fax: 765-646-8462

4631 St. Joseph Behavioral Medicine Network

861 Corporate Drive
Suite 103
Lexington, KY 40503-5433   606-232-4202
                            Fax: 606-224-2024

4632 St. Joseph Hospital: Health Promotion Network

80 E Chestnut Street
Suite 1A
Bellingham, WA 98225   360-647-3847
                                 800-244-6142
                            Fax: 360-715-6567

4633 Stamos Associates

353 Sacramento Street
Suite 600
San Francisco, CA 94111-3604   650-234-9501
                            Fax: 650-234-9505

4634 Steven A Wright Consulting

288 Scenic Avenue
Piedmont, CA 94611-3417   510-428-2800
                            Fax: 510-658-2888

4635 Strategic Advantage

3414 Peachtree Road NE
Suite 1400
Atlanta, GA 30326-1114   612-331-8700
Fax: 612-331-8181
E-mail: info@stradv.com
www.stradv.com

4636 Stresscare Behavioral Health

3306 Executive Parkway
Suite 201
Toledo, OH 43606-1335   419-531-3500
Fax: 419-531-1877

4637 Suburban Psychiatric Associates

600 N Jackson Street
Media, PA 19063-2561   610-891-9024
Fax: 610-892-0399

4638 Sue Krause and Associates

15 Jutland Road
Binghamton, NY 13903-1336   607-771-8009
Fax: 607-651-9236

4639 SunRise Health Marketing

1104 Marquis Trce
Louisville, KY 40223-3750   502-254-5695
Fax: 502-254-5387

4640 Supportive Systems

25 Beachway Drive
Suite C
Indianapolis, IN 46224   317-788-4111
800-660-6645
Fax: 317-788-7783

Pamela Ruster ACSW LCSW, President/CEO

4641 Synergestic Consultants

PO Box 634
Solomons, MD 20688-0634   202-965-8251

4642 Syratech Corporation

185 McClellan Highway
E Boston, MA 02128-1146   617-561-2200
Fax: 617-568-1361

4643 Systems In Focus

11230 Gold Express Drive
Suite 310-157
Gold River, CA 95670-4484   707-554-4914
Fax: 707-544-2657

4644 T Kendall Smith

690 Hopewell Road
Downingtown, PA 19335-1219
Fax: 215-269-4530

4645 TASC

1500 N Halsted Street
Chicago, IL 60622-2517   312-787-0208
Fax: 312-787-9663

4646 Tailored Computers Consultants

3240 W 7 Mile Road
Detroit, MI 48221-2282   313-861-1444

4647 Towers Perrin Integrated HeatlhSystems Consulting

335 Madison Avenue
New York, NY 10017   212-309-3400
www.tower.com/towers

Managed behavorial health care consultants specializing in strategy and operations, clinical effectiveness, actuarial and reimbursement and human resources for both the provider and the payer sides.

4648 Trachy Healthcare Management Company

9288 E Hillery Way
Scottsdale, AZ 85260-2849   602-314-9280
Fax: 602-384-7570

4649 Tribrook Management Consultants

999 Oakmont Plaza Drive
Suite 600
Westmont, IL 60559-5517   708-990-8070
Fax: 708-325-0337

4650 US Behavioral Health

2000 Powell Street
Suite 1180
Emeryville, CA 94608-1860   510-601-2209
Fax: 510-601-4536

4651 US Healthcare

980 Jolly Road
Suite 21 F
Blue Bell, PA 19422-1957   215-283-6551
Fax: 215-654-6007

4652 US Quality Algorithms

980 Jolly Road
Suite 21 F
Blue Bell, PA 19422-1963   215-654-5624
Fax: 215-283-6825

4653 Underwriters and Administrators

6345 Flank Drive
Harrisburg, PA 17112-2765   717-652-8040
Fax: 717-652-8328

4654 United Behavioral Health

425 Market Street
Suite 27
San Francisco, CA 94105-2406   415-547-5201
Fax: 415-547-5999

4655 United Behavioral Health

4170 Ashford Dunwoody Road NE
Suite 100
Atlanta, GA 30319-1457
Fax: 404-231-0125

Clinical Management/Management Companies

4656 United Correctional Managed Care

12647 Olive Boulevard
Saint Louis, MO 63141-6345   770-989-0002

4657 United Health Care

9900 Bren Road E
Hopkins, MN 55343-9664   612-936-6838
Fax: 612-936-6814

4658 Unity Health Network

12409 Powers Court Drive
Saint Louis, MO 63131   314-364-3646
800-413-8008
Fax: 314-364-2036
E-mail: Bultmb@STLO.SMHS.com

Mary Beth Bulte, Director

4659 Univera

130 Empire Drive
W Seneca, NY 14224-1320   716-668-9765
Fax: 716-668-5862

4660 Universal Behavioral Service

820 Fort Wayne Avenue
Indianapolis, IN 46204-1309   317-684-0442
Fax: 317-684-0679

4661 University Behavioral Health Care

57 Route 1 S
Suite 3060
Iselin, NJ 08830   732-283-6100
732-283-6060

4662 University of North Carolina School of Social Work, Behavioral Healthcare

301 Pittsboro Street
Suite 3550
Chapel Hill, NC 27516-2911   919-962-4372
Fax: 919-962-6562
E-mail: amsheye@email.unc.edu
www.unc.edu/depts.ssw

4663 VJT Associates

26 Diaz Plaza
Staten Island, NY 10306-5600   718-627-0700
Fax: 718-375-3389

4664 Value Health

22 Waterville Road
Avon, CT 06001-2066   860-678-3472
Fax: 860-678-3469

4665 ValueOptions

3110 Fairview Park Drive
Falls Church, VA 22042-4503
800-824-7762
Fax: 703-208-8850
E-mail: info@valueoptions.com
www.valueoptions.com

Designs and operates innovative administrative and full-risk services for a wide range of behavioral health and chemical dependency programs, Medicaid, child welfare and other human services, and Employee Assistance Programs. Develops collaborative relationships with government agencies, community providers, consumer groups, health plans, insurers, and others to foster a deeper understanding of the needs of the various populations they serve. Develops child welfare programs based upon the principles of managed care.

4666 Vance Messmer and Butler

1853 S Horne
Suite 2
Mesa, AZ 85204-6501   602-497-1250

4667 Vanderveer Group

520 Virginia Drive
Fort Washington, PA 19034-2795   215-283-5373
Fax: 215-646-5547

4668 Vasquez Management Consultants

100 S Greenleaf Avenue
Gurnee, IL 60031-3378   847-249-1900
800-367-7378
Fax: 847-249-2772

4669 Vedder, Price, Kaufman, and Kammholz

222 N Lasalle Street
Suite 2500
Chicago, IL 60601-1003   312-609-7654
Fax: 312-609-5005

4670 Veri-Trak

179 Niblick Road
Suite 149
Paso Robles, CA 93446-4845   805-550-1443

4671 VeriCare

47415 Viewridge Avenue
Suite 230
San Diego, CA 92123-1680   858-454-3610
800-257-8715
Fax: 800-819-1655
www.seniorpsycholoyservices.com

4672 Virginia Beach Community Service Board

Pembroke 6
Suite 208
Virginia Beach, VA 23462   757-437-5770
Fax: 804-490-5736

4673 Watson Wyatt Worldwide

15303 Ventura Boulevard
Suite 700
Sherman Oaks, CA 91403-3197   818-906-2631
Fax: 808-906-2097

4674 Webman Associates

4 Brattle Street
Cambridge, MA 02138-3714   617-864-6769
Fax: 617-492-3673

531

4675 Weimer Associates

1560 E Chevy Chase Drive
Suite 320
Glendale, CA 91206-4140   213-662-5798
Fax: 213-913-0260

4676 WellPoint Behavioral Health

11200 Westheimer Road
Suite 928
Houston, TX 77042-3227   713-914-3677
Fax: 713-787-9701

4677 William M Mercer

133 Peachtree Street NE
3700 Georgia Pacific Center
Atlanta, GA 30303-1808   404-527-4728
Fax: 404-523-1458

4678 Working Press

2525 Main Street
Suite 205
Santa Monica, CA 90405-3538   310-314-8600

4679 Wyatt Company, Research and Information

1850 M Street NW
Suite 400
Washington, DC 20036-5815   202-887-4600

Software Companies

4680 ACC

12500 San Pedro
Suite 460
San Antonio, TX 78216-2867
800-880-4222
Fax: 210-545-5545

4681 ADAPS

1154 Fort Street Mall
Suite 209
Honolulu, HI 96813-2712   808-528-1184
Fax: 808-566-1885

4682 AHMAC

140 Allens Creek Road
Rochester, NY 14618-3307   716-461-4236
Fax: 716-461-0059

4683 AIMS

485 Underhill Boulevard
Syosset, NY 11791-3434   516-496-7700
Fax: 516-496-7069

4684 AMCO Computers

750 W Golden Grove Way
Covina, CA 91722-3255   626-859-6292
E-mail: amco@aol.com

4685 APPC Data Processing

3 Maryland Farms
Suite 350
Brentwood, TN 37027-5082   615-221-4450

4686 ASP Software

1031 E Duane Avenue
Suite M
Sunnyvale, CA 94086-2625   408-733-7831
800-822-7832

4687 Accreditation Services

Glen E Philmon Sr
PO Box 73270
Metairie, LA 70033-3270   504-469-4285
Fax: 504-467-7688
www.accreditationservices.com

Multiple software programs dedicated to the support of health care industry's needs for training, continuing education, work order processing and inventory control and the various demands placed upon the system by regulatory boards. Services are completely confidential and available for almost every department of the hospital, nursing home, ICF/MR facilities and many others. Each software program can be customized to be site-specific.

4688 Accumedic Computer Systems

11 Grace Avenue
Great Neck, NY 11021-2417   516-466-6800
800-765-9300
Fax: 516-466-6880
E-mail: sales@accumedic.com
www.accumedic.com

Sean Doolan, Director Sales/Marketing

Practice management solutions for mental health facilities: scheduling, billing, EMR, HIPAA.

4689 Ada S McKinley

16603 Paulina Street
Harvey, IL 60426-5849   312-434-5577

4690 Adam Software

3110 Bonnell Avenue SE
Grand Rapids, MI 49506-3136
800-788-4774

4691 Advanced Data Systems

700 Mount Hope Avenue, Suite 100
Bangor, ME 04401-6295   207-947-4494
800-779-4494
Fax: 207-947-0650
E-mail: info@adspro.com
www.adspro.com

Advanced Data Systems (ADS) is a New England-based software developer and reseller of accounting information systems with over 23 years of experience. We specialize in developing, implementing and supporting administrative software. As a complement to our software we also provide technical services. Advanced Data Systems is your "total accounting solution".

4692 Agilent Technologies

3000 Minuteman Road
Andover, MA 01810-1032   978-687-1501
                               Fax: 978-794-7646

4693 Algorithms for Behavioral Care

PO Box 10889
Tampa, FL 33679-0889
                               800-357-1200
                               Fax: 203-866-9614

PC software application supports test administration and produces reports relating to outcomes tracking, intake measurement of symptom severity, index of risk factors, individual profiling and case mix outcomes reporting.

4694 Alliance Underwriters

155 Franklin Road
Suite 250
Brentwood, TN 37027-4646   615-377-2000
                               Fax: 615-377-2025
                               www.allianceu.com

4695 American Health Management and Consulting

140 Allens Creek Road
Rochester, NY 14618-3307   716-461-4236
                               Fax: 716-461-0059

4696 American Medical Software

1180 S State Highway 157
PO Box 236
Edwardsville, IL 62025-0236   618-692-1300
                               800-423-8836
                               Fax: 618-692-1809
           E-mail: sales@americanmedical.com
                   www.americanmedical.com

W David Scott, President

Practice management software for billing, electronic claims, appointments and electronic medical records.

4697 American Pediatric Medical Association

9312 Old Georgetown Road
Bethesda, MD 20814-1698   301-571-9200
                               Fax: 301-530-2752

4698 American Psychiatric Press Reference Library CD-ROM

American Psychiatric Publishing
1000 Wilson Boulevard
Suite 1825
Arlington, VA 22209-3901   703-907-7322
                               800-368-5777
                               Fax: 703-907-1091
                      E-mail: appi@psych.org
                               www.appi.org

Katie Duffy, Marketing Assistant

$395.00

Year Founded: 1998

4699 Anasazi Software

9831 S 51st Street
Suite C117
Phoenix, AZ 85044-5673   480-598-8833
                               800-651-4411
                               Fax: 480-496-8089
                      www.anasazisoftware.com

4700 Andrew and Associates

PO Box 9226
Winter Haven, FL 33883-9226   941-299-4767
                               Fax: 941-293-9678

4701 Applied Behavioral Technologies

2050 S Clinton Avenue
Rochester, NY 14618-5703   716-244-5590

4702 Aries Systems Corporation

200 Sutton Street
N Andover, MA 01845-1656   978-975-7570
                               Fax: 978-975-3811
                               www.kfinder.com

4703 Ascent

PO Box 230
Naples, ID 83847-0239   208-267-3626
                               Fax: 208-267-5711

4704 Askesis Development Group

325 W Huron Street
Suite 506
Chicago, IL 60610-3640   312-951-0302
                               Fax: 312-951-0493
                               www.psychconsult.org

Askesis Development Group's PsychConsult is a complete informatics solution for behavioral health organizations: inpatient or outpatient behavioral health facilities, managed care organizations, and provider networks. PsychConsult is Windows NT based, and Y2K compliant. ADG development is guided by the PsychConsult Consortium, a collaborative effort of leading institutions in behavioral health.

4705 Aspen Tree Software

709 Grand Avenue
Laramie, WY 82070-3945   307-721-5888
                               Fax: 307-721-2135

4706 Assist Technologies

16267 S 13th Street
Phoenix, AZ 85048-9212   602-460-4125

4707 Austin Travis County Mental Health Mental Retardation Center

1430 Collier Street
Austin, TX 78704-2911   512-447-4141
                               Fax: 512-440-4081
                      E-mail: help@atcmhmr.com
                               www.atcmhmr.com

Provides mental health, mental retardation and substance services to the Austin-Travis County community.

4708 Aware Resources

96 Graham Road
Suite C
Cuyahoga Falls, OH 44223-1205   330-940-4383
                                  Fax: 330-940-4393
            E-mail: info@awareresources.com
                    www.awareresources.com

Susan Searl, Director Clinical Services

Provides behavior management consultation, staff training and client counseling.

4709 Beaver Creek Software

525 SW 6th Street
Corvallis, OR 97333-4323   541-752-5039
                                  800-895-3344
                             Fax: 541-752-5221
            E-mail: sales@beaverlog.com
                    www.beaverlog.com

Powerful, yet easy to use practice management and billing software for IBM compatible computers. Updated regularly. *$249.00*

Year Founded: 1989

4710 Beechwood Software

975 Ebner Drive
Webster, NY 14580-9398   716-872-6450
                           Fax: 716-872-0862

4711 Behavior Data

994 San Antonio Road
Palo Alto, CA 94303-4951   650-843-1850
                                  800-627-2673
                             Fax: 408-554-0481

4712 Behavior Graphics Division of Supervised Lifestyles

106 Brewster Square
Department 279
Brewster, NY 10509-1118   845-228-4328
                                  800-448-6975
                             Fax: 845-279-7678
                             www.slshealth.com

Fully intergrated informatics software solutions; clinical, billing/AR, administration, outcomes.

4713 Behavior Therapy Software

890 Biddle Road
Suite 280
Medford, OR 97504-6117
                                  800-838-9173
                             Fax: 541-773-3621

4714 Behavioral Health Advisor

McKesson Clinical Reference Systems
335 Interlocken Parkway
Broomfield, CO 80021-3484   303-664-6485
                                  800-237-8401
                             Fax: 303-460-6282
            E-mail: crs-info@cliniref.com
                    www.patienteducation.com

The Behavioral Health Advisor software program provides consumer health information for more than 600 topics covering pediatric and adult mental illness, disorders and behavioral problems. Includes behavioral health topics from the American Academy of Child and Adolescent Psychiatry. Many Spanish translations available. *$4.75*

Year Founded: 1998

4715 Behavioral Health Partners

2200 Century Parkway NE
Suite 675
Atlanta, GA 30345-3156   404-315-9325
                           Fax: 404-315-0786

4716 Behavioral MAPS

21900 Greenfield Road
Oak Park, MI 48237-2577   248-968-3887
                           Fax: 248-968-2886

4717 Bellefaire Jewish Children's Bureau

22001 Fairmount Boulevard
Shaker Heights, OH 44118-4819   216-932-2800
                                       800-879-2522
                                  Fax: 216-932-6704
            E-mail: contact@bellefairejcb.org
                    www.bellefairejcb.org

Adam G Jacobs PhD, Director
Deborah W Cowan, Associate Director
Jamie Cole, Director Communications

A nonprofit mental health agency committed to serving the needs of children, youth and their families through an array of child welfare and behavioral health services. Provides its services without regard to race, religion, sex or national origin.

4718 BetaData Systems

3137 E Greenlee Road
Tucson, AZ 85716-1225   520-733-5656

4719 Blackberry Technologies

430 Park Avenue
Floor 3
New York, NY 10022-3505   212-217-9200
                            Fax: 212-246-7282

4720 Body Logic

PO Box 162101
Austin, TX 78716-2101   512-327-0050
                               800-285-8212
                          Fax: 512-328-9234

4721 Brand Software

500 W Cummings Park
Woburn, MA 01801-6503   781-937-0404
                               800-343-5737
                          Fax: 781-937-3232
            E-mail: sporter@helper.com
                    www.helper.com

Shobhan Porter, Director Marketing

Therapist Helper, the leading practice management software program, processes patient and insurance billing transactins, accounts receivable, statements, and tracks payments. Therapist Helper will also assist in scheduling managed care tracking, and electronic claims submission. Will network at no additional charge. All you'll need is IMB or compatible Pentium with 16 MB RAM and at least 25 MB available hard drive space. Download a free, full working demo at our website.

4722 Bull Worldwide Information Systems
300 Concord Road
Billerica, MA 01821-3465
978-294-6675
Fax: 978-294-5164

4723 CARE Computer Systems
636 120th Avenue NE
Bellevue, WA 98005-3039
425-451-8272
800-426-2675
Fax: 425-455-4895

4724 CASCAP, Continuous Quality
678 Massachusetts Avenue
Floor 10
Cambridge, MA 02139-3355
617-492-5559
Fax: 617-492-6928

4725 CDS
PO Box 691145
Houston, TX 77269-1145
713-320-9797

4726 CLARC Services
5919 Beneva Road
Sarasota, FL 34236
941-924-5488
800-246-5488
Fax: 941-924-7940
E-mail: dclaise@clarc.com
www.clarc.com

Dave Claise, Sales Consultant

Computer consultancy which provides software, software training and support, custom programming, modifacations to packaged products and education. We help your business with hardware and software installation and setup as well as data migration, integration and data conversion. Creators of Mental Health Organizational System Interface (MHOSI).

4727 CMHC Systems
570 Metro Place N
Dublin, OH 43017-1300
614-764-0143
Fax: 614-799-3159

4728 COMPSYCH Software Information Services
Peter Hornby and Margaret Anderson, SUNY
101 Broad Street
Plattsburgh, NY 12901
www.plattsburgh.edu.compsych/

Provides information about psychological software, arranged in topical categories such as statistics, cognitive, physiological, and personality testing.

4729 CORE Management
200 Wheeler Road
Suite 5
Burlington, MA 01803-5501
781-229-9400
Fax: 781-229-9429

4730 CSI Software
24 E Greenway Plaza
Suite 606
Houston, TX 77046-2486
713-572-8322
800-247-3431

4731 Cardiff Software: San Marcos
1782 La Costa Meadows Drive
San Marcos, CA 92069-5106
760-752-5200
Fax: 760-936-4800

4732 Cardiff Software: Vista
3220 Executive Road
Vista, CA 92083-8527
760-936-4500
Fax: 760-936-4800
www.cardiff.com

4733 Center for Clinical Computing
350 Longwood Avenue
Beth Israel Hospital
Boston, MA 02115-5726
617-732-5925

4734 Center for Health Policy Studies
10400 Little Patuxent Parkway
Suite 10
Columbia, MD 21044-3518
410-715-9400
Fax: 410-715-9718

4735 Center for Human Development
332 Birnie Avenue
Springfield, MA 01107-1106
413-733-6624
Fax: 413-746-4657

4736 Ceridian Corporation
3311 E Old Shackopee Road
Minneapolis, MN 55425
612-853-8100

4737 Chartman Software
PO Box 551
Santa Barbara, CA 93102-0551
800-500-0893
Fax: 805-563-1977

4738 Chattanooga State Tech Community Colle
4501 Amnicola Highway
Chattanooga, TN 37406-1097
423-697-2417
Fax: 423-697-3131

4739 Cincom Systems
55 Merchant Street
Cincinnati, OH 45246-3732
513-662-2300
Fax: 513-612-2000

4740 Cirrus Technology

5301 Buckeystown Pike
Floor 4
Frederick, MD 21704-8370   301-698-1900
                                  Fax: 301-698-1909

4741 Clermont Counseling Center

1088 Hospital Street
Suite C
Batavia, OH 45013   513-732-5475
                                  Fax: 513-732-5467

4742 Client Management Information System

WilData Systems Group
4995 Bradenton Avenue
Suite 140
Dublin, OH 43017-3551   614-734-4719
                                  800-860-4222
                             Fax: 614-734-1063
          E-mail: jeffwilt@wildatainc.com
                     www.wildatainc.com

Jeffrey D Wilt, President

Complete software package designed as a total solution for the information and reporting requirements of behavioral health care centers, drug and alcohol abuse centers, human service organizations and family service agencies. CMIS is easy to use with graphical user input screens allowing point and click capabilities under Microsoft Windows.

4743 CliniSphere version 2.0

Facts and Comparisons
111 Westport Plaza
Suite 300
Saint Louis, MO 63146-3014
                                  800-223-0554
                             Fax: 314-878-1574
                             www.drugfacts.com

Access to all information in a clinical drug reference library, by drug, disease, side-effects; thousands of drugs (prescription, OTC, investigational) all included; contains information from Drug Facts and Comparisons, most definitive and comprehensive source for comparative drug information.

4744 Clinical Nutrition Center

7555 E Hampden Avenue
Suite 301
Denver, CO 80231-4834   303-750-9454
                                  Fax: 303-750-1996

4745 Communications Media

1 Tower Bridge
Suite 250
Conshohocken, PA 19428   610-825-1100
                                  Fax: 610-825-8660

4746 Community Sector Systems PsychAccess Chart

700 5th Avenue
Suite 6100
Seattle, WA 98104-5061   206-467-9061
                                  Fax: 206-467-9237

Patient-centered documentation for problem-focused care; the electronic answer to more descriptive and reliable patient charts.

4747 Community Solutions

123 Moultrie Street
San Francisco, CA 94110-5615   415-512-7768
                                  Fax: 415-512-0181

4748 Companion Technologies

633 Davis Drive
Suite 600
Morrisville, NC 27560   919-286-5509
                                  Fax: 919-484-1850

4749 Comprehensive Review Technology

781 NW Boulevard
Columbus, OH 43212-3858   614-291-7071

4750 Compu-Care Management and Systems

13740 Research Boulevard
Suite U4
Austin, TX 78750-1841   512-219-8025
                                  Fax: 512-249-1258

4751 CompuLab Healthcare Systems Corporation

PO Box 11739
Fort Lauderdale, FL 33339-1739   954-564-1200

4752 CompuSystems

1 Science Court
Carolina Research Park
Columbia, SC 29203-9356   803-735-7700
                                  800-800-6472
                             Fax: 800-800-8355
                             www.medic.com

4753 Computer Applications in Clinical Psychology

10070 Pasadena Avenue
Cupertino, CA 95014-5942   408-446-3322
                                  Fax: 408-446-4233

4754 Computer Assisted Treatment Systems

8306 Wilshire Boulevard
Beverly Hills, CA 90211-2382   323-731-7900
                                  800-274-9027
                             Fax: 213-653-1429

4755 Computer Business Solutions

8007 S Meridian Street
Suite 2A
Indianapolis, IN 46217-2901   317-888-6916
                                  800-729-6916
                             Fax: 317-888-6945

4756 Computer Scheduling Services

103 Roxbury Street
Suite 305
Keene, NH 03431-3800   301-356-2953

4757 Computer Transition Services

3223 S Loop 289
Lubbock, TX 79423-1337   806-793-8961
                                Fax: 806-793-8968

4758 Computers and High Tech in Behavioral Practice Special Interest Group

Association for Advancement of Behavior Therapy
116 N Robertson Boulevard
Suite 905
Los Angeles, CA 90048   310-652-4252
                                Fax: 310-652-4913
                                E-mail: bgalephd@aol.com
                        www.luna.cas.usf.edu/~rrusson/chip

Bruce M Gale PhD, President

This organization is composed of individuals interested in the experimental and clinical application of computers and other technology in the psychological and behavioral sciences. It fosters discussion and collaboration, disseminating information among its members and AABT's broader membership. While most members belong to AABT, nonmembers of AABT are invited to apply as well.

4759 Computers for Medicine

2900 Adams Street
Suite 420
Riverside, CA 92504-4335   909-687-6465
                                Fax: 909-687-6698

4760 Concord-Assabet Family and Adolescent Services

380 Massachusetts Avenue
Acton, MA 01720-3745   978-263-3006
                                Fax: 978-263-3088

4761 Confidential Data Services

14828 W 6th Avenue
Golden, CO 80401-5000   303-278-1501

4762 Consultec, Managed Care Systems

9040 Roswell Road
Suite 700
Atlanta, GA 30350-7530   813-784-7947
                                Fax: 813-789-6136

4763 Control-0-Fax Corporation

3070 W Airline Highway
Waterloo, IA 50703-9591   319-234-4651
                                Fax: 319-236-7350

4764 CoolTalk

Netscape Communicatons
PO Box 7050
Mountain View, CA 94039-7050   650-254-1900
                                800-784-3348
                                Fax: 650-528-4124
                                www.netscape.com

Intergrated telephone application, allows connected users to draw or sketch ideas cooperatively onto the same area on each person's computer screen.

4765 Cornucopia Software

PO Box 6111
Albany, CA 94706-0111   510-528-7000
                                www.practicemagic.com

4766 Creative Computer Applications

26115 Mureau Road
Suite A
Calabasas, CA 91302-3128   818-880-6700
                                Fax: 818-880-4398
                                www.ccaine.com

4767 Creative Socio-Medics Corporation

146 Nassau Avenue
Islip, NY 11751-3216   516-968-2000
                                800-421-7503
                                Fax: 516-968-2123

Member of the National Leadership Council.

4768 DB Consultants

198 Tabor Road
Ottsville, PA 18942-9606   610-847-5065
                                Fax: 610-847-2298

4769 DISC Systems

3055 Old Highway 8
Minneapolis, MN 55418-2500   612-782-9373
                                800-879-3472
                                Fax: 612-782-7500

4770 Data Flow Companies

4214 Beechwood Drive
Suite 105
Greensboro, NC 27410-8107   919-275-3324

4771 Data General

255 Washington Street
2 Newton Place
Newton, MA 02458-1637   508-366-8911
                                Fax: 508-898-4052

4772 DataBreeze

2151 W Hillsboro Boulevard
Suite 307
Deerfield Beach, FL 33442-1100
                                800-929-3076
                                Fax: 954-427-0280

4773 DataMark

30233 Southfield Road
Suite 201
Southfield, MI 48076-1363   248-203-1240
                                Fax: 248-203-1243

4774 Datamedic

20 Oser Avenue
Hauppauge, NY 11788-3825   516-435-8880
                                800-446-4021
                                Fax: 516-435-1062

4775 Dataminder Systems
PO Box 191224
San Diego, CA 92159-1224   619-464-5193
                                  Fax: 619-464-5403

4776 Datasys/DSI
4125 Keller Springs Road
Suite 166
Dallas, TX 75244   214-931-9195
                                  Fax: 214-931-9619

4777 Delta Health Systems
PO Box 1824
Altoona, PA 16603-1824   814-944-1651
                                  Fax: 814-942-0125

4778 DeltaMetrics
225 Market Street
Suite 1120
Philadelphia, PA 19106-4502
                                  800-238-2433
                                  Fax: 215-665-2892

4779 DeltraMetrics Treatment Research Institute
2005 Market Street, Suite 1020
One Commerce Square
Philadelphia, PA 19103-7042   215-665-2880
                                  Fax: 215-665-2892

4780 Digital Medical Systems
185 Berry Street
San Francisco, CA 94107-1729   650-866-4466
                                  Fax: 415-866-4477

4781 Distance Learning Network
111 W Main Street
Boalsburg, PA 16827   814-466-7808
                                  800-326-9166
                                  Fax: 814-466-7509
E-mail: dlnstaff@dlnetwork.com
www.dlnetwork.com

Eric Porterfield, President/CEO
Sandy Weaver, VP Program Development
Sheri Mills, Marketing

Broadcast and multimedia company dedicated solely to meeting the medical education and communications needs of physicians through the use of both traditional and innovative media formats. More than 150,000 physicians, nurses and pharmacists turn to DLN each year for their medical education.

Year Founded: 1996

4782 Docu Trac
20140 Scholar Drive
Suite 218
Hagerstown, MD 21742-2562   301-766-9397
                                  800-850-8510
                                  Fax: 301-766-4097
E-mail: info@quicdoc.com
www.quicdoc.com

Brenda K Shirk, Account Manager

Offering Quic Doc clinical documentation software, a comprehensive software system designed specifically for behavioral healthcare providers.

4783 DocuMed
8101 N High Street
Suite 370
Columbus, OH 43235-1442   614-786-7650
                                  800-321-5595
                                  Fax: 612-645-0019

4784 E Care
1510 Portola Road
Redwood City, CA 94062-1227   650-851-3037

4785 EAP Information Systems
PO Box 1650
Yreka, CA 96097-1650
                                  800-755-6965

4786 Earley Corporation
130 Krog Street NE
Atlanta, GA 30307-2478   404-370-1212
                                  800-297-3270
                                  Fax: 404-378-0346

4787 East Oregon Human Services Consortium
100 K Avenue
La Grande, OR 97850   541-962-3430
                                  Fax: 541-962-3427

4788 Eastern Computer
6711 Kingston Pike
Knoxville, TN 37919-4830   423-588-6491
                                  Fax: 423-588-7822

4789 Echo Group
1700 Broadway
Suite 800
Oakland, CA 94612-2116   510-238-2727
                                  Fax: 510-238-2730

4790 Eclipsys Corporation
141 Stony Circle
Suite 150
Santa Rosa, CA 95401   707-528-7300
                                  Fax: 707-528-4500

4791 Eclipsys Corporation
777 E Atlantic Avenue
Suite 200
Delray Beach, FL 33483-5360   561-243-1440
                                  Fax: 561-243-8850

4792 Eldorado Computing
5353 N 16th Street
Suite 400
Phoenix, AZ 85016-3200   602-493-0288
                                  Fax: 602-687-7920

4793 Electronic Healthcare Systems
100 Brookwood Plaza
Suite 410
Birmingham, AL 35209-6831   205-871-1031
Fax: 205-871-1185

4794 Engineered Data Products
2550 W Midway Boulevard
Broomfield, CO 80020-1633   303-465-2800
Fax: 303-404-5849

4795 Enterprise Health Solutions
2 Alba Avenue
Salem, MA 01970   978-740-0381
800-745-8123
Fax: 978-744-9860
E-mail: EHealth@aol.com

David R Selden, President

Operational consulting services for behavioral organizations.

4796 Enterprise Systems
1400 S Wolf Road
Wheeling, IL 60090-6573   708-537-4800

4797 Enterprize Management Systems
207 Hidden Springs Lane
Covington, LA 70433-5575   423-282-5049
Fax: 423-282-3604

4798 Entre Computer Center of Billings
PO Box 7157
Billings, MT 59103-7157   406-256-5700
Fax: 406-256-0201

4799 Experior Corporation
5710 Coventry Lane
Fort Wayne, IN 46804-7141   219-432-2020
Fax: 219-432-4753

4800 Facts Services
1575 San Ignacio Avenue
Suite 406
Coral Gables, FL 33146-3000   305-284-7400
Fax: 305-661-6710

4801 Family Service Agency
123 W Gutierrez Street
Santa Barbara, CA 93101-3424   805-965-1001
Fax: 805-965-2178
E-mail: info@fsacares.org
www.fsacares.org

William EG Batty III, Executive Director
Caroline Baker, Development Director

Non profit, non sectarian human service agency whose mission is to strengthen and to advocate for families and individuals of all ages, thereby creating a strong community. Programs are either free of charge or available on a sliding fee schedule based on ability to pay.

4802 Family Services of Delaware County
806 W Jackson Street
Muncie, IN 47305-1551   765-284-7789
Fax: 765-281-2733

4803 Ferguson Software
12444 Powerscourt Drive
Suite 272
Saint Louis, MO 63131-3619   314-822-0081
Fax: 314-822-1994

4804 Filipino American Service Group
135 N Park View Street
Los Angeles, CA 90026-5215   213-487-9804
Fax: 213-487-9806

4805 First Data Bank
1111 Bayhill Drive
San Bruno, CA 94066-3027   650-266-4808
800-633-3453

4806 Florida Health Information Management Association
5901 Augusta National Drive
Suite 110
Orlando, FL 32822-3244   407-647-4677

4807 Focus Services
800 E Wardlow Road
Suite A
Long Beach, CA 90807-4651   562-981-2101
800-540-1200
Fax: 562-981-2104
www.focusservicesinc.com

Charles Ume, Consultant
Dom Domingo, Manager Buisness Development

Provides integrated practice management solutions using The Medical Manager Software which helps providers control costs while improving the quality of care they deliver.

4808 Gadrian Corporation
5680 Greenwood Plaza Boulevard
Suite 260
Englewood, CO 80111-2404   303-930-2663
Fax: 800-789-9328

4809 Gateway Healthcare
160 Beechwood Avenue
Pawtucket, RI 02860-5402   401-722-5523
Fax: 401-722-5630

4810 GenSource Corporation
25572 Stanford Avenue
Valencia, CA 91355   661-294-1300
Fax: 661-294-1310

4811 Genelco
9735 Landmark Parkway Drive
Saint Louis, MO 63127   314-525-9000
888-436-3526
Fax: 314-525-9922

4812 Great Lakes Medical Computer Clinic

3930 Sunforest Court
Suite 180
Toledo, OH 43623-4441   419-473-1444
Fax: 419-473-2437

4813 HBOC

5995 Windward Parkway
Alpharetta, GA 30005-4184   404-338-6000
Fax: 404-338-6101

4814 HCA Information Services

2555 Park Plaza
Nashville, TN 37203-1512   615-320-6489
Fax: 615-320-6997

4815 HCIA Response

950 Winter Street
Suite 3450
Waltham, MA 02451-1486

800-522-1440
Fax: 781-768-1811

4816 HCIA-RESPONSE

300 E Lombard Street
Baltimore, MD 21202-3219   410-895-7300
Fax: 410-547-8297

4817 HMS Healthcare Management Systems

3401 W End Avenue
Suite 290
Nashville, TN 37203   615-383-7300
Fax: 615-383-6093
www.hmstn.com

4818 HMS Software

14875 Landmark Boulevard
Dallas, TX 75240-6786   212-960-6036

4819 HSA-Mental Health

1080 Emeline Avenue
Santa Cruz, CA 95060-1966   831-454-4000
Fax: 831-454-4770
TDD: 831-454-2123
E-mail: info@santacruzhealth.org
www.santacruzhealth.org

Rama Khalsa PhD, Health Services Administrator
David McNutt MD, County Health Officer

Exists to protect and improve the health of the people in Santa Cruz County. Provides programs in environmental health, public health, medical care, substance abuse prevention and treatment, and mental health. Clients are entitled to information on the costs of care and their options for getting health insurance coverage through a variety of programs.

4820 HZI Research Center

150 White Plains Road
Tarrytown, NY 10591-5535   914-631-3315
Fax: 914-616-5905

4821 Habilitation Software

Betsy Rasmussen
204 N Sterling Street
Morganton, NC 28655-3345   828-438-9455
Fax: 828-438-9488
E-mail: paulehabsoft.com
www.habsoft.com

Personal Planning System, Windows-based computer program which assists agencies serving people with developmental disabilities with the tasks of person-centered planning; tracks outcomes, services and supports, assists with assesments and quarterly reviews, and maintains a customizable library of training programs. Also includes a census system for agencies which must maintain an exact midnight census, as well as an Accident/Incident system.

4822 Habilitative Systems

415 S Kilpatrick Avenue
Chicago, IL 60644-4923   773-261-2252
Fax: 773-854-8300

4823 Healing for Survivors

PO Box 4698
Fresno, CA 93744-4698   559-442-3600
Fax: 559-442-0187

4824 Health Data Sciences Corporation

268 W Hospitality Lane
San Bernardino, CA 92408-3241   909-888-3282
Fax: 909-885-0124

4825 Health Ed Resources and Medical Extracts

82 Seacliff Drive
Aptos, CA 95003-4542

Fax: 408-622-0755

4826 Health Management

3687 Mount Diablo Boulevard
Suite 200
Lafayette, CA 94549-3717   510-631-6750
Fax: 510-299-7010

4827 Health Resource

209 Katherine Drive
Conway, AR 72032-8891   501-329-5272
Fax: 501-329-8700

4828 HealthLine Systems

11423 W Bernardo Court
San Diego, CA 92127-1639   619-673-1700
800-733-8737

4829 HealthSoft

620 E Livingston Street
Orlando, FL 32803   407-648-4857
800-235-0882
Fax: 407-426-7440
E-mail: healthsoft@bellsouth.net
www.nursingresourcecenter.com

Mary Alice Willis MS, RN, President

CD - ROM and web based software for professionals on mental health nursing and developmental disabilities nursing.

4830 Healthcafe Software Solutions

636 Grand Avenue
Suite 217
Des Moines, IA 50309-2502   515-237-6602

4831 Healthcare Data

5693 S Bear Wallow Road
Suite 100
Morgantown, IN 46160-9315   317-887-1326
                                Fax: 314-887-1326

4832 Healthcare Management Systems

3102 W End Avenue
Suite 400
Nashville, TN 37203-6866   615-383-7300
                           Fax: 615-383-6093
                    E-mail: hms@hmstn.com
                            www.hmstn.com

Carl N Schneider, VP Sales/Marketing

4833 Healthcare Strategy Associates

1815 H Street NW
Suite 400
Washington, DC 20006-3604   202-463-7551
                                Fax: 202-463-7549

4834 Healthcare Vision

2601 Scott Avenue
Suite 600
Fort Worth, TX 76103-2307   817-923-0173
                                888-836-7428
                           Fax: 817-531-2360

4835 Healthcheck

3954 Youngfield Street
Wheat Ridge, CO 80033-3865   916-556-1880
                                Fax: 916-447-0444

4836 Healthware Systems

298 Robertson Boulevard
Suite 485
Beverly Hills, CA 90211   310-550-1145

4837 Hill Associates Healthcare Management Services

A Industrial Drive
PO Box 4070
Windham, NH 03087-4070   603-898-3115
                                Fax: 603-893-4856

4838 Hogan Assessment Systems

PO Box 521178
Tulsa, OK 74152   918-749-0632
                                Fax: 918-749-0639

4839 Horizon Systems

3050 Royal Boulevard S
Suite 100
Alpharetta, GA 30022-4484   770-410-5900
                                800-366-0593
                           Fax: 770-410-5910

4840 Human Services Assessment

110 Virginia Street
Luverne, MN 56156
                                800-477-1675
                           Fax: 507-283-9523

4841 Humanitas

3416 Olandwood Court
Suite 208
Olney, MD 20832-1373   301-570-3403
                                Fax: 301-570-4023

4842 IBM Corporation

3200 Windy Hill Road SE
Atlanta, GA 30339-5610   770-835-7917
                           Fax: 770-835-7972

4843 IBM Corporation Health Industry Marketing

PO Box 2150
Atlanta, GA 30301-2150   404-238-4420

4844 IBM Global Healthcare Industry

404 Wyman Street
Waltham, MA 02451-1264   781-768-1806
                           Fax: 781-768-1811

4845 IDX Systems Corporation

116 Huntington Avenue
Boston, MA 02116-5749   802-862-1022
                           Fax: 617-277-3426

4846 IMNET Systems

5995 Windward Parkway
Alpharetta, GA 30005-4184   770-521-5727
                           Fax: 770-521-5702

4847 IMS Medacom Networks

15000 W 6th Avenue
Suite 400
Golden, CO 80401-5047   303-279-6116

4848 InStream Corporation

67 S Bedford Street
One Burlington Business Center
Burlington, MA 01803-5152   781-221-7800
                           Fax: 781-935-2103

4849 InfoCapture

121 Meadowlook Way
Boulder, CO 80304-0431   303-607-9830

4850 InfoMC

2009 Renaissance Boulevard
Suite 100
King of Prussia, PA 19406-2763   610-292-8002
Fax: 610-292-9702

4851 InfoMed

1180 SW 36th Avenue
Pompano Beach, FL 33069-4837   954-343-8500

4852 InfoWorld Management Systems

95 Great Valley Parkway
Malvern, PA 19355-1309   610-647-2210
Fax: 610-272-4891

4853 Infocure Corporation

2970 Clairmont Road NE
Suite 930
Atlanta, GA 30329-1638   404-633-0066
Fax: 404-636-7525

4854 Information Architects

175 Highland Avenue
Needham, MA 02494-3034   781-449-0086

4855 Information Concepts

222 E Huntington Drive
Suite 225
Monrovia, CA 91016-3523   626-305-7200
Fax: 626-305-7213

4856 Information Management Solutions

1600 W Broadway Road
Suite 385
Tempe, AZ 85282-1181   602-921-0469
Fax: 602-921-7469

4857 Information Network Corporation (INC)

7600 N 16th Street
Suite 230
Phoenix, AZ 85020-4498   602-957-7670
Fax: 602-957-4307

Member of the National Leadership Council.

4858 Informational Medical Systems

2445 Park Avenue
Minneapolis, MN 55404-3790   612-941-1600
800-326-7833

4859 Informed Access

335 Interlocken Parkway
Broomfield, CO 80021-3484   303-443-4600
Fax: 303-443-3909

4860 Informix Software

4100 Bohannon Drive
Building 4300
Menlo Park, CA 94025-1032   650-926-6313
Fax: 650-926-6172

4861 Inforum

424 Church Street
Suite 2600
Nashville, TN 37219-2379   615-780-7236
800-829-0600
Fax: 615-780-7201

4862 Inner Health

1260 Lincoln Avenue
San Diego, CA 92103-2322   619-299-7273
800-283-4679

4863 Innovative Computer Consulting

PO Box 488
Sonora, CA 95370-0488   209-532-4278
Fax: 209-532-3750

4864 Innovative Data Solutions

5311 Northfield Road
Suite 400
Bedford, OH 44146-1135   216-587-9440
Fax: 216-587-9480

4865 Innovative Health Systems/SoftMed

8950 Cal Center Drive
Suite 201
Sacramento, CA 95826-3225   916-368-4676
800-695-4447
Fax: 916-368-4984

4866 Innovative Systems Development

3361 Executive Parkway
Toledo, OH 43606-1377   419-531-4442
Fax: 419-539-6234
E-mail: JFisher@innSystems.com
www.innSystems.com

PsychServ incorporates the necessary tools to ensure
outcomes measurement in a proactive environment,
ensure the most efficient workflow, and ensure the
highest level of automation.

4867 Institute for Healthcare Quality

8000 W 78th Street
Minneapolis, MN 55439-2534   612-829-3639
800-241-9611
Fax: 612-829-3506
E-mail: qual1st@hrmi.com
www.ihqi.com

4868 Institute for the Study of Children and Families

102 King Hall
Eastern Michigan University
Ypsilanti, MI 48197-2239   313-487-7607

4869 Integra

1060 1st Avenue
Suite 410
King of Prussia, PA 19406-1336   610-992-5493
Fax: 610-992-7046
E-mail: edwynl@integra-ease.com
www.integra-ease.com

Ed Lackey, Director Communications

Pioneered the use of outcomes measurement in behavioral healthcare with the development of COMPASS and Index of Special Services (ISS) informatics tools, which are widely recognized as unique, scientifically validated methods that ensure quality of care during treatment. Provides full and shared risk arrangements to health plans in addition to employee assistance programs and managed care services for corporations and unions.

4870 Integrated Business Services
118 W Streetsboro Street
Suite 150
Hudson, OH 44236-2711 216-656-1100
Fax: 216-656-1106

4871 Integrated Computer Products
125 Commerce Drive
Fayetteville, GA 30214-7336 770-719-1500

4872 Integrative Technical Services
2675 Windmill Parkway
Apartment 3321
Henderson, NV 89014-1945 702-898-9322

4873 InterQual
293 Boston Post Road W
Marlborough, MA 01752-4615 508-481-1181
Fax: 508-481-2393

4874 Interactive Health Systems
1337 Ocean Avenue
Suite C
Santa Monica, CA 90401-1009 310-451-8111
Fax: 310-470-6685

4875 InternetPhone
VocalTec
1 Executive Drive
Fort Lee, NJ 07024-3309 201-228-7000
Fax: 201-363-8986
E-mail: info@vocaltec.com
www.vocaltec.com

Telephone solution with availability on multiple platforms; one week free trial period for mental health related software is available.

4876 Intertec Publishing
9800 Metcalf Avenue
Overland Park, KS 66212-2216 913-967-1872
Fax: 913-967-1897

4877 JJO Enterprises
12651 S Dixie Hwy
Miami, FL 33156-5975 305-251-7267
Fax: 305-251-0303

4878 Jess Wright Communication
502 Plum Island
Newbury, MA 01951 208-462-3611
Fax: 208-462-6778

4879 Jewish Family Service
111 Prospect Street
Stamford, CT 06901-1208 203-921-4161
Fax: 203-921-4169

4880 Jewish Family Service of America
12500 NW Military Highway
Suite 250
San Antonio, TX 78231-1871 210-349-5481
Fax: 210-349-4634

4881 Juliette Fowler Homes
200 Fulton Street
Dallas, TX 75014 214-827-0813
Fax: 214-827-7021

4882 Kaiser Technology Group
PO Box 339
Brighton, CO 80601-0339 303-659-2446
Fax: 303-659-7995

4883 Kennedy Computing
55 Colonial Drive
Shrewsbury, MA 01545-1545
800-367-5369
Fax: 508-757-2266

4884 Kennedy Krieger Family Center
2917 E Middle Street
Baltimore, MD 21213 410-550-9669
Fax: 410-550-9135

4885 LINC Case Management Services
424 N Lake Avenue
Pasadena, CA 91101-1200 626-585-4100

4886 Lan Vision
4700 Duke Drive
Suite 170
Mason, OH 45040-8472
800-878-5262
Fax: 513-794-7272

4887 Lexical Technologies
1000 Atlantic Avenue
Suite 3106
Alameda, CA 94501-1160 501-865-8500

4888 LifeCare Management Systems
700 W Linda Vista Boulevard
Tucson, AZ 85737-5019 602-544-2902

4889 Lifelink Corporation: Bensenville Home Society
331 S York Road
Suite 206
Bensenville, IL 60106-2600 630-766-5800
Fax: 630-860-5130

4890 Lotus Development Corporation
55 Cambridge Parkway
Cambridge, MA 02142-1234   617-693-8627
Fax: 617-693-5474

4891 M/MGMT Systems
9261 Folsom Boulevard
Suite 503
Sacramento, CA 95826-2560   916-856-1960
Fax: 916-856-1964

4892 MEDCOM Information Systems
2117 Stonington Avenue
Hoffman Estates, IL 60195-2016   847-885-1553
800-424-0258
www.http://idt.net/~medcom19

4893 MEDIC Computer Systems
8529 Six Forks Road
Raleigh, NC 27615-2981   919-847-8102
Fax: 919-846-1555
www.medic.com

4894 MEDecision
724 W Lancaster Avenue
Suite 200
Wayne, PA 19087-2587   610-254-0202
Fax: 610-254-5100

4895 MHS
908 Niagara Falls Boulevard
N Tonawanda, NY 14120-2016   716-754-7401
800-465-3003
Fax: 416-424-1736

4896 MSJ Communications Corporation
42580 Caroline Court
Suite B
Palm Desert, CA 92211-5139   760-773-9453
Fax: 760-773-1194

4897 MULTUM Information Services
3200 Cherry Creek S Drive
Suite 300
Denver, CO 80209-3245   303-733-4447
Fax: 303-733-4434

4898 Magnus Software Corporation
2233 Lake Park Drive SE
Suite 400
Smyrna, GA 30080-8856   404-431-0554

4899 Main Street Software
292 Glen Drive
Sausalito, CA 94965-1819   415-331-6627
800-548-2256

4900 Managed Care Software
PO Box 18245
Columbus, OH 43218-0245   614-442-1115
800-841-2660
Fax: 614-888-2240

4901 McHenry County M/H Board
620 Dakota Street
Crystal Lake, IL 60012   815-455-2828
Fax: 815-455-2925
www.mc708.org

Our misson is to provide leadership and be accountable for the provision of prevention and treatment of mental illness, developmental disabilities, and chemical abuse by coordinative, developing and contracting services for all citizens of McHenry County.

4902 Med Assist
2420 NW 39th
Suite 100
Oklahoma City, OK 73112   405-946-3118
800-637-2251
Fax: 405-949-1295

4903 Med Data Systems
110 Escondido Avenue
Suite 203
Vista, CA 92084-6038   760-536-1074

4904 Med-ai
602 Courtland Street
Suite 400
Orlando, FL 32804-1342   407-644-5011
Fax: 407-644-8175

4905 MedPLUS
205 Reidhurst Avenue
Suite N-104
Nashville, TN 37203-1618   615-329-2016
Fax: 615-329-0250

4906 MedPLus Relations
8805 Governors Hill Drive
Cincinnati, OH 45249-3314   513-697-2200
800-444-6235
Fax: 513-583-8884

4907 Medcomp Software
PO Box 7847
Colorado Springs, CO 80933-7847   719-266-6159
Fax: 719-575-0272
www.medcompsoftware.com

4908 Medi-Span
8425 Woodfield Crossing Boulevard
Indianapolis, IN 46240-7315   765-469-5200
Fax: 765-469-5252

4909 Media International
5900 San Fernando Road
Glendale, CA 91202-2765   818-242-5314

4910 Medic Computer Systems
1633 Bayshore Highway
Suite 160
Burlingame, CA 94010-1515   650-259-7542

4911 Medical Data Partners

410 W Fallbrook Avenue
Suites 105, 106
Fresno, CA 93711-6197   209-486-4750

4912 Medical Documenting Systems

8101 N High Street
Suite 370
Columbus, OH 43235-1442   612-645-9500

4913 Medical Electronic Data Procesing

411 E Huntington Drive
Suite 302
Arcadia, CA 91006-3736   626-446-5700

4914 Medical Group Systems

601 E Corporate Drive
Lewisville, TX 75057-6403   214-613-1190

4915 Medical Information Systems

201 E University Parkway
Baltimore, MD 21218-2829   410-321-5478
Fax: 410-321-5479

4916 Medical Manager Corporation

562 E Weddell Drive
Suite 8
Sunnyvale, CA 94089-2108   408-541-0390
800-222-7701
Fax: 415-969-0118
www.medicalmanager.com

4917 Medical Manager Web MD

135 W Lake Drive
Springfield, IL 62703-4960   217-529-8700
800-879-2240
Fax: 217-529-8701

4918 Medical Records Institute

567 Walnut Street
PO Box 600700
Newton, MA 02460   617-964-3923
Fax: 617-964-3926
www.tepr.com

4919 Medical Records Solution

Creative Solutions Unlimited
203 Gilman Street
PO Box 550
Sheffield, IA 50475-0550   641-892-4466
800-253-7697
Fax: 641-892-4333

Reliable, comprehensive, intuitive, fully-integrated clinical software able to manage MDS 2.0 electronic submission, RUGs/PPS, triggers, Quick RAP's, survey reports, QI's, assessments, care plans, Quick Plans, physician orders, CQI, census, and hundreds of reports. Creative Solutions Unlimited provides outstanding toll-free support, training, updates, user groups, newsletters, and continuing education.

4920 Medipay

521 SW 11th Avenue
Suite 200
Portland, OR 97205-2620   800-842-1973
Fax: 503-299-6490
E-mail: medipay@medipay.com

Medipay's information technology products and services monitor and control quality, manage clinical and financial risk, collaborate and integrate with external stakeholders, and empower front line staff.

4921 Mediplex

70 Granite Street
Lynnma, MA 01904   781-592-5227
Fax: 781-581-3080
www.sunh.com

4922 Medix Systems Consultants

17050 S Park Avenue
S Holland, IL 60473-3374   708-331-0203
800-732-9280
Fax: 708-331-1272

4923 Medware

1055 N Dixie Freeway
Suite 2
New Smyrna Beach, FL 32168-6200   904-427-0558
Fax: 904-423-2571

4924 Mental Health Connections

21 Blossom Street
Lexington, MA 02421-8103   781-863-1583
800-788-4743
Fax: 781-890-6635

4925 Mental Health Outcomes

1500 Waters Ridge Drive
Lewisville, TX 75057-6011   972-420-8220
800-266-4440
Fax: 972-420-8215
www.mhoutcomes.com

Johan Smith, VP Operations/Development

Designs and implements custom outcome measurement systems specifically for behavioral helath programs through its CQI Outcomes Measurement System. This system provides information for a wide range of patient and treatment focused variables for child, adolesent, adult, geriatric and substance abuse programs in the inpatient, partial hospital, residential treatment and outpatient settings.

4926 MeritCare Health System

Child/Adolescent Services
700 1st Avenue S
Fargo, ND 58103-1802   701-234-4171
800-437-4010
Fax: 701-234-4037
www.meritcare.com

4927 Meritcare Health System

720 4th Street N
Fargo, ND 58122-0002   701-234-6956
Fax: 701-234-6979

Clinical Management/Software Companies

4928 Micro Design International
1375 S Semoran Boulevard
Suite 1350
Winter Park, FL 32792-5513   407-677-8333
Fax: 407-677-8365

4929 Micro Psych Software: Medical Management Software Corporation
4425 N Wildwood Avenue
Milwaukee, WI 53211-1408   414-964-4789
800-964-4789
Fax: 414-964-2974

Bob Miller, President

Medical billing software that is easy to use and is in more than 19,000 practices nationally. *$1499.00*

4930 Micro-Office Systems
3825 Severn Road
Cleveland, OH 44118-1910   216-289-1666
800-929-1170

4931 MicroHealth Corporation
PO Box 98471
Raleigh, NC 27624-8471   919-954-0807

4932 MicroScript
99 Rosewood Drive
Suite 220
Danvers, MA 01923-1300   978-777-5202
Fax: 978-750-8295

4933 Micromedex
6200 S Syracuse Way
Suite 300
Englewood, CO 80111-4705   303-486-6400
Fax: 303-486-6464

4934 Mind
PO Box 597
Palo Alto, CA 94302-0597   650-326-3890

4935 Montgomery County Project SHARE
538 Dekalb Street
Norristown, PA 19401-4931   610-272-7997
Fax: 610-272-4891

4936 Motorola
1500 Gateway Boulevard
Suite 110
Boynton Beach, FL 33426-8292   407-739-2000
Fax: 407-364-3815

4937 Multidata Computer Systems
251 5th Avenue
New York, NY 10016-6515   212-545-7070
Fax: 212-545-8784

4938 Mutual Alliance
440 Linc Street
Allmerica Financial
Worcester, MA 01653-0001   508-855-1000
Fax: 508-855-2877

4939 Mutual of Omaha Companies' Integrated Behavioral Services
Mutual of Omaha Plaza
S-3 Integrated Behavioral Services
Omaha, NE 68175-0001   402-342-7600
800-488-7706
Fax: 402-351-2880

4940 NYNEX Information Resources
35 Village Road
Middleton, MA 01949-1202   978-762-1483
Fax: 978-762-1848

4941 National Consortium on Telepsychiatry
MCMR-AT
Building 1054
Frederick, MD 21702   301-619-7928
Fax: 301-619-2518

4942 National Data Corporation
National Data Plaza
Atlanta, GA 30329   404-728-3817
Fax: 404-728-3911

4943 National Families in Action
2957 Clairmont Road NE
Suite 150
Atlanta, GA 30329-1647   770-934-6364
Fax: 770-934-7137

4944 National Medical Computer Systems
8928 Terman Court
San Diego, CA 92121-3296   619-566-5800

4945 National Medical Health Card Systems
26 Harbor Park Drive
Port Washington, NY 11050-4688   516-625-5317
800-645-3332
Fax: 516-621-4793
www.nmhcrx.com

4946 National Mental Health Self-Help Clearinghouse
1211 Chestnut Street
Suite 1000
Philadephia, PA 19017   215-751-1810
Fax: 215-636-6310

4947 National Technology Group
112 S Tryon Street
Suite 1100
Charlotte, NC 28284-2191   704-384-7288

4948 NetMeeting
Microsoft Corporation
Customer Advocate Center
One Microsoft Way
Redmond, WA 98052
800-936-5700
www.microsoft.com/ie/download/ieadd.htm

Allows users to share Microsoft-based documents and spreadsheets with one another in a 'whiteboard' area.

4949 Network Behavioral Health

265 North Street
Harrison, NY 10528-1524

888-224-2273
Fax: 914-925-5175

4950 Network Medical

1863 Technology Drive
Troy, MI 48083-4244

248-583-3100
Fax: 248-583-9877

4951 New Standards

4663 Chatsworth Street N
Suite 101
Shoreview, MN 55126-5813

800-755-6299
Fax: 612-690-1303

4952 Next Computer

1 Infinite Loop
Cupertino, CA 95014-2083

650-366-0900

4953 North American Computer Services

14828 W 6th Avenue
Suite 16B
Golden, CO 80401-5000

303-278-1501
Fax: 303-278-1173

4954 Northpointe Behavioral Healthcare Systems

715 Pyle Drive
Kingsford, MI 49802-4456

906-774-9522
Fax: 906-774-1570
E-mail: info@nbhs.org
www.nbhs.org

Michigan Community Health agency serving Dickinson, Menominee, and Iron counties. Provides a full spectrum of managed behavioral healthcare services to the chronically mentally ill and developmentally disabled. A corporate services division provides employee assistance programs both in Michigan and outside the state.

4955 Northwest Analytical

519 SW Park Avenue
Portland, OR 97205-3207

503-224-7727
Fax: 503-224-5236
E-mail: nwa@nwasoft.com
www.nwasoft.com

Provides comprehensive SPC software tools meeting technically stringent mental health industry requirements.

4956 OPTAIO-Optimizing Practice Through Assessment, Intervention and Outcome

Psychological Corporation
555 Academic Court
San Antonio, TX 78204

888-467-8246
Fax: 888-200-4880
www.tpcweb.com

Provides the clinical information necessary for proactive decision making.

4957 Occupational Health Software Systems

6609 NE Tara Lane
Bainbridge Island, WA 98110-4030

206-842-5838
800-234-6477

4958 Omni Data Sciences

220 Colrain Street SW
Grand Rapids, MI 49548-1013

616-246-1600
Fax: 616-246-1633

4959 On-Line Psych Services

90 Sutton Street
N Andover, MA 01845-1655

978-685-4329

4960 Optaio Software

4800 River Green Parkway
Duluth, GA 30096-2568

770-283-8500
Fax: 770-283-8699

4961 Optimed Medical Systems

20 Maguire Road
Lexington, MA 02421-3112

781-863-2000
Fax: 781-863-0464

4962 Oracle Corporation

500 Oracle Parkway
Redwood City, CA 94065-1675

650-506-7000

4963 Oracle Federal

3 Bethesda Metro Center
Suite 1400
Bethesda, MD 20814-6306

301-657-7860
Fax: 301-913-5155

4964 Orion Healthcare Technology

1823 Harney Street
Suite 101
Omaha, NE 68102

402-341-8880
800-324-7966
Fax: 402-341-8911
E-mail: info@orionhealthcare.com
www.orionhealthcare.com

Orion provides technology solutions to meet the ever changing needs of the healthcare industry. To accomodate the behavioral health field, Orion developed the AccuCare software system, a highly integrated and adaptive approach to the clinical practice environment. AccuCare enables clinicians to quickly realize value, effiency and standardization without disrupting their primary focus to provide excellence in health care.

4965 Orion Systems Group

PO Box 426
Sayville, NY 11782-0426

631-467-8844
Fax: 631-471-0739

4966 Outer Montana Systems

PO Box 661
Nevada City, CA 95959-0661

916-265-5612

4967 Output Technologies
2534 Madison Avenue
Kansas City, MO 64108-2335   816-435-3070
800-252-4541

4968 P and W Software
5655 Lindero Canyon Road
Suite 403
Westlake Village, CA 91362-4046   818-707-7690
Fax: 818-707-9097

4969 PATHware
7111 Moorland Drive
Clarksville, MD 21029-1734   410-997-4588

4970 PC Consulting Group
PO Box 69382
Portland, OR 97201-0382   503-246-7858

4971 PSI Computer Systems
7231 Boulder Avenue
Suite 539
Highland, CA 92346-3313   909-370-1943

4972 PSIMED Corporation
1221 E Dyer Road
Suite 260
Santa Ana, CA 92705-5654
800-374-4292
Fax: 949-432-8256

4973 Pacific Management Group-PMG
Penguin Putnam
100 Brook Creek Road
Suite 201
Santa Rosa, CA 95404   707-539-6634
Fax: 707-539-8234
E-mail: mriley@sonic.net
www.midmanagers.com

Mary Riley PhD, Partner
JoAnne Kennedy, Office Manager

PMG provides tools and courses for the creation and maintenance of mentally and financially healthy workplaces.

4974 Parrot Software
6505 Pleasant Lake Court
W Bloomfield, MI 48322-4709   248-788-3223
800-727-7681

4975 Pathware
12105 Gold Ribbon Way
Columbia, MD 21044-2786   860-225-8245
Fax: 860-223-7080

4976 Patient Infosystems
46 Prince Street
Rochester, NY 14607-1023   716-242-7271
Fax: 716-244-1367

4977 Patient Medical Records
901 Tahoka Road
Brownfield, TX 79316-3817   806-637-2556
899-285-7627
Fax: 806-637-4283

4978 Perot Systems
12404 Park Central Drive
Dallas, TX 75251-1808   972-340-5000
Fax: 972-383-5895
www.perotsystems.com

4979 Perot Systems Corporation
12377 Merit Drive
Dallas, TX 75251-2224   214-663-7000

4980 Pheonix Programs
1875 Willow Pass Road
Suite 300
Concord, CA 94520-2527   510-825-4700
Fax: 510-825-2610

4981 Point of Care Technologies
6 Taft Court
Suite 150
Rockville, MD 20850-5361   301-610-2421

4982 Policy Management Systems Corporation
PMSC Court
Monticello, SC 29106-9999   803-735-4382
Fax: 803-735-4131

4983 Policy Resource Center
1555 Connecticut Avenue NW
Suite 200
Washington, DC 20036-1126   202-775-8826
Fax: 202-659-7613

4984 Preferred Health Care Systems
1513 16th Street NW
Suite 4
Washington, DC 20036-1480   301-941-8055
Fax: 301-941-8080

4985 Primary Care Medicine on CD
Facts and Comparisons
111 Westport Plaza
Suite 300
Saint Louis, MO 63146-3014
800-223-0554
Fax: 314-878-1574
www.drugfacts.com

Current, comprehensive coverage of what's happening in the discipline; quarterly updates include summary, analysis and critique of relevant studies on ambulatory care, family medicine, internal medicine, pharmacology, cardiology, therapeutic advances, plus twelve critical reviews of major new studies in the field of medical practice.

4986 ProMetrics

480 American Avenue
King of Prussia, PA 19406-1405   610-265-6344
                                   Fax: 610-265-8377

4987 Professional Information Planning Corporation

6820 Delmar Boulevard
Suite 100
Saint Louis, MO 63130-3155   314-863-0767

4988 Professional Software Solutions

2520 NW 39th Street
Suite 113
Oklahoma City, OK 73112-3759   405-949-1200
                                  800-637-2251

4989 Psybernetics

26 Eastern Avenue
Augusta, ME 04330-5722   207-622-3197
                                  Fax: 207-623-5195

4990 PsychCare Alliance

423 S Pacific Coast Highway
Suite 102
Redondo Beach, CA 90277-3731   310-540-5864
                                  Fax: 310-540-8904

4991 PsychConsult Consortium

3030 Ashby Avenue
Suite 109B
Berkeley, CA 94705-2439   510-843-0321
                                  Fax: 510-704-7579

4992 PsychReport

507 W Drive
Severna Park, MD 21146   410-647-4403
                                  Fax: 410-647-1941

4993 PsychSolutions

41 William Fairfield Drive
Wenham, MA 01984-1012   978-468-2290
                                  888-779-7658
                                  Fax: 888-779-7658
                                  E-mail: psyol@aol.com
                                  www.psychsolotions.com

Provides the AdvantaSoft Suite of software for office, clinical, and performance management. Help providers skillfully use software to maximize profits and satisfaction, and minimize expenses.

4994 Psychemedics Corporation

1280 Massachusetts Avenue
Suite 200
Cambridge, MA 02138-3840   617-868-7455
                                  www.corporatedrugtesting.com

4995 Psychiatric Research Institute

1100 N St. Francis Street
Suite 200
Wichita, KS 67214-2878   316-291-4774
                                  800-362-0070
                                  Fax: 316-291-7975
                                  www.pri-research.org

4996 Psycho Medical Chirologists

11612 Lockwood Drive
Apartment 103
Silver Spring, MD 20904-2314   316-816-614
                                  Fax: 301-681-0738

4997 Psychological Assessment Resources

PO Box 998
Odessa, FL 33556-0998   813-754-8081
                                  800-331-8378
                                  Fax: 800-727-9329
                                  www.parinc.com

This program produces normative-based interpretive hypotheses based on your client's scores. It produces a profile of T scores, a listing of the associated raw and percentile scores, and interpretive hypotheses for each scale. Although this program is not designed to produce a finished clinical report, it allows you to integrate BRS and SRI data with other sources of information about your client. The report can be generated as a text file for editing.

4998 Psychological Corporation

555 Academic Court
San Antonio, TX 78204-2498   210-299-1061
                                  888-467-8246
                                  Fax: 888-200-4800

4999 Psychological Health Tech

800 N Haven Avenue
Suite 259
Ontario, CA 91764-4915   626-305-7200
                                  Fax: 626-948-9387

5000 Psychological Resource Organization

950 S Cherry Street
Suite 200
Denver, CO 80246-2663   303-758-3700

5001 Psychological Software Services

6555 Carrollton Avenue
Indianapolis, IN 46220-1664   317-257-9672
                                  Fax: 317-257-9674
                                  E-mail: obracy@inetdirect.net
                                  www.neuroscience.center.com

Nancy Bracy, Sales/Production

Comprehensive and easy-to-use multimedia cognitive rehabilitation software. Packages include 64 comuputerized therapy tasks with modifiable parameters that will accommodate most requirements. Exercises extend from simple attention and executive skills, through multiple modalities of visuospatial and memory skills. For clinical and educational use with head injury, stroke, LD/ADD and other brain compromises. Price range: $260-$2,500.

5002 Psychometric Software

2210 Front Street
Department AD
Melbourne, FL 32901-7360   407-729-6390

5003 Public Health Service

4350 E Highway
Suite 7-D41
Bethesda, MD 20857   301-594-4060
                           Fax: 301-594-4984

5004 QS

Nationsbank Plaza 1106
PO Box 847
Greenville, SC 29602-0847   864-232-2666
                           Fax: 864-370-2230

5005 QuadraMed Corporation

12110 Sunset Hills Road
Reston, VA 20190   703-709-2300
                          800-393-0278
                   Fax: 703-709-2490
                   www.quadramed.com

5006 Qualifacts Systems

9180 Oakhurst Road
Suite 1
Seminole, FL 33776-2109   813-596-9960
                           Fax: 813-593-1784

5007 Quesix Software

28521 Warm Springs Boulevard
Suite 307
Freemont, CA 94539   408-288-3939
                           Fax: 415-321-7345

5008 R&L Software Associates

65 Federal Street
Salem, MA 01970-3436   978-744-6750
                           Fax: 978-740-5182

5009 RCF Information Systems

4200 Colonel Glenn Highway
Suite 100
Beavercreek, OH 45431-1670   937-427-5680
                           Fax: 937-427-5689

5010 Raintree Systems

12842 Valley View Street
Suite 4-204
Garden Grove, CA 92845-2515   760-509-9000
                           Fax: 760-509-9001
                           www.raintreeinc.com

5011 Redtop Company

350 5th Avenue
Suite 5124
New York, NY 10118-5124   212-244-6868
                           Fax: 212-244-2107
              E-mail: bgoldhagen@redtop.com
                           www.redtop.com

Benjamin Goldhagen, CEO/Founder

Supports the mental health community by developing electronic tools for clinicians, researchers, educators and administrators. Products include the Redtop Clinical Environment, a paperless patient record which is medically valid and technologically advanced. It is designed to satisfy MCO and government demands for more complete and detailed clinical records.

5012 Research Information Systems

2355 Camino Vida Roble
Carlsbad, CA 92009-1572   760-438-5526
                          800-544-3049
                   Fax: 760-438-5573
                   www.risinc.com

5013 Research Media

9090 Chilson Road
Brighton, MI 48116-5142   810-231-3211
                           Fax: 810-231-3912

5014 Resource Information Management Systems

500 Technology Drive
PO Box 3094
Naperville, IL 60566-7094   630-369-5300
                           Fax: 630-369-5813

5015 Right On Programs/PRN Medical Software

778 New York Avenue
Huntington, NY 11743-4413   631-424-7777
                           Fax: 631-424-7207
         E-mail: friends@rightonprograms.com
                   www.rightonprograms.com

David Farren, VP

Computer software for mental health, medical and other organizations requiring cataloging and searching a wide range of materials. Software is especially easy to learn and use. Programs include The Circulation Desk for cataloging and circulation of books, CDs, videos, photos, booklets, etc., Computer Acess Catalog for cataloging without the circulation module, and Periodical Manager for periodicals including supplements.

5016 SHS Computer Services

600 Sarah Street
Stroudsburg, PA 18360-2120   717-424-7437
                           Fax: 717-424-7437

5017 SLA Consulting

1008 Balmoral Drive
Silver Spring, MD 20903-1303   301-445-6548
                           Fax: 301-445-6548

5018 SPSS

444 N Michigan Avenue
Chicago, IL 60611-3903   312-494-3277
                           Fax: 312-329-3668

5019 SRC Software
PO Box 1569
Portland, OR 97207-1569   503-221-0448
800-544-3477

5020 STM Technology: Health Care Company Systems
147 Main Street
Maynard, MA 01754   978-897-0002
Fax: 978-897-6417

Jerold Budinoff, President

Mental health and substance abuse administration, billing and medical records systems.

5021 Saner Software
37 W 222 Route 64
Suite 253
Saint Charles, IL 60175   630-513-5599
Fax: 630-513-4210

5022 Santa Cruz Operations
PO Box 1900
Santa Cruz, CA 95061-1900   408-427-7112
Fax: 408-425-3544

5023 Seaquest Health Care Resources
Two Trans Am Plaza Drive
Suite 280
Oakbrook Terrace, IL 60181   630-853-1548
Fax: 630-853-0896

5024 Seinet
11117 Mockingbird Drive
Omaha, NE 68137   402-331-6660
Fax: 402-331-8055

5025 Sentient Systems
10410 Kensington Parkway
Kensington, MD 20895-2943   301-929-7600
Fax: 301-929-7680

5026 Sierra Health Services
PO Box 15645
Las Vegas, NV 89114-5645   702-242-7000
Fax: 702-242-6559

5027 Skypek Group
2528 W Tennessee Avenue
Tampa, FL 33629-6255   813-254-3926
Fax: 813-254-3926

5028 Softouch Software
5200 SW Macadam Avenue
Suite 255
Portland, OR 97201-3838   503-241-1841
Fax: 513-223-6240

5029 Source One Systems (Health Records)
5076 Winters Chapel Road
Suite 200
Atlanta, GA 30360-1832   770-455-9076

5030 Southeastern Data Systems
1324 Centerpoint Boulevard
Knoxville, TN 37932-1959   423-584-1507

5031 Spangler Automated Medical Services
PO Box 9169
Chattanooga, TN 37412-0169   800-722-7267

5032 Spurling and Cohan
110 Marsh Drive
Suite 105
Foster City, CA 94404-1184   650-513-0979

5033 Star Systems Corporation
2143 Green Acres Road
PO Box 1744
Fayetteville, AR 72702-1744   501-587-0882
Fax: 501-587-9449

5034 Stephens Systems Services
267 5th Avenue
New York, NY 10016   212-545-7788
Fax: 212-545-9081
E-mail: stephenssys@cs.com

5035 Strategic Advantage
3414 Peachtree Road NE
Suite 1400
Atlanta, GA 30326-1114   Fax: 612-871-1151

5036 Strategic Healthcare Solutions
2848 Good Hope Church Road
New Market, TN 37820-3002   423-475-1088

5037 Stratus Computer
111 Powder Mill Road
Maynard, MA 01754   978-461-7000
Fax: 978-461-5210

5038 Sumtime Software
3748 N Causeway Boulevard
Suite 300
Metairie, LA 70002-7229   504-828-2551
Fax: 504-837-0495

5039 Sun Microsystems
2550 Garcia Avenue
Mountain View, CA 94043-1100   650-960-1300
Fax: 650-786-3530

5040 Sunquest Information Systems
4801 E Broadway Boulevard
Tucson, AZ 85711-3609   602-570-2450
Fax: 602-570-2492

5041 Superior Consultant Company
2 E 8th Street
Suite 2511
Chicago, IL 60605-2133   312-851-6465
Fax: 312-427-7874

5042 Supported Living Technologies

1607 4th Street
Bay City, MI 48708-6137   517-893-6453
Fax: 517-893-6453
E-mail: irreronov@aol.com
www.hometechsystems.com/commliv

James Irrer, President

Advanced telecommunications products designed to promote and enhance independence for consumers while greatly reducing staffing cost. Our proven technology significantly increases the independence of consumers, allows them a better night's sleep and the ability for more progress during daytime hours. Also reduces department expenditures for perrsonnel costs. *$7.99*

5043 Sweetwater Health Enterprises

3939 Belt Line Road
Suite 600
Dallas, TX 75244   972-888-5638
Fax: 972-620-7351
E-mail: mktg@sweetwaterhealth.com
www.sweetwaterhealth.com

Cherie Holmes-Henry, VP Sales/Marketing

5044 Synergistic Office Solutions (SOS Software)

17445 E Apshawa Road
Clermont, FL 34711-9049   352-242-9100
Fax: 352-242-9104
www.sosoft.com

Katherine E Panes PhD, VP

Produce patient management software for behavioral health service providers, including billing, scheduling and clinical records.

5045 SysteMetrics

777 E Eisenhower Parkway
Ann Arbor, MI 48108-3273   313-996-3782
Fax: 313-996-2000

5046 System One

2900 Green Court S
Boulder, CO 80301   303-786-9951
Fax: 303-786-9960

5047 TASS

Association Software Comapany
480 S Washington Street
Suite 220
Falls Church, VA 22046-4414   703-237-3155
800-858-8272
Fax: 703-532-4916
E-mail: marketing@tass.com
www.tass.com

5048 TDS Healthcare Systems

200 Ashford Center N
Atlanta, GA 30338-2668   404-847-5000

5049 TEI Computers

11311 N Central Expressway
Suite 300
Dallas, TX 75243-6716   214-750-1144
Fax: 214-750-0224

5050 TKI Computer Center

103 N East Street
Benton, AR 72015-3760   501-778-4869
Fax: 501-778-0094
E-mail: tkicc@tkicc.com
www.tkicc.com

5051 Tasmin NAMI Affiliates Program

180 S Washington Street
Suite 220
Falls Church, VA 22046-2900   703-237-3155
Fax: 703-532-4916

Tasmin provides automation control in the essential area of: membership, committees, meetings, NAMI data synchronization, cash receipts, and reporting.

5052 Tempus Software

225 Water Street
Suite 2250
Jacksonville, FL 32202-5181   904-355-2900
800-583-6787
Fax: 904-355-3322
E-mail: information@tempus.com
www.tempus.com

5053 Therapists Genie

811 SW 58th Avenue
Portland, OR 97221-1558   503-297-2717
888-297-2717

5054 Trego Systems

1001 4th Avenue
Suite 1500
Seattle, WA 98154-1144   708-359-6910

5055 Turbo-Doc

771 Buschmann Road
Suite G
Paradise, CA 95969-5848   916-877-8650
Fax: 916-877-8621

5056 UNI/CARE Systems

150 Preston Executive Drive
Suite 202
Cary, NC 27513-8485   919-467-9295
Fax: 919-467-3005
E-mail: sales@unicaresys.com
www.unicaresys.com

Michelle Means, VP Sales/Marketing

Provides fully-integrated software solutions for all facets of Behavioral Healthcare. Our software is designed for use in every setting, from Inpatient to Outpatient, from Day Treatment and Partial Hospitalization to Case Management. The Uni/Care Information System is a flexible and user-friendly network of software modules that support integrated clinical and financial data with powerful reporting capabilities. Uni/Care is an industry leader with a track record of responding to the ever-changing behavioral health environment.

5057 UNI/CARE: National Resource Consultants

1200 Westheimer Road
Suite 8
Houston, TX 77006-2613   713-914-3677
                                Fax: 713-914-8175

5058 United Way of Chicago

221 NlaSalle Street
Floor 9
Chicago, IL 60601   312-906-2388

5059 Universal Behavioral Service

820 Fort Wayne Avenue
Indianapolis, IN 46204-1309   617-684-0442
                                Fax: 617-684-0679

5060 Universal Software Associates

12422 Wirt Street
Omaha, NE 68164-2594   402-496-7339

5061 Value Health Management

5400 Legacy Drive
Suite A3-1D-12
Plano, TX 75024-3105   203-676-3679

5062 Valumed Systems

4405 E West Highway
Suite 501
Bethesda, MD 20814-4536   301-652-7773
                                800-374-2216
                                Fax: 301-651-7614

5063 Vann Data Services

PO Box 10989
Daytona Beach, FL 32120-1989   904-677-5607

5064 Velocity Healthcare Informatics

8441 Wayzata Boulevard
Suite 105
Minneapolis, MN 55426-1349   612-797-9997
                                Fax: 612-797-9993

5065 VersaForm Systems Corporation

591 W Hamilton Avenue
Suite 210
Campbell, CA 95008-0521
                                800-678-1111
                                Fax: 408-370-3393
                                E-mail: debby@versaform.com
                                www.versaform.com

Debra Atlas, Sales Manager

Electronic medical records and practice management.

5066 Virtual Software Systems

PO Box 815
Bethel Park, PA 15102-0815   412-835-9417
                                Fax: 412-835-9419
                                E-mail: sales@vss3.com
                                www.vss3.com

Thomas Palmquist, Partner

Easy to use practice management, billing, and scheduling software. *$3500.00*

5067 Wang Software

290 Concord Road
Billerica, MA 01821-3499   770-594-9473

5068 Wellness Integrated Network

3435 Ocean Park Boulevard
Suite 108
Santa Monica, CA 90405-3309   310-452-4946
                                Fax: 310-581-8151

5069 Woodlands

68 W Church Street
Suite 305
Newark, OH 43055-5050   740-349-9384
                                Fax: 740-345-6028

5070 Work Group for the Computerization of Behavioral Health

4 Brattle Street
Suite 207
Cambridge, MA 02138-3714   617-864-6769
                                Fax: 617-492-3673
                                www.workgroup.org

5071 Worldwide Healthcare Solutions: IBM

404 Wyman Street
Waltham, MA 02451-1264   781-895-2486
                                Fax: 781-895-2235

5072 XI Tech Corporation

34 Regis Avenue
Pittsburgh, PA 15236   412-655-2120
                                Fax: 412-655-2405

5073 Zy-Doc Technologies

1455 Veterans Memorial Highway
Hicksville, NY 11749   631-273-1963
                                Fax: 631-273-1988
                                www.zydoc.com

Information Services

5074 3M Health Information Systems

575 Murray Boulevard
PO Box 7900
Murray, UT 84123-4611 801-265-4247
Fax: 801-263-3658

5075 ADL Data Systems

20 Livingstone Avenue
Dobbs Ferry, NY 10522-3400 914-591-1800
Fax: 914-591-1818
E-mail: sales@mail.adldata.com
www.adldata.com

The most comprehensive software solution for MH/MRDD and the continuum of care. 38 modules to choose from. Designed to meet all financial, clinical, and administrative needs. For organizations requiring greater flexiblity and processing power. Ask about new Windows-based products utilizing the latest in technology, including bar coding, scanning, etc.

Year Founded: 1977

5076 Accumedic Computer Systems

11 Grace Avenue
Great Neck, NY 11021-2417 516-466-6800
800-765-9300
Fax: 516-466-6880
E-mail: sales@accumedic.com
www.accumedic.com

Practice management solutions for mental health facilities: scheduling, billing, EMR, HIPAA.

5077 American Institute for Preventive Medicine

30445 Northwestern Highway
Suite 350
Farmington Hills, MI 48334-3107 248-539-1800
Fax: 248-539-1808

Don R Powell, President
Sue Jackson, VP

5078 American Nurses Foundation: National Communications

8332 Tuckaway Shores Drive
Franklin, WI 53132-9730 414-427-0437

5079 Apache Medical Systems

1650 Tysons Boulevard
Suite 300
McLean, VA 22102-3915 703-847-1400
800-634-9379
Fax: 703-847-1401

5080 Applied Computing Services

2764 Allen Road W
Elk, WA 99009-9548 509-292-0500
800-553-4055

5081 Applied Informatics (ILIAD)

295 Chipeta Way
Salt Lake City, UT 84108-1220 801-584-6485

5082 Arbour Health System-Human Resource Institute Hospital

227 Babcock Street
Brookline, MA 02446 617-731-3200
800-828-3934
Fax: 617-738-6800
E-mail: arbourhealth@mindspring.com
www.arbourhealth.com

Charles Rossignol, CEO
Michael Caplan MD, Medical Director
Judith Merel, Director Marketing

5083 Arbour-Fuller Hospital

200 May Street
S Attleboro, MA 02703-5515 508-761-8500
800-828-3934
Fax: 508-761-4240
TTY: 800-974-6006
E-mail: arbourhealth@mindspring.com
www.arbourhealth.com

Gary Gilberti, CEO
Frank Kahr MD, Medical Director
Judith Merel, Director Marketing

Psychiatric hospital providing services to adults, adolesents and adults with developmental disabilities.

5084 Artificial Intelligence

345 Upland Drive
Seattle, WA 98188-3802 206-575-2135

5085 Association for Ambulatory Behavioral Healthcare

11240 Waples Mill Road
Suite 200
Fairfax, VA 22030 703-934-0160
Fax: 703-359-7562
E-mail: info@aabh.org
www.aabh.org

Karla Gray, President
Jerry Galler, Executive Director

Powerful forum for people engaged in providing mental health services. Promoting the evolution of flexible models of responsive cost-effective ambulatory behavioral healthcare.

5086 Automation Research Systems

4480 King Street
Alexandria, VA 22302-1300 703-998-5090
800-666-8737
Fax: 703-820-9106

5087 Behavioral Intervention Planning: Completing a Functional Behavioral Assessment and Developing a Behavioral Intervention Plan

Pro-Ed Publications
8700 Shoal Creek Boulevard
Austin, TX 78757-6816 512-451-3246
800-897-3202
Fax: 800-397-7633
E-mail: info@proedinc.com
www.proedinc.com

Provides school personnel with all tools necessary to complete a functional behavioral assessment, determine whether a behavior is related to the disability of the student, and develop a behavioral intervention plan. *$22.00*

5088 Breining Institute College for the Advanced Study of Addictive Disorders

8880 Greenback Lane
Suite A
Orangevale, CA 95662-4019 916-987-2007
Fax: 916-987-8823
E-mail: college@breining.edu
www.breining.edu

Kathy Breining, Dean of Students

5089 Brief Therapy Institute of Denver

8791 Wolff Court
130
Westminster, CO 80030 303-426-8757
800-598-8120
Fax: 303-426-1390
www.btid.com

Lawrence Nelson MSW, LCSW, Therapist
Lisa Sydow MA, LPC, Therapist
Tracy Todd PhD, LMFT, Therapist

Our form of psychotherapy emphasizes goals, active participation between therapist and client, client strengths, resources, resiliencies and accountability of the therapy process.

5090 Buckley Productions

238 E Blithedale Avenue
Mill Valley, CA 94941-2032 415-383-2009
Fax: 415-383-5031
E-mail: buckleypro@aol.com
www.buckleyproductions.com

Richard Buckley, President
Beth Popson, National Sales Director

Alcohol and drug education handbooks, videos, and web-based products for safety sensitive employers, supervisiors and employees who are covered by the Department of Transportaion rules. We provide training materials for Substance Abuse Professional (SAPs) and urine collectors. We distribute Truth about...Series that includes drinking, drugs, marijuana, sex, violence, and hate for young adults.

5091 CBI Group

100 S Prospect Avenue
Park Ridge, IL 60068-4057 847-698-1090
Fax: 847-698-1146

5092 CMHC Systems

570 Metro Place N
Dublin, OH 43017-1300 614-764-0143
800-528-9025
E-mail: info@@cmhcsys.com
www.mis.cmhc.com

5093 COMPSYCH Software Information Services

Peter Hornby and Margaret Anderson, SUNY
101 Broad Street
Plattsburgh, NY 12901
www.plattsburgh.edu.compsych/

Provides information about psychological software, arranged in topical categories such as statistics, cognitive, physiological, and personality testing.

5094 CambridgM02138142617495266174962hup.harvare Sacramento

11130 Sun Center Drive
Suite E
Rancho Cordova, CA 95670-6112 916-638-5037
Fax: 916-638-2926

5095 CareCounsel, LCC

68 Mitchell Boulevard
Suite 200
San Rafael, CA 94903-2018 415-472-2366
Fax: 415-456-3131

5096 Catholic Community Services of Western Washington

100 23rd Avenue S
PO Box 22608
Seattle, WA 98122-0608 206-328-5696
Fax: 206-328-5699

5097 Center for Creative Living

40 Central Avenue
Glen Rock, NJ 07452-1837 201-251-8224
Fax: 201-818-5027

5098 Central Washington Comprehensive M/H

PO Box 959
Yakima, WA 98907-0959 509-575-4084
Fax: 509-575-4811

5099 Choice Health

12000 Pecos Street
Suite 350
Denver, CO 80234-2079 303-252-1120
Fax: 303-252-1194

5100 Cirrus Technology

5301 Buckeystown Pike
Floor 4
Frederick, MD 21704-8370 301-698-1900
Fax: 301-698-1909

5101 Community Sector Systems

700 5th Avenue
Suite 6100
Seattle, WA 98104-5061
206-521-2588
800-988-6392
Fax: 206-467-9237
www.cssi.com

5102 Community Solutions

123 Moultrie Street
San Francisco, CA 94110-5615
415-512-7768
Fax: 415-512-0181
E-mail: info@community-solutions.com
www.community-solutions.com

5103 Compass Information Systems

1060 1st Avenue
Suite 410
King of Prussia, PA 19406-1336
610-992-7060
Fax: 610-992-7070
E-mail: quality@compass-is.com
www.compass-is.com

Compass Treatment Assessment System is a scientifically-based system of measuring and managing a the course of behavioral health treatment.

5104 Compucare Company

12110 Sunset Hills Road
Reston, VA 20190-3223
703-709-2424
Fax: 703-709-2490

5105 Computer Billing and Office Managment Programs

Ed Zuckrman

www.cmch.com/guide/pro24.html

Includes a detailed review of computer billing and office management programs, where to buy or use electronic claims submission, other computer programs of interest to clinicians, resources, references and readings, and programs for writing assistance.

5106 Consultec Managed Care Systems

9040 Roswell Road
Suite 700
Atlanta, GA 30350-7530
813-784-7947
Fax: 813-789-6136

5107 Consumer Health Information

3852 NW 90th Place
Polk City, IA 50226-2072
515-964-4000
Fax: 515-964-5479

5108 Control-O-Fax Corporation

3070 W Airline Highway
Waterloo, IA 50703-9591
319-234-4651
Fax: 319-236-7350

5109 DCC/The Dependent Care Connection

400 Nyla Farms
PO Box 2783
Westport, CT 06880-0783
203-226-2680
Fax: 203-226-2852

5110 Dean Foundation for Health, Research and Education

2711 Allen Boulevard
Middleton, WI 53562-2215
608-827-2300
Fax: 608-827-2399
www.deancare.com

The Dean Foundation is the non-profit research and education entity of DHS. The Foundation currently encompasses Dean's Educational Services Department, supports community service and health education projects, funds research grants, and cunducts its own ancillary research including several outcomes management studies and computer-assisted, voice-activated programs for behavioral medicine.

5111 Distance Learning Network

111 W Main Street
Boalsburg, PA 16827
814-466-7808
800-326-9166
Fax: 814-466-7509
E-mail: dlnstaff@dlnetwork.com
www.dlnetwork.com

Eric Porterfield, President/CEO
Sandy Weaver, VP Program Development
Sheri Mills, Marketing

Broadcast and multimedia company dedicated solely to meeting the medical education and communications needs of physicians through the use of both traditional and innovative media formats. More than 150,000 physicians, nurses and pharmacists turn to DLN each year for their medical education.

Year Founded: 1996

5112 Dorland Healthcare Information

1500 Walnut Street
Suite 1000
Philadelphia, PA 19102
215-875-1212
800-784-2332
Fax: 949-752-8433
E-mail: info@dorlandhealth.com
www.dorlandhealth.com

5113 Drug and Crime Prevention Funding News

Government Information Services
4301 Fairfax Drive
Ste 875
Arlington, VA 22203-1635
703-920-7600
800-876-0226
Fax: 800-426-2012
www.grantsandfunding.com

Provides federal and private drug and crime funding information, including congressional legislation and appropriations. Also features grant alert a weekly compilation of federal grants and contracts. Recurring features include a collection, reports of meetings, and notices of publications available. *$289.00*

10-12 pages 56 per year ISSN 1076-1519

5114 FOCUS: Family Oriented Counseling Services

PO Box 921
Rolla, MO 65402-0921
573-364-7551
Fax: 573-364-4898

5115 Federation of Families for Children's Mental Health

1101 King Street
Suite 420
Alexandria, VA 22314 703-684-7710
Fax: 703-836-1040
E-mail: ffcmh@ffcmh.org
www.ffcmh.org

Barbara Huff, Executive Director

National family-run organization dedicated exclusively to children and adolesents with mental health needs and their families. Our voice speaks through our work in policy, training and technical assistance programs. Publishes a quarterly newsletter and sponsors an annual conference and exhibits.

5116 HSA-Mental Health

1080 Emeline Avenue
Santa Cruz, CA 95060-1966 831-454-4000
Fax: 831-454-4770
TDD: 831-454-2123
E-mail: info@santacruzhealth.org
www.santacruzhealth.org

Rama Khalsa PhD, Health Services Administrator
David McNutt MD, County Health Officer

Exists to protect and improve the health of the people in Santa Cruz County. Provides programs in environmental health, public health, medical care, substance abuse prevention and treatment, and mental health. Clients are entitled to information on the costs of care and their options for getting health insurance coverage through a variety of programs.

5117 Hagar and Associates

1848 Commercenter E
San Bernardino, CA 92408-3406 909-888-8821
Fax: 909-384-9852
E-mail: dhagar5@aol.com

Deborah Hagar, CEO

Provides clients with data, from national databases, of outcomes, patient demographics, and benchmark data. Can provide technology and/or automated data connection. Provides support in objective outcomes measurement.

5118 HealthOnline

PO Box 339
Brighton, CO 80601-0339 303-659-2252
Fax: 303-659-7995

5119 Healthcare Management Systems

3401 W End Avenue
Suite 290
Nashville, TN 37203-6866 615-383-7300
Fax: 615-383-6093

5120 Healthcheck

3954 Youngfield Street
Wheat Ridge, CO 80033-3865 916-556-1880
Fax: 916-447-0444

5121 Healtheast Crisis Intervention

69 Exchange Street W
Saint Paul, MN 55102-1004 612-232-3222
Fax: 612-291-5422

5122 Human Resources Consulting Group

1202 Dover Drive
Provo, UT 84604-5240 801-765-4417
Fax: 801-765-4418
E-mail: hrconsultinggroup@msn.com
www.hrconsultinggroup.com

Consultants in Human Resources and benefits plan design. Software systems and evolutions nation wide.

5123 INMED/MotherNet America

45449 Severn Way
Suite 208
Sterling, VA 20166-8918 703-444-4477
Fax: 703-444-4471

5124 InfoNation Systems

2701 University Avenue
Suite 465
Madison, WI 53705 608-209-1950
www.infonat.com

Info Nation Systems is a team of experienced health care and computer professionals offering consulting services to help healthcare providers implement solutions to their data management needs. Our team delivers fast, cost effective systems that are easy to learn, use and customize. We feature an architecture that allows maximum performance, flexibility and access to information at a significantly lower cost than other approaches.

5125 Information Access Technology

1100 E 6600 S
Suite 300
Salt Lake City, UT 84121-7411 801-265-8800
800-574-8801
Fax: 801-265-8880

5126 Informedics

4000 Kruse Way Place
Building 3, Suite 300
Lake Oswego, OR 97035 503-697-3000
Fax: 503-697-7671
www.mediware.com

5127 Lad Lake

PO Box 158
Dousman, WI 53118-0158 414-342-0607
Fax: 414-965-4107

5128 Lanstat Resources

PO Box 259
Southworth, WA 98386-0259 800-672-3166
Fax: 360-769-7308

5129 Liberty Healthcare Management Group

300 Hamilton Avenue
Suite B
White Plains, NY 10601-1816   914-328-0422
                                      800-662-5800

Liberty provides individualized programs and a continuum of services for psychiatric and substance abuse treatment at our centers located throughout the Northeast, Oklahoma and Florida. Liberty's commitment to medical excellence within an environment of results-oriented care is evident in our outstanding record of clinical success.

5130 Lifelink Corporation/Bensenville Home Society

331 S York Road
Suite 206
Bensenville, IL 60106-2673   630-766-5800
                                      Fax: 630-860-5130

5131 MADNESS

146-5 Chrystal Terrace
Suite 5
Santa Cruz, CA 95060   408-426-5335
                                      Fax: 408-426-5335

5132 Managed Care Local Market Overviews

Dorland Healthcare Information
1500 Walnut Street
Suite 1000
Philadelphia, PA 19102   215-875-1212
                                      800-784-2332
                                      Fax: 215-735-3966
                          E-mail: info@dorlandhealth.com
                                www.dorlandhealth.com

Delivers valuable intelligence on local health and managed care marekts. Each of these 71 reports describes key market participants and competitive environment in one US market, including information on: local trends in events, key players, alliances among MCOs and providers, legislative developments, regulatory development, statistics on Managed Penetration. *$475.00*

5133 Managed Care Washington

4319 Stone Way N
Seattle, WA 98103-7420   206-441-1722
                                      Fax: 206-441-4823

5134 Manisses Communication Group

Manisses Communications Group
208 Governor Street
Providence, RI 02906-3246   401-831-6020
                                      800-333-7771
                                      Fax: 401-861-6370
                        E-mail: manissescs@manisses.com
                                www.manisses.com

5135 Mayo HealthQuest/Mayo Clinic Health Information

200 1st Street SW
Rochester, MN 55905-0001   507-284-2511
                                      800-430-9699
                                      Fax: 507-284-5410

5136 Medical Data Research

5225 Wiley Post Way
Suite 500
Salt Lake City, UT 84116-2899   801-536-1110

5137 Medical Online Resources

67 Shaker Road
Suite 8
Gray, ME 04039-9640   207-729-6228

5138 Medicine Shoppe InerNet

1100 N Lindbergh Boulevard
Saint Louis, MO 63132-2992   314-993-6000
                                      800-325-1397
                                      Fax: 314-872-5500

5139 Medipay

521 SW 11th Avenue
Suite 200
Portland, OR 97205-2620   503-274-7841
                                      800-879-6334
                                      Fax: 503-299-6490

Complete information technology solutions for integrated continuum of managed behavioral health care.

5140 Meridian Resource Corporation

401 W Michigan Street
Milwaukee, WI 53203-2804   414-226-6732
                                      Fax: 414-226-5109

5141 Microsoft Corporation

1 Microsoft Way
Redmond, WA 98052-8300   425-882-8080
                                      Fax: 425-936-7329

5142 Multimedia Medical Systems

400 Ray C Hunt Drive
Suite 380
Charlottesville, VA 22903   804-977-8710
                                      Fax: 804-979-3022

5143 NASW West Virginia Chapter

1608 Virginia Street E
Charleston, WV 25311-2114   304-345-6279
                                      Fax: 304-343-3295

5144 National Child Support Network

PO Box 1018
Fayetteville, AR 72702-1018
                                      800-729-5437
                                      www.childsupport.org

5145 National Clearinghouse on Child Abuse & Neglect

Children's Bureau
330 C Street SW
Washington, DC 20447   703-385-2000
                                      800-394-3366
                                      Fax: 703-385-3206
                          E-mail: nccanch@calib.com
                                www.calib.com/nccanch

Mary Sullivan, Project Director

The clearinghouse serves as a facilitator of information and knowledge exchange; the Chilren's Bureau and its training and technical assistant network; the child abuse and neglect, child welfare, and adoption communities; and allied agencies and professions.

5146 National Council on Alcoholism and Drug Dependence

20 Exchange Place, Suite 2902
New York, NY 10005   212-269-7797
Fax: 212-269-7510
E-mail: national@ncadd.org
www.ncadd.org

5147 National Families in Action

2957 Clairmont Road NE
Suite 150
Atlanta, GA 30329-1647   770-934-6364
Fax: 770-934-7137

5148 National Mental Health Self-Help Clearinghouse

1211 Chestnut Street
Suite 1000
Philadelphia, PA 19107-4103   215-751-1810
Fax: 215-636-6310

5149 North Bay Center for Behavioral Medicine

1100 Trancas Street
Suite 244
Napa, CA 94558-2908   707-255-7786
Fax: 707-252-1092
E-mail: nbcbm@napanet.net
www.behavioralmed.org

Frank Lucchetti, Psychologist

Represents comprehensive assessment and a balanced schedule of medical and/or psychological treatments for individuals with disabilities needing relief from chronic pain, disabling conditions and stress related to depression, anxiety, and unhealthy work, community or family conditions.

5150 On-Line Information Services

1187 Coast Village Road
Suite 207
Montecito, CA 93108-2737   805-565-5115
Fax: 805-565-5114

5151 Open Minds

Behavioral Health Industry News
10 York Street
Suite 200
Gettysburg, PA 17325-2301   717-334-1329
Fax: 717-334-0538
E-mail: openminds@openminds.com
www.openminds.com

Provides information on marketing, financial, and legal trends in the delivery of mental health and chemical dependency benefits and services. Recurring features include interviews, news of research, a calendar of events, job listings, book reviews, notices of publications available, and industry statistics. *$185.00*

12 pages 12 per year ISSN 1043-3880

5152 Optaio: The Psychological Corporation

Harcourt Brace & Company

888-467-8246
Fax: 888-200-4880

Provides quality assessment tools for behavioral health care providers and clinical decision-support system.

5153 Optum

Mail Route MN010-S203
6300 Olson Memorial Highway
Golden Valley, MN 55427   612-797-4169
888-262-4614
Fax: 612-797-2730
www.optumcare.com

Colleen Dillon, Sr Director Marketing
Judy Tacyn, Marketing Communications Manager

A market leader in providing comprehensive information, education and support services that enhance quality of life through improved health and well-being. Through multiple access points-the telephone, audio tapes, print materials, in-person consultations and the Internet-Optum helps participants address daily living concerns, make appropriate health care decisions, and become more effective managers of their own health and well-being.

5154 Our Town Family Center

3830 E Bellevue
PO Box 26665
Tucson, AZ 85726-6665   520-323-1708
800-537-8696
Fax: 520-323-9077
E-mail: jacquelynlc@hotmail.com
www.ourtownfamilycenter.org

Sue Krahe-Eggleston, Executive Director
Jacquelyn Lesure-Croteau, Development Director
Karen Pugh, Assistant Director

A general social services agency which focuses on serving children, youth, and their families. We offer low or no cost assistance with counseling, prevention, services for homeless youth and runaways (their families too) mediation, services for at risk youth, residential programs, parent mentoring, and much more. Our Town has made a conscious decision to keep its services focused in Pima County, in order to better serve our community. We are nonprofit, and funded by United Way, private donations, and grants with the state, county and city.

5155 Ovid Online

Ovid Technologies
333 7th Avenue
New York, NY 10001-5004   212-563-3006
                                 800-950-2035
                            Fax: 212-563-3784
                     E-mail: sales@ovid.com
                               www.ovid.com

Online reference and database information provider.
$.50/record

5156 Patient Medical Records

901 Tahoka Road
Brownfield, TX 79316-3817   806-637-2556
                                 800-285-7627
                            Fax: 806-637-4283

5157 Penelope Price

4900 Blazer Parkway
Dublin, OH 43017-3305   614-766-3633
                            Fax: 614-793-0443

5158 Physicians' ONLINE

560 White Plains Road
Tarrytown, NY 10591-5113   914-332-6100
                            Fax: 914-332-6445

5159 Piedmont Community Services

208 Cleveland Avenue
Martinsville, VA 24112-3715   540-632-4669
                            Fax: 540-632-9998

5160 Point of Care Technologies

6 Taft Court
Suite 150
Rockville, MD 20850-5361   301-610-2420
                            Fax: 703-713-3474

5161 Preferred Medical Informatics

1251 W Glen Oaks Lane
Suite 201
Mequon, WI 53092-3356   414-790-9339
                                 800-868-7859

5162 PsychAccess

700 5th Avenue
Sutie 5500
Seattle, WA 98104-5016   206-521-2588
                            Fax: 206-467-9237

5163 RTI Business Systems

5622 Ox Road
Suite 220
Fairfax Station, VA 22039-1018   703-503-9600
                            Fax: 703-503-9696

5164 Servisource

104 S Freya Street
Suite 209
Spokane, WA 99202-4866   509-532-9144
                                 888-532-9144

5165 SilverPlatter Information

100 River Ridge Drive
Norwood, MA 02062-5030   781-769-2599
                            Fax: 781-769-8763

5166 Stress Management Research Associates

10609-B Grant Road
Houston, TX 77070   281-890-8575
                     E-mail: relax@stresscontrol.com
                           www.stresscontrol.com

5167 Supervised Lifestyles

106 Brewster Square
Department 279
Brewster, NY 10509-1118   845-228-4328
                                 888-822-7348
                            Fax: 845-279-7678
                     E-mail: sls@slshealth.com
                               www.slshealth.com

5168 Technical Support Systems

775 E 3300 S
Salt Lake City, UT 84106-4077   801-484-1283

5169 Telepad Corporation

PO Box 1909
Herndon, VA 20172-1909   703-834-9000
                            Fax: 703-834-1235

5170 Traumatic Incident Reduction Association

13 NW Barry Road, PMB 214
Kansas City, MO 64155-2728   816-468-4945
                                 800-499-2751
                            Fax: 816-468-6656
                     E-mail: info@tir.org
                               www.tir.org

5171 UNISYS Corporation

8008 Westpark Drive
Suite NH3C
McLean, VA 22102-3197   703-847-2412
                            Fax: 704-362-9787

5172 Universal Behavioral Service

820 Fort Wayne Avenue
Indianapolis, IN 46204-1309   317-684-0442
                            Fax: 617-684-0679

5173 Virginia Beach Community Service Board

Pembroke 6
Suite 208
Virginia Beach, VA 23462   757-437-5770
                            Fax: 804-490-5736

5174 Well Mind Association

4649 Sunnyside Avenue N
Suite 344
Seattle, WA 98103   206-547-6167
                     E-mail: wma@speakeasy.org
                               www.speakeasy.org

Well Mind Association distributes information on current research and promotes alternative therapies for mental illness and related disorders. WMA believes that physical conditions and treatable biochemical imbalances are the causes of many mental, emotional and behavioral problems.

5175 WordPerfect Corporation

1555 N Technology Way
Suite A337
Orem, UT 84097-2395   801-222-4050
                             Fax: 801-222-4077

Manufacturers A-Z

5176 Abbott Laboratories

100 Abbott Park Road
Abbott Park, IL 60064-6400   847-937-6100
Fax: 847-937-1511
www.abbott.com

Manufactures the following psychological drugs:
Cylert, Desoxyn, Depakote, Nembutal, Placidyl,
Prosom, Tranxene.

5177 Akzo Nobel

525 W Van Buren Street
Chicago, IL 60606   312-544-7000
www.akzonobelusa.com

Manufactures the following psychological drugs:
Remeron, Tolvon.

5178 Astra Zeneca Pharmaceuticals

1800 Concord Pike
PO Box 15437
Wilmington, DE 19850   302-886-3000
Fax: 302-886-3119
www.astrazeneca-us.com

Full range of products in six therapeutic areas; gastrointestinal, oncology, anesthesia, cardiovascular, central nervous system and respiratory.

5179 Bristol-Myers Squibb

345 Park Avenue
New York, NY 10154-0037   212-546-4000
www.bms.com

Manufactures the following psychological drugs:
Serzone, BuSpar.

5180 Cephalon

145 Brandywine Parkway
West Chester, PA 19380   610-344-0200
Fax: 610-738-6590
www.cephalon.com

Manufactures the following pharmaceutical: Provigil.

5181 Eisai

Glenpointe Centre W
500 Frand W Burr Boulevard
Teaneck, NJ 07666   201-692-1100
www.eisai.com

Manufactures the following psychological drug:
Aricept.

5182 Eli Lilly and Company

Lilly Corporate Center
Indianapolis, IN 46285   317-276-2000
Fax: 317-277-6579
www.lilly.com

Manufactures pharmaceuticals for Schizophrenia.

5183 First Horizon Pharmaceutical

6195 Shiloh Road
Alpharetta, GA 30005   770-442-9707
Fax: 770-442-9594
www.horizonpharm.com

Manufactures the following psychological drug:
Cognex.

5184 Forest Laboratories

909 Third Avenue
New York, NY 10022-4731   212-421-7850
Fax: 212-750-9152
www.frx.com

Manufactures the following psychological drugs:
Lexapro, Benicar.

5185 Glaxo-SmithKline

5 Moore Drive
PO Box 13398
Research Triangle Park, NC 27709   888-825-5249
Fax: 919-483-5249
www.gsk.com

Manufactures the following psychological drugs:
Wellbutrin, Eskalith, Lamictal, Paxil, Parnate,
Compazine.

5186 Hoffman-La Roche

340 Kingsland Street
Nutley, NJ 07110   973-235-5000
Fax: 973-235-7605
www.rocheusa.com

Manufactures the following psychological drugs:
Aurorix, Lexotan, Valium, Kloropin.

5187 Johnson & Johnson

One Johnson & Johnson Plaza
New Brunswick, NJ 08933   732-524-0400
Fax: 732-524-3300
www.jnj.com

Manufactures the following psychological drugs:
Reminyl, Risperdal, Concerta.

5188 Mallinckrodt

Corporate Headquarters
675 McDonnell Boulevard
Hazelwood, MO 63042   314-654-2000
Fax: 314-654-5380
www.mallinckrodt.com

Manufactures the following psychological drugs:
Dexedrine, Methylin.

5189 Novartis Institutes for BioMedical Research

400 Technology Square
Cambridge, MA 02139   617-871-8000
Fax: 617-551-9540
www.novartis.com

Manufactures the following psychological drugs: Exelon, Clozaril, Ritalin, Anafranil, Leponex, Tegretol.

5190 Organon

56 Livingston Avenue
Roseland, NJ 07068   973-325-4500
Fax: 973-325-4589
www.organon-usa.com

Manufactures the following psychological drugs: Remeron.

5191 Ortho-McNeil Pharmaceutical

1000 US Route 202 S
Raritan, NJ 08869   877-323-2200
www.ortho-mcneil.com

Manufactures the following psychological drugs: Topomax.

5192 Pfizer

235 E 42nd Street
New York, NY 10017-5755   212-733-2323
Fax: 212-733-7851
www.pfizer.com

Manufactures the following psychological drugs: Aricept, Zoloft, Geodon.

193 Sanofi-Synthelabo

90 Park Avenue
New York, NY 10016   212-551-4000
Fax: 212-551-4903
www.sanofi-synthelabous.com

Manufactures the following psychological drugs: Dogmatil, Solain. Also the sleeping medication: Ambien.

194 Shire Richwood

One Riverfront Place
Newport, KY 41071   859-669-8000
Fax: 859-669-8414
www.shire.com

Manufactures the following psychological drugs: Adderall, DextroStat.

195 Solvay Pharmaceuticals

901 Sawyer Road
Marietta, GA 30062   800-241-1643
www.solvaypharmaceuticals.com

Manufactures the following psychological drugs: Klonopin, Lithobid, Lithonate.

96 Somerset Pharmaceuticals

5415 W Laurel Street
Tampa, FL 33607   813-288-0040
www.somersetpharm.com

Manufactures the following psychological drug: Eldepryl.

5197 Wyeth

5 Giralda Farms
Madison, NJ 07940   973-660-5500
Fax: 973-660-7026
www.wyeth.com

Manufactures the following psychological drugs: Effexor, Ativan, Equanil, Surmontil.

Drugs A-Z

5198 Adderall

Used to manage anxiety disorders and some cases of attention deficit hyperactivity disorder. This product is manufactured by Shire Richwood. See Manufacturers section for company information.

5199 Ambien

Used to manage sleeping disorders. This product is manufactured by Sanofi-Synthelabo. See Manufacturers section for company information.

5200 Anafranil

Used to manage obsessive-compulsive disorder. This product is manufactured by Novartis Consumer Health Corporation. See Manufacturers section for company information.

5201 Aricept

Used to help manage Alzheimer's disease. This product is manufactured by Pfizer and Eisai. See Manufacturers section for company information.

5202 Ativan

Used to help sleeping disorders and as a tranquilizer. This product is manufactured by Wyeth-Ayerst Laboratories and American Home Products Corporation. See Manufacturers section for company information.

5203 Aurorix

Used to manage depression. This product is manufactured by Hoffman-La Roche. See Manufacturers section for company information.

5204 BuSpar

Used to help manage anxiety. This product is manufactured by Bristol-Myers Squibb. See Manufacturers section for company information.

5205 Celexa

Used to help manage depression. This product is manufactured by Forest Laboratories. See Manufacturers section for company information.

5206 Clozaril

Used to help manage schizophrenia. This product is manufactured by Norvartis Consumer Health Corporation. See Manufacturers section for company information.

5207 Cognex

Used to help manage Alzheimer's disease. This product is manufactured by First Horizon Pharmaceutical. See Manufacturers section for company information.

5208 Compazine

Used to help manage psychotic episodes. This product is manufactured by Glaxco-SmithKline. See Manufacturers section for company information.

5209 Concerta

Used to manage attention deficit disorder. This product is manufactured by Johnson and Johnson. See Manufacturers section for company information.

5210 Cylert

Used to help manage attention deficit hyperactive disorder. This product is manufactured by Abbott Laboratories. See Manufacturers section for companys information.

5211 Depakote

Used to help manage the manic episodes associated with bipolar disorder and mania. This product is manufactured by Abbott Laboratories. See Manufacturers section for companys information.

5212 Desoxyn

Used to help manage attention deficit hyperactive disorder. This product is manufactured by Abbott Laboratories. See Manufacturers section for company information.

564

5213 Dexedrine

Used to help manage attention deficit hyperactive disorder. This product is manufactured by Mallinckrodt. See Manufacturers section for company information.

5214 DextroStat

Used to help manage attention deficit disorder. This product is manufactured by Shire Richwood. See Manufacturers section for company information.

5215 Dogmatil

Used to help manage depression. This product is manufactured by Sanofi-Synthelabo. See Manufacturers section for company information.

5216 Effexor

Used to help manage depression. This product is manufactured by Wyeth-Ayerst Laboratories and American Home Products Corporation. See Manufacturers section for company information.

5217 Elavil

Used to help manage depression. This product is manufactures by Astra Zeneca Pharmaceuticals. See Manufacturers section for company information.

5218 Eldepryl

Used to help manage Parkinson's disease. This product is manufactured by Somerset Pharmaceuticals. See Manufacturers section for company information.

5219 Equanil

Used to help manage anxiety. This product is manufactured by Wyeth-Ayerst Laboratories and American Home Products. See Manufacturers section for company information.

5220 Exelon

Used to help manage Alzheimer's disease. This product is manufactured by Novartis. See Manufacturers section for company information.

5221 Geodon

Used to help manage psychotic episodes. This product is manufactured by Pfizer. See Manufacturers section for company information.

5222 Kloropin

Used to help manage panic disorder. This product is manufactured by Hoffman-La Roche. See Manufacturers section for company information.

5223 Lamictal

Used to help manage bipolar disorder. This product is manufactured by Glaxo-SmithKline. See Manufacturers section for company information.

5224 Leponex

Used to help manage psychotic episodes. This product is manufactured by Novartis Consumer Health Corporation. See Manufacturers section for company information.

5225 Lexapro

Used to help manage depression. This product is manufactured by Forest Laboratories. See Manufacturers section for company information.

5226 Lexotan

Used to help manage depresion. This product is manufactured by Hoffman-La Roche. See Manufacturers section for company information.

5227 Lithobid

Used to help manage bipolar disorder and depression. This product is manufactured by Solvay Pharmaceuticals. See Manufacturers section for company information.

5228 Luvox

Used to help manage obsessive compulsive disorder. This product is manufactured by Solvay Pharmaceuticals. See Manufacturers section for company information.

5229 Methylin

Used to help manage attention deficit disorder. This product is manufactured by Mallinckrodt. See Manufacturers section for company information.

5230 Nembutal

Used to help manage insomnia and other sleeping disorders, used as sedatives and/or hypnotics. This product is manufactured by Abbott Laboratories. See Manufacturers section for company information.

5231 Neurontin

Used to help manage bipolar disorder. This product is manufactured by Parke-Davis Pharmacutical Company. See Manufacturers section for company information.

5232 Parnate

Used to help manage depression. This product is manufactured by Glaxo-SmithKline. See Manufacturers section for company information.

5233 Paxil

Used to help manage depression and social anxiety. This product is manufactured by Glaxo-SmithKline. See Manufacturers section for company information.

5234 Placidyl

Used to help manage insomnia in short-term hypnotic therapy. This product is manufactured by Abbott Laboratories. See Manufacturers section for company information.

5235 Prosom

Used to help manage insomnia in short-term uses. This product is manufactured by Abbott Laboratories. See Manufacturers section for company information.

5236 Provigil

Used to help manage sleep disorders. This product is manufactured by Cephalon. See Manufacturers section for company information.

5237 Prozac

Used to help manage depression. This product is manufactured by Eli Lilly and Company. See Manufacturers section for company information.

5238 Reboxetine

Used to help manage depression. This product is manufactured by Pharmacia & Upjohn. See Manufacturers section for company information.

5239 Remeron

Used to help manage depression. This product is manufactured by Organon and Akzo Nobel. See Manufacturers section for company information.

5240 Reminyl

Used to help manage Alzheimer's disease. This product is manufactured by Johnson and Johnson. See Manufacturers section for company information.

5241 Risperdal

Used to help manage schizophrenia and other mental illnesses such as psychosis. This product is manufactured by Johnson & Johnson. See Manufacturers section for company information.

5242 Ritalin

Used to help manage attention deficit disorders and in some forms of treating narcolepsy. This product is manufactured by Novartis Consumer Health Corporation. See Manufacturers section for company information.

5243 Sermion

Used to help manage dementia. This product is manufactured by Pharmacia & Upjohn. See Manufacturers section for company information.

5244 Seroquel

Used to help manage the manifestations of psychotic disorders. This product is manufactured by Astra Zeneca Pharmaceuticals. See Manufacturers section for company information.

5245 Serzone

Used to help manage depression. This product is manufactured by Bristol-Myers Squibb. See Manufacturers section for company information.

5246 Solian

Used to help manage schizophrenia. This product is manufactured by Sanofi-Synthelabo. See Manufacturers section for company information.

5247 Surmontil

Used to help manage depression. This product is manufactured by Wyeth-Ayerst Laboratories and American Home Products Corporation. See Manufacturers section for company information.

5248 Tegretol

Used to help manage bipolar disorder. This product is manufactured by Novartis Consumer Health Corporation. See Manufacturers section for company information.

5249 Tolvon

Used to help manage depression. This product is manufactured by Akzo Nobel. See Manufacturers section for company information.

5250 Topamax

Used to manage bipolar disorder. This product is manufactured by Ortho-McNeil Pharmacutical. See Manufacturers section for company information.

5251 Tranxene

Used to help manage sleeping disorders or as a tranquilizer. This product is manufactured by Abbott Laboratories. See Manufacturers section for company information.

5252 Valium

Used to help manage anxiety. This product is manufactured by Hoffman-La Roche. See Manufacturers section for company information.

5253 Wellbutrin

Used to help manage depression. This product is manufactured by Glaxo-SmithKline. See Manufacturers section for company information.

5254 Xanax

Used to help manage anxiety. This product is manufactured by Pharmacia & Upjohn. See Manufacturers section for company information.

5255 Zoloft

Used to help manage depression and post traumatic stress disorder.This product is manufactured by Pfizer. See Manufacturers section for company information.

5256 Zyprexa

Used to manage the manifistations of psychotic disorders. This product is manufactured by Eli Lilly and Company. See Manufacturers section for company information.

ADHD

Adjustment Disorders

Alcohol Abuse & Dependence

Anxiety Disorders

Autistic Disorder

Bipolar Disorder

Cognitive Disorders

Conduct Disorder

Depression

Gender Identification Disorder

Impulse Control Disorders

Movement Disorders

Obsessive Compulsive Disorder

Pediatric & Adolescent Issues

Personality Disorders

Post Traumatic Stress Disorder

Psychosomatic (Somatizing) Disorders

Substance Abuse & Dependence

Suicide

Tic Disorders

A

B

D

G

I

Meharry Medical College, 3595
Memory and Dementia, 677
Memory, Trauma and the Law, 3072
Memphis Alcohol and Drug Council, 2472
Memphis Business Group on Health, 2062
Memphis Mental Health Institute, 4207
Men and Depression, 796
Mendota Mental Health Institute, 4252
Menninger Care Systems, 4527
Menninger Clinic, 1745
Menninger Clinic Department of Research, 706, 3297, 3596
Menninger Division of Continuing Education, 3596
Mental & Physical Disability Law Reporter, 3408
Mental Affections Childhood, 3193
Mental Disability Law: Primer, a Comprehensive Introduction, 2863
Mental Health Aspects of Developmental Disabilities, 3409
Mental Health Association, 2074
Mental Health Association in Albany County, 1987
Mental Health Association in Dutchess County, 1988
Mental Health Association in Illinois, 2284
Mental Health Association in Marion County Consumer Services, 1883
Mental Health Association in Michigan, 1293
Mental Health Association in South Carolina, 2458
Mental Health Association of Arizona, 1807
Mental Health Association of Colorado, 1837
Mental Health Association of Delaware, 1846
Mental Health Association of Greater St. Louis, 1950
Mental Health Association of Maryland, 1913
Mental Health Association of Montana, 1955
Mental Health Association of New Jersey, 1972
Mental Health Association of South East Pennsylvania, 2032
Mental Health Association of Summit, 2013
Mental Health Association of West Florida, 1856
Mental Health Association: Connecticut, 1841
Mental Health Board of North Central Alabama, 1799
Mental Health Center, 3597
Mental Health Center of North Central Alabama, 1800
Mental Health Connections, 4924
Mental Health Consultants, 3254
Mental Health Corporations of America, 2696
Mental Health Council of Arkansas, 2219
Mental Health Directory, 3933
Mental Health Law News, 3410
Mental Health Law Reporter, 3411
Mental Health Materials Center (MHMC), 2697
Mental Health Net, Eating Disorders, 970
Mental Health Outcomes, 4925
Mental Health Rehabilitation: Disputing Irrational Beliefs, 2864
Mental Health Report, 3412
Mental Health Resources Catalog, 2865
Mental Health Services Training Collaborative, 3598
Mental Health Special Interest: Section Quarterly, 3413
Mental Health Views, 3414

Mental Health Weekly, 3415
Mental Health and Aging Network (MHAN) of the American Society on Aging (ASA), 1746
Mental Health and Developmental Disability Division: Department of Human Services, 2433
Mental Health and Social Work Career Directory, 3934
Mental Health and Substance Abuse Corporations of Massachusetts, 1923
Mental Illness Education Project, 1747, 3706, 595, 1294, 1295, 3702
Mental Retardation, 3416
Mental Retardation: Definition, Classification, and Systems of Supports, 2866
Mental, Emotional, and Behavior Disorders in Children and Adolescents, 704, 1626
Mentalhelp, 1302
Mentally Disabled and the Law, 3417
Mentally Ill Kids in Distress, 1584, 1748
Menu for Understanding Panic Attacks, 238
Mercer, Meidinger and Hansen, 4528
Meridian Resource Corporation, 4529, 5140
Merit Behavioral Care Tricare, 4530
Merit Behavioral Care of California, 3963
Merit Behavorial Care Corporation, 4531
MeritCare Health System, 4926
Meritcare Health System, 4927
Mertech, 2544
Mesa Mental Health, 4532
Metaphor in Psychotherapy: Clinical Applications of Stories and Allegories, 2867
Methamphetamine: Decide to Live, 1472
Methamphetamine: a Methamphetamine Prevention Video, 1473
Methylin, 5229
Metro Intergroup of Overeaters Anonymous, 1989, 917
Metro Regional Treatment Center: Anoka, 4094
Metropolitan Area Chapter of Federation of Families for Children's Mental Health, 1932
Metropolitan Family Services, 1879
Metropolitan Saint Louis Psychiatric Center, 4105
Metropolitan State Hospital, 3964
Michael J Fox Foundation, 1042
Michael Reese Hospital and Medical Center, 944, 946
Michigan Alliance for the Mentally Ill, 1933
Michigan Association for Children with Emotional Disorders: MACED, 1934
Michigan Association for Children's Mental Health, 1585
Michigan Association for Children's Mental Health, 1935
Michigan Department of Community Health, 2342
Michigan Department of Community Health: Prevention Policy, 2343
Michigan Department of Community Health: System Development and Monitoring, 2341
Michigan Department of Community Health: Treatment Policy Section, 2340
Michigan Department of Mental Health, 2344
Michigan Department of Mental Health Bureau of Community Mental Health Services, 2345

Michigan Department of Public Health, 2346
Michigan Department of Social Services, 2347
Michigan Division of Substance Abuse Quality & Planning, 2348
Michigan State Representative: Co-Chair Public Health, 2349
Micro Design International, 4928
Micro Psych Software: Medical Management Software Corporation, 4929
Micro-Office Systems, 4930
MicroHealth Corporation, 4931
MicroScript, 4932
Microcounseling: Innovations in Interviewing, Counseling, Psychotherapy, and Psychoeducation, 2868
Micromedex, 4933
Microsoft Corporation, 5141, 4948
Mid-Hudson Forensic Psychiatric Center, 4145
Mid-Missouri Mental Health Center, 4106
Middle Tennessee Mental Health Institute, 4208, 2479
Middletown Psychiatric Center, 4146
Mihalik Group, 4533
Mildred Mitchell-Bateman Hospital, 4247
Miles of Heart, 103
Millcreek Children's Services, 4168
Milliman and Robertson, 4534
Mills-Peninsula Hospital: Behavioral Health, 3965
Mind, 4934
Mind Body Connection, 4535
Mind of its Own, Tourette's Syndrome: Story and a Guide, 1552
Mind-Body Problems: Psychotherapy with Psychosomatic Disorders, 1228
Mindblindness: An Essay on Autism and Theory of Mind, 496
Minimize & Manage Risk, 4536
Minnesota Association for Children's Mental Health, 1940
Minnesota Department of Human Services, 2352
Minnesota Department of Mental Health and Human Services, 2353
Minnesota National Alliance for the Mentally Ill, 1941
Minnesota Psychiatric Society, 1942
Minnesota Psychological Association, 1943
Minnesota Youth Services Bureau, 2354
Mirror, Mirror, 971, 3796
Missed Opportunity: National Survey of Primary Care Physicians and Patients on Substance Abuse, 3123
Mississippi Alcohol Safety Education Program, 2356
Mississippi Alliance for the Mentally Ill, 1947
Mississippi Bureau of Mental Retardation, 2357
Mississippi Department of Human Services, 2358
Mississippi Department of Mental Health, 2360
Mississippi Department of Mental Health: Division of Medicaid, 2359, 2361
Mississippi Families as Allies, 1948
Mississippi State Hospital1, 4098
Missouri Alliance for the Mentally Ill, 1951
Missouri Department of Mental Health, 2362
Missouri Department of Public Safety, 2363
Missouri Department of Social Services, 2365

N

O

P

Q

R

S

U

X

Y

Z

Alabama

Alabama Alliance for the Mentally Ill, 1796
Alabama Department of Human Resources, 2197
Alabama Department of Mental Health and Mental Retardation, 2198
Alabama Department of Public Health, 2199
Alabama Disabilities Advocacy Program, 2200
Alabama State Department of Mental Health, 2201
Association of State and Provincial Psychology Boards, 2649
Behavioral Health Systems, 4301, 2652
Birmingham Psychiatry, 1797
Center for Family Counseling, 3534
Corporate Benefit Consultants, 4359
Daniel and Yeager Healthcare Staffing Solutions, 3547
Electronic Healthcare Systems, 4793
Horizons School, 1798
MCC Behavioral Care, 2690
Mental Health Board of North Central Alabama, 1799
Mental Health Center of North Central Alabama, 1800

Alaska

Alaska Alliance for the Mentally Ill, 1801
Alaska Department of Health & Social Services, 2202
Alaska Division of Medical Assistance/DHSS, 2203
Alaska Division of Mental Health and Developmental Disabilities, 2204
Alaska Division of Mental Health and Developmental Disabilities, 2205
Alaska Mental Health Association, 1802, 2206
Alaska Mental Health Board, 2207

Arizona

Action Healthcare, 4266
American Psychological Association Division of Independent Practice (APADIP), 2616
Anasazi Software, 4699
Arizona Alliance for the Mentally Ill, 1803
Arizona Center For Mental Health PC, 4285
Arizona Department of Health Services, 2208
Arizona Department of Health Services: Behavioral Services, 2209
Arizona Department of Health Services: Child Fatality Review, 2210
Arizona Department of Health: Substance Abuse, 2211
Assist Technologies, 4706
BetaData Systems, 4718
CARF: The Rehabilitation Accreditation Commission, 2533
Commission on Accreditation of Rehabilitation Facilities, Behavioral Health: CARF, 2661
Community Partnership of Southern Arizona, 1804

Contact, 4358
DeLair Systems, 4373
Devereux Arizona Treatment Network, 1805
Eldorado Computing, 4792
Governor's Division for Children, 2212
Healthcare Southwest, 1806, 4434
Information Management Solutions, 4856
Information Network Corporation (INC), 4857
Life Development Institute, 1743
LifeCare Management Systems, 4888
Managed Care Consultants, 4514
Mental Health Association of Arizona, 1807
Mentally Ill Kids in Distress, 1584, 1748
Merit Behavioral Care Tricare, 4530
National Behavioral Health Consulting Practice, 4541
National Health Enhancement, 2720
Navajo Nation K'E Project: Children & Families Advocacy Corporation, 1808
Navajo Nation K'E Project: Chinle Children & Families Advocacy Corporation, 1809
Navajo Nation K'E Project: Tuba City Children & Families Advocacy Corporation, 1810
Navajo Nation K'E Project: Winslow Children & Families Advocacy Corporation, 1811
Northern Arizona Regional Behavioral Health Authority, 2213
Pinal Gila Behavioral Health Association, 4569
Professional Horizons, Mental Health Service, 3615
SJ Hughes Consulting, 4603
Sunquest Information Systems, 5040
Trachy Healthcare Management Company, 4648
Vance Messmer and Butler, 4666
WorldatWork, 2762

Arkansas

Arkansas Alliance for the Mentally Ill, 1812
Arkansas Department of Health, 2214
Arkansas Department of Human Services, 2215
Arkansas Division of Children & Family Service, 2216
Arkansas Division on Youth Services, 2217
Arkansas State Mental Hospital, 2218
Center for Outcomes Research and Effectiveness, 4328
Centers for Mental Healthcare Research, 4332
Health Resource, 4827
IMC Studios, 4459
Mental Health Council of Arkansas, 2219
National Child Support Network, 1586, 1758
Star Systems Corporation, 5033
TKI Computer Center, 5050

California

ADA/EAP Consulting, 4259
AMCO Computers, 4684
ASP Software, 4686
Academy of Managed Care Providers, 4262

Adult Children of Alcoholics World Services Organization, 108
American Association of Mental Health Professionals in Corrections (AAMHPC), 2577
American Board of Examiners of Clinical Social Work Regional Office, 2531
American College of Psychiatrists, 2590
American College of Psychiatrists Annual Meeting, 3230
American Holistic Health Association, 1705
American Psychological Association: Applied Experimental and Engineering Psychology, 2617
American Society on Aging, 2629
Annual Summit on International Managed Care Trends, 3237
Arthur S Shorr and Associates, 4286
Assistance League of Southern California, 1813
Associated Claims Management, 4287
Association for Humanistic Psychology: AHP, 2640
Association for Pre- & Perinatal Psychology and Health, 2641
Association of Community Mental Health Agencies, 2648
Autism Research Institute, 423
BB Consulting Group, 4290
Barbanell Associates, 4293
Behavior Data, 4711
Behavioral Healthcare Tomorrow: Spring Calender of Events, 3240
BehavioralCare, 4303
Breining Institute College for the Advanced Study of Addictive Disorders, 3528
Bright Consulting, 4306
CPP Incorporated, 4319
California Alliance for the Mentally Ill, 1814
California Association of Marriage and Family Therapists, 1815
California Association of Social Rehabilitation Agencies, 1816
California Department of Alcohol and Drug Programs, 2220
California Department of Alcohol and Drug Programs: Mentor Resource Center, 2221
California Department of Corrections: Health Care Services, 2222
California Department of Education: Healthy Kids, Healthy California, 2223
California Department of Health Services: Medicaid, 2224
California Department of Health Services: Medi-Cal Drug Discount, 2225
California Department of Mental Health, 2227
California Health & Welfare Agency, 2228
California Health Information Association, 1817
California Health and Welfare Agency, 2229
California Hispanic Commission on Alcohol Drug Abuse, 2230
California Institute for Mental Health, 1818, 2231
California Institute of Behavioral Sciences, 3530
California Mental Health Directors Association, 2232
California Psychiatric Association: CPA, 1819
California Psychological Association, 1820

United Behavioral Health, 4654
University of California at Davis, 3656
Veri-Trak, 4670
VeriCare, 4671
VersaForm Systems Corporation, 5065
Watson Wyatt Worldwide, 4673
We Insist on Natural Shapes, 879
Weimer Associates, 4675
Wellness Integrated Network, 5068
Working Press, 4678

Colorado

Adolescent and Family Institute of Colorado, 1832
American Humane Association: Children's Services, 2599
Asian Pacific Development Center, 3520
Association for Applied Psychophysiology & Biofeedback, 2635
Association for the Advancement of Psycholog y: AAP, 2646
Behavioral Health Advisor, 4714
Behavioral Health Care, 4295
CAFCA, 4309
CHINS UP Youth and Family Services, 1833
Centennial Mental Health Center, 4326
Clinical Nutrition Center, 4744
Colorado Department of Health Care Policy and Finance, 2234
Colorado Department of Human Services: Alcohol and Drug Abuse Division, 2235
Colorado Department of Institions, 2236
Colorado Department of Social Services, 2237
Colorado Division of Medical Assistance, 2238
Colorado Division of Mental Health, 2239
Colorado Health Networks-Value Options, 1834
Confidential Data Services, 4761
Craig Counseling & Biofeedback Services, 1835
Denver County Department of Social Services, 2240
El Paso County Human Services, 2241
Employee Benefit Specialists, 4383
Engineered Data Products, 4794
Federation of Families for Children's Mental Health, 1836
Gadrian Corporation, 4403, 4808
Healthcheck, 4835
IMS Medacom Networks, 4847
InfoCapture, 4849
Informed Access, 4859
Integrated Behavioral Health Consultants, 2679
John Maynard and Associates, 4480
Kaiser Technology Group, 4882
MULTUM Information Services, 4897
Medcomp Software, 4907
Medical Group Management Association, 2694
Mental Health Association of Colorado, 1837
Micromedex, 4933
Milliman and Robertson, 4534
NASW JobLink, 4540
National Academy of Neuropsychology (NAN), 2699
North American Computer Services, 4549, 4953

PRO Behavioral Health, 1772, 4560
Pragmatix, 4576
Psychological Resource Organization, 5000
System One, 5046
University of Colorado Health Sciences Center, 3658

Connecticut

Aetna-US HealthCare, 4271
American Academy of Clinical Psychiatrists, 2560
American Academy of Psychiatry & Law Annual Conference, 3222
American Academy of Psychiatry and the Law (AAPL), 2562
American Academy of Psychoanalysis Preliminary Meeting, 3223
American Academy of Psychoanalysis and Dynam ic Psychiatry, 2563
American Association of Chairs of Department s of Psychiatry, 2568
American Association of Directors of Psychiatric Residency Training, 2572
CARE, 4310
Casey Family Services, 4325
Connecticut Department of Mental Health and Addiction Services, 2242
Connecticut Department of Children and Families, 2243
Connecticut Department of Mental Health, 2244
Connecticut Families United for Children's Mental Health, 1838
Connecticut National Association of Mentally Ill, 1839
Consumer Credit Counseling, 4356
Family & Community Alliance Project, 1840
Gaynor and Associates, 4405
Infoline, 1458
Institute of Living Anxiety Disorders Center, 1738
Jewish Family Service, 2072, 4879
Largesse, The Network for Size Esteem, 869
Mental Health Association: Connecticut, 1841
Obsessive Compulsive Foundation, 1059
Obsessive-Compulsive Foundation, 1095
Roger Rose Consulting, 4601
Sarmul Consultants, 4610
Stonington Institute, 3640
Thames Valley Programs, 1842
University of Connecticut Health Center, 3659
Value Health, 4664
Women's Support Services, 1843
Yale University School of Medicine: Child Study Center, 3694
Yale University: Depression Research Program, 806

Delaware

Astra Zeneca Pharmaceuticals, 5178
Delaware Alliance for the Mentally Ill, 1844
Delaware Department of Health & Social Services, 2245
Delaware Division of Child Mental Health Services, 2246

Delaware Division of Family Services, 2247
Delaware Guidance Services for Children and Youth, 1845
Mental Health Association of Delaware, 1846

District of Columbia

AAMR-American Association on Mental Retardation Conference: Annual Meeting at the Crossroads, 2552, 3218
AAMR: American Association on Mental Retardation, 1697
Administration for Children and Families, 2145
Administration for Children, Youth and Families, 2146
Administration on Aging, 2147
Administration on Developmental Disabilities US Department of Health & Human Services, 2148
Alliance of Genetic Support Groups, 1700
American Academy of Child and Adolescent Psychiatry (AACAP): Annual Meeting, 3219
American Academy of Child & Adolescent Psychiatry Annual Conference, 2559, 3221
American Academy of Child and Adolescent Psychiatry, 1575, 1701, 3514, 3514
American Association for Behavioral Healthcare, 2564
American Association for World Health, 2566
American Association of Health Plans, 2574
American Association of Homes & Services for the Aging Annual Convention, 3227
American Association of Homes and Services for the Aging, 2576
American Association of Psychiatric Services for Children (AAPSC), 1704
American Association of Retired Persons, 2580
American Association of Suicidology, 1500
American Health Care Association, 2596
American Health Care Association Annual Meeting, 3232
American Managed Behavioral Healthcare Association, 1706, 4282, 2600, 2600
American Nurses Association, 2608
American Pharmacists Association, 2609
American Psychologial Association: Division of Family Psychology, 2614
American Psychological Association, 1710, 2615
American Psychological Society (APS), 2618
American Public Human Services Association, 58
Association of Black Psychologists Annual Convention, 3239
Association of Black Psychologists: ABPsi, 2647
Association of Maternal and Child Health Programs (AMCHP), 2150
Bazelon Center for Mental Health Law, 1714, 2651
California Department of Health and Human Services, 2226
Center for Mental Health Services, 1219, 1238, 1320, 1320, 1347, 1376, 1503, 1720

Florida

Research Center for Children's Mental Health, Department of Children and Family, 3625
Research and Training Center for Children's Mental Health, 1592
Skypek Group, 4621, 5027, 2550, 2550
Somerset Pharmaceuticals, 5196
Suncoast Residential Training Center/Developmental Services Program, 153, 575, 687, 687, 732, 1005, 1061, 1128, 1172, 1225, 1245, 1385
Synergistic Office Solutions (SOS Software), 5044
Tempus Software, 5052
United Families for Children's Mental Health, 1595, 1787
University of Miami - Department of Psychology, 3668
Vann Data Services, 5063
Youth Services International, 1597, 1794

Georgia

Advanced Healthcare Services Group, 4270
American Board of Professional Psychology (ABPP), 2583
American Nouthetic Psychology Association: A NPA, 2607
Anxiety Disorders Institute, 140
Behavioral Health Partners, 4298, 4715
Calland and Company, 4320
Cameron and Associates, 4321
Centers for Disease Control & Prevention, 2153
Consultec, Managed Care Systems, 4762
Earley Corporation, 4786
Emory University School of Medicine, Psychology and Behavior, 3553
Emory University: Psychological Center, 3554
First Horizon Pharmaceutical, 5183
Fowler Healthcare Affiliates, 4398
Georgia Association of Homes and Services for Children, 1858
Georgia Department Human Resources: Behavioral Health Plan, 2257
Georgia Department of Human Resources, 2258
Georgia Department of Health and Human Services, 2259
Georgia Department of Human Resources, 2260
Georgia Department of Medical Assistance, 2261
Georgia Division of Mental Health and Mental Retardation, 2262
Georgia Division of Mental Health: Mental Retardation and Substance Abuse, 2263
Georgia National Alliance for the Mentally Ill, 1859
Georgia Parent Support Network, 1860
Grady Health Systems: Central Fulton CMHC, 1861
HBO and Company, 4411
HBOC, 4813
Health Capital Consultants, 4418
Horizon Systems, 4839
Human Resources Projects/Consulting, 4453
IBM Corporation, 4842
IBM Corporation Health Industry Marketing, 4843

IMNET Systems, 4846
Infocure Corporation, 4853
Integrated Computer Products, 4871
Locumtenens.com, 3581
MACRO International, 4500
MCG Telemedicine Center, 4502, 3582
MDA, Staffing Consultants, 3584
MSI International, 4506
MTS, 4507
Magellan Health Services, 4510
Magnus Software Corporation, 4898
McManis Associates, 3253
Medical College of Georgia, 3589
Murphy-Harpst-Vashti, 4539
National Center of HIV, STD and TB Prevention, 2161
National Data Corporation, 4942
National Families in Action, 4943
Optaio Software, 4960
Quality Management Audits, 4594
REC Management, 4596
Society for the Advancement of Social Psychology (SASP), 2753
Solvay Pharmaceuticals, 5195
Source One Systems (Health Records), 5029
Southeast Nurse Consultants, 4624
Strategic Advantage, 4635, 5035
TDS Healthcare Systems, 5048
United Behavioral Health, 4655
William M Mercer, 4677

Hawaii

ADAPS, 4260, 4681
Hawaii Alliance for the Mentally Ill, 1862
Hawaii Department of Adult Mental Health, 2264
Hawaii Department of Health, 2265
Hawaii Families As Allies, 1863
John A Burns School of Medicine Department of Psychiatry, 3575
National Alliance for the Mentally Ill in Hawaii, 1864
Villages, Program Administration, 1884

Idaho

Ascent, 4703
College of Southern Idaho, 4344, 3539
Department of Health and Welfare: Medicaid Division, 2266
Department of Health and Welfare: Community Rehab, 2267
Idaho Department of Health & Welfare, 2268
Idaho Alliance for the Mentally Ill, 1865
Idaho Bureau of Maternal and Child Health, 2269
Idaho Bureau of Mental Health and Substance Abuse, Division of Family & Community Service, 2270
Idaho Department of Health and Welfare: Family and Child Services, 2271
Idaho Mental Health Center, 2272

Illinois

ARRISE, 419

Abbott Laboratories, 5176
Academy of Psychosomatic Medicine, 2554
Ada S McKinley, 4689
Advocate Behavioral Health Partners, 2556
Advocate Ravenswood Hospital Medical Center, 3506
Akzo Nobel, 5177
Alexander Consulting Group, 4273
Allendale Association, 1866
Alzheimer's Association National Office, 614
Alzheimer's Disease and Related Disorders Association, 616
Alzheimer's Hospital Association, 617
American Academy of Medical Administrators, 2561
American Academy of Pediatrics, 1576, 1702
American Academy of Sleep Medicine, 1345
American Association of Healthcare Consultants, 2575
American Board of Psychiatry and Neurology (ABPN), 2584
American College of Healthcare Executives, 2587, 3229, 3516, 3516
American College of Psychoanalysts: ACPA, 2591
American College of Women's Health Physicians, 3517
American Health Information Management Association Annual Exhibition and Conference, 2597, 3233
American Hospital Association: Section for Psychiatric and Substance Abuse, 2598
American Medical Association, 2601
American Medical Association Annual and Interim Conferences, 3234
American Medical Software, 4696
Anorexia Nervosa and Associated Disorders National Association (ANAD), 861
Anxiety & Mood Disorders Clinic: Department of Psychiatry & Behavioral Medicine, 3519
Askesis Development Group, 4704
Association for Psychological Type: APT, 2643
Attention Deficit Disorder Association, 266
Baby Fold, 1867
CANDU Parent Group, 1629
CBI Group, 4311
Center for the Study of Adolescence, 944
Chaddock, 1868
Chicago Child Care Society, 1869
Children's Home Association of Illinois, 1870
Coalition of Illinois Counselors Organization, 1871
College of Dupage, 4343
ComPsych, 4347
Community Service Options, 1726
Compassionate Friends, 21
DD Fischer Consulting, 4369
Depression & Bi-Polar Support Alliance, 717
Depression & BiPolar Support Alliance, 570
Depression and Bi-Polar Alliance, 720
Dupage County Health Department, 4379
Eating Disorders Research and Treatment Program, 946
Employee Assistance Society of North America, 2669
Enterprise Systems, 4796
Family Service Association of Greater Elgin Area, 1872
Finch University of Health Sciences, 3560
G Murphy and Associates, 4401

Indiana

Iowa

Kansas

Kentucky

FCS, 4390
KAMFT/Managed Care Coordinators, 4484
KY-SPIN, 1894
Kentucky Alliance for the Mentally Ill, 1895
Kentucky Cabinet for Human Resources, 2301
Kentucky Department for Medicaid Services, 2302
Kentucky Department for Social Services, 2303
Kentucky Department of Mental Health and Mental Retardation, 2304
Kentucky IMPACT, 1896
Kentucky Justice Cabinet: Department of Juvenile Justice, 2305
Kentucky Psychiatric Association, 1897
National Anxiety Foundation, 149
Project Vision, 1899
River Valley Behavioral Health, 3255
SPOKES Federation of Families for Children's Mental Health, 1900
Shire Richwood, 5194
St. Joseph Behavioral Medicine Network, 4631, 3638
SunRise Health Marketing, 4639
University of Louisville School of Medicine, 3664

Louisiana

Accreditation Services, 4687
Active Intervention, 3505
Alton Ochsner Medical Foundation, Psychiatry Residency, 3513
Enterprize Management Systems, 4797
Family Managed Care, 4392
Integrated Behavioral Health, 4466
Louisiana Alliance for the Mentally Ill, 1901
Louisiana Commission on Law Enforcement and Administration, 2306
Louisiana Department of Health and Hospitals: Office of Mental Health, 2307
Louisiana Department of Health and Hospitals: Division of Programs, 2308
Louisiana Department of Health, 2309
Louisiana Department of Health & Hospitals, 2310
Louisiana Department of Health & Human Services, 2311
Louisiana Department of Health and Hospitals: Office of Alcohol and Drug Abuse, 2312
Louisiana Division of Mental Health, 2313
Louisiana Federation of Families for Children's Mental Health, 1902
Louisiana Office for Prevention and Recovery, 2314
SUPRA Management, 2548
Sumtime Software, 5038
West Jefferson Medical Center: Behavioral Medical Center, 3691

Maine

Advanced Data Systems, 4691
Counseling and Consultation Services, 4362
Familes United for Children's Mental Health, 1903
Maine Alliance for the Mentally Ill, 1904

Maine Department Mental Health and Bureau of Children, 2315
Maine Department Services for Children with Special Needs, 2316
Maine Department of Behavioral and Developmental Services, 2317
Maine Department of Human Services: Children's Emergency Services, 2318
Maine Division of Mental Health, 2319
Maine Office of Substance Abuse: Information and Resource Center, 2320
Maine Psychiatric Association, 1905
Northland Health Group, 4550
Psybernetics, 4989
Spring Harbor Hospital, 4628

Maryland

Agency for Health Care Policy & Research Center for Health Information, 2557
Agency for Healthcare Research and Quality: Office of Communications and Knowledge Transfer, 2149
Alzheimer's Disease Education and Referral Center, 615
American Association for Geriatric Psychiatry, 1577, 1703
American Association of Children's Residential Center Annual Conference, 2569, 3224
American Association of Geriatric Psychiatry (AAGP), 2573
American Association of Geriatric Psychiatry Annual Meetings, 3225
American Association of University Affiliate Programs for Persons With Developmental Disabilities, 2581
American College Health Association, 2585
American Health Assistance Foundation, 618
American Medical Directors Association, 2602
American Medical Informatics Association, 2604
American Pediatric Medical Association, 4697
American Society of Addiction Medicine, 3249
American Society of Health System Pharmacist s, 2626
American Society of Psychoanalytic Physicians: ASPP, 2627
Annie E Casey Foundation, 2630
Anxiety Disorders Association of America, 139
Association of Behavioral Healthcare Management, 59
Autism Society of America, 425, 539
Black Mental Health Alliance (BMHA), 1717
Bonny Foundation, 2653
CHADD: Children and Adults with AD/HD, 367, 1630
Center for Mental Health Services Homeless Programs Branch, 2151
Center for Health Policy Studies, 4734, 3535
Center for Substance Abuse Treatment, 2152
Centers for Medicare & Medicaid Services: Office of Research/Demonstration, 2321
Centers for Medicare & Medicaid Services, 2322
Centers for Medicare & Medicaid Services: Division of Payment Policy, 2154, 2323

Chemically Dependent Anonymous, 1456
Children and Adults with AD/HD, 269
Children and Adults with Attention Deficit Disorders, 270
Cirrus Technology, 4740
Community Behavioral Health Association of Maryland: CBH, 1906
Community Services for Autistic Adults and Children, 430
Comsort, 4354
Council on Quality and Leadership, 1728
Counseling Associates, 4361
David Group, 4372
Docu Trac, 4782
Epidemiology-Genetics Program in Psychiatry, 594
Families Involved Together, 1908
Goucher College, 4408
Green Spring Health Services, 4409
Green Spring Health Services' AdvoCare Program, 4410
HCIA-RESPONSE, 4816
Health Resources and Services Administration, 1909
Humanitas, 4841
Information Resources and Inquiries Branch, 2159
Institute of Psychiatry and Human Behavior: University of Maryland, 1910
International Association of Psychosocial Rehabilitation Services, 2681
International Critical Incident Stress Foundation, 146
Jeri Davis Marketing Consultants, 4479
Johnson, Bassin and Shaw, 4481
KAI Associates, 4483
Kennedy Krieger Family Center, 4884
Magellan Health Service, 4509
Management Recruiters of Washington, DC, 3586
Maryland Health Care Financing Administration: Divison of Coverage Policy, 2324
Maryland Alcohol and Drug Abuse Administration, 2325
Maryland Alliance for the Mentally Ill, 1911
Maryland Department of Health and Mental Hygiene, 2326
Maryland Department of Human Resources, 2327
Maryland Division of Mental Health, 2328
Maryland Health Care Financing Administration: Division of Eligiblity Policy, 2329
Maryland Health Care Financing Administration, 2330
Maryland Health Systems Financing Administration, 2331
Maryland Office of State Healthcare Reform, 2332
Maryland Psychiatric Research Center, 1912
Medical Information Systems, 4915
Mental Health Association of Maryland, 1913
Mental Health Services Training Collaborative, 3598
National Institutes of Mental Health Division of Extramural Activities, 2160
National Association of School Psychologists, 2708, 3602
National Clearinghouse for Alcohol and Drug Information, 63, 1381
National Clearinghouse for Alcohol and Drug Information, 1454

National Clearinghouse for Drug & Alcohol, 2162
National Consortium on Telepsychiatry, 4941
National Council for Community Behavioral Healthcare, 1759
National Eldercare Services Company, 2719
National Family Caregivers Association, 623
National Institute of Alcohol Abuse and Alcoholism: Treatment Research Branch, 2163
National Institute of Alcohol Abuse and Alcoholism: Homeless Demonstration and Evaluation Branch, 2164
National Institute of Alcohol Abuse and Alcoholism: Office of Policy Analysis, 2165
National Institute of Drug Abuse: NIDA, 1762, 2166
National Institute of Health (NIH): Division Research, 2167
National Institute of Mental Health Information Resources and Inquiries Branch, 727, 875, 985, 985, 1763
National Institute of Mental Health: Schizophrenia Research Branch, 2168
National Institute of Mental Health: Office of Science Policy and Program Planning, 2169
National Institute of Neurological Disorders and Stroke, 624
National Institute on Alcohol Abuse and Alcoholism, 64
National Institute on Drug Abuse Science: Policy and Analysis Division, 2170
National Institute on Drug Abuse: Division of Clinical Research, 2171
National Institutes of Mental Health: Office on AIDS, 2172
National Institutes of Mental Health: Mental Disorders of the Aging, 2173
National Library of Medicine, 2174
National SIDS Foundation, 6
New Hope Foundation, 1771
Office of Applied Studies, SA & Mental Health Services, 2175
Office of Program and Policy Development, 2181
Office of Science Policy, 2182
Oracle Federal, 4963
PATHware, 4969
PSC, 4561
Pathware, 4975
Point of Care Technologies, 4981
Professional Services Consultants, 4583
Protection and Advocacy Program for the Mentally Ill, 2186
PsychReport, 4992
Psycho Medical Chirologists, 4588, 4996
Public Health Service, 5003
SLA Consulting, 4604, 5017
Schizophrenia Research Branch: Division of Clinical and Treatment Research, 1289
Sentient Systems, 5025
Sentinent Systems, 4617
Sheppard Pratt Health Plan, 4619
Sheppard Pratt Health System, 1915
Sidran Traumatic Stress Institute, 1784
Substance Abuse & Mental Health Services Adminstration (SAMHSA), 2188
Substance Abuse and Mental Health Services Administration, 2189
Substance Abuse and Mental Health Services Administration: Homeless Program, 2190

Sudden Infant Death Syndrome Alliance, 7
Survey & Analysis Branch, 1916
Synergestic Consultants, 4641
Taylor Health System, 2758
US Department of Health and Human Services Bureau of Primary Health, 2193
US Department of Public Health: Indian Services, 2195
University of Maryland Medical Systems, 3665
University of Maryland School of Medicine, 3666
VA Medical Center, 3688
Valumed Systems, 5062
Warren Grant Magnuson Clinical Center, 1789

Massachusetts

ABE, 4257
AD-IN: Attention Deficit Information Network, 366
Advocates for Human Potential, 1698
Agilent Technologies, 4692
American Association of General Hospital Psychiatrists, 3515
American Board of Examiners in Clinical Social Work, 2530, 2582
American Society of Psychopathology of Expression (ASPE), 2628
Analysis Group Economics, 4283
Aries Systems Corporation, 4702
Associated Counseling Services, 4288
Association for Academic Psychiatry: AAP, 2631
Autism Research Foundation, 422
Autism Treatment Center of America Sun-Rise Program, 540
B&W Associates Health and Human Services Consultants, 4289
BMC Division of Psychiatry, Boston University, 3521
BROOKS and Associates, 4291
Baystate Medical Center, 3522
Behavioral Healthcare Center, 3523
Behavioral Healthcare Consultants, 4302
Boylston Group, 4305
Brand Software, 4721
Brandeis University/Heller School, 3527
Bull Worldwide Information Systems, 4722
CASCAP, Continuous Quality, 4724
CORE Management, 4317, 4729
CORE/Peer Review Analysis, 4318
Cambridge Hospital: Department of Psychiatry, 3531
Center for Clinical Computing, 4733
Center for Human Development, 4735
Choate Health Management, 4339
Concord-Assabet Family and Adolescent Services, 1917, 4760
Data General, 4771
Dougherty Management Associates, 4378
Enterprise Health Solutions, 4795, 3555
Entropy Limited, 4385
Evaluation Center at HSRI, 4388
Executive Consulting Group, 4389
Federation for Children with Special Needs (FCSN), 1581, 1733
Glazer Medical Solutions, 4407
Greater Lynn Mental Health & Retardation Association, 1919

HCIA Response, 4815
Healthcare Value Management Group, 4435
Hellman Health Strategies, 4441
Human Services Research Institute, 1736, 4455
IBM Global Healthcare Industry, 4844
IDX Systems Corporation, 4845
InStream Corporation, 4848
Information Architects, 4854
Institute for Health Policy, 3572
InterQual, 4873
International Society for Developmental Psychology: ISDP, 2684
Jean Piaget Society: Society for the Study of Knowledge and Development (JPSSSKD), 2688
Jennings Ryan and Kolb, 4478
Jess Wright Communication, 4878
Jewish Family and Children's Services, 1920
Judge Baker Children's Center, 1740
KPMG Peat Marwick, 4485
Kennedy Computing, 4883
Lotus Development Corporation, 4890
MEDA, 951
Magellan Public Solutions, 4511
Massachusetts Alliance for the Mentally Ill, 1921
Massachusetts Behavioral Health Partnership, 1922
Massachusetts Bureau of Substance Abuse Services, 2333
Massachusetts Department of Mental Health, 2334
Massachusetts Department of Public Health, 2335
Massachusetts Department of Public Welfare, 2336
Massachusetts Department of Social Services, 2337
Massachusetts Division of Medical Assistance, 2338
Massachusetts Executive Office of Public Safety, 2339
May Mental Health Service, 4523
Medical Records Institute, 4918
Mediplex, 4921
Mental Health Connections, 4924
Mental Health and Substance Abuse Corporations of Massachusetts, 1923
Mental Illness Education Project, 1747
Mercer, Meidinger and Hansen, 4528
Mertech, 2544
MicroScript, 4932
Mutual Alliance, 4938
NYNEX Information Resources, 4940
National Empowerment Center, 1760, 4542
National Managed Health Care Congress, 2721
National Mental Illness Screening Project, 2723
New England Center for Children, 437
New England Psych Group, 4546
Novartis Institutes for BioMedical Research, 5189
On-Line Psych Services, 4959
Optimed Medical Systems, 4961
Parent Professional Advocacy League, 1924
Porras and Associates, Healthcare Consulting, 4570
PsychSolutions, 4993
Psychemedics Corporation, 4994
Public Consulting Group, 4590
R&L Software Associates, 5008

Refuah, 1781
SADD-Students Against Drunk Drivers, 115
SADD: Students Against Drunk Drivers, 1637
STM Technology: Health Care Company Systems, 5020
Scheur Mangement Group, 4613
Sleep Disorders Unit of Beth Israel Hospital, 1352
Son-Rise Autism Treatment Center of America, 439
Stratus Computer, 5037
Syratech Corporation, 4642
University of Massachusetts Medical Center, 3667
Wang Software, 5067
Webman Associates, 4674
Windhorse Associates, 1791
Women Helping Agoraphobia, 155
Work Group for the Computerization of Behavioral Health, 5070
Worldwide Healthcare Solutions: IBM, 5071

Michigan

Adam Software, 4690
Adult Learning Systems, 4268
Agoraphobics in Motion, 138
Ameen Consulting and Associates, 4277
American College of Osteopathic Neurologists & Psychiatrists, 2589
Ann Arbor Consultation Services Performance & Health Solutions, 1925
Annual AAMA Conference & Convocation, 3236
Association for Behavior Analysis, 2636
Behavioral MAPS, 4716
Borgess Behavioral Medicine Services, 1926, 2532
Boysville of Michigan, 1927
Christian Horizons, 1723
DataMark, 4773
First Corp-Health Consulting, 4395
Harper House: Change Alternative Living, 3566
Health Alliance Plan, 4416
Health Decisions, 4421
Institute for the Study of Children and Families, 4868
JGK Associates, 4475
Justice in Mental Health Organizations, 1928
Lapeer County Community Mental Health Center, 1929
Macomb County Community Mental Health, 1930
Manic Depressive and Depressive Association of Metropolitan Detroit, 1931
Metropolitan Area Chapter of Federation of Families for Children's Mental Health, 1932
Michigan Alliance for the Mentally Ill, 1933
Michigan Association for Children with Emotional Disorders: MACED, 1934
Michigan Association for Children's Mental Health, 1585, 1935
Michigan Department of Community Health: Treatment Policy Section, 2340
Michigan Department of Community Health: System Development and Monitoring, 2341

Michigan Department of Community Health, 2342
Michigan Department of Community Health: Prevention Policy, 2343
Michigan Department of Mental Health, 2344
Michigan Department of Mental Health Bureau of Community Mental Health Services, 2345
Michigan Department of Public Health, 2346
Michigan Department of Social Services, 2347
Michigan Division of Substance Abuse Quality & Planning, 2348
Michigan State Representative: Co-Chair Public Health, 2349
Mississippi Alliance for the Mentally Ill, 1947
National Association to Advance Fat Acceptance (NAAFA), 873
National Council on Alcoholism and Drug Dependence of Michigan, 1382, 2350
Network Medical, 4950
Northpointe Behavioral Healthcare Systems, 1936, 4551, 4954, 4954
Omni Data Sciences, 4958
Parrot Software, 4974
Posen Consulting Group, 4572
Psychiatric Society of Informatics, 2735
Psychological Diagnostic Services, 3621
Rapid Psychler Press, 2743
Research Media, 5013
SIGMA Assessment Systems, 4602
Sandra Fields-Neal and Associates, 4609
Schizophrenics Anonymous Forum, 1293
Society for the Psychological Study of Social Issues (SPPI), 2755
Southwest Counseling & Development Services, 1937
Supported Living Technologies, 5042
SysteMetrics, 5045
Tailored Computers Consultants, 4646
University of Michigan, 3669
University of Psychiatric Center, 3681
Wayne State University School of Medicine, 3690
Woodlands Behavioral Healthcare Network, 1938

Minnesota

Affiliated Counseling Clinic, 3507
Allina Hospitals & Clinics Behavioral Health Services, 4276
American Guidance Service (AGS), 4280
Behavioral Health Services, 4299
Behavioral Health Services - Allina Health, 4300
CIGNA Behavioral Care, 4313
Centre for Mental Health Solutions: Minnesota Bio Brain Association, 1939
Ceridian Corporation, 4736
Changing Your Mind, 3536
Corporate Health Systems, 4360
DISC Systems, 4769
Department of Human Services: Chemical Health Division, 2351
Emotions Anonymous International Service Cen ter, 721
Gerard Treatment Programs, 3565
Health Risk Management (HRM), 4427
HealthPartners, 4429

Healtheast Behavioral Care, 2540
Human Services Assessment, 4840
Informational Medical Systems, 4858
Institute for Healthcare Quality, 4867
MMHR, 4504
McGladery and Pullen CPAs, 4525
Minnesota Association for Children's Mental Health, 1940
Minnesota Department of Human Services, 2352
Minnesota Department of Mental Health and Human Services, 2353
Minnesota National Alliance for the Mentally Ill, 1941
Minnesota Psychiatric Society, 1942
Minnesota Psychological Association, 1943
Minnesota Youth Services Bureau, 2354
NASW Minnesota Chapter, 1944
National Association for Rural Mental Health, 1752
New Standards, 4547, 4951
North American Training Institute: Division of the Minnesota Council on Compulsive Gambling, 1945
Pacer Center, 1946
River City Mental Health Clinic, 3626
United Health Care, 4657
University of Minnesota Health Systems, 3670
University of Minnesota Press Test Division, 3671
University of Minnesota, Family Social Science, 3672
University of Minnesota-Media Distribution, 3673
Velocity Healthcare Informatics, 5064

Mississippi

Advanced Psychotherapy Association, 2555
Department of Rehabilitation Services: Vocational Rehab, 2355
Mississippi Alcohol Safety Education Program, 2356
Mississippi Bureau of Mental Retardation, 2357
Mississippi Department of Human Services, 2358
Mississippi Department of Mental Health: Division of Alcohol and Drug Abuse, 2359
Mississippi Department of Mental Health, 2360
Mississippi Department of Mental Health: Division of Medicaid, 2361
Mississippi Families as Allies, 1948

Missouri

Anorexia Bulimia Treatment and Education Center, 860
Blue Springs Psychological Service, 3526
CliniSphere version 2.0, 4743
College of Health and Human Services: SE Missouri State, 3538
Depressive and Manic-Depressive Association of St. Louis, 1918, 1949
Ferguson Software, 4803
Genelco, 4811
Health Capital Consultants, 4419

New Mexico Behavioral Health Services Division, 2403
New Mexico Children: Youth and Families Department, 2404
New Mexico Department of Health, 2405
New Mexico Department of Human Services, 2406
New Mexico Department of Human Services: Medical Assistance Programs, 2407
New Mexico Health & Environment Department, 2408
Overeaters Anonymous, 954
University of New Mexico, School of Medicine, 3675

New York

AHMAC, 4682
AIMS, 4683
Accumedic Computer Systems, 4688
Ackerman Institute for the Family, 3504
Alcoholics Anonymous (AA): Worldwide, 56, 112
Aldrich and Cox, 4272
Alfred Adler Institute (AAI), 3509
Alliance for the Mentally Ill: Friends & Advocates of the Mentally Ill, 1980
American Anorexia/Bulimia Association, 859
American Behavioral Systems, 4279
American Foundation for Psychoanalysis and Psychoanalysis in Groups: AFPPG, 2593
American Foundation for Suicide Prevention, 1501
American Geriatrics Society, 2594
American Group Psychotherapy Association Annual Conference, 2595, 3231
American Health Management and Consulting, 4695
American Healthware Systems, 4281
American Parkinson's Disease Association, 1029
American Psychoanalytic Association (APsaA), 2613
American Suicide Foundation, 1502
Anxiety and Phobia Treatment Center, 141
Applied Behavioral Technologies, 4701
Association for Advancement of Behavior Therapy, 682
Association for Advancement of Behavioral Therapy, 2632
Association for Advancement of Psychoanalysi s: Karen Horney Psychoanalytic Institute and Center: AAP, 2633
Association for Birth Psychology: ABP, 2637
Association for Psychoanalytic Medicine (APM), 2642
Association for Research in Nervous and Ment al Disease: ARNMD, 2644
Association for the Help of Retarded Children, 1579, 1712
Autism Network International, 421
Autistic Services, 426
Babylon Consultation Center, 1981, 4292
Beechwood Software, 4710
Behavior Graphics Division of Supervised Lifestyles, 4712
Berkshire Farm Center and Services for Youth, 3525
Blackberry Technologies, 4719

Boys Town National Hotline, 1628
Bristol-Myers Squibb, 5179
CG Jung Foundation for Analytical Psychology, 2654
CHPS Consulting, 4312
CLF Consulting, 4315
COMPSYCH Software Information Services, 4728
Capital Behavioral Health Company, 4322
Caregivers Consultation Services, 4323
Center for Family Support (CFS), 2, 60, 143, 143, 267, 427, 568, 619, 684, 715, 836, 863, 981, 1001, 1030, 1054, 1114
Center for the Study of Anorexia and Bulimia, 945
Center for the Study of Issues in Public Mental Health, 1721
Center for the Study of Psychiatry and Psychology, 2656
Children's Home of the Wyoming Conference, Quality Improvement, 4338
Coalition of Voluntary Mental Health Agencies, 1724
Committee for Truth in Psychiatry: CTIP, 2156
Commonwealth Fund, 2662
Community Access, 1725
Compeer, 1982
Corporate Counseling Associates, 2664
Council on Accreditation (COA) of Services for Families and Children, 2537
Council on Size and Weight Discrimination (CSWD), 866
Creative Management Strategies, 4366
Creative Socio-Medics Corporation, 4767
Datamedic, 4774
Downstate Mental Hygiene Association, 3550
Eating Disorder Council of Long Island, 1983
Employee Network, 4384
Facilitated Learning at Syracuse University, 536
Families Together in New York State, 1984
Finger Lakes Parent Network, 1985
Forest Laboratories, 5184
Freedom From Fear, 145, 722
Gam-Anon Family Groups, 1012
HZI Research Center, 4820
Healthcare Association of New York State, 1986
Heartshare Human Services, 3568
Institute for Contemproary Psychotherapy, 1222
Integrated Behavioral Systems, 4468
International Association for the Scientific Study of Intellectual Disabilities, 2680
International Society for Adolescent Psychiatry, 2682
JM Oher and Associates, 4476
Julia Dyckman Andrus Memorial, 3576
Juniper Healthcare Containment Systems, 4482
LMS Consultation Network, 4491
Legend Pharmaceutical, 2689
Liberty Healthcare Management Corporation, 4497
Life Science Associates, 3579
Lifespire, 1583, 1744
MHS, 4895
McGraw Hill Healthcare Management, 4526
Mental Health Association in Albany County, 1987
Mental Health Association in Dutchess County, 1988

Mental Health Materials Center (MHMC), 2697
Metro Intergroup of Overeaters Anonymous, 1989
Multidata Computer Systems, 4937
NADD: Association for Persons with Developmental Disabilities and Mental Health Needs, 147, 272, 434, 434, 572, 621, 685, 723, 839, 870, 983, 1003, 1032, 1056, 1116, 1125, 1169
Nathan S Kline Institute for Psychiatric Research, 1750, 3600
National Alliance for Research on Schizophrenia and Depression, 724, 802, 1241, 1241, 1288
National Association for the Advancement of Psychoanalysis: NAAP, 2701
National Association for the Dually Diagnosed: NADD, 4
National Center for Learning Disabilities, 1756
National Center for Overcoming Overeating, 953
National Center on Addiction and Substance Abuse at Columbia University, 1757
National Foundation for Depressive Illness: NAFDI, 726
National GAINS Center for People with Co-Occurring Disorders in the Justice System, 1761
National Medical Health Card Systems, 4945
National Psychological Association for Psychoanalysis (NPAP), 2727
National Resource Center on Homelessness & Mental Illness, 1768
National Self-Help Clearinghouse Graduate School and University Center, 1769
Network Behavioral Health, 4544, 4949
New York Association of Psychiatric Rehabilitation Services, 1991
New York Business Group on Health, 1992
New York City Depressive & Manic Depressive Group, 730
New York County Department of Social Services, 2409
New York Department of Mental Health, 2410
New York Department of Social Services, 2411
New York Office of Alcohol & Substance Abuse Services, 2412
New York State Alliance for the Mentally Ill, 1993
New York University Behavioral Health Programs, 3603
Newbride Consultation, 4548
NineLine, 1525, 1635
Obesity Research Center, 947
Obsessive Compulsive Anonymous, 1058
Obsessive-Compulsive Anonymous, 1094
Orange County Mental Health Association, 1994
Orion Systems Group, 4965
PMCC, 4559
Parents United Network: Parsons Child Family Center, 1995
Paris International Corporation, 4563
Pass-Group, 219
Patient Infosystems, 4976
Pfizer, 5192
Postgraduate Center for Mental Health, 3613
Prime Care Consultants, 4578
Project LINK, 1996

Psychological Services Index, 2737
Psychology Society (PS), 2738
Radical Caucus in Psychiatry (RCP), 2742
Redtop Company, 5011
Resource Center for Systems Advocacy, 2744
Resources for Children with Special Needs, 1594, 1783
Right On Programs/PRN Medical Software, 5015
Risk and Insurance Management Society, 2745
Rockland Children's Psychiatric Center, 3629
SUNY, 3632
Salud Mangement Associates, 4608
Sanofi-Synthelabo, 5193
Schizophrenic Biologic Research Center, 1290
Schools for Children With Autism Spectrum Disorders: A Directory of Educational Programs in NYC and The Lower Hudson Valley, 438
Sciacca Comprehensive Service Development for MIDAA, 4615
Sciacca Comprehensive Services Development, 2746
Selective Mutism Foundation, 151
Sigmund Freud Archives (SFA), 2747
Special Interest Group on Phobias and Related Anxiety Disorders (SIGPRAD), 152
State University of New York at Stony Brook: Mental Health Research, 1997
Stephens Systems Services, 5034
Success Day Training Program, 3641
Sue Krause and Associates, 4638
Tourette Syndrome Association, 1546, 1562
Towers Perrin Integrated HeatlhSystems Consulting, 4647
Ulster County Mental Health Department, 3652
Univera, 4659
VJT Associates, 4663
Westchester Alliance for the Mentally Ill, 1998
Westchester Task Force on Eating Disorders, 1999
YAI/National Institute for People with Disabilities, 3248
Yeshiva University: Soundview-Throgs Neck Community Mental Health Center, 2000
Young Adult Institute and Workshop (YAI), 1596, 1793
Zy-Doc Technologies, 5073

North Carolina

Companion Technologies, 4748
Counseling Services, 3545
Data Flow Companies, 4770
East Carolina University Department of Psychiatric Medicine, 3551
Elon Homes for Children, 4381
Glaxo-SmithKline, 5185
Habilitation Software, 4821
MEDIC Computer Systems, 4893
Managed Healthcare Consultants, 4516
MicroHealth Corporation, 4931
National Board for Certified Counselors, 2545
National Technology Group, 4947

North Carolina Alliance for the Mentally Ill, 2002
North Carolina Department of Human Resources: Mental Health Developmental Disabilities & Substance Abuse Division, 2413
North Carolina Department of Human Resources, 2414
North Carolina Department of Mental Health, 2415
North Carolina Division of Mental Health: Drug Dependency and Substance Abuse Services, 2416
North Carolina Division of Social Services, 2417
North Carolina Governor's Office of Substance Abuse Policy, 2418
North Carolina Mental Health Consumers Organization, 2003
North Carolina Mental Health Services, 2419
North Carolina Substance Abuse Profession Certification Board, 2420
Onslow County Behavioral Health, 3607
TEACCH, 537
UNI/CARE Systems, 5056
University of North Carolina School of Social Work, Behavioral Healthcare, 4662
University of North Carolina School of Social Work, Behavioral Healthcare, 3676
University of North Carolina, School of Medicine, 3677
Wake Forest University, 3689
Western North Carolina Families CAN (Children and Adolescents Network), 2004

North Dakota

MeritCare Health System, 4926
Meritcare Health System, 4927
National Association of Social Workers: North Dakota Chapter, 1847, 1898, 1914, 1914, 1959, 2001, 2005
North Dakota Federation of Families for Children's Mental Health: Region II, 2006
North Dakota Alliance for the Mentally Ill, 2007
North Dakota Department of Human Services: Medicaid Program, 2421
North Dakota Department of Human Services: Mental Health Services Division, 2422
North Dakota Department of Human Services: Division of Mental Health and Substance Abuse, 2423
North Dakota Department of Mental Health, 2424
North Dakota Federation of Families for Children's Mental Health: Region V, 2008
North Dakota Federation of Families for Children's Mental Health: Region VII, 2009
North Dakota Federation of Families for Children's Mental Health, 2010
South Valley Mental Health Association, 2011

Ohio

Alliance Behavioral Care, 4274

Alliance Behavioral Care: University of Cincinnati Psychiatric Services, 3511
Aware Resources, 4708
Bellefaire Jewish Children's Bureau, 4717
Brown and Associates, 4308
CMHC Systems, 4727
Central Behavioral Healthcare, 4333
ChoiceCare, 4341
Cincom Systems, 4739
Clermont Counseling Center, 4741
Client Management Information System, 4742
Compass Information Services, 4350
Comprehensive Review Technology, 4749
Comprehensives Services, 4353
Concerned Advocates Serving Children & Families, 2012
Crystal Clinic, 4368
DocuMed, 4783
Findley, Davies and Company, 4393
Geauga Board of Mental Health, Alcohol and Drug Addiction Services, 4406
Great Lakes Medical Computer Clinic, 4812
Human Affairs International: Ohio, 4449
Innovative Data Solutions, 4864
Innovative Systems Development, 4866
Integrated Business Services, 4870
Lan Vision, 4886
Laurelwood Hospital and Counseling Centers, 3578
Managed Care Software, 4900
Marsh Foundation, 3587
MedPLus Relations, 4906
Medical College of Ohio, Psychiatry, 3590
Medical Documenting Systems, 4912
Mental Health Association of Summit, 2013
Micro-Office Systems, 4930
Mount Carmel Behavioral Healthcare, 2014
NE Ohio Universities College of Medicine, 3599
National Anorexic Aid Society, 952
National Association of Social Workers: Ohio Chapter, 2015
Ohio Alliance for the Mentally Ill, 2016
Ohio Association of Child Caring Agencies, 2017
Ohio Community Drug Board, 2425
Ohio Council of Behavioral Healthcare Providers, 2018
Ohio Department of Mental Health, 2019, 2426
Parents of Murdered Children, 23
Penelope Price, 3610
Planned Lifetime Assistance Network of Northeast Ohio, 2020
Positive Education Program, 2021
PsychTemps, 3617
Psychology Department, 3622
QualChoice Health Plan, 4593
RCF Information Systems, 5009
Rosemont Center, 3630
SAFY of America, 3631
SAFY of America: Specialized Alternatives for Families and Youth, 2547
Self Management and Recovery Training, 116, 1464
Six County, 2022
Specialized Alternatives for Families & Youth of America (SAFY), 4625
Stresscare Behavioral Health, 4636
University of Cincinnati College of Medical Department of Psychiatry, 3657
Woodlands, 5069

Oklahoma

Child & Adolescent Network, 2023
Hogan Assessment Systems, 4838
Med Assist, 4902
Medical Group Management Association: Assemblies & Society, 2695
Oklahoma Alliance for the Mentally Ill, 2024
Oklahoma Department of Human Services, 2427
Oklahoma Department of Mental Health and Substance Abuse Service, 2428
Oklahoma Healthcare Authority, 2429
Oklahoma Mental Health Consumer Council, 2025, 4555
Oklahoma Office of Juvenile Affairs, 2430
Oklahoma Psychiatric Physicians Association, 2026
Oklahoma's Mental Health Consumer Council, 2431
Professional Software Solutions, 4988
St. Anthony Behavioral Medicine Center, Behavioral Medicine, 4629
Utica Psychiatric Service, 3687

Oregon

Anorexia Nervosa & Related Eating Disorders, 2027
Anorexia Nervosa and Related Eating Disorders, 862
Beaver Creek Software, 4709
Behavior Therapy Software, 4713
Center for the Study of Autism (CSA), 429
Deborah MacWilliams, 1221
East Oregon Human Services Consortium, 4787
Healthwise, 4438
Interlink Health Services, 4472
Marion County Health Department, 2432
Medipay, 4920
Mental Health and Developmental Disability Division: Department of Human Services, 2433
Multnomah Co. Behavioral Health, 4538
Nickerson Center, 3604
Northwest Analytical, 4955
Office of Mental Health and Addiction Services Training & Resource Center, 2434
Oregon Alliance for the Mentally Ill, 2028
Oregon Commission on Children and Families, 2435
Oregon Department of Human Resources: Medical Assistance Program, 2436
Oregon Department of Human Resources: Health Service Section, 2437
Oregon Department of Mental Health, 2438
Oregon Family Support Network, 2029
Oregon Health Plan Unit, 2439
Oregon Psychiatric Association, 2030
PC Consulting Group, 4970
People First of Oregon, 1775
Providence Behavioral Health Connections, 4584
Regional Research Institute for Human Services of Portland University, 3624
Research and Training Center on Family Support and Children's Mental Health, 1593, 1782

Riverside Center, 3628
SRC Software, 5019
Softouch Software, 5028
Therapists Genie, 5053

Pennsylvania

100 Top Series, 4256
ACORN Behavioral Care Management Corporation, 4258
APOGEE, 4261
Access Behavioral Care, 4263
Acorn Behavioral Healthcare Management Corporation, 4265
Allegheny Behavioral Health Services, 3510
American College of Mental Health Administration: ACMHA, 2588
American Psychology- Law Society (AP-LS), 2619
Association for Hospital Medical Education, 2639
CIGNA Corporation, 4314
Center For Prevention And Rehabilitation, 4327
Cephalon, 5180
Chi Systems, 4337
Communications Media, 4745
Consumer Satisfaction Team, 2536
Counseling Program of Pennsylvania Hospital, 3544
Craig Academy, 4365
DB Consultants, 4768
Dauphin County Drug and Alcohol, 2440
Deloitte and Touche LLP Management Consulting, 4375
Delta Health Systems, 4777
DeltaMetrics, 4376, 4778
DeltraMetrics Treatment Research Institute, 4779
Distance Learning Network, 4781, 3549
GMR Group, 4402
Hay/Huggins Company: Philadelphia, 4415
Health Federation of Philadelphia, 2031
Health Net Services, 4425
Healthcare America, 4430
Human Affairs International, 4447
Human Affairs International: Pennsylvania, 4450
InfoMC, 4850
InfoWorld Management Systems, 4852
Integra, 4869
International Society of Psychiatric-Mental Health Nurses, 1739
International Technology Corporation, 4473
JS Medical Group, 4477
Jefferson Drug/Alcohol, 3574
Kid Save, 1633
Learning Disability Association of America, 271, 1742
MCF Consulting, 4501
MEDecision, 4894
MS Hershey Medical Center, 3585
Mayes Group, 4524
Medical College of Pennsylvania, 3591
Mental Health Association of South East Pennsylvania, 2032
Mental Health Consultants, 3254
Montgomery County Project SHARE, 2033, 4935
National Association of Addiction Treatment Providers, 2703

National Association of Therapeutic Wilderness Camps, 1755
National Attention Deficit Disorder Association, 274
National Healthcare Solutions, 4543
National Mental Health Consumer's Self-Help Clearinghouse, 65, 150, 276, 276, 436, 1224
National Mental Health Consumer's Self-Help Clearinghouse, 5, 574, 625, 625, 686, 728, 840, 876, 986, 1004, 1033, 1057, 1117, 1127, 1171, 1244, 1323
National Mental Health Self-Help Clearinghouse, 4946
National Psychiatric Alliance, 2726
National Summit of Mental Health Consumers and Survivors, 3244
North American Society of Adlerian Psychology (NASAP), 2731
Open Minds, 4556
Parents Involved Network, 2034
Pennsylvania Alliance for the Mentally Ill, 2035
Pennsylvania Bureau of Community Program Standards, 2441
Pennsylvania Chapter of the American Anorexia Bulimia Association, 2036
Pennsylvania Department of Health: Office of Drug and Alcohol Programs, 2442
Pennsylvania Department of Mental Health, 2443
Pennsylvania Department of Public Welfare, 2444
Pennsylvania Department of Public Welfare: Office of Mental Health, 2445
Pennsylvania Deputy Secretary for Public Health Programs, 2446
Pennsylvania Division of Drug and Alcohol Training: Information, 2447
Pennsylvania Division of Drug and Alcohol Program: Monitoring, 2448
Pennsylvania Division of Drug and Alcohol Prevention: Intervention and Treatment, 2449
Pennsylvania Medical Assistance Programs, 2450
Pennsylvania Society for Services to Children, 2037
Persoma Management, 4564
Philadelphia Health Management, 4566
Philadelphia Mental Health Care Corporation, 4567
Pittsburgh Health Research Institute, 3612
Practice Integration Team, 4573
Pressley Ridge Schools, 3614
ProMetrics, 4986
ProMetrics CAREeval, 4580
ProMetrics Consulting & Susquehanna PathFinders, 4581
Psych-Med Association, St. Francis Medical, 3616
Risk Management Group, 4600
SHS Computer Services, 5016
Schafer Consulting, 4612
Society for the Advancement of the Field Theory (SAFT), 2754
Southwestern Pennsylvania Alliance for the Mentally Ill, 2038
St. Francis Medical Center, 3637
Suburban Psychiatric Associates, 4637
Systems Advocacy, 1785
T Kendall Smith, 4644
US Healthcare, 4651

Datasys/DSI, 4776
Depression and Bipolar Support Alliance of
    Houston and Harris County, 2070
Education Research Laboratories, 3552
Eye Movement Desensitization and
    Reprocessing International Association
    (EMDRIA), 1729
Fox Counseling Service, 2071
Group for the Advancement of Psychiatry:
    GAP, 2674
HMS Software, 4818
Harris County Mental Health: Mental
    Retardation Authority, 2483
Healthcare Vision, 4834
Horizon Behavioral Services, 4442
Horizon Mental Health Management, 4444
INTEGRA, 4460
Inroads Behavioral Health Services, 4463
Interface EAP, 4469
Jewish Family Service of America, 4880
Jewish Family Service of San Antonio, 2073
Juliette Fowler Homes, 4881
Medical Group Systems, 4914
Menninger Care Systems, 4527
Menninger Clinic, 1745
Mental Health Association, 2074
Mental Health Outcomes, 4925
Meridian Resource Corporation, 4529
Mothers Against Drunk Drivers, 113
OPTAIO-Optimizing Practice Through
    Assessment, Intervention and Outcome,
    4956
OPTIONS Health Care-Texas, 4554
PRIMA A D D, 3608
Parent Connection, 2075
Patient Medical Records, 4977
Perot Systems, 4978
Perot Systems Corporation, 4979
ProAmerica Managed Care, 4579
Psychological Associates-Texas, 3619
Psychological Corporation, 4998
Psychonomic Society, 2741
Reclamation, 1779
SUMMIT Behavioral Partners, 4606
Sid W Richardson Institute for Preventive
    Medicine of the Methodist Hospital, 803
Specialty Healthcare Management, 4627
Sweetwater Health Enterprises, 5043, 2551
TEI Computers, 5049
Tarrant County Mental Health: Mental
    Retardation Services, 2484
Texas Alliance for the Mentally Ill, 2076
Texas Commission on Alcohol and Drug
    Abuse, 2485
Texas Counseling Association, 2077
Texas Department of Human Services, 2486
Texas Department of Mental Health:
    Retardation, 2487
Texas Department of Protective Services,
    2488
Texas Federation of Families for Children's
    Mental Health, 2078
Texas Health and Human Services
    Commission, 2489
Texas Psychological Association, 2079
Texas Society of Psychiatric Physicians, 2080
Texas Tech Health Sciences
    Center-Department of Corrections,
    Education Resources, 3642
UNI/CARE: National Resource Consultants,
    5057
University of Texas Medical Branch
    Managed Care, 3683

University of Texas Southwestern Medical
    Center, 2081
University of Texas, Southwestern Medical
    Center, 3684
University of Texas-Houston Health Science
    Center, 3685
University of Texas: Mental Health Clinical
    Research Center, 805
Value Health Management, 5061
WellPoint Behavioral Health, 4676

Utah

Allies for Youth & Families, 2082
CompHealth Credentialing, 2535
Copper Hills Youth Center, 3542
DMDA Southern Utah and Nevada, 2083
Healthwise of Utah, 2084
Human Affairs International, 4446
Human Affairs International: Utah, 4451
IHC Behavioral Health Network, 4458
Ramsay Health Care, 4597
University of Utah Neuropsychiatric, 3686
Utah Alliance for the Mentally Ill, 2085
Utah Commission on Criminal Justice, 2490
Utah Department of Health, 2491
Utah Department of Health: Health Care
    Financing, 2492
Utah Department of Mental Health, 2493
Utah Department of Social Services, 2494
Utah Division of Substance Abuse, 2495
Utah Health Care Financing Administration,
    2496
Utah Parent Center, 2086
Utah Psychiatric Association, 2087

Vermont

Brattleboro Retreat, 2088
Fletcher Allen Health Care, 2089, 3561
Spruce Mountain Inn, 2090
Vermont Alliance for the Mentally Ill, 2091
Vermont Department of Developmental and
    Mental Health Services, 2497
Vermont Department of Social Welfare:
    Medicaid Division, 2498
Vermont Employers Health Alliance, 2092
Vermont Federation of Families for
    Children's Mental Health, 2093
Vermont Office of Alchol and Drug Abuse
    Programs, 2499

Virginia

APA-Endorsed Psychiatrists Professional
    Liability Insurance Program, 2553
Accountable Oncology Associates, 4264
Agoraphobics Building Independent Lives,
    217
Al-Anon Family Group Headquarters, 109
Al-Anon Family Group National Referral
    Hotline, 110
Alateen, 1455
Alateen and Al-Anon Family Groups, 111,
    1627
AmeriChoice, 4278

American Association for Marriage and
    Family Therapy, 2565
American Association of Health Care
    Consultants Annual Fall Conference, 3226
American Association of Pastoral
    Counselors, 2578
American Association of Pharmaceutical
    Scientists, 2579
American College of Health Care
    Administrators: ACHCA Annual Meeting,
    2586, 3228
American Council on Alcoholism, 57
American Counseling Association, 2592
American Medical Group Association, 2603
American Mental Health Counselors
    Association: AMHCA, 2605
American Network of Community Options
    and Resources (ANCOR), 1707
American Psychiatric Association, 1709
American Psychiatric Association: APA,
    2610
American Psychiatric Nurses Association,
    2611
American Psychiatric Press Reference
    Library CD-ROM, 4698
American Psychiatric Publishing, 2612
American Psychosomatic Society, 2620
American Psychosomatic Society Annual
    Meetin g, 2621
American Society for Clinical Pharmacology
    & Therapeutics, 2623
American Society of Consultant Pharmacists,
    2624
Association for Ambulatory Behavioral
    Healthcare: Training Conference, 2634,
    3238
Center for State Policy Research, 4330
Children and Adolescents with Emotional
    and Behavioral Disorders, 3537
Clinical Social Work Federation, 2660
Colonial Services Board, 3540
Community Anti-Drug Coalitions of
    America: CADCA, 2663
Council for Learning Disabilities, 1727
Council on Social Work Education, 2538,
    2666
Employee Assistance Professionals
    Association, 4382, 2668
Essentials of Clinical Psychiatry: Based on
    the American Psychiatric Press Textbook
    of Psychiatry, 3556
Essentials of Consultation-Liaison
    Psychiatry: Based on the American
    Psychiatric Press Textbook of
    Consultation-Liaison Psychiatry, 3557
Family-to-Family: National Alliance for the
    Mentally Ill, 1291
Federation of Families for Children's
    Mental Health, 1582, 1734
First Hospital Corporation, 2094
Garnett Day Treatment Center, 2095
Hay Group:Washington, DC, 4414
Institute on Psychiatric Services: American
    Psychiatric Association, 2678
Lewin Group, 4496
MHM Services, 3252
Managed Networks of America, 4517
Medical College of Virginia, 3592
Minimize & Manage Risk, 4536
NAMI, 2096
NAMI Convention, 3242
National Academy of Certified Clinical
    Mental Health Counselors, 2698

National Alliance for the Mentally Ill, 148, 273, 435, 435, 573, 725, 871, 1126, 1170, 1242, 1350, 1379, 1505, 1544, 1751
National Association of Alcholism and Drug Abuse Counselors, 3601
National Association of Alcohol and Drug Abuse Counselors, 62
National Association of State Mental Health Program Directors (NASMHPD), 2710
National Association of State Mental Health Program Directors, 1754, 2711
National Mental Health Association, 1243, 1462, 1764, 1764, 2722
National Niemann-Pick Disease Foundation, 626
National Nurses Association, 2724
National Pharmaceutical Council, 2725
National Rehabilitation Association, 1767
Newport News Support Group, 2097
Options Health Care, 4558
Parent Resource Center, 2098
Parents & Children Coping Together: PACCT, 2099
Parents & Children Coping Together: Roanoke Valley, 2100
Parents Information Network, 1774
Parents Information Network FFCMH, 1590
Parents and Children Coping Together, 2101
Pharmaceutical Care Management Association, 2732
Piedmont Behavioral Health Center, 2102
QuadraMed Corporation, 5005, 3623
Richmond Support Group, 2103
SOLOS-Survivors of Loved Ones' Suicides, 26
Society for Personality Assessment: SPA, 2750
Society of Multivarative Experimental Psychology (SMEP), 2756
Survivors of Loved Ones' Suicides (SOLOS), 1526
TASS, 5047
Tasmin NAMI Affiliates Program, 5051
Trigon BC/BS of Virginia, 2104
ValueOptions, 4665
Virginia Alliance for the Mentally Ill, 2105
Virginia Beach Community Service Board, 2106, 4672
Virginia Department of Medical Assistance Services, 2500
Virginia Department of Mental Health, 2501
Virginia Department of Mental Health, Mental Retardation and Substance Abuse Services, 2502
Virginia Department of Social Services, 2503
Virginia Federation of Families for Children's Mental Health, 2107
Virginina Office of the Secretary of Human Resources, 2504
World Federation for Mental Health, 1792

Washington

Association for Women in Psychology: AWP, 2645
Bellevue Alliance for the Mentally Ill, 2108
CARE Computer Systems, 4723
Carewise, 4324
Children's Alliance, 1891, 2109
Common Voice for Pierce County Parents, 2110

Community Sector Systems PsychAccess Chart, 4746
Developmental Disabilities Nurses Association, 2667
Eating Disorders Awareness and Prevention, 867
Family Support Group Alliance for the Mentally Ill, 2111
Good Sam-W/Alliance for the Mentally Ill Family Support Group, 2112
Gray's Harbour Alliance for the Mentally Ill, 2113
Healthcare in Partnership, LLC, 4436
Integrated Behavioral Healthcare, 4467
King County Federation of Families for Children's Mental Health, 2114
Kitsap County Alliance for the Mentally Ill, 2115
Lanstat Incorporated, 2542
Lanstat Resources, 4494
Living Center, 3580
Managed Care Washington, 2116
National Eating Disorders Association, 874
NetMeeting, 4948
North Sound Regional Alliance for the Mentally Ill, 2117
North Sound Regional Support Network, 2118
Nueva Esperanza Counseling Center, 2119
Occupational Health Software Systems, 4957
Pierce County Alliance for the Mentally Ill, 2120
Seattle University District Alliance for the Mentally Ill, 2121
Sharing & Caring for Consumers, Families Alliance for the Mentally Ill, 2122
South King County Alliance for the Mentally Ill, 2123
Southwest Alliance for the Mentally Ill, 2124
Spanish Support Group Alliance for the Mentally Ill, 2125
Spokane Mental Health, 2126
St. Joseph Hospital: Health Promotion Network, 4632
Tardive Dyskinesia: Tardive Dystonia National Association, 1035
Trego Systems, 5054
Washington Alliance for the Mentally Ill, 2127
Washington Department of Alcohol and Substance Abuse: Department of Social and Health Service, 2505
Washington Department of Mental Health, 2506
Washington Department of Social & Health Services, 2507
Washington Department of Social and Health Services: Mental Health Division, 2508
Washington Institute for Mental Illness Research and Training, 1790
Washington State Psychological Association, 2128
Well Mind Association, 2760
Western State Hospital Alliance for the Mentally Ill, 2129
Whidbey Island Alliance for the Mentally Ill, 2130

West Virginia

Autism Services Center, 424, 538

Behavioral Health Management Group, 4296
Mountain State Parents Children Adolescent Network, 2131
Process Strategies Institute, 4582
West Virginia Alliance for the Mentally Ill, 2132
West Virginia Department of Health, 2509
West Virginia Department of Health & Human Resources, 2510
West Virginia Department of Mental Health and Human Services, 2511
West Virginia Department of Welfare, 2512
West Virginia Governor's Commission on Crime, 2513
West Virginia Office of Behavioral Health Services, 2514
West Virginia University Department Family Medicine, 2133

Wisconsin

Alliance for Children and Families, 2558
American Foundation of Counseling, 3518
Bethesda Lutheran Homes and Services, 1716
Bipolar Disorders Treatment Information Center, 566
CNR Health, 4316
Charter BHS of Wisconsin/Brown Deer, 2134
Child and Adolescent Psychopharmacology Information, 2135
Dane County Mental Health Center, 2515
Department of Health and Social Service: Southern Region, 2516
Employer Health Care Alliance Cooperative, 2670
First Things First, 4396
Information Centers for Lithium, Bipolar Disorders Treatment & Obsessive Compulsive Disorder, 1737
Lithium Information Center, 571
MCW Department of Psychiatry and Behavioral Medicine, 4503, 3583
Medical College of Wisconsin, 3593
Micro Psych Software: Medical Management Software Corporation, 4929
Obsessive Compulsive Information Center, 1060
Society for Behavioral Medicine, 2748
Stoughton Family Counseling, 2136
TOPS Club, 878
University of Wisconsin Center for Health Policy and Program Evaluation, 2517
We Are the Children's Hope, 2137
Wisconsin Alliance for the Mentally Ill, 2138
Wisconsin Association of Family and Child Agency, 2139
Wisconsin Bureau of Community Mental Health, 2518
Wisconsin Bureau of Health Care Financing, 2519
Wisconsin Bureau of Substance Abuse Services, 2520
Wisconsin Department of Health and Family Services, 2521
Wisconsin Department of Mental Health, 2522
Wisconsin Division of Community Services, 2523
Wisconsin Family Ties, 2140

Wyoming

ADHD

Adjustment Disorders

Alcohol Abuse & Dependence

Anxiety Disorders

It's Not All In Your Head: Now Women Can Discover the Real
Causes of their Most Misdiagnosed Health Problems, 183
  adaa.org
Journal of Anxiety Disorders , 209
  elsevier.nl/locate/janxdis
Let's Talk Facts About Anxiety Disorders , 210
  appi.org
Let's Talk Facts About Panic Disorder , 211
  appi.org
Master Your Panic and Take Back Your Life , 184
  adaa.org
Master Your Panic and Take Back Your Life: Twelve Treatment
Sessions to Overcome High Anxiety, 185
  impactpublishers.com
NADD: Association for Persons with Developmental Disabilities
and Mental Health Needs, 147
  thenadd.org
National Alliance for the Mentally Ill , 148
  nami.org
National Anxiety Foundation , 149
  lexington-on-line.com/naf.html
National Mental Health Consumer's Self-Help Clearinghouse, 150
  mhselfhelp.org
No More Butterflies: Overcoming Shyness, Stagefright, Interview
Anxiety, and Fear of Public Speaking, 186
  newharbinger.com
Panic Attacks , 212
  etr.org
Panic Disorder and Agoraphobia: A Guide , 187
  miminc.org
Panic Disorder: Critical Analysis , 188
  guilford.com
Perfectionism: What's Bad About Being Too Good, 189
  freespirit.com
Real Illness: Generalized Anxiety Disorder , 213
  nimh.nih.gov
Real Illness: Panic Disorder , 214
  nimh.nih.gov
Real Illness: Social Phobia Disorder , 215
  nimh.nih.gov
Recovery , 221
  recovery-inc.com
Relaxation & Stress Reduction Workbook , 190
  newharbingcr.com
Selective Mutism Foundation , 151
  selectivemutismfoundation.org
Self-Esteem Revolutions in Children: Understanding and
Managing the Critical Transition in Your Child's Life, 191
  addwarehouse.com
Shopping in a Supermarket , 232
  newharbinger.com
Social Anxiety Disorder: A Guide , 192
  miminc.org
Social Phobia: From Shyness to Stage Fright , 193
  adaa.org
Special Interest Group on Phobias and Related Anxiety Disorders
(SIGPRAD), 152
  cyberpsych.org
Stop Obsessing: How to Overcome Your Obsessions and
Compulsions, 194
  adaa.org
Stress , 216
  etr.org
Stress and Mental Health: Contemporary Issues and Prospects for
the Future, 195
  kluweronline.com
Stress-Related Disorders Sourcebook , 196
  omnigraphics.com
Suncoast Residential Training Center/Developmental Services
Program, 153
  goodwill-suncoast.org
Textbook of Anxiety Disorders , 197
  appi.org

Treatment Plans and Interventions for Depression and Anxiety
Disorders, 198
  guilford.com
Trichotillomania: A Guide , 201
  miminc.org
Triumph Over Fear: a Book of Help and Hope for People with
Anxiety, Panic Attacks, and Phobias, 199
  adaa.org
Worry Control Workbook , 200
  newharbinger.com

Associations & Organizations

AAMR: American Association on Mental Retardation, 1697
  aamr.org
Adolescent and Family Institute of Colorado , 1832
  aficonline.com
Alaska Alliance for the Mentally Ill , 1801
  nami-alaska.org
Alaska Mental Health Association , 1802
  alaska.net/~mhaa
Aleppos Foundation , 1699
  aleppos.org
Allendale Association , 1866
  allendale4kids.org
Alliance for the Mentally Ill: Friends & Advocates of the Mentally
Ill, 1980
  nami-nyc-metro.org
Alliance of Genetic Support Groups , 1700
  geneticalliance.org
American Academy of Child and Adolescent Psychiatry, 1701
  aacap.org
American Academy of Pediatrics , 1702
  aap.org
American Association for Geriatric Psychiatry, 1703
  aagpgpa.org
American Holistic Health Association , 1705
  ahha.org
American Managed Behavioral Healthcare Association, 1706
  ambha.org
American Network of Community Options and Resources
(ANCOR), 1707
  ancor.org
American Pediatrics Society , 1708
  aps-spr.org
American Psychiatric Association , 1709
  psych.org
American Psychological Association , 1710
  apa.org
Anorexia Nervosa & Related Eating Disorders , 2027
  anred.com
Arizona Alliance for the Mentally Ill , 1803
  az.nami.org
Arkansas Alliance for the Mentally Ill , 1812
  nami.org
Assistance League of Southern California , 1813
  assistanceleague.net
Association for Children of New Jersey , 1969
  acnj.org
Association for the Help of Retarded Children, 1712
  ahrcnyc.org
Association of Mental Health Librarians (AMHL), 1713
  fmhi.usf.edu/amhl
Babylon Consultation Center , 1981
  kindesigns.com
Bazelon Center for Mental Health Law , 1714
  bazelon.org
Bellevue Alliance for the Mentally Ill , 2108
  nami.org
Best Buddies International (BBI) , 1715
  bestbuddies.org

Florida Federation of Families for Children' s Mental Health, 1853
  fifionline.org
Florida Health Care Association , 1854
  fhca.org
Florida National Alliance for the Mentally Ill, 1855
  namifl.org
Georgia Association of Homes and Services for Children, 1858
  gahsc.org
Georgia National Alliance for the Mentally Ill, 1859
  nami.org
Georgia Parent Support Network , 1860
  gspn.org
Gold Coast Alliance for the Mentally Ill , 1824
  nami.org
Good Sam-W/Alliance for the Mentally Ill Family Support Group, 2112
  nami.org
Gray's Harbour Alliance for the Mentally Ill , 2113
  nami.org
Greater Lynn Mental Health & Retardation Association, 1919
  glmh.org
Hawaii Alliance for the Mentally Ill , 1862
  nami.org
Hawaii Families As Allies , 1863
  mentalhealth.org
Healing for Survivors , 1735
  hfshope.org
Health Resources and Services Administration , 1909
  hrsa.gov
Health Services Agency: Mental Health , 1825
  santacruzhealth.org
Healthcare Association of New York State , 1986
  hanys.org
Horizons School , 1798
  horizonsschool.org
Human Resources Development Institute , 1873
  hrdi.org
Human Services Research Institute , 1736
  hsri.org
Huron Alliance for the Mentally Ill , 2059
  sd.nami.org
Idaho Alliance for the Mentally Ill , 1865
  nami.org
Illinois Alcoholism and Drug Dependency Association, 1874
  iadda.org
Illinois Alliance for the Mentally Ill , 1875
  il.namil.org
Illinois Federation of Families for Children's Mental Health, 1876
  iffcmh.ner/contact.htm
Indiana Alliance for the Mentally Ill , 1881
  nami.org
Information Centers for Lithium, Bipolar Disorders Treatment & Obsessive Compulsive Disorder, 1737
  miminc.org
Institute of Living Anxiety Disorders Center, 1738
  instituteofliving.org/ADC
Institute of Psychiatry and Human Behavior: University of Maryland, 1910
  medschool.umaryland.edu
International Society of Psychiatric-Mental Health Nurses, 1739
  ispn-psych.org
Iowa Alliance for the Mentally Ill , 1885
  nami.org
Iowa Federation of Families for Children's Mental Health, 1886
  ffcmh.org/local.htm
Jewish Family Service of Atlantic County and Cape, 1971
  jfsatlantic.org
Judge Baker Children's Center , 1740
  jbcc.harvard.edu
KY-SPIN , 1894
  kyspin.com
Kansas Alliance for the Mentally Ill , 1888
  nami.org

Kent County Alliance for the Mentally Ill , 2043
  nami.org
Kentucky Alliance for the Mentally Ill , 1895
  nami.org
Kentucky IMPACT , 1896
  mhmr.chs.ky.gov
Kentucky Psychiatric Association , 1897
  icypsych.org
Keys for Networking: Federation Families for Children's Mental Health, 1890
  keys.org
King County Federation of Families for Children's Mental Health, 2114
  ffcmh.org/local.htm
Kitsap County Alliance for the Mentally Ill , 2115
  nami.org
Lapeer County Community Mental Health Center , 1929
  countylapeer.org
Larkin Center , 1877
  larkincenter.org
Learning Disability Association of America , 1742
  ldanatl.org
Life Development Institute , 1743
  life-development-inst.org
Lifespire , 1744
  lifespire.com
Little City Foundation (LCF) , 1878
  LittleCity.org
Louisiana Alliance for the Mentally Ill , 1901
  la.nami.org
Louisiana Federation of Families for Children's Mental Health, 1902
  laffcmh.com
Maine Alliance for the Mentally Ill , 1904
  me.nami.org
Manic Depressive and Depressive Association of Metropolitan Detroit, 1931
  mdda-metro-detroit.org
Maryland Alliance for the Mentally Ill , 1911
  nami.org
Maryland Psychiatric Research Center , 1912
  mprc.umaryland.edu
Massachusetts Alliance for the Mentally Ill , 1921
  namimass.org
Menninger Clinic , 1745
  menninger.edu
Mental Health Association in Dutchess County, 1988
  mhadc.com
Mental Health Association in Marion County Consumer Services, 1883
  mcmha.org
Mental Health Association of Arizona , 1807
  mhaaz.com
Mental Health Association of Colorado , 1837
  mhacolorado.org
Mental Health Association of Delaware , 1846
  mhinde.org
Mental Health Association of Greater St. Louis, 1950
  mhagstl.org
Mental Health Association of Maryland , 1913
  mhamd.org
Mental Health Association of Montana , 1955
  mhamontana.org
Mental Health Association of New Jersey , 1972
  naminj.org
Mental Health Association of South East Pennsylvania, 2032
  mhasp.org
Mental Health Association of Summit , 2013
  mentalhealthassociationofsummitcounty.org
Mental Health Association: Connecticut , 1841
  mhct.org
Mental Health Board of North Central Alabama , 1799
  mhcnca.org

Mental Health Center of North Central Alabama, 1800
mhcnca.org

Mental Health and Aging Network (MHAN) of the American Society on Aging (ASA), 1746
asaging.org

Mental Illness Education Project , 1747
miepvideos.org

Mentally Ill Kids in Distress , 1748
mikid.org

Metropolitan Area Chapter of Federation of Families for Children's Mental Health, 1932
ffcmh.org/local.htm

Metropolitan Family Services , 1879
metrofamily.org

Michigan Alliance for the Mentally Ill , 1933
mi.nami.org

Michigan Association for Children with Emotional Disorders: MACED, 1934
michkids.org

Michigan Association for Children's Mental Health, 1935
ffcmh.org

Minnesota Association for Children's Mental Health, 1940
macmh.org

Minnesota National Alliance for the Mentally Ill, 1941
nami.org/namimn

Minnesota Psychiatric Society , 1942
mnpsychoc.org

Minnesota Psychological Association , 1943
mnpsych.org

Mississippi Alliance for the Mentally Ill , 1947
nami.org

Mississippi Families as Allies , 1948
cecp.air.org

Missouri Institute of Mental Health , 1952
mimh.edu

Missouri Statewide Parent Advisory Network: MO-SPAN, 1953
mo.span.org

Monadnock Family Services , 1966
mfs.org

Montana Alliance for the Mentally Ill , 1956
mt.nami.org

Mount Carmel Behavioral Healthcare , 2014
mcbh.com

Mountain State Parents Children Adolescent Network, 2131
mspcan.org

NADD: Association for Persons with Developmental Disabilities and Mental Health Needs, 1749
thenadd.org

NAMI , 2096
nami.org

NASW Minnesota Chapter , 1944
naswmn.org

Nathan S Kline Institute for Psychiatric Research, 1750
rfmh.org/nki

National Alliance for the Mentally Ill , 1751
nami.org

National Association for Rural Mental Health , 1752
narmh.org

National Association for the Mentally Ill of New Jersey, 1973
naminj.org

National Association of Mental Illness: California, 1826
namicalifornia.org

National Association of Protection and Advocacy Systems, 1753
protectionandadvocacy.com

National Association of Social Workers Florida Chapter, 1857
naswfl.org

National Association of Social Workers New York State Chapter, 1990
naswnys.org

National Association of Social Workers: Delaware Chapter, 1847
naswdc.org

National Association of Social Workers: Kentucky Chapter, 1898
naswky.org

National Association of Social Workers: Maryland Chapter, 1914
nasw-md.org

National Association of Social Workers: Nebraska Chapter, 1959
naswne.org

National Association of Social Workers: North Carolina Chapter, 2001
naswnc.org

National Association of Social Workers: Ohio Chapter, 2015
naswoh.org

National Association of State Mental Health Program Directors, 1754
nasmhpd.org

National Association of Therapeutic Wilderness Camps, 1755
natwc.org

National Center for Learning Disabilities , 1756
CD.org

National Center on Addiction and Substance Abuse at Columbia University, 1757
casacolumbia.org

National Child Support Network , 1758
childsupport.org

National Council for Community Behavioral Healthcare, 1759
nccbh.org

National Empowerment Center , 1760
power2u.org

National GAINS Center for People with Co-Occurring Disorders in the Justice System, 1761
gainsctr.com

National Health Foundation , 1827
hasc.org

National Institute of Drug Abuse: NIDA , 1762
nida.nih.gov

National Institute of Mental Health Information Resources and Inquiries Branch, 1763
nimh.nih.gov

National Mental Health Association , 1764
nmha.org

National Mental Health Consumer's Self-Help Clearinghouse, 1765
mhselfhelp.org

National Organization on Disability , 1766
nod.org

National Rehabilitation Association , 1767
nationalrehab.org

National Resource Center on Homelessness & Mental Illness, 1768
nrchmi.samsa.gov

National Self-Help Clearinghouse Graduate School and University Center, 1769
selfhelpweb.org

National Technical Assistance Center for Children's Mental Health, 1770
dml.georgetown.edu/research/gucdc/cassp.html

Nebraska Alliance for the Mentally Ill , 1960
ne.nami.org

Nevada Alliance for the Mentally Ill , 1964
nami-nevada.org

Nevada Principals' Executive Program , 1965
nvpep.org

New Avenues Alliance for the Mentally Ill , 2044
nami.org

New Hampshire Alliance for the Mentally Ill , 1967
naminh.org

New Hope Foundation , 1771
newhopfoundationinc.org

New Jersey Association of Mental Health Agencies, 1974
njamha.org

New Jersey Protection and Advocacy , 1975
njpanda.org

New Mexico Alliance for the Mentally Ill , 1979
naminm.org

New York Association of Psychiatric Rehabilitation Services, 1991
nyaprs.org

New York Business Group on Health , 1992
nybgh.org

Bipolar Disorder

Clinical Management

Accreditation Services , 4687
  accreditationservices.com
Accumedic Computer Systems , 4688
  accumedic.com
Accumedic Computer Systems , 5076
  accumedic.com
Advanced Data Systems , 4691
  adspro.com
Aetna-US HealthCare , 4271
  aetna.com
Alliance Underwriters , 4694
  allianceu.com
Allina Hospitals & Clinics Behavioral Health Services, 4276
  allina.com
AmeriChoice , 4278
  americhoice.com
American Guidance Service (AGS) , 4280
  agsnet.com
American Managed Behavioral Healthcare Association, 4282
  ambha.org
American Medical Software , 4696
  americanmedical.com
American Psychiatric Press Reference Library CD-ROM, 4698
  appi.org
Anasazi Software , 4699
  anasazisoftware.com
Arbour Health System-Human Resource Institute Hospital, 5082
  arbourhealth.com
Arbour-Fuller Hospital , 5083
  arbourhealth.com
Aries Systems Corporation , 4702
  kfinder.com
Askesis Development Group , 4704
  psychconsult.org
Association for Ambulatory Behavioral Healthcare, 5085
  aabh.org
Austin Travis County Mental Health Mental Retardation Center, 4707
  atcmhmr.com
Aware Resources , 4708
  awareresources.com
Barry Associates , 4294
  barry-online.com
Beaver Creek Software , 4709
  beaverlog.com
Behavior Graphics Division of Supervised Lifestyles, 4712
  slshealth.com
Behavioral Health Advisor , 4714
  patienteducation.com
Behavioral Health Partners , 4298
  bhpi.com
Behavioral Health Services , 4299
  allina.com
Behavioral Health Systems , 4301
  bhs-inc.com
Behavioral Intervention Planning: Completing a Functional Behavioral Assessment and Developing a Behavioral Intervention Plan, 5087
  proedinc.com
Bellefaire Jewish Children's Bureau , 4717
  bellefairejcb.org
Brand Software , 4721
  helper.com
Breining Institute College for the Advanced Study of Addictive Disorders, 5088
  breining.edu
Brief Therapy Institute of Denver , 5089
  btid.com
Brown and Associates , 4308
  danbrownconsulting.com
Buckley Productions , 5090
  buckleyproductions.com
CBI Group , 4311
  cbipartners.com

CIGNA Behavioral Care , 4313
  apps.cignabehavioral.com
CLARC Services , 4726
  clarc.com
CMHC Systems , 5092
  mis.cmhc.com
COMPSYCH Software Information Services , 4728
  plattsburgh.edu.compsych/
COMPSYCH Software Information Services , 5093
  plattsburgh.edu.compsych/
CPP Incorporated , 4319
  cpp.com
Cardiff Software: Vista , 4732
  cardiff.com
Casey Family Services , 4325
  caseyfamilyservices.org
Cherokee Health Systems , 4336
  cherokeehealth.com
Chi Systems , 4337
  chiinc.com
Client Management Information System , 4742
  wildatainc.com
CliniSphere version 2.0 , 4743
  drugfacts.com
College Health IPA , 4342
  chipa.org
College of Southern Idaho , 4344
  csi.edu
Columbia/HCA Behavioral Health , 4346
  medtropolis.com/behavioralhealth
ComPsych , 4347
  compsych.com
Community Sector Systems , 5101
  cssi.com
Community Solutions , 5102
  community-solutions.com
Compass Health Systems , 4349
  compasshealthsystems.com
Compass Information Services , 4350
  compassinformation.com
Compass Information Systems , 5103
  compass-is.com
Comprehensive Behavioral Care , 4351
  compcare.com
Comprehensive Care Corporation , 4352
  comprehensivecare.com
CompuSystems , 4752
  medic.com
Computer Billing and Office Managment Programs, 5105
  cmch.com/guide/pro24.html
Computers and High Tech in Behavioral Practice Special Interest Group, 4758
  luna.cas.usf.edu/~rrusson/chip
Comsort , 4354
  comsort.com
CoolTalk , 4764
  netscape.com
Cornucopia Software , 4765
  practicemagic.com
Coventry Health Care of Iowa , 4364
  chia.cvty.com
Craig Academy , 4365
  craigacademy.org
Creative Computer Applications , 4766
  ccaine.com
DML Training and Consulting , 4370
  dmlmd.com
Dean Foundation for Health, Research and Education, 5110
  deancare.com
Deloitte and Touche LLP Management Consulting, 4375
  deloitte.com
Devon Hill Associates , 4377
  devonhillassociates.com

Cognitive Disorders

Conduct Disorder

Depression

Dissociative Disorders

Eating Disorders

Facilities

Crossroad: Fort Wayne's Children's Home , 4022
crossroad-fwch.org
Dominion Hospital , 4234
dominionhospital.com
Eastern State Hospital , 4050
bluegrass.org/easternst.html
Elmbrook Memorial Hospital , 4251
http://207.198.127.147/affiliat/elmbr.shtml
Evansville Psychiatric Children's Center , 4023
epcckids.com
Fremont Hospital , 3961
fremonthospital.com
Good Will-Hinckley Homes for Boys and Girls , 4064
gwh.org
Hamilton Center , 4026
hamiltoncenter.org
Hampstead Hospital , 4124
hampsteadhospital.com
Highland Hospital , 4246
highlandhosp.com
Indiana Family Support Network, MHA Indiana, 4027
nmha.org
John L. Gildner Regional Institute for Children and Adolescents, 4069
dhmh.state.md.us/jlgrica/
Klingberg Family Centers , 3978
klingberg.org
Laurel Regional Hospital , 4070
dimensionshealth.org
Life Transition Therapy , 4125
lifetransition.com
Lincoln Child Center , 3962
lincolncc.org
MacNeal Hospital , 4015
macnealfp.com/hospital.htm
Manatee Glens , 3984
manateeglens.com
Mendota Mental Health Institute , 4252
dhfs.state.wi.us/MH_Mendota/
Mills-Peninsula Hospital: Behavioral Health , 3965
mills-peninsula.org/behavioralhealth
Mississippi State Hospital1 , 4098
msh.state.ms.us
Nathan S Kline Institute , 4148
rfmh.org/nki
New England Home for Little Wanderers: Planning and Programs, 4081
thehome.org
New Horizons Ranch and Center , 4219
newhorizonsinc.com
North Star Centre , 3987
northstar-centre.com
Orange County Mental Health , 3967
mhaoc.org
Oregon State Hospital: Portland , 4183
omhs.mhd.hr.state.or.us
Our Lady of Bellefonte Hospital , 4052
olbh.com
PacifiCare Behavioral Health , 3968
pbhi.com
Parkview Hospital Rehabilitation Center , 4034
parkview.com
Piedmont Geriatric Hospital , 4238
pgh.state.va.us
Pine Grove Hospital , 3970
pinegrovehospital.com
Presbyterian Intercommunity Hospital Mental Health Center, 3971
whittierpres.com
Rainbow Mental Health Facility , 4045
kumc.edu/rainbow
Renfrew Center Foundation , 4190
renfrew.org
Renfrew Center Foundation , 4255
renfrew.org

Richmond State Hospital , 4035
richmondstatehospital.org
River Oaks Hospital , 4060
riveroakhospital.com
Rockland Children's Psychiatric Center , 4153
omh.state.ny.us/omhweb/facility/rcph/facility
Ryther Child Center , 4244
ryther.org
Salem Children's Home , 4018
salemhome.org
Samaritan Counseling Center , 4089
samaritancounselingmichigan.com
San Antonio State Hospital , 4222
mhmr.state.tx.us/hospitals/sanantonioSH
Silver Hill Hospital , 3979
silverhospital.com
South Beach Psychiatric Center , 4156
omh.state.ny.us/omhweb/facilities/sbpc/facilit
Southern Virginia Mental Health Institute , 4239
svmhi.state.va.us
Southwestern Virginia Mental Health Institute, 4240
swvmhi.state.va.us
Spring Harbor Hospital , 4065
springharbor.org
Spring Lake Ranch , 4229
springlakeranch.org
St. Mary's Home for Boys , 4185
stmaryshomeforboys.org
Transitions Mental Health Rehabilitation , 4020
transrehab.org
University Pavilion Psychiatric Services , 3992
uhmchealth.com
Western State Psychiatric Center , 4180
odmhsas.org
William C Weber and Associates , 4036
webereap.com
Willough Healthcare System , 3993
thewillough.com
Willow Crest Hospital , 4181
willowcresthospital.com
Woodridge Hospital , 4211
frontierhealth.org

Gender Identification Disorder

Center for Family Support (CFS) , 981
cfsny.org
Center for Mental Health Services Knowledge Exchange Network, 982
mentalhealth.org
Gender Identify Disorder and Psychosexual Problems in Children and Adolescents, 988
booknews.com
Identity Without Selfhood , 989
cup.org
NADD: Association for Persons with Developmental Disabilities and Mental Health Needs, 983
thenadd.org
National Gay and Lesbian Task Force , 984
ngltf.org
National Institute of Mental Health , 985
nimh.nih.gov
National Mental Health Consumer's Self-Help Clearinghouse, 986
mhselfhelp.org
Parents and Friends of Lesbians and Gays , 987
pflag.org

Government Agencies

Administration for Children, Youth and Families, 2146
os.dhhs.gov

Administration on Aging , 2147
  aoa.gov
Administration on Developmental Disabilities US Department of
Health & Human Services, 2148
  acf.dhs.gov/programs/ada
Agency for Healthcare Research and Quality: Office of
Communications and Knowledge Transfer, 2149
  ahrq.org
Alabama Department of Mental Health and Mental Retardation,
2198
  mh.state.al.us
Alabama Disabilities Advocacy Program , 2200
  adap.net
Alaska Department of Health & Social Services, 2202
  hss.state.ak.us/dmhdd/
Alaska Mental Health Board , 2207
  alaska.net/~amhb
Alcohol and Drug Council of Middle Tennessee, 2469
  adcmt.org
Arizona Department of Health Services , 2208
  webmaster@hs.state.az.us
Arizona Department of Health: Substance Abuse, 2211
  http://www.hs.state.az.us/bhs/bsagmh.htm
Association of Maternal and Child Health Programs (AMCHP),
2150
  amchp.org
Austin Travis County Mental Health: Mental Retardation Center,
2481
  atcmhmr.com
California Department of Education: Healthy Kids, Healthy
California, 2223
  californiahealthykids.org
California Department of Health Services: Medicaid, 2224
  dhs.ca.gov
California Health & Welfare Agency , 2228
  dmh.cahwnet.gov
California Institute for Mental Health , 2231
  cimh.org
California Mental Health Directors Association, 2232
  cmhda.org
Center for Mental Health Services Homeless Programs Branch,
2151
  mentalhealth.org
Centers for Medicare & Medicaid Services , 2322
  cms.hhs.gov
Committee for Truth in Psychiatry: CTIP , 2156
  harborside.com/~equinox/ect.htm
Connecticut Department of Mental Health, 2244
  state.ct.us/
Dane County Mental Health Center , 2515
  mhcdc.org
Department of Human Services: Chemical Health Division, 2351
  dhs.state.mn.us
Georgia Department of Health and Human Services, 2259
  hcfa.gov
Georgia Department of Human Resources , 2260
  dmh.dhr.state.ga.us
Information Resources and Inquiries Branch , 2159
  nimh.nih.gov
Kansas Department of Mental Health and Retardation and Social
Services, 2299
  ink.org
Maine Department of Behavioral and Developmental Services,
2317
  STATE.ME.US/dmhmrsa/
Maine Office of Substance Abuse: Information and Resource
Center, 2320
  maine.gov/bds/osa
Maryland Department of Health and Mental Hygiene, 2326
  dhmh.state.md.us/
Maryland Department of Human Resources , 2327
  dhr.state.mdus
Massachusetts Department of Public Welfare , 2336
  spat.ma.us/dta

Mental Health Association in Illinois , 2284
  mhai.org
Mississippi Alcohol Safety Education Program , 2356
  ssrc.misstate.edu/
Missouri Department of Mental Health , 2362
  modhmg.state.mo.us
National Institute of Alcohol Abuse and Alcoholism: Treatment
Research Branch, 2163
  nimh.nih.gov
National Institute of Drug Abuse: NIDA , 2166
  nida.nih.gov
Nebraska Mental Health Centers , 2381
  mmhc-clinics.com
Nevada Division of Mental Health & Developme ntal Services,
2386
  mhds@dhr.state.nv.us
New Jersey Department of Social Services , 2398
  state.nj.us/humanservices/dhsmahl.html
New Jersey Division Of Mental Health Services, 2399
  state.nj.us/humanservices/dmhs
New Mexico Behavioral Health Services Division, 2403
  health.state.nm.us
New Mexico Department of Health , 2405
  health.state.nm.us
North Carolina Governor's Office of Substance Abuse Policy, 2418
  dhhs.state.nc.us
North Dakota Department of Human Services: Medicaid Program,
2421
  state.dd.us/humanservices
Office of Mental Health and Addiction Services Training &
Resource Center, 2434
  open.org/~oprc/
Oklahoma Department of Mental Health and Substance Abuse
Service, 2428
  odmhsas.org
Oklahoma Office of Juvenile Affairs , 2430
  oja.state.ok.us
Oklahoma's Mental Health Consumer Council , 2431
  okmentalhealth.org
President's Committee on Mental Retardation , 2183
  acf.dhhs.gov/programs/pcmr
Presidents Committee on Mental Retardation: Administration for
Children & Families, 2185
  acf.dhhs.gov/programs/pcmr
Rhode Island Department of Mental Health: Mental Retardation
and Hospital, 2454
  hrh.state.ri.us
South Carolina Department of Alcohol and Other Drug Abuse
Services, 2460
  daodas.state.sc.us
South Dakota Department of Human Services: Division of Mental
Health, 2464
  state.sd.us/dhs/dmh/
Substance Abuse and Mental Health Services Administration, 2189
  samsha.org
Substance Abuse and Mental Health Services Administration:
Center for Mental Health Services, 2191
  mentalhealth.org
Tennessee Commission on Children and Youth , 2473
  state.tn.us/teey
Tennessee Department of Mental Health and Mental Disabilities,
2478
  state.tn.us/mental
Texas Department of Mental Health: Retardation, 2487
  mhmr.state.tx.us
Vermont Department of Developmental and Mental Health
Services, 2497
  state.vt.us/dmh/
Wisconsin Bureau of Substance Abuse Services , 2520
  dhfs.state.wi.us/substance/index.htm
Wyoming Mental Health Division , 2526
  mentalhealth.state.wy.us

Paraphilias (Perversions)

Pediatric & Adolescent Issues

Personality Disorders

Pharmaceutical Companies

Organon , 5190
organon-usa.com
Ortho-McNeil Pharmaceutical , 5191
ortho-mcneil.com
Pfizer , 5192
pfizer.com
Sanofi-Synthelabo , 5193
sanofi-synthelabous.com
Shire Richwood , 5194
shire.com
Solvay Pharmaceuticals , 5195
solvaypharmaceuticals.com
Somerset Pharmaceuticals , 5196
somersetpharm.com
Wyeth , 5197
wyeth.com

Post Traumatic Stress Disorder

After the Crash: Assessment and Treatment of Motor Vehicle
Accident Survivors, 1174
apa.org
Aging and Post Traumatic Stress Disorder , 1175
appi.org
Anxiety Disorders , 1195
mentalhealth.org
Association of Traumatic Stress Specialists , 1164
ATSS-HQ.com
Career Assessment & Planning Services , 1165
goodwill-suncoast.org
Center for Family Support (CFS) , 1166
cfsny.org
Center for Mental Health Services Knowledge Exchange Network,
1167
mentalhealth.org
Coping with Post-Traumatic Stress Disorder , 1177
rosenpublishing.com
Coping with Trauma: a Guide to Self-Understa nding, 1178
appi.org
EMDR: Breakthrough Therapy for Overcoming Anxiety, Stress
and Trauma, 1179
sidran.org
Effective Treatments for PTSD , 1180
guilford.com
Helping Children and Adolescents Cope with Violence and
Disasters, 1196
nimh.nih.gov
Herbs for the Mind: What Science Tells Us about Nature's
Remedies for Depression, Stress, Memory Loss and Insomnia, 1181
guilford.com
International Society for Traumatic Stress Studies, 1168
istss.org
Let's Talk Facts About Post-Traumatic Stress Disorder, 1197
appi.org
NADD: Association for Persons with Developmental Disabilities
and Mental Health Needs, 1169
thenadd.org
National Alliance for the Mentally Ill , 1170
nami.org
National Mental Health Consumer's Self-Help Clearinghouse,
1171
mhselfhelp.org
Post-Traumatic Stress Disorder: Additional Perspectives, 1183
ccthomas.com
Post-Traumatic Stress Disorder: Assessment, Differential
Diagnosis, and Forensic Evaluation, 1184
prpress.com
Post-Traumatic Stress Disorder: Complete Treatment Guide, 1185
sidran.org
Posttraumatic Stress Disorder in Litigation: Guidelines for
Forensic Assessment, 1186
appi.org

Posttraumatic Stress Disorder: A Guide , 1194
miminc.org
Psychological Trauma , 1187
appi.org
Real Illness: Post-Traumatic Stress Disorder, 1198
nimh.nih.gov
Rebuilding Shattered Lives: Responsible Treatment of Complex
Post-Traumatic and Dissociative Disorders, 1188
wiley.com
Risk Factors for Posttraumatic Stress Disorder, 1189
appi.org
Suncoast Residential Training Center/Developmental Services
Program, 1172
goodwill-suncoast.org
Take Charge: Handling a Crisis and Moving Forward, 1190
HealthyLife.com
Traumatic Incident Reduction Association , 1173
tira.org
Traumatic Stress: Effects of Overwhelming Experience on Mind,
Body and Society, 1191
guilford.com
Treating Trauma Disorders Effectively , 1199
rossinst.com
Trust After Trauma: a Guide to Relationships for Survivors and
Those Who Love Them, 1192
newharbinger.com
Understanding Post Traumatic Stress Disorder and Addiction, 1193
sidran.org

Professional

A Family-Centered Approach to People with Mental Retardation,
2764
aamr.org
A Guide to Consent , 2765
aamr.org
A History of Nursing in the Field of Mental Retardation, 2766
aamr.org
A Primer on Rational Emotive Behavior Therapy, 2767
researchpress.com
A Research Agenda for DSM-V , 2768
appi.org
AACAP News , 3256
aacap.org
AAHP/Dorland Directory of Health Plans , 3894
dorlandhealth.com
AAMI Newsletter , 3257
az.nami.org
AAMR-American Association on Mental Retardation: Religion
Division, 2552
aamr.org
AAMR-American Association on Mental Retardation Conference:
Annual Meeting at the Crossroads, 3218
aamr.org
AAPL Newsletter , 3258
aapl.org
ADHD in Adolesents: Diagnosis and Treatment , 2966
guilford.com
ADHD in Adulthood: Guide to Current Theory, Diagnosis and
Treatment, 2967
healthsourcebooks.org
AJMR-American Journal on Mental Retardation , 3260
aamr.org
AMIA News , 3261
amia.org
APA Monitor , 3263
apa.org/monitor
APA-Endorsed Psychiatrists Professional Liability Insurance
Program, 2553
psychprogram.com
Abusive Personality: Violence and Control in Intimate
Relationships, 3028
guilford.com

American Society of Psychoanalytic Physicians: Membership Directory, 3902
aspp.net

American Society on Aging , 2629
asaging.org

Americans with Disabilities Act and the Emerging Workforce, 2777
aamr.org

An Elephant in the Living Room: Leader's Guide for Helping Children of Alcoholics, 2942
hazelden.org

Anatomy of a Psychiatric Ilness: Healing the Mind and the Brain, 3084
appi.org

Anitdepressant Fact Book: What Your Doctor Won't Tell You About Prozac, Zoloft, Paxil, Celexa and Luvox, 2996
perseusbooksgroup.com

Annie E Casey Foundation , 2630
aecf.org

Annual AAMA Conference & Convocation , 3236
aameda.org

Annual Summit on International Managed Care Trends, 3237
aihs.com

Antipsychotic Medications: A Guide , 2997
miminc.org

Anxiety & Mood Disorders Clinic: Department of Psychiatry & Behavioral Medicine, 3519
uicomp.uic.edu/psychiatry

Anxiety Disorders: a Scientific Approach for Selecting the Most Effective Treatment, 2947
prpress.com

Applied Relaxation Training in the Treatment of PTSD and Other Anxiety Disorders, 2948
newharbinger.com

Arts in Psychotherapy , 3278
elsevier.nl/locate/artspsycho

Asperger Syndrome: a Practical Guide for Teachers, 2980
addwarehouse.com

Assesing Problem Behaviors , 2778
aamr.org

Assessment and Prediction of Suicide , 3279
guilford.com

Assessment and Treatment of Anxiety Disorders in Persons with Mental Retardation, 3472
thenadd.org

Assessment of Neuropsychiatry and Mental Health Services, 3473
appi.org

Assimilation, Rational Thinking, and Suppression in the Treatment of PTSD and Other Anxiety Disorders, 2949
newharbinger.com

Association for Academic Psychiatry: AAP , 2631
academicpsychiatry.org

Association for Advancement of Behavior Therapy: Membership Directory, 3903
aabt.org

Association for Advancement of Behavioral Therapy, 2632
aabt.org

Association for Ambulatory Behavioral Healthcare, 2634
aabh.org

Association for Ambulatory Behavioral Healthcare: Training Conference, 3238
aabh.org

Association for Applied Psychophysiology & Biofeedback, 2635
aapb.org

Association for Behavior Analysis , 2636
abainternational.org

Association for Birth Psychology: ABP , 2637
birthpsychology.org

Association for Child Psychoanalysts: ACP , 2638
childanalysis.org

Association for Hospital Medical Education , 2639
ahme.org

Association for Humanistic Psychology: AHP , 2640
ahpweb.org

Association for Pre- & Perinatal Psychology and Health, 2641
birthpsychology.org

Association for Psychological Type: APT , 2643
aptcentral.org

Association for Research in Nervous and Ment al Disease: ARNMD, 2644
ammd.org

Association for Women in Psychology: AWP , 2645
awpsych.org

Association for the Advancement of Psycholog y: AAP, 2646
AAPNet.org

Association of Black Psychologists Annual Convention, 3239
abpsi.org

Association of Black Psychologists: ABPsi , 2647
abpsi.org

Association of State and Provincial Psychology Boards, 2649
asppb.org

Association of the Advancement of Gestalt Therapy: AAGT, 2650
aagt.org

At Health Incorporated , 3904
athealth.com

At-Risk Youth in Crises , 3149
proedinc.com

Attachment and Interaction , 2940
taylorandfrancis.com

Attachment, Trauma and Healing: Understanding and Treating Attachment Disorder in Children and Families, 3150
sidran.org

Attention Deficit Disorder ADHD and ADD Syndromes, 2969
proedinc.com

Attention Deficit Disorder and Learning Disabilities: Realities, Myths and Controversial Treatments, 2970
addwarehouse.com

Attention Deficit/Hyperactivity Disorder: Cl inical Guide to Diagnosis and Treatment for Health and Mental Health Professionals, 2971
appi.org

Attention-Deficit Hyperactivity Disorder: a Handbook for Diagnosis and Treatment, 2972
guilford.com

Attention-Deficit/Hyperactivity Disorder Test: a Method for Identifying Individuals with ADHD, 3474
proedinc.com

Attention-Deficit/Hyperactivity Disorder in the Classroom, 2973
proedinc.com

Bad Boys, Bad Men: Confronting Antisocial Personality Disorder, 3044
oup-usa.org

Basic Child Psychiatry , 3151
appi.org

Basic Personal Counseling: Training Manual for Counslers, 2779
ccthomas.com

Bazelon Center for Mental Health Law , 2651
bazelon.org

Because Kids Grow Up , 3281
nami.org

Before It's Too Late: Working with Substance Abuse in the Family, 3107
wwnorton.com

Behavior Modification for Exceptional Children and Youth, 3152
proedinc.com

Behavior Rating Profile , 3153
proedinc.com

Behavior Research and Therapy , 3282
elsevier.nl/locate/bbr

Behavioral & Cognitive Psychotherapy , 3283
cup.org

Behavioral Approach to Assessment of Youth with Emotional/Behavioral Disorders, 3154
proedinc.com

Behavioral Approaches: Problem Child , 3155
cup.org

Behavioral Brain Research , 3284
elsiver.nl/locate/bbr

Psychosomatic (Somatizing) Disorders

Schizophrenia

Sexual Disorders

Sleep Disorders

Substance Abuse & Dependence

Your Brain on Drugs , 1433
hazelden.org

Suicide

Adolescent Suicide , 1508
appi.org
Adolescent Suicide: A School-Based Approach to Assessment and Intervention, 1509
researchpress.com
American Association of Suicidology , 1500
suicidology.org
American Foundation for Suicide Prevention , 1501
afsp.org
Anatomy of Suicide: Silence of the Heart , 1510
ccthomas.com
Center for Mental Health Services , 1503
mentalhealth.org
Center for Mental Health Services Knowledge Exchange Network, 1504
mentalhealth.org
Choosing to Live: How to Defeat Suicide through Cognitive Therapy, 1511
newharbinger.com
Consumer's Guide to Psychiatric Drugs , 1512
newharbinger.com
Harvard Medical School Guide to Suicide Assessment and Intervention, 1513
wiley.com
In the Wake of Suicide , 1514
wiley.com
Left Alive: After a Suicide Death in the Family, 1515
ccthomas.com
National Alliance for the Mentally Ill , 1505
nami.org
National Mental Health Consumer's Self-Help Clearinghouse, 1506
mhselfhelp.org
NineLine , 1525
covenanthouse.org/nineline/kid.html
Suicidal Adolescents , 1516
ccthomas.com
Suicidal Patient: Principles of Assesment, Treatment, and Case Management, 1517
appi.org
Suicide (Fast Fact 3) , 1521
mentalhealth.org
Suicide Over the Life Cycle , 1518
appi.org
Suicide Prevention Advocacy Network (SPAN) , 1507
spanusa.org
Suicide Talk: What To Do If You Hear It , 1522
etr.org
Suicide: Who Is at Risk? , 1523
etr.org
Survivors of Loved Ones' Suicides (SOLOS) , 1526
1000deaths.com
Understanding and Preventing Suicide: New Perspectives, 1519
ccthomas.com
Youth Suicide: Issues, Assesment and Intervention, 1520
ccthomas.com

Tic Disorders

Adam and the Magic Marble , 1547
hopepress.com
After the Diagnosis...The Next Steps , 1563
tsa-usa.org
Center for Family Support (CFS) , 1541
cfsny.org

Center for Mental Health Services Knowledge Exchange Network, 1542
mentalhealth.org
Children with Tourette Syndrome: A Parent's Guide, 1548
addwarehouse.com
Clinical Counseling: Toward a Better Understanding of TS, 1564
tsa-usa.org
Complexities of TS Treatment: Physician's Roundtable, 1565
tsa-usa.org
Don't Think About Monkeys: Extraordinary Stories Written by People with Tourette Syndrome, 1549
hopepress.com
Echolalia: an Adult's Story of Tourette Syndrome, 1550
hopepress.com
Family Life with Tourette Syndrome... Personal Stories, 1566
tsa-usa.org
Hi, I'm Adam: a Child's Story of Tourette Syndrome, 1551
hopepress.com
Mind of its Own, Tourette's Syndrome: Story and a Guide, 1552
oup-usa.org/orbs/
NADD: Association for Persons with Developmental Disabilities and Mental Health Needs, 1543
thenadd.org
National Alliance for the Mentally Ill , 1544
nami.org
National Mental Health Consumer's Self-Help Clearinghouse, 1545
mhselfhelp.org
RYAN: a Mother's Story of Her Hyperactive/Tourette Syndrome Child, 1553
hopepress.com
Raising Joshua , 1554
hopepress.com
Teaching the Tiger, a Handbook for Individuals Involved in the Education of Students with Attention Deficit Disorders, Tourette Syndrome, or Obsessive - Compulsive Disorder, 1555
hopepress.com
Tourette Syndrome Association , 1546
tsa-usa.org
Tourette Syndrome Association , 1562
tsa-usa.org
Tourette Syndrome and Human Behavior , 1557
hopepress.com
Tourette's Syndrome, Tics, Obsession, Compulsions: Developmental Psychopathology & Clinical Care, 1558
wiley.com
Tourette's Syndrome: The Facts , 1559
oup-usa.org/orbs/
Tourette's Syndrome: Tics, Obsessions, Compulsions, 1560
addwarehouse.com
Understanding and Treating the Hereditary Psychiatric Spectrum Disorders, 1567
hopepress.com
What Makes Ryan Tic?: a Family's Triunph Over Tourette's Syndrome and Attention Deficit Hyperactivity Disorder, 1561
hopepress.com

The Complete Mental Health Directory

Available Formats

Online Database

The Complete Mental Health Directory is available in Print and in an Online Database. Subscribers to the Online Database can access their subscription via the Internet and do customized searches that instantly locate needed resources of information. It's never been faster or easier to locate just the right resource. Whether you're searching for a Support Group in your area or a Disorder Description, the information you need is only a click away with *The Complete Mental Health Directory – Online Database.*

Online Database (annual subscription): $215.00
Online Database & Print Directory combo: $300.00

Visit www.greyhouse.com and explore the subscription site free of charge or call (800) 562-2139 for more information.

Mailing List Information

This directory is available in mailing list form on mailing labels or diskettes. Call (800) 562-2139 to place an order or inquire about counts. There are a number of ways we can segment the database to meet your mailing list requirements.

Licensable Database on Disk

The database of this directory is available on diskette in an ASCII text file, delimited or fixed fielded. Call (800) 562-2139 for more details.

Call (800) 562-2139 for more information

To preview any of our Directories Risk-Free for 30 days, call (800) 562-2139 or fax to (518) 789-0556

Sedgwick Press
Health Directories

The Complete Directory for People with Disabilities, 2004

A wealth of information, now in one comprehensive sourcebook. Completely updated for 2004, this edition contains more information than ever before, including thousands of new entries and enhancements to existing entries and thousands of additional web sites and e-mail addresses. This up-to-date directory is the most comprehensive resource available for people with disabilities, detailing Independent Living Centers, Rehabilitation Facilities, State & Federal Agencies, Associations, Support Groups, Periodicals & Books, Assistive Devices, Employment & Education Programs, Camps and Travel Groups. Each year, more libraries, schools, colleges, hospitals, rehabilitation centers and individuals add *The Complete Directory for People with Disabilities* to their collections, making sure that this information is readily available to the families, individuals and professionals who can benefit most from the amazing wealth of resources cataloged here.

"No other reference tool exists to meet the special needs of the disabled in one convenient resource for information." –Library Journal

1,200 pages; Softcover ISBN 1-59237-007-1, $165.00 ◆ Online Database $215.00 ◆ Online Database & Directory Combo $300.00

The Complete Directory for People with Chronic Illness, 2003/04

Thousands of hours of research have gone into this completely updated 2003/04 edition – several new chapters have been added along with thousands of new entries and enhancements to existing entries. Plus, each chronic illness chapter has been reviewed by an medical expert in the field. This widely-hailed directory is structured around the 90 most prevalent chronic illnesses – from Asthma to Cancer to Wilson's Disease – and provides a comprehensive overview of the support services and information resources available for people diagnosed with a chronic illness. Each chronic illness has its own chapter and contains a brief description in layman's language, followed by important resources for National & Local Organizations, State Agencies, Newsletters, Books & Periodicals, Libraries & Research Centers, Support Groups & Hotlines, Web Sites and much more. This directory is an important resource for health care professionals, the collections of hospital and health care libraries, as well as an invaluable tool for people with a chronic illness and their support network.

"A must purchase for all hospital and health care libraries and is strongly recommended for all public library reference departments." –ARBA

1,200 pages; Softcover ISBN 1-930956-83-5, $165.00 ◆ Online Database $215.00 ◆ Online Database & Directory Combo $300.00

The Complete Learning Disabilities Directory, 2003/04

The Complete Learning Disabilities Directory is the most comprehensive database of Programs, Services, Curriculum Materials, Professional Meetings & Resources, Camps, Newsletters and Support Groups for teachers, students and families concerned with learning disabilities. This information-packed directory includes information about Associations & Organizations, Schools, College & Testing Materials, Government Agencies, Legal Resources and much more. For quick, easy access to information, this directory contains four indexes: Entry Name Index, Subject Index and Geographic Index. With every passing year, the field of learning disabilities attracts more attention and the network of caring, committed and knowledgeable professionals grows every day. This directory is an invaluable research tool for these parents, students and professionals.

"Due to its wealth and depth of coverage, parents, teachers and others… should find this an invaluable resource." –Booklist

900 pages; Softcover ISBN 1-930956-79-7, $145.00 ◆ Online Database $195.00 ◆ Online Database & Directory Combo $280.00

The Directory of Drug & Alcohol Residential Rehabilitation Facilities, 2004

This brand new directory is the first-ever resource to bring together, all in one place, data on the thousands of drug and alcohol residential rehabilitation facilities in the United States. *The Directory of Drug & Alcohol Residential Rehabilitation Facilities* covers over 6,000 facilities, with detailed contact information for each one, including mailing address, phone and fax numbers, email addresses and web sites, mission statement, type of treatment programs, cost, average length of stay, numbers of residents and counselors, accreditation, insurance plans accepted, type of environment, religious affiliation, education components and much more. It also contains a helpful chapter on General Resources that provides contact information for Associations, Print & Electronic Media, Support Groups and Conferences. Multiple indexes allow the user to pinpoint the facilities that meet very specific criteria. This time-saving tool is what so many counselors, parents and medical professionals have been asking for. *The Directory of Drug & Alcohol Residential Rehabilitation Facilities* will be a helpful tool in locating the right source for treatment for a wide range of individuals. This comprehensive directory will be an important acquisition for all reference collections: public and academic libraries, case managers, social workers, state agencies and many more.

1,000 pages; Softcover ISBN 1-59237-031-4, $165.00

To preview any of our Directories Risk-Free for 30 days, call (800) 562-2139 or fax to (518) 789-05

Older Americans Information Directory, 2004/05

Completely updated for 2004/05, this Fifth Edition has been completely revised and now contains 1,000 new listings, over 8,000 updates to existing listings and over 3,000 brand new e-mail addresses and web sites. You'll find important resources for Older Americans including National, Regional, State & Local Organizations, Government Agencies, Research Centers, Libraries & Information Centers, Legal Resources, Discount Travel Information, Continuing Education Programs, Disability Aids & Assistive Devices, Health, Print Media and Electronic Media. Three indexes: Entry Index, Subject Index and Geographic Index make it easy to find just the right source of information. This comprehensive guide to resources for Older Americans will be a welcome addition to any reference collection.

"Highly recommended for academic, public, health science and consumer libraries..." –Choice

1,200 pages; Softcover ISBN 1-59237-037-3, $165.00 ◆ Online Database $215.00 ◆ Online Database & Directory Combo $300.00

The Complete Directory for Pediatric Disorders, 2002/03

This important directory provides parents and caregivers with information about Pediatric Conditions, Disorders, Diseases and Disabilities, including Blood Disorders, Bone & Spinal Disorders, Brain Defects & Abnormalities, Chromosomal Disorders, Congenital Heart Defects, Movement Disorders, Neuromuscular Disorders and Pediatric Tumors & Cancers. This carefully written directory offers: understandable Descriptions of 15 major bodily systems; Descriptions of more than 200 Disorders and a Resources Section, detailing National Agencies & Associations, State Associations, Online Services, Libraries & Resource Centers, Research Centers, Support Groups & Hotlines, Camps, Books and Periodicals. This resource will provide immediate access to information crucial to families and caregivers when coping with children's illnesses.

"Recommended for public and consumer health libraries." –Library Journal

1,120 pages; Softcover ISBN 1-930956-61-4, $165.00 ◆ Online Database $215.00 ◆ Online Database & Directory Combo $300.00

The Complete Directory for People with Rare Disorders, 2002/03

This outstanding reference is produced in conjunction with the National Organization for Rare Disorders to provide comprehensive and needed access to important information on over 1,000 rare disorders, including Cancers and Muscular, Genetic and Blood Disorders. An informative Disorder Description is provided for each of the 1,100 disorders (rare Cancers and Muscular, Genetic and Blood Disorders) followed by information on National and State Organizations dealing with a particular disorder, Umbrella Organizations that cover a wide range of disorders, the Publications that can be useful when researching a disorder and the Government Agencies to contact. Detailed and up-to-date listings contain mailing address, phone and fax numbers, web sites and e-mail addresses along with a description. For quick, easy access to information, this directory contains two indexes: Entry Name Index and Acronym/Keyword Index along with an informative Guide for Rare Disorder Advocates. The Complete Directory for People with Rare Disorders will be an invaluable tool for the thousands of families that have been struck with a rare or "orphan" disease, who feel that they have no place to turn and will be a much-used addition to the reference collection of any public or academic library.

"Quick access to information... public libraries and hospital patient libraries will find this a useful resource in directing users to support groups or agencies dealing with a rare disorder." –Booklist

726 pages; Softcover ISBN 1-891482-18-1, $165.00

Sedgwick Press
Education Directories

Educators Resource Directory, 2003/04

Educators Resource Directory is a comprehensive resource that provides the educational professional with thousands of resources and statistical data for professional development. This directory saves hours of research time by providing immediate access to Associations & Organizations, Conferences & Trade Shows, Educational Research Centers, Employment Opportunities & Teaching Abroad, School Library Services, Scholarships, Financial Resources, Professional Consultants, Computer Software & Testing Resources and much more. Plus, this comprehensive directory also includes a section on Statistics and Rankings with over 100 tables, including statistics on Average Teacher Salaries, SAT/ACT scores, Revenues & Expenditures and more. These important statistics will allow the user to see how their school rates among others, make relocation decisions and so much more. In addition to the Entry & Publisher Index, Geographic Index and Web Sites Index, our editors have added a Subject & Grade Index to this 2003/04 edition – so now it's even quicker and easier to locate information. *Educators Resource Directory* will be a well-used addition to the reference collection of any school district, education department or public library.

"Recommended for all collections that serve elementary and secondary school professionals." –Choice

000 pages; Softcover ISBN 1-59237-002-0, $145.00 ◆ Online Database $195.00 ◆ Online Database & Directory Combo $280.00

To preview any of our Directories Risk-Free for 30 days, call (800) 562-2139 or fax to (518) 789-0556

Sedgwick Press
Hospital & Health Plan Directories

The Directory of Hospital Personnel, 2004

The Directory of Hospital Personnel is the best resource you can have at your fingertips when researching or marketing a product or service to the hospital market. A "Who's Who" of the hospital universe, this directory puts you in touch with over 150,000 key decision-makers. With 100% verification of data you can rest assured that you will reach the right person with just one call. Every hospital in the U.S. is profiled, listed alphabetically by city within state. *The Directory of Hospital Personnel* is the only complete source for key hospital decision-makers by name. Whether you want to define or restructure sales territories... locate hospitals with the purchasing power to accept your proposals... keep track of important contacts or colleagues... or find information on which insurance plans are accepted, *The Directory of Hospital Personnel* gives you the information you need – easily, efficiently, effectively and accurately.

"Recommended for college, university and medical libraries." -ARBA

2,500 pages; Softcover ISBN 1-59237-026-8 $275.00 ◆ Online Database $545.00 ◆ Online Database & Directory Combo, $650.00

The Directory of Health Care Group Purchasing Organizations, 2004

This comprehensive directory provides the important data you need to get in touch with over 1,000 Group Purchasing Organizations. By providing in-depth information on this growing market and its members, *The Directory of Health Care Group Purchasing Organizations* fills a major need for the most accurate and comprehensive information on over 1,000 GPOs – Mailing Address, Phone & Fax Numbers, E-mail Addresses, Key Contacts, Purchasing Agents, Group Descriptions, Membership Categorization, Standard Vendor Proposal Requirements, Membership Fees & Terms, Expanded Services, Total Member Beds & Outpatient Visits represented and more. With its comprehensive and detailed information on each purchasing organization, *The Directory of Health Care Group Purchasing Organizations* is the go-to source for anyone looking to target this market.

"The information is clearly arranged and easy to access...recommended for those needing this very specialized information." –ARBA

1,000 pages; Softcover ISBN 1-59237-036-5, $325.00 ◆ Online Database, $650.00 ◆ Online Database & Directory Combo, $750.00

The HMO/PPO Directory, 2004

The HMO/PPO Directory is a comprehensive source that provides detailed information about Health Maintenance Organizations and Preferred Provider Organizations nationwide. This comprehensive directory details more information about more managed health care organizations than ever before. Over 1,100 HMOs, PPOs and affiliated companies are listed, arranged alphabetically by state. Detailed listings include Key Contact Information, Prescription Drug Benefits, Enrollment, Geographical Areas served, Affiliated Physicians & Hospitals, Federal Qualifications, Status, Year Founded, Managed Care Partners, Employer References, Fee & Payment Information and more. Plus, five years of historical information is included related to Revenues, Net Income, Medical Loss Ratios, Membership Enrollment and Number of Patient Complaints. *The HMO/PPO Directory* provides the most comprehensive information on the most companies available on the market place today.

"Helpful to individuals requesting certain HMO/PPO issues such as co-payment costs, subscription costs and patient complaints. Individuals concerned (or those with questions) about their insurance may find this text to be of use to them." -ARBA

600 pages; Softcover ISBN 1-59237-022-5, $250.00 ◆ Online Database, $495.00 ◆ Online Database & Directory Combo, $600.00

The Directory of Independent Ambulatory Care Centers, 2002/03

This first edition of *The Directory of Independent Ambulatory Care Centers* provides access to detailed information that, before now, could only be found scattered in hundreds of different sources. This comprehensive and up-to-date directory pulls together a vast array of contact information for over 7,200 Ambulatory Surgery Centers, Ambulatory General and Urgent Care Clinics, and Diagnostic Imaging Centers that are not affiliated with a hospital or major medical center. Detailed listings include Mailing Address, Phone & Fax Numbers, E-mail and Web Site addresses, Contact Name and Phone Numbers of the Medical Director and other Key Executives and Purchasing Agents, Specialties & Services Offered, Year Founded, Numbers of Employees and Surgeons, Number of Operating Rooms, Number of Cases seen per year, Overnight Options, Contracted Services and much more. Listings are arranged by State, by Center Category and then alphabetically by Organization Name. *The Directory of Independent Ambulatory Care Centers* is a must-have resource for anyone marketing a product or service to this important industry and will be an invaluable tool for those searching for a local care center that will meet their specific needs.

"Among the numerous hospital directories, no other provides information on independent ambulatory centers. A handy, well-organized resource that would be useful in medical center libraries and public libraries." –Choice

986 pages; Softcover ISBN 1-930956-90-8, $185.00 ◆ Online Database, $365.00 ◆ Online Database & Directory Combo, $450.00

To preview any of our Directories Risk-Free for 30 days, call (800) 562-2139 or fax to (518) 789-0556

Universal Reference Publications
Statistical & Demographic Reference Books

The Hispanic Databook: Statistics for all US Counties & Cities with Over 10,000 Population

The Hispanic Databook brings together a wide range of data relating to the Hispanic population for over 10,000 cities and counties. This second edition has been completely updated with figures from the latest census and has been broadly expanded to include dozens of new data elements. The Hispanic population in the United States has increased over 42% in the last 10 years. Persons of Hispanic origin account for 12.5% of the total population of the United States. These 35 million people are represented across the country, in every state. For ease of use, *The Hispanic Databook* is arranged alphabetically by state, then alphabetically by place name. More than 20 statistical data points are reported for each place, including Total Population, Percent Hispanic, Percent who Speak Spanish, Percent who Speak Only Spanish, Hispanic and Overall Per Capita Income, Hispanic and Overall Percent High School Graduates and Percent of Hispanic Population by Ancestry. A useful resource for those searching for demographics data, career search and relocation information and also for market research. With data ranging from Ancestry to Education, *The Hispanic Databook* presents a useful compilation of information that will be a much-needed resource in the reference collection of any public or academic library along with the marketing collection of any company whose primary focus in on the Hispanic population.

,000 pages; Softcover ISBN 1-59237-008-X, $150.00

Ancestry in America: A Comparative Guide to Over 200 Ethnic Backgrounds

This brand new reference work pulls together thousands of comparative statistics on the Ethnic Backgrounds of all populated places in the United States with populations over 10,000. Never before has this kind of information been reported in a single volume. *Ancestry in America* is divided into two sections: Statistics by Place and Comparative Rankings. Section One, Statistics by Place, is made up of a list of over 200 ancestry and race categories arranged alphabetically by each of the 5,000 different places with populations over 10,000. The population number of the ancestry group in that city or town is provided along with the percent that group represents of the total population. This informative city-by-city section allows the user to quickly and easily explore the ethnic makeup of all major population bases in the United States. Section Two, Comparative Rankings, contains three tables for each ethnicity and race. In the first table, the top 150 populated places are ranked by population number for that particular ancestry group, regardless of population. In the second table, the top 150 populated places are ranked by the percent of the total population for that ancestry group. In the third table, those top 150 populated places with 10,000 population are ranked by population number for each ancestry group. These easy-to-navigate tables allow users to see ancestry population patterns and make city-by-city comparisons as well. Plus, as an added bonus with the purchase of *Ancestry in America*, a free companion CD-ROM is available that lists statistics and rankings for all of the 35,000 populated places in the United States. This brand new, information-packed resource will serve a wide-range or research requests for demographics, population characteristics, relocation information and much more. *Ancestry in America: A Comparative Guide to Over 200 Ethnic Backgrounds* will be an important acquisition to all reference collections.

500 pages; Softcover ISBN 1-59237-029-2, $225.00

The American Tally, 2003/04   Statistics & Comparative Rankings for U.S. Cities with Populations over 10,000

This important statistical handbook compiles, all in one place, comparative statistics on all U.S. cities and towns with a 10,000+ population. *The American Tally* provides statistical details on over 4,000 cities and towns and profiles how they compare with one another in Population Characteristics, Education, Language & Immigration, Income & Employment and Housing. Each section begins with an alphabetical listing of cities by state, allowing for quick access to both the statistics and relative rankings of any city. Next, the highest and lowest cities are listed in each statistic. These important, informative lists provide quick reference to which cities are at both extremes of the spectrum for each statistic. Unlike any other reference, *The American Tally* provides quick, easy access to comparative statistics – a must-have for any reference collection.

"A solid library reference." –Bookwatch

0 pages; Softcover ISBN 1-930956-29-0, $125.00

The Value of a Dollar – Millennium Edition

A guide to practical economy, *The Value of a Dollar* records the actual prices of thousands of items that consumers purchased from the Civil War to the present, along with facts about investment options and income opportunities. The first edition, published by Gale Research in 1994, covered the period of 1860 to 1989. This second edition has been completely redesigned and revised and now contains two new chapters, 1990-1994 and 1995-1999. Each 5-year chapter includes a Historical Snapshot, Consumer Expenditures, Investments, Selected Income, Income/Standard Jobs, Food Basket, Standard Prices and Miscellany. This interesting and useful publication will be widely used in any reference collection.

"Recommended for high school, college and public libraries." –ARBA

pages; Hardcover ISBN 1-891482-49-1, $135.00

preview any of our Directories Risk-Free for 30 days, call (800) 562-2139 or fax to (518) 789-0556

Working Americans 1880-1999
Volume I: The Working Class, Volume II: The Middle Class, Volume III: The Upper Class

Each of the volumes in the *Working Americans 1880-1999* series focuses on a particular class of Americans, The Working Class, The Middle Class and The Upper Class over the last 120 years. Chapters in each volume focus on one decade and profile three to five families. Family Profiles include real data on Income & Job Descriptions, Selected Prices of the Times, Annual Income, Annual Budgets, Family Finances, Life at Work, Life at Home, Life in the Community, Working Conditions, Cost of Living, Amusements and much more. Each chapter also contains an Economic Profile with Average Wages of other Professions, a selection of Typical Pricing, Key Events & Inventions, News Profiles, Articles from Local Media and Illustrations. The *Working Americans* series captures the lifestyles of each of the classes from the last twelve decades, covers a vast array of occupations and ethnic backgrounds and travels the entire nation. These interesting and useful compilations of portraits of the American Working, Middle and Upper Classes during the last 120 years will be an important addition to any high school, public or academic library reference collection.

"These interesting, unique compilations of economic and social facts, figures and graphs will support multiple research needs. They will engag and enlighten patrons in high school, public and academic library collections." —Booklist (on Volumes I and I

Volume I: The Working Class ◆ 558 pages; Hardcover ISBN 1-891482-81-5, $145.00
Volume II: The Middle Class ◆ 591 pages; Hardcover ISBN 1-891482-72-6; $145.00
Volume III: The Upper Class ◆ 567 pages; Hardcover ISBN 1-930956-38-X, $145.00

Working Americans 1880-1999 Volume IV: Their Children

This Fourth Volume in the highly successful *Working Americans 1880-1999* series focuses on American children, decade by decade from 1880 to 1999. This interesting and useful volume introduces the reader to three children in each decade, one from each of the Working, Middle and Upper classes. Like the first three volumes in the series, the individual profiles are created from interviews, diaries, statistical studies, biographies and news reports. Profiles cover a broad range of ethnic backgrounds, geographic area and lifestyles – everything from an orphan in Memphis in 1882, following the Yellow Fever epidemic of 1878 to an eleven-year-old nephew of a beer baron and owner of the New York Yankees in New York City in 1921. Chapters also contain important supplementary materials including News Features as well as information on everything from Schools to Parks, Infectious Diseases to Childhood Fears along with Entertainment, Family Life and much more to provide an informative overview of the lifestyles of children from each decade. This interesting account of what life was like for Children in the Working, Middle and Upper Classes will be a welcome addition to the reference collection of any high school, public or academic library.

600 pages; Hardcover ISBN 1-930956-35-5, $145.00
Four Volume Set (Volumes I-IV), Hardcover ISBN 1-59237-017-9, $540.00

Working Americans 1880-2003 Volume V: Americans At War

Working Americans 1880-2003 Volume V: Americans At War is divided into 11 chapters, each covering a decade from 1880-2003 and examines the lives of Americans during the time of war, including declared conflicts, one-time military actions, protests, and preparations for war. Each decade includes several personal profiles, whether on the battlefield or on the homefront, that tell the stories of civilians, soldiers, and officers during the decade. The profiles examine: Life at Home; Life at Work; and Life in the Community. Each decade also includes an Economic Profile with statistical comparisons, a Historical Snapshot, News Profiles, loc News Articles, and Illustrations that provide a solid historical background to the decade being examined. Profiles range widely nc only geographically, but also emotionally, from that of a girl whose leg was torn off in a blast during WWI, to the boredom of bei stationed in the Dakotas as the Indian Wars were drawing to a close. As in previous volumes of the *Working Americans* series, information is presented in narrative form, but hard facts and real-life situations back up each story. The basis of the profiles com from diaries, private print books, personal interviews, family histories, estate documents and magazine articles. For easy referenc *Working Americans 1880-2003 Volume V: Americans At War* includes an in-depth Subject Index. The *Working Americans* series has become an important reference for public libraries, academic libraries and high school libraries. This fifth volume will be a welcom addition to all of these types of reference collections.

600 pages; Hardcover ISBN 1-59237-024-1; $145.00
Five Volume Set (Volumes I-V), Hardcover ISBN 1-59237-034-9, $675.00

To preview any of our Directories Risk-Free for 30 days, call (800) 562-2139 or fax to (518) 789-05

Profiles of America: Facts, Figures & Statistics for Every Populated Place in the United States

Profiles of America is the only source that pulls together, in one place, statistical, historical and descriptive information about every place in the United States in an easy-to-use format. This award winning reference set, now in its second edition, compiles statistics and data from over 20 different sources – the latest census information has been included along with more than nine brand new statistical topics. This Four-Volume Set details over 40,000 places, from the biggest metropolis to the smallest unincorporated hamlet, and provides statistical details and information on over 50 different topics including Geography, Climate, Population, Vital Statistics, Economy, Income, Taxes, Education, Housing, Health & Environment, Public Safety, Newspapers, Transportation, Presidential Election Results and Information Contacts or Chambers of Commerce. Profiles are arranged, for ease-of-use, by state and then by county. Each county begins with a County-Wide Overview and is followed by information for each Community in that particular county. The Community Profiles within the county are arranged alphabetically. *Profiles of America* is a virtual snapshot of America at your fingertips and a unique compilation of information that will be widely used in any reference collection.

A Library Journal Best Reference Book   "An outstanding compilation." –Library Journal

0,000 pages; Four Volume Set; Softcover ISBN 1-891482-80-7, $595.00

America's Top-Rated Cities, 2004

America's Top-Rated Cities provides current, comprehensive statistical information and other essential data in one easy-to-use source on the 100 "top" cities that have been cited as the best for business and living in the U.S. This handbook allows readers to see, at a glance, a concise social, business, economic, demographic and environmental profile of each city, including brief evaluative comments. In addition to detailed data on Cost of Living, Finances, Real Estate, Education, Major Employers, Media, Crime and Climate, city reports now include Housing Vacancies, Tax Audits, Bankruptcy, Presidential Election Results and more. This outstanding source of information will be widely used in any reference collection.

"The only source of its kind that brings together all of this information into one easy-to-use source. It will be beneficial to many business and public libraries." –ARBA

500 pages, 4 Volume Set; Softcover ISBN 1-59237-038-1, $195.00

America's Top-Rated Smaller Cities, 2004

A perfect companion to *America's Top-Rated Cities, America's Top-Rated Smaller Cities* provides current, comprehensive business and living profiles of smaller cities (population 25,000-99,999) that have been cited as the best for business and living in the United States. Sixty cities make up this 2004 edition of *America's Top-Rated Smaller Cities*, all are top-ranked by Population Growth, Median Income, Unemployment Rate and Crime Rate. City reports reflect the most current data available on a wide-range of statistics, including Employment & Earnings, Household Income, Unemployment Rate, Population Characteristics, Taxes, Cost of Living, Education, Health Care, Public Safety, Recreation, Media, Air & Water Quality and much more. Plus, each city report contains a background of the City, and an Overview of the State Finances. *America's Top-Rated Smaller Cities* offers a reliable, one-stop source of statistical data that, before now, could only be found scattered in hundreds of sources. This volume is designed for a wide range of readers: individuals considering relocating a residence or business; professionals considering expanding their business or changing careers; general and market researchers; real estate consultants; human resource personnel; urban planners and investors.

"Provides current, comprehensive statistical information in one easy-to-use source… Recommended for public and academic libraries and specialized collections." –Library Journal

00 pages; Softcover ISBN 1-59237-043-8, $160.00

Crime in America's Top-Rated Cities, 2000

This volume includes over 20 years of crime statistics in all major crime categories: violent crimes, property crimes and total crime. *Crime in America's Top-Rated Cities* is conveniently arranged by city and covers 76 top-rated cities. *Crime in America's Top-Rated Cities* offers details that compare the number of crimes and crime rates for the city, suburbs and metro area along with national crime trends for violent, property and total crimes. Also, this handbook contains important information and statistics on Anti-Crime Programs, Crime Risk, Hate Crimes, Illegal Drugs, Law Enforcement, Correctional Facilities, Death Penalty Laws and much more. A much-needed resource for people who are relocating, business professionals, general researchers, the press, law enforcement officials and students of criminal justice.

"Data is easy to access and will save hours of searching." –Global Enforcement Review

pages; Softcover ISBN 1-891482-84-X, $155.00

preview any of our Directories Risk-Free for 30 days, call (800) 562-2139 or fax to (518) 789-0556

The Comparative Guide to American Elementary & Secondary Schools, 2004/05

The only guide of its kind, this award winning compilation offers a snapshot profile of every public school district in the United States serving 1,500 or more students – more than 5,900 districts are covered. Organized alphabetically by district within state, each chapter begins with a Statistical Overview of the state. Each district listing includes contact information (name, address, phone number and web site) plus Grades Served, the Numbers of Students and Teachers and the Number of Regular, Special Education, Alternative and Vocational Schools in the district along with statistics on Student/Classroom Teacher Ratios, Drop Out Rates, Ethnicity, the Numbers of Librarians and Guidance Counselors and District Expenditures per student. As an added bonus, *The Comparative Guide to American Elementary and Secondary Schools* provides important ranking tables, both by state and nationally, for each data element. For easy navigation through this wealth of information, this handbook contains a useful City Index that lists all districts that operate schools within a city. These important comparative statistics are necessary for anyone considering relocation or doing comparative research on their own district and would be a perfect acquisition for any public library or school district library.

"This straightforward guide is an easy way to find general information. Valuable for academic and large public library collections." –ARB

2,400 pages; Softcover ISBN 1-59237-047-0, $125.00

The Comparative Guide to American Suburbs, 2004

The Comparative Guide to American Suburbs is a one-stop source for Statistics on the 2,000+ suburban communities surrounding the 50 largest metropolitan areas – their population characteristics, income levels, economy, school system and important data on how they compare to one another. Organized into 50 Metropolitan Area chapters, each chapter contains an overview of the Metropolitan Area, a detailed Map followed by a comprehensive Statistical Profile of each Suburban Community, including Contact Information, Physical Characteristics, Population Characteristics, Income, Economy, Unemployment Rate, Cost of Living, Education, Chambers of Commerce and more. Next, statistical data is sorted into Ranking Tables that rank the suburbs by twenty different criteria, including Population, Per Capita Income, Unemployment Rate, Crime Rate, Cost of Living and more. *The Comparative Guide to American Suburbs* is the best source for locating data on suburbs. Those looking to relocate, as well as those doing preliminary market research, will find this an invaluable timesaving resource.

"Public and academic libraries will find this compilation useful…The work draws togeth figures from many sources and will be especially helpful for job relocation decisions." – Bookl

1,700 pages; Softcover ISBN 1-59237-004-7, $130.00

The Environmental Resource Handbook, 2004

The Environmental Resource Handbook, now in its second edition, is the most up-to-date and comprehensive source for Environment Resources and Statistics. Section I: Resources provides detailed contact information for thousands of information sources, includir Associations & Organizations, Awards & Honors, Conferences, Foundations & Grants, Environmental Health, Government Agencies, National Parks & Wildlife Refuges, Publications, Research Centers, Educational Programs, Green Product Catalogs, Consultants and much more. Section II: Statistics, provides statistics and rankings on hundreds of important topics, including Children's Environmental Index, Municipal Finances, Toxic Chemicals, Recycling, Climate, Air & Water Quality and more. This kind of up-to-date environmental data, all in one place, is not available anywhere else on the market place today. This vast compilation of resources and statistics is a must-have for all public and academic libraries as well as any organization with a prima focus on the environment.

"…the intrinsic value of the information make it worth consideration by libraries w environmental collections and environmentally concerned users." –Book

1,000 pages; Softcover ISBN 1-59237-030-6, $155.00 ◆ Online Database $300.00

Weather America, A Thirty-Year Summary of Statistical Weather Data and Rankings, 200

This valuable resource provides extensive climatological data for over 4,000 National and Cooperative Weather Stations through the United States. *Weather America* begins with a new Major Storms section that details major storm events of the nation and a National Rankings section that details rankings for several data elements, such as Maximum Temperature and Precipitation. Th main body of *Weather America* is organized into 50 state sections. Each section provides a Data Table on each Weather Station, organized alphabetically, that provides statistics on Maximum and Minimum Temperatures, Precipitation, Snowfall, Extreme Temperatures, Foggy Days, Humidity and more. State sections contain two brand new features in this edition – a City Index an narrative Description of the climatic conditions of the state. Each section also includes a revised Map of the State that includes n only weather stations, but cities and towns.

"Best Reference Book of the Year." –Library Jou

2,013 pages; Softcover ISBN 1-891482-29-7, $175.00

To preview any of our Directories Risk-Free for 30 days, call (800) 562-2139 or fax to (518) 789-0

Grey House Publishing
Business Directories

The Directory of Business Information Resources, 2003/04

With 100% verification, over 1,000 new listings and more than 12,000 updates, this 2003/04 edition of *The Directory of Business Information Resources* is the most up-to-date source for contacts in over 98 business areas – from advertising and agriculture to utilities and wholesalers. This carefully researched volume details: the Associations representing each industry; the Newsletters that keep members current; the Magazines and Journals - with their "Special Issues" - that are important to the trade, the Conventions that are "must attends," Databases, Directories and Industry Web Sites that provide access to must-have marketing resources. Includes contact names, phone & fax numbers, web sites and e-mail addresses. This one-volume resource is a gold mine of information and would be a welcome addition to any reference collection.

"This is a most useful and easy-to-use addition to any researcher's library." –The Information Professionals Institute

2,500 pages; Softcover ISBN 1-59237-000-4, $250.00 ◆ Online Database $495.00

Nations of the World, 2004 A Political, Economic and Business Handbook

This completely revised Third Edition covers all the nations of the world in an easy-to-use, single volume. Each nation is profiled in a single chapter that includes Key Facts, Political & Economic Issues, a Country Profile and Business Information. In this fast-changing world, it is extremely important to make sure that the most up-to-date information is included in your reference collection. This 2004 edition is just the answer. Each of the 200+ country chapters have been carefully reviewed by a political expert to make sure that the text reflects the most current information on Politics, Travel Advisories, Economics and more. You'll find such vital information as a Country Map, Population Characteristics, Inflation, Agricultural Production, Foreign Debt, Political History, Foreign Policy, Regional Insecurity, Economics, Trade & Tourism, Historical Profile, Political Systems, Ethnicity, Languages, Media, Climate, Hotels, Chambers of Commerce, Banking, Travel Information and more. Five Regional Chapters follow the main text and include a Regional Map, an Introductory Article, Key Indicators and Currencies for the Region. New for 2004, an all-inclusive CD-ROM is available as a companion to the printed text. Noted for its sophisticated, up-to-date and reliable compilation of political, economic and business information, this brand new edition will be an important acquisition to any public, academic or special library reference collection.

"A useful addition to both general reference collections and business collections." –RUSQ

700 pages; Print Version Only Softcover ISBN 1-59237-006-3, $145.00 ◆ Print Version and CD-ROM $180.00

International Business and Trade Directories, 2003/04

Completely updated, the Third Edition of *International Business and Trade Directories* now contains more than 10,000 entries, over 1,000 more than the last edition, making this directory the most comprehensive resource of the worlds business and trade directories. Entries include content descriptions, price, publisher's name and address, web site and e-mail addresses, phone and fax numbers and editorial staff. Organized by industry group, and then by region, this resource puts over 10,000 industry-specific business and trade directories at the reader's fingertips. Three indexes are included for quick access to information: Geographic Index, Publisher Index and Title Index. Public, college and corporate libraries, as well as individuals and corporations seeking critical market information will want to add this directory to their marketing collection.

800 pages; Softcover ISBN 1-930956-63-0, $225.00 ◆ Online Database (includes a free copy of the directory) $450.00

Sports Market Place Directory, 2004

For over 20 years, this comprehensive, up-to-date directory has offered direct access to the Who, What, When & Where of the Sports Industry. With over 20,000 updates and enhancements, this 2004 *Sports Market Place Directory* is the most detailed, comprehensive and current sports business reference source available. In 1,800 information-packed pages, *Sports Market Place Directory* profiles contact information and key executives for: Single Sport Organizations, Professional Leagues, Multi-Sport Organizations, Disabled Sports, High School & Youth Sports, Military Sports, Olympic Organizations, Media, Sponsors, Sponsorship & Marketing Event Agencies, Event & Meeting Calendars, Professional Services, College Sports, Manufacturers & Retailers, Facilities and much more. *The Sports Market Place Directory* provides organization's contact information with detailed descriptions including: Key Contacts, physical, mailing, email and web addresses plus phone and fax numbers. Plus, nine important indexes make sure that you can find the information you're looking for quickly and easily: Entry Index, Single Sport Index, Media Index, Sponsor Index, Agency Index, Manufacturers Index, Brand Name Index, Facilities Index and Executive/Geographic Index. For over twenty years, *The Sports Market Place Directory* has assisted thousands of individuals in their pursuit of a career in the sports industry.

1,800 pages; Softcover ISBN 1-59237-048-9, $225.00 ◆ CD-ROM $479.00 ◆ Online Database $479.00

preview any of our Directories Risk-Free for 30 days, call (800) 562-2139 or fax to (518) 789-0556

The Directory of Venture Capital Firms, 2004

This edition has been extensively updated and broadly expanded to offer direct access to over 2,800 Domestic and International Venture Capital Firms, including address, phone & fax numbers, e-mail addresses and web sites for both primary and branch locations. Entries include details on the firm's Mission Statement, Industry Group Preferences, Geographic Preferences, Average and Minimum Investments and Investment Criteria. You'll also find details that are available nowhere else, including the Firm's Portfolio Companies and extensive information on each of the firm's Managing Partners, such as Education, Professional Background and Directorships held, along with the Partner's E-mail Address. *The Directory of Venture Capital Firms* offers five important indexes: Geographic Index, Executive Name Index, Portfolio Company Index, Industry Preference Index and College & University Index. With its comprehensive coverage and detailed, extensive information on each company, *The Directory of Venture Capital Firms* is an important addition to any finance collection.

"The sheer number of listings, the descriptive information provided and the outstanding indexing make this directory a better value than its principal competitor, Pratt's Guide to Venture Capital Sources. Recommended for business collections in large public, academic and business libraries." —Choic

1,300 pages; Softcover ISBN 1-59237-025-X, $450.00 ◆ Online Database (includes a free copy of the directory) $889.00

The Directory of Mail Order Catalogs, 2004

Published since 1981, this Eighteenth Edition features 100% verification of data and is the premier source of information on the mai order catalog industry. Details over 12,000 consumer catalog companies with 44 different product chapters from Animals to Toys & Games. Contains detailed contact information including e-mail addresses and web sites along with important business details such as employee size, years in business, sales volume, catalog size, number of catalogs mailed and more. Four indexes provide quick access to information: Catalog & Company Name Index, Geographic Index, Product Index and Web Sites Index.

"This is a godsend for those looking for information." —Reference Book Revie
"The scope and arrangement make this directory useful. Certainly the broad coverag of subjects is not available elsewhere in a single-volume format." —Bookl

1,700 pages; Softcover ISBN 1-59237-027-6, $250.00 ◆ Online Database (includes a free copy of the directory) $495.00

The Directory of Business to Business Catalogs, 2004

The completely updated 2004 *Directory of Business to Business Catalogs*, provides details on over 6,000 suppliers of everything from computers to laboratory supplies… office products to office design… marketing resources to safety equipment… landscaping to maintenance suppliers… building construction and much more. Detailed entries offer mailing address, phone & fax numbers, e-ma addresses, web sites, key contacts, sales volume, employee size, catalog printing information and more. Jut about every kind of product a business needs in its day-to-day operations is covered in this carefully-researched volume. Three indexes are provided fo at-a-glance access to information: Catalog & Company Name Index, Geographic Index and Web Sites Index.

"Much smaller and easier to use than the Thomas Register or Sweet's Catalog, it is excellent choice for libraries… wishing to supplement their business supplier resources." —Bookl

800 pages; Softcover ISBN 1-59237-028-4, $165.00 ◆ Online Database (includes a free copy of the directory) $325.00

Thomas Food and Beverage Market Place, 2004

Thomas Food and Beverage Market Place is bigger and better than ever with thousands of new companies, thousands of updates to existing companies and two revised and enhanced product category indexes. This comprehensive directory profiles over 18,000 Food & Beverage Manufacturers, 12,000 Equipment & Supply Companies, 2,200 Transportation & Warehouse Companies, 2,000 Brokers & Wholesalers, 8,000 Importers & Exporters, 900 Industry Resources and hundreds of Mail Order Catalogs. Listings include detailed Contact Information, Sales Volumes, Key Contacts, Brand & Product Information, Packaging Details and much more. *Thomas Food and Beverage Market Place* is available as a three-volume printed set, a subscription-based Online Database via the Internet, on CD-ROM, as well as mailing lists and a licensable database.

"An essential purchase for those in the food industry but will also be useful in public libraries where needed. Much of the informat will be difficult and time consuming to locate without this handy three-volume ready-reference source." —AR

8,500 pages, 3 Volume Set; Softcover ISBN 1-59237-018-7, $495.00 ◆ CD-ROM $695.00 ◆
CD-ROM & 3 Volume Set Combo $895.00 ◆ Online Database $695.00 ◆ Online Database & 3 Volume Set Combo, $895.00

To preview any of our Directories Risk-Free for 30 days, call (800) 562-2139 or fax to (518) 789-05

The Grey House Safety & Security Directory, 2004

The Grey House Safety & Security Directory is the most comprehensive reference tool and buyer's guide for the safety and security industry. Published continuously since 1943 as *Best's Safety & Security Directory*, Grey House acquired the title in 2002. Arranged by safety topic, each chapter begins with OSHA regulations for the topic, followed by Training Articles written by top professionals in the field and Self-Inspection Checklists. Next, each topic contains Buyer's Guide sections that feature related products and services. Topics include Administration, Insurance, Loss Control & Consulting, Protective Equipment & Apparel, Noise & Vibration, Facilities Monitoring & Maintenance, Employee Health Maintenance & Ergonomics, Retail Food Services, Machine Guards, Process Guidelines & Tool Handling, Ordinary Materials Handling, Hazardous Materials Handling, Workplace Preparation & Maintenance, Electrical Lighting & Safety, Fire & Rescue and Security. The Buyer's Guide sections are carefully indexed within each topic area to ensure that you can find the supplies needed to meet OSHA's regulations. Six important indexes make finding information and product manufacturers quick and easy: Geographical Index of Manufacturers and Distributors, Company Profile Index, Brand Name Index, Product Index, Index of Web Sites and Index of Advertisers. This comprehensive, up-to-date reference will provide every tool necessary to make sure a business is in compliance with OSHA regulations and locate the products and services needed to meet those regulations.

,500 pages, 2 Volume Set; Softcover ISBN 1-59237-033-0, $225.00

The Grey House Homeland Security Directory, 2004

This brand new directory features the latest contact information for government and private organizations involved with Homeland Security along with the latest product information and provides detailed profiles of nearly 1,000 Federal & State Organizations & Agencies and over 3,000 Officials and Key Executives involved with Homeland Security. These listings are incredibly detailed and include Mailing Address, Phone & Fax Numbers, Email Addresses & Web Sites, a complete Description of the Agency and a complete list of the Officials and Key Executives associated with the Agency. Next, *The Grey House Homeland Security Directory* provides the go-to source for Homeland Security Products & Services. This section features over 2,000 Companies that provide consulting, Products or Services. With this Buyer's Guide at their fingertips, users can locate suppliers of everything from Training Materials to Access Controls, from Perimeter Security to BioTerrorism Countermeasures and everything in between – complete with contact information and product descriptions. A handy Product Locator Index is provided to quickly and easily locate suppliers of a particular product. Lastly, an Information Resources Section provides immediate access to contact information for hundreds of Associations, Newsletters, Magazines, Trade Shows, Databases and Directories that focus on Homeland Security. This comprehensive, information-packed resource will be a welcome tool for any company or agency that is in need of Homeland Security information and will be a necessary acquisition for the reference collection of all public libraries and large school districts.

00 pages; Softcover ISBN 1-59237-035-7, $195.00 ◆ Online Database (includes a free copy of the directory) $385.00

The Grey House Performing Arts Directory, 2004

The Grey House Performing Arts Directory is the most comprehensive resource covering the Performing Arts. This important directory provides current information on over 8,500 Dance Companies, Instrumental Music Programs, Opera Companies, Choral Groups, Theater Companies, Performing Arts Series and Performing Arts Facilities. Plus, this edition now contains a brand new section on Artist Management Groups. In addition to mailing address, phone & fax numbers, e-mail addresses and web sites, dozens of other fields of available information include mission statement, key contacts, facilities, seating capacity, season, attendance and more. *The Grey House Performing Arts Directory* pulls together thousands of Performing Arts Organizations, Facilities and Information Resources into an easy-to-use source – this kind of comprehensiveness and extensive detail is not available in any source on the market place today.

> *"An immensely useful and user-friendly new reference tool... recommended for public, academic and certain special library reference collections."* –Booklist

00 pages; Softcover ISBN 1-59237-023-3, $170.00 ◆ Online Database $335.00

Research Services Directory, 2003/04 Commercial & Corporate Research Centers

This Ninth Edition provides access to well over 8,000 independent Commercial Research Firms, Corporate Research Centers and Laboratories offering contract services for hands-on, basic or applied research. *Research Services Directory* covers the thousands of types of research companies, including Biotechnology & Pharmaceutical Developers, Consumer Product Research, Defense Contractors, Electronics & Software Engineers, Think Tanks, Forensic Investigators, Independent Commercial Laboratories, Information Brokers, Market & Survey Research Companies, Medical Diagnostic Facilities, Product Research & Development Firms and more. Each entry provides the company's name, mailing address, phone & fax numbers, key contacts, web site, e-mail address, as well as a company description and research and technical fields served. Four indexes provide immediate access to this wealth of information: Research Firms Index, Geographic Index, Personnel Name Index and Subject Index.

> *"An important source for organizations in need of information about laboratories, individuals and other facilities."* –ARBA

00 pages; Softcover ISBN 1-59237-003-9, $395.00 ◆ Online Database (includes a free copy of the directory) $850.00

preview any of our Directories Risk-Free for 30 days, call (800) 562-2139 or fax to (518) 789-0556